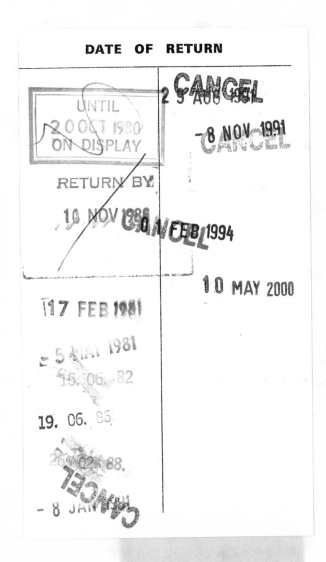

DATE OF RETURN

UNTIL
2 0 OCT 1980
ON DISPLAY

2 5 AUG 1981

CANCEL

- 8 NOV 1991

CANCEL

RETURN BY

10 NOV 1986

CANCEL

0 1 FEB 1994

1 0 MAY 2000

17 FEB 1981

- 5 MAY 1981

15. 06. 82

19. 06. 86

26. 02. 88.

CANCEL

- 8 JAN

CARDIAC ARREST & RESUSCITATION

CARDIAC ARREST
& RESUSCITATION

HUGH E. STEPHENSON, Jr.
M.D., F.A.C.S., A.B., B.S.

Professor of Surgery,
University of Missouri School of Medicine,
Columbia, Missouri

FOURTH EDITION

with 379 illustrations

THE C. V. MOSBY COMPANY
SAINT LOUIS 1974

1 597875 /25
26 IX 80

FOURTH EDITION

Copyright © 1974 by The C. V. Mosby Company

Previous editions copyrighted 1958, 1964, 1969

Printed in the United States of America

Distributed in Great Britain by Henry Kimpton, London

Library of Congress Cataloging in Publication Data

Stephenson, Hugh E
   Cardiac arrest and resuscitation.

   Bibliography: p.
   1. Cardiac resuscitation. 2. Heart failure.
I. Title. [DNLM: 1. Heart arrest. 2. Resuscitation.
WG205 S836c 1974]
RC682.S78 1974   616.1'2   73-16163
ISBN 0-8016-4780-0

CB/CB/B 9 8 7 6 5 4 3 2

CONTRIBUTORS

ELWYN L. CADY, Jr., J.D., B.S.Med.

Medicolegal Consultant of the Independence, Kansas City, and St. Louis, Missouri, bars

STEPHEN W. CARVETH, M.D.

Medical Director of Mobile Heart Unit, Lincoln, Nebraska

DENTON A. COOLEY, M.D.

Surgeon-in-Chief, Texas Heart Institute, St. Luke's Episcopal and Texas Children's Hospitals, Houston, Texas

CLARENCE D. DAVIS, M.D.

Professor of Obstetrics and Gynecology, Yale University School of Medicine, New Haven, Connecticut

EDWARD B. DIETHRICH, M.D.

Director and Chief of Cardiovascular Surgery, Arizona Heart Institute, St. Joseph's Hospital and Medical Center, Phoenix, Arizona

ALEX L. FINKLE, M.D., Ph.D.

Associate Clinical Professor of Urology, University of California Medical School, San Francisco, California

ARCHER S. GORDON, M.D., Ph.D.

Research Physiologist, Department of Anesthesiology, UCLA Medical Center, Los Angeles, California

HAROLD H. HILLMAN, M.D., B.Sc., Ph.D.

Reader in Physiology, University of Surrey, Guilford, Surrey; Editor of "Resuscitation," England

ROBERT HOOK, M.D.

Associate Clinical Professor of Anesthesiology; Chief of Obstetrical Anesthesia, Yale–New Haven Hospital, Yale University School of Medicine, New Haven, Connecticut

ADRIAN KANTROWITZ, M.D.

Professor and Chairman, Surgical Services, Wayne State University College of Medicine, Detroit, Michigan

DAVID G. KILPATRICK

President, Kilpatrick Associates, Inc., Consulting Biomedical Engineers, Bala Cynwyd, Pennsylvania

WILLEM J. KOLFF, M.D., Ph.D.

Professor and Chairman, Division of Artificial Organs, Department of Surgery, University of Utah Medical Center, and Director, Institute for Biomedical Engineering, University of Utah, Salt Lake City, Utah

CLIFFORD S. KWAN-GETT, M.D.

Associate Research Professor in Surgery; Assistant Research Professor in Electrical Engineering, College of Engineering, University of Utah; Associate Director of Engineering—Division of Artificial Organs, University of Utah College of Medicine, Salt Lake City, Utah

B. G. B. LUCAS, M.D., F.F.A., R.C.S., C.I. Mech.E.

Consultant Anesthetist to the National Heart Hospital, the Brompton Hospital, the Hospital for Sick Children, Great Ormond Street, and University College Hospital, London, England

RICHARD H. MARTIN, M.D.

Professor of Medicine and Director, Division of Cardiology, University of Missouri School of Medicine, Columbia, Missouri

JACK M. MARTT, M.D.

Professor of Medicine, Department of Cardiology, Scott-White Clinic, Temple, Texas

HERBERT L. McDONALD, M.D.

Kansas City, Missouri

TONY A. DON MICHAEL, M.D., F.A.C.C.

Chairman, Department of Internal Medicine, and Director of Cardiology, Kern General Hospital; Associate Professor of Medicine, the UCLA School of Medicine, and Associate Cardiologist, Cedars-Sinai Medical Center, Los Angeles, California

FRANK L. MITCHELL, B.S., M.D., F.A.C.S.

Professor of Surgery and Director, Emergency Medical Services, University of Missouri School of Medicine, Columbia, Missouri

VLADIMIR A. NEGOVSKII, M.D.

Director, Laboratory of Experimental Physiology on Resuscitation of the Organism, Academy of Medical Sciences of the U.S.S.R., Moscow, U.S.S.R.

WERNER OVERBECK, Professor Dr. Med.

Stadtisches Krankenhaus, Chirurgische Klinik, Kaiserslautern, Germany

JOHN C. SCHUDER, Ph.D.

Professor of Surgery (Biophysics), Department of Surgery, University of Missouri School of Medicine, Columbia, Missouri

WILLIAM A. SODEMAN, M.D.

Professor Emeritus and Dean Emeritus, Jefferson Medical College, Thomas Jefferson University, Philadelphia, Pennsylvania

GLENN O. TURNER, M.D.

The Clinic of Internal Medicine, Springfield, Missouri

JURO WADA, M.D.

Professor and Chairman, Department of Cardio-Thoracic Surgery, Sapporo Medical College and Hospital, Sapporo City, Japan

VALLEE L. WILLMAN, M.D.

Professor and Chairman, Department of Surgery, St. Louis University School of Medicine, St. Louis, Missouri

DON C. WUKASCH, M.D.

Associate Surgeon, Texas Heart Institute, St. Luke's Episcopal and Texas Children's Hospital, Houston, Texas

Dr. Werner Overbeck's contribution translated from German to English by

CARL H. IDE, M.D.

Professor of Ophthalmology, University of Missouri School of Medicine, Columbia, Missouri

With the editorial assistance of

ROBERT S. KIMPTON, A.B., B.S., M.Ed.

Journalistic Consultant, Columbia, Missouri

FOREWORD

The status of this authoritative volume on cardiac arrest and resuscitation and the great activity in this field have demanded a new, fourth edition. The fact that over 90 percent of sudden deaths (those occurring within one hour of onset of illness) result from cardiovascular disease in our country, and especially the fact that over half of those so afflicted die before entrance to a hospital make the problem of cardiac arrest an issue of broad concern, not only in the hospital and the operating room, but also in the home and elsewhere throughout the community. It is indeed one of our most important health problems.

While of special importance to the surgeon, this volume brings up-to-date concepts and approaches to a problem that is vitally important to everyone: the physician, the patient, the public. As a source book for such information it is superb—well written, clear, informative in depth, and understandable for all. The new edition comes at a critical time in this field. It comes with authority. It comes when we need updated information.

W. A. Sodeman, M.D.

Professor Emeritus and Dean Emeritus,
Jefferson Medical College

PREFACE

Sudden unexpected death, in terms of absolute loss of life, poses our greatest single medical problem today. It is the most common mode of death in our adult population. Some have suggested that the actual incidence of sudden death represents 30 percent of all natural deaths.

Many of our earlier concepts concerning the frequency and significance of ventricular arrhythmias in the early stages of acute myocardial infarction are now outdated, particularly those regarding ventricular tachyarrhythmias. The enhanced automaticity of some of the Purkinje fibers with resultant ectopic beats is now being rather effectively managed.

Almost two decades ago Beck and Leighninger, in urging the application of cardioresuscitation techniques, repeatedly referred to hearts that were "too good to die." The soundness of their perception has been borne out increasingly by many studies showing an essentially normal myocardium with minimal disease of the coronary arteries and no evidence of thrombotic occlusion at the time of autopsy in patients dying suddenly.

We continue to be indebted to the pioneering efforts of Kowenhoven, Jude, and Knickerbocker. Unquestionably, a new era in cardiac resuscitation was begun by their efforts and its immediate by-products are visible in a host of major changes in the approach to the patient, such as utilization of the intensive care and mobile coronary care units.

Since the publication of the third edition in 1969, significant contributions have been made toward a broader understanding of the mechanisms of ventricular fibrillation and cardiac asystole. This, the fourth edition, supplements and updates material in the previous editions. Once again the bibliography is practically all new. Because of the tremendous volume of bibliographical material, it is suggested that the reader refer to previous editions for references not included here. The scope and volume of scientific information on cardiac arrest and resuscitation have expanded far beyond the easy accessibility of even those with more than a casual interest in the field. As one of our objectives in this revision, we have endeavored to condense, collate, and categorize much of this information in a manner that may provide easier access to the reader.

It is estimated that fibrillation in structurally good hearts occurs over 900 times a day in the United States in victims outside a hospital. Ventricular fibrillation is a major cause of death from coronary heart disease. This fatal ventricular dysrhythmia occurs most frequently shortly after the onset of infarction. Although the concept of mobile coronary care has yet to obtain universal support among members of the medical profession, it seems obvious that means must be found to monitor and prevent ventricular fibrillation outside the hospital and during transportation to the hospital. More than half of those who die of heart attacks each year never reach a hospital, but serious attempts are being made to reduce this figure. The chapter on a mobile coronary care unit and resuscitation outside the hospital represents a considerable change in the approach to the problem over the last few years. The lifesaving benefits of cardiac monitoring in resuscitation of the coronary infarction patient outside the hospital are now well documented. Spain and Bradess estimate that there are approximately 500,000 deaths in the United States every year from acute myocardial infarction with about 50 percent of these patients dying before adequate medical care is available. The presence of a recent coronary thrombus in these sudden and unexpected fatalities (approximately 20 percent) lends encouraging support to the concept of mobile coronary care.

Approximately 70 percent of deaths from arteriosclerotic heart disease occur in persons who die outside a hospital or who are dead on arrival. This book reflects the advancements and refinements in resuscitation information that are coming from an increasingly wider variety of disciplines: the engineering sciences, medical systems developers, psychiatrists, sociologists, nurses, lawyers, biochemists, statisticians, and others.

As our knowledge of the mechanisms of cardiac arrest continues to increase, it is encouraging to note how it can be applied to clinical situations. A good example is the well-documented story of succinylcholine-induced hyperkalemia and the propensity of patients with severe trauma and burns to develop cardiac arrest. It is our hope that hospital cardiac resuscitation committees will find the book valuable as a continuing source of reference to aid them in their periodic evaluation of cases occurring in the hospital.

There seems to be little question that an effective committee can contribute significantly to a reduction in mortality from sudden death within the hospital.

Few individuals have contributed so significantly to the further extension of successful resuscitation efforts as has the nurse. With the active defibrillation of patients by nursing personnel in intensive care and coronary care units, a major breakthrough in resuscitation has occurred.

A new addition to the book is the chapter by Dr. Carveth concerning the "spectator heart." His studies, as well as others, are providing worthwhile experience and information from the management of resuscitation among high-density populations, such as those experienced at football games.

It is encouraging to note the increasing emphasis given to cardiopulmonary resuscitation by a wide variety of organizations, including the American College of Chest Physicians, American College of Cardiology, American Heart Association Committee on Cardiopulmonary Resuscitation and Emergency Cardiac Care, American College of Emergency Care Physicians, Society of Critical Care Medicine, American National Red Cross, Industrial Medical Association, and United States Public Health Service.

The Registry of Emergency Medical Technicians—Ambulance is strongly committed to improved medical care through better emergency transportation facilities and well-trained ambulance attendants. The Ambulance Association of America, International Association of Chiefs of Police, International Association of Fire Chiefs, International Rescue and First Aid Association, National Ambulance and Medical Supplies Association, National Funeral Directors' Association, and the National Sheriffs' Association are all committed to the goals of the Registry and each provides a director to its board.

Other organized groups interested in this problem include the Equipment Committee of the American Society of Anesthesiologists and the Association for the Advancement of

Medical Instrumentation. Numerous types of equipment have been advocated in the management of cardiopulmonary resuscitation. Fortunately, the effectiveness of most of these has been scrutinized by the Cardiopulmonary Resuscitation Committee of the American Heart Association or the National Science Council. For example, the Emergency Care Research Institute at Philadelphia under Dr. Nobel maintains a full-time interdisciplinary scientific staff to evaluate acute care devices. Since the medical device field has become extremely complex, it is imperative that qualified biomedical engineers or physicians trained in engineering disciplines be actively involved.

Numerous reports indicate that electronic devices used in hospitals in the United States in the care of cardiac patients have significant deficiencies. The need for regular inspection of equipment, uniform standards, and increasing familiarity with medical electronics has prompted the inclusion of Chapter 7, by David Kilpatrick. The magnitude of the problem of excessive leakage of electrical current appears to be significant.

The first cardiac transplantation was undertaken on December 3, 1967. In the following two years, approximately 147 heart recipients were recorded. While the tempo of this activity has decreased considerably, it seems likely that a resumption will occur once major progress in coping with the rejection phenomena occurs. The chapters on preservation of the heart and on resuscitation of transplanted hearts should prove of interest to many readers. By including as much

material as possible relevant to the field of cardiac resuscitation in this book, we hope that our efforts will give added perspective to workers in this field. To those readers not actively involved, it is our hope that this edition will provide an updated and reliable account of the "state of the art."

A chapter on the historical aspects of cardiac resuscitation is again included. Readers tell us that they enjoy the chapter and that it effectively places the progress of resuscitation in its proper perspective.

We have continued to devote considerable space to the variety of factors influencing the mechanism of cardiac arrest, as it is our conviction that the relatively low rate of successful resuscitation in hospitals is partially due to a lack of realization of therapeutic requirements for specific situations. Broad generalizations are helpful for educational purposes, but the field of cardiac resuscitation has become sufficiently sophisticated to require in-depth knowledge of modifications in resuscitation efforts as individually required.

If one views the significant contributions made to the field of cardiac resuscitation over a span of years it is apparent that advances seem to be the product of different disciplines and different times. For example, after the advances by Shiff and other physiologists, there evolved a long era dominated by surgeons and subsequently by anesthesiologists. Certainly, it would seem that the last decade belongs to the cardiologist.

Hugh E. Stephenson, Jr., M.D.

CONTENTS

PART ONE

INTRODUCTORY

Chapter 1

INTRODUCTION: REANIMATOLOGY—THE SCIENCE OF RESUSCITATION

Vladimir A. Negovskii

The Laboratory of Experimental Physiology on the Resuscitation of the Organism was founded in Moscow in 1936 in connection with the N. N. Burdenko Institute of Neurosurgery.

The laboratory was organized by Professor V. A. Negovskii, who has served as its director since it was founded. A small group of young scientists (six or seven) began working with him at that time. They set as their goal the study of the general pathophysiologic regularities of the processes of the extinction and restoration of the vital functions, that is, the heart, the respiration, and the central nervous system (CNS), and also the research of scientifically based methods of resuscitation.

In 1948, in line with a decision of the Council of Ministers of the U.S.S.R., the laboratory was reorganized as an independent scientific research department under the auspices of the Academy of Medical Sciences.

Over the course of 37 years, the laboratory's staff has grown considerably (to sixty-five), and the scope of the work that is carried out has been broadened. The functions of the cardiovascular system, the respiratory center, and the CNS during terminal states and in the restorative period and also the functions of such interior organs as the liver, the kidneys, and the endocrine system as well as biochemical changes arising from the disturbance of metabolic processes and related considerations—all are subjected to detailed study with the help of modern research methods.

Along with its purely experimental department, the laboratory also maintains a clinical department of resuscitation at the S. P. Botkin Hospital. Patients in terminal or near-terminal conditions are brought there from the hospital's various departments. The department of resuscitation also maintains a mobile center, which ensures treatment of terminal patients in hospitals where there is a lack of personnel well-qualified in the area of resuscitation.

Along with applied work in the department of resuscitation, scientific research work dedicated to the study of various clinical aspects of resuscitology is carried out.*

One of the important facts of contemporary science is the ever deeper and more attentive study of the mechanisms of death and resuscitation. Now we are fully justified in speaking of the appearance of a special science dedicated to the study of this question. Cessation of cardiac activity, cessation of respiration, extinction of the functions of the CNS, suppression of the cortical regulation of the physiologic functions, the dynamics of the restoration of functions in the process of resuscitation, and a series of other similar matters make up the content of this science.

Historically it has come about that, along with the rapid development of our knowledge in the treatment of the most varied diseases, we were, even recently, using purely empirical methods thousands of years old regarding the treatment of the dying organism. Attempts at resuscitation were made in ancient times. Apparently, however, only the modern level of development of biologic and medical knowledge provides the prerequisites for a comprehensive study of all the problems relating to resuscitation. Detailed study of the processes of the extinction and restoration of the organism's vital functions, elucidation of

_____
*The Laboratory of Experimental Physiology on the Resuscitation of the Organism, Academy of Medical Sciences of the U.S.S.R., Moscow, U.S.S.R.

the essence of transitional states between life and death, and specifics of the organism's life in terminal states and in the so-called post-reanimation period, and, likewise, elaboration of more modern methods of reanimation—such are the basic problems which, arisen from the needs of life, appealed for their solution to a new medical science: the science of reanimatology.

One of the factors that contributed to the development of reanimatology was the necessity to reconsider fundamentally the concept that had previously been accepted regarding the absolute impossibility of a battle with a "groundless" death. Theoretically the idea was corroborated regarding the reversibility of the death processes when the viable organism is still perishing and the possibility of prevention and, in indicated cases, treatment of terminal states (agony and clinical death).

Although closely linked with a series of such experimental and clinical disciplines as pathophysiology, surgery, anesthesiology, obstetrics and gynecology, and therapeutics (particularly emergency therapeutics), reanimatology, at the same time, finds its own place among these disciplines. Reanimatology generalizes from the material of the above disciplines, not infrequently employing methods already used in them to find a solution to its specific problems. In turn reanimatology enriches these sciences with the results of its own theoretical and clinical investigations. Yet, all the same, reanimatology poses quite original problems for itself, problems whose solutions it approaches from the positions of those theoretical concepts it has elaborated.

Later I shall examine the main problems of the dynamics of the extinction and restoration of the organism's vital functions, consider some debatable questions regarding various methods of resuscitation, and touch on some of the current problems in reanimatology such as the treatment of a resuscitated patient, prognosis, and so forth.

I would like to point out here the differ-ence in the meaning of the two words *reanimatology*—a theoretical science, and *reanimation*—practical measures used for the restoration of vital functions of the organism.

Extinction of functions of cerebral cortex—the first stage of CNS dying

Complete restoration of the functions of the cerebral cortex after terminal states is often impossible because of death of the cerebral neurons, which are extremely sensitive to anemia, hypoxia, intoxication by incompletely oxidized substances of metabolism, and other noxious influences. Relative resistance of ancient, life-ensuring systems (vegetative nervous formation), formed during phylogenesis, and increased sensitivity to pathogenic factors of the highly developed systems (cortex of the hemispheres and some subcortical formations) control the regular sequence of extinction of functions of the central nervous system.

In the very early period of dying, hypoxia causes reflex stimulation of chemoreceptors, angioreceptors, and cerebral vegetative formations including the respiratory and the vasomotor centers and the reticular formation of the brainstem. This reflex stimulation, one of the body's important defense-adaptive factors, is aimed at compensating for failing functions, ensuring homeostasis, and preserving the higher sectors of the central nervous system. It causes accelerated and deeper respiration, acceleration of cardiac contractions, increase of the minute volume of the heart and of arterial blood pressure, constriction of the peripheral blood vessels and of the blood vessels of the abdominal cavity, and dilatation of the capillary network of the brain. Activation of function of the central nervous system is manifested by excitation, motor anxiety, partial restoration of consciousness (in animals, restoration of some conditioned reflexes), the reaction of desynchronization evidenced on electroencephalogram, and other signs. However, in the dying process the activation of the compensatory-defensive process is followed by the equally important activation of the defensive inhibition of the brain cortex, which defends the higher structures of the central nervous system from maximum exhaustion.

It has been proved that this latter signal system is especially sensitive to hypoxia and anemia. Abrupt and considerable hypoxia caused by acute arrest of cerebral circulation or abrupt cardiac arrest leads to almost instant loss of consciousness and, in animals, to loss of conditioned reflexes.

Following the extinction of the cerebral cortex functions, the pupils' reaction to light and corneal, skin, and tendon reflexes decrease and then disappear; paralytic mydriasis supervenes; defense reflexes and reflexes of oral automaticity appear and then disappear; often, tonic paroxysm or decerebrate rigidity is observed; function of the pelvic organs is upset; body temperature falls by 1 or 2° C.; and arterial pressure falls considerably.

Electroencephalographic data point to the earlier extinction of the bioelectrical activity of the cortical structures and adjacent subcortical formations. Follow-up observations of the EEG show that after a transient exaltation of alpha activity, there is slower activity of beta rhythm and in the delta range. In oxygen hunger of the brain, predominance of high-amplitude delta waves of sinusoidal form is typical; they gradually lose their regular form, and the rate and amplitude of biopotentials drop. Later on, "bioelectrical silence" of the cortex supervenes also in the adjacent subcortical formations, but the electrical activity of the nuclei of the amygdaloid complex (archipallium) of the brainstem and its reticular formation is still retained.

Extinction of functions of medulla oblongata during agony

During that period of agony in which the coordinated influences of the brain cortex are inhibited, but the reflex and neurohumoral actions of the brainstem are retained, excitation of the latter is sharply accentuated.

With the bioelectrical silence in the background of the upper segments of the brain, quite often one can observe exaltation of electrical activity of the caudal segment of the brain, especially of its reticular formation. However, control of neurophysiologic functions regulated by the vegetative centers becomes primitive and chaotic. There is pronounced upset in metabolism and in the vitally important functions.

Gross excitation of the vegetative formations of the brainstem (sympathoadrenal structures of the reticular formation, the respiratory and vasomotor centers, and nuclei of the vagus) is especially clear-cut during agony in death from acute hemorrhage. Respiration becomes agonal, cardiac activity increases, and arterial blood pressure increases somewhat, at times leading to the return of bioelectrical activity of the cerebral cortex and even to consciousness, and, in animals, to the return of certain conditioned reflexes. However, progressing influence of the factors of dying leads eventually to extinction of the central (bulbar) control and to inhibition of compensatory-adaptive mechanisms.

On the whole, progressive extinction of the functions of the central nervous system depends mainly on their phylogenetic conditioned complexity, on the degree of resistance to hypoxia of individual formations, on the type of hypoxia, and on the rate of evolution of oxygen hunger in the cerebral structures.

Restoration of the functions of the central nervous system

Evolution of the restoration of the functions of the central nervous system after clinical death depends on the absence or presence of morphologic changes, on the functional relations of structures that have sustained damage from hypoxia, and on the type of pathophysiologic factors acting on the brain during the restorative period. Restoration of the cerebral functions takes place mainly along the functional pathways of individual systems, the links of which are found at different levels of the nervous system. As a rule, function returns first to the functional systems that are phylogenetically more ancient and that are vitally indispensable for the survival of the species.

In the early period of resuscitation, the first to be restored are (1) the automatic activity of the heart and of spinal respiratory centers and (2) the systems that influence muscular tonus. Then the bulbar vegetative centers (vasomotor and respiratory) and the parasympathetic formations (systems of the vagus and oculomotor nerves) begin to function. Although muscular tonus is generally increased, it becomes most predominant in the extensor groups (decerebrate rigidity). Then the functions of nuclear formations, in the systems of the pons varolii, in the midbrain, and the mesencephalon are restored. Return of functions of the body is completed by restoration of the function of the higher nervous system and of the brain cortex, which is confirmed by electroencephalographic data. Biopotentials of the brain begin to be recordable on EEG soon after reappearance of spontaneous respiration and corneal reflexes, during the period of restoration of the muscular tonus and contraction of pupils. Electrical activity of the reticular formation reappears much earlier than in the subcortical formations and the brain cortex. Phases of restoration of the electrical activity of the brain are not always identical with the phases of its extinction.

Animals that survive subcritical periods of clinical death often exhibit paradoxical evolution of electrical activity of the brain. Twenty-four hours after resuscitation, during the period of awakening, the animal's EEG differs little from the normal, although gross changes of function of the higher analyzor and incoordination of movements are present. In the following days, when the neurologic status gradually improves, the electrical activity of the brain may progressively deteriorate. Special investigations have shown that critical periods in the evolution of the EEG

appear between the third and the seventh days of the restorative period. If they occur during the first 3 to 4 days, there are but slight deviations from normal. In a week's time (the critical period), despite restoration of the neurologic status, the amplitude of biopotentials decreases significantly in the range of high frequency rhythms.

The presence of the higher amplitude of brain potentials 1 to 3 days after resuscitation as compared with their low amplitude a week later suggests that the neurons that take part in electrogenesis of the brain are able to function for several days. It is also plausible that even 3 to 6 days after clinical death, which in time is very close to biological death, some pathogenic factors continue to exert their influence and lesions in the brain substance are increased. As a result, we see secondary deterioration of neurologic status, which sometimes occurs in resuscitated patients precisely at the end of the first week after revival and can be lethal.

Extinction and restoration of cardiac activity

In response to the unfavorable factor that provokes hypoxia, the organism's compensatory reactions begin to be manifested. These are implemented at the expense of the excitation of different divisions of the nervous system. On the ECG at this time, along with increased frequency of rhythm and the appearance of other signs of excitation of the sympathetic nervous system (increase of the P wave and quickening of the atrioventricular conduction), only insignificant signs of hypoxia of the myocardium are detected.

According to the depth of hypoxia, the compensatory reactions acquire an opposite character—a state of general inhibition occurs: respiration ceases, and the heart stops as a result of the cessation of the sinus activity. The cessation of the heartbeat in this case is linked with the abrupt elevation of the tonus of the vagus nerves during marked hypoxia. The above observation is corroborated by the effect of atropine in negating the inhibition (Binet and Strumza, 1951). Observation of the ECG shows that, as a result of the inhibition of the sinus activity, the foci of the automatic activity of the second or third order begin to function. Respiration is completely absent during the course of this entire stage, which normally lasts from 2 to 5 minutes.

Next, the agonal stage of dying is characterized by a weakening of the inhibition of the vital functions. This is first manifested on the ECG by a restoration of the sinus activity and by a corresponding increase in the work of the heart, as a result of which a noticeable increase of the arterial pressure may occur. Simultaneously, respiratory movements of the agonal type appear, then systole is gradually slowed and weakened.

During clinical death, sharp changes of bioelectrical activity are not always evidenced on the ECG. Only in the case of a rapid death from exsanguination is a sudden lengthening of the time of atrioventricular conduction noted. This lengthening may serve as a sign of secondary strengthening of vagal inhibition (after the terminal pause). The sinus activity normally persists in the course of the first 2 to 3 minutes of clinical death. Then a complete blockage of atrioventricular conductivity develops, and the pacemaker is the nodal or, more often, the idioventricular focus of slow sinus activity. In some experimental dogs, even during clinical death, it is possible to observe the interchange between periods of the restoration of sinus activity and periods of its retardation.

The normal form of the ventricular complex is preserved for 3 to 5 minutes of clinical death. Later, biopotentials of the heart acquire a character of monophasic deviation, the amplitude of which is gradually lowered. An interesting fact is the sudden shortening of the continuance of the ventricular complex (to 0.18 second) during a clinical death that follows a rapid dying process.

The described sequence of ECG changes is typical for death from acute hemorrhage. With other causes of death, the general trends of ECG evolution are retained; however, changes in the shape of biopotentials have their specific characteristics. Thus, dying from mechanical asphyxia is accompanied by rapid change of sinus rhythm into nodal rhythm even during the agonal stage or in the first minute of clinical death. Amplitude of the T wave soars (the "gigantic" T's). Formation of biphasic and monophasic complexes occurs during the second and third minutes of clinical death, and after 3 minutes bioelectrical activity of the heart generally ceases.

Extinction of bioelectrical activity of the heart in ventricular fibrillation runs a very peculiar course when the condition is caused by electrical trauma. Taking into consideration the presence of two kinds of oscillations —the rhythmic (sinusoidal) and the arrhythmic (polymorphous)—it is possible to describe a number of main stages of the evolution of ventricular fibrillation from the moment of its inception to the marked decrease of the amplitude of ECG potentials. Analysis of ECG data 7 to 10 minutes after electrical trauma permits an assessment of the degree of cardiac hypoxia and consequently of the heart's capacity to function in case defibrillation is decided upon.

The preservation of bioelectrical activity of the heart during clinical death allows the presence of some reflex reactions of the heart. They consist of a disorder in the rhythm of the biopotentials of the heart and the appearance of grouped extrasystolic ventricular complexes in response to irritations of the mucosa in the upper respiratory tract.

Restoration of a normal form of bioelectrical activity of the heart during resuscitation occurs as a kind of reversed (mirror) reflection of the development of the impairment of this activity, which occurred during clinical death. First to be restored is the characteristic form of the ventricular complexes, followed by a restoration of atrioventricular conduction and sinus activity. Subsequently, effective systole occurs. In the case of a short clinical death, the spontaneous work of the heart is restored within 25 to 35 seconds after artificial circulation is established in the organism by using a perfusion apparatus, by forcing the blood into the arteries from ampules, or by external cardiac massage.

As an example of a peculiar phenomenon observed during dying and resuscitation, we can note the short duration of the electrical systole during clinical death and its significant prolongation at the time effective systoles appear. The presence of moments of suddenness in these changes allows us to consider them a consequence of the suppression of several components of the myocardium by the process of stimulation due to the impairment of conductivity during clinical death.

Control from the vasomotor center on the cardiovascular system is normally restored simultaneously with the appearance of the first spontaneous inspiration—within 3 to 4 minutes after resuscitation begins. This is manifested by corresponding changes in the heart's rhythm, synchronized with respiratory movements of the thorax (respiratory arrhythmia).

Earlier or later restoration of the normal appearance of the ECG can serve, in a measure, as an indicator of the degree of preservation of liquidation of the aftereffects that the experience of hypoxia has left on the organism and, correspondingly, as a prognostic sign of the outcome of resuscitative measures.

Respiration

One of the fundamental conditions for resuscitation of the organism is restoration of gaseous interchange in the lungs and early restoration of spontaneous respiration. The appearance of a focus of excitation in the area of the respiratory center promotes the "awakening" of the higher divisions of the brain, which is of fundamental importance for the final outcome of resuscitation (Negovskii, 1943).

Pathophysiologic trends of changes in respiration during the terminal state and the type of its restoration in the postresuscitation period are now fairly well known after experiments on animals (Negovskii, 1943, 1954; Petrov, 1949; Smirenskaya, 1967; Tolova, 1965, 1967, 1971). Patients resuscitated after the terminal state are subjected to the study of their ventilatory indices, which, together with data regarding their acid-base balance, undoubtedly provide much material for assessment of respiratory function, although they do not always indicate respiratory insufficiency. Forced activity of respiratory muscles, even with satisfactory blood gas levels, can be a sign of respiratory insufficiency if pulmonary ventilation is obtained at the expense of profound excitation of the respiratory center that eventually leads to its complete exhaustion. Thus study of the electrical activity of respiratory muscles enables indirect determination of the functional state and functional organization of the respiratory center.

In experiments on dogs the dynamics of the structure of the respiratory act (that is, the correlation of the electrical activity of the inspiratory, the expiratory, and the supplementary respiratory muscles—EMG) were studied, both in the process of the development of a terminal state brought on by massive blood loss and in the period of restoration after clinical death lasting 3 to 8 minutes (Tolova, 1965, 1966, 1967). Besides the EMG of the respiratory muscles, a pneumogram, the volumes of pulmonary ventilation, arterial pressure, the EEG and the ECG were registered, and observation of the animals' general condition was carried out.

An analysis of this experimental material indicates that the structure of the respiratory act—in the process of death from massive exsanguination—undergoes regular changes: the electrical activity of the inspiratory muscles is strengthened, and expiratory and supplementary respiratory muscles are engaged in the act of breathing. During agony, in the inspiration phase, the expiratory muscles contract simultaneously with the inspiratory and the auxiliary respiratory muscles because of the upset of reciprocal interrelationships between the inspiratory and expiratory centers. Because of the potent excitation of the respiratory center, the amplitude of oscillations of biocurrents of the respiratory muscles during agony greatly exceeds the initial level. During this period, impulses from the respiratory center radiate not only to the expiratory center but also to the motor neurons of other skeletal muscles; as a result, electrical activity during the inspiration phase is recorded in all the muscles of the trunk and extremities.

With a long-term death, the character of contractions of the respiratory muscles at the end of agony changes; sustained tetanic contraction is broken up into a series of clonic volleys, repeating the oscillatory rhythm in discharges of the reticular formation of the medulla oblongata. With deepening agony the moment arrives when the discharges in the reticular formation still go on, while signs of activity of the respiratory center, according to the electromyogram of the respiratory muscles, disappear entirely and discharges in the reticular formation of the medulla oblongata become the last reflection of activity of the respiratory center (Gurvich, 1966).

Agonal breathing forms at the expense of the autonomous mechanisms of the medulla oblongata and does not depend on the influence of the higher-lying segments of the central nervous system (Lumsden, 1923; Negovskii, 1943; Breckenridge and Hoff, 1953; Hukuhara and Nakayama, 1959; Arshavsky, 1966; Tolova, 1971). Agonal respiration in terminal states is caused not only by hypoxic exclusion of central control over respiration by the respiratory center of the medulla oblongata, but by this or other degree of hypoxic alteration of the mechanisms in the brainstem (Gurvich, 1966; Tolova and Sidora, 1971).

The respiratory center during agony does not react to the afferent impulses coming from pulmonary receptors and the upper respiratory tract. Section of the afferent nerves (the vagi and the glossopharyngeus)

or stimulation of their central segments produces no effect on the rhythm or rate of respirations or on the electrical activity of the respiratory muscles.

At the end of agony, the first muscles to stop the respiratory rhythm are the expiratory muscles. Next, in 60% of cases, there is simultaneous arrest of diaphragmatic and intercostal respiration; in 40% of cases cessation of intercostal respiration precedes diaphragmatic arrest. In 60% of cases neck muscles switch themselves off from inspiration at the same time as the diaphragm and in 40% of cases after it.

Efficacy of external respiration during agony is extremely low. Minute pulmonary ventilation is only 15% of the initial level. This can be explained by the fact that expiratory muscles (muscles of the anterior abdominal wall), contracting at the same time as the inspiratory muscles, hinder the movements of the diaphragm, which is the main muscle of inspiration, ensuring three fourths of the respiratory volume (Wade, 1954).

In the restorative period after clinical death, the inspiratory center is the first to function—inspiratory and auxiliary respiratory muscles begin to take part in the act of respiration. Expiratory muscles come into play a few minutes later, the time depending on the duration of clinical death. As external breathing becomes normalized, the auxiliary respiratory muscles gradually recede from the respiratory act, but active inspiration is retained for a long time. Thus, on the strength of electromyograms of the respiratory muscles in the postresuscitation period, three types of normalization of structure of the respiratory act have been isolated, which, along with other symptoms of hypoxic lesions of the brainstem, can serve for prognosis of the resuscitation.

At the initial stages of resuscitation, contractions of muscles taking part in respiration are clonic in character. Sustained clonus on electromyogram of respiratory muscles during the restorative period after clinical death for over 20 minutes points to severe hypoxic lesions of the brainstem (Gurvich, 1966).

Nervous mechanisms ensuring active expiration are more sensitive to hypoxia than those controlling inspiration. Restoration of active expiration is often simultaneous with the reappearance of the corneal reflexes, just as during the period of dying, there is also a definite relationship between the time of extinction of corneal reflexes and exclusion of expiratory muscles from the act of respiration. Section of the medulla oblongata at the border between it and the pons varolii produces extinction of electrical activity in the expiratory muscle in the expiratory phase. All these facts allow one to think that the formations of the brainstem taking part in the formation of active expiration are located on the border dividing the medulla oblongata and pons varolii.

During the restorative (postresuscitation) period, the respiratory center begins to react to afferent impulses coming from the lung receptors a few minutes after restoration of respiration. Hering-Breuer reflexes have no significant importance for the appearance of the first inspiration. This is proved, in particular, by results of experiments on vagotomized dogs. After a 5-minute clinical death following hemorrhage, respiration in these dogs was reestablished in the same amount of time as in animals with the vagi intact—in the first 4 minutes after resuscitation had been started (Tolova, 1967; Smirenskaya, 1967). Moreover, in resuscitation with artificial blood circulation apparatus, 10 minutes after circulation had been stopped by ventricular fibrillation (and with the fibrillation still continuing) activity of the respiratory center was restored 3 to 4 minutes from the start of perfusion, even though artificial respiration was not used in these experiments. Delays in restoration of excitability of the respiratory center as related to the afferent impulses depend on the duration of hypoxia. Afferent impulses going to the respiratory center through the vagi, besides influencing the respiration rate, exert a stimulating influence

on the expiratory center. They help restore active expiration, and consequently more effective and less energy-requiring breathing, since with the restoration of active expiration, the oscillation amplitude of biocurrents diminishes both in the inspiratory and in the auxiliary respiratory muscles.

For reflex stimulation of activity of respiratory muscles in the postresuscitation period, respiratory reflexes interlocking at the level of the spinal cord have a definite significance —their intensity depending on the magnitude of the respiratory volume.

In the postterminal period, the nucleus of the diaphragmatic nerve can serve not only to transmit impulses from the respiratory center of the medulla oblongata but also to generate its own rhythmic activity.

Study of the structure of the respiratory act during the restorative period allows an objective criterion of the completeness of the restoration of the functions of central and effector components of the apparatus of external respiration to be established. Intensified work of the respiratory muscles demands an accessory expenditure of energy, which is especially undesirable when hypoxia has not been effectively removed. Hence, artificial respiration should be stopped only when the structure of the respiratory act has become completely normalized, that is, after electrical activity in the auxiliary respiratory muscles has disappeared.

Disturbances of metabolism

The main cause of oxygen budget and acid-base balance disturbances seen in terminal states is hypoxia. However, such disturbances are aggravated by the upset in the function of systems ensuring the control of acid-base balance (central nervous system, respiration, kidneys).

There is a definite trend in the sequence of disturbances of acid-base balance in terminal states produced by different causes (Bulanova, 1966). These disturbances pass through two phases. The first phase—specific —depends on the cause producing the terminal state; it embraces the period of dying and the first 10 to 20 minutes of the restorative period. Changes during this phase can vary greatly. Thus in asphyxia one can see acidosis of a mixed type—gaseous and metabolic; in hemorrhage and electric trauma, gaseous alkalosis in the arterial blood is coupled with metabolic acidosis in the venous blood. However, in all cases, independent of the cause of the terminal state, increasing hypoxia leads to accumulation of suboxidized products of metabolism, lactic acid included, and to the drop of pH in the venous blood.

After 10 to 20 minutes, the specific features of acid-base disturbances, depending on the noxious factor, are smoothed down and the second phase sets in, monotypic in all cases, conditioned by maximum severe hypoxia endured during the dying period and during clinical death. Noncompensated metabolic acidosis is seen at the beginning of this period with the pH falling to 7.0 and lower. The quantity of suboxidized products of metabolism accumulated in the tissues during the clinical death soars, and they enter the bloodstream as the circulation is restored. Concentration of lactate rises to 70 to 80 mg./100 ml. Noncompensated metabolic acidosis, coupled with a low tension of carbon dioxide in the blood, remains unaltered for 1½ to 3 hours after resuscitative measures have been applied, independent of the cause of the circulation arrest.

On the other hand, compensated disturbances of acid-base balance in revived animals are retained much longer. Relative normalization of metabolism seen after 4 to 5 hours after resuscitation is replaced by a new wave of its disturbances; noncompensated gaseous alkalosis develops gradually (pH exceeds initial figures) and arterial hypoxemia is often encountered. It deserves mention that although the concentration of lactate and pyruvate falls below the initial figures after 3 hours following resuscitation, production of lactate exceeds that of pyruvate. The presence of the "lactate excess" and also the increased level of organic acids allow the

hypoxic features of metabolism to be detected (Zaks, 1972).

Even in those animals where restoration of functions after clinical death was prompt, normalization of metabolism occurred roughly 72 hours following resuscitation.

In clinical practice, during urgent resuscitation metabolic or respiratory acidosis predominates, usually compensated or subcompensated. With correct treatment, prompt removal of hemodynamic disturbances and of respiratory distress removes acidosis.

Practical resuscitation frequently also leads to alkalosis, both gaseous and metabolic. Metabolic alkalosis is more often seen at the end of the first 24 hours—at the beginning of the following day of treatment when disturbances of the vitally important functions are already gone. Here base excess is coupled with increased content of organic acids in the blood plasma and with activation of ammoniogenesis in the kidneys. The causes of base excess with the simultaneous presence of hypoxia are not altogether clear: apparently there is a direct relationship to deficit of the volume of circulating blood, total water in the body, and accumulation of bases in the blood plasma.

The study of metabolism of the brain during dying and resuscitation showed that during the process of dying the oxidative pathway of carbohydrate utilization is replaced by the glycolytic pathway (Gaevskaya, 1964). In the condition of clinical death, the brain manages to survive at the expense of the energy of the residual processes of glycolytic transformation of carbohydrate-phosphorus compounds.

Toward the end of a clinical death caused by exsanguination and lasting 5 minutes, glycolysis in the cortex of the brain is slowly extinguished. This process is manifested by a cessation of lactic acid accumulation and the preservation of a constant level of carbohydrates. In the cortex of the brain, PK is absent, there is very little ATP, and a quantity of ammonia accumulates. Along with this, the content of the majority of the free amino acids does not significantly change. The impossibility of subsequent reception of energy to maintain the viability of the brain tissue predetermines the impossibility of resuscitation after a more prolonged period of clinical death.

At the beginning of resuscitation, processes of aerobic glycolysis are in operation in the brain; because of this, the brain tissues restore their reserves of energy and, primarily, of phosphorus chemical compounds rich in energy (PK and ATP). Under these conditions the content of ADP is abruptly lowered. AMP completely disappears, and the level of inorganic phosphate returns to its initial point, but the synthesis of glycogen is still not realized. At this time a sharp change in the content of the free amino acids is observed.

Only after 1 to 2 hours following resuscitation is the brain metabolism transferred into the oxidizing route. The restoration of the oxidative processes and also of the processes of synthesis requires restoration not only of phosphorus chemical combinations rich with energy and of reserves of carbohydrates but also of glutamine as well, with the simultaneous lowering of ammonia in the brain. The content of the free amino acids is also normalized.

A complete normalization of the carbohydrate-phosphorus brain metabolism is observed approximately 72 hours after resuscitation.

Urinary, excretory, and digestive systems

In chronic and acute tests (Kidanov, 1966), the fundamental indicators of the functions of the kidneys (glomerular filtration, maximal secretion, effective renal blood flow, reabsorption and secretion in the canaliculi, and so on) were studied. An analysis of the facts that were gathered in both acute and chronic tests shows that, in the early and late recovery period, diuresis, glomerular filtration, effective renal blood flow, and maximal secretion are significantly lowered. To a lesser extent, the reabsorbing function of the canaliculi is impaired.

One of the fundamental functions of the kidneys, that is, maintenance of the osmotic balance of the inner medium of the organism, suffers very significantly. This is linked with an acute disturbance of the permeability of the cellular membranes and with a slowing of the processes of reabsorption in the renal canaliculi.

However, the function of the kidneys (according to the facts of chronic tests) is gradually normalized after a series of oscillations. The process of restoration is extended over a period of 2 to 4 months, depending on the type of clinical death (electrotrauma, exsanguination) and the length of the dying process (the duration of hypoxia). It is interesting that the degree of injury to the renal functions and the time span of their restoration are correlated with the disturbance and restoration of the functions of the CNS.

In investigations of the function of the stomach (Usievich, 1957), it became apparent that the amount of secretion, acidity, and digestive strength of the gastric juices are lowered during the first several days of the recovery period. Subsequently, the oscillations of these indicators tend to be raised or lowered. Simultaneously, an abrupt rise in the stimulation of the musculature of the stomach is observed. Meanwhile, the excretory function of the stomach suddenly begins to slow down. These disturbances gradually disappear, and the function of the stomach is normalized within 3 months after the patient was resuscitated.

The liver

In the study of the question of the changes of proteinogenic and prothrombinogenic function of the liver in terminal states, it was shown (Shapiro, 1966, 1967) that after a rapid dying process, for example, from electrotrauma, the overall quantity of protein in the blood is not altered. Nonessential changes in the prothrombinogenic function of the liver are manifested.

More significant disorders of the proteinogenic and prothrombinogenic function of this organ occur during a lengthy dying period. With dogs in which, with the use of bleeding, the arterial pressure is maintained at a level of 40 mm. Hg in the course of 2 hours, hypoproteinemia is noted, with a reduction in the quantity of albumins and an increase in the quantity of globulins, possibly caused by the entrance into the bloodstream of the liver's own proteins. The quantity of fibrinogen is reduced during the period of hypotension and is restored directly after resuscitation.

The quantity of prothrombin is significantly reduced in the blood flowing from the liver, both in the period of hypotension and immediately after resuscitation. This testifies to the depression of the prothrombinogenic function of the liver. Also noticeable is the depression of the excretory function of the liver by bromsulphalein (BSP), particularly when the dying process occurs in conjunction with prolonged hypotension. The study of the dynamics of the process of the removal of BSP by Bradley's method reveals a higher threshold for the removal of BSP after the period of clinical death. This can be explained by the suppression of the excretory function of the hepatic cells. A significant increase of the difference in the content of BSP in the arterial blood and in the blood of the hepatic veins is manifested. This apparently depends on the reduced speed of the hepatic blood flow. Doubtless, such extensive and severe impairment of the functions of the liver cannot be without importance for the subsequent restoration of the vital functions of the organism and reflects the essential role of the functional state of the liver in the pathogenesis of terminal conditions. In reality, a sufficiently evident parallelism can be established between the severity of liver lesions, as has been described, and the prognosis for resuscitation.

The role of the liver in the irreversibility of terminal states is seen also in the fact that when, during clinical death, the liver is protected from hypoxia by the aid of isolated perfusion of the organ with oxygenated blood, the prognosis significantly improves during resuscitation (Shapiro, 1970).

The endocrine system

The initial hormonal profile of the body and the endocrine reaction during the development of the terminal state exert vital influence on the resistance of the organism to hypoxia and on the possibility of subsequent resuscitation (Volkov, 1964, 1966; Volkov and Kozhura, 1970). Persistent thyrotoxicosis, diabetes, hypoparathyroidism, and excessive sympathoadrenal reaction diminish the body's resistance to hypoxia in terminal states and make resuscitation more difficult. On the other hand, transient hypothyrosis, administration of insulin with glucose and potassium, and inhibition of pronounced sympathoadrenal reaction contribute toward complete resuscitation after protracted periods of clinical death.

Currently, special attention is being paid to the hypophysis-adrenal cortex systems and its relation to other glands of internal secretion. Preliminary removal of the hypophysis and of the adrenal cortex (but not the medulla) leads to marked deterioration during the terminal state, enhancing the body's sensitivity to hypoxia and rendering more difficult the restoration of functions. The high content of glucocorticoids and ACTH in the body during the period of dying and in the initial period of resuscitation exerts a protective effect on the body, in particular on all the segments of the central nervous system, which is itself hypoxic. After resuscitation, the changes of the adrenocortical functions are closely connected to the character of restoration of the central nervous system. A favorable course of the postresuscitation period is accompanied by a periodic change of inhibition and activation of the adrenal cortex, with inhibition of thyroid function in the background. In severe neurologic disturbances with unfavorable outcome of resuscitation in the posthypoxic period, one notes excessive sympathoadrenal reaction and a prolonged, slow activation of the adrenal cortex and of the thyroid gland with simultaneous inhibition of the insular function of the pancreas. In such conditions, inception and maintenance of the activation of adrenal cortex functions are conditioned to a great extent by modulating influences on the hypothalamus from amygdaloid nuclei of the limbic system of the brain. In addition, parahypophyseal pathways of activation of glucocorticoid secretion predominate and the metabolism of hormones in the liver is upset.

With the use of exogenous glucocorticoids in the initial stages of dying and during resuscitation, it is possible, within certain limits, to direct the course of the terminal state. Administration of small doses of hydrocortisone (1 to 2 mg./kg.) in the initial relative glucocorticoid insufficiency retards agony and clinical death; when the initial reactivity of the adrenal cortex is high, it significantly improves resuscitation results after protracted periods of clinical death. High doses of hydrocortisone (10 to 20 mg./kg.) exert a favorable effect after resuscitation only when there is a relative adrenal insufficiency.

Further investigation of endocrine reactions in terminal states can provide better understanding of the interaction of the nervous and humoral control in dying and in resuscitation. Such investigation can bring out the role of interendocrine relationships in the compensatory and restorative processes. This will permit rational use of hormonal agents in the prophylaxis and treatment of agony and clinical death.

Changes in the blood coagulating system

Disturbances in the coagulating system of the blood contribute to the beginning of massive hemorrhages and to thromboembolic complications. Such complications in the postresuscitation period aggravate the severity of the patient's condition and decrease the efficacy of treatment. Study of the coagulating system and of causes of disorders constitutes one of the main tasks of reanimatology.

On the strength of experiments with circulatory arrest caused by electric trauma, phasic changes were found in the coagulating system of the blood and in fibrinolytic activity, as were the relations of these changes with the functional state of the sympathoadrenal system.

With the cessation of blood circulation, coagulation of the blood is significantly accelerated, and the coagulogram, which includes fifteen different indices, manifests the traits characteristic of hypercoagulation. During resuscitation, the phase of hypercoagulation gives way to a phase of hypocoagulation, and about 1 hour after resuscitation and restoration of the blood circulation, the time of coagulation of the blood is normalized. However, some changes of the coagulogram do not disappear, and these changes are characteristic for prethrombosis state. It is noteworthy that with the change of several indicators of the coagulogram toward hypercoagulation (factors of coagulation), other indicators may have an opposite direction (protective activation of the anticoagulatory factors). Regarding the reaction of the sympathoadrenal system, it is activated simultaneously with the appearance of signs of hypercoagulation (Trusov; Kozhura, 1966). The recovery period (up to 7 hours of observation) is characterized by undulating and multidirectional changes in the indices of the coagulogram, but with a tendency toward normalization.

The intensity of the disturbances in the blood's coagulation as just described is found to depend directly upon the duration of the circulatory arrest and, consequently, upon the severity of hypoxia. Changes in the coagulability of the blood may be laid out as a diagram of the thrombohemorrhagic syndrome (Negovskii and co-workers, 1967; Machabely, 1962). They probably are conditioned by partial intravascular coagulation during the circulatory arrest with a rather rapid activization of the systems and processes directed to the prevention of generalized thrombosis.

Neurohistology

After periods of terminal states in the cerebrum, constantly diffused changes in the nerve cells, glia, fibers, and vessels are noted. They are identical with different causes provoking the clinical death and carry a marked hypoxic character (total tigrolysis; a nucleus hyperchromatosis; swelling of the nerve cells; cariocytolysis; vacuolation of the protoplasm; swelling of the bodies and appendices of the astrocytes; enlargement, agglutination, and unequal distribution of the argyrophilic granules; a thickening of the argyrophilic fibers; and a central tinctorial acidophilia).

Experiments with dogs showed that the development of these lesions has a definite dynamics: directly after coming out of clinical death, changes affected separate cells and vessels, grew during the first days of life, and attained their maximum level in 2 to 3 days. In investigations of the brains of revived animals over a more prolonged period (up to 1 year), it has been shown that a significant portion of the disturbances manifested in the first days of life turn out to be reversible in the course of time. Thus acute hypoxic changes were not noticed after 5 to 7 days of life; vacuolation of the protoplasm and changes of the argyrophilic fibers persisted up to 30 days of life. However, despite the reversed development, part of the nerve cells perish all the same. Most vulnerable are the cortex of the brain, the hippocampus major, and the cerebellum; the brainstem is significantly less harmed, and changes in the nucleus amygdalus are practically not observed

The intensity of histopathologic changes depends on the severity of hypoxia, on the prolongation of the period of dying and clinical death, and also on the rapidity of the restoration of cardiac activity and respiration.

The methods of treatment used also exert an influence on the preservation of the morphologic structure. Morphologic disturbances are significantly less marked under conditions of a high level of arterial pressure established with the help of heart massage, more complete neutralization of the incompletely oxidized products of metabolism, and appropriate employment of artificial respiration using oxygen and air (Romanova, 1962).

Metabolic and toxemic aspects of resuscitation

Complete restoration of the functions of the organism that has experienced clinical death is determined in significant measure by the course of the early period of restoration, since pathologic changes are, for the most part, formed after the restoration of respiration and blood circulation. Precisely in this period specific interrelations of the disturbances of hemodynamics and metabolism are observed. Even in the presence of good indicators of general hemodynamics, injuries of the vitally important systems of the organism may continue to develop or may arise again.

It is known that bringing the organism out of a terminal state, even after cardiac arrest, is often easier than saving the life of a person who has been resuscitated. Thus careful observation of the hemodynamics and respiratory function of patients who have been revived, prolonged application of artificial respiration (sometimes over the course of many days), normalization of the acid-base balance, restoration of the electrolytic and aqueous balance, and so on, are fundamental and absolutely necessary. Along with this arises the important question of the battle with toxemic factors, which can fundamentally worsen the course of the recovery period in patients who have been resuscitated. It has been established that even clinical death with a duration of 3 to 5 minutes, brought on by electrotrauma, and preceded by a period of rapid dying (fibrillation of the heart) leads to a significant suppression of the functions of the liver and kidneys. Along with this, these organs (especially the liver) are in no condition to ensure a sufficient level of disintoxication. Moreover, in this period they can themselves serve as a source for the production of toxic substances. Thus, for a comparatively long period after the restoration of the blood circulation and respiration, the organism is suffering from severe intoxication caused by the products of the disturbed metabolism.

Naturally, it is impossibe to regard disintoxicating methods of treatment of terminal states as universal means suitable for all cases of irreversibility. The pathogenic approach was and remains the fundamental cure for terminal states in all instances. However, the pathologic shifts noticed in these states, which are usually provoked by disturbances of the metabolism with an accumulation of toxic products in the resuscitated organism, always demand the application of disintoxicating therapeutics.

Methods for disintoxicating the organism in early recovery period

An appreciable effect in the resuscitation program after a more prolonged period of clinical death was noted in an experiment where such radical methods as the administration of sodium bicarbonate, the exchange transfusion of blood, and plasmapheresis were used. In dogs resuscitated using these methods after 15 minutes of clinical death provoked by fibrillation of the heart, changes in the CNS were no more marked than in animals that were resuscitated after 10 minutes of fibrillation without supplementary measures. Such a period equals roughly 5 to 6 minutes of clinical death provoked by exsanguination. The active removal of toxic products from the organism by means of exchange transfusion of the blood and plasmapheresis, even more than the application of sodium bicarbonate, helps normalize the metabolism and restore vital activity after 15 minutes of clinical death caused by electrotrauma, and with the use of cross blood transfusion up to 20 minutes. In later experi-

ments an apparatus for artificial circulation was applied (Gerya and co-workers, 1965). At the present time it has still not been established to what extent morphologic changes (which appear after clinical death lasting 15 to 20 minutes in those dogs that outwardly had been fully restored) are "indifferent" for humans; so perhaps it is not yet possible to claim the complete resuscitation of an organism that has endured such a prolonged clinical death. Other means of disintoxication of the organism also deserve attention (drainage of the patient's blood through the specially prepared, insulated pig's liver, the use of an artificial liver, and so on).

PLASMAPHERESIS

The search for a method by which toxic products could be most quickly removed necessitated a detailed study of such comparatively new means of disintoxication of the organism as plasmapheresis. This method allows removal of the blood plasma, in which the toxic products are chiefly concentrated, and the quick administration of washed red cells.

Particular attention was given to the dynamics of restoration of the functions of the CNS after a prolonged cessation of the blood circulation brought on by electrotrauma. It has been shown in experiments (Shikunova, 1966, 1967) that plasmapheresis significantly lengthens the periods of complete circulatory arrest, after which a functional restoration of the CNS is more easily attained. Thus in control experiments in which the heart was stopped for 12 minutes, only 30% of the dogs survived, while in experiments using plasmapheresis, full restoration of the functions of the CNS occurred in 75% of the animals (nine of the twelve dogs in this series) after 14 to 15 minutes of circulatory arrest. Plasmapheresis exercised a favorable influence not only on the duration but also on the nature of the functional restoration of the CNS as well. In the animals to which plasmapheresis was administered, the appearance of uninterrupted electrical activity was noticed earlier than in the control animals. Pathologic sinusoidal activity according to the EEG data was retained in the average by 20 minutes less than in experiments without plasmapheresis (P 0.05). Thus plasmapheresis helped to restore EEG in animals in an easier way.

Over the course of 1 year, in order to study the peculiarities of the restoration of cerebral cortical functions and the possibility of compensation, the acidic defensive method was used to investigate conditioned-reflex activity in two animals that had experienced clinical death lasting 14 to 15 minutes. The formation of both positive- and negative-conditioned reflexes in the resuscitated dogs passed quickly. The positive-conditioned reflexes were strong and high, attesting to the sufficient strength of the stimulating process. Inhibition, according to the elaborated dif-

ferentiation and according to the animal's behavior during and after the experiment, was also suitably strong and well-concentrated.

Several methods of resuscitation

There is no reason to dwell on such methods of resuscitation as external cardiac massage and expiratory artificial respiration. At the present time these methods occupy the leading position in the system of measures for resuscitating the organism and have, by right, gained broad acceptance in the medical profession.

I would like to discuss some techniques that are subject to contradictory opinions in published material (intra-arterial transfusion of the blood and defibrillation) or that have not yet been sufficiently discussed in the literature (electrostimulation of the uterus in the treatment of fatal atonic hemorrhages).

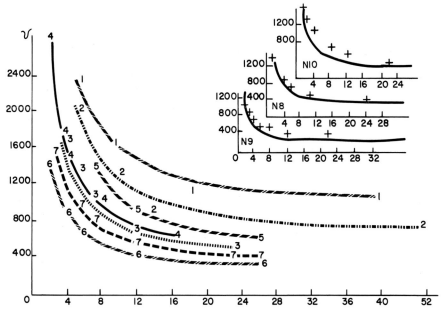

Fig. 1-1. Curved dependencies of the amount of defibrillating tension on the capacity of the condenser (discharge without induction). The capacity, in microfarads (μf.), is plotted on the abscissa and the tension, in volts, on the ordinate. In the upper-right diagram the curves are plotted according to facts gathered in experiments on cats; in the lower diagram the curves are plotted according to facts gathered in experiments on dogs. (From Negovskii, V. A.: Moscow, 1957, Medigiz.)

DEFIBRILLATION

The first defibrillator with a direct current was designed as early as 1900 by Prevost and Batelli. The extremely high tension and insufficient effectiveness of the condenser discharge in these experiments led to an underestimation of the single impulse, with the result that later investigations on defibrillation were conducted primarily with alternating current (Hooker, Kouwenhoven, and Langworthy, 1933; Ferris and co-workers, 1936; Wiggers, 1940). However, the experimental investigations of N. L. Gurvich and G. S. Yuniev (1939, 1946, 1947) show that the effectiveness of the discharge can be significantly increased with an increase of the capacity of the condenser. With a capacity of 10 to 15 μf. for external defibrillation of the heart, a tension of 2 to 3 kv. is necessary (with the energy of the discharge between 20 to 60 watt-seconds). Further research made it possible to establish the now well-known fact that the success of electrical defibrillation of the heart depends on the strength and the duration of the stimulation. Of particular interest is the fact of the coincidence of the temporal characteristic of the curves that reflects this dependence for the defibrillation of the heart and for its stimulation during diastole. When the threshold is of a different value, the value of the chronaxy in either case is about 1 msec. (Fig. 1-1).

On the basis of these facts, it became clear that the defibrillation of the heart is a corollary of the excitatory action of electrical stimulation. This method was later brought up to date, and the effectiveness of the discharge was raised through the inclusion of an inductance in the electric circuit. Induction is valuable because it increases the duration of the impulse, since the initial high-voltage portion of the discharge current is eliminated. This leads to an increase in the effectiveness of the discharge while, simultaneously, the current is three to four times lower and consequently there is much less danger of heart damage. The minimal cur-

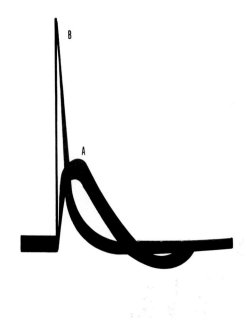

Fig. 1-2. Comparative size of the amplitude of the current in defibrillation of a dog's heart with discharges having a differing form: *A,* 5.25, with a condenser discharge of 24 μf. through an induction of 0.28 henry, and *B,* 19, with a discharge of the same capacity as in *A* but without induction in the electrical circuit of the discharge. The scale is divided into time spans of 0.002 second (a photocomposition of two oscillograms received in two successive experiments). (From Negovskii, V. A.: Moscow, 1957, Medigiz.)

rent for defibrillation of the heart is attained by lengthening the impulse order to 8 to 10 msec.—a prolongation roughly equal to the "useful time span" of heart stimulation. An impulse of this duration is used with a condenser capacity of approximately 20 μf. and an induction of 0.3 henry (active resistance of the induction is 25 to 30 ohms, while that of the animal's thorax is 60 to 70 ohms). In the latest model of the Soviet impulse defibrillator (ID-66) the capacity is lowered somewhat (16 μf.), which gives under the same inductivity 0.3 henry, a more optimal form of impulse.

Inclusion of induction in the electric circuit considerably alters the form of the dis-

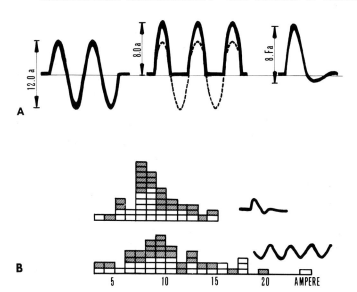

Fig. 1-3. A, Liminal volumes of defibrillating current: alternating current (oscillogram on the left); direct pulsating current (center); solitary impulse with an oscillating discharge (right). **B,** Diagrams of the determined liminal volumes of defibrillating current with a solitary impulse (upper diagram) and with an alternating current (lower diagram). The volumes of the current are plotted horizontally; the number of experimental dogs is plotted vertically. Shaded rectangles correspond to liminal volume of defibrillating current; unshaded rectangles correspond to maximal volume of nondefibrillating current (subliminal).

charge current: instead of a momentary increase in the strength of the current to its maximal amplitude, as with a discharge where induction is absent, an oscillating discharge is received, appearing as a rapidly extinguished sinusoid (Fig. 1-2). This permits a visual comparison of the values of the single impulse and the sinusoidal alternating currents. Such measurings show the approximate coincidence of the current strength in both cases despite varying duration of influence—between 0.01 and 0.2 second (Fig. 1-3). From this, it follows that applying an alternating current for a prolonged time is useless, since the defibrillatory effect occurs in its first period. Further use of the current is superfluous and may only harm the heart. The tension on the patient (and the current that passes through him) is exactly the same with a defibrillation discharge of 4,000 volts and with an alternating current of 440 volts. This is explained by the fact that in the first instance the tension of the subject (in the presence of induction) is three to four times lower than the tension on the condenser (1,000 to 1,300 volts). In the case of the alternating current, the opposite correlation is found: the tension of the full (peak-to-peak) amplitude of the alternating current exceeds its effective value 2.82 times, making up not 440 volts, but 1,240 volts—as many as are received with a discharge from the condenser.

In recent years many authors have used the transient action of the alternating current with the duration of a single period of 0.02 second. Such a method of using A.C. is reasonable, although technically it is more difficult to accomplish.

The use of alternating current to stop arrhythmia in the presence of fibrillation of the auricles may provoke fibrillation of the ventricles. The possibility of such a dangerous complication underlines the greater value of using the single impulse (Mackay and Leeds, 1953; Lown and associates, 1962).

In the Soviet impulse defibrillator ID-1-VEI, the tension of the discharge to the patient is three to four times lower than the tension of the charge on the condenser. With Lown's cardioverter, which has an induction of less than 0.1 henry, the tension on the patient makes up 40% of the tension of the charge on the condenser; and with the equipment of West German firms, the value reaches 65%. For this reason, the defibrillating current is much less in conditions of the same tension of charge and the same energy with the use of the ID-1-VEI apparatus, which has more induction (Fig. 1-4).

In several models of defibrillators the scale of the instrument is not gradated according to tension but according to the energy of the discharge in watt-seconds. This evaluation seems less valuable, since the energy of the discharge in the presence of induction in the electric circuit is distributed differently than it is with a direct discharge (without induction). Besides that, any given quantity of watt-seconds in the presence of an inadequate form of impulse does not ensure the effectiveness of the latter (that is, of the

direct discharge). The basic problem is in maintaining an optimal impulse length (7 to 8 msec.); therefore, only one of the two parameters of the impulse is subject to calibration, namely, tension. It is regulated by the doctor, depending upon specific conditions.

In line with the previous discussion, it seems not entirely correct to use the term "direct current" with respect to the impulse defibrillator and the impulse that it generates. This term came into use as a result of contrasting the single impulse as a "direct current" to the alternating current. Considerable amplitude of the second half-period is a necessary component of the defibrillatory effect. Investigations in recent years (Gurvich, 1966; Makarychev, 1967) have shown that the stimulating action of two peak-to-peak half-waves is summarized in the effect of defibrillation. With the removal of the second half-wave, which reaches 40% to 50% of the amplitude of the first, it is necessary to strengthen the current of the first half-wave by the same value (Fig. 1-5). It is obvious that the summation of the stimulating action of the current's two directions is an important condition for the optimum effect of the oscillating discharge, since this lowers the absolute value of the current. Thus the two-phase impulse has more of a resemblance to one period of the alternating current and consequently the use of the term "direct current" in the strict sense of this word is not justified.

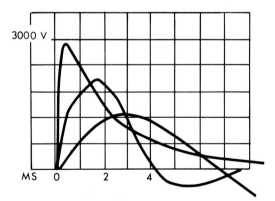

Fig. 1-4. Varying volumes of tension on a patient with an impulse of 200 watt-seconds depending on the form of impulse generated by the apparatus: 3,000 volts—from the apparatus Defi-card FRG; 2,000 volts—from the Lown cardioverter; and 1,300 volts—from the ID-66 apparatus.

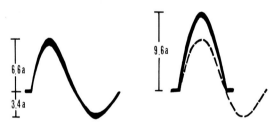

Fig. 1-5. Comparative volumes of defibrillating current with a two-phase impulse of an oscillating discharge (left) and without a second half-wave (right).

The importance of lowering the strength of the defibrillating current becomes evident upon calculation of the volume of current needed for defibrillation. A measurement of this volume in the clinic (Makarychev, Tsukerman, and Gurvich, 1966) shows that even with a relatively low tension of the discharge (up to 4 kv., 100 watt-seconds) the amplitude of the current of the first half-period attains 20 to 25 amperes; and with 5 kv. (200 watt-seconds) it attains up to 30 amperes. The resistance of the patient's thorax to the discharge current was 30 to 50 ohms, and the indicated values of the current were applied with a discharge tension of 800 to 1,300 volts directly on the patient.

Occasionally it is mistakenly supposed that the stronger the current, the more reliable its action and the more stable the effect. Furthermore, a result of such a supposition is that, with a relapse of arrhythmia, the discharge tension is increased. The basic value of electropathy lies in the fact that it eliminates arrhythmia, not by means of a change in the functions of the heart, but as a result of the effect of a single moment—the electrical stimulation of the entire heart. The less the accessory influence of current strength (suppression of conductivity, extrasystoles), the more reliable and effective the electropathy.

In clinics in the Soviet Union, an impulse defibrillator of the type ID-1-VEI has been used since 1952 in heart operations. More recently it has been used for external defibrillation of the ventricles and for the counteracting of other arrhythmias (Vishnevskii and co-workers, 1959; Radushkevich, 1966; Lukoshevichute, 1965).

In later years a single electrical impulse found its place in obstetrics for treatment of atonic postpartum hemorrhages. The method is based on the marked increase of the tonus of the uterus under the influence of an electrical impulse. In clinics, the defibrillator of N. L. Gurvich is usually used. The advantages of this method, suggested by Z. A. Chiladze (1964) together with scientists of our laboratory (Negovskii, Berman, Gurvich, 1966), are its simplicity in use, the possibility of offering aid to the woman with maximum speed, and, especially important, the ability to avoid amputation or extirpation of the womb, a method that is usually resorted to.

INTRA-ARTERIAL BLOOD TRANSFUSION

Although indications for arterial infusion of blood have become more restricted in more recent years, this method still occupies a leading place among measures for prophylaxis and treatment of terminal states.

Arterial blood infusion is exceptionally important for treatment of prolonged hypotension, when intravenous transfusions are ineffective. It is known that protracted hypotension, especially when preceded by unreplaced blood loss, can lead to irreversible damage of vitally important organs even before clinical death has set in. In hypotension caused by massive unreplaced blood loss repeated arterial transfusions help not only to reestablish the volume of the circulating blood more rapidly, but also to normalize hemodynamics, thus preventing further negative action of hypotension on the body. If hypotension persists despite replacement of blood loss, good results can be obtained with fractional arterial infusions combined with administration of corticosteroids and agents tending to normalize body metabolism Zolotokrylina, 1966).

In treating clinical death, external massage of the heart is justifiably preferred as a more simple, accessible, and effective method. However, external massage coupled with artificial ventilation of the lungs does not always produce the level of arterial pressure that is necessary to reestablish cardiac activity, respiration, and functions of the higher segments of the brain. It is especially difficult to maintain arterial pressure at a sufficiently high level when the heart stops from massive blood loss. Under these conditions, in our opinion, external cardiac massage must be combined with transfusion therapy (Negovskii, 1966).

However, the question of the best means of reestablishing the volume of the circulating blood continues to be discussed (Kirimli and Safar). Experiments on dogs in our laboratory show the advantages of arterial infusion over the intravenous method. The combination of external cardiac massage with arterial blood transfusion (at the rate of 15 ml./kg./min.) started after 5 minutes of clinical death produced rise of arterial pressure in the first 15 seconds from the beginning of resuscitation, sinus rhythm appeared on ECG, cardiac activity reappeared after 68 ± 19.3 seconds, respiration after 4 minutes, 38 ± 38 seconds, and the concentration of the sum of organic acids fell by the end of the first hour to 13.7 ± 0.6 mEq. per liter. Complete and stable restoration of the functions of the central nervous system was recorded in 72% of the animals. When external cardiac massage was combined with intravenous blood transfusions at the same rate of administration after identical periods of dying and clinical death, arterial pressure began to rise at the end of the first minute of resuscitation, ventricular fibrillation appeared as a rule, and cardiac activity was restored after defibrillation (sometimes repeated) after 4 minutes, 19 ± 40.3 seconds, respiration after 10 minutes, 34 seconds ± 2 minutes, 12 seconds and the concentration of the sum of organic acids remained at 23.9 ± 0.81 mEq. per liter at the end of the first hour of resuscitation. Complete and stable restoration of the functions of the higher segments of the central nervous system, could be recorded in only 20% of the animals in this group.

There is every reason to believe that higher efficacy of external cardiac massage with arterial infusion as compared with the intravenous method results from the different mechanisms of the action of these measures. Inception of arteriovenous gradient in the beginning of resuscitation with arterial transfusion of the blood contributes to an earlier restoration of circulation in the body and, in particular, in the coronary vessels.

With removal or decrease of hypoxia, the reflex stimulation of the cardiovascular system from angioreceptors is of great significance.

A special role is played by arterial infusion of the blood when blood loss is coupled with traumatic shock. In this condition the pain stimulus becomes ultrastrong and, even with a relatively small blood loss, leads to disruption of compensatory mechanisms.

The possibility of various complications while the arteries are being manipulated is often used as an argument against the use of intra-arterial transfusions. This danger, however, must not be exaggerated. Extensive clinical experience and literature data show that, with careful operative technique of isolation of the artery, such complications are extremely rare. In any case, we believe this possible danger cannot serve as a motive to ban from the arsenal of resuscitation measures such an effective means of resuscitation as intra-arterial transfusion. The more severe the condition, the wider are the indications for the use of this method.

The period of restoration

When it has experienced prolonged agony of clinical death of any duration, the organism is in a state of the most severe morbidity. Practically all the systems and organs are gripped by a complex interaction of the processes of restitution, compensation, and the appearance of new injuries. The period of restoration after resuscitation may least of all be called restorative in the true sense of this word. The patient who has just been resuscitated experiences a special disease that probably should be classified as an independent disease entity that we might label disease of a resuscitated patient.

Among pathologic changes that entail particularly severe sequelae for the body, disturbances of metabolism and, above all, of the acid-base balance must be mentioned. Every hypoxia is accompanied by acidosis, but postterminal acidosis runs an especially severe course and exerts an unfavorable influence on the outcome of resuscitation. Content of suboxidized products in the blood after restoration of cardiac activity rises 2.5 to 3.5 times as they are washed out of tissues. However, this does not mean that the concentration of suboxidized products in tissues diminishes. Their accumulation results from the disparity between the increasing demand for oxygen on the part of tissues and the limited possibilities for its utilization, conditioned by cardiovascular and respiratory insufficiency. Thus, in brain tissues, concentration of organic acids continues to be as high 20 to 30 minutes after resuscitation as it is at the end of the period of clinical death. Accumulation of suboxidized products of metabolism at the beginning of the restorative period leads to noncompensated metabolic acidosis. If the condition of patients deteriorates (labile arterial pressure, acute deficit of circulating blood volume in the early period of restoration) the pH of the blood drops to 7.19 ± 0.03 and deficit of bases is 11.8 ± 1.9 mEq. per liter. With a favorable course, in 6 to 7 hours noncompensated metabolic acidosis becomes compensated.

Later on (at the end of 24 hours and in the beginning of the next day), bases accumulate and metabolic acidosis is transformed into alkalosis. Subcompensated and decompensated forms of metabolic alkalosis are seen more often with the more severely ill patients.

However, data that we possess indicates that an increase of sodium bicarbonate in plasma does not always point to a great reserve of bases in the vascular sector. Development of metabolic alkalosis is the consequence of hypovolemia.

Disturbances in the acid-base balance are accompanied by upset of electrolyte balance in the cells, that is, the accumulation of sodium ions and the loss of potassium ions. Sustained hypokalemia, as well as progressing kaliuresis, points to the severity of electrolyte metabolism disturbance and constitutes a bad prognostic sign. It must be noted that a fairly good level of arterial pressure during the restorative period does not yet mean complete well-being. Histophysiological investigations (Levin, 1966) showed that in the initial period of resuscitation, considerable disturbances of microcirculation exist (aggregation of the formed elements of the blood; occlusion of capillary lumen), which are aggravated by the spasm of peripheral vessels. As a result of this, inflow of oxygen to tissues takes place unevenly and in those areas where the capillaries do not function, cells continue to suffer from oxygen want. These disturbances of hemodynamics aggravate shifts in the acid-base balance, which in turn exert unfavorable influence on the circulation. Thus a vicious circle is formed.

In the restorative period severe secondary changes have already developed in the body; these are most pronounced in the central nervous system (as a result of microcirculatory upset) or in the parenchymatous organs —liver and kidneys (as a result of circulatory centralization)—and often lead to a fatal outcome.

It is well known that after periods of clinical death slightly exceeding the "permissible" duration in dogs, electrical activity of the cerebral cortex is almost completely restored 1 to 2 days after resuscitation. In this period, however, paresis, impairment of coordination, and impairment of the functions of such analyzors as vision and hearing may be observed. After 4 to 7 days, despite apparent restoration of the neurologic functions, there is a clear and irreversible depression of the electrical activity of the brain. An extremely flattened curve is registered on the EEG. Morphologically, in such dogs killed 3 to 4 weeks after resuscitation, very severe atrophic processes in the higher divisions of the cerebral hemispheres and in the cerebellum are manifested. These facts thus demonstrate a parallel course of both processes: on the one hand, restitution and compensation, and, on the other, appearance of new disturbances.

In clinical literature dedicated to the dynamics of neurologic changes in resuscitated patients, many observations have been accumulated regarding secondary deterioration of the neurologic status 2 to 4 days after the functions of the CNS were initially restored quickly. In a brain section of such patients, widespread, very severe changes in the subcortical nuclei are most often manifested.

The nature of secondary changes in the brain in the postreanimation period is still not sufficiently clear. Probably these changes are provoked by the joint action of the disturbance of the microcirculation, by intoxication from incompletely oxidized metabolic products, by the action of a hypoxic edema, and by the disturbance of the midcentral relations accompanied by the development of motor excitation and convulsions. However, neither the developmental mechanism nor the significance of the posthypoxic edema of the brain is entirely clear. Unfortunately very little is known about the nature of the intimate changes that are developed in the neurons after the restoration of gas exchange and circulation. Apparently it is impossible to explain these changes by a privation of oxygen alone; supplementary and detailed investigations are needed.

In relation to the above, treatment of disease of a resuscitated organism must be directed in the first place against hypoxia (circulatory, anemic, and hypoxic), intoxication, and the developing metabolic disturbances caused by them.

Prognosis

To arrive at a prognosis we attempt to evaluate pathologic changes that arise in many organs and systems, namely, in the heart, the regulatory system of ventilation, the endocrine system, and the liver, the blood, the CNS, and the enzyme spectrum. Since changes that arise in the CNS have the greatest meaning in the final analysis of restoration, particular attention is now being devoted to the development of systems for neurologic prognosis.

It has been found that resistance of the brain to hypoxia has definite limits, and if its viability has been retained, cerebral functions are reestablished without fail under the influence of a current of afferent impulses and humoral effects after resumption of circulation and gaseous exchange.

Systems of criteria for an early prognosis are, for the time being, worked out in experiments on laboratory animals. Prognosis is based for the most part on the EEG and EMG data (Gurvich, 1966a, b, and c; Tolova, 1965, 1966, 1967).

Because functions of the phylogenetically more ancient parts of the brain, its stem in particular, possess resistance to hypoxia to a greater degree and are restored much earlier than the functions of other younger parts, the earliest evidence of the severity of injuries appearing in the brain can be expected from the EMG of the respiratory muscles, which reflect changes in the neural regulation of respiration. The prognostic meaning, as has been shown, is correlated with the interrelation between inspiratory, expiratory, and auxiliary respiratory muscular activity in the very earliest stages when spontaneous respiration is restored. Particular changes in the EMG of the inspiratory and auxiliary muscles appear on the "summarized" EMG. Instead of the normal asynchronous, tetanic discharge, a clonic discharge of excitation with a rhythm of clonic contractions of nine to twelve per second is registered. This is a reliable negative prognostic sign in a death caused by exsanguination and sudden cardiac arrest. The presence of these changes allows a foundation for prognosis only within 15 to 20 minutes after the beginning of resuscitation.

The severity of injuries to the CNS may be judged by the time of the restoration of respiration and by some neuroreflex reactions. Thus the delay of the appearance of spontaneous respiration beyond 4 to 10 minutes (depending on the causes of death), the absence of the corneal reflex for more than 20 minutes, and the appearance of decerebration, rigidity, and general convulsions all serve as unfavorable prognostic signs.

Electroencephalographic criteria of prognosis are particularly valuable and reliable, but only if the technical requirements of EEG recording are strictly adhered to and follow-up observations are made; the earlier the first record is made, the more reliable the prognosis (Gurvich, 1966; Pampiglione and Harden, 1968; Kurtz et al., 1970).

The sudden restitution of uninterrupted polymorphous electrical activity of the brain of sufficient amplitude (more than 25 to 50 μv.) within 5 minutes after the beginning of resuscitation is favorable to the functional restoration of the CNS. Lengthening the time of latent restoration (electrical silence) of the EEG to 25 to 30 minutes and lengthening the period of restoration of uninterrupted activity to 50 minutes (without the appearance of convulsive potentials or synchronous sinusoidal activity along the entire surface of the hemispheres) with a frequency of 7 to 14 oscillations per second are compatible with a complete restoration of the CNS, but they indicate that the latter will proceed with difficulties and delay. An unfavorable prognostic meaning lies in prolongation of the latent recovery period beyond 30 minutes or delay beyond 50 minutes in restoring uninterrupted activity, combined with the appearance in the EEG of the pathologic oscillations mentioned. The functions of the CNS in this case are not usually restored.

The types and variants of EEG restoration, which were described above, are conditioned by the duration of the circulatory arrest and by the severity of the injuries to the CNS. This dependence, along with the simultaneous registration of the rate of restoration of the EEG, can be used for prognosis.

These criteria are reliable when one is dealing with unanesthetized animals dying under normothermia as well as for animals dying under conditions of superficial ether anesthesia. To make a prognosis of restoration of functions of the central nervous system of a resuscitated man is a considerably more complicated matter. Early prognostic criteria found experimentally can be carried over to clinical practice with utmost care. In clinical practice, according to the majority of authors, the following symptom complexes have decisive significance.

The most serious prognostic symptom complex is the persistent coma (coma depassé) in which all signs of the organism's vital activity are completely lacking except cardiac activity, which is maintained by pharmacologic stimulants and artificial respiration. In this state the tonus of all the muscles and all forms of reflex reactions (including the reflexes involving the heart) are absent; there is no reaction of cardiac activity to the atropine, and all electrical manifestations of brain activity are absent. If such a condition persists for 24 hours or longer, further treatment of the patient is hopeless (Mollaret and Goulon, 1959; Jouvet, 1959; Schwab, 1967).

In irreversible coma the level of metabolic processes in the brain drops violently as shown by the exceedingly low arteriovenous difference in oxygen, lower 2.0 to 2.4 vol.% (Raudam et al., 1969; Gerand et al., 1969), and decrease to lower than 10% of the normal of oxygen utilization by the brain (Hoyer and Wawerisk, 1968; Shalit et al., 1970). The "nonfilling phenomenon" in total cerebral angiography (Gros et al., 1970; Vlachovitch et al., 1971; Negovskii, 1971) as well as marked decrease of volume blood flow in the brain (5 to 10 ml./100 g./min.) measured after Kety or with the aid of Xe^{133} clearance (Brock et al., 1969; Bes et al., 1969) is a convincing proof of "brain death." However, it must be noted that to prove brain death, stoppage of blood flow in all four main arteries must be ascertained. In presence of other clinical signs of brain death (areflexia, atony, absence of respiration, and bioelectric silence on EEG), absence of cerebral circulation for 20 to 30 minutes is apparently sufficient for a corresponding diagnosis.

In less serious cases where the restoration of the functions of the CNS is still hopeless, maintenance of complete electrical silence in the EEG for 45 to 60 minutes after the beginning of resuscitation serves as a manifestation of irreversible brain damage. In a later period, damage is attested to by the persistence over the span of many hours of EEG delta waves that are broken by intervals of electrical silence and/or convulsion potentials registered when the patient is completely immobilized and transferred to controlled ventilation. Manifestations of this damage are: (1) delay in restoring spontaneous respiration for a period of more than 1 to 1.5 hours; (2) the absence of corneal reflexes for more than 4 to 6 hours; (3) persistent disturbances of the oculomotor innervation (absence of the reaction of the pupils to light, anisocoria, deformations and displacement of the pupils, natatorial movements of the eyes, deviation of one or both eyeballs) lasting many hours; and (4) persistent, generalized clonic contractions and general convulsions, particularly when they appear 12 hours or more after resuscitation and hyperthermia (Gurvich, 1966; Hockaday and associates, 1965).

Favorable signs include rapid restoration of spontaneous respiration and eye reflexes (within 3 to 10 minutes) and the appearance of uninterrupted polymorphous electrical activity of the brain within 10 to 15 minutes after the beginning of resuscitation and its rapid enrichment by frequent oscillation.

If initially favorable restoration of the neurologic functions is disturbed in the first hours after resuscitation, even by momentary worsening of hemodynamics and the gaseous interchange, and is accompanied by a repeated development of electrical silence on the EEG, the prognosis is severely worsened and normally becomes hopeless (Arfel, 1963, 1970).

It has been mentioned that rapid restoration of the neurologic functions within 1 to 3 days in patients who have suffered clinical death does not provide a basis for an absolutely favorable prognosis. In cases of apparently complete well-being for 2 to 5 days after resuscitation, a sudden, serious worsening of the neurologic status, which usually turns out to be fatal, is possible. Thus control over the state of such patients must be preserved for no less than 1 week.

For later prognosis of restoration besides the criteria previously described, the duration of coma may also be used. Clinical practice shows that when the recovery period has a favorable course the length of deep coma does not usually exceed 48 hours. Duration of a coma of such depth for a period of more than 4 days is followed by complete recovery only in isolated cases.

The foregoing criteria of prognosis were established for patients who had suffered clinical death in conditions of normothermia and without the use of large doses of barbiturates. In terminal states that have developed as a result of intoxication, particularly under the effect of barbiturates, and also as a result of trauma, complete restoration is possible after much more prolonged periods of deep coma and a low electrical activity of the brain. A reliable system of prognosis for these states has still not been worked out.

Prolonged hypotension, often preceding the onset of clinical death, has an extremely negative influence on the outcome of reanimation. The prolongation of hypotension for a period of many hours, during which maximal arterial pressure does not exceed 40 mm. Hg, can lead to irreversible disturbance to the CNS and to serious injuries of the liver and kidneys even before the onset of clinical death. It is also difficult to effect the complete restoration of the functions of the CNS, even in the absence of hypotension in patients who have previously experienced injuries of the liver and kidneys.

As a result of discussions on the question of brain death by national (United States, France, Federated German Republic, Switzerland, Czechoslovakia, Great Britain) and international commissions of specialists, in particular by the Commission on Transplantation of the Heart of the Council of International Medical Organisations (C.J.O.M.S., 1968), the Committee on Brain Death of the International Federation of Societies on

EEG and Clinical Neurophysiology, and by others (Negovskii, 1971; Penin, Kaufer, 1969) the following criteria of brain death may be considered as generally recognized:

1. Complete and prolonged absence of consciousness
2. Prolonged absence of spontaneous respiration
3. Disappearance of all reactions to external stimulation and of all types of reflexes
4. Atony of all muscles
5. Disappearance of control of body temperature
6. Preservation of vascular tonus only by administration of vascular analeptics
7. Complete and persistent absence of spontaneous or induced electrical activity of the brain

All these criteria are valid only in normothermia (body temperature not lower than 93.2° F. [34° C.]) and when action of narcotics has been excluded.

Thorough experimental and clinical study of these and many other problems of reanimatology, a contribution that brings to this question scholars from all nations (A. A. Vishnevskii, B. V. Petrovskii, V. A. Korolev, I. R. Petrov, V. P. Radushkevich, H. Stephenson, P. Safar, C. Beck, R. Hosler, E. Ciocatto, A. Larcan, U. Strahl, B. Peleska, E. Racenberg, M. Holmdahl, O. Norlander, and many others) provides us with a basis to hope for correct solutions to the main problems of this young science. A more effective battle to return life to those who are dying or who have just died depends on this.

Chapter 2

DEATH

Harold H. Hillman

Despite the fact that "death lays his icy hand on all," it is remarkable how little is understood of the phenomenon. Yet fundamental advance in resuscitation must involve, at some stage, greater comprehension of death's pathology and biochemistry. Furthermore, all over the world, the lives of thousands of hypothermic old people, shipwrecked sailors, avalanche victims, and exposed mountaineers might be saved if knowledge that is already available were applied to their treatment.

There has been a great resistance to the study of death, some of it irrational. Probably part of this resistance originates from the feeling that in an overpopulated world, it would be mischievous even to attempt to keep alive a large number of aged senile patients with multiple pathologic conditions. A discussion of the desirability of this is outside the interest of this chapter, which is concerned mainly with the acute death in the otherwise relatively healthy patient.

Definition

Much of the confusion about death in recent years has risen from the failure to understand that it is a continuous loss of body organization. Death is defined at different levels.

THE GENERAL PRACTITIONER'S CRITERIA

For practical purposes, the general practitioner wants to know when he can instruct the undertaker to proceed with the burial.

Several criteria must be used, as no single one is pathognomonic; they are briefly described in the following paragraphs.

Absence of heartbeat and radial and carotid pulses is the first criterion. However, in hypothermia and fainting, the pulses may be absent and in the rare condition, Takayusu's disease, the peripheral pulses are absent and the carotid body is hypersensitive. In emphysema and in pneumothorax, the heartbeat sometimes cannot be heard, and in hypotension, from any cause, and arteriosclerosis, the peripheral pulses may not be easily palpable. Furthermore, on auscultation of the chest in recently dead patients a rumbling sound, probably caused by redistribution of the blood, may be mistaken for weak heartbeats or respiratory sounds.

In hospitals, an electrocardiogram or cardioscope may be used to see if the heart is still beating. The atrium usually continues for minutes or hours after the ventricle has stopped, and as the QRS complex diminishes in amplitude it becomes impossible to distinguish from the P wave, which remains at fairly constant amplitude of about 0.5 mv. until the atria stop.

Apnea is the second sign the general practitioner normally uses. It is detected by absence of movement of lips, nostrils, and chest and by auscultation for the respiratory sounds. The old-fashioned mirror test shows deposit of moisture from the expired air. Apnea is present in the conditions of cardiac arrest, but it may also occur in barbiturate or morphia overdosage and in high cervical lesions. It is important to appreciate that apnea during dying or hypothermia occurs many valuable minutes before cardiac arrest; within one minute of apnea, serious damage has occurred to the control of the heart (Feldman and Hillman, 1969).

Cyanosis and *blotchy skin* also occur in cor pulmonale, exposure, malnutrition, drug addiction, and as a result of beating or torture.

"Glassy eyes" are also seen in dehydration and malnutrition and occasionally in psychosis.

Dilated fixed pupils are a sign of death, but it also occurs in brain damage, drug addiction, and occasionally after epilepsy. Some cosmetic preparations used by women also cause this.

Areflexia is a sign of deep hypothermia and deep coma due to any cause, particularly intoxication. General paralysis of the insane or any lower motor neuron lesion can produce local loss of reflexes.

Lowered body temperature, besides being a sign of death, may be seen in hypothermia, malnutrition, exposure, drug intoxication, anesthesia, and phenothiazine or Rauwiloid ingestion; the skin temperature may not reflect the core temperature accurately, and the body temperature may not appear to have fallen if the patient had hyperpyrexia previously or if the ambient temperature was near body temperature.

Patients who have died recently often defecate or micturate, but this rarely occurs in hypothermic animals (Hillman, Loupekine, and Fullbrook, 1972).

I would like to conclude this list by saying that the absolute criterion for death is its irreversibility, because there are many cases in the literature of patients who have had all the previously listed signs, yet have subsequently recovered.

DEATH AND TRANSPLANTATION

Corneas and kidneys can be taken out of dead patients, but transplant surgeons prefer to use as donors patients who have their circulations physiologically intact but their nervous systems grossly and irreversibly damaged. Obviously, such patients have relatively normal respiratory and cardiovascular systems even if they have to be supported by artificial respiration or extracorporeal circulation. Transplants are considered only from patients who have, as evidence of drastically diminished cerebral function, a flat electroencephalogram for at least several hours; many surgeons also will not excise organs unless there is radiologic evidence of cerebral damage. It is thus clear that many transplant teams do not wait as long as the general practitioner to consider a patient dead, because the longer a patient has been dead by any criteria, the less likely his organs are to be recovered to subsequent complete function in the recipient.

The legal situation. The law in regard to death and transplantation is in a very ambivalent situation. Since donors at the time of transplant have relatively normal cardio-respiratory function, they could be considered to be alive. In a certain sense, then, excision of their organs may be illegal.

There is a great deal of public apprehension lest organs be excised prematurely, preventing recovery of a patient who might have had some chance. Legal aspects are beyond the ambit of this chapter, but it may be worth noting that, both in the United States and Britain, it has been suggested that a legal basis be established for the intermediate condition (Capron and Kass, 1972; Hillman and Aldridge, 1972). Hillman and Aldridge propose that a condition of "irreversible brain damage" be certifiable by doctors not connected with the transplant team and nominated by the relatives of the potential donor; the certification, given only after tests had proved conclusively the existence of irreversible brain damage, would permit excision of the donor organs. It is hoped that this would allay public anxiety. The proposed new legal definition would not include the term "death," and would not disturb the current legal definition, involved as it is in questions of inheritance, partnership, compensation, and so forth.

Organ death. Even if the general practitioner's definition of death is used, a cornea, kidney, or blood vessel can still be excised and transplanted. For nearly 100 years biochemists have been perfusing isolated hearts and for 50 years they have been setting up heart-lung preparations, all taken from dead animals. The isolated muscle contracts on stimulation of its nerve and the isolated brain has virtually normal electrical activity (White, Albin, and Verdura, 1964) long after the animals from which these organs have been taken have been discarded. Therefore, although the animal is dead in that it has lost a major degree of organization, its organs can still function relatively normally; death of these organs is a further loss of organization.

Stages of dying

As an animal dies, it goes through several stages, which have been classified in the following way: First, there is an excitatory stage, probably caused initially by a stress and pain reaction. At a later stage, the excitatory state can be attributed to hypoxia stimulating the motor area of the brain or the cut ends of nerves initiating a train of excitatory depolarization. A second stage may be called the autonomic stage, when the hair erects, the pupils dilate, and the animals defecate or micturate. The final disorganization of the whole animal occurs when the temperature, blood pressure, and reflexes disappear, still, however, leaving the organs potentially functional.

Biochemistry of death

Relatively little is known about the biochemistry of the body during dying, although the brain has been studied more than other organs (Gaevskaya, 1964; Negovskii, 1962; Leonard and Hillman, 1973). There is probably a massive stress reaction resulting in the release of catecholamines and corticosteroids, although this has yet to be demonstrated

biochemically. The cerebral adenosine triphosphate, phosphocreatine, and glucose levels fall dramatically, the latter almost to zero. The cerebral lactate level rises, although animals can subsequently recover from a high venous lactate level (Rogers and Hillman, 1972). The cerebral Na^+ and K^+ concentrations both fall slightly, probably because of cerebral swelling. The serum K^+ level rises and Na^+ level falls, since the extracellular concentrations of these ions are dependent on the supply of substrate and oxygen (Hillman, 1964). Nevertheless, all the cerebral changes can be mimicked during convulsions or stimulation of cerebral slices (McIlwain and Rodnight, 1962) and are reversible. Thus is seen the paradox that the overall death of the animal is irreversible by definition, but the apparent physiologic and biochemical changes within the individual organs are not.

Hypoxia

There are several clues to the physiologic nature of death. At the tissue level, it is probably caused by hypoxia for a period of tens of minutes. Hypoxia normally not only "stops the machine, but wrecks the machinery." However, even this is a generalization that should be tempered. Andjus and Smith (1955) froze down rats that had been narcotized by their own expired carbon dioxide, and were almost certainly extremely hypoxic. Within a week, they recovered completely even their ability to find their way through mazes (Mrosovsky, 1967). We have frozen pentobarbital-anesthetized rats down to cardiac arrest in which they had no oxygen in the venous blood (Rogers and Hillman, 1970a), yet such animals could subsequently be induced to recover (Rogers and Hillman, 1970b). Of course, it is generally held among clinicians that about 4 minutes' cardiac arrest causes irreversible brain damage and this has been detected on electron microscopy (Brown and Brierley, 1968). Hypothermic animals have been shown to recover completely from 30 minutes' cardiac arrest, but that is not death, and the experimental animals were young and healthy. Infarcted patients are not. Also, the cold may have protected the animals used. Nevertheless, it would be wrong to be too dogmatic about hypoxia being the final cause of death.

Physiologic nature of death

In a series of experiments on rats cooled to hypothermic cardiac arrest and held thus for 30 minutes, it was found that in the hypoxic rats that would not survive, the blood pressure fell about half a minute *before* the heart stopped; in the much less hypoxic rats, the heart stopped and *then* the blood pressure fell immediately (Rogers and Hillman, 1970a). The following theory for the mechanism of death was put forword. Anoxia plus cold causes irreversible blockage, both of the synapses involved in baroreceptor reflexes and in the chemical reactions involved in the local vasomotor tone. There is thus a massive vasodilatation, as is found in normothermic shock. The blood is pooled peripherally, as has been shown to occur in death (Dickinson and Secker-Walker, 1970), and there is not enough in the central circulation. So, although cardiac contractility may return, there is too little blood in the system to prime the pump. The ineffectiveness of drugs, other than those injected intracardially, fits in with this hypothesis. It also explains the fact that dying may be delayed by administration of oxygen or Adrenalin, by blood transfusion, or by the coupling of an extracorporeal circulation.

Resuscitation from hypothermic asystole

In clinical practice, it has usually been accepted, despite the classic experiments of Niazi and Lewis (1954, 1956a and b, 1958) on human beings, monkeys, dogs, and rats, as well as the many individual and anecdotal cases of patients reported (Brooks, 1967; Keatinge, 1969), that a patient found in cardiac arrest is necessarily dead. Following a recent tragedy in the Cairngorm mountains of Scotland, in which six children were found frozen and in cardiac arrest, the question was

again raised as to whether or not attempts should be made to resuscitate such cases (Hillman, 1971; Lancet editorial, 1972; Lemire and Johnson, 1972). The practical problems of applying resuscitation procedures while on a frozen mountainside cannot be ignored, but neither can the question of the desirability of attempting to do so in more optimum conditions be evaded. The main fear of resuscitation is that the result might be a "mindless vegetable." Against this lie two barriers of ignorance. In such circumstances as the one above, it cannot be known how long their hearts had stopped before the patients were discovered, nor do we know how long a young, healthy human being (or, for that matter, an old, ill one) can survive in cardiac arrest (Lemire and Johnson, 1972). However, it is well known that children can make remarkable recoveries from acute brain damage, and reference has already been made to the protection afforded by cold. Even if—as is by no means certain—such patients were to recover as "vegetables," the circumstances may well give guidance in the future as to when resuscitation should be attempted. It would thus seem incumbent upon a physician to attempt to revive any patient (a) found in cardiac arrest without an apparent cause and whose history is not known, (b) whose heart is beating, however weakly, and (c) in whom it is suspected that hypothermia, narcotics, or alcohol is relevant to the physical condition.

Although there are slight physiologic differences detectable in experimental animals between hypothermic cardiac arrest and death, these are not clinically evident. The former state passes imperceptibly into the latter, and the only real distinction between the two is that cardiac arrest is reversible, death is not. The only way to find out if the condition is reversible is to try to reverse it as early and as vigorously as possible.

Clinical history of recovery

Extreme care, similar to that used for patients in coma or deep anesthesia, must be taken during resuscitation from apparent death to prevent corneal damage, skin abrasions, and bone fractures. Signs of recovery—if it is going to occur—are usually seen within 15 to 20 minutes, although vigorous efforts should probably be continued for at least 60 minutes before they are abandoned. The first sign of recovery is a change of color from cyanosis or pallor to pink. Second, the pupils, which were previously dilated, constrict. Third, occasional weak heartbeats can be detected; a regular, even if slow, initial rhythm is a good sign. At this stage there is a considerable danger of the circulation restarting with no oxygen being supplied to the lungs. The warming tissues consume more oxygen, but there is no pulmonary ventilation. It is of the utmost importance to start artificial respiration *before* cardiac massage, defibrillation, or warming; otherwise the patient is circulating more and more hypoxic blood, and this may kill him.

The next sign usually seen is that the tone of the pyloric sphincter returns and the patient may vomit. This has sometimes been regarded as a contraindication for particular techniques of resuscitation. On the contrary, it is a sign of recovery but, nevertheless, there is a clear danger of the patient inhaling the vomitus. It is a medical and professional tragedy to lose a patient who has been resuscitated to this extent; powerful suction may be needed if a patient has recently consumed a large meal. Respiration returns minutes after restarting of the heart, initially as single, deep sighs, then as a Cheyne-Stokes rhythm, and subsequently becomes normal; an occasional chest compression may help a rather weak rhythm.

Postresuscitation syndrome

The postresuscitation syndrome has been extensively studied (Negovskii, 1971). The dangers during the first 24 hours arise from incomplete recovery. They include sudden cardiac or respiratory arrest, cerebral edema, and hypothermia from poor temperature regulation. Later complications are pneumonia, renal failure, and irreversible brain damage as well as other diseases arising from immobility. The treatment is largely beyond the scope of this chapter but, clearly, oxygen must be kept at hand, antibiotics must be given to prevent pneumonia, physiotherapy often may be indicated, and dehydration may be necessary for threatened cerebral edema.

Summary

In summary, death may be thought of as a syndrome. Its study has already raised several questions: First, what is the biochemical change that occurs when anoxia proceeds to death? Second, how much can death be delayed or reversed by manipulating body biochemistry? Third, can we make a differential diagnosis between death and cardiac arrest? Fourth, will we ever be able to know at the time of death whether successful resuscitation would result in a healthy or a severely brain-damaged patient? Last, but not least, is death really irreversible?

PART TWO

DETECTION AND AVOIDANCE OF RISK FACTORS IN CARDIAC ARREST

Chapter 3

PREVENTION OF CARDIAC ARREST

Prevention of cardiac arrest at last has assumed paramount importance. It is for this reason that the early part of this fourth edition of *Cardiac Arrest and Resuscitation* is devoted to the preventive aspects of cardiac asystole and ventricular fibrillation. Whereas cardiac arrest has usually been considered a totally unexpected occurrence in most situations, new and evolving information seems to hold the promise that a great number of potential cases will be prevented by further application of our knowledge of mechanisms involved in the production of ventricular asystole and ventricular fibrillation. Patients known to be in risk of these conditions are being identified with increasing accuracy. Notable, of course, is the evolution of the coronary care unit and the contribution these units have made in providing knowledge about the arrhythmias preceding the development of ventricular fibrillation. Although the patient with myocardial infarction represents the number one indication for continued preventive efforts, there are dozens of other clinical situations that, if understood by the physician, can add to that pool of patients diverted from a collision course with cardiac arrest.

The purpose of this chapter is to call attention to generalities and specifics that may aid the physician in his day-to-day contact with the potential cardiac arrest patient.

Periods of increased hazard

Although generalizations, the following are examples from the Cardiac Arrest Registry of circumstances that often require increased alertness for the appearance of cardiac arrhythmias or arrest.

1. During passage of endotracheal tubes, particularly in the patient under light anesthesia and in the burn patient
2. During extubation
3. While employing tracheal suction
4. During downward traction of the stomach or manipulation of abdominal viscera
5. During manipulation of gallbladder or common bile duct
6. During positional changes such as moving the patient to cart or onto bed
7. Elevation of the kidney rest or turning the patient on one side
8. At the time of peritoneal closure (About one third of all cases occurred near the completion of the procedure and frequently at about the time the traction was being placed under the peritoneum in order to allow closure.)
9. During operations for strabismus or with pressure on the eye
10. In the patient with obstructive jaundice
11. In the patient arriving on the operative floor with an undue amount of fear and apprehension
12. At time of injection of dye during angiocardiography
13. At time of removal of aortic clamps following surgical correction of coarctation of the aorta
14. While positioning cardiac catheter in outflow tract of right ventricle

General preventive measures

Metabolic disturbances are particularly common to the critically ill patient and lead to many of the life-threatening ventricular and supraventricular arrhythmias. From their extensive experience with intensive care units, Ayres and Grace conclude that the likelihood of metabolically induced arrhythmias can be markedly reduced by preventing arterial hypoxemia through the administration of oxygen mixtures, adjustment of ventilatory rates to prevent respiratory alkalosis or acidosis, and adequate replacement of electrolyte deficiencies. As stressed elsewhere in this book, arterial blood should frequently be analyzed for oxygen pressure, carbon dioxide pressure, and pH in all clinically ill patients.

The following general preventive measures have been suggested by Turk and Glenn as being applicable before, during, and after any operative or diagnostic procedure.

1. Adequate oxygenation and ventilation
2. Close observation of changes in cardiac rate or rhythm: withdrawal of all stimuli in the presence of rapid runs of ectopic ventricular beats or bradycardia
3. Preoperative vagal inhibition with atropine: repetition during operation indicated
4. Repression of myocardial response to local stimuli in selected cases
5. Gentle manipulation during all surgery, particularly in the region of the heart and great vessels
6. Drug sensitivity: careful testing for sensitivity, with adequate sedation
7. Careful cardiac stimulation in the presence of an acutely failing circulation (by means of levarterenol bitartrate and calcium chloride)
8. Careful evaluation and treatment of cardiac disorders
9. Constant reminders to the staff of the causes, methods of prevention, and treatment of cardiac arrest*

Following a concerted effort, the incidence of cardiac arrest in one hospital was lowered to less than half that of the previous year. West reports that in this hospital the reduction was due to (1) reemphasis of the necessity for adequate oxygenation of the patient throughout anesthesia, (2) discontinuance of thiopental sodium (Pentothal) on one surgical service, and (3) the use of atropine or

*From Turk, L. N., III, and Glenn, W. W. L.: Cardiac arrest; results of attempted cardiac resuscitation in forty-two cases, N. Engl. J. Med. 251: 795, 1954.

hyoscine as a preoperative medication for children as well as adults.

Preventive measures before and during surgery

PREOPERATIVE EVALUATION

A number of considerations are of much importance in the preoperative evaluation of the patient. The presence of cardiac arrhythmias is thought to be significant. Holden has called attention repeatedly to the predisposing influence of cardiac arrhythmias toward cardiac arrest.

Casten and Bardenstein call attention to chronic respiratory acidosis produced by chronic pulmonary disease in which interference with respiratory exchange has occurred.

Although compensation may have been accomplished prior to surgery, the added effect of anesthetic induced, uncompensated respiratory acidosis may be sufficient to cause cardiac arrest. In these patients, preparation is best accomplished by intermittent oxygen therapy over a period of several days. Sudden flooding of the alveoli with oxygen may cause the same posthypercapnic phenomenon observed after anesthesia. Finally, as has been pointed out, restoration of normal fluid and electrolytic balance is essential, both as regards osmolarity and composition. Acid-base balance should certainly be restored before subjecting the patient to anesthesia and surgery, and, in most instances, this can be accomplished in a matter of hours.

During surgery, blood and fluids should be replaced as lost, since hemorrhage and shock potentiate the noxious effects of hypercapnia. Anesthetic agents which predispose to respiratory acidosis should be avoided whenever possible and muscle relaxants which inhibit respiratory excursion should be administered only under the most careful supervision, if at all. The utilization of nonrebreathing techniques which diminish the dead space and which "wash out" carbon dioxide is most desirable. Finally, it is highly desirable, though rarely practical to utilize continuous electrocardiographic tracings throughout the operative procedure, since in experimental animals, the first warning of cardiac arrest is a prolongation of the QRS interval. If this is observed, immediate attempts to correct respiratory acidosis and diminish serum potassium should be instituted. The latter is best accomplished by the intravenous administration of glucose and insulin, or glucose alone, since in the metabolism of glucose, potassium is taken from the plasma.*

PREVENTIVE MEASURES IN THE OPERATING ROOM

It seems logical to assume that many potential cases of cardiac arrest are prevented by the usual monitoring of premonitory signs of cardiac problems and their management as outlined elsewhere in this book. Poor-risk patients are watched carefully for any acid-base imbalance and alterations in central venous pressure. Electrolyte, fluid, and warm blood replacement have added significantly to the safety of the patient in surgery.

MONITORING

Despite obvious advantages of techniques for constantly monitoring patients under anesthesia, there still seems to be some hesitancy in their widespread acceptance. Pierce notes that in twenty-two cardiac arrests occurring in a large community hospital there were only three instances in which ECG oscilloscopy was employed. He believes that it would have been helpful in at least eight additional cases. This is an area of sophistication in patient management, and I certainly agree with Pierce's philosophy that ancillary equipment of a monitoring nature is mandatory in every patient receiving general anesthesia. When a critical situation arises, the electrical status of the heart is immediately known. Such aids need not be distracting, nor should they replace proved, careful clinical observation of the anesthetized patient. The instruments available are small, compact, easy to operate, and relatively free of maintenance problems.

By use of the cathode ray oscillograph and the pulse tachometer or the direct-writing continuous ECG tracing, early recognition of

---

*From Casten, D. F., and Bardenstein, M.: Cardiac arrest in children, Bull. Hosp. Joint Dis. **16**:13-21, 1955.

occult irregularities of the heart's action can be detected. It seems logical to assume that the incidence of cardiac arrest should be somewhat decreased by careful following of the heart's action by these methods. Especially are they valuable during the induction phases of anesthesia and during intubation, when ectopic beats are particularly prone to occur.

It seems certain that, with increased use of the oscillograph, pulse tachometer, or continuous ECG recordings, the number of successful cardiac resuscitations should increase. With the oscillograph, no longer should there be reason for delay in instituting treatment, since this instrument provides immediate and almost certain evidence of cardiac arrest. Not only does it tell that the heart's action has ceased being effective, but it also defines the type of arrest that has occurred, including ventricular fibrillation.

Cardiac arrest occurred during direct recordings of the ECG in two cases reported by Turk and Glenn. In one case, the asystole spontaneously resulted in a resumption of cardiac retractions after approximately 36 seconds. In a second instance, cardiac arrest occurred while the pericardium was being grasped so that incision could be made.

ANESTHESIA AND THE ANESTHESIOLOGIST

The anesthesiologist today cannot be too impressed with his responsibility in the prevention of sudden death of patients under anesthesia. From a total of 307 cases studied by the Anesthesia Study Commission, forty-seven of the group were considered to be preventable, and the majority of these were preventable under situations controllable by the anesthesiologist or the individual giving the anesthesia. The Anesthesia Study Commission was appointed by the Philadelphia County Medical Society to review the fatalities occurring under anesthesia. These were not necessarily cases of cardiac arrest, but they can be discussed from the broad aspect of prevention. Factors listed by this commission as contributing to the preventable fatalities were the following:

1. Either inadequate or excessive preoperative medication
2. Errors in judgment
3. Poor choice of anesthetic agent
4. Excessive dose of agent
5. Respiratory obstruction during operation
6. Laryngospasm during operation
7. Inadequate oxygenation
8. Improper management of the case in general
9. Error in technique
10. Inadequate supervision
11. Inefficient resuscitation
12. Respiratory obstruction in the postoperative period

This report emphasized that not only is the injudicious selection of the anesthetic agent a main factor to be considered but also, and perhaps of more importance, is the skill of the anesthesiologist in administering that particular agent.

Prolonged anesthesia with closed system. Prolonged anesthesia, particularly with closed systems, may be accompanied by poor absorption of carbon dioxide by the apparatus, allowing this substance to build up to high levels in the alveoli and producing high levels in the blood; the blood pH can shift to 7.2 or even as far as 7.0. Such temporary and extreme acidosis almost certainly accounts for many of the cardiac irregularities or even arrests that have occurred in patients under anesthesia.

Prevention of death under local anesthesia. In a symposium on anesthesia at the 1948 meeting of the American Academy of Ophthalmology and Otolaryngology, Seevers is quoted as having made the point that "There are probably more deaths from local anesthetics than from any other single class of compounds in common use today." He asked for a show of hands of those present who had witnessed a toxic reaction or death from topical anesthesia during the past 5 years. An estimated 30% to 40% of the audience responded in a positive nature.

A careful anesthetic history must be taken in all cases when local anesthesia is to be used. If a history of a possible reaction is obtained, then another agent of a different chemical group or, better yet, the complete avoidance of local anesthesia is to be urged. It is important that the physician always inform the patient experiencing a reaction to a local anesthetic so that he may be aware of his idiosyncrasy.

Since the toxicity of a local anesthetic drug is believed to increase in geometric, not arithmetic, progression, it is of great importance that the weakest possible solution be used whenever possible. In general, the more concentrated solutions are needed only for the blocking of large nerve trunks and plexus blocks. A dilute solution can be more easily used for cutaneous anesthesia.

Since the rapid establishment of a high dosage level of a local anesthetic is intimately related with the likelihood of a toxic reaction, the vascularity of the area that is being injected must be considered. Absorption from the respiratory and intestinal tract as well as the mouth, nose, and throat is extremely fast. When the drug is sprayed into the throat, the patient should be cautioned to spit out any excess solution and not to swallow it. It goes without saying that scrupulous attention to the avoidance of intravascular injection must be made by aspirating several times during an injection. The dosage of the anesthetic agent may be reduced in patients whose metabolic rate is low, such as the aged or debilitated patient or the patient in shock.

Since cocaine intoxication is usually caused by either an overdosage or an unpredictable increase in the rate of absorption, this complication is difficult to control. Fundamentally, only the first of these two predisposing factors can be influenced to any great degree. The prophylactic use of barbiturates for control of excessive stimulation in respiratory failure from cocaine intoxication has been recommended.

The sequence of events in toxic reactions may vary. In general, the respiratory center seems to be more susceptible than the cardiovascular system. The apparent susceptibilities of the two systems often approximate each other and, in many instances, the failure of the cardiovascular system may come first, particularly if there is preexisting cardiac pathology and if barbiturates have been given.

Local anesthetic agents may have a variety of adverse reactions. In addition to local reactions, systemic reactions may center in CNS effects, cardiovascular effects, allergenic reactions, and various other idiosyncrasies. Tetracaine (Pontocaine) is an example of a drug whose first manifestations may be syncope caused by myocardial depression or asystole prior to CNS excitation.

Lamberts and co-workers were able to successfully resuscitate a 19-year-old boy following two separate episodes of cardiac arrest approximately 6 weeks apart. Topical cocaine had been instilled over the vocal cords immediately prior to each of the episodes of cardiac arrest.

Prevention of vagovagal reflex from endotracheal intubation. A most common initiating factor in the production of the vagovagal reflex in modern surgery is introduction of the endotracheal tube for anesthesia. Beecher and Todd, in their analysis of death associated with anesthesia and surgery from ten large teaching hospitals over a 5-year period, observe an increase (more than double) in the use of endotracheal intubation as an adjunct of intravenous anesthesia. They also call attention to the markedly increased tendency of using inflatable cuffs on the endotracheal tube.

Many groups of investigators have reported on the incidence of arrhythmias produced during introduction of the endotracheal tube. The frequency with which they are produced has been well documented. ECG changes have been observed after simply spraying the throat with cold water (Reid and Brace). The complete abolition of this reflex by atropine is of marked significance.

That ECG disturbances involved in association with the irritation of the respiratory tract by the passage of the endotracheal tube

are of a reflex nature is also substantiated by the fact that the changes occur at the very instant that the tube is passed through the larynx into the trachea. Burstein took ECG determinations during endotracheal intubation in 109 cases following anesthesia with the various and usual techniques. He demonstrated ECG disturbances in 68% of the patients at the time of intubation. These disturbances varied from mild transitory sinus tachycardia to premature ventricular contraction, nodal rhythm, sinus bradycardia, decrease in the voltage of the T waves, depression of the S-T segment, increase in the P-R interval, sinus arrhythmia, ventricular tachycardia, and auricular fibrillation. Burstein found that insufficient depth of anesthesia, prolonged laryngoscopy with numerous attempts at intubation, respiratory obstruction before intubation, and tracheal irritation after intubation were the important factors in production of these ECG disturbances. In addition, he called attention to his belief that topical cocainization of the pharynx and larynx during general anesthesia seems to enhance these disorders. Burstein attributes these additional arrhythmias to sympathetic stimulation from the systemic absorption of cocaine with potentiation of these effects during the state of general anesthesia.

In another group of patients studied by Burstein and co-workers during intrathoracic surgery, an incidence of 73% was noted regarding cardiac irregularities occurring at the time of the passage of the endotracheal tube. Rib and intercostal nerve stimulations produced by periosteal rib scraping, direct intercostal nerve stimulation prior to rib resection, and wide rib spreading by rib retractors were also shown to cause various types of ECG changes. Pleural incision produced significant electrocardiographic changes in over 20% of the cases. Burstein, in addition, notes that manipulation or incision of the pericardium (in patients who appear to have inflammatory pericarditis) is usually attended by severe circulatory response. He recommends topical application of 2% procaine solution as well as rapid intravenous injection of 100 mg. of procaine solution in a 1% or 2% concentration. He reasons that the procaine tends to overcome cardiac irritability caused by pericardial and cardiac manipulation during the phase of general anesthesia.

Prevention of hypercapnia. The posthypercapnic phenomenon, or sudden lowering of the carbon dioxide concentration, can be prevented by avoiding any sudden carbon dioxide "blow off." Should various atrial and ventricular arrhythmias occur at this stage, they may be counteracted by the intravenous administration of sodium bicarbonate (Graham). Since hypercapnia exerts a detrimental effect on the conduction system of the heart in augmenting the vagovagal reflex and prolonging the conduction time of the heart, every effort should be made to keep the blood pH at a constant level by preventing the accumulation of carbon dioxide in the alveolar air and blood. If a rebreathing machine is used for anesthesia administration, the soda lime should be changed at frequent intervals.

Gibbon and Stayman have pointed out that acidosis will produce cardiac arrest and that the asystole generally occurs in diastole. They point to the wealth of recently elicited material showing the importance of avoiding accumulations of carbon dioxide in the body during the course of prolonged intrapleural operations, or, for that matter, any operation. Such an accumulation raises the tension of carbon dioxide in the arterial blood, with the resultant fall in the blood pH. Severe acidosis in the course of prolonged intrathoracic operations is well known. This has a particularly deleterious effect on the heart musculature and on the conduction of cardiac impulses through the atrioventricular bundle. Acidosis favors relaxation of the cardiac muscle and reduces its contractility. It also reduces the conductivity of the bundle of His. In the closed gas circuit, the soda lime, if of a good quality and in adequate amount, will remove the accumulated carbon dioxide satisfactorily—provided that there is

a continuous movement of gas between the lungs and the anesthesia apparatus. This cause of acidosis can be avoided by maintaining a good tidal exchange and intermittent compression of the anesthetic bag.

In posthypercapnic periods during and following surgery, major alterations in the cardiac rhythm and ECG pattern may occur (Young, Sealy, and Harris). Among these changes are a disappearance of P waves, alterations in height and direction of QRS and T waves, and broadening of the QRS complex. Bradycardia, atrioventricular block, ventricular extrasystoles, ventricular tachycardia, and ventricular fibrillations and arrest may also make up the sequence of events. Of particular importance is the observation that "widening of the QRS complex precedes fibrillation or arrest by several minutes in almost every instance."

Therefore, in order to identify QRS prolongation, it seems logical that a continuous ECG pattern be observed during periods of lengthy operative procedures so that ventricular fibrillation or cardiac asystole may be prevented.

As discussed under etiologic aspects of cardiac arrest, considerable available evidence indicates that the underlying mechanism is related to a disturbed sodium-potassium ratio. Should signs of cardiac arrhythmias develop during hyperventilation with 100% oxygen, preventive measures against accentuation of the character of the arrhythmia may be instituted by administration of sodium chloride or by the intravenous injection of calcium salt. The high potassium level that develops following correction of hypercapnia necessitates an accompanying high level of sodium ion.

Finch and others have called attention to the usefulness of hypertonic sodium chloride and glucose in correcting ECG abnormalities caused by hyperpotassemia in uremia. Young and associates have found that hypertonic sodium chloride in glucose solutions (20% glucose and 3% saline) have been equally effective in preventing fatal cardiac arrhythmias in the posthypercapnic dog. They are unable to explain the mode of action, however. It is important that the hypertonic glucose-saline solution be given sufficiently early if a reversal of the ECG disturbance is to be expected.

Prevention of cardiac arrhythmias during tracheal suctioning. Shim and others were able to eliminate transient cardiac arrhythmias in hypoxic patients by administering 100% oxygen for 5 minutes before suctioning and by limiting the suctioning period to less than 10 seconds at a time. Patients not being treated by this routine had a variety of disturbances of the cardiac rhythm during and after tracheal suctioning while breathing air. Their arrhythmias included frequent atrial premature contractions, nodal tachycardia, transient sinus arrest, incomplete heart block, and frequent premature ventricular contractions.

PREVENTIVE MEASURES FOR THE
PATIENT UNDERGOING CARDIAC SURGERY

Cardiac arrest in the surgical patient with known, preexisting cardiac disease is, as pointed out elsewhere, not as frequent as one would imagine. Even so, a definitely increased risk is present in the patient with cardiac disease undergoing surgery. A number of precautions should be mentioned. Nearly all investigators agree that the danger of cardiac arrest in patients undergoing cardiac surgery is materially decreased when a minimum of anesthetic agents is used. Harken, in over 800 mitral valvuloplasties, states that a total volume of over 15 to 30 ml. of ether should not be used during an operation of 1 to 1½ hours.

Harken, who has had extensive experience with mitral stenosis, has discontinued the use of cyclopropane because of its increased tendency to accentuate cardiac irritability. Harken advises against the routine prophylactic use of procaine before or during cardiac surgery because of the resulting depressant effect on the myocardium. He believes that this is true of the procainamide in hydrochloride solutions. It is his experience that hearts depressed by such drugs go into arrest more frequently. In addition, every effort should be made to prevent the myocardial ischemia that occurs with hypotension by controlling the tachycardia and by use of vasoconstrictors and blood replacement (by intravenous or intra-arterial route).

Black and Harken state:

> Experience with hundreds of patients abundantly demonstrates that safety lies in prevention rather than treatment. This prevention is complex and begins with the selection of the patient. It includes his optimal medical preparation, the bolstering of his confidence, proper premedication, impeccable anesthetic induction, ample pulmonary ventilation and careful, rapid surgery.*

Patients with aortic stenosis or first-degree heart block deserve special note.

Patients with aortic stenosis. A number of individuals have noted the increased likelihood of sudden death during surgical procedures on patients with aortic stenosis. This is particularly true when the blood volume is lowered considerably by hemorrhage. General anesthesia or prolonged anoxia may contribute to a lowering of the peripheral resistance with resulting hypotension and ineffective coronary artery circulation. Patients in whom aortic stenosis has been diagnosed should receive special attention during the entire operative procedure. They are particularly good candidates for close observation with the oscillograph or continuous ECG tracings. Levine has called attention to the apparent increased likelihood of a sensitive carotid sinus condition with aortic stenosis.

Patients with first-degree heart block. First-degree heart block, as determined by measurements of the P-R interval on the ECG tracing, adds to the likelihood of complete atrioventricular disassociation and ventricular standstill during an operative procedure, or under anesthesia. Lyons believes that

---

*From Black, H., and Harken, D. E.: Safe conduct of the patient through cardiac surgery, N. Engl. J. Med. **251**:45-51, 1954.

digitalis, quinidine, and procaine (Novocain) contribute to the likelihood of these complications.

Ziegler studied ECG tracings of 175 patients during procedures for pulmonic stenosis at the Johns Hopkins Hospital, and noted that certain changes in cardiac activity preceded cardiac arrest in most cases. Bradycardia of 30 to 40 beats per minute during anesthesia was the most serious of these changes. Unexplained tachycardia or extrasystoles also served as a warning in his series. It would therefore seem obvious that, in spite of direct observation of the heart's activity, ECG tracings should be followed, since many of the arrhythmias of the heart are not quickly picked up on direct observation.

The advisability of employing drugs to reduce the irritability of the heart during cardiac procedures accompanied by obvious manipulation is a question that is raised. In my limited experience, I have not used such a drug. Gross states that he has used procainamide (Pronestyl) in the past but that he now believes that it was a factor in producing serious fall of the peripheral arterial pressure. He employs this drug only if there is a ventricular tachycardia during the procedure or if frequent extrasystoles precede the operation. He no longer injects procaine into the pericardial sac during operations. This would seem to be the general sentiment of cardiovascular surgeons.

Prevention of atrial fibrillation. Because of the considerable frequency with which atrial fibrillation develops postoperatively in patients who undergo mitral surgery (patients who previously had normal sinus rhythm), mechanisms regarding the etiology and prevention of atrial fibrillation have been considered (Kittle and Crockett). Local trauma to the left atrium at the time of atriotomy is considered the most important factor. Even without left atrial hypertension, atrial fibrillation frequently follows atriotomy. It would appear that trauma is a factor in lowering the fibrillary threshold of the atria and that the prophylactic use of

digitalis and quinidine is of considerable value in prevention of this deleterious arrhythmia.

Prevention of heart block during open-heart surgery. Knowledge of the anatomic location of the bundle of His will prevent many instances of surgically induced heart block during repair of ventricular septal defects, either isolated cases or those associated with tetralogy of Fallot as well as in patients with endocardial cushion defects. In most instances, the bundle runs along the posteroinferior margin of the ventricular defect in a subendocardial position—when viewed from the right side. I have not employed cardioplegia or hypothermia in repair of ventricular septal defects. By careful monitoring of the ECG pattern with each suture placement, heart block has been prevented. Vital staining of the bundle (5% iodine dissolved in 10% sodium iodide) can be effected—but not without possible damage to the tissue from the dye.

Gerbode encountered only two permanent heart blocks in 112 patients by placing the sutures as shown in Fig. 3-1. Interrupted mattress sutures are placed several millimeters away from the defect and include only the right side of the muscular septum. The septal leaflet of the tricuspid valve is used to buttress the repair. A conduction system locator utilizing an electronic depth probe is available and can indicate the presence of the conduction system within an accuracy of 1 mm. The triaxial gold electrodes are effective on both the beating and the arrested heart. Audible tone signals change pitch according to the proximity of the bundle of His.

An improved electrophysiologic technique developed by G. A. Kaiser and colleagues at New York's Presbyterian Hospital provides an accurate method of localizing the atrioventricular (A-V) conduction system during surgery. Although the increasing experience of cardiac surgeons is resulting in a decreased incidence of permanent complete heart block from ventricular septal defect (VSD) closures

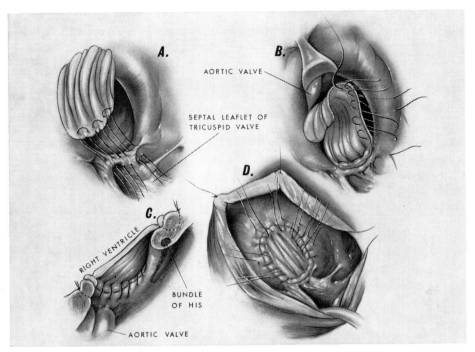

Fig. 3-1. Gerbode method of closing ventricular septal defect to avoid conduction bundle. (From Gerbode, F., and Keen, G.: Dis. Chest. **42**:635, 1962.)

or from correction of a tetralogy of Fallot and repair of ostium primum–type VSD repairs, the complication is life threatening when it does occur and every step should be taken to prevent it. The technique requires a conducted supraventricular atrial rhythm. This technique for demonstrating the anatomical position of the cardiac conduction system during surgery is as follows: an electrode probe is used to record electrograms from the bundle of His or bundle branches to identify the anatomic position of the specialized A-V conduction system. To ensure a conducted supraventricular rhythm and thus a predictable P-R interval and QRS configuration, the heart is simultaneously paced from an atrial site.

The atria are paced through an electrode plaque sewn to or held in position beneath the superior vena cava near the sino-atrial node. The paced rate is slightly in excess of the spontaneous rate and the stimulus is provided by a digital threshold stimulator

and delivered through a stimulus isolator (Electrace system, Electro-Catheter Corporation, Rahway, New Jersey). The paced rhythm is continuously monitored on the electrocardiogram. Atrial pacing permits beat-to-beat observation of changes in P-R interval or changes in QRS duration and shape that might result from any surgical manipulation. Constant antegrade conduction to the ventricles is assured by atrial pacing. Both supraventricular and ventricular arrhythmias are thus suppressed, and a bradycardia often associated with any induced hypothermia is avoided. Bipolar electrograms and simultaneous standard and augmented ECG leads are monitored on an 8-channel, switched beam oscilloscope and recorded on photographic paper moving at 100 mm. per second. During the paced rhythm, the anatomic course of the bundle of His and bundle branches is delineated by recording bipolar electrograms from the region of the A-V conduction pathways in the atria and ventricles with electrode probes and observing the appearance of a typical "His spike" during the P-R interval in the recorded ECG.

PREVENTION OF REFLEX CARDIOVASCULAR REACTION DURING ABDOMINAL SURGERY

As pointed out elsewhere in this book, numerous procedures within the abdomen at the time of abdominal surgery elicit a marked reflex cardiovascular reaction manifested first by sudden bradycardia, followed by fall in mean blood pressure and decreased pulse amplitude. If vagal inhibition of the sinus nodes is prolonged and the ventricle is unable to originate its own ectopic beat, then cardiac arrest, of course, ensues. Minimizing traction and using a more general approach to exploration of the upper abdomen are helpful. In patients with already evident increased vagal tone, such as patients with obstructive jaundice, large doses of atropine should be given and repeated frequently. Increasing the depth of anesthesia apparently does not change the extent of the reflex response. The exceptions to this would include halothane anesthesia, which is said to abolish the signs of reflex sympathetic inhibition. Atropine will be helpful in abolishing the initial bradycardia, but small amounts of sympathomimetic drugs should be given to provide adequate tonic sympathetic discharge.

Blockage of the regional sympathetic plexus by infiltration with local anesthetic provides an additional means of dealing with the reflexly inhibited tonic sympathetic discharge. Such inhibition is possibly involved in the reflex cardiovascular reaction during abdominal surgery (Folkow and associates).

PREVENTION IN PATIENTS WITH ATRIOVENTRICULAR BLOCK

Special precautions are indicated for preventing episodes of cardiac arrest in those patients with complete atrioventricular block, as recognized by a ventricular rate below 45 beats per minute. This is also true in those patients with first-degree atrioventricular block as manifested by a long P-R interval.

Patients with atrioventricular block usually receive careful evaluation prior to surgery. Throughout surgery and into the postoperative period, these patients should be continuously monitored. In addition, an electric pacemaker should be attached and ready for use if not already functioning.

Proper administration of atropine sulfate will greatly reduce likelihood of arrest. Atropine sulfate, 1 to 2 mg. every 4 hours during anesthesia, is indicated. Sympathomimetic drugs, by improving atrioventricular conduction and increasing the heart rate, decrease chances of Adams-Stokes attack. Ephedrine sulfate and isoproterenol hydrochloride are two such useful drugs.

Quinidine and procainamide are generally conceded to be contraindicated during heart block in patients with Adams-Stokes syndrome because they may depress the idioventricular pacemaker and may produce ventricular fibrillation. Quinidine has undesirable side effects, and attempts at resuscitation of and arrested heart after administration of quinidine often have proved refractory.

PREVENTION DURING POSITIONAL CHANGES OF THE PATIENT

It has been shown by several workers that the effect on the autonomic nervous system by a sudden positional change can be avoided, to a large extent, by the use of a parasympathetic blocking agent such as atropine or methantheline (Banthine). The prophylactic value of an intravenous dose of methantheline (5 mg.) prior to movement of the patient or of an intravenous injection of atropine will be such that cardiac arrest will largely be prevented.

PREVENTION OF PROFOUND BRADYCARDIA AND CARDIAC ARREST DURING OPHTHALMOLOGIC PROCEDURES

Most oculocardiac reflexes encountered during surgery on the eye are, fortunately, preventable. Anesthetists are well aware that arrhythmias, with marked slowing of the heart and even asystole, are an ever present source of real danger. These arrests constitute one of the most easily preventable groups of cardiac arrests—simply by the use of atropine and the usual efforts to administer adequate oxygenation. Kirsch and co-workers have demonstrated that this reflex can be completely abolished by anesthetic (2% lidocaine [Xylocaine]) retrobulbar injection and recommend that retrobulbar injection be a routine safeguard in all cases of strabismus surgery.

Sorenson and Gilmore have demonstrated that cardiac arrest may occur from tension or traction on either of the rectus muscles during strabismus surgery. Particularly is tension on the medial rectus muscle likely to produce a vagovagal effect. Therefore manipulation of the rectus muscles during these squint corrections should involve considerable care. An oculocardiac reflex is present in approximately 90% of children (Sabena and Posteli).

Because of the frequency of observed oculocardiac reflexes in children undergoing operations to correct strabismus, Taylor, Wilson, Roesch, and Stoelting compare the relative benefits of preventing this reflex by the two most commonly used techniques: retrobulbar local anesthetic block and intravenous injection of atropine. Table 3-1 shows the results of this study, which indicate that retrobulbar block appears to be more effective in preventing the oculocardiac reflex than is atropine—at least in the doses used by Taylor and co-workers (0.0025 mg. per pound). It is significant that retrobulbar

block with lidocaine prevented the reflex in all of their cases. In using the retrobulbar block, 1 to 2 ml. of 2% lidocaine was given. The block was considered successful if dilatation of the pupil was produced. It should be noted that 58% of thirty-two control patients showed an oculocardiac reflex. Deliberate pressure on the globe before blocking agents were used in thirty-four patients showed a 67% incidence of ECG changes.

The vagovagal effect produced by the oculocardiac reflex from tension or traction on the lateral or medial rectus muscle is difficult to abolish with the usual premedication dose of atropine. Sorenson and Gilmore found that doses of 0.3 to 0.4 mg. were generally ineffective in preventing bradycardia. Larger doses of atropine are recommended (0.0025 mg. per pound, intravenously).

Total vagal blockage may not always be necessary to relieve the detrimental effect of vagal stimulation. Howland and colleagues record the case of a patient being operated upon 6 months after the first operation during which cardiac arrest had taken place. Both operations were neck resections. During the second procedure, as the local tumor recurrence was being removed, a severe hypotensive episode with an almost imperceptible pulse occurred. An intravenous injection of 0.4 mg. of atropine was given, and the blood pressure and pulse immediately returned to normal tensive levels.

It seems evident that during any procedure on the eye, particularly in children, when

Table 3-1. The development of the oculocardiac reflex in relation to the type of protection offered to the eye*

	Total number	Strabismus operations	
		Number associated with reflex	Percentage incidence of reflex
Group A atropine for preanesthetic medication	55	32	58
Group B			
(1) Retrobulbar block	51	0	0
(2) Intravenous atropine	51	14	28

*From Taylor, C., et al.: Prevention of the oculocardiac reflex in children, Anesthesiology **24**:646-649, 1963.

there is increased physiologic vagotonia and when general anesthesia is employed, constant ECG monitoring is indicated.

Most of the oculocardiac reflexes resulting in fatalities have been in persons from younger age groups, particularly children and adolescents. This probably is to be expected because of the physiologic vagotonia present in younger persons.

PREVENTION OF AIR EMBOLISM

In open-heart surgery. Unless measures for prevention of air embolism are taken, open-heart surgery can end in disaster when air is not completely displaced by the blood returned to the heart. I generally let the coronary sinus flow fill the heart and displace the air gradually. Flooding the wound with carbon dioxide, elevating and venting the apex of the left ventricle, and electively fibrillating the heart are additional aids in prevention, although carbon dioxide is less frequently used today.

It should be pointed out that flooding of the chest with carbon dioxide during open-heart surgery to decrease the incidence of cerebral air embolism carries the potential risk of producing hypercapnic acidosis (Burbank and associates).

Closure of ostium secundum atrial septal defects in 150 consecutive patients is reported by Stansel and other. In each patient, ventricular fibrillation was electrically induced to minimize the possibility of air embolism, which is a significant hazard in closing atrial septal defects in a beating heart. In no instance was cerebral embolism of air recognized. In addition, the suction catheter was never allowed to lower the pool of blood in the atrium so as to expose the mitral valve. The lungs were ventilated vigorously to flush any air that might have been kept in the pulmonary veins prior to placement of the last suture in the defect. Blood from the coronary sinus was then allowed to fill the right atrium and the final sutures were tied down in the depths of this pool of blood to prevent air from getting to the left ventricle.

After the right atrium had been closed and air had been evacuated, the heart was defibrillated with the patient in a moderate Trendelenburg position so that any air that could possibly have been overlooked would be unlikely to get to the cerebral vessels and more likely to pass through an aortic vent made just above the right coronary cusp.

In craniotomy. Because of the high incidence of air emboli during craniotomies, especially posterior fossa craniectomies, Tisovec and Hamilton suggest three prophylactic measures:

1. Place a catheter in or near the right side of the heart for measuring central venous pressure and for the aspiration of gas if it accumulates.
2. Use a continuous monitor of cardiac sounds.
3. Avoid nitrous oxide or use it in low concentrations (50% or less).*

If actual embolization is suspected, nitrous oxide administration should probably be discontinued completely.

In Rubin test for pregnancy. There are at least ten deaths on record of fatal air emboli following oxygen or carbon dioxide insufflation in performing the Rubin test. (Carbon dioxide is almost always used in preference to oxygen because of the irritating effect of oxygen.) Oil insufflation is now considered the method of choice (Davis).

In phlebotomy. Under certain conditions, air embolization may occur to the donor undergoing phlebotomy. Fig. 3-2 demonstrates the mechanism of that occurrence. In a review of this problem, Schmidt and Kevy emphasize the necessary precaution of clamping the phlebotomy tubing before releasing the pressure of the tourniquet on the donor's arm.

Other precautions. Knowledge of etiologic aspects of air embolism will allow one to avoid some of the pitfalls. If air is being used and it is suspected that air has entered the

---

*From Tisovec, L., and Hamilton, W. K.: Newer considerations on air embolism during operation, J.A.M.A. **201**:376-377, 1967.

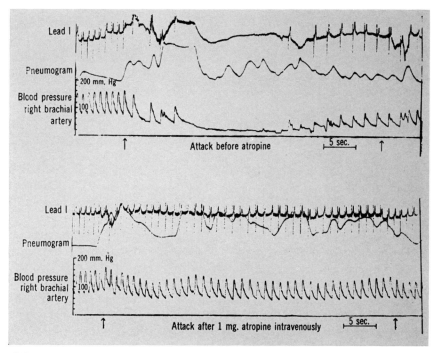

Fig. 3-2. Pneumogram illustrating use of atropine sulfate in preventing cardiac arrest from glossopharyngeal neuralgia. (From Kjellin, K., Müller, R., and Widén, L.: Neurology 9:527, 1959.)

circulation, the patient should be placed in a left-side-down or a head-down position, depending on whether it is a right or left heart embolism. The coronary orifices should be below the aortic valve.

PREVENTION OF FAT EMBOLISM

After closed-chest resuscitation. It appears evident that fat is released into the circulation at the site of injury, that is, the sternum. Although a sizeable percentage of patients coming to autopsy after closed chest cardiac compression have fat embolization to the lungs, the percentage, of course, is not known in those surviving. It is certainly possible that the confusion and diminished pulmonary oxygenation may have some contribution from the fat embolism syndrome. Perhaps all patients with prolonged closed chest compression should be emperically treated with steroids in the postresuscitative period, as-

suming that fat embolism has occurred. Unfortunately, it is difficult to monitor the effluent from the mediastinum in order to detect the fat emboli by the ultrasonic Doppler principle. Ultrasound has been used to detect fat emboli in the venous drainage from long bones (Kelly and others).

The overall prognosis after posttraumatic pulmonary fat embolism is generally related to the amount of respiratory failure that ensues and is not usually related to the cerebral fat embolism. The pulmonary arteriolar network will stop the larger quantities of fat. These particles induce inflammatory changes and are responsible for the pulmonary insufficiency, which sometimes is fatal.

PREVENTION IN GALLBLADDER SURGERY

Biliary-induced abnormalities of ECG tracings have been well documented. Presumably, reflex coronary artery spasm, mediated by stimulation of the vagus nerve, occurs rather commonly with diseases of the gall-bladder and the common bile duct.

The vagolytic effect of atropine has been effectively used to establish that reflex coronary artery spasm does have a major role in the genesis of these changes. Kaufman and Lubera report on patients with biliary disease, gallstones, and profound T wave inversion of the ECG. An ECG taken 45 minutes after an intramuscular injection of 2 mg. of atropine sulfate showed marked improvement in the T wave abnormalities. As soon as the atropine effect had worn off, the ECG tracings reverted to a normal pattern. Furthermore, the T wave abnormality was permanently abolished following cholecystectomy.

Kaufman and Lubera utilized this important observation in differentiating S-T and T waves accompanying abnormalities secondary to reflex vagal stimulation of biliary disease from those same changes due to true myocardial ischemia. Patients with myocardial ischemia caused by coronary artery disease showed no improvement in ECG tracings after a 2 mg. intramuscular injection of atropine.

Vagal and sympathetic fibers originating from cells of the first to the fourth segments of the spinal cord innervate the heart. Fibers from the sixth thoracic through the first lumbar segments, ending in the celiac plexus, innervate the gallbladder. These represent fibers from the right vagus and splanchnic nerves. It is well established that many interconnections involve the impulses transmitted between the gallbladder and heart. Equally well established is the fact that atropine sulfate will block many of the effects of vagal reflexes initiated in the gallbladder as well as in other abdominal viscera.

There now seems little doubt that reflex vagal stimulation from the biliary tree may exert a detrimental effect on the myocardium through reflex coronary artery spasms. That these changes can be so readily abolished after atropine administration gives strong support to recommendation for the use of atropine in such cases.

PREVENTION IN JAUNDICED PATIENTS

It is suggested that patients with obstructive jaundice who undergo surgery should routinely receive atropine sulfate preoperatively and during anesthesia induction. A dosage schedule greater than that given normally is recommended. Atropine sulfate should be given to the adult patient within 15 to 20 minutes of the induction, and atropine should be given intravenously during the course of operative procedure if signs of vagal irritation appear or if maneuvers likely to produce a vagovagal reflex are to be attempted. In Johnstone's case, a patient with rather marked bradycardia and partial A-V block, it was not until a large dose of atropine was given that a beneficial effect on the cardiac conduction mechanism could be observed. Experimentally, the intravenous injection of atropine almost completely eliminates the dangers from this possibility, and its use is strongly recommended.

The investigative work done within the past 35 years on frogs, turtles, and dogs shows that distension of the gallbladder usually produces an inhibition of the heart. However, a definite pattern can seldom be presented purely by distension of the biliary passages in dogs. In order for a vagovagal reflex of a marked clinical nature to occur regularly, it is usually necessary to sensitize the cardiac center to this reflex effect, and such sensitization occurs in obstructive jaundice.

What about nonobstructive jaundice? Among my collected cases, I have noted no single case of cardiac arrest in an individual with nonobstructive jaundice. However, my attention has been called to a case of cardiac arrest in an individual having this disease. Undoubtedly, there are others, but their relative incidence is extremely small compared with patients with obstructive jaundice.

The vagotonic aspects of excessive bile-acid concentration in the blood and skin are not clear. An agent for relief of the pruritus of jaundice is now available in the form of a bile-acid-sequestering resin. A resin appears to be effective in removing the bile-acids from the enterohepatic circulation and increasing their excretion in the feces, thereby lowering the concentration in the serum.

SUDDEN CARDIOVASCULAR COLLAPSE AFTER TRACHEOSTOMY

It should be recognized that sudden removal of tracheal and bronchial secretions and resultant respiratory obstruction, along with a sudden decrease in ventilatory dead space, all contribute to increased pulmonary ventilation with a resultant rapid washout of accumulated carbon dioxide and reversal of respiratory acidosis. Approximately 3% to 4% of all emergency tracheostomies will subsequently show a profound cardiovascular effect, including numerous arrhythmias and arterial hypotension. Ventricular fibrillation may occur. To prevent this sequence of events, which is discussed elsewhere in the book, it is, first of all, important to recognize that it can occur. Second, the use of vasopressors to help maintain an adequate coronary and cerebral flow should be resorted to, if necessary. The Trendelenburg position has been recommended by Green. Blood pressures should be monitored. An intravenous route must be open and ready to receive a vasopressor. Ideally, tracheostomies should be done before asphyxia is severe.

PREVENTION DURING HYPOTHERMIA

Cardiac arrest in ventricular standstill, or particularly in ventricular fibrillation, still represents the most common complication of hypothermia. Swan lists the most likely periods during hypothermia when ventricular fibrillation may occur.

1. During cooling, but below 26° C. without cardiac manipulation or circulatory arrest
2. During cardiac manipulation, particularly, ventricular incision
3. Immediately following restoration of circulation after occlusion*

---

*From Swan, H., et al.: Cessation of circulation in generalized hypothermia; physiologic changes and their control, Ann. Surg. **138**:360, 1953.

From these observations, it appears likely that the ventricular fibrillation under hypothermia can be prevented, at least to a degree. Many surgeons prefer not to allow the temperature to go below 30° C. Cardiac manipulation is maintained at a minimum. Rapid changes in tissue pH are prevented by forced respirations during the preceding cooling efforts. It appears likely that prevention of carbon dioxide accumulation is of definite benefit. As mentioned elsewhere, neostigmine (Prostigmin) is being used as a prophylactic agent against ventricular fibrillation. This is done by coronary artery perfusion.

AN ORTHOPEDIC SAFEGUARD

Although it is an admitted rarity, S. R. Gaston of New York City reported on a patient with a large body spica cast applied for the treatment of scoliosis who suffered cardiac arrest while the body spica cast was in place. The delay in removing the plaster cast was, of course, serious, and he recommended: "No patient who requires a chest spica should be allowed in the operating room in specialty surgery without a previous large area having been made available for entrance into the heart." This type of complication has been reported on three different occasions. In one instance, it was discovered to the dismay of the operator that in the rush of opening the cast, the right side had been selected instead of the left. So far, none of the patients with this complication has been resuscitated.

POSTOPERATIVE RECOVERY ROOM

A recovery room with supervision by particularly well-trained nursing personnel and under the direction of the chief of the anesthesia department or otherwise capable personnel, with all the necessary resuscitative equipment at hand, should greatly increase the safety of the operative patient in a period long recognized as a most dangerous one. A considerable number of cases of cardiac arrest have occurred in the immediate postoperative period. The chances of immediate recognition of the acutely arrested heart are much greater when the patient is being constantly observed under such a controlled environment. The possibilities of successful resuscitation are much greater in such a situation. The chances of permanent survival are obviously also substantially increased.

At the University of Missouri Hospital, patients are often moved from the recovery room to the "special care" room, where they are observed for an additional period of time.

Preventive measures in medical situations

PREVENTION OF GLOSSOPHARYNGEAL TIC DOULOUREUX (NEURALGIA)

Two trigger zones are identified by Kjellin. One zone is in the upper part of the supratonsillar fossa, on the left side. An attack can be elicited by rubbing with a cotton applicator. The second trigger zone is found at the entrance of the bony part of the external auditory canal. If these areas are topically anesthetized with lidocaine (Xylocaine), the attack can be prevented. Most significantly, however, the intravenous administration of 0.5 to 1 mg. of atropine entirely eliminates the attack and even prevents pain. An intracranial section of the glossopharyngeal nerve was done after atropinization in Kjellin's patient, who has had no further attacks of glossopharyngeal neuralgia. Fig. 3-3 clearly demonstrates the effect of atropine, given intravenously, on the clinical course of glossopharyngeal neuralgia.

PREVENTION OF SUDDEN DEATH IN ANURIC PATIENTS

A considerable number of sudden deaths in anuric patients have been reported. Although not a clear-cut consideration, many observers believe that this is caused by potassium "intoxication." Darrow stresses that

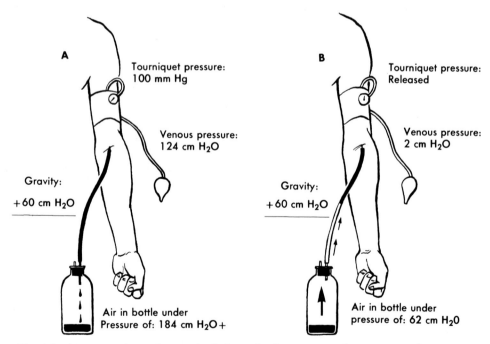

Fig. 3-3. Failure to clamp donor tube before releasing arm tourniquet may produce an embolism. **A,** Formation of positive pressure in phlebotomy container without patent air vent. **B,** Air traveling up phlebotomy tubing into circulation when tourniquet is released without first clamping shut of donor tubing. (Redrawn after Schmidt, P. J., and Kevy, S. V.: N. Engl. J. Med. 258:424, 1958.)

when there is oliguria as a result of circulatory failure, dehydration, or shock, the administration of solutions containing potassium should be preceded by the injection of an appropriate mixture of solutions containing sodium chloride, or sodium chloride and sodium lactate, together with glucose in water. The amount of potassium freed by tissue catabolism must be reduced as far as possible by the administration of glucose, and any food taken should be low in nitrogen and practically free of potassium.

PREVENTION DURING TREATMENT OF BURNS

Because of the frequency of cardiovascular collapse following succinylcholine administration in the burn patient, it has been recommended that succinylcholine be avoided in patients with burns. Lowenstein, however, reports only one cardiac arrest in 406 consecutive administrations of anesthetics in which succinylcholine was used in 188 burn patients. He stresses the fact that hypovolemia should be suspected in all burn patients and must be ruled out as a cause of cardiovascular collapse during anesthesia.

Nevertheless, the evidence does suggest that drastic cardiovascular responses induced by succinylcholine are real. Rapid administration of succinylcholine in a single bolus whether injected intravenously or intramuscularly or given intralingually should be discouraged. The endogenous catecholamine release incident upon the massive injection of succinylcholine may increase serum potassium to levels that can endanger the patient's life. Atropine and thiopental may be beneficial in preventing the hypotensive and subsequent dysrhythmic effect of succinylcholine upon the cardiovascular system. Atropine blocks the muscarinic effect of succinylcholine. Thiopental decreases the myocardial irritability and may thus prevent the onset of dangerous arrhythmia.

Succinylcholine should not be administered before electrocardiographic leads are applied

or else cardiac irregularity may not be noted early.

In eighteen orthopedic casualties returned from Vietnam, elevated potassium levels occurred after succinylcholine injections. Cardiac arrest occurred in two instances. The average potassium increase for the eighteen patients was more than 80% above preanesthetic values. Control patients increased only 12%.

In addition to the mechanisms described, Hirshowitz and co-workers consider other factors that also contribute to the high incidence of cardiac arrest in burns. They include a low hemoglobin and serum albumin level and lowered resistance of the patient because of toxemia, septicemia, and hypovolemia. Positional changes must be viewed with added concern.

PROGRESSIVE EXTERNAL OPHTHALMOPLEGIA

Progressive external ophthalmoplegia complicated by Adams-Stokes attacks (with a ventricular rate as low as 16 per minute) has been reported by Ross and colleagues, from the University of Colorado Medical Center. A 23-year-old male, who had previously experienced multiple attacks of syncope, was successfully treated by the use of a permanent, fixed-rate pacemaker. Drachman has reported a second case so treated. Although this poorly understood disease entity is not always associated with heart block, it should alert the clinician to search for electrocardiographic evidence of delayed conduction.

PREVENTION OF SUDDEN DEATH DURING ARTERIOGRAPHY AND ANGIOCARDIOGRAPHY

Deaths from angiocardiography are occurring with a sufficient frequency to warrant planning of active measures for resuscitation by the available personnel well in advance. All too often, when the first case of cardiac arrest is encountered under such conditions, inadequate attempts at resuscitation are made, improper drugs in inadequate doses are used, and unsuccessful resuscitation is the rule rather than the exception. It is imperative that all precautions be taken to ensure successful resuscitation under such circumstances.

The incidence of death following angiocardiography has been estimated from a large study done by Dotter and Jackson. In the United States and Canada, in 5,961 angiocardiographic studies performed, there were eighteen deaths. This was an incidence of one death in 309 procedures. In Great Britain there were seven deaths in 413 examinations, a ratio of one death in every fifty-nine examinations. In Sweden, one death was reported in 450 examinations. Diamond and co-workers report two deaths in 100 examinations.

The most common form of death following angiocardiography is the sudden cardiorespiratory one, immediately or shortly following the injection of the constrast medium. In an analysis of twenty-six reported deaths during angiocardiography, Dotter and Steinberg mention that almost half the fatalities appeared after the second injection of the contrast medium. The risk of multiple injections of the dye should therefore be emphasized and avoided. I have noted at least one additional case of such a sequence of events after the second injection of iodopyracet (Diodrast).

Atropine sulfate should be given in all such cases when dye is injected into the bloodstream.

PREVENTION IN OBSTETRIC PATIENTS

Excluding the patient with cardiac disease, the incidence of cardiac arrest in obstetric patients is unusually low. However, in a review of this subject, Gold urges that several prophylactic measures be observed in the obstetric patient, including measures to relieve the patient's apprehension and anxiety, measures to guard against aspiration of vomitus, and proper timing and judicious use of premedication. He suggests atropine to allay the depressing effect or scopolamine

for its amnesic and mild sedative effects as well as its ability to reduce secretions. Rapid induction by inhalation anesthesia should not be used in patients admitted to the hospital with a fully dilated cervix and delivery imminent.

PREVENTION ASSOCIATED WITH EXTRACORPOREAL HEMODIALYSIS

With an elevated serum potassium level associated with various stages of renal insufficiency, the likelihood of cardiac arrest is considerably increased. Lawton and Lardner treated a 31-year-old white male who had acute renal failure accompanied by serum potassium level of 9.32 mEq. per liter. While the patient was being prepared for a second dialysis, cardiac standstill suddenly occurred. A thoracotomy was performed, and the heart action was restored. In addition, 5 gm. of calcium gluconate was administered intravenously and the patient was rapidly digitalized with 0.8 mg. of lanatoside C (Cedilanid). A 3½-hour period of dialysis was subsequently employed, following which all evidence of potassium intoxication disappeared. The patient did not, however, recover.

PREVENTIVE MEASURES DURING TRANSFUSION

Cardiac arrest associated with massive transfusions. Boyan and Howland, at Memorial Hospital in New York City, no longer are concerned about the ionic changes in stored blood and their effect on the heart during massive blood transfusions. Instead, their experiences indicate that the incidence of cardiac arrest during massive blood transfusions can be markedly decreased if the stored blood is warmed to near normal temperature.

Fig. 3-4 shows one type of blood warmer. This apparatus consists of a 24-foot coil of sterile plastic tubing, 4.5 mm. in diameter, immersed in a 20 liter waterbath. The temperature is maintained at 37° C. by adding warm water. This device will warm cold bank

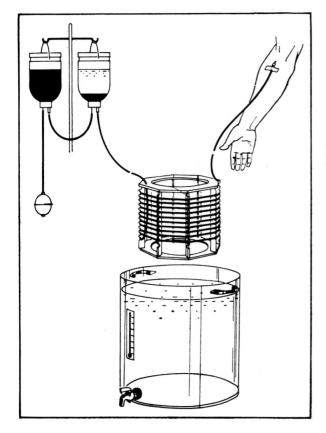

Fig. 3-4. Blood warmer for use when large amounts of blood are required. (From Boyan, C. P.: J.A.M.A. **183**:58, 1963.)

blood from 4° to 36° C. at transfusion rates of 50 to 150 ml. per minute.

In support of this apparatus, Boyan and Howland cite twenty-one cases of cardiac arrest in the operating room among thirty-six patients receiving 3,000 ml. or more of citrated blood at a rate of 50 ml. or more per minute. These patients all received cold stored blood. In contrast, only one case of cardiac arrest occurred among forty-five patients receiving 3,000 ml. or more of warmed stored blood at a rate of 50 ml. or more per minute. Nine of the eleven patients receiving in excess of 6,000 ml. of cold stored blood at a rate in excess of 100 ml. per minute experienced cardiac arrest. Temperatures as low as 27.5° C. have been recorded in cardiac arrest patients receiving large amounts of cold stored blood. These temperatures were esophageal recordings taken behind the heart.

The ECG changes observed during the administration of large amounts of cold stored blood are not reproduced if warmed stored blood is used. Furthermore, less increase in peripheral vascular resistance is noted, and intravascular agglutination of blood is less prominent. With the resultant increased tissue perfusion, the cardiovascular complications resulting from sudden shifts in potassium, calcium, and acid-base balance can more readily be combated.

In a more recent communication, Howland and co-workers suggest that exogenous sodium bicarbonate be employed to counteract a high theoretic acid load from massive transfusions. They therefore recommend the use of sodium bicarbonate in a ratio of 44.6 mEq. to every 5 units of bank blood. This procedure resulted in a reduction in mortality rate from 38% to 8% in the patients who were transfused with 20 or more units of blood.

The rapid cooling of the heart by massive

blood transfusions has a profound effect on cardiac function and can lead to ventricular fibrillation or asystole. Boyan has placed esophageal thermocouples directly behind the cardiac atria to measure heart temperatures in patients during massive bleeding and has correlated these changes with the amount of blood transfused (Fig. 3-5). A marked lowering of temperature was recorded, and in two patients cardiac arrest was observed at 27.5° C. and 32° C., respectively, although the blood loss was properly replaced. There will be prolongation of the S-T segment, distorted QRS complexes, peaked T waves, premature ventricular contractions, and, finally, bradycardia followed by standstill.

Massive transfusions of cold blood cause a reduction of cardiac output, coronary blood flow, heart rate, and blood pressure. The blood pH falls in spite of adequate ventilation. The acidosis is thought to be of a metabolic origin produced by vasoconstriction leading to inadequate tissue perfusion and hypoxia. The lowered body temperature will decrease the rate of citrate metabolism. According to Boyan, bank blood kept refrigerated at 4° C. has a pH of 6.9 because of citric acid and an excess of carbon dioxide. It is deficient in calcium ions, the potassium-sodium ratio in red blood cells is reversed with an increase of extracellular potassium, and there is absence or a decrease of blood clotting factors.

The intra-arterial route of rapid cold blood transfusions carries a lower morbidity than does the intravenous route, since the blood circulates through the body and is warmed and buffered and the citrate is removed before it reaches the right side of the heart (Smith and Stetson).

The incidence of cardiac arrest during massive blood replacement (3,000 ml. or more per hour) was reduced from 58.3% to 6.8% by warming the cold bank blood to body temperature while it was being transfused (Boyan).

ECG monitoring during transfusion. ECG monitoring seems particularly valuable be-

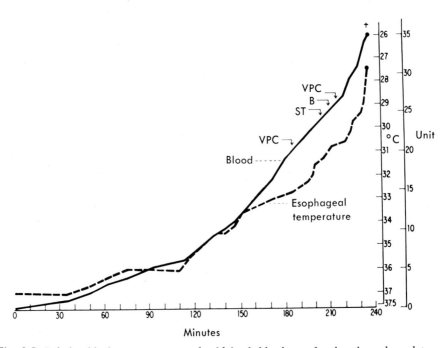

Fig. 3-5. Relationship between amount of cold bank blood transfused and esophageal temperatures showing onset of ventricular premature contractions, *VPC;* prolonged *S-T* segment, *ST;* bradycardia, *B;* cardiac arrest†. (From Boyan, C. P.: Ann. Surg. **160:**282, 1964.)

cause of the previously mentioned dangers encountered during transfusion, particularly in the use of old blood, large quantities of blood, cold blood, or concentrated blood preparations such as triple-strength plasma.

In exchange transfusion. The frequency of sudden death during or immediately following transfusion was studied by Diamond at the Little Company of Mary Hospital in Evergreen Park, Illinois. During the 3-year period, a total of 120 exchange transfusions was performed at this private institution. Four deaths from sudden cardiac arrhythmia or cardiac arrest occurred during the exchange transfusions.

In the event of an exchange transfusion, donor blood should be warmed. The danger of using cold blood for massive transfusions is presented in the preceding discussion. If the blood used has been stored for a considerable period, the risk of hyperkalemia adds to the possibility of cardiac arrhythmia and arrest. Hyperkalemia may be reduced by the use of fresh donor blood, and an adequate ionized calcium level may be maintained by using heparinized blood or by injecting calcium gluconate during the exchange transfusion. Since stored blood is acidotic, the likelihood of increased acidosis in the infant is raised. Fifteen milliliters of THAM buffer may be added to each 500 ml. of whole blood.

Since attention has been called to the increased frequency of cardiac arrhythmias and cardiac arrest during exchange transfusions in infants, it may be wise to perform such transfusion either in the operating room or in a similar area where resuscitative equipment is readily available. Certainly, constant monitoring of the vital signs is in order in all of these cases. Cardiac arrest generally occurs without warning.

PREVENTION OF SUDDEN DEATH
DURING CARDIAC CATHETERIZATION

Certain precautions will lower both the incidence and the severity of arrhythmias during cardiac catheterization. Adequate ventilation is essential. If the catheter is in an arrhythmia-producing area of the myo-

cardium, the rhythm will usually be restored to normal if the catheter is rapidly moved. Atropine sulfate should be administered if bradycardia is persistent. If supraventricular tachycardia is present, intra-atrial manipulation of the catheter will often reinstate a sinus rhythm. For a persistent tachycardia, electrical cardioversion is usually preferred.

Rigid precautions must be employed to ensure adequate grounding of patients during cardiac catheterization studies when low-resistance electrode catheters are used, since the delivery of a dangerous electrical current directly to the heart becomes a real danger. The minimum fibrillating current and the amount of current potentially deliverable to the heart by an electrode catheter are not far apart. Obviously, these patients should, in addition, be carefully monitored. Fortunately, this is usually done.

Sudden cardiac standstill or ventricular fibrillation occurs with sufficient frequency during cardiac catheterization procedures that it is of the utmost importance that the cardiac physiology laboratory be equipped for prompt and effective resuscitative measures. A listing of the most frequent arrhythmias associated with cardiac catheterization would include atrial extrasystoles, ventricular extrasystoles, supraventricular tachycardia, and ventricular tachycardia. It is my belief that a direct-writing electrocardiograph, a Cardi-Cator, or similar device should be employed with every catheterization procedure. Unless specifically contraindicated, atropine sulfate should always be given prior to insertion of the catheter.

With the cardiac catheterization and angiocardiography being performed with increasing frequency in larger and larger numbers of institutions, it is important that attention be directed to the adequate protective safety measures that should surround each procedure. Ideally, an anesthetist, endotracheal equipment, and some sort of mobile resuscitation unit should be present. It is wise for a continuous ECG reading to be carried out with each angiocardiogram. In the opinion of Dimond and Gonlubol: "The risk to the patient's life that is brought into play the instant the dye is thrust into the blood stream must be justified by an imperative need for diagnostic information; the information must have value in terms of the patient's welfare—value that offsets the risk to his life."

PACEMAKERS AND THE POSSIBILITY OF VENTRICULAR FIBRILLATION

Bilitch reports on a group of 86 patients paced with permanent transvenous pacemakers. Forty-six of the group had unipolar lead systems and demand pulse generators. The others had fixed-rate generators with bipolar electrodes. In the fixed-rate group, an immediate postoperative mortality of 20% is recorded as compared with a 4.3% mortality in the demand pacemaker group. Ventricular fibrillation was documented in 5 of the 8 deaths in the fixed-rate group. In all of this group competitive rhythms had developed. Two deaths occurred in patients with demand pacemakers with competitive rhythm. Bilitch concludes that competitive rhythm is detrimental in artificially paced patients and that it should be circumvented by the use of R wave demand-type pulse generators.

Zoll and his associates are not in agreement with the degree of risk involved with fixed-rate pacemakers in the production of ventricular fibrillation. In a group of 204 patients treated with fixed-rate pacemakers since 1960, their results indicate that competition carries little if any risk of producing repetitive response, of causing ventricular tachycardia or fibrillation, or of increasing the total mortality or sudden death. Competitive rhythms were documented in only 108 of the 204 patients. In 16 patients ventricular tachycardia or fibrillation was observed, and the onset was documented electrocardiographically in 12. In every instance repetitive response was clearly absent. Altogether there were 72 deaths in the series. Thirty-six (33%) of the 108 with and 36 (38%) of the 96 without competition died. Thirty of the 72 patients died suddenly; one half of

those who died were in the group without competitive rhythms.

In a detailed presentation in the Annals of the New York Academy of Sciences, Chardack and others reviewed the problems of pacing and ventricular fibrillation. It seems clear that competitive pacing stimuli during acute coronary ischemia are capable of triggering ventricular fibrillation, especially if the electrode is placed in an ischemic area of the heart. Chardack's experimental work does not conclusively suggest that competition from asynchronous pacemakers during acute coronary ischemia will increase the risk of fibrillation if the electrode is placed in non-ischemic territory. Generally speaking, it seems that the danger of electrical parasystole is remote in stable patients in whom the pacemaker electrode has been implanted for some time. It is pointed out that during electrical parasystole approximately 3,000 stimuli can be expected to fall into the vulnerable period in a 24-hour stretch. With the advent of demand pacemakers it became obvious that they are particularly indicated in patients who are predominantly in normal sinus rhythm and who experience only intermittent block (Chardack), in patients with intermittent sinus arrest or bradycardia, and in patients in whom a sinus rhythm has returned after instillation of a fixed-rate system and who are symptomatic because of competitive rhythm or require a periodic change of their pulse generator.

WOLFF-PARKINSON-WHITE SYNDROME AND VENTRICULAR FIBRILLATION

Although Wolff-Parkinson-White syndrome is often regarded as a relatively benign condition, it appears that some normal hearts cannot tolerate the rapid supraventricular arrhythmias, especially if repetitive or sustained. Kaplan and Cohen report a case of ventricular fibrillation in a woman with this syndrome and speculate that the arrhythmia may have led to foci of hypoxia and, hence, to ventricular fibrillation. They stress that the Wolff-Parkinson-White anomaly should be viewed as a potentially fatal condition and that all episodes of paroxysmal heart action should be carefully documented whenever possible.

PROLONGED Q-T INTERVAL

It is now apparent that approximately 1% of children born deaf have an additional bizarre prolongation of the Q-T interval. From infancy to adolescence, these persons are in particular jeopardy in that single or multiple ventricular premature beats falling in the Q-T interval may lead to ventricular fibrillation. Certainly, every infant or child with syncopal attacks, breath-holding spells, or any form of unexplained unconsciousness should be suspected of this syndrome and should have an electrocardiogram. Identification of these children may prevent some of the tragic potential sequelae. The family should be well schooled in the principles of cardiopulmonary resuscitation since these hearts respond quickly if treatment is applied promptly. It might be particularly worthwhile for all persons, including teachers who work in schools of the deaf, to have an ability in performing cardiopulmonary resuscitation. At this point it is unclear as to the best therapeutic regime to follow in order to shorten the Q-T interval or to prevent ventricular arrhythmias. Since many of these attacks are associated with excitement and fright with a subsequent further prolongation of the Q-T interval, phenobarbital and diphenylhydantoin may be worthwhile since they have fewer untoward effects than some of the antiadrenergic drugs.

PREVENTION DURING ELECTROSHOCK THERAPY

The number of patients receiving electroshock therapy (ECT) is sufficiently high to warrant that the psychiatrist possess an adequate knowledge of resuscitative techniques. In addition, careful monitoring of the patient's cardiovascular system is warranted, both during and immediately after ECT. Because of the marked vagal discharge occur-

ring after the grand mal seizure, vagolytic agents should be employed—particularly atropine sulfate. Conventional doses of atropine do not appear sufficient. In addition, ECT is seldom used for patients on phenothiazine medication. Sympatholytic tranquilizers appear to compound the increased likelihood of an occasional cardiac arrest.

What is a sufficient dose of atropine premedication for electroshock therapy? Rich and associates in the Department of Psychiatry at Washington University School of Medicine, studied by electrocardiography the effects of atropine in association with electroshock therapy. After a systematic study of four doses of atropine (1.0, 1.5, 2.0, and 2.5 mg.) as premedication for electroshock therapy, they concluded that there were no differences in side effects, ECG abnormalities, or postelectroshock apnea. They found no apparent advantages in the higher doses and subsequently recommend that 1.0 mg. of atropine be given subcutaneously as premedication for routine electroshock therapy.

PREVENTION IN PATIENTS WITH RHEUMATOID SPONDYLITIS

Patients with rheumatoid spondylitis require additional precautions. Cardiac conduction disturbances are frequent. Sobin and Hagstrom report such a case that included the destruction of the atrioventricular bundle by lesions characteristic of rheumatoid disease.

PREVENTION OF DEATH FOLLOWING CAROTID SINUS PRESSURE

Whenever carotid massage is applied in the elderly patient or in the patient with abnormal electrocardiographic tracing, one must be prepared for the possibility of asystole. Should asystole occur it may often respond immediately to the use of a single midsternal blow to the patient's chest. Smiddy and associates performed carotid massage on a group of 24 asymptomatic men over 65 years of age who had abnormal base line

ECGs. Five developed asystole and syncope following carotid massage, but each returned to normal sinus rhythm after a single mid-sternal blow to the chest.

Sudden death caused by carotid sinus stimulation is well documented. For example, in cases cited by Greenwood and Dupler, ventricular fibrillation occurred after less than 4 seconds of diagnostic carotid sinus pressure in a 66-year-old man, and asystole occurred after rather gentle pressure to the carotid sinus in a 70-year-old woman.

While a generally safe, reliable, and worthwhile procedure under certain circumstances, carotid sinus pressure can be lethal. It may cause complete asystole or sudden slowing of the pulse, or it may cause marked fall of the blood pressure.

Greenwood and Dupler's excellent review of this subject merits attention. They make the following recommendations in an effort to prevent many untoward reactions to ill-advised use of carotid sinus pressure:

1. Bilateral carotid sinus stimulation should *never* be used.
2. Pressure should be limited to the briefest effective period, preferably less than 5 seconds.
3. Electrocardiographic monitoring should always be used. (Possible exceptions include emergency patients and persons known to have paroxysmal supraventricular tachycardia.)
4. Auscultatory monitoring should be maintained without exception.
5. With systolic blood pressures below 100 mm. Hg, carotid sinus pressure should be avoided.
6. Much discretion should be used when treating any patient receiving cardiotonic drugs.
7. Use of cardiotonic drugs is seldom indicated in elderly patients, especially those with cerebral vascular disease.
8. ECG and EEG monitoring should be used when carotid sinus pressure or carotid artery occlusion is considered necessary for the diagnosis of carotid vascular disease.*

---

*From Greenwood, R. J., and Dupler, D. A.: Death following carotid sinus pressure, J.A.M.A. 181:605-609, 1962.

PREVENTION OF ANAPHYLACTIC DEATH

Although sudden death from anaphylactic shock may occur without suggestive antecedent history, a careful inquiry will frequently reveal pertinent information regarding an obvious drug allergy and previous drug reactions. Rosenthal, in his report of thirty penicillin fatalities in a 5-year period in New York City, established that a previous history of penicillin sensitivity could possibly have been detected in approximately 24%. Kern lists the following rules of prevention against sudden fatal anaphylactic drug reaction:

1. Stress is placed upon prevention which begins with the avoidance of unnecessary sensitization.
2. Particular care is urged in avoidance of sensitization in those with an allergic history or strong allergic heredity.
3. The routine use of depot penicillins by parental injection in rheumatic fever prophylaxis is challenged.
4. Topical application of antibiotics is condemned.*

The most common cause of sudden fatal anaphylactic responses to drug sensitivity is penicillin. Testing for drug sensitivity fortunately is of greater usefulness with penicillin than with many other drugs, with the exception of serums. Certainly, all patients with a strong history of allergy, and who have received penicillin, should be tested before being given penicillin. A conjunctival test may also be performed. When receiving drugs likely to cause a sudden reaction, all patients should be given medication where emergency resuscitative equipment is available, including hydrocortisone, airways, and a tourniquet.

Penicillin sensitivity is being tested with the penicilloyl-polylysine reagent. The Public Health Service has reported a 1% penicillin sensitivity reaction in 2,542 patients who did not react to the test. Of 330 patients who did have known evidence of sensitivity, 36% reacted positively to the test.

---

*From Kern, R. A.: Anaphylactic drug reactions, J.A.M.A. **179**:19-21, 1962.

Unfortunately, the simultaneous injection of antihistamines fails to protect the patient.

PREVENTION IN PATIENTS WITH ENDOCRINE IMBALANCE

In 1952 Reid and his colleagues called attention to the possible need for endocrine substitution therapy as a good preoperative measure in patients with obvious endocrine imbalance, such as those in the climacteric, especially if any disturbance in cardiac dynamics is present. King and associates (in a series of experiments designed to study the effects of estrogen on the composition and function of cardiac muscle) conclude that the contractile system of the cardiac muscle is greatly dependent upon estrogen. Apparently the hormone is thought to directly influence the specific synthesis of contractile cardiac protein. By increasing the estrogen level, a corresponding increase in the actomyosin concentration is accomplished.

Preventive measures associated with untoward response to drugs

PREVENTION DURING USE OF NEOSTIGMINE TO NEUTRALIZE RELAXANTS

As mentioned elsewhere, neostigmine (Prostigmin) is a potent vagal stimulant, and, unless guarded against, marked slowing of the heart and even arrest will occur when neostigmine is administered by the anesthesiologist to neutralize the curare-like relaxants. Prior use of atropine and careful monitoring are essential to avoid this complication.

PREVENTION OF SUDDEN DEATH FOLLOWING MERCURIAL DIURETICS

Mention should be made of the occasional sudden death following mercurial diuretics, most of which may result in ventricular fibrillation. The drug should particularly be cautioned against when evidence of intraventricular conduction deformities are present. The weight-dosage ratio should be carefully observed, and large doses should not be given to small patients.

CAUTION AGAINST RAPID INJECTION OF POTASSIUM

Since occasional cases of sudden death have followed the inadvertent intravenous injection of concentrated solutions of potassium chloride, caution should be continually observed. When potassium salts are added to fluids for infusion, they should be already prepared with the necessary concentration of potassium. Potassium additions should never be made to the tube leading to the patient's vein. The maximum effects of potassium toxicity are usually observed immediately after the time of their administration if normal renal function is present.

PRECAUTIONS WITH CORTISONE, RESERPINE, AND CHLORPROMAZINE

Circulatory collapse may be prevented in the operating room in those patients receiving cortisone by increasing the dosage of the drug before and after surgery. If the patient is receiving reserpine, hypotensive reactions may also occur in patients under general anesthesia who are being treated with chlorpromazine.

Alexander suggests that steroids may affect cell membrane permeability, concentration of potassium, and resultant formation of action potentials. Spontaneous defibrillation during closed-chest cardiac massage was documented by Hur and co-workers in Jerusalem, Israel. Unfortunately, several days after the patient's successful resuscitation, he began to bleed from a preexisting duodenal ulcer; he died of hemorrhagic shock. Hur recommends that patients with peptic ulcers who happen to be subjects of cardiac resuscitation should have antiulcer treatment instituted as soon as possible. He also suggests that corticosteroids, even in small doses, be avoided.

AVOIDANCE OF CNS STIMULANTS

During any period of cerebral anoxia associated with cardiac arrest and resuscitation, it is imperative that CNS stimulants such as pentylenetetrazol (Metrazol), picrotoxin, caffeine, and strychnine be avoided because the likelihood of permanent cerebral damage will apparently be increased.

Drugs used in prevention

ATROPINE

Preventive effects. Reid has repeatedly stressed the preventive effect of atropine as related to the problem of cardiac arrest and as would apply in a large percentage of cases. Perhaps he more than anyone else is responsible for the recent popularity in the choice of atropine sulfate as a preoperative medication.

Wilson, in 1915, pointed out that atropine has a most selective action on the A-V node in protecting it from the effects of vagal stimulation. He demonstrated the occurrence of A-V nodal escape during orbital pressure in atropinized subjects, and he suggested that the escape occurs because the period of the S-A node is depressed below the period of the A-V node, with the result that the latter node becomes the pacemaker.

Johnstone, in England, has reported on an ECG study carried out on sixty healthy subjects. He states that cardiac inhibition to the point of complete cardiac arrest may result from inhaling cyclopropane or ether.

He believes that the degree of inhibition varies directly with the irritativeness of the inhaled vapors and that the stimulation causes reflex inhibition of the heart through the pulmocardiac reflexes. He was able to prevent, by atropine, the more serious degrees of inhibition in all except the most vagotonic subjects. Doses of 1.2 mg. or less did not prevent the occurrence of A-V nodal rhythm during anesthesia. He warns against simultaneous administration of atropine and neostigmine (Prostigmin), and suggests that the latter may potentiate the sympathomimetic effect of atropine with fatal results. Fig. 3-6 is a representative ECG tracing showing the effect of atropine as a parasympathetic (vagal) blocking agent.

Schwartz and co-workers reported on the beneficial effect of atropine sulfate administered intramuscularly in 0.6 mg. daily doses in the prevention of premature ventricular beats in one patient with transient ventricular fibrillation during established A-V disassociation. It was possible in this manner to avoid the onset of transient seizures in the patient. In Schwartz's opinion, the action of atropine sulfate in abolishing these spontaneously developing mechanisms leaves little doubt that the "idiovascular" pacemaker is at all times

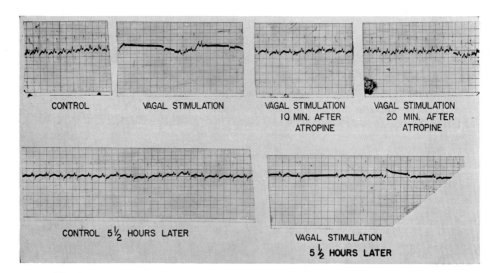

Fig. 3-6. ECG showing abolition of vagal inhibition after atropine administration.

under the influence of vagal nerves or the carotid sinus mechanism. Wiggers reports that atropine and scopolamine afford the heart some degree of protection against reflexes that may precipitate cardiovascular arrest. The mechanism of action is by the blocking of the vagal effects on the sino-auricular pacemaker.

In discussing the Adams-Stokes syndrome, Weiss and Ferris conclude that atropine, in doses that produce only slight depression of the vagomotor endings, abolishes the symptoms as well as the heart block. Paralysis of either of the vagal sheaths in the neck with procaine hydrochloride also abolishes the fainting and the block.

The pharmacologic action of atropine sulfate lies in its activity as a cholinergic blocking agent. Atropine sulfate will block the effect of acetylcholine. Acetylcholine is thought to be produced by stimulation of the vagal nerves. Its action is as brief as it is highly unstable, but over the course of a few minutes it may produce dramatic effects. The effect on the heart is to cause a decrease in the rate and force of contraction. This may go on to complete heart block. Since all vagal activity in general results in the release of acetylcholine from nerve endings and the diffusion of this substance to or on the effector organ, this drug provides the mechanism by which the break in protoplasmic continuity between nerve and organ is bridged. Acetylcholine is absorbed on a very small area of the cell surface. This active path may well be described as a patterned cell receptor. Acetylcholine is unable to locate in the cell area where an effect can take place. Atropine minimizes or actually prevents the undesirable reactions potentially present in autonomic reflexes. Thus, by interfering with the action of acetylcholine on the patterned cell receptor or that patch of the cell surface where it would ordinarily be absorbed, atropine prevents the rare vagovagal reflex from taking effect through its release of acetylcholine. Particularly should it be used before procedures

likely to elicit a vagovagal reflex, such as during angiocardiography, during downward traction of the stomach, during insertion of an endotracheal tube, or before a major positional change, to mention but a few examples. Where vagal tone is increased, as in the patient with obstructive jaundice, large doses of atropine should be used. Too often, atropine is given preoperatively but in insufficient amounts and too long before it is needed.

Johnstone reports from England that, after completing 2,000 intubations, he has never observed any evidence of reflex cardiac inhibition following the intubation of atropinized patients.

Gross states in his book *The Surgery of Infancy and Childhood* that atropine is preferable for infants because it does not depress respirations. He also believes that atropine is the desirable premedication for all thoracic surgery because of its better vagolytic action.

Johnstone recommends that atropine sulfate, 0.6 mg. intravenously, be given before operations and states that sinus bradycardia, ventricular standstill, and atrioventricular block can be prevented. When there is evidence of increased vagal tone, such as in patients with jaundice, simple sinus bradycardia, and peptic ulceration, Johnstone emphasizes the importance of simultaneous intravenous administration of atropine.

Adequate blocking of reflex arcs concerned with vagal discharges to the heart is still not an easy matter, despite the years that we have been concerned with the problem. It is generally considered that complete blockage of the vagus nerve in the human being requires nearly 2 mg. of atropine administered intravenously. Howland and colleagues recommend intravenous administration of atropine in doses of 0.5 to 1 mg. or more as a preventive dose.

While this discussion is not intended as a compendium of examples of vagal inhibitory action on the heart, its purpose is to stress the important preventive action afforded by atropine in blocking the vagal reflex. Instead of giving atropine intramuscularly an hour before operation, many anesthesiologists now prefer its intravenous administration immediately prior to anesthesia induction in order to ensure a high atropine effect when its action is most needed. Then, also, the patient's response to atropine can easily be monitored.

How much atropine should be given? When the atropine dose is calculated on the basis of weight, children should receive a proportionately larger dose than adults. A representative adult dose intramuscularly is 0.6 or 0.7 mg. Three fourths of this amount can safely be given as a rapid intravenously injected dose. For a newborn infant, 0.1 mg. atropine sulfate can be given intramuscularly. A fully adequate dose of atropine is advisable since some patients react to a small dose of atropine by a slower heart rate and an occasional atrial arrhythmia or period of A-V disassociation.

It seems clear that in the operating room there is an increased incidence of vagovagal responses under specific conditions. Therefore, atropine should be given, especially in children, for example, prior to the use of succinylcholine and particularly when combined with halothane anesthesia and before certain activities such as orotracheal intubation, bronchoscopy, and muscle correction procedures on the eye. The chief of anesthesia at a large metropolitan otolaryngology institute told me that at least 80% of children being anesthetized during adenoidectomy incur arrhythmias unless they are given 0.01 mg. of atropine per kilogram of body weight. Certainly, patients with obstructive jaundice require atropine, often in repeated doses, to reduce vagotonia during operation. Atropine prior to intubation is usually indicated, since approximately 75% of patients will demonstrate cardiac irregularities at the time of passage of an endotracheal tube.

However, Kuner and co-workers inject a note of caution regarding the use of atropine. In their study of cardiac arrhythmias during anesthesia, it is noted that atropine apparently causes occasional cardiac arrhythmias.

A-V disassociation was seen by this group and was believed to be related to individual differences in the balance between the early vagotonic affect of atropine (depressing the supranodal focus) and an early selective action of the anticholinergic effect of atropine on the ventricular conduction system.

Routine administration of atropine as a protective measure in acute myocardial infarction, in order to increase the heart rate to theoretically suppress ventricular arrhythmias, should be cautioned against. In fact, animal laboratory work with experimentally produced coronary artery occlusion indicates that atropine may actually tend to increase the incidence of arrhythmias during acute myocardial infarction.

Use during urography. An intravenous injection of atropine during the compression phase of urography reduces the incidence of severe cardiovascular reactions. Svendsen, reporting on the use of atropine in 393 of 726 urographic examinations, recommends that an intravenous injection of 1 mg. of atropine by given. The incidence of severe reactions dropped from 6% to 1% with this dose. An injection of 0.5 mg. of atropine reduced the incidence from 6% to 3%.

Effect on ventricular fibrillation. DiPalma and Schultz point out the antifibrillary properties of atropine by stating:

> The chemical structure while lacking a phenyl or quinoline radical does possess a property substituting nitrogen for its antifibrillatory effect. Also its formula is closely related to cocaine whose marked local anesthetic and antifibrillation properties are well known. It will be recalled that quinidine appears to antagonize acetylcholine in skeletal muscle and in this respect resembles atropine. Of considerable importance is the fact that acetylcholine and vagus stimulation predisposed to auricular fibrillation and atropine can counteract this effect.*

In the animal laboratory, we have found ventricular fibrillation difficult to induce in a dog after a therapeutic dose of atropine. Similarly, once ventricular fibrillation is pro-

---

*From DiPalma, J. R., and Schultz, J. E.: Antifibrillatory drugs, Medicine **29**:123-163, 1950.

duced, defibrillation seems easier to accomplish.

QUINIDINE

Cardiotoxicity. Hurt and Myerburg warn against the serious side effects that may be produced (or provoked) by the use of quinidine sulfate in the treatment of supraventricular and ventricular ectopic activities. They believe that many instances of sudden death attributed to toxic effects of quinidine on the CNS are actually the result of a quinidine-induced cardiac arrhythmia. Cardioversion, in their opinion, is generally safer than the use of quinidine in the conversion from atrial fibrillation and flutter to a normal rhythm.

The incidence of mortality associated with cardioversion with the use of quinidine is estimated to be about 4%. When electrical cardioversion is used, a mortality of approximately 1% is encountered. In instances of quinidine cardiotoxicity, supportive treatment is indicated until the major effect of the drug is removed by excretion (approximately 2 hours). Molar lactate may help antagonize the effects of the drug.

Patients receiving quinidine for the first time or those who evidence any of the clinical manifestations of cinchonism should be watched carefully for the onset of ventricular extrasystoles, ventricular tachycardia, and even ventricular fibrillation. Since quinidine inhibits conduction in all portions of the heart, the ECG can alert the physician to the potential danger of ventricular fibrillation, particularly if widening of the QRS complex is appreciable. Widening of the QRS complex by 50% is considered a distinct forerunner of ventricular fibrillation (Marriott). Should undue widening of the QRS complex be noted in addition to lengthening P-R and Q-T intervals, therapeutic measures may need to be started to reverse the cardiotoxic effects of quinidine. Since isoproterenol increases the speed of cardiac conduction and shortens the refractory period of the heart, it will frequently be the drug of choice. More frequent use of sodium lac-

tate and epinephrine may also be made in this connection.

Role in ventricular fibrillation. The exact role played by quinidine in possibly preventing ventricular fibrillation has been one of considerable dispute. Wegria summarized his work with quinidine by stating that he believe it raises the fibrillation threshold of the dog's ventricle to protect against the fibrillation induced by the combination of benzol and epinephrine hydrochloride. If properly administered, he believes that quinidine has definite preventive properties in the treatment of ventricular fibrillation.

MacKay and associates find that animals receiving preoperative doses of quinidine are more difficult to fibrillate by electrical means and are also easier to defibrillate electrically once ventricular fibrillation has occurred. In those animals not receiving quinidine, about 60% of the defibrillation attempts require serial shock, whereas those animals having the benefit of quinidine require serial shocks in only 30% of the cases. They even suggest the routine administration of quinidine preoperatively in those patients undergoing thoracic surgery—particularly surgery of the heart. The use of quinidine as a preventive measure has, however, not received widespread support.

Quinidine probably exerts its inhibitory vagal influence because of its atropine-like anticholinergic effect. A variety of dose schedules has been suggested. The desired effect may be accomplished by 0.2 to 0.4 gm. given three or four times a day. Larger doses may be needed, however.

Role in hypersensitive carotid sinus syndrome. Quinidine, by its vagolytic effect, may be employed to prevent syncope and cardiac asystole in those patients with a hypersensitive carotid sinus.

LIDOCAINE

The remarkable effectiveness of lidocaine as an antiarrhythmic agent when administered during the early hours after an acute myocardial infarction is illustrated in a 6-year study of patients treated at the San Pedro

Community Hospital in California (Wyman). Only one episode of primary ventricular fibrillation occurred in 735 patients treated prophylactically, an incidence of 0.1%. Wyman calls attention to a California cooperative investigation of 15,782 myocardial infarctions in which there were 761 cases of primary ventricular fibrillation. There was an eventual mortality of 48%. He extrapolates from this data to suggest that there are at least 12,000 hospital deaths each year from ventricular fibrillation in association with acute myocardial infarction.

The remarkable protection given by lidocaine in this hospital's program has prompted the adoption of a plan calling for prophylactic administration of lidocaine to every suspected myocardial infarction patient upon admission to the hospital. A 75 mg. bolus of lidocaine is given, followed by 2 mg. per minute. The amount administered is controlled by an infusion pump. A 2 mg. per minute drip of lidocaine is given for a 24-hour period; the dosage is then decreased to 1 mg. per minute in the following 6 hours if premature ventricular beats are absent. If, however, the premature ventricular beats continue, a second or third 50 mg. bolus of lidocaine is given and the drip infusion is increased to 4 mg. per minute. Procainamide, 100 mg., is injected intravenously if the latter therapy is ineffective, which is rare. Procainamide was required in 8% of the cases. In a group of 139 patients who received no initial intravenous suppressive therapy, a 6% incidence of ventricular fibrillation occurred.

PROCAINE

In 1936 Beck and Mautz utilized the properties of procaine during cardiac surgery as a topical agent to the heart and observed a decreased incidence of cardiac arrhythmias. Burstein, who has done much clinical and experimental work on procaine, introduced the intravenous administration of procaine for its antiarrhythmic action, and subsequently the drug has been employed by some anesthetists during cardiac and thoracic operations. Procainamide was later introduced, and among its advantages were its qualities of producing less CNS stimulation and of being unaffected by the enzyme responsible for the rapid hydrolysis of procaine. The use of procainamide has been particularly valuable in the treatment of recurrent premature ventricular contractions and in the suppression of extrasystoles. Particularly valuable was its control of ventricular tachycardias. Procainamide is effective by oral administration.

Considerable disagreement arises on the advisability of using procaine to reduce the irritability of the heart during procedures in and around the heart. Gross states:

We employed Pronestyl (procaine amide) in about half of our cases, but have often felt that it was a factor in producing a serious fall of peripheral arterial pressure. We now use it but rarely; it is given only if there have been frequent extrasystoles before operation or ventricular tachycardia during the procedure. While some have advocated the injection of procaine into the pericardium before opening it, we have abandoned this.*

In making a right ventriculotomy for surgical correction of a stenotic pulmonic valve, some cardiac surgeons have injected a procaine solution locally at the point of the proposed incision into the ventricle. In this way, they believe that a generalized myocardial depression can be avoided.

In spite of much literature to the contrary, Converse and colleagues were unable to note that intravenous procaine provided much prophylaxis against cardiac arrhythmias. They also noted that the application of topical tetracaine (Pontocaine) to the larynx does not alter the changes occurring during endotracheal intubation. It is their belief that the practice of ventilating the patient's lungs with oxygen before intubation seems to offer the greatest protection against the occurrence of cardiac arrhythmias.

---

*From Gross, R. E.: The surgery of infancy and childhood, Philadelphia, 1953, W. B. Saunders Co., p. 907.

Chapter 4

CARDIAC ARREST AND MYOCARDIAL INFARCTION

Cardiac arrhythmias

Because an arrhythmia associated with an acute myocardial infarction is most commonly the specific fatal mechanism responsible for the death of the patient, the question arises as to what is the mechanism of arrhythmia production in acute myocardial infarction. James (1967) has contributed significantly to the understanding of arrhythmias occurring during myocardial infarction. In stating that the depressed or disorganized function of the sinus node is usually a major contributing factor to arrhythmias during acute myocardial infarction, he suggests that three anatomic features of the sinus node contribute: blood supply of the node, proximity of the node to the epicardium, and the large number of local nerve endings and ganglia. Because of the blood supply to the sinus node (originating from the proximal few centimeters of the right coronary artery in about 55% of hearts and from the proximal few millimeters of the left circumflex artery in the remaining 45%), atrial arrhythmias developing during acute myocardial infarction indicate an occlusion proximal to the origin of the sinus node artery. In fatal instances of myocardial infarction with recent onset of atrial arrhythmias, James states that there is regularly an infarction at the junction of the sinus node and the right atrium.

In the presence of pericarditis, the sinus node is often involved because of the associated edema and inflammation, since the human sinus node is normally located less than 1 mm. from the epicardium.

When the sinus node tissue becomes hypoxic because of partial or complete coronary artery occlusion, local tissue acidosis and liberation of certain normal intracellular constituents take place (James, 1967). The rate of sinus impulse formation is lowered with acidosis, and the local ganglia may become stimulated to repetitive firing and may give rise to certain neuroflexes. The marked sinus bradycardia seen in patients with acute myocardial infarction is extremely detrimental to the heart. The minute output of the heart cannot be well maintained since the stroke volume cannot be appreciatively increased during a slow rate. The sinus bradycardia associated with acute myocardial infarction is often caused by a vagal reflex.

In his excellent discussion on arrhythmias associated with myocardial infarction, James calls attention to the observation of Imai and co-workers, who found that adenosine is liberated by the ischemic myocardium. Adenosine, a normal intracellular substance, has a profound negative chronotropic action. Liberation of the adenosine from an ischemic myocardial cell may be anticipated to exert a profound influence on at least the immediately neighboring cells. In addition, potassium liberated from injured cells will also effect adjacent cells.

Because of the blood supply to the A-V node and the bundle of His, an acute heart block during myocardial infarction is thought to almost always indicate a complication of posterior (diaphragmatic) infarcts. The A-V node and the bundle of His are supplied, in 90% of instances, from the right coronary artery by a branch entering from the diaphragmatic surface of the heart (James,

1967). Nerves and ganglia are numerous near the A-V node, particularly around its posterior margin, thus lying between the coronary sinus and the node. The sinus bradycardia, an often vagus-mediated phenomenon commonly observed in acute posterior myocardial infarction, is most likely caused by reflexes originating in such extracardiac neural centers.

A sinus bradycardia, usually less than 60 per minute, may have serious prognostic features after a myocardial infarction. Not only is there a decreased cardiac output and a subsequently reduced coronary flow with the slowed heart, but there is also a decrease in the flow through any anastomotic vessels that may be carrying the flow. More significantly, however, a slow heart is often the precursor of more intense vagal discharge, which may then lead to complete heart block or cessation of sinus activity. Since the sinus bradycardia is often vagus-mediated, the patient should be treated with atropine in an attempt to abolish the bradycardia (James, 1967). Drugs with a vagomimetic action such as morphine should *not* be employed without atropine. As morphine is a drug of choice to relieve pain and anxiety, it should be combined with atropine.

The majority of deaths from acute myocardial infarction occur within 12 hours of the onset of symptoms and, according to Pantridge, 60% are seen within the first hour. For this reason, when patients come under observation in coronary care units, the period of greatest risk often has passed.

In Belfast, deaths from myocardial infarction during 1965 were studied, and, of 901 patients with fatal coronary attacks, only 414 reached the hospital. Of these 414, there were 102 fatalities by the time of hospital arrival.

Considerable emphasis has been placed on the oxygen differential to which various portions of the ventricular myocardium are subjected in patients with coronary artery disease as the principal mechanism of the sudden death. Adelson agrees that the ventricular fibrillation is initiated by electrical instability caused by varying degrees of oxygenation in various parts of the myocardium. Nickel and Gale report two patients successfully resuscitated by thoracotomy following acute myocardial infarction. My own experience adds support to the theory that the mechanism of arrest in myocardial infarction results from the electrical instability produced by oxygen differentials in various areas of the myocardium.

Beck calls attention to the various effects of the "two-color heart." Due to uneven coronary artery distribution, neither oxygenation nor permeability of cell membranes is uniform. Because of this, electrical potentials of different magnitudes result. He likens this to self-electrocution. This "checkerboard" distribution of coronary artery blood flow is thought considerably more likely to result in ventricular fibrillation than is an overall hypoxia of the heart.

In dog hearts made ischemic by ligation of a coronary artery and subsequently allowed to go into ventricular fibrillation, further changes were observed before and after defibrillation. Following defibrillation, Senderoff and co-workers note that the color contrast increases in magnitude as the cardiac contractions become more effective. They believe that effective cardiac contraction without fibrillation can be maintained in the presence of unequal blood distribution and unequal myocardial oxygenation.

By perfusing the coronary arteries with a nonoxygenated solution, Danese attempted to learn more of the role of localized anoxia as a trigger mechanism in the production of ventricular fibrillation that occurs soon after myocardial infarction. By perfusing with homologous serum obtained by bleeding a dog 1 day in advance and separating the serum from the clot prior to the perfusion procedure, a solution could be injected into the artery distal to the occlusion to eliminate the stasis that would occur in the anoxic area if other methods were employed, for example, ligation. The circumflex branch of the left coronary artery was used because of the high incidence of ventricular fibrillation with its occlusion. Interestingly enough, Danese found that ventricular fibrillation did not occur in any of the perfused hearts in ten dogs. In a group of thirty control animals, ventricular fibrillation occurred in 60% following the ligation of the circumflex branch of the left coronary artery. This study led Danese to question the role of oxygen concentration differential as the mechanism responsible for ventricular fibrillation following occlusion.

The oxygen differential theory of ventricular fibrillation could not be verified experimentally by Warren and associates. By means of epicardial electrocardiograms performed with the use of bare platinum microelectrodes, tissue oxygen tension was measured polarographically and recorded simultaneously. Ischemia of the myocardium was produced by occlusion of the right coronary or the descending coronary arteries. By ventilation with 4% oxygen, hypoxia was produced. Arterial and venous pressure were monitored; carbon dioxide and oxygen pressure, pH, and rectal temperature were determined. Warren and co-workers concluded that a difference in oxygen content between myocardial areas is not the factor producing the current of injury and subsequent ventricular fibrillation when the coronary artery is occluded in the dog. Other factors related to inadequate perfusion of the tissues must be of primary importance. It is possible to demonstrate this by producing a diffuse hypoxia from ventilation with 4% oxygen prior to the coronary artery occlusion and subsequent release of the occlusion during diffuse hypoxia.

When the current of injury in the ischemic area is fully developed and there is maximal hypoxia of all areas, the occlusion is relieved. No change in the oxygen content of either the ischemic or the surrounding area occurs. Nevertheless, there is rapid clearing of the pattern of injury on the EKG.*

Beck and Leighninger, although emphasizing the dangers of adjacent areas of myo-

---

*From Warren, W. D., Saurbrey, J., and Wandall, H. H.: Experimental study of the oxygen differential theory of ventricular fibrillation, Surg. Forum **13**:177-179, 1962.

cardium with different degrees of oxygenation, demonstrate that the myocardium that is almost entirely anoxic is more resistant to the spontaneous development of fibrillation.

Huffnagel and his associates (Pifarré and co-workers) at Georgetown University report data from an experimental study of ventricular fibrillation after acute coronary artery occlusion and conclude that the presence of an ischemic area next to a well-oxygenated area will not, in itself, always result in ventricular fibrillation. Other factors must be related to the myocardial mass that is deprived of its blood supply, and these factors seem to be in direct proportion to the size and flow of the artery occluded. They point out that graded reduction in perfusion of the anterior descending artery results in a proportionate reduction in the fibrillation threshold.

INCREASED VULNERABILITY TO FIBRILLATION AFTER CORONARY OCCLUSION

Numerous clinical studies indicate that from 40% to 60% of a 30-day mortality from myocardial infarction occurs within 1 hour of the onset of symptoms. During the initial 4 hours after a myocardial infarction, ventricular fibrillation is 25 times more frequent than during the ensuing 24 hours (Lown and Wolf) and most evidence points to ventricular fibrillation as the major cause of early death in myocardial infarction patients.

Studies in dogs indicate that the frequency of ectopic beats immediately after coronary occlusion correlates closely with this extremely high early mortality rate observed in patients. In all animals studied, vulnerability to fibrillation increased within 2 minutes of coronary occlusion and usually reached a maximal level 5 minutes after the occlusion (Burgess and co-workers). In dogs there is a restoration of approximate control levels within 30 minutes of the occlusion. Burgess speculates that the reason for the decrease in vulnerability may be caused by clearing of potassium from the ischemic area, release of catecholamines, altered hemodynamic state, or possibly the cooling of the surface of the heart.

In humans, an additional factor lowering the fibrillatory threshold is represented by the high incidence of bradyarrhythmias seen in the first hour of a coronary occlusion. Lown reports 61% of patients with inferior myocardial infarction exhibited bradyarrhythmia within the first hour of care. There is also a lowering of the fibrillation threshold associated with an increase in disparity in the functional refractory periods at slow heart rate (Han).

PREDICTABILITY OF VENTRICULAR FIBRILLATION

The predictability of ventricular tachycardia is considerably increased if the electrocardiogram includes (1) supraventricular or ventricular extrasystoles preceding the irregularity, (2) in fibrillation, extrasystoles occurring early after a normal cycle, (3) concomitant S-A block and changes in the configuration of the P waves, and (4) an increased number of ventricular extrasystoles characterized by their degree of prematurity. A prematurity index is derived from the ratio between the interval from the normal to the extrasystolic beat and the Q-T interval of the preceding normal beat (Buchner). If the prematurity index is less than 0.7, the likelihood of a dangerous arrhythmia is increased and it signals the need for an antiarrhythmic drug.

Over three years ago, Lawrie, at the Royal Infirmary in Edinburgh, Scotland, cautioned against the optimistic belief that many cases of ventricular fibrillation are predictable and therefore preventable so that the incidence of ventricular fibrillation in an efficient cardiac care unit should be low. In 12 of his patients who developed primary ventricular fibrillation and on whom adequate monitoring information was available, only 2 had premonitory arrhythmias detected and were on suppressive therapy at the time of their first arrest. As other authors have subsequently noted, ventricular fibrillation occurring later in the course of a myocardial infarction is more predictable. Premonitory arrhythmias usually provide adequate time to prevent the fibrillation. Unfortunately, ventricular fibrillation after 48 hours is uncommon compared with early fibrillation.

In 851 individuals with proved myocardial infarction, a premonitory cardiac arrhythmia was missing in five patients of twenty who developed primary ventricular fibrillation. Because the monitoring system consisted of a permanent record of every heartbeat, a precise identification of all arrhythmias was possible.

Continuous, close monitoring of the post-myocardial infarction patient in the coronary care unit is most rewarding in the prevention of cardiac arrest in that frequent ventricular extrasystoles may herald the possibility of a forthcoming ventricular fibrillation. In such cases there is adequate time to administer antiarrhythmic drugs. Unfortunately, a considerable number of myocardial infarction patients suffer arrest within the first hour or so of admission without the usual warning of ventricular extrasystoles or short bursts of ventricular tachycardia. Bennett and Pentecost have documented, in a group of twenty-seven patients experiencing their first arrest after admission to the coronary care unit, five instances of arrest caused by ventricular tachyarrhythmia that had no warning. Additionally, two had warning beats for less than 5 minutes, and twenty had ventricular premature beats for more than 5 minutes before the arrest. The degree of warning was usually less than five ventricular premature beats per minute. In contrast, the patients readmitted to the coronary care unit after late cardiac arrest had numerous ventricular extrasystoles before their next arrest and short episodes of ventricular tachycardia often preceded the second arrest.

SIGNIFICANCE OF VENTRICULAR PREMATURE SYSTOLE

Electrocardiograms of 5,129 persons over 16 years of age were studied by Ching and colleagues at the University of Michigan; premature systoles were present in 5.1%. Almost one third of these were supraventricular in origin, and there did not seem to be any correlation with the prevalence of coronary artery disease in this group. In persons over 30 with ventricular premature systoles, however, there was a considerably greater likelihood of coexisting coronary artery disease. Six times as many persons dying suddenly outside the hospital within an hour of the onset of symptoms had an antecedent ventricular premature systole known long before the fatal attack.

OTHER RISK FACTORS

Certainly bradycardia and bundle branch block should be included as important risk factors in association with sudden death. In addition, men over age 45 with ECG records of ventricular extrasystoles show as much as a 10 times increase in the risk of sudden death as compared to men in whom such beats are absent.

Killip would also include cardiac enlargement as an additional risk factor. For example, a patient may experience ventricular fibrillation from an extrasystole originating in the left ventricle that encounters delayed conduction caused by bundle branch block or ventricular enlargement with patchy fibrosis that will arouse reentry.

Forty percent of sudden deaths in middle-aged males occur in persons with at least two of the following characteristics: hypertension, hypercholesterolemia, and cigarette smoking.

PREVENTION OF VENTRICULAR FIBRILLATION DURING MYOCARDIAL INFARCTION

In the Belfast experience mentioned earlier, fifteen of a group of 155 patients developed ventricular fibrillation within 4 hours after onset of symptoms. Nine survived to leave the hospital. Pantridge believes that an even higher incidence of ventricular fibrillation would have occurred had it not been for a liberal use of antiarrhythmic drugs. If an ECG pattern observed by the physician with the mobile intensive care unit reveals the ominous QRS-on-T pattern, no attempt is made to transfer the patient to the ambulance until this and other evidence of ventricular irritability have been dealt with by antiarrhythmic drugs.

Corday and Vyden observed more than 300 patients with acute myocardial infarction in coronary care units. Lidocaine or procainamide was used as soon as ventricular irritability occurred, and only two subsequent cardiac arrests ensued. They state that they would have anticipated forty-eight cases of cardiac arrest. It is their recommendation that, when signs of cardiac irritability occur, lidocaine hydrochloride should be administered in intravenous doses of 25 mg. to terminate the irritability. If this is not successful, then 50 mg. may be given intravenously. Once the ectopic beat stops, an intravenous drip of 2% lidocaine hydrochloride is given in a concentration of 1 to 2 ml. per minute. They believe that if lidocaine fails, procainamide hydrochloride (50 mg.) should be given intravenously and repeated every 2 minutes, and, at the same time, 250 to 500 mg. should be given intramuscularly or orally every 4 hours. Should lidocaine or procainamide fail, diphenylhydantoin sodium, propranolol hydrochloride, or quinidine sulfate should be tried, in this order.

There is increasing evidence that most instances of ventricular fibrillation occurring as a primary electrical event in acute myocardial infarction can be prevented by the prompt use of proper pharmacologic agents for the prevention of ventricular extrasystoles, which often precede fibrillation.

VENTRICULAR FIBRILLATION AND CARDIAC STANDSTILL

In the first edition of this book we reported a predominance of asystole as encountered in the operating room in patients requiring open-chest resuscitation. Today roughly two thirds to three fourths of all cases requiring cardiopulmonary resuscitation within the hospital are patients whose primary dysrhythmia is ventricular fibrillation. The recognition that ventricular fibrillation in association with acute myocardial infarction may be reversible has markedly altered the ratio of the incidence of ventricular fibrillation to asystole. There is clearly a much better prognosis in the patient whose heart initially fibrillates than one in whom asystole is the initial problem.

It must be understood that there can be a time relationship between the two rhythms of fibrillation and asystole in that fibrillation will progress to a straight-line pattern after several minutes of circulatory arrest. Similarly, however, we have frequently seen short straight-line patterns quickly move into fibrillation.

INTRAVENTRICULAR CONDUCTION ABNORMALITIES IN MYOCARDIAL INFARCTION

The propensity to sudden death is considerably increased in acute myocardial infarction with intraventricular conduction abnormalities. In one large series of 212 consecutive cases of acute myocardial infarction (Col and Weinberg), there was a mortality rate of 47% in those patients with intraventricular conduction defects as compared with the hospital mortality rate of 21.2% in the entire series. Of the 212 myocardial infarction cases, 24% had some type of intraventricular conduction defect during sinus mechanisms. Left anterior hemiblock was the most common intraventricular defect associated with myocardial infarction, probably because of the unique blood supply from septal branches of the anterior descending artery and the delicate structure of the left anterior fascicle that makes it vulnerable to ischemia and subsequent necrosis. On the other hand, the posterior division of the left bundle branch is relatively invulnerable to these changes since it has a double blood supply from the anterior and posterior descending arteries, has the largest diameter of the three fascicles, and has the shortest pathway

to the angle of the intraventricular system. Fortunately, the most benign or innocuous intraventricular conduction defect appears to be left anterior hemiblock. The second most common conduction defect is incomplete bilateral bundle branch block followed by isolated complete bundle branch block and complete left bundle branch block. Of the twenty-four conduction defects, nine resulted in a sudden death (ventricular fibrillation).

RESUSCITATION AFTER CARDIAC ARREST FROM MYOCARDIAL INFARCTION

Since the third edition of this book, considerable strides have been made in the resuscitation of the acute myocardial infarction patient whose heart has suddenly stopped in ventricular asystole or is in ventricular fibrillation. In fact, sudden death from myocardial infarction undoubtedly represents the most common indication for cardiac resuscitation as employed today.

Chiocca reviewed the first sixty-two documented instances in which either closed- or open-cardiac compression attempts in such patients were successful. The largest number of patients were men in the 40- to 60-year age span. Males predominated in a ratio of almost six to one. Cardiac arrest most commonly occurred in association with infarctions of the posterior wall of the ventricle. Ventricular fibrillation was apparently the initial mechanism of arrest in 74% of the cases.

The history of the progress of medicine is replete with examples of advances that have been made, both experimentally and clinically, despite clear-cut warnings that such could not be accomplished. The number of patients who have been successfully resuscitated following the onset of ventricular fibrillation or asystole after sudden coronary artery occlusion is sufficiently great to give considerable support to the proponents of resuscitative attempts in such instances.

It is noted that many people who die suddenly from coronary artery disease may have only a relatively restricted stenosis of the coronary circulation. Adelson studied the records of 500 persons who died suddenly because of coronary artery disease. Of this group, 316 hearts failed to indicate recent increase in the stenosis or indications of an acute myocardial infarct. Recent coronary thrombi were present in twenty of the patients. Acute myocardial infarction without coronary thrombi was present in twenty of the patients.

If Adelson's series of 500 patients who died suddenly from coronary artery disease is indicative of other such relatively large groups of cases, then one can conclude that sudden deaths from coronary disease are primarily deaths occurring in men; only 12% of Adelson's series were women. It is interesting to note that 13% of the 500 persons were under 39 years of age.

No longer is it accurate to conclude that ventricular fibrillation subsequent to an acute coronary occlusion represents an irreversible situation. Successful defibrillations in such instances are now commonplace. Senderoff and others ligated coronary arteries in twenty-one dogs, and after ventricular fibrillation had subsequently developed, all dogs were subjected to cardiac massage and oxygen administration. Defibrillation, without removal of the occluding ligatures, resulted in a 52% resuscitation rate.

Probably the first successful case of electrical defibrillation in acute myocardial infarction by means of externally applied electrodes is that reported by Nast and co-workers. While an ECG was recording the electrical impulses from the heart *(it is interesting to note how many cases of ventricular fibrillation appear to develop during the actual recording of the ECG!),* the changes appeared to be diagnostic of a recent posterior myocardial infarct. Suddenly the patient cried out, became unconscious, and developed opisthotonos and apnea. The ECG revealed that ventricular fibrillation was occurring. After electrical countershock of 0.15 second's duration with 350 volts of 60-cycle A.C., repeated twice more with 10-second intervals, the ventricular fibrillation reverted

to a complete atrial ventricular block and atrioventricular rhythm. Twelve minutes later, the heart had regained its sinus rhythm and the patient was conscious. Premature contractions were frequent, and 200 mg. quinidine gluconate was administered intramuscularly as well as 0.4 mg. atropine sulfate. Atropine was continued every 6 hours for the first day, and 200 mg. quinidine was given by mouth every 6 hours for several weeks. Several months later the patient was reported to be again employed as a school librarian with only an occasional complaint referable to her cardiac status.

Nast and associates mention that they had previously treated eight patients with ventricular fibrillation in acute myocardial infarctions by thoracotomy, cardiac massage, and direct defibrillation. There were no survivals in any of these cases.

Since one of the first successful cases was a 65-year-old physician, it seems unlikely that advanced age in itself is a contraindication.

An acute anteroseptal myocardial infarction resulted in ventricular fibrillation during an ECG tracing in a 60-year-old man in the emergency ward of the Beth Israel Hospital in 1961. The case is of particular interest in that a successful outcome was achieved by the combined use of external cardiac massage, external cardiac defibrillation (250 volts), and external electrical cardiac stimulation. In their report on this case, Shohet and Sweet emphasize the need for electrical stimulation when the intrinsic cardiac pacemaker fails to respond.

With the advent of external cardiac massage and external electrical defibrillation, a rapid increase in the number of successful resuscitative attempts in myocardial infarction cases occurred. Moss and others relate the histories of three patients whose cardiac output was maintained satisfactorily with closed-chest compression and subsequent defibrillation.

Since successful resuscitative efforts in cases of cardiac arrest occurring after an acute myocardial infarct are being reported with increasing frequency, it is obvious that the question of selection of the patients be entertained. Crum and Harris go so far as to state that cardiac massage should be attempted in all cases of cardiac arrest caused by myocardial infarction, provided that the physician can arrive within 5 minutes of the arrest.

MANAGEMENT OF VENTRICULAR ASYSTOLE IN ASSOCIATION WITH ACUTE MYOCARDIAL INFARCTION

Corday and Vyden state that ventricular asystole occurs as a complication in approximately 6% of myocardial infarctions. (For the most part the problem is one of ventricular defibrillation.) If, however, ventricular asystole is a complication of myocardial infarction, initial treatment should be precordial concussion; this alone may serve to pace the heart. I have seen this demonstrated graphically on the electrocardiogram in several instances. An external pacemaker may be applied through the use of subcutaneous electrodes; or preferably, a transvenous catheter may be used. Because it takes considerable time to place in operation, closed-chest resuscitation should be promptly instituted. As mentioned above, a transvenous pacemaker should be positioned in the heart whenever a second- or third-degree heart block is noticed so that the pacemaker may be automatically or manually switched on should cardiac arrest occur. Corday and Vyden recommend that the drugs of choice in ventricular asystole complicating myocardial infarction are isoproterenol hydrochloride, 0.02 to 0.1 mg. (or epinephrine, 0.5 mg.), injected intravenously or directly into the heart every 3 to 5 minutes as required. They mention that atropine sulfate, 0.4 mg., given intravenously, is also of value in restoring normal rhythm. Glycoside toxicity may be the cause of the ventricular asystole and therefore chelating agents such as sodium and potassium citrate salts or antiarrhythmic drugs such as diphenylhydantoin sodium may prevent recurrence of the asystole. As in all

types of cardiac arrest, metabolic acidosis must be combated; perhaps this may be best accomplished by giving 50 ml. of bicarbonate (3.75 gm. or 44.6 mEq.) intravenously. This may be repeated every 5 to 8 minutes.

CORONARY CARE UNITS

The coronary care unit no longer exists solely for the purpose of providing on-the-spot resuscitative efforts. Because of the use of well-accepted and reliable monitoring techniques, many of the cardiopulmonary emergencies will be *prevented* by the recognition and treatment of arrhythmias after onset.

Ventricular fibrillation in the coronary care unit. The incidence of arrhythmias following myocardial infarction is, of course, high. The reported frequency depends upon several factors, among which must be included the time interval between myocardial infarction and admission to the coronary care unit. In addition, the frequency of arrhythmias detected will obviously depend upon the monitoring devices used. In many series, the incidence of ventricular fibrillation approximates 10%. In the coronary care unit at the Royal Melbourne Hospital in Melbourne, Australia, 200 consecutively admitted patients with myocardial infarction were studied by Stock and co-workers. One hundred sixty-five patients (82.5%) developed arrhythmias. Twenty of the patients had ventricular fibrillation. There was a survival rate of 50% in this group, including all six patients who suffered mild infarction and ventricular fibrillation. The mortality was high in patients with severe infarction and ventricular fibrillation.

Seventy-three percent of a group of thirty patients were continuously monitored with an electronic device for an average of 52 hours after myocardial infarction, as reported by Spann and co-workers at the Massachusetts General Hospital. It is interesting that nine patients (who had twenty arrhythmias during their acute myocardial infarctions) were restudied an average of 7 months after infarction and were found to have only two arrhythmias, neither of ventricular origin.

An analysis of the ECG rhythm at the time of arrest in forty-three patients with myocardial infarction is reported by Hofkin. Ventricular fibrillation was present in twenty-five of forty-three patients (58%).

In Kaplan's series of 100 consecutively treated patients with cardiac arrest, there were thirty-two patients with acute myocardial infarction. Of these thirty-two patients, eighteen experienced ventricular fibrillation.

During the first year in a coronary care unit at the Community Hospital Coronary Intensive Care Unit of Greenwich, Connecticut, thirteen patients (18%) developed ventricular fibrillation.

NEED FOR SPECIAL OBSERVATION ROOM AFTER THE CORONARY CARE UNIT

For administrative and economic reasons it is not always easy to retain the patient in the coronary care unit beyond the fifth or sixth postoperative day. For this reason, there may be a real need for a unit to which patients may be discharged from the coronary care unit but in which some monitoring can be maintained and trained personnel and adequate equipment are present.

The danger of persistent electrical instability of the heart muscle or the progression of a previous ischemic episode persists even after discharge from the coronary care unit. Grace notes that approximately 10% of patients discharged from the coronary care unit have life-threatening arrhythmias. Killip in 1967 found that 20% of deaths from myocardial infarction occurred after transfer to regular care units. Numerous authors have reported their experience with "late ventricular fibrillation." Restieaux was able to resuscitate five of ten patients who developed ventricular fibrillation between the sixth and twenty-fourth days after onset of an infarction.

It probably is not possible at this point to clearly identify the patients who are most likely to die nor are there many studies that lend support to any clear-cut guidelines to determine the duration of administration of antiarrhythmic drugs. However, it is certain that especially those patients whose initial course is complicated by left ventricular failure, hypotension, or ventricular arrhythmias should be continuously followed in a special observation area after discharge from the coronary care unit.

An analysis made of ventricular dysrhythmias both in and after discharge from the coronary unit at London's St. Mary's Hospital is reported by Spracklen and colleagues. Of 163 patients diagnosed as having had a myocardial infarction and subsequently transferred to a general ward after 5 days in the coronary care unit, a total of 142 patients were discharged from the coronary care unit with a stable rhythm. Subsequent "late" cardiac arrest occurred in nine of these patients (6.3%) while still in the hospital. Ventricular fibrillation was present in eight of the nine. In contrast 16.6% had cardiac arrest caused by ventricular fibrillation or asystole while in the coronary care unit. Although it is generally recognized that the greatest incidence of ventricular arrhythmias occurs within the first 48 hours after an infarction, the patients still remain in some risk. Ventricular fibrillation within the first 4 weeks of a myocardial infarction is not uncommon and the work of Spracklen would lend encouragement to continuation of cardiac monitoring in infarction patients after discharge from the coronary care unit.

Chapter 5

THE CORONARY CARE UNIT

Jack M. Martt

Each year approximately two million Americans sustain acute myocardial infarctions, and more than 30% of them succumb during the acute phase. The coronary care unit (CCU) concept provides a potential for reducing this mortality rate by approximately 50%.

The objectives of a CCU are:

1. To prevent, detect, and treat cardiac arrhythmias
2. To observe patients in whom myocardial infarction is suspected
3. To provide cardiac defibrillation and cardiopulmonary resuscitation
4. To measure physiologic parameters relating to myocardial infarction (generally applied in a research setting)

More than a decade of experience with CCUs has indicated that a reduction in the mortality rate usually can be attributed to prevention of serious changes in cardiac rhythm. In contrast, intensive therapy in the CCU has not influenced the number of deaths caused by cardiogenic shock. Although most of the serious arrhythmias associated with myocardial infarction occur during the first day, an arbitrary minimal stay of 5 to 7 days in the CCU is recommended. However, it is now evident that a significant percentage of patients die during the succeeding days of hospitalization following transfer from the CCU. This realization is responsible for the intermediate coronary care unit (ICCU) concept that now seems essential to the overall care of patients with myocardial infarction. The ICCU provides monitoring of the cardiac rhythm during convalescence and ambulation, but it gives less emphasis to intensive nursing care.

Basic requirements for a CCU include:

1. Quiet, temperature-controlled, individual rooms
2. Electrocardiographic monitoring devices with automatic alarm systems
3. Resuscitative equipment
4. Trained personnel

Even small community hospitals, many of which may already have the necessary equipment and space, can establish a CCU. Location of the unit near the emergency or admitting department is desirable. The number of required beds can be established by determining the annual number of patients admitted with proved or suspected myocardial infarction and allotting 1 bed per 25 patients. Trained personnel is the chief deficiency in most hospitals.

A quiet environment is a major physical objective of a CCU, and this cannot be attained by draperies forming partitions between beds. The use of glass in wall and door panels will provide good visibility from the nurses' station without complete loss of privacy for the patient (Fig. 5-1). Closed circuit television with a camera for each room affords direct observation of each patient and may be preferable and more economical than reconstruction of existing facilities.

A large screen, multichannel oscilloscope that is mounted at the nurses' station and visible from all parts of the unit allows bold display of the electrocardiograms. Individual small oscilloscopes mounted in a "bank" will suffice for the smaller CCU. A small bedside

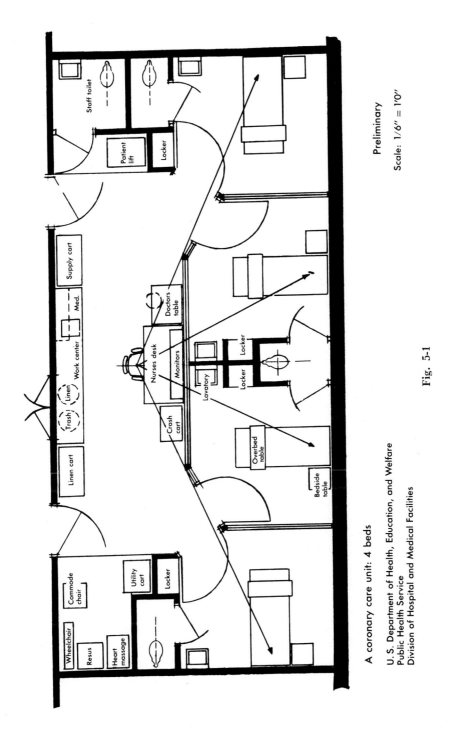

A coronary care unit: 4 beds

Preliminary

Scale: 1/6" = 1'0"

Fig. 5-1

U. S. Department of Health, Education, and Welfare
Public Health Service
Division of Hospital and Medical Facilities

oscilloscope, mounted above the patient's eye level, is desirable for monitoring during crises and while administering drugs during urgent situations. Each oscilloscope should provide an outlet for the recorder so that ECGs can be evaluated at the patient's bedside as well as at the central nursing station. An alarm that automatically triggers at extremes in heart rate or with ventricular fibrillation (audible and visible at the central desk) is a requirement for each bed. Another alarm system is desirable linking the nurses' station to the hospital switchboard to summon assistance during emergencies. A simple buzzer or a designated telephone number can be used to signal the operator that help is needed.

The prerequisites for cardiac monitoring therefore are:

1. An individual oscilloscope with ECG amplifier at each bedside
2. Central oscilloscope at the nurses' station
3. An ECG recorder linked to the oscilloscope
4. A rate meter with automatic alarm for each assigned bed

For dealing with cardiac emergencies, a nearby portable cart should contain:

1. Resuscitation board
2. Airway
3. Direct current defibrillator with synchronizer
4. Suction apparatus
5. Positive pressure ventilator
6. Venous cutdown set
7. Bipolar venous pacemaker catheters
8. Battery-powered cardiac pacemaker
9. Laryngoscope and endotracheal tube
10. Emergency drugs in ampules
    a. Epinephrine
    b. Sodium bicarbonate
    c. Calcium chloride
    d. Lidocaine
    e. Procainamide
11. Portable ECG recorder.

A fluoroscope, preferably a portable unit, facilitates insertion of a temporary transvenous cardiac pacemaker for treatment of patients with heart block or ventricular arrest. Smaller pacemaker electrodes may be "floated" from a peripheral arm vein or the subclavian vein. The catheter tip can be guided by recording an electrocardiogram from the proximal end of the catheter; a characteristic high voltage QRS complex indicates when the tip enters the right ventricle. Proper grounding of all electrical equipment in a CCU is important to minimize the risk of inducing ventricular fibrillation by inadvertent flow of current through the cardiac electrode employed for pacing.

A direct current defibrillator is essential for dealing with ventricular fibrillation and drug refractory ventricular tachycardia. Every hospital with a CCU must determine as a matter of policy whether or not the nursing staff is to be authorized to administer defibrillatory shock prior to a physician's attendance.

Personnel

The nursing staff plays a big role in the successful functioning of a CCU as a nurse usually will be the first to recognize a complication and to initiate therapy. A ratio of one nurse per two patients is satisfactory although one nurse may be adequte for three patients in a large unit.

Special instruction courses for the nursing staff should include (1) basic electrocardiography, especially the recognition of cardiac arrhythmias; (2) principles and methods of cardiac resuscitation, including use of a defibrillator; (3) manifestations and complications of myocardial infarction; and (4) operation of monitoring equipment and cardiac pacemakers. To be comprehensive, such instruction requires approximately 4 weeks. Training can be provided by local physicians or through special courses at medical centers. It is suggested that nurses who work in such units be recognized by higher salaries, time off for continuing education, and visits to CCUs at other institutions.

A staff cardiologist should assume overall direction of the CCU. He should be responsible for designating physician coverage at all times. In addition, he must determine the policies and procedures of the unit.

Chapter 6

ELECTIVE CONVERSION OF CARDIAC ARRHYTHMIAS WITH PRECORDIAL SHOCK

Richard H. Martin

History

Zoll and his co-workers first demonstrated in 1956 that external A.C. shock would terminate experimental atrial arrhythmias. The use of this method in patients was reported in 1961 by several groups of investigators. In 1962, Lown and his colleagues presented to the American Society for Clinical Investigation their results with conversion of arrhythmias using synchronized D.C. precordial shock. This technique, which is now commonly referred to as cardioversion, has gained widespread acceptance and is now considered the method of choice for emergency as well as for elective conversion of many arrhythmias.

General indications for cardioversion

The ideal method for abolishing arrhythmias should meet the following requirements:

1. The ectopic mechanism should be instantly abolished in all cases.
2. There should be depression of the normal cardiac pacemaker, no impairment of A-V or intraventricular conduction, and no depression of myocardial performance.
3. There should be no adverse effects on the heart or on other organ systems.
4. The method should be simple to apply, readily available to all patients, and inexpensive.

Cardioversion falls somewhat short of several of these objectives. However, there is little question that the method, when properly applied, is highly effective, safe, and relatively free of adverse side effects (see Table 6-1). It will convert approximately 90% of all arrhythmias caused by rapid, repetitively depolarizing foci or reentrant rhythms. These facts stand in rather striking contrast to the results of high dosage quinidine therapy for the conversion of atrial fibrillation, for example, where the success rate in unselected cases is approximately 60% to 70%, and where as many as 4% of patients treated require resuscitation because of toxic effects of the drug (Rokseth and Storstein, 1963).

At present, cardioversion is considered to be indicated for any susceptible arrhythmia that is judged to be undesirable in the context of a specific patient's total state of illness or health if the following requirements are met: (1) there is a reasonable chance that the rhythm can be prevented from recurring; (2) a trained staff and adequate equipment are available to perform cardioversion and to manage any potential complications; and (3) the rhythm fails to respond to safer, simpler, or less costly forms of therapy. The last requirement is commonly waived if the arrhythmia is deemed too threatening to permit time for other measures that have only limited chances for success.

Specific arrhythmias

ATRIAL FIBRILLATION

Atrial fibrillation has provided the largest experience with cardioversion in most clinics. The serious problems that may be encoun-

Table 6-1. Immediate results of attempted electrical conversion of atrial fibrillation*

Published series	Attempts	Successes	Complications		
			Ventricular arrhythmias	Systemic emboli	Other†
Lown and others, 1963	65	58	0	1	0
Killip, 1963	59	53	2	0	0
Hurst and others, 1964	158	151	0	2	0
Rabbino and others, 1964	65	59	3	1	1
Oram and Davies, 1964	129	108	0	1	1
Lemberg and others, 1964	101	92	0	0	0
McDonald and others, 1964	40	33	0	0	4
Morris and others, 1966	167	159	1	4	2
Total	784	713	6	9	8
		(91%)	(0.8%)	(1.1%)	(1.0%)

*Adapted from Morris, J. J., Peter, R. H., and McIntosh, H. D.: Electrical conversion of atrial fibrillation. Immediate and long-term results and selection of patients, Ann. Intern. Med. **65:**216-231, 1966.
†Includes pulmonary embolism (2), transient hypotension (4), ST-T changes (1), and pneumonitis (1).

tered with the use of quinidine for conversion have been alluded to previously. With most conventional quinidine conversion regimens, the patient and his ECG are observed only every 2 hours. Thus respiratory arrest, cardiac arrest, or quinidine-induced ventricular fibrillation may go undetected and may be fatal. Because of this risk of death from the therapy itself, it is no longer justifiable to treat this arrhythmia with doses of quinidine higher than those required for maintenance of sinus rhythm after conversion occurs (up to 0.4 gm. every 6 hours), unless the arrhythmia presents an immediate and distinct threat of mortality or serious morbidity and cardioversion is not available to the patient. This does not imply that all patients with atrial fibrillation should be cardioverted, but only that those patients who are deemed candidates for conversion should be cardioverted unless sinus rhythm appears during 1 or 2 days of relatively low-dose, "maintenance" quinidine therapy.

Although 90% of patients receiving shock energies up to 400 joules will convert, a disappointingly low percentage of patients remains in sinus rhythm for significant periods of time following cardioversion (see Table 6-2). In addition, recent evidence has challenged the concept that atrial fibrillation is always hemodynamically less effective than sinus rhythm, both in the experimental animal (Martin and others, 1967) and in patients with mitral stenosis (Carleton and Graettinger, 1967; Graettinger and others, 1964) and idiopathic atrial fibrillation (Killip and Baer, 1966). For these reasons, the initial enthusiasm for attempting cardioversion of virtually all fibrillating atria has cooled. Universally agreed upon criteria for selection of candidates for conversion have yet to emerge. However, several studies, particularly that of Morris and his colleagues (1966), have indicated that long-term maintenance of sinus rhythm is particularly unlikely in certain groups. These include patients with significant heart failure (New York Heart Association functional classes III and IV); with ischemic, hypertensive, or valvular heart disease other than pure mitral stenosis; and with atrial fibrillation present for over 1 year. When two or three of these risk factors were present, Morris found that a significantly reduced percentage of patients remained in sinus rhythm for 1 year after the initial cardioversion, even though multiple conversions were performed during this period.

Table 6-2. Long-term results of cardioversion for chronic atrial fibrillation

Published series	Number of patients converted	Persistent sinus rhythm (%)	Minimum follow-up (months)
Hurst and others, 1964	121	53	3
Futral and McGuire, 1967	42	45	3
Ebert and others, 1967	35	54	4
Kastor and DeSanctis, 1967	44	27	5
Jensen and others, 1965	42	40	6
Szekely and others, 1966	97	7	6
Bell and others, 1967	44	30	6
Korsgren and others, 1965	100	43	6
Halmos, 1966	137	42	9
Killip and others, 1965	115	23	12
Radford and Evans, 1968	119	15	24
Total	896	33	

I currently attempt cardioversion in all patients with atrial fibrillation who fail to convert after 2 days of quinidine therapy sufficient to maintain a serum concentration of 4 to 6 mg. per liter and are at significant risk from arterial emboli (particularly patients with mitral stenosis or with previous embolic episodes) or have limited cardiac reserve and may benefit from the booster-pump effect of atrial systole. I believe at least one conversion attempt is worthwhile in any patient meeting the above requirements, even though his prognosis for long-term maintenance may be poor, unless the patient is to undergo heart surgery in the near future or unless untreated hyperthyroidism or one or more contraindications listed below are present. I do not generally attempt cardioversion for 8 to 12 weeks after a cardiac operation, unless atrial fibrillation or flutter first occurred during the operation. I prefer to anticoagulate for at least 3 weeks after a recent arterial embolus before converting, in the hope that residual atrial thrombi will be organized by that time. However, I do not routinely anticoagulate all patients prior to conversion.

Absolute contraindications to attempting conversion are:

1. The presence of suspected digitalis intoxication

2. Complete A-V block (in which conversion of the atrial mechanism will do no good and anesthesia may produce asystole)
3. A past history of episodes of rapid atrial tachycardia that were symptomatic, impossible to prevent, and stabilized by the appearance fibrillation

The following are relative contraindications that must be considered in assessing the chances that conversion will be of significant benefit or may do harm:

1. Intolerance to quinidine (propranolol or procainamide may be substituted, but data on the prophylactic effect of these agents are meager)
2. Previous early recurrence of fibrillation after cardioversion
3. Failure to note significant symptomatic improvement during previous episodes of sinus rhythm
4. The presence of a slow ventricular response to fibrillation in the absence of digitalis therapy (this generally is associated with ischemic heart disease; such patients may manifest asystole or slow nodal or atrial rhythms following conversion)

Investigators in the United States generally agree that prophylactic therapy with quinidine is worthwhile after reestablishment of sinus rhythm. Several British investigators, however, believe the drug to be too dangerous for use in this situation (Oram and Davies, 1964; Radford and Evans, 1968). One recent

British study indicates that 1 gm. of quinidine per day, a dose that produced a mean serum concentration of 2.2 mg. per liter, does not alter the risk of reversion from that present without prophylactic drug therapy (Hall and Wood, 1968). However, we have found a statistically significant improvement in prognosis for long-term sinus rhythm in patients who maintain serum quinidine concentrations above 4 mg. per liter when compared with those receiving comparable doses of the drug whose serum levels are below 4 mg. per liter (Martin and others, 1968). Quinidine sulfate should be given every 6 hours to minimize fluctuations in concentration of the drug. If 12 hours elapse between doses, the blood level will fall to less than half of the peak concentration. Since atrial fibrillation is likely to persist once it recurs, even though the quinidine concentration later returns to the prophylactic range (4 to 6 mg. per liter), it appears important to avoid even transient inadequate blood levels. I currently administer quinidine for at least 1 year after cardioversion unless intolerance develops or fibrillation recurs and further attempts to convert are not deemed advisable.

ATRIAL FLUTTER

In most respects the treatment of atrial flutter can be considered to be identical with that of atrial fibrillation. There is one important exception to this rule. Whereas the patient with a fast ventricular response to atrial fibrillation will usually improve during digitalis therapy, which increases A-V block and slows the ventricular rate, the usual doses of digitalis may have no effect on the ventricular response to atrial flutter. Indeed, attempts to "push" digitalis to slow the ventricular rate may lead to digitalis intoxication, a situation that makes subsequent cardioversion hazardous. When slowing of heart rate is urgent in a patient with atrial flutter (for example, a patient with myocardial infarction complicated by acute atrial flutter with 2:1 A-V conduction), cardioversion, without any preliminary drug therapy, is the most appropriate form of treatment.

SUPRAVENTRICULAR TACHYCARDIA

Supraventricular tachycardias generally respond readily to simpler measures such as carotid sinus massage, other vagal maneuvers, sedation, and digitalis therapy, singly or in combination. These measures should be tried before attempting cardioversion, although in life-threatening situations, such as the presence of associated severe valvular heart disease with pulmonary edema, the speed and high probability of success of cardioversion warrant its use before beginning a potentially time-consuming titration of various drugs. Cardioversion may induce more serious arrhythmias in the presence of digitalis intoxication; thus digitoxicity must be excluded as the cause of any arrhythmia before cardioversion is attempted. A specific indication for cardioversion without first attempting digitalization is the presence of serious decompensation or anginal pain during tachyarrhythmias associated with the Wolff-Parkinson-White syndrome. This is particularly true in the case of atrial fibrillation associated with the Wolff-Parkinson-White syndrome. Here, digitalis fails to yield the expected slowing of the ventricular response because impulses from the atria bypass the A-V node where the drug exerts its depressant effect on conduction. During digitalis therapy, the ventricular rate, which is often alarmingly rapid in this condition, may increase to levels in excess of 350 with resultant hypotension and a near-fatal outcome.

VENTRICULAR TACHYCARDIA

Ventricular tachycardia is generally associated with more severe depression of cardiac function than those arrhythmias discussed previously. For this reason, therapy with myocardial depressants such as procainamide and quinidine is less desirable than cardioversion if the latter therapy is readily available. Lidocaine and diphenylhydantoin have less profound effects on contractility but may cause CNS irritability, heart block, and other complications if administered improperly. Cardioversion will revert at least 90% of episodes of ventricular tachycardia and should be used early if intravenous lidocaine is not effective. This is particularly true when ventricular tachycardia follows successful resuscitation. In this circumstance, however, drug therapy is generally necessary to prevent further recurrences; for this a slow intravenous drip of lidocaine is the treatment of choice.

It should be emphasized that the lack of a synchronizing unit on a defibrillator should not deter one from the use of precordial shock in life-threatening ventricular tachycardia. Even in the absence of synchronization, induction of ventricular fibrillation is an unusual event; should it appear, a defibrillating shock can be administered before any serious effect has occurred.

Contraindications to cardioversion

The only general contraindication to the use of cardioversion for any of the previously discussed arrhythmias is the presence of digitalis intoxication. Serious arrhythmias, including ventricular fibrillation, may follow cardioversion in this setting, sometimes several hours later. This risk may be reduced by administration of lidocaine or potassium salts (in the absence of high degrees of A-V block), but cardioversion should be attempted only as a last resort when rapid transvenous atrial pacing, potassium, or propranolol has failed to convert or control the rhythm and the situation is desperate. Such patients should be closely monitored until digitalis intoxication is clearly alleviated.

Multiple premature atrial or ventricular contractions will not respond to cardioversion. These arrhythmias should be treated, if necessary, with suppressing drugs.

Technique of cardioversion

The procedure of cardioversion is essentially the same, regardless of the type of rhythm. Minor variations are made depending upon the specific situation; for example, anesthesia or analgesia may be omitted if death is imminent or if the sensorium is profoundly depressed, such as after a previous resuscitative effort or major operation. Since atrial fibrillation is the most commonly

treated arrhythmia, the steps described apply to it.

PATIENT PREPARATION

The patient should be in the postabsorptive state. Premedication may be given with pentobarbital, either alone or in combination with narcotic agents; however, care should be taken to avoid respiratory depression that may produce myocardial hypoxia and may increase the possibility of postcardioversion arrhythmias. Digitalis glycosides are omitted for at least 24 hours prior to the procedure. This measure has been found to essentially eliminate postcardioversion arrhythmias resembling digitalis intoxication, which are seen not infrequently in fully digitalized but nontoxic patients. Quinidine is administered for 2 days before cardioversion to ascertain whether it can be tolerated, to obtain blood and tissue levels adequate to help prevent a recurrence of atrial fibrillation, and to convert the 5% to 10% of patients who will respond to the drug alone. In addition, this permits time for determination of the serum quindine concentration attained by the dose chosen and adjustment of the dose if levels above 6 or below 4 mg. per liter are present.

Electrodes are applied to the extremities for recording the ECG before and after conversion, for synchronization, and for postconversion monitoring. Unless a high resistance is present in the leads, they should be placed distally on the arms and legs, because a significant amount of current may pass from the "hot" defibrillator paddle to one of these small electrodes and produce a serious burn. Monitoring of the ECG, preferably on both an oscilloscope and a strip-chart recorder, is essential (even if synchronization is not possible with the equipment available) in order to determine the rhythm following the shock and to assess the need for further therapy.

SYNCHRONIZATION

The cardioverter triggering circuit is set to respond to a component of the QRS complex, and it is adjusted so that it will dis-

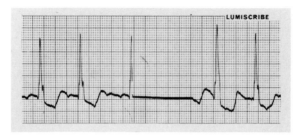

Fig. 6-1. ECG demonstrating test synchronization of cardioverter discharge. Test shock, which was not transmitted to patient, fell on downslope of third R wave. The instrument employed automatically shorts out ECG for 1.06 seconds after the shock to protect the circuitry of ECG recorder.

charge within a safe portion of the cardiac cycle. It has been shown that shocks delivered during the vulnerable period (near the apex of the T wave of the ECG) may induce ventricular fibrillation. Avoiding this area does not completely eliminate the risk of this complication, but it is generally believed to reduce it significantly. Most instruments of recent design no longer allow adjustment of the delay between QRS detection and capacitor discharge, which is set to be only a few milliseconds. Care must be taken to avoid the possibility that the instrument may accidentally trigger on a T wave. This is best done by choosing an ECG lead that shows a low-voltage T wave and, if possible, one with the major QRS deflection opposite in polarity to the T wave. The proper trigger polarity should then be chosen and the trigger sensitivity slowly increased from zero until triggering just occurs consistently on the QRS complex. The timing of the shock is then tested by recording a low-voltage test shock with the defibrillator paddles shorted internally in the instrument or by touching them together. This will produce a discharge artifact on the ECG, as shown in Fig. 6-1.

ANESTHESIA, ANALGESIA, AND MUSCLE RELAXANTS

Although it is possible to deliver a low-energy D.C. shock (100 joules or less) without severe discomfort to some patients, I have not found this to be a generally worth-while endeavor. For elective procedures I routinely use intravenous thiopental (administered by an anesthesiologist) sufficient to induce hypnosis and amnesia in all conscious patients. By paying adequate attention to patency of the airway and by administering supplemental ventilation and oxygen when respiration appears depressed, I have encountered no significant problems with this agent. Intravenous diazepam, with or without a narcotic drug, will also provide amnesia in the majority of patients. However, some patients will remember the shock after this premedication. If high energies are used, this memory may be sufficiently unpleasant to seriously impair future efforts to treat recurrent arrhythmias, particularly if cardioversion is again required. Muscle relaxants are not routinely necessary, although their use is advisable in elderly patients with osteoporosis of the spine; compression fractures have resulted from the skeletal muscle contraction that accompanies precordial shock in such patients.

APPLICATION OF SHOCK

Conventional defibrillator paddles may be applied the same as for external ventricular defibrillation. It has been shown that less energy is required for conversion of atrial fibrillation when paddles are placed in the anteroposterior plane, with one centered over the sternum at the level of the third intercostal space and a special paddle positioned

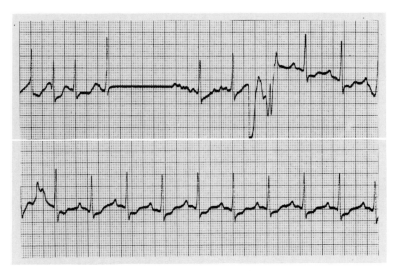

Fig. 6-2. Continuous ECG demonstrating conversion of atrial fibrillation by 100-joule shock delivered during fourth R wave (upper panel). Baseline artifact was caused by skeletal muscle contraction resulting from shock.

under the patient's left scapula. The initial shock energy chosen is dependent upon the patient's body size and other variables, such as previous history of energy requirement for conversion. Generally, I begin with 100 joules unless the patient's chest is very thin. The ECG is recorded during administration of the shock, as shown in Fig. 6-2. If the arrhythmia persists, the energy is increased in 100 joule increments until conversion occurs or 400 joules is given without effect.

POSTCARDIOVERSION CARE

The patient generally awakens within 1 to 5 minutes, having no recollection of the shock(s). A brief examination is performed to search for cerebral or arterial embolization. The patient is monitored for a variable period, depending upon the circumstances of the case; 1 hour generally suffices for routine conversion of atrial fibrillation unless a possibility of digitalis-induced arrhythmias is present. Ventricular ectopic beats may be seen for a variable period after cardioversion. These are usually easily suppressed with intravenous lidocaine and subside within several minutes.

Hazards of cardioversion

ELECTRICAL SHOCK AND BURNS

The high electrical energy delivered by this method carries with it the usual hazards to the patient and the operators of the equipment; these hazards, and the precautions to be taken, are described elsewhere in this book.

MYOCARDIAL DAMAGE

There are few experimental data bearing upon the question of myocardial damage from precordial shock as administered for cardioversion in human subjects. Serum creatine phosphokinase rises after cardioversion but appears to come from skeletal muscles in the shock pathway. S-T segment elevation suggestive of acute epicardial injury has been described on occasion. No serious residual myocardial damage has been reported. It is the general practice to limit the maximum energy delivered during elective procedures to 400 joules and the total number of shocks delivered to four at any one conversion attempt. However, more than 200 shocks have been administered to one patient over a 2-year period with no apparent adverse effects (Giannelli et al., 1967).

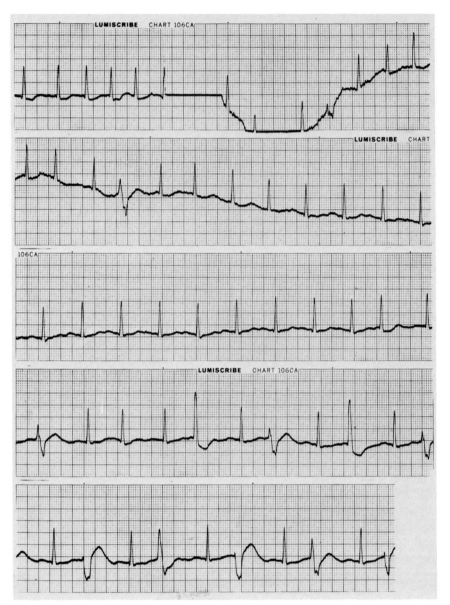

Fig. 6-3. Continuous lead II ECG illustrating postcardioversion arrhythmias. A 100-joule shock was administered during sixth R wave (top panel). Baseline artifact obscured the record for several beats, which were irregular in rhythm and presumably represent wandering atrial mechanism. Poorly developed P waves are present (second panel) with P-R interval of 0.24 second. Occasional atrial and ventricular premature beats then appeared, followed by multi-focal ventricular premature beats occurring in bigemini. Patient had undergone mitral valve replacement 8 weeks before cardioversion. Digoxin had been withheld for 48 hours, and serum quinidine was 4.8 mg. per liter at time of conversion. Premature beats subsided 5 minutes after cardioversion, but atrial fibrillation recurred 12 hours later.

INDUCTION OF ARRHYTHMIAS

Potential causes for arrhythmias are:

1. Delivery of discharge during the vulnerable period (generally results in ventricular tachycardia or fibrillation)
   a. Improper adjustment of delay between trigger and discharge
   b. Improper triggering on T wave of ECG
2. Liberation of catecholamines and acetylcholine from cardiac autonomic nerve endings in the heart, and stimulation of sympathetic ganglia by the cardioversion shock
3. Myocardial hypoxia caused by inadequate ventilation or arterial oxygenation (may cause premature beats, ventricular tachycardia, or ventricular fibrillation)
4. Digitalis intoxication (may cause any type of abnormal rhythm)
   a. Already clinically or electrocardiographically demonstrable before cardioversion
   b. Unmasked by shock, perhaps mediated by liberation of intracellular potassium
5. Possible arrhythmic effect of drugs, such as thiopental, used during procedure (may cause premature ventricular beats)

The precautions to be taken in avoiding these arrhythmias have been discussed previously. It must be stressed that, in spite of these precautions, a variety of arrhythmias, including ventricular fibrillation, may still occur immediately after the shock (see Fig. 6-3) or after a delay of as much as several hours. Immediate ventricular fibrillation presents only a minor problem, since the team performing the cardioversion is optimally prepared to deal with this complication. The rhythm is recognizable at once and may generally be terminated by a second shock delivered within a matter of several seconds without any intervening cardiac massage. The synchronizing circuit of the cardioverter must be inactivated in order to defibrillate, since no QRS complexes are present to trigger the shock during ventricular fibrillation. The extremely small, but nonetheless real, risk of delayed ventricular arrhythmias warrants close supervision and ECG monitoring of the patient during the postcardioversion period.

EMBOLI

Systemic arterial embolization occurs with an incidence of about 1% to 3% at the time of conversion of atrial fibrillation, regardless of whether this event is spontaneous, drug-induced, or the result of cardioversion. Will routine anticoagulation of all patients before conversion reduce this risk? The best data relative to this question are those of Bjerkelund and Orning (1969). These authors concluded that oral anticoagulation does provide some prophylaxis against systemic embolization. However, a well-controlled trial of anticoagulation for this purpose has not been performed. It seems reasonable to assume that the risk of spontaneous embolization from a fibrillating atrium in a patient who may potentially embolize at the time of cardioversion is at least as great as it would be during and immediately after conversion. There is moderately conclusive evidence that conversion and maintenance of sinus rhythm does reduce the risk of future emboli. Thus embolization, in itself, cannot legitimately be considered as a specific risk of cardioversion.

PULMONARY EDEMA

Acute pulmonary edema is a relatively rare complication of cardioversion of both ventricular tachycardia and atrial fibrillation. The mechanism of this complication has not been clearly defined. In patients with mitral stenosis, it may result from a sudden increase in right ventricular output (Resnekov and McDonald, 1965) or from retrograde pumping of blood into the pulmonary veins by left atrial contractions that are relatively ineffective in forcing blood across the fixed valvular obstruction (Carleton and Graettinger, 1967). Myocardial injury has been postulated as a cause in some cases. Therapy consists of the usual measures for pulmonary edema.

Chapter 7

DETECTION AND CORRECTION OF ELECTRICAL HAZARDS WITHIN THE HOSPITAL

David G. Kilpatrick

The impact of electromedical devices on patient care has indeed been significant. Utilization of life- and labor-saving instrumentation and appliances has accelerated, particularly during the short interval since the last edition of this book. Some insight into the present clinical significance of such devices may be gained by surveying the other chapters of this edition. The increasing utilization of electrically powered equipment has increased awareness and concern among both engineering and medical professionals.

Electrical safety was identified as a severe and growing (if not generally recognized) problem in the late 1960s. The rapidly increasing quantity and complexity of electrically powered instruments and appliances used within a patient's environment have created new hazards. Probability theory indicates that hazard will increase at a rate greater than the rate of increase of the quantity of devices as they are used in combination. Among these hazards is "microshock," a subtle and often misunderstood cause of death, which results in little or no pathology. Consequently, invalid statistics and controversy have added much confusion relating to hazard.

In medical facilities we must be prepared to cope with a vast variety of hazards. For there we encounter the usual hazards of general industry and the explosion and fire hazards of the petrochemical industry, as well as those associated with the private residence. But even more important are those hazards, primarily electrical, completely unique to the delivery of health care. There are even specific hazards caused by modern medical procedures such as cardiac catheterization.

In engineering practice, the need for cost-effective protective methodology becomes evident early. The basic problem is that of achieving a reasonable level of electrical safety for patients and personnel, within the constraints of our resources. Therefore, I will emphasize my experience and techniques, as I develop practical guidelines.

The role of clinical biomedical engineering

Biomedical engineering began as an adjunct to medical research. In the early 1960s, it became obvious that the professional engineering needs of clinical medicine were acute. As a direct result, efforts have been directed primarily to those technologic needs that are unique to the delivery of health care.

SYSTEMS ENGINEERING

A primary characteristic of effective engineering of any form is the ability to apply economics and the sciences in a practical plan of action and to carry out that plan. Integration of subsystems, such as power, communications, monitoring, and lighting, is essential to achieving a reasonable level of safety. An obvious side benefit has been a more efficient facility.

I have characterized biomedical engineering as simply a multidiscipline form of classic systems engineering. An important goal is fuller use of this vital, new branch of engineering that applies both life sciences and physical sciences. My emphasis is on the generalist in engineering rather than on the superspecialist. Near mastery, necessary for useful, coordinated application, of the many contributing disciplines is needed.

The basic task has been to integrate the physical and procedural environment. In addressing the complex problems of operation and design of medical facilities, we have found that cost-effectiveness can be achieved by considering the three major interacting elements of the health care delivery system: personnel, environment (plant and equipment), and organization and controls.

Perhaps the most important element is personnel, and the most effective means of reducing hazard is the education of these people. It is necessary to carefully consider their "initial ability" and the "needed ability" in order to devise appropriate training programs. Although the search continues, no hardware method of protection completely eliminates the consequences of human error in utilization or maintenance of electromedical devices. Therefore, some level of tutorial effort is always indicated.

Hardware, the plant, and the medical appliances and instruments make up the gross electrical environment. Codes and standards are primarily addressed to reducing hazards through controlling hardware and construction. However, with few exceptions it is impractical to provide protection from all the consequences of human failure solely by means of hardware. We may, however, look on hardware providing complete protection as a worthy goal. In areas with many transient personnel, as in teaching hospitals, this becomes an extremely worthwhile goal. Hardware costs are an important factor in

our decisions regarding protection. In old facilities there are many unknowns, greatly complicating design of correction, rehabilitation, and renovation.

The third and last element of the system, the organization and control of people and equipment, is often neglected. An important part of the joint responsibilities of the medical staff and the administration is the regulation of the facility, including personnel as well as hardware. The control of electricity is very much like the control of sepsis or of dangerous drugs. The trend is toward more formal organization of these functions under the aegis of a responsible engineering professional.

THE ENGINEER AND THE PHYSICIAN

The medical profession should be concerned in initiating programs in facilities but electrical safety is a complex technical problem requiring responsible engineering guidance. The practice of engineering, like the practice of medicine, is not a matter for the unqualified, particularly where matters of public safety are involved. There are stringent legal regulations to protect the public, requiring that only registered engineers perform "any professional service wherein the safeguarding of life, health, or property is concerned or involved when such professional service requires the application of engineering principles and data." These generally unrecognized legal requirements should be kept in mind.

The much-publicized "communications gap" of the last twenty years is not entirely one of differing scientific vocabularies but also the lack of emphasis of the similarities between the two professions of engineering and medicine. Obvious similarities include: (1) rigorous scientific training, (2) internship (the engineer in training), (3) experience plus board examination leading to the M.D. and the P.E., (4) rigorous ethical codes, and (5) specialization. Electrical safety and other problems of mutual concern can be effectively addressed in consort by utilizing the aggregate knowledge of the two professions.

CARDIAC ARREST AND RESUSCITATION

In a way, this chapter runs counter to the rest of the book. Its major purpose is to prevent some of the need for the techniques of cardiac resuscitation. However, this preventive methodology tends to be interactive and complex. An assumption of responsible knowledgeability on the reader's part is necessary in applying this methodology, and the glossary at the end of this chapter is intended to assist in understanding. If there is the slightest doubt regarding the reader's personal understanding, it is strongly recommended that a qualified consultant be retained. His necessary functions are to determine the situation by analysis and measurement and to determine a coordinated course of corrective action. Such a consultant should have extensive experience in both the unique equipment and the special power systems utilized in hospitals.

Hazards

Two major hazards involve electricity: (1) ignition or detonation of flammables and (2) the effects of electrical currents passing through the body. Static electricity or power-distribution current can cause either ignition or electrical shock.

IGNITION OR DETONATION

A few decades ago, the danger to life from explosions and fires of flammable anesthetics, in the very places where we were trying to save lives was acute. However, the regulation of flammable anesthetics as a precautionary measure has now become standard practice. Today, accidents do not occur often, but they do occur and are often caused by improper use of spark- or heat-producing devices such as cautery instruments rather than accidental sparking.

Electrical sparks. The most common cause of ignition is a high-energy electrical spark although any flame or hot object can cause ignition. There are two sources of electrical sparks: *static electricity* and *faults* in a piece of electrical equipment or in the power system itself. Initially, the phenomenon of static electricity sparking was considered virtually unpredictable. We have now found many practical, simple measures we can take to prevent the generation of static electricity or permit its harmless dissipation in the event generation cannot be avoided. These protective measures are apparent in the regulations for the safe use of flammable anesthetics and the handling of petrochemicals, hydrogen, and other flammables.

The control of sparking electrical equipment has been more difficult to achieve as more and more electrically powered equipment has been brought into operating and induction rooms. Isolated power systems have been designed and installed for the purpose of limiting the energy when a first fault occurs. If this energy is effectively limited to a low enough level, any sparking that occurs will not ignite the flammables.

Combinatory hazard. Electrical shock hazards also exist in anesthetizing locations. These hazards must be evaluated in combination with the ignition-preventing measures that we have adopted. Patients with artificial conductive invasion in or near the heart are likely to be present. Consequently, the hazard of "microshock," or ventricular fibrillation caused by very small electrical currents, is often acute. The protective systems required for the use of flammable anesthetics both increase and reduce shock hazard. The isolated power system can prevent macroshock, or large-current shock, up to the time of the first fault. However, the system hazard current of such power systems can be a thousand times the electrical current threshold of ventricular fibrillation of those patients who are particularly susceptible to electrical current. The "conducting" floor is designed to provide a resistive path to ground for dissipation of static electricity. This electrical resistance can create a hazard. Consider a faulty piece of portable equipment without a grounding connection but connected to the power system. This equipment can then inject a fault current into the partially conducting floor, creating potential differences between other pieces of equipment in the room that may not be electrically powered. The faulty piece of equipment need not be in use or turned on to cause a potential difference.

EFFECTS OF ELECTRICAL CURRENT

In simplified electrical terms, the human body consists of a core of low resistance encased by the skin, a relatively high-resistance outer boundary. The core of relatively conductive blood and tissues permits the free passage of electrical current. The skin is somewhat insulating, particularly when dry, providing some protection. Three factors determine the effects of an electric current: (1) the path of the current through the body, (2) the amount and nature of the electrical current, and (3) the length of time that the current flows through the body. The serious effects, in order of increasing current, may be summarized as follows:

1. Circulatory failure from ventricular fibrillation or other serious cardiac arrhythmias. This can be caused by a relatively small quantity of current passing through the heart. (No pathologic evidence is present.)
2. Paralysis of the respiratory muscles. The lungs fail to function normally because of the continuous contraction of the muscles of the chest. (This, alone, may be the cause of death or it may be associated with other effects.)
3. Respiratory failure caused by neural inhibition or damage to the central nervous system. This usually results from passage of large amounts of current. (Pathologic evidence may be present.)
4. Skin and flesh burns resulting from localized high current at the point of contact. (Pathologic evidence is present.)
5. Hemorrhage from increasing the temperature of the blood and increasing pressure on the walls of the vessels causing them to rupture. (Pathologic evidence may be present.)

Except in the case of ventricular fibrillation, the effects are likely to be combined and the result of very large electric currents.

Although neural stimulation is often a factor in industrial accidents, in a medical situation death is more likely to be caused by electrical induction of serious cardiac arrhythmias. It is obvious that if we protect patients and personnel from ventricular fibrillation, the effect requiring lowest electrical energy, we will also protect them from the high current effects. Since ignition of flammables also requires higher energy, this hazard is also minimized.

VENTRICULAR FIBRILLATION THRESHOLD

A variable. In order to design protective measures, we must know the smallest electrical current that can possibly induce ventricular fibrillation. In the human, ventricular fibrillation threshold (VFT) is not a single value of current. It is quite variable, depending on many factors. We must base our standards, such as maximum-equipment-leakage current, on situations and factors that are likely to be present in a clinical situation. The factors known to affect VFT are summarized in Table 7-1. Note that the data include large ranges of current. We are without completely valid data on the VFT of the human heart. We must depend on extrapolation of animal data and poorly reported human incidents. For the most part, reports of human accidents cover only those where resuscitation efforts have been successful. Without a valid data base we have had to determine minimum lethal current in the same manner that we adduce "minimum lethal doses" for drugs: primarily from animal studies.

Body weight. Studies of VFT of animals of differing body weights have shown conclusively that lower body weight implies lower threshold. It has not been generally recognized that children are probably much more susceptible than adults. However, both the Underwriters Laboratory and the Canadian Standards Association have taken this into account in their choice of 5 milliamperes as the maximum leakage current of household appliances. Based on intact dry skin as

Table 7-1. Clinical factors affecting ventricular fibrillation threshold (lowering VFT increases susceptibility)

Factor	Variable	Examples	Reference
Body weight	VFT proportional to weight (transthoracic)	30 kg. child—VFT about 30 ma. 90 kg. adult—VFT about 95 ma.	Whitaker, 1939
Current path and impedance of circuit	Insulated natural and artificial conductors direct or concentrate the electrical current (the electrically sensitive patient)	Aorticorenal path—VFT about 5 ma. Cardiac catheter—VFT about 0.02 ma. (Low-impedance catheter 0.01 v., difference for 0.02 ma., fluid-filled catheter greater than 0.5 v. difference for 0.02 ma.)	Kilpatrick, 1970
Period of cardiac cycle	Coincidence of current with vulnerable phase of systole	The longer the duration of electrical shock, the greater the likelihood of fibrillation	Stephenson, 1958
Quality of electrical current	Frequency	Direct current—VFT about 28 ma. 60 Hz. power—VFT about 20 ma. 500 Hz. power—VFT about 40 ma.	Dalziel, 1968
Other clinical factors reducing VFT	Patient's condition	Acidosis, anoxia, coronary occlusion, hypothermia, cardiac catheterization	Chapter 18
	Medical procedures	Circumvention of skin barrier, competitive artificial pacing	
	Drugs	Some anesthetics and diuretics in combination with cardiac drugs	

a protective mechanism, we would expect the maximum allowable safe voltage to be between 10 and 25 volts.

Current path. A second major factor relates to the current path. Not only is the route that the current takes important but also important is the impedance or resistance of that path. In an effort to explain fibrillation caused by dropping a low-voltage nurse-call switch in the lap and urinating on the switch, we have considered the "aorticorenal path." A similar current path is probably involved in incidents related to some electrically powered devices like proctosigmoidoscopes. Blood and urine are highly conductive electrolytes and the descending aorta, like all great vessels, has walls that act as relative insulators. When a hazardous current is directed or concentrated by an insulated conductor with a small-area

contact of the myocardium, VFT is much lower. In cardiac catheterization the conducting fluid in the catheter lumen, or a wire in the case of an electrode catheter, forms the conductor. With such concentration or localization of the electrical current stimulating the myocardium, we expect a VFT between 10 and 30 microamperes. The electrical impedance of the total circuit, including the current path through the heart, determines the role of the electrical quantity —voltage.

The current that can actually flow through a hazardous path through the heart is determined by the basic relationships between impedance or resistance, voltage difference, and current flow. Current may be calculated by simply dividing voltage by circuit or path resistance. Hence, the larger the resistance, the smaller the current that can flow for a given source of voltage. In cardiac catheterization, this becomes important. The very low impedance of an electrode catheter intended for pacing the heart becomes the most dangerous to the patient. If we are to limit the possible current through the heart to 10 microamperes, we must limit potential differences within the patient's environment to 5 millivolts under probable fault conditions. However, with a fluid-filled catheter of relatively high impedance, potential or voltage differences within the environment of one-half volt or more can be tolerated.

Ventricular fibrillation threshold also varies with the frequency of the hazardous current. The examples of Table 7-1 make it obvious that a particularly hazardous frequency was chosen for the power distribution systems.

Other factors. We should recognize that a patient is often further compromised. Clues abound in the medical literature and in examples of wet environments in industrial safety regulations. These data are largely nonquantitative. However, we can be aware of these factors and continually question whether the patient's condition, the therapeutic and diagnostic procedures, and drugs involved in his treatment are possibly lowering the threshold of ventricular fibrillation and making individual patients more susceptible to small electrical currents.

Electrical defibrillation has become the most effective means of reversing ventricular fibrillation. A paradox is involved since this procedure incurs a large electrical shock directed through the heart. Uncorrelated data, largely animal, suggests that under similar situations of heart condition, electrical current path, and waveform characteristics, the threshold of defibrillation is 500 to 1,000 times the threshold of ventricular fibrillation. The same common clinical factors that decrease VFT or increase susceptibility seem also to decrease the threshold of defibrillation, requiring less energy to achieve depolarization of the myocardium, or defibrillation.

HUMAN SUSCEPTIBILITY

The information that we have regarding human susceptibility to very small electrical currents is largely tenuous, primarily because there is no pathologic evidence and engineering studies of the electrical environment at the time of an incident are rare. However, animal data are valid, and research in electrophysiology has provided much factual information. Those of us who have accepted a degree of responsibility for defining safe current levels have been well aware of the lack of hard data regarding various clinical situations. As a consequence, such standards are vulnerable to criticism chiefly related to the definition of "minimal lethal current" for the "electrically sensitive patient" or patient with cardiac catheterization. Since canine experiments with typical catheters have been repeatable with VFT currents as low as 20 microamperes, we must accept 10 microamperes as the "minimum lethal current" for humans. (We are also influenced by the two-to-one lower pacemaker current threshold that was observed in humans in the late 1950s.) VFT for transthoracic current paths, such as limb-to-limb, can be better defined. For many years 5 milliamperes, or 5000 microamperes, has been accepted as the "minimum lethal current" for this situation.

In summary, the three components of the hospital population—the nonpatient, the general patient, and the "electrically sensitive patient"—differ in their susceptibility to electric current. I have found the presentation of Fig. 7-1 a useful summary based on our aggregate knowledge. The three components of the hospital population are related to possible ventricular fibrillation thresholds. The general patient level of susceptibility is extrapolated from "wet-bed" incidents involving low-voltage devices. The current path is believed to have been through urine, the renal system, the descending aorta, and into the heart. Skin electrodes are believed to cause a similar threshold. The "electrically sensitive patient" is the patient with conduc-

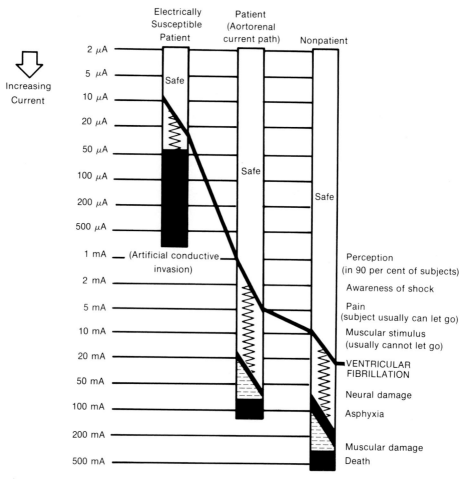

Fig. 7-1. Susceptibility of the electrically susceptible patient, the general patient, and the nonpatient to electric current. (From Kilpatrick, D. G.: Med. Clin. North Am. 55:1095, 1971.)

tive invasion in or near the heart. (Until recently this patient was referred to as "electrically susceptible.") Information regarding the effects of electrical current on the nonpatient is, of course, the most complete.

THE HAZARDOUS CIRCUIT

There is always a finite hazard associated with electrically powered equipment. The hazard can range from virtually nonexistent, as in low-voltage battery-operated devices, to extremely dangerous, as in poorly designed equipment powered from a poorly maintained power distribution system within the building. We can quantify the shock hazard

by measuring the amount of current that can possibly pass through the victim's body from a specific electrical device. This can be measured in nanoamperes when the power source is low energy and an integral part of the equipment, and in amperes in the worst case—when faulty line-powered equipment is involved, a range of a billion to one is possible.

In recent years, equipment used in the hospital, particularly electronic instrumentation, has increased very rapidly in quantity and variety as well as in complexity and sophistication. For the most part, the equipment has become essential. More

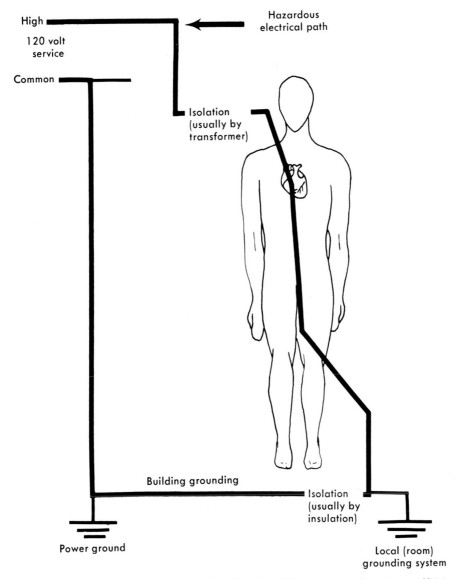

Fig. 7-2. The hazardous electrical path. (Copyright Kilpatrick Associates, Inc., 1971.)

and more electrically powered instruments and appliances are being connected to a patient or used in the immediate environment.

The source of power. Most instruments and appliances must, as a practical matter, be powered from the general distribution system of the hospital structure. The power distribution system is referenced to the building ground. This means that of the two wires completing the work or load circuit, one, the return or common connection, is connected to ground at the building electrical service entrance. Consequently, the other wire, known as the "high" side of the line, is at 120 volts with respect to all grounded objects. Electrical safety is largely concerned with preventing completion of the circuit between the "high" side of the line and a grounded object by way of an electrical path including a human body. As explained earlier, an electrical path including the heart is particularly hazardous.

A current path. It is useful in analyzing shock hazards to consider a single hazardous electrical path, as in Fig. 7-2. The patient is usually grounded by the many conducting surfaces of his immediate environment (Fig. 7-4) or by sensitive instrumentation that requires a reference ground in order to function. In the case of the ordinary wall recepta-

cle, 120 volts is available with respect to ground.

The line-frequency impedance between the "high" side of the line and some point on the victim's body and ground determines the quantity of current that will flow. If either impedance is infinitely large, no current can flow. If both impedances are zero ohms, amperes of current will flow. Accepting that the patient is grounded, we usually increase

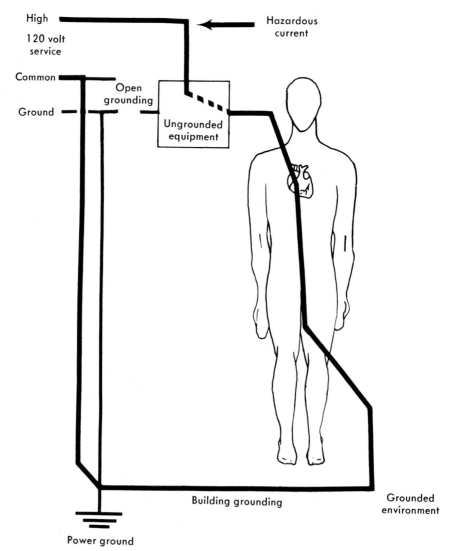

Fig. 7-3. Hazardous current from equipment. (Copyright Kilpatrick Associates, Inc., 1971.)

the first impedance or "isolation" between the high side of the line and the equipment contacting the patient. For example, if we increase this impedance to 120 million ohms, the maximum current that can flow from a 120 volt source, returning to ground, is 1 microampere. This is one tenth of the lowest current known to have caused a human heart to fibrillate. Thus, we can begin to quantify isolation and insulation.

In the clinical situation, there are as many hazardous current paths as there are line-powered devices within the patient's environment plus many other intentional and unintentional connections, usually to ground. These hazardous current paths add up quickly. I identified 51 possibly hazardous paths for one CCU patient. This particular situation is not as atypical as might be expected.

Equipment leakage and fault currents. Under some conditions leakage current contributed by individual pieces of equipment to the hazardous electrical path can be additive. (An additional risk of many pieces of equipment connected to one patient is the increasing probability of a faulty or ungrounded device.) Therefore, the single piece of equipment shown in Fig. 7-3 should be viewed as several connected to, or contacting, the patient. Hazardous current may be the leakage current of one device or several combined, the total systems hazard current of an isolated power system, a very large fault current caused by a short circuit within a defective piece of equipment, or any possible combination of the above. If grounding connections are intact and of low enough impedance, these hazardous currents are conducted harmlessly to ground, hence, the importance of grounding.

Present clinical environment

Much progress is being made in meeting safety requirements particularly in new or renovated facilities. Unfortunately, the majority of our medical facilities are old and many do not meet minimal electrical code requirements for even ordinary residential wiring. Our most pressing problem, then, is rehabilitating these older facilities to meet the safety requirements imposed by increased electrical susceptibility and exposure of patients. There are seldom standard solutions. Earlier, I introduced the notion of three interacting elements of the health care delivery system. The differences between hospitals is most evident in the ability of personnel and the condition of plant and equipment. These differences require individual solutions.

CLINICAL EMPHASIS

In actual clinical practice, we find illogical and dangerous emphasis. Where there is a traditional concern for spark ignition, as in surgical facilities, emphasis is on protection designed to prevent rapid discharge of static electricity. Ignition or detonation of flammables is dependent on creation of an energetic spark. Faulty electrically powered equipment is also likely to provide that spark. The amount of electrically powered equipment utilized in a given "anesthetizing location" is increasing rapidly. However, the greatest emphasis is usually on protective measures directed at controlling static electricity. Hazard-conscious personnel tend to believe their facility is "safe" if the conductive floors passed the "test" last week, while the ground fault detector monitoring the isolated power system may have been in "alarm" for as long as a month. There is often little or no concern regarding possible injury by electrical shock. And yet, in some instances these same personnel have complained of receiving distracting or startling shocks.

In special facilities where there is a strong medical concern over serious cardiac arrhythmias, we find the reverse situation. Elaborate systems are often installed to protect the patient against macroshock or even microshock, yet there is often no protection against shock caused by electrostatics. We often find static-electricity-generating carpeting in new coronary care units. These new facilities seldom have adequate humidity controls or other measures intended to minimize generation of static electricity. A basic fact is often over-looked—ignition energy is about a thousand times greater than the microshock hazard. Electrical cardiac stimulation by static electricity is certainly possible, given an appropriate combination of electrical capacitance and resistance (the apparent cause of an unreported case of accidental defibrillation). The problem of emphasis in both types of areas is educational and involves professionals in many fields including medicine, architecture, engineering, and hospital administration.

INDICATIONS OF EXPERIENCE

Several engineering firms routinely evaluate medical facilities for electrical safety. Although not statistically valid because of the relatively small sample of hospitals, my experience, in the form of an automated "data bank," provides some clues to existing hazards. These data, relating to identifying and correcting hazards, permit some general conclusions. My investigations considered three classes of hazards: (1) ignition, (2) macroshock, and (3) microshock, as well as combinations of the three.

ANESTHETIZING LOCATIONS

Ignition of flammables and macroshock are hazards with similar minimum energy thresholds. If available energy is maintained below that necessary to cause ignition or detonation, it is unlikely that current will be above the threshold of ventricular fibrillation for attendants or for patients uncompromised by conductive invasion. Anti-ignition protective measures do not mitigate the microshock or electrically sensitive patient hazard except when combined with an equipotential grounding system.

At this time, the hazard of ignition or detonation of flammable medical gases or vapors is generally believed to be completely controlled, and in our more modern facilities,

it is. However, I have found that some hospitals have never installed conductive floors or isolated power systems. Another, more important, observation has been the gross deterioration of older isolated systems. Many of these isolated and ground-fault detection systems are no longer providing the intended protection against either sparking or macroshock. Although system hazard current usually is not quite enough to injure personnel, it is a sufficiently large current to startle, which adds greatly to surgical risk. These old systems have often deteriorated to the point where there is more than enough energy available to cause ignition. The questionable age seems to be 5 years. If more than 8 years old, the system is likely to be defective. I have not examined one system over 12 years old that was working as intended.

A common failure mode provides a false indication of a safe condition. Self-checking test buttons still indicate that the defective fault detector is functional. In more than one case, the detector has been indicating a fault and someone has transposed the red and green lamp lenses and turned off the audible alarm; a clever but very dangerous "medical" procedure. In my opinion, the only factor preventing serious accidents in these completely unprotected facilities is the widespread use of closed or semiclosed anesthetizing systems, preventing the escape into the atmosphere of substantial amounts of flammable anesthetic gases. It is essential that these old systems be cleared of faults and the ground fault detectors repaired and maintained. System hazard currents as high as half an ampere (500 milliamperes) have been measured, which constitutes a macroshock as well as a high hazard of ignition.

Perhaps the greatest latent danger in these older facilities is the false confidence of the personnel. They are conscientiously following all the precautions for preventing the generation of static electricity, and the green light indicates that the power system and connected equipment is safe. There is also confidence in the portable equipment that has served well for many years without any trouble. This equipment may have been deteriorating for many years without preventive maintenance or even inspection for defective insulation. When faulty equipment is connected to a defective isolated power system, the hazards in the entire area served by this power system become enormous. However, when functioning as intended and combined with an effective local grounding system, these isolated and fault-monitored power systems will protect personnel and patients from gross electrical shock, as well as keeping static electricity below the ignition level. When they are combined with an "equipotential" local grounding system, microshock protection may be achieved.

OTHER HIGH-RISK AREAS

Special procedure or catheterization facilities are often adapted from general-purpose radiology rooms. Consequently, cardiac catheterization may be performed with little or no electrical precaution. Often there is inadequate grounding. Use of poorly grounded or ungrounded wall receptacles to power devices such as dye injector is very common. Sometimes temporary grounding by spring clamps and heavy flexible cables is not included in the preparation for a procedure. Several volts of potential difference may exist between the table contacting the patient and ancillary equipment or nearby exposed conducting surfaces. (In older buildings, the fault currents causing these voltage differences may be from unidentified faults quite remote from the room.) Ungrounded and two-wire electrical equipment is very likely to be used. Overhead x-ray sources and image intensifiers are often poorly grounded.

All cardiac catheterization implies a patient susceptibility in the ten to thirty microampere range. This imperceptible current may be injected into the heart by the external end of the catheter contacting any electrical conductor, including those manipulating the catheter. From my discussion of the hazardous current path it should be clear that the catheters with a conductive wire in the lumen are the most dangerous because of their low impedance. The ordinary open-lumen catheter is as hazardous as a pacemaker electrode catheter during the time it is directed with an uninsulated guide wire. This common practice creates an unnecessary hazard. Teflon-coated guide wires are available and will reduce this hazard, providing the insulating coating is continuous and includes the ends of the wire.

Acute care units are likely to include patients with cardiac catheterization, or electrically sensitive patients. Except for those units constructed or renovated in the last few years, most facilities have little or no special provision for the high electrical susceptibility of these patients. In many units grounding, the elimination of two-wire receptacles and cords, the control of portable equipment, and other fundamental protection cannot be considered adequate even for areas serving general patients.

Wet diagnostic and therapeutic procedures involve somewhat lower, but important, electrical risks. These procedures include: (1) placing of skin and needle electrodes, (2) hemodialysis, (3) internal examinations (G.I., renal, proctologic, E.N.T., and so forth), and (4) any procedure in which electrolyte (blood, urine, saline, and so forth) spills are likely. In general, our present precautions are not equal to the industrial standards for wet work areas. For example, hemodialysis units are often installed in a room because it happens to have adequate plumbing. Electrical grounding is whatever happens to be in the room and seldom includes the plumbing. Typical pump motors have very high leakage current and grounding of the metal tanks is undependable.

GENERAL PATIENT AREAS AND GROUNDING

Much of a hospital serves patients without conductive invasion, and the electrical hazards to patients are not much greater than to the attendants. With aging plant and equipment, the degree of hazard becomes dependent on their maintenance and the most important protection becomes the grounding. Our electrical surveys indicate that the "average" hospital has at least one section, the oldest wing building, or floor with two-wire or ungrounded receptacles. For example, in one case of an old wing with no grounding, an administrative problem became evident. Enough three-to-two wire adaptors were never available. (These adaptors or "cheaters" permit a three-wire grounding plug to be inserted in a two-wire receptacle.) This prob-

lem was "solved" by installing three-wire receptacles *without* any connection to the grounding contacts of the receptacles. Fortunately, this situation was corrected beginning with the surgical recovery room.

There are difficulties in just providing functional three-wire grounding for power receptacles, a minimal protection. I have found the following conditions prevalent:

1. A section has no grounding except for plumbing. (Conduits were not used in the original wiring.)
2. Conduits have provided adequate grounding

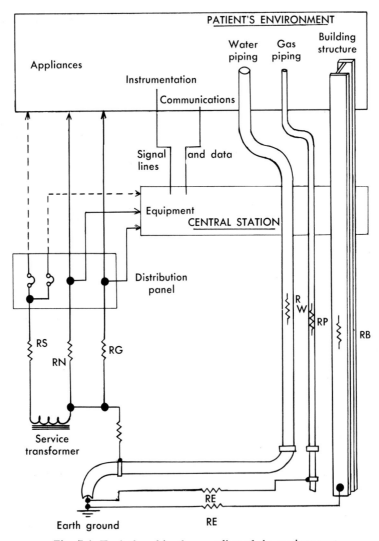

Fig. 7-4. Typical multipath grounding of the environment.

for less than 5 years because of corrosion at each joint. (Much of the existing grounding is solely by conduit.)

3. Existing conduits or raceways are not large enough to allow installation of grounding wires.

4. For one reason or another, the receptacle grounding impedance is greater than 5 ohms (code maximum).

5. In new construction or renovation, up to 10% of the three-wire receptacles are miswired, sometimes with a hot wire on an insulated grounding contact of a receptacle.

In general, the importance of three-wire grounding receptacles and plugs is usually not completely understood by hospital electricians and, occasionally, electrical contractors.

The patient's environment is likely to include many independent paths to ground, as shown in Fig. 7-4. Since each path has a finite resistance, a fault current flowing in any one path will cause potential or voltage differences to develop within a patient's environment. In older buildings, we often find large potential differences within a patient's environment caused by undiscovered faults of hundreds of amperes in combination with multiple paths to "earth ground."

PORTABLE ELECTRICAL EQUIPMENT

Medical instrumentation and appliances present a continuing safety problem. Unlike any other industry, we have selected equipment rather than specifying it. Recently, "incoming inspection" has been required by some hospitals. However, the bulk of the equipment in patient areas has never had the most cursory examination. Ben-Zvi reported a new equipment rejection rate of nearly 40% over a 2-year period.* His acceptance criteria were reasonable safety and the manufacturer's published performance data. Lubin (see references at the end of the chapter) found that the common soft-molded-plastic line-cord three-wire plug did not provide reliable grounding after about 2 years of

*Ben-Zvi, S.: The lack of safety standards in medical instrumentation, Trans. N. Y. Acad. Sci. 31(6):737, 1969.

hospital service. There is often a break between the grounding pin and the line-cord wire with no external visual evidence.

REPORTING OF ELECTRICAL INCIDENTS

A basic difficulty in determining the magnitude of the hazards in a given medical facility is in the usual practice of reporting, or rather the lack of complete reporting, possible electrical accidents. Indeed, reporting is often crucial to convincing the medical staff that any unidentified electrical hazards exist and that corrective action is indicated in their hospital. Accidents involving obvious injury from fire, explosion, and the passage of large electrical currents through the body are always investigated. When there are no burns, as in many electrical shock cases, it is not always obvious that electrical current has been the cause of injury. "Microshock," related to the passage of a very small electrical current through the heart, is even more subtle. Pathologic evidence is nonexistent unless the electrical current through the victim is quite large. Engineering evidence can be obtained only by examining the precise electrical environment extant at the time of the suspected accident. Consequently, the existence of real hazard has been the subject of debate within the individual hospitals. Protection of electrically sensitive patients usually is considered only in extensive renovation or new construction. Personnel in hospitals that have installed isolated power centers often believe that the patient is safe without any other protection. This safety depends on an intact grounding system including *all* plug and line-cord equipment. Much equipment used in these areas lacks ground connections. All incidents, particularly those involving serious cardiac arrhythmias, should be reported and investigated.

PRESENT CONDITIONS IN A FACILITY

The only method of determining actual conditions is a room-by-room electrical survey of power and grounding systems and all electrically powered devices. Generally, records, such as equipment-control inventories and "as-built" drawings of the building, are incomplete and often inaccurate. Consequently, the electrical survey must include measurements and tests as well as inspection to provide a meaningful evaluation of actual conditions.

Particularly in hospitals with few electrically sensitive patients, it seems appropriate to address the neglected protection of the majority of the population, the general patients and personnel. The needed "modernization" of plant and equipment involves meeting codes and standards that have been effective for more than a decade. Even universal compliance with past standards will appreciably reduce electrical hazards. The most important part of this compliance is in providing adequate grounding in all patient areas.

SUMMARY

The situation may be summarized as *unknowing utilization of unknowns*. The equipment and the power systems teem with unknowns. Regardless of the condition of the plant and the built-in protection, known or unknown, knowledgeable utilization of equipment by attendants is essential to safety. When the very existence of hazards is sincerely doubted by some of the medical staff, feasibility of corrective action becomes the subject of controversy and debate. Some of this disagreement has spilled into the lay press in promoting or discrediting various protective methods.

Our medical facilities are overwhelmed with advice (often conflicting), new standards, and added inspections—all intended to protect the patient or the employee from unnecessary hazards. These demands on our resources come at a time of increasing costs. Therefore, the economics of safety becomes an important consideration in attempts to cope with the situation. It must be recognized that absolute safety is unlikely to be achieved within reasonable economic constraints. *A reasonable level of safety can be achieved*

if we insist on a maximum return in protection for each expenditure of our resources. We cannot afford to add to the increasing hazards of utilizing more and more electromedical equipment the real and costly hazard of confusion.

Modern technology, often highly sophisticated, has been applied in a fragmented form to medicine. Technology has not been properly integrated into rational combinations of disciplines except in rare instances. Because of this, we find dangerous, but generally unrecognized, situations in our hospitals. This piecemeal utilization of, often, modish ideas and fragmented technology has created a conflicting hodgepodge. In adopting new methodology, the questions of safety, efficacy, and "cost effectiveness" are seldom properly considered. We must find the means to cope with hazard-generating traditions.

Evolving a pragmatic program

Human susceptibility to electricity and the energy necessary for ignition have been reduced to physical quantities. The condition of equipment and of plant in medical facilities can be determined in the necessary detail and corrective action taken. We can educate physicians, nurses, technicians, architects, engineers, and administrators to understand and prevent the hazards. We can anticipate that the health care delivery system will become more technologically complex. A practical coordinated plan of action is needed to apply our knowledge. It is important that a safety program be total, including personnel, equipment, electrical and other systems, and procedures. No method of protection provides safety by itself. There will always be the consequences of human failure in design, utilization, or maintenance.

We must cope with two forms of electricity: that derived from generation of electrostatic charge and that derived from the power distribution system. Both forms of electricity can ignite flammables and both can injure people directly. Electrostatics can be controlled by preventing appreciable generation of charge differences or by conducting any unavoidable charge slowly to ground. Basic control of electricity from the power distribution is by insulating conductors and conducting small leakage currents caused by imperfect insulation and large fault currents caused by insulation failure harmlessly to ground. Thus, grounding or providing a harmless path to ground is important in protection from both forms of electricity. Since we cannot reduce the value of spark

A continuing electrical safety program

PERSONNEL
Tutorial sessions directed at the specific needs of:
  Physicians and surgeons
  Acute-care nursing
  General nursing
  Ancillary services
  Engineering and maintenance
  Administration
Procedures
  Time-of-use safety checks
  Reporting of questionable situations and incidents
  Medical procedures requiring special precautions
  Provision of coordinated procedural, operational, and maintenance manuals for high-risk areas
  Specification rather than selection of new equipment
ENVIRONMENT (HARDWARE)
Electrical surveys to determine the detailed condition and necessary corrective action for:
  The plant and built-in equipment
  Portable equipment
Action to meet minimal standards
ORGANIZATION AND CONTROLS
Institute and require practical regulations and procedures
Organize a program of efficacy based on clearly defined policies
Control people and environment with delegation of authority to match responsibility
  Day-to-day operations
  Acquiring new facilities and capabilities

energy or shock current to zero, we direct our efforts to limiting energy and current to a low enough value to prevent ignition or injury to a person, under likely clinical conditions.

An effective and continuing safety program for existing medical facilities must address the interacting health care delivery system elements of personnel, environment, and administrative controls. The outline to the left gives my program based on this systems approach. It is not economically feasible (or necessary) to provide in all areas the same level of safety as that required by the electrically sensitive patient. Table 7-2 illustrates a classification scheme that I have found effective since 1968. The primary objectives of the program have been to reduce the hazards to acceptable levels as quickly as possible and to achieve a viable safety program under the aegis of the administration. A program initiated by a consultant must be continuing within the resources of the hospital.

There is always a finite hazard inherent in electrically powered equipment. We can quantify the hazard by measuring the amount of electrical current that can possibly pass through the body or through a spark. Through many techniques, the hazard can be reduced by any degree that is necessary in a given situation. Determination of what is "necessary" involves practical engineering and medical "trade-off" between very small, but acceptable, risks and costs. Our primary constraint is economic, not in any way the available technology.

We must avoid expenditure of time and money on relatively low-yield safety activities. As in fire prevention, it is worthwhile considering the causes of electrical accidents before allocating resources. Our criteria must be what efforts will have the highest yield in reduced risk. Analysis of hundreds of medical electrical accidents by several researchers has clearly indicated that more than half are caused by human failure, carelessness, and misuse of equipment. We have no way of knowing how many accidents could

Table 7-2. Electrical risk by areas

		Maximum Current	Maximum Voltage	Minimum humidity	Temporal exposure
Risk A	**Electrically sensitive patient areas**	10 μa.	5 mv.	60%	
	Catheterization facilities				Moderate
	Special procedures facilities				Moderate
	Coronary care units				Long
	Intensive care units				Long
	Operating rooms				Moderate
	Recovery rooms (including neonatal)				Short
	Delivery rooms				Moderate
	Dialysis facilities				Very long
	Other conductive invasive procedures facilities				Moderate
	Probable sites of medical emergency				Short
	(Services to these areas, e.g., ECG, EEG, x-ray, inhalation, housekeeping, etc.)				Short
Risk B	**General patient areas**	500 μa.	500 mv.	40%	
	General areas involving electrolyte spills				Moderate
	Renal invasive procedures				Moderate
	Intravenous therapy				Short
	Internal examination rooms (G.I., proctology, dental, etc.)				Short
	Screening and testing facilities				Short
	Electrophysiological examining rooms				Short
	Physical therapy facilities				Long
	Nurseries				Long
	General care bedrooms				Long
	Emergency rooms				Short
	Treatment rooms				Moderate
	Examining rooms				Short
	Clinics				Short
Risk C	**Nonpatient areas**	3 ma.	1.5 v.	30%	
	Lounges and waiting areas				
	Kitchen				
	Wet laboratories				
	Maintenance and mechanical areas				
	Offices				

be avoided by moderate efforts to improve equipment and procedures. However, it is obvious that we should direct most of our efforts to personnel training, the distribution system, and the condition of portable equipment.

A safety program must incorporate sufficient redundance to tolerate the carelessness inherent in human behavior. Training, preventive maintenance methods, and acquisition methods each contribute. Codes and standards tend to emphasize hardware because equipment and plant wiring are easier (but more costly) to control than people. To achieve continued safe operation, greater emphasis must be placed on training, inspection, and maintenance.

PERSONNEL

Initial ability. In spite of the increasing use of electromedical devices singly or in complex combinations in clinical medicine, there seems to be little basic knowledge of their basic use. Medical and nursing schools fully cover traditional tools of medicine, such as pharmacology and sepsis control but seldom include instrumentation or even a good physics course. Consequently, we often find only a vague notion of the nature of electricity. Important concepts, such as conductivity, insulation, current, and the electrical circuit, are usually completely lacking. Some understanding of electricity is necessary in order to address electrical safety.

Training. By recognizing the differing needs of the personnel involved, it is practical to provide a slide-illustrated course in electrical safety in about 1 hour. Such brevity is particularly desirable for the nursing staff since only a part of each duty tour can be spared from the floor at one time. Those working in electrically sensitive patient areas require additional training, as do those working in anesthetizing locations because of the additional hazards of flammables ignition. Typical subjects covered in such courses include the following:

1. Electricity (completing the circuit)
2. The mechanism of electrocution
3. The mechanism of ignition
4. Electrical susceptibility
5. The electrically sensitive patient
6. "Time-of-use testing" and methodology
7. Special safety devices and systems
8. Areas and situations of specific risk
9. The facility operational manual
10. Electrically sensitive patient area and procedure
11. Legal aspects
12. Control of equipment

The greatest reduction of hazards per unit cost is achieved by education of personnel. A first concern is for those connecting and using equipment in the immediate vicinity of patients. Their awareness must include recognition of developing faults in equipment and early reporting of these incipient faults.

Needed ability. The understanding of basic principles must be sufficient for the personnel to alertly respond to the everyday hazards. They will display a confidence that comes from this understanding. Not every situation can be covered in brief courses. Therefore,

the basic principles must be used to improve common practices evolving medical procedures that are safe. Provision should be made for organizing similar in-service courses for new personnel and as refresher courses. The following procedures apply particularly to the staffs of intensive care units:

1. Insulation
   a. *Inspect power cords, attachment to equipment,* etc., for damage—cracked or missing insulation material, exposed conductors (never depend on make-shift [adhesive tape] repairs)—*before every use* of the equipment. Inspection must be particularly rigorous when equipment is brought from other areas. Questionable equipment should not be used in electrically susceptible patient areas. *No ungrounded or "two-wire" equipment may be used.*
   b. *Inspect power receptacles* for mechanical damage—cracked or missing insulation material, exposed contacts—before each use.
   c. *Report every incident* of perceptible electrical shock, no matter how minor, and immediately remove the equipment from service for engineering evaluation. (Patients may be harmed by leakage currents much smaller than the perception threshold.)
2. Grounding, required of all equipment
   a. *Inspect power cords and plugs* for missing or damaged grounding connections before *each* use of the equipment. Inspection must be particularly rigorous when equipment is brought from other areas. Grounding connections of equipment used by housekeeping, ECG, inhalation therapy, EEG, and other external services must be suspect.
   b. *Equipment that is questionable* in any way should have redundant grounding cord sets permanently attached to the frame or cabinet. These cord sets should be plugged into a grounding receptacle before plugging in the power cord. Included in this questionable category are all appliances and instruments that have unknown inherent leakage currents or known leakage currents in excess of 10 microamperes and all equipment with no or unreliable (such as molded plastic three-wire plugs) grounding connections.
3. Multiple connections to the patient
   It should be noted that it is difficult to prevent the patient from becoming "grounded." When several pieces of equipment are connected to the same patient at one time, a current path to ground is likely to be provided by one

instrument and a source of current may be provided by a faulty second instrument. When skin electrodes are utilized, the considerable protection of the high impedance of normal dry skin is deliberately circumvented. It is therefore prudent to avoid connecting a second power line–operated machine to the patient whenever possible. For example, when a special electrocardiogram is to be obtained, we recommend that the patient cable be disconnected from the cardiac monitor at the multiple-pin connector. Turning the monitor off does not open this current pathway.

4. *Avoid extension cords* if possible. Plug all equipment into the same receptacle cluster. A line cord or extension cord over 8 feet long may present danger because of the long, relatively small-sized grounding connection. *Never use two-wire line cords or extension cords.*

5. *Insulate the proximal or exposed end of all indwelling catheters or electrodes,* particularly from grounded objects like bedrails. (Rubber surgical gloves are useful electrical protection when manipulating catheters.) Battery-powered pacemakers insulated from ground are preferred. Dye injectors and pressure transducers should be the isolated type.

6. *Be aware of possible current paths.* Touch only *one* thing or person at a time. Rules cannot cover all situations. You cannot perceive currents that could fibrillate the patient. Be continuously alert.

7. *Check and record the relative humidity three times a day.* A practical method of minimizing generation of static electricity is maintenance of humidity at 60%. Inexpensive vaporizers (such as Hankscraft) may be used to supplement the built-in systems.

8. *Control electrically powered equipment;* know what is in use and its condition; report all equipment with any question—smoke, odors, strange sounds are often precursors of failure leading to hazard or reduced performance. Degraded performance is not only indicative of possible shock hazard but introduces another hazard. Equipment that does not perform as expected can be as dangerous as electrically unsafe equipment.

ENVIRONMENT

In existing facilities, the first concern must be to determine the actual condition of the power distribution systems and the portable electrical equipment on a room-by-room basis throughout the entire medical facility. Condition is determined by detailed inspection and measurement.

Portable appliances and instruments are each identified by a unique (nonrepeating) survey number. Permanent features of a room or area are identified by a number related to location in that room. The numbering rule is from top to bottom and left to right; for example, a room's power receptacles are numbered clockwise, beginning with 1 to left as one enters by the main entrance to the room.

"Risk A areas" (electrically sensitive patient areas) are given priority, employing direct engineering supervision. Emphasis should be on the local grounding systems, which are most often inadequate. The presence of an engineer during surveys of these areas facilitates subsequent design of specific corrective measures.

As built. A first step is a study of available architectural and engineering drawings. Emphasis is on special power systems including emergency power sources. Critical details must be checked on site. Available drawings are never absolutely "as built." More important is determining the year of construction or renovation of each section of the hospital so that conditions may be correlated with codes and standards in force at the time.

Electrical outlets. A minimum of two tests is performed on each 120-volt receptacle. An outlet tester is inserted to determine whether the receptacle is wired correctly and whether some sort of grounding (less than 5 ohms) does exist. Fig. 7-5 illustrates this procedure. The common 3-neon-lamp receptacle tester does not check grounding with sufficient rigor. High grounding-connection resistances (up to 40,000 ohms) are indicated as "OK" or satisfactory.

Electrical equipment (portable). The first step is to determine the integrity of the line-cord and plug-grounding connection to the equipment's frame, panel, or chassis. This is checked by a "go-no-go" test, indicating if this connection has a resistance of 5 ohms or less.

If the electrical equipment cannot be conveniently removed from an area that is

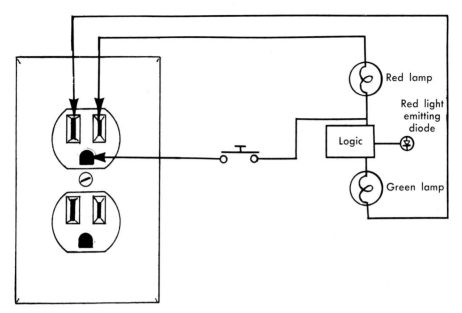

Fig. 7-5. Checking receptacle wiring and grounding impedance.

supplied with isolated power, the leakage current is measured by a portable isolated power system shorted to ground (simulated first fault). The second step is to measure the leakage current in four modes: with and without line reversal and with the device "on" and "off" (Fig. 7-6, *A* and *B*).

When equipment has been examined and tested, a color tag is attached to designate the classification and the action required. The meanings of the color tags are defined in Table 7-3. The 5-digit survey number is printed on the colored tag. The first digit of the survey number corresponds to the color of the tag.

Electrically sensitive patient areas. In especially hazardous areas such as ICUs, CCUs, or operating and recovery rooms, a standard of 5 millivolts maximum is established under probable fault current conditions. Depending on the current available at a given receptacle, the fault current can range between fifty and several hundred amperes before protective devices open the circuit. Consequently, correct methodology for electrically susceptible patient areas includes

engineering supervision and requires local grounding systems with impedances in the milliohm range.

Local equipotential grounding system impedances. Grounding connections are measured by application of 16.5 to 22 amperes of regulated alternating current to the grounding connection (see Fig. 7-7). The open circuit voltage is limited to 3 volts rms. The choice of this relatively high measurement current permits detection of broken strands in grounding wires. When it is necessary to make these measurements with patients in the area, voltage is limited to 5 millivolts. The measurement current is applied between the patient ground point and the conductive surface or receptacle grounding connection to be measured. By measuring the voltage difference caused by application of the current, we compute the actual impedance of the grounding system between the two points. Impedances are measured in this manner between the patient ground point and all conductive objects within 15 feet of the bed location. Acceptable

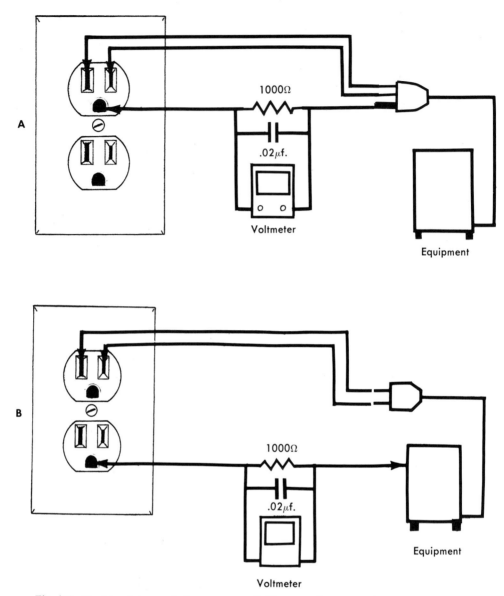

Fig. 7-6. Checking inherent leakage current. **B,** No grounding connection in the line cord.

impedances depend on the magnitude of estimated probable fault currents and anticipated patient susceptibility.

In Risk A areas where an equipotential grounding system has never been designed and installed, meaningful testing can only determine intactness or continuity of the local grounding systems. We use go-no-go testers with thresholds of 0.1 ohm (100 milliohms) and 1.0 ohm. Estimates must be made of maximum probable fault current for each area. Usually an equipotential grounding system is indicated, on a priority basis.

Isolated power systems. In spite of indica-

Table 7-3. Tagging code

Tag color	Measured leakage*	Class of use	Action
Green	Less than 10μa.	U.L. "Professional use A" (grounded equipment)	Use in electrically sensitive areas
Yellow	Less than 100 μa.	U.L. "Professional use B" (double-insulated equipment)	Use in general areas only
Orange	Less than 500 μa.	U.L. "Professional use B" (grounded equipment)	Use in general areas only
Red	Less than 5 ma.	Hazardous	Must correct immediately
No tag	More than 5 ma.	Lethal	Must disable to prevent use

*Multiply upper limits by 1.4 if measured leakage current is direct current. (Limits shown in the table are for rms 60 Hz. current.)

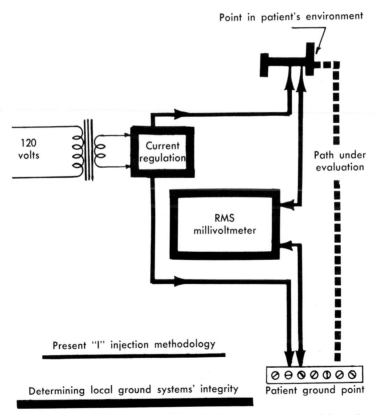

Fig. 7-7. A known high current (simulating a fault current) is injected into the grounding path of question. The cause voltage difference is measured and converted to grounding impedance. It is practical to limit voltage to a few volts for personnel and instrumentation protection.

tion of "safe" condition, I have learned to be suspicious of isolated power systems and their fault detectors. Consequently, my survey instrument carts have a built-in isolation transformer to protect the surveyor.

Line isolation monitor (dynamic fault detector) or ground fault detector (static fault detector) function and system hazard current are determined by introducing a calibrated fault at one of the receptacles. The calibrated fault is introduced sequentially to each side of the line and the resistance recorded for both alarm thresholds. Net system hazard (leakage) current is measured from both sides of the isolated line to ground. The monitor readings and the loaded secondary voltage are recorded. Functioning of audible and visual indication are also checked.

The minimal tests and measurements are the following:

1. System hazard currents for both sides of line
2. Equivalent fault currents to alarm for both sides of the line
3. Detection function for standard faults to each side of the line and balances using equivalent faults that are (a) resistive, (b) reactive, and (c) hybrid. A dynamic fault detector must alarm under all nine equivalent fault conditions.

Corrective action. One or more priority reports are submitted during the electrical survey, sometimes on a day-to-day basis. In this way, extremely hazardous situations are corrected immediately. Following automated data processing, the detailed condition of electrical systems and equipment becomes known. Print-outs are in order of priority, that is, most hazardous in Risk A areas first.

ORGANIZATION AND CONTROLS

Management. Industrial safety programs can provide some guidance. Although we can learn from industrial experience, direct detailed application of this experience is limited to the "industrial" areas of the hospital such as machinery spaces and maintenance shops and cannot be applied to the

safety problems unique to medical care. However, the general principles of industrial safety management can be profitably adapted, as below:

1. *A primary commitment* by the governing body is necessary. Authority as well as responsibility should be delegated. Adequate resources, people as well as financial, must be made available.
2. *The safety director* should be given the authority of an executive officer. In addition to management capability, there should be safety and broad engineering experience available, directly or through outside consultation.
3. *Technical consultation* is usually necessary to deal with the increasingly complex and interrelated systems of modern medical facilities.
4. *The selection of the safety committee* is crucial and should be determined by interest, motivation, departmental authority, education, and teaching ability. The best role includes advisory, line management, and training functions for the director.
5. *Training action* is the core of any safety program. Training of hospital personnel is an essential part of a safety program. Personnel must understand the hazards to patients and themselves in the application of electrically powered equipment. The indoctrination should be provided for personnel from the nursing and medical staffs as well as for the maintenance and administrative staffs. Each group has a role in electrical safety.
6. *Control of personnel, plant, and equipment* is the goal of any safety program and is essential to good overall management of a facility. Continuity, under the aegis of the administration, can be achieved only by initiating and never relaxing these controls. Functions include surveys, regular inspection, specification and testing of all acquisitions of plant and equipment, investigation of all incidents, and keeping of records.

A system of reporting is necessary, in order for those responsible to monitor the program. Reporting should cover, as a minimum, all incidents or possible incidents, present condition of all equipment and the plant systems, and corrective action taken with follow-up results.

Equipment control. Existing equipment is

a current maintenance problem. We must bring this equipment up to present standards and so maintain it. A numbered property label with a corresponding file card on all equipment is an excellent beginning to controlling equipment and its utilization. The first step of effective preventive maintenance is the *control inventory*. This inventory can be generated by a properly performed hospital-wide electrical survey and include quantitative equipment-condition information.

Another general category of hazards pertains to *equipment operability*. The proper operation must be checked to ascertain that malfunctions in this category do not represent a hazardous condition. Checking the operability on a periodic basis can provide the indications of possible malfunction so that the equipment may be repaired before the hazardous conditions manifest themselves. Hospital equipment is scattered throughout the various sections of the hospital under control of the local area or central supply. It is often impossible (without extensive searching) to determine how many ECG monitors are in the hospital let alone know the operability status of each because frequently no centralized list or "control inventory" of equipment exists.

A computerized program for clinical equipment control may be utilized. The data is entered on standard punched cards of 80 columns. The recorded data includes:

1. Type of equipment (ECG monitor, lamp, x-ray, etc.)
2. Location (room number or area)
3. Manufacturer and model/serial number
4. Leakage current category
5. Performance or operability

Such a system, which provides a ready method for finding the status of any equipment or sorting in groups by types of equipment, is of great assistance in determining the record of a particular manufacturer. It is also beneficial for safety status and maintenance and for management inventory control, that is, *control of utilization.*

Another item of concern to hospital administrators is the need for properly trained personnel to carry out *preventive maintenance*. The administration must evaluate the allocation of its resources, based not only on present needs but also on those of the immediate future. Indications strongly imply that the hospital of the future will require a more permanent maintenance program for delivering an adequate health care program to its patients.

A policy of preventive maintenance must be established so that every piece of equipment, including those on standby or backup, is *regularly* inspected for both *performance* and *safety,* and this particularly includes the hospital's power system down to every receptacle. Records must be kept and periodic reports made to the administrator. Besides ensuring that the job is being done, these reports will indicate, by the frequency of repairs, which equipment is becoming unreliable and must be replaced. The administration should exercise control of the equipment and its utilization.

Risk A areas should receive priority. It is these areas where the electrically sensitive patient will be treated and where microshock can result in fatalities; consequently measurements of leakage current are necessary. Increase in leakage current can be an indication of insulation deterioration even before it can be visually detected.

In addition to the regularly scheduled preventive maintenance there is necessary repair of malfunctions. Because this is dependent on reporting of faults by the user, there must be a good reporting system as well as a fast and accurate repair cycle. Good rapport among the personnel is essential because safety is a team effort.

New equipment should be purchased only after careful technical evaluation of candidate equipment. The criteria of equipment evaluation should include:

1. Probability of filling the medical or other requirement
2. Initial safety
3. Safety in service

4. Initial cost
5. Maintainability
6. Operating cost
7. Probability of early obsolescence

It is important that equipment be *specified* rather than *selected*. Specifications should be nonproprietary and emphasize necessary performance and safety requirements. When practical and the equipment is sophisticated, independent laboratory evaluation of candidate equipment is useful and economically justified.

The medical staff is capable of effectively determining the general efficacy of the equipment. However, determining whether the equipment is well-constructed, correctly designed, intrinsically safe, easy to maintain, and capable of being interconnected with the entire "hospital system" must be decided by a capable engineer.

Aside from the obvious economics of selecting and purchasing the right equipment at the best price at the right time, there is the contingent responsibility of assuring that the equipment purchased is safe and operating properly when received and that it will continue to be as long as it is in use.

Furthermore, there is the responsibility that the equipment will be safe and operate properly when connected to the hospital system. The hospital system, as used here, includes not only the electrical wall receptacles into which equipment is plugged, but also such other "systems" as will become "attached" to it. These systems include personnel as well as mechanical systems. Personnel systems include the engineers and technicians who inspect and maintain the equipment, the medical and nursing staffs who utilize the equipment, and the all-important patients whose life may depend on it. Mechanical systems, other than the more obvious power systems, would include the grounding systems, chemical and gas systems, the structural system, and the equipment that may have to function and react with the particular item in question.

It is of paramount importance to remember that *every* piece of equipment in the hospital, from the lowly power scrubber to equipment in the most elaborate CCU, comes into contact with many of these "systems," and their selection, purchase, inspection, operation, maintenance, and even storage capabilities must be considered as part of the overall hospital system.

It is quite obvious, then, that the process—from the selection of a particular piece of equipment through its operational life to the decision to dispose of it—is much more than consideration only of medical application.

A rigid incoming inspection should be instituted to ensure that equipment received is operating properly and safely *before it is released for use*. Unfortunately, as much as 40% of all electrical equipment purchased by a hospital is defective in either safety or performance when it is received. When there are no requirements and procedures for checking every piece of equipment purchased, many useless and dangerous instruments are accepted, paid for, and, worst of all, permitted to jeopardize human life. An essential component of any piece of equipment is the accompanying instructions. No new equipment should be accepted without complete, accurate manuals documenting *operation, maintenance,* and *repair* procedures.

Many of the hazards I have discussed can be assessed and corrected or prevented by incoming inspections. The problem of maintaining equipment in a safe condition is greatly simplified by a sound engineering inspection. Such an approach is customary in other industries. I recommend this for the medical industry.

Inspections allow only equipment that meets the safety requirements to become part of the hospital inventory. Guidance in specifications can be obtained from Underwriters Laboratories, Melville, New York (for example, Subject 544, Standard for Medical and Dental Equipment) and Veterans Administration, Washington, D. C. (for example, Spec. X1414 amended).

Responsibility for the maintenance of safe conditions and practices falls mutually upon:

1. The governing body of the facility
2. All personnel using the facility
3. The administration of the facility
4. Those responsible for approval and inspection (such as those accrediting or licensing the medical facility)

Since the governing body of the facility has the primary responsibility for safety of as well as care of patients, they should determine that adequate regulations have been adopted by the medical staff and that adequate regulations for inspection and maintenance are in use by the administrative, engineering, nursing, and ancillary personnel of the facility. These regulations should be prominently posted in anesthetizing locations and areas of special electrical shock risk. However, the authority to properly utilize, correct, and maintain existing equipment and the authority to select, purchase, and accept new equipment must be shared.

Safety by design

At the time of acquisition of new equipment, new construction, rehabilitation, or renovation, there is opportunity and also an obligation to avoid past mistakes. Corrective action is expensive even with a cost-effective safety program. Therefore, it is useful to become familiar with the available protective devices, techniques, and systems before planned changes are made in the plant or equipment.

GROUNDING

Grounding in combination with over-current protection is the best means of reducing the dangers of electrocution or fire. Simply stated, this means that the situation is safe if all exposed conductors in an area are connected electrically to one point, preferably the earth or true ground. Plumbing and other metal structural parts of a building are usually at true ground potential. The ground connections must have very low impedance and must also be capable of conducting to

ground any fault currents that exist without appreciable voltage drop along the grounding connection. If the impedance of these connections is not sufficiently low, that is, if the connections have an appreciable resistance, there will be a potential difference between various "grounded" objects, including those at true ground.

An equipotential grounding system is the primary protection for the electrically sensitive patient, and to be effective the system must be carefully designed.

Systems engineering is useful in integrating the interacting factors. The following subdisciplines must be utilized for effective design:

1. Instrumentation engineering provides the single point ground concept, adapted as the "patient grounding point."
2. Power electrical engineering provides the basic concept of low-impedance grounding for large fault-current protection.
3. From physics, electrostatics contributes resistive or high-impedance grounding techniques, as in the partially conducting operating room floor.

Although many factors must be considered, one design factor, that of multiple grounding paths, is particularly difficult to define in renovation, as indicated by Fig. 7-4. A common error relates to the designer's con-

---

Primary design factors

Localized grounding subsystems

I. Anticipated patient susceptibility level to:
   A. Currents
   B. Potential differences
II. Maximum probable fault current to ground ("source impedance") for:
   A. First fault
   B. Subsequent faults
III. Personnel capabilities in:
   A. Equipment utilization
   B. Maintenance
IV. Multiple grounding paths that can cause potential differences within the patient's electrical environment

cern for connecting a local grounding system to true ground or the earth. This can be costly and can involve very large wire, which must run down through the building to below ground level. The potential difference between the local grounding system making up the patient's environment and true ground is relatively unimportant. Instead, the emphasis must be on preventing appreciable potential differences within the patient's electrical environment.

Differential voltages between exposed conductive surfaces or loss of ground connection can cause currents through a victim via attached electrodes or internal probes to ground, even though some of the attached instruments are not in operation. A very localized ground should be used, connecting everything with any possibility of contact with the patient to a common ground but not necessarily to true ground. In short, grounding of the patient environment is effective only as long as all points in the environment are actually at the same potential at all times and no grounds, including the grounding of the line cords and plugs of portable equipment, have been lost through connection failure.

EQUIPMENT ACCESSORIES

Several techniques have been developed that provide protection with older, high-leakage current equipment. These techniques are also applied in the design of new equipment.

Loss-of-grounding detectors. If one can be certain that grounding is intact and of sufficient current-carrying capability, protection from leakage current and fault current is achieved. Many loss-of-grounding detectors have been devised, sometimes as parts of power systems and instrumentation. In the latter case, we must concern ourselves with the current required to detect loss of grounding since this current can pass through the patient.

The most common detector of loss of grounding is a neon lamp connected between the high side of the line and the ground connection. This lamp is lighted as long as the ground connection is intact. The current through the lamp is usually limited to between 2 and 5 ma. When the grounding connection is broken, this current, which is a significant current to an electrically sensitive patient, can pass through the patient. Similarly, we find that relatively large sensing current flows in the redundant grounding connection when it is broken to devices with built-in audible alarms, such as dye injectors.

Some current must be passed to determine if the connections exist; however, we must not permit such "safety" devices to introduce new hazards. The paradox is in the physical fact that a large sensing current is necessary to determine if the resistance of the grounding connection is low enough to be effective protection.

Loss of ground, power interruption. Many loss-of-grounding detectors, particularly when built into the equipment, interrupt power as well as provide an indication or alarm.

The best answer seems to be to break the grounding connection to the equipment case or frame as well as the two power connections. This prevents the relatively large loss-of-grounding sensing current from becoming a hazard in the event of loss of equipment grounding. The available three-wire devices require installation on the equipment case or the frame at the line-cord entrance and replacement of the equipment's original line cord and plug.

Ground fault circuit interrupters. In the event a dangerous current is conducted to ground by any path, this device interrupts or opens the power circuit. The current to ground may be either a fault current or a large leakage current in a defective device. Power interruption occurs when the current to ground exceeds 5 to 10 ma., and since it occurs quite rapidly, it affords considerable protection against macroshock. With an effective local grounding system it affords some protection against microshock because the fault current is quickly interrupted.

There are two disadvantages in using the ground fault circuit interrupter in medical situations. Although attendants are protected, patient protection is marginal because of the time required to interrupt the circuit and the relative insensitivity of present fault current detection.

The second disadvantage is economic. An interrupter would be needed for each device in use. If one interrupter is used for a number of appliances or instruments, a fault in any one will disconnect all equipment from the power source. Many medical procedures are dependent on uninterrupted power.

Since the device continually monitors and compares the current in the conductors carrying the work or load current, it is effective with two-wire appliances such as electric hand tools. There is no dependence on the third grounding conductor for fault protection as in isolated power systems and their fault detectors.

Leakage current monitors. A typical device rapidly scans all the electrically powered equipment within the area, measuring leakage current with respect to ground. Should leakage or fault current in any equipment within the patient's area exceed a threshold, usually 10 microamperes, an audiovisual alarm is actuated. The piece of equipment with the relatively high current is identified. The usual cause of alarm is loss of grounding, making the inherent leakage current of the appliance or instrument available from its case or frame.

Again, a major disadvantage is economic. It is necessary to connect a sensing wire to the case or frame of every piece of equipment in the patient area and run these wires to a central point where the current monitoring device is located. This labor would be more effectively expended by using heavier wires connected to each piece of equipment and running them to a central grounding point. Redundant grounding of this type eliminates the hazard of loss of grounding.

Devices breaking the hazardous current path. The hazardous electrical path, as illus-trated in Fig. 7-3, may be broken by isolation or insulation. Use of these techniques in new facilities is shown in Table 7-4. However, two important applications of these techniques are available as accessories for older equipment.

The connections to skin electrodes can provide a path for hazardous current. It is practical to place a discontinuity in the leads connecting the skin electrodes to an instrument such as a cardiac monitor. To be effective, these devices must place a discontinuity in each of all leads connected to the patient, including the indifferent or ground-reference electrode. Early lead isolators were very large resistors or field-effect diodes in series with the electrode limiting the current that could flow in the lead. Some of the early field-effect devices did not limit current when the potential difference exceeded about 70 volts. This dangerous characteristic was corrected in later isolators. More recently, instrument manufacturers have developed true iso-lated patient-lead circuitry and built it into instruments. Most of these are light coupled, with no electrical connection between the in-strument power supply and the patient. Simi-lar isolation is achieved with radio frequency coupling.

The second important technique in obtain-ing protection in older equipment is adding an isolation transformer and a special low-leakage line cord. The leakage current of the equipment can be reduced to less than 5 microamperes. The transformer is enclosed in a metal box and permanently attached to the instrument or appliance at an inconspicous point. This is included in Table 7-4 as method III. Since modification costs average 10% of the original equipment cost, this presents an economical solution for somewhat unsafe older equipment that is otherwise satisfactory in performance or function.

ISOLATION AND INSULATION

Recognizing that in the usual situation the patient is, intentionally or unintentionally, grounded through many conducting paths

Table 7-4. Comparison of typical parameters of protective methods

Method	System hazard current (at time of first fault in area) (ma.)	Achieved isolation from power ground (ohms)	First fault current in area grounding system (ma.)	Subsequent faults current in area grounding system (ma.)	Protection against				Advantages	Disadvantages
					Micro-shock	Macro-shock	Igni-tion	Line		
I. Insulated area grounding system (faults monitored; area isolated)	1.0	10^5	1.0	Amps	None	Good	None	Fair	Low cost, permits reduced ampacity in area (local) grounding system	Faults accumulative, grounding system must be intact
IIA. Double-insulated instrument or appliance ungrounded	As low as 0.01	10^7	As low as 0.01	As low as 0.03	Fair	Good	None	None	Lower cost than III, applicable to many appliances with inherent hazard due to function	Exposed conductive surfaces may be electrified by contacting other faulty equipment.
IIB. Double-insulated instrument or appliance exposed metal grounded	As low as 0.03	10^6	5	Amps	Good	Good	None	Some		Failure of primary insulation is not detected by functioning of over-current protection
III. Isolation in instrument or appliance (individual transformers)	As low as 0.005	10^7	As low as 0.005	As low as 0.005	Good	Good	None	None	Protection is in all portable equipment not in permanent facility	Requires addition of special line cord and transformer to older equipment (all equipment in use)
IV. Area isolated power system (faults monitored; area transformer)	1.0	10^5	1.0	Amps	None	Good	Good	Fair	Permits reduced ampacity in area (local) grounding system	Faults accumulative, grounding system must be intact
V. Receptacle isolated power systems (individual transformer)	0.005	10^7	0.005	0.005	Good	Good	Good	Good	Permits safe use of faulty equipment, grounding not critical; no interaction or fault accumulation	High cost; if unnecessary fault monitoring is required, can be circumvented by deliberate action

(Figs. 7-2, 7-3, and 7-4), we must consider methods of preventing hazardous currents from returning to ground through the patient. His complex environment, including his bed and instrumentation, presents variously grounded surfaces that can contact both the patient and other persons in the immediate vicinity. Furthermore, there are conductive fluids—blood, saline, urine, and so forth —that can electrically bridge materials that are normally nonconductive. One side of the building's power system is, of course, grounded. We must prevent the completion of the circuit from the high, or "hot," side of the power line, through the victim, to the common, or grounded, side of the line. This is prevented by isolation or insulation.

Although some of the protective methods considered in Table 7-4 are built in or part of the structure, they all are intended to provide protection from faulty equipment. This comparison is based on measurements and estimates of typical hazard currents and other performance parameters. Achieved protection is evaluated with respect to *microshock, macroshock,* possible *ignition* of flammables, and possible line cord insulation damage as the wires enter the equipment.

In new facilities, it is often necessary to use combinations of the five methods. In general, we must depend on the integrity of the local grounding system for primary protection. A first step in design of a new facility must be obtaining an overview that includes the detailed medical needs and all the constraints.

Summary

Education and control of all personnel reduce unknowing utilization of electromedical equipment. Quantitative measurements reduce the *unknowns* in the hardware. The condition of the medical equipment and the hospital plant can no longer be taken for granted. Initially, extensive measurement and inspection are necessary. Once a hospital is "current," records, control procedures, preventive maintenance, and incoming inspec-

tion of new equipment all act, at reasonable cost, to keep the equipment and plant at an acceptable level of safety. The electrical safety program must be an active program in order to be effective. As such, the program must be organized and administered as an integral part of the normal operation of the hospital. Personnel and hardware control for electrical safety may be addressed in ways similar to those used to control sepsis and dangerous drugs.

We know enough about electrical shock to prevent it. We know the conditions of plant and equipment and we know the medical procedures and the conditions of the patients. We can assess objectively an individual patient's response to electrical currents. Those who are most likely to have an adverse response represent a small proportion of the patient population and can be assigned to specially protected areas.

There is no single solution in the design of new facilities, such as "isolated power centers" or "isolated patient leads." A reasonable level of safety can be created only by integrating all the system elements into a functional whole.

There is no longer any excuse for poorly explained death or cardiac arrhythmia. Fortunately, ventricular fibrillation is reversible if discovered quickly and if resuscitation equipment is immediately available. Procedures of some risk, such as cardiac catheterization, may require reconsideration. The greatest need, now, is for the education of physicians, nurses, engineers, and administrators in order to convince them that a real hazard exists and is growing and that prevention is practical. We cannot permit the problem to be given a low priority simply because there is no pathology or because the hazards cannot be perceived except by interpretation of sensitive instrumentation by capable technical personnel.

System science has been neglected as a pragmatic tool to the disadvantage of the health-care industry. This neglect has included the subdiscipline of cost-benefit analysis, as well as subsystems integration. Safety, efficacy, and efficiency can be achieved. Our existing technology can answer medical needs, but rational, professional, and integrated application of the physical and life sciences is a necessity. Safety is not an "end" or even a discrete objective, but a part of the overall tasks of appropriate design and utilization of medical facilities and equipment.

Glossary of terms

anesthetizing location Any area in which it is intended to utilize any flammable or nonflammable inhalation anesthetic agents in the course of examination or treatment. The hazardous location includes the volume defined by the floor of the room and 5 feet above the floor.

electrical quantities Current (volume of flow): 1,000 milliamperes = 1 ampere; 1,000,000 microamperes = 1 ampere; 1,000 microamperes = 1 milliampere. Impedance (resistance to flow): 1,000 milliohms = 1 ohm. Voltage (pressure causing flow): 1,000 millivolts = 1 volt (A 150 watt lamp operated on a 120 volt A.C. line has a current of 1.25 amperes flowing through its impedance of 96 ohms.)

electrically sensitive patient (formerly electrically susceptible patient) A human being whose life is threatened by exposure to alternating current at commercial power frequencies of magnitudes less than 30 volts. In some cases, the patient's life may be jeopardized by voltage as low as 5 millivolts. Basis is a possible 10 microamperes fibrillation threshold (500 ohm heart/body impedance). This is usually a patient who has an unprotected artificial electrical conductor (liquid or solid) connecting his environment with a vital organ in such a manner that substantially all of the current applied to the external end of the conductor will be delivered to the patient's heart. Examples are angiography, cardiac catheterization for measurements of physical parameters, and artificial cardiac pacemaker electrodes. The last example is the most hazardous, because the current path impedance can be as low as 500 ohms.

electrically sensitive patient area A location in a health care facility where "electrically sensitive patients" are cared for individually or collectively.

fault An undesired or accidental current path, usually to ground. The impedance of the fault determines the amount of current that can flow. This can range from hundreds of amperes when the fault is a direct "short circuit" to a few microamperes (leakage current) when the fault impedance is in the millions of ohms.

fault, first (and second) The first fault usually refers to the first accidental fault of major consequence to occur. (When an isolated power system is involved, the net leakage current or system "hazard current" of all connected equipment can flow.) The second fault is the next fault. (When an isolated power system is involved, the higher impedance of the two faults tends to determine the fault current that can flow, providing the two faults are on opposite sides of the isolated line.)

fault, probable The result of one or more failures of the following: (1) any single component, (2) any components that might fail without detection during normal use, including interruption of the grounding conductor, (3) any components that might fail as a result of the failure of any or all of the components above.

flammable agents Many liquid or aerosol-dispensed medicaments and germicidal, defatting, cleaning, or adhesive materials are flammable, as well as the more obvious materials. Agents involving a flammable volatile solvent or vehicle are also classed as flammables.

flammable anesthetics Gases or vapors, such as cyclopropane, divinyl ether, ethyl chloride, ethyl ether, ethylene, and fluroxene, that may form flammable or explosive mixtures with air, oxygen, or nitrous oxide.

flammable anesthetizing location Any operating room, delivery room, anesthetizing room, corridor, utility room, or other area if used or intended for utilization of flammable anesthetics.

ground fault (circuit) interrupter A device interposed between the power source and the load that automatically disconnects the load when a macrofault occurs to ground. Important parameters are the minimum fault current causing interruption and the time delay of interruption.

grounding, equipotential A local grounding system designed to minimize the potential difference between exposed conducting surfaces (including instrumentation and appliances) within the patient's environment during a fault. Potential difference is determined by the impedance and the routing of the grounding conductors, for example, assume an impedance of 0.5 milliohm between the site of a fault, which injects a 10 ampere current into the grounding connection, and the patient grounding bus. The potential difference between the site of the fault and other grounded surfaces in the patient's environment would be 5 millivolts, the maximum permitted in an electrically sensitive patient area when low-impedance cardiac catheters may be used.

grounding, redundant An additional grounding connection. (Redundant grounding wires should be added to equipment used in electrically sensitive patient areas if it has a leakage current in excess of 10 microamperes.)

grounding bus, patient (also reference grounding point) The terminal grounding bus with a conductivity at least that of copper that serves as the single focus for grounding the electrical equipment connected to an individual patient or for grounding the metal or conductive furniture or other equipment within reach of the patient or a person who may touch the patient.

grounding impedance That very low impedance, predominantly resistive, between points in a grounding system; for example, the electrical resistance between a cardiac monitor outer case and the patient grounding bus or point.

grounding point, patient Idealized patient grounding bus. The focus of the grounding system of a patient's environment. (The single "focal point" of a local grounding system.)

grounding system, local The combination of grounding buses, grounding wires (including line cords on portable equipment) and straps, and exposed conductive surfaces that should be nearly equipotential (at the same voltage) under all probable fault conditions. The local grounding system refers to a patient's or small group of patients' immediate area, and is not necessarily equipotential with the building's ground.

health care facilities These include, but are not limited to, hospitals, sanitariums, clinics, nursing homes, and medical and dental offices, whether fixed or mobile.

intrinsically safe Refers to parts of or complete devices employing circuitry limiting energy so that it is incapable of releasing sufficient electrical energy, under any conditions, to ignite flammables in an oxygen-enriched atmosphere. This *energy* limitation, preventing ignition or detonation, is *several hundred times the minimal energy* that can cause *ventricular fibrillation*.

isolated power center An assembly of electrical devices, including local isolating power transformer, a line isolation monitor, a single grounding point, and multiple parallel-connected power and grounding receptacles.

isolated power system Supplies power without a conductive connection to the "high side" of the ground-referenced building power system and may supply power to many pieces of equipment (as in isolated power center) or to a single appliance or instrument.

isolating transformer Provides isolated-from-ground power by means of an inductively coupled device wherein the primary and secondary windings are not conductively connected. Usually operated at power distribution frequency (60 Hz.).

leakage current Any small unintended current, including a capacitively coupled current, that flows from a line-powered piece of equipment or assembly to ground, possibly through the victim.

line, high side (and return side) The "high side" of a ground-referenced power line is at 120 volts or more with respect to ground. The "return side," or "neutral," or "common," is connected to ground, usually at a service entrance, and carries the same large work current as the high side of the power line. A third wire of the distribution system provides grounding and is connected to ground, usually at a service entrance, and carries no current (except small leakage-currents) until a fault occurs (and then only for the time required for a protective device to open the circuit).

line isolation monitor (LIM, dynamic ground fault detector) An instrument designed to continually check the balanced and unbalanced impedance from each line of an isolated circuit to ground and equipped with a built-in test circuit to exercise the alarm without adding to the leakage or system hazard current. Purpose is to detect faults in the power system or connected equipment when they occur.

macrofault A low impedance fault permitting relatively large currents in excess of 1 milliampere to flow to ground creating a macroshock hazard.

macroshock Large currents (in excess of 1 milliampere) passing through the victim's body. In addition to cardiac arrhythmia, other vital functions, such as respiration, may be affected. At high currents there are burns and other thermal effects.

measurement current (LIM) A small current passed in order to determine if a fault has occurred. This current is injected into the system in series with the fault and during the first fault and limits the fault current to the measurement current. Consequently, this measurement current should be as small as possible. Present devices require from 2 microamperes to 2 milliamperes.

microfault A high impedance fault permitting small leakage currents, between 5 microamperes and 1 milliampere, to flow to ground creating a microshock hazard.

microshock Small currents (in excess of 10 microamperes but less than 1 milliampere) passing through the victim's body. The victim's high resistance (dry) skin protection has been circumvented, often by prepared skin electrodes or by conductive invasion, such as catheter. Resulting ventricular fibrillation usually has no pathology.

shield, interwinding A conductive shield placed between the primary and secondary windings of an isolated transformer, connected to the transformer enclosure and core and/or to ground. It provides additional protection against insulation failure between the windings and additional isolation from high frequency transients introduced in the primary.

system hazard current That leakage current that flows to ground from an isolated power system. It is the total of transformer leakage, line isolation monitor measuring current, and wiring leakage current. Often, connected portable and fixed equipment leakage currents are also included in this index of hazard. It is simply the current that is normally flowing in any part of the local grounding system. It is measured by sequentially grounding each side of the line through a low known value of resistance and measuring the voltage across that resistance.

Annotated references

The physicians and engineers cited below have contributed to the literature of medical electrical safety. The articles listed are introductory examples of their work and have been selected for their utility.

Bruner, J. M. R.: Hazard of electrical apparatus, Anesthesiology 28:396, 1967. An early coordinated analysis of equipment hazards in the clinical environment, specific to the operating room—technical and medical factors.

Dalziel, C. R.: Reevaluation of lethal electric currents, IEEE Trans. Ind. Gen. Applications, IGA-4, 5, 1968. A review of prior studies of human "let-go" currents and comparison with fibrillation data from many sources. Fibrillating current, shock duration, and other factors are related.

Keesey, J. C.: Bibliography on human thresholds to extra-low-frequency electrical current, Project MR005.08-0030B Report No. 2, Naval Medical Research Inst., 1970. Over a thousand references, well organized into seven major categories, most from 1944 to mid-1969 period.

Kilpatrick, D. G., and Kilpatrick, L. B.: Electrical

safety standards in the health care delivery system, Critical Reviews in Bioengineering, Vol. 1, No. 3, C.R.C., 1972. Discusses the nature of the clinical hazards and present protective methodology, an extensive review, including 49 references.

Kusters, N. L.: The ground detector problem in hospital operating rooms, Trans. Eng. Ins. Can. 2(1), 1958. Establishes the technical requirements for monitoring the degree of isolation of ungrounded power systems.

Staewen, W. S., Lubin, D., and Mower, M. M.: The significance of leakage currents in hospital electrical devices, Sinai Hosp. (Baltimore) J. 15(1), 1969. Describes canine experimentation with an electric bed and transvenous electrode catheterization causing ventricular fibrillation with a leakage current of 20 microamperes.

Stanley, P. E.: Electrical shock hazards, 1. and 2., Hospitals 45:58, 73, 1971. Part 1 defines the problem, the two categories of shock, and the various sources of hazard. Part 2 discusses the requirements in hospital plant and equipment for patient safety.

Walter, C. W.: Safe electric environment, Bull. Am. Coll. of Surg. 54:177, 1969. Develops the criteria for safe use of electricity in the care of patients.

Weinberg, D. A.: Electrical safety in the operating room and at bedside. In Segal, B. L., and Kilpatrick, D. G., editors: Engineering in the Practice of Medicine, Baltimore, 1967, The Williams & Wilkins Co. Discusses types of hazard, causes, and some reductive methodology; includes an analysis of specific patient-connected equipment incidents.

Whalen, R. E., Starmer, D. F., and McIntosh, H. D.: Electrical hazards associated with cardiac pacemaking, Ann. N. Y. Acad. Sci. 3:922, 1964. Identifies the special hazards of cardiac catheterization through canine experimentation. Minimum ventricular fibrillation threshold was 35 microamperes.

Whitaker, H. B.: Electric shock as it pertains to the electric fence, Bull. Res., No. 14, Underwriters' Laboratories, December, 1939, 5th printing, June, 1967. An intensive investigation of the effects of electricity on animals and humans; the basis for much of the following work.

Chapter 8

WARNING SIGNS AND EARLY DETECTION
OF CARDIAC ARREST

It is true, as other authors have empha-sized, that cardiac arrest has become less often a completely unexpected event. Much information has now been accumulated from intensive care and coronary care units to alert the physician or nurse to conditions likely to produce ventricular fibrillation or cardiac standstill. Nevertheless, even in these carefully controlled areas, cardiac arrest frequently appears in a completely unannounced fashion.

A committee representing both the American Heart Association and International Society of Cardiology (Paul) decided to establish certain guidelines for clinicians. They agreed on a definition of sudden death as an unexpected death that occurs within an estimated 24 hours of onset of acute symptoms and signs. An instantaneous death is one that occurs within seconds or minutes. In Paul's series of 64 coronary deaths occurring within a 10-year period among 2,000 middle-aged men (40 to 55 years), 31 of the victims died almost instantaneously or within 15 minutes of onset of acute episode. In a Baltimore study, approximately half of patients dying suddenly of coronary disease had been free of cardiac symptomology until the fatal event.

In discussing problems related to the acutely arrested circulation, the term "cardiac arrest" has continued to be used. One author entitled his editorial "Stamp Out Cardiac Arrest!" He did not, however, suggest a more appropriate term for the state of an acutely arrested heart, whether it be in ventricular fibrillation or in asystole. In fact, in the majority of instances requiring cardio-pulmonary resuscitation today, a precise de-

lineation of the etiology of the arrest is not known prior to the institution of resuscitative efforts. Certainly, we would be delighted to see a better term for the sudden, unexplained, and unexpected cessation of cardiac activity, a catastrophe that afflicts the child and adult alike.

Many different words have been substituted to imply a more precise situation, but without success. It can be easily argued that the term "cardiac arrest" is sometimes used as a waste-basket diagnosis and, for this reason, has become meaningless and should be discarded. Perhaps the term "cardiac arrest" is comparable to the term "cystosarcoma phylloides." The latter, a tumor of the breast, has been given at least fifty-five to sixty new and different names; but after more than 100 years most doctors well know what is meant when the diagnosis of cystosarcoma phylloides is applied. Similarly, cardiac arrest serves an equally useful purpose, despite some obvious disadvantages inherent in this title.

Many authors have suggested a definition of cardiac arrest. "Failure of the heart action to maintain an adequate cerebral circulation, in the absence of a causative and irreversible disease" is the definition used by Milstein.*

Safar, in reporting on the International Symposium on Resuscitation in Vienna, defines cardiac arrest as the clinical picture of cessation of circulation (unconsciousness; pulselessness of large arteries; apnea; and gray color) in a person who is not expected to die at the time.

---

*From Milstein, B. B.: Cardiac arrest and resuscitation, Chicago, 1963, Year Book Publishers.

119

In addition to cardiac asystole and ventricular fibrillation, extremes of tachycardia and bradycardia may be included. Cardiovascular collapse caused by a diminished myocardial contractility or hypovolemia may be so severe that acute circulatory arrest is, for all practical purposes, present.

An additional strong point in favor of the term "cardiac arrest" is that it tends to emphasize features that are paramount in effective diagnosis and successful treatment of the condition, that is, urgency and action.

Some clinicians dispute the fact that cardiac arrest often represents a "sudden and unexplained" occurrence in a hospital setting. It is true that as the years pass there is a clearer understanding of the conditions most likely to predispose to sudden ventricular arrhythmias. Nevertheless, even on very sophisticated intensive care wards, a life-threatening arrhythmia may occur without warning. Osborn, Gerbode, and their staff at the Presbyterian Medical Center in San Francisco completed a very thorough study of 150 patients in the cardiopulmonary intensive care ward with advanced instrumentation and an information system that allowed for measurements to be computed, stored, and displayed by means of an IBM 1800 digital computer. Their parameters included systolic and diastolic arterial blood pressure, mean arterial pressure, first derivative of arterial pressure, central venous pressure, respiratory rate, tidal volume, minute volume, total compliance, nonelastic resistance, peak airway pressure, end-expiratory P_{CO_2}, CO_2, minute output, inspired and end-expiratory P_{O_2}, O_2, minute intake, and three temperatures. Arterial and venous blood gases were measured routinely several times a day on the sickest patient. At irregular intervals, measurement of cardiac output was recorded. The entire group was on pressure-controlled or volume-controlled respirators, usually connected by an endotracheal tube, with some kind of tracheostomy or tight-fitting face mask.

Despite these excellent control studies, six instances of ventricular fibrillation occurred suddenly and unexpectedly and there were two cases of sudden ventricular tachycardial shock. No important physiologic changes previous to the events could be identified as etiologic in three of the eight patients; in five, however, serious disturbances in pulmonary function or ventilation were shown on the record prior to occurrence of the arrhythmia and probably contributed to it. This usually consisted of an unrecognized hypoventilation and hypercardia resulting from maladjustment or malfunction of a pressure-controlled, patient-triggered respirator. It is important to note that clinical signs are usually inadequate for a diagnosis. Blood gases probably would have been diagnostic but were not being taken frequently enough to indicate the sudden changes. Hypoventilation and hypercardia may not be as easy to diagnose as some would think, since few patients show classic signs of the condition. Long-term respiratory movements are often weak or absent. Many of the patients were heavily sedated and the normal responses were attenuated or weak from prolonged illness or surgery. From the study it is concluded that respiratory abnormalities of many kinds are common during the use of positive pressure respirators and that these abnormalities are often unrecognized without continuous measurements of respiratory parameters. A more frequent reliance on respiratory gas analyses would seem to offer one possible hope in suspecting the likelihood of sudden death in these individuals.

Fortunately, with knowledge of cardiac arrest and resuscitation becoming more widespread, generally there seems to be earlier recognition of the problem. Yet it is the delay in diagnosis, with the subsequent delay in instituting efforts at cardiac resuscitation, that is responsible for an overwhelming proportion of the unsuccessfully resuscitated patients. *Unless it is realized that cardiac arrest continues to be basically a 3-minute emergency and unless a proper evaluation of the TIME FACTOR is continually before the physician during any consideration of cardiac arrest and resuscitation, the opportunity for successful resuscitation will be severely hampered, despite hypothermia and other aids in the postresuscitative period.*

More patients lose their chance for total recovery during the crucial period between arrest and diagnosis than at any other time in the resuscitative period. It must be remembered that in almost every case of cardiac arrest there is a period during which reversibility and resuscitation are possible. To allow this short period to pass in pursuing needless diagnostic procedures, by questioning the accuracy of monitoring devices, by the use of various ineffective stimulants and other pharmacologic agents, by a frantic search for a stethoscope, or by an attempt to locate a consultant, is to add disaster to an already serious tragedy.

Monitoring

Since ventricular fibrillation is twenty-five times more likely to occur within the first 4 to 6 hours following an acute myocardial infarction than during the following 24 hours, it is absolutely essential that proper monitoring be instituted at the earliest possible moment. If such monitoring is not available through the mobile coronary unit, certainly it should be instituted immediately upon arrival in any emergency room and should be continued until the patient arrives in the coronary care unit.

Rapid advances in engineering and electronics have almost inundated the physician with newer methods of monitoring, some of which are sophisticated to the point of requiring considerable specialized knowledge. As one views the general field of resuscitation over a period of almost 25 years, it is indeed apparent that equipment and techniques once regarded as being too sophisticated for the average physician or community hospital frequently become commonplace within a short time. In my opinion, a good example of this will be provided by a follow-up in the near future of the status of blood-gas monitoring of the patient. While it is not available in all medical centers today, I believe that its use will eventually be regarded as an essential feature of hospital care of the seriously ill.

The rapidity with which the concept of the coronary care unit has covered the country is ample testimony to the willingness of the public to pay for such worthwhile adjuncts.

A questionnaire relative to their current practices in cardiac monitoring was sent to ninety-two anesthesiologists in the United States and Canada by Nicholson of the Lahey Clinic. The group of seventy-four replies included those from anesthesiologists practicing in medical centers, large metropolitan charity or private hospitals, large clinics, pediatric hospitals, and community hospitals. Of some surprise was the finding that only four of the seventy-four routinely used the ECG with the oscilloscope in monitoring their patients. With regard to the monitoring methods proved most practical, the majority indicated the pulse, blood pressure, precordial or esophageal stethoscope, or the ECG with

Table 8-1. Survival rate after cardiac arrest*

Year	Routine use of precordial stethoscope—14 hospitals		No special monitoring routine—22 hospitals	
	Number of arrests	Complete recovery	Number of arrests	Complete recovery
1958	54	26	105	30
1959	59	26	100	35
1960	62	32	102	30
Total	175	84 (47%)	307	95 (30.8%)

*From Nicholson, M. J., and Crehan, J. P.: Cardiac monitoring on clinical anesthesia: current status, Anesth. Analg. 43:109, 1964.

the oscilloscope. Of interest is the comparison of survival rates in those hospitals monitoring patients at operation and those not monitoring patients (see Table 8-1).

Monitoring in the operating room, the recovery room, and the ward has expanded to the extent that many aspects of cardiovascular, nervous, and respiratory function can be constantly observed. Monitoring of body temperature is a common practice. Because of the wide choice of available monitoring systems and because of the considerable expense required to purchase some of them, the decision by a physician or a hospital regarding adequate monitoring equipment is not always easy. Ideally, monitoring should be kept relatively simple and should answer specific questions that are of practical consideration unless investigative studies are being conducted. Monitoring of blood pressure by the indirect method is still quite satisfactory, even though the direct method will have certain indications. Heart sounds can be recorded by various photocardiographic techniques, but the anesthesiologist can audit the heart sound constantly. By means of a Ploss earpiece connected to the stethoscope by a length of 18-gauge plastic catheter, the anesthetist will have a comfortable means for continual surveillance of heart sounds. Esophageal stethoscopes are now available. Simple pulse indicators applied to the thumb provide an inexpensive and worthwhile monitor.

Failure to use available monitoring devices in the operating room may be inexcusable. The few seconds needed for attachment to the patient should not be a deterrent to the busy anesthesiologist.

Cardiac monitors may give false information as a result of inadequate initial contact of the skin electrodes, excessive perspiration resulting in loss of contact of the electrodes, displacement of electrodes under the drapes, or inadequate setting of the sensitivity on the monitor.

Advances in the effectiveness and versatility of cardiac monitoring have been dramatic. Monitors adaptable for the ward, the intensive care unit, the operating room, the emergency room, or the recovery room are now in frequent operation. Some of the more refined units include the following features: (1) a cardiac arrest alarm that sounds a loud, high-pitched tone when the heart rate falls to a preset minimum level or when cardiac arrest occurs; (2) a warning device that indicates when the heart rate reaches an alarming degree of tachycardia; (3) audible as well as visual indication of ventricular contraction; (4) a dial that indicates the heart rate per minute; (5) a built-in oscilloscope that allows continuous observation of the QRS complex.

Efforts to monitor some aspects of cardiac activity have become routine in the operating room and often in the recovery room. In addition, increasing efforts are being made to monitor cardiac activity in the patient's room (Fig. 8-1). Wilburne and Fields described a central coronary care unit that will reduce the element of chance in cardiac resuscitation of patients with known coronary involvement. *Random assignment of patients with acute coronary disease to scattered areas of the hospital is rapidly becoming an inadequate method of management.*

Monitoring activity is generally concerned with measurements of arterial pressure, peripheral pulse, electroencephalography, or electrocardiography. As an index of cardiac function, certain disadvantages are inherent in most monitoring systems. Due to vasoconstrictive effects, cardiac output may be decreased even though it is not reflected in the blood pressure reading. The drawback in an evaluation of cardiac function from ECGs is well known. An additional method of monitoring cardiac function has been suggested by Hopkins and Simeone. By positioning a balloon at the end a length of plastic tubing behind the heart and in the esophagus, cardiac impulses can be recorded. A satisfactory means of dampening the respiratory action so as not to interfere with the cardiac impulse recording has not, however, been worked out.

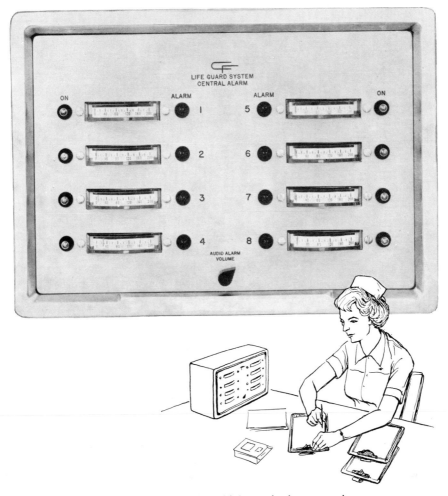

Fig. 8-1. Nursing station equipped with multiple monitoring system in coronary care area.

The rapid and accurate determination of the degree of oxygen transport in the circulating blood is a most valuable adjunct in the monitoring of the patient. In making a strong editorial plea for blood-gas monitoring in the operating room, Spencer predicts that the addition of a round-the-clock blood-gas technician to the operating room staff will soon be considered essential—as much so as is a 24-hour-a-day blood bank technician. Among all monitoring systems, serial monitoring of blood-gas tensions during operative procedures may prove to be the most useful in preventing fatal arrhythmias during surgery and in the recovery room.

Of the blood-gas measurements needing determination, arterial pH, oxygen tension, and carbon dioxide tension are essential. Oxygen and carbon dioxide tensions, as primary indices of ventilation, reflect pulmonary gas exchange. Venous oxygen tensions may be of value as a reflection of the ratio between metabolic requirements for oxygen and oxygen transport by the circulating blood. In listing the usual causes for a decrease in oxygen tension, Spencer mentions low cardiac output resulting from cardiac failure, hypovolemia, or anemia. The pH of the mixed venous blood reflects the accumulation of acids from anaerobic metabolism.

Since present-day technology allows complex determinations of blood pH, oxygen tension, and carbon dioxide tension to be rapidly run in the laboratory, serial determinations can be made at intervals as often as 30 minutes. In Spencer's opinion, cardiac arrest almost never occurs in the presence of a normal pH in the central venous blood, unless a coronary occlusion develops or a cardiac rhythm disturbance produces ventricular fibrillation.

Despite the many advances in monitoring devices, it is my belief that none begins to replace the judgment and technical skill of a competent anesthesiologist and surgeon who are both alert to any possible deviation from an accepted physiologic state.

With more widespread application of resuscitative technique brought about particularly by the use of external electrical defibrillation and closed-chest massage, the advantages of a portable cardiac monitoring device seem obvious (Trotman). One such monitor, described by Fields and co-workers, fits into a small aluminum case weighing 3 pounds. Four standard-size 1.5-volt flashlight battery cells supply the power. Standard-size ECG electrodes may be strapped directly onto the surface of each arm. A uniform, pulsatile deflection of a constant amplitude is visualized on the galvanometer. The deflection corresponds to the major wave of depolarization occurring immediately before contraction of the ventricular muscle and is comparable to the QRS complex. The unit is able to feed into a recording device, if desired. Because of the inexpensiveness, small size, portability, and self-contained power supply, such a monitor should find widespread use, particularly with a trend toward employment of resuscitative techniques by more and more lay groups and rescue squads. It would seem that police and fire departments and ambulance services would be particularly desirous of such a unit.

Small portable cardioscopes that provide adequate tracings of cardiac activity are available. Using needle-type electrodes that can be inserted subcutaneously in the deltoid region, the cardioscope can be employed with speed.

A particularly small and relatively inexpensive miniature cardiac monitor has been described by Veling. Plug-and-jack type connections have been avoided to minimize faulty electrical contact resulting in "false alarms." The unit is said to be relatively durable. It provides a "beep-beep" that coincides with each R wave.

One cardiac arrest "detector" (Edmark) utilizes the contraction of the QRS complex to cause a light on the machine to blink. In addition, a dial indicates the instantaneous heart rate in beats per minute. The sensitivity to the QRS waves can be increased or decreased at will. Unquestionably, the various cardiac monitors developed over the last several years have added considerably to the rapidity and accuracy of diagnosing cardiac arrest.

The ECG is an excellent monitor for signaling dramatic electrical dysfunctions of the heart, such as ventricular fibrillation. Unfortunately, the ECG does not always correlate with cardiac output or oxygenation sufficiently to ensure cerebral function. Mazzia and associates, in an excellent study, call attention to the dissociation between the electrical and contractile cardiac activity. In nineteen deaths associated with anesthesia during which the ECG was monitored, electrocardiographic changes failed to occur during the period of time in which cardiac output was critically depressed in at least nine patients. Mazzia and his co-workers strongly emphasize the fact that ECG monitors are not indicative of cardiac hemodynamic competence. It is not enough to assume that there is a 4-minute grace period after all cessation of cardiac activity occurs, as recorded on the ECG. Reestablishment of an adequate flow of oxygenated blood may be resumed too late if the ECG is relied upon as the sole indicator of cerebral oxygenation. As an example of this, they cite the case of a 40-year-old woman on whom a thyroidectomy was being performed. During endotracheal intubation, the patient became cyanotic and her pupils dilated. In spite of the fact that the electro-cardioscope showed no change, no pulse or blood pressure could be obtained. During the next 2 minutes, the location of the endo-tracheal tube was checked; phenylephrine and atropine were also administered. It was not until the lapse of 2 minutes that cardiac standstill was diagnosed on the basis of the ECG. Even though external cardiac massage was then immediately instituted, the patient's color improved, the pupils became miotic, and spontaneous respirations returned, the patient never regained consciousness and she died 2 weeks later. *In the presence of clinical evidence of anoxia, there is no place for procrastination in the decision to institute manual systole because of a normal-appearing ECG complex.*

While the ECG does, of course, have real value, its limitations must be realized, and it must be combined with other monitoring methods such as the EEG, an earlobe oxim-eter, a pulse pickup monitor on the earlobe or nasal septum, or other means that indi-cate cardiac activity and cerebral oxygena-tion.

Since the ECG may continue to appear fairly normal for several minutes after car-diac arrest, anesthesiologists at the Sick Chil-dren's Hospital in Toronto, Canada, perform closed-chest cardiac compression for 1 to 2 minutes at any time the circulation appears to be grossly inadequate, without waiting to see if the heart has arrested. In many in-stances, complete cardiac standstill may be avoided (Conn, as quoted by Nicholson).

ECG monitoring of the activity of the heart is certainly not foolproof. Many studies are available to support the fact that ECG activity may be present for some time after the onset of a completely ineffective heart-beat. Usually these tracings are abnormal. This may not always be the case, however, as brought out in a number of reports. For example, Sabawala and his colleagues ob-tained an apparently normal ECG from a heart that was not performing effectively as a pump.

MONITORING OF SURGICAL PATIENTS

Although the value of monitoring all sur-gical patients would seem obvious, the feasi-bility of such monitoring has been questioned. Is it practical to do so? Do monitors consti-tute an unjustified distraction? At the Lahey Clinic, the home of the first successful case of cardiac defibrillation using drugs, in 1941, concern arose because of failure to improve the recovery rate in patients with cardiac standstill and ventricular fibrillation. A de-cision to obtain more factual information concerning the role of cardiac monitoring in clinical anesthesia prompted a 6-month study during which 500 consecutive patients were monitored. All patients were included in the study except those undergoing open-heart operations. Of particular significance is the occurrence of eight episodes of cardiac standstill that were promptly recog-nized, with seven successfully resuscitated (88%). All seven were discharged from the hospital without a neurologic deficit. In all eight patients, a monitor-pacemaker de-vice was used to provide immediate external electric stimulation and pacing. If the pacing was unsuccessful after 2 minutes, either closed-chest cardiac massage or thoracotomy with manual systole was the plan.

In the years between 1941 and 1962 the usual rate of successful resuscitation of car-diac arrest in patients during anesthesia re-mained around 30% at the Lahey Clinic. Since the use of the monitor-pacemaker, the recovery rate has risen to almost 83%.

MISTAKES IN DIAGNOSIS

Although oscilloscopic monitoring of the electrocardiogram is extremely valuable, dis-tortions do occur that may lead to serious errors in interpretation of the ECG. This prompted Arbeit and co-workers to urge that conventional tracings be taken directly from the patient and not through the monitor before definitive therapy based on electrocardiographic abnormalities is instituted. The rapid sweep of the scope, the evanescent character of the display, the unstable base line, movement of the patient, shifting of electrodes, and introduction of artifacts by the electronic filtering circuits all contribute to possible errors of interpretation.

It is difficult to estimate how often closed-chest compression is used when, in actuality, cardiac arrest is not really present. Hopefully, this is not frequent, since closed-chest compression is not a benign procedure—even in the hands of a trained surgeon. As with the open-chest approach, accurate knowledge of the presence of cardiac arrest is desirable.

How often will a mistake in diagnosis occur? In the cases originally reviewed, there were six instances where, when a thoracotomy was performed, the heart was found, not in standstill or ventricular fibrillation, but beating weakly. Such cases will occasionally be encountered, but it will usually be that the output of the heart is of inadequate strength to supply the necessary amount of oxygen to the cerebral cortex. Manual massage will be of value in restoring the myocardial tone to its normal cardiac output. On two occasions the heart was in complete standstill and was started upon opening the chest. In no case have I seen a thoracotomy performed on a heart that was still beating when a detrimental reaction was encountered. Recoveries were made in all cases. The fear of an occasional mistaken diagnosis should not be a deterring influence on prompt, immediate resuscitative measures.

It is now known that closed-chest compression or cardiac massage is of some value in "assisting the heart"—especially during periods of prolonged bradycardia and/or shock. Furthermore, there will be times when mistaken diagnosis can hardly be avoided. These mistakes must be accepted if the survival rate of the actual cases of cardiac arrest is to be improved. Also, it is true that all cases that are eligible for cardiac resuscitation are not true cases of cardiac arrest per se. The exact mechanism of a sudden, fatal, so-called anaphylactic response to a penicillin injection is not well understood at present. Circulatory and respiratory failure that occurs with sudden allergic responses can be aided by the usual cardiac resuscitative procedures until such time as the anaphylactic response has subsided. Periods of asystole lasting 30 seconds or so are well known, and spontaneous recovery without massage or stimulants occasionally may be encountered.

Periods of asystole associated with Adams-Stokes attacks may persist for 20 to 30 seconds. Unless the pulse of such an individual is being checked at the exact time the arrest occurs, considerably longer than 30 seconds will usually pass before a diagnosis of cardiac arrest has been made. Therefore, in these cases of transient standstill of the heart (very rarely, ventricular fibrillation), a return to a spontaneous contraction will have occurred before efforts at resuscitation have begun.

Turk and Glenn report having found the heart beating in two cases at the time of thoracotomy for cardiac arrest. This was from a collection of forty-two cases. In one patient, cardiac compression was instituted because the heartbeat was feeble and slow; a rapid recovery ensued. In another patient, the cardiac arrest was diagnosed in the outpatient clinic where the patient was undergoing local anesthetization with tetracaine (Pontocaine) for bronchography. In spite of septic technique, the patient recovered completely, with no ill effects from the thoracotomy. The heart was found to be contracting slowly on exposure.

From Toronto, Canada, at St. Michael's Hospital, Mullens reports a case in which the chest was opened and the heart was found beating with normal rhythm but very weakly. I agree with his statement that: "No surgeon should apologize for such an eventuality. The hesitant surgeon can convince himself of a distant beat in what is actually a silent chest. Thoracotomy is a much safer procedure than spending precious time at prolonged auscultation." This statement was made in 1955. With closed-chest compression, the heart could probably have been effectively assisted.

Mistakes as to the mechanism of the arrest may lead to difficulties. For example, unless a cardiac tamponade or a right-sided air embolus is suspected, the most effective method of treatment may be neglected.

PORTABLE ELECTROCARDIOGRAPH

There is increasing use of portable electrocardiographs. Such instruments do not have a warm-up period and can thus be utilized more quickly. In some states, the highway patrol uses portable electrocardiographs as a means of confirming death.

THE PULSE MONITOR

The value of the pulse monitor as an early indicator of a general systemic circulatory disturbance—even in the face of a normal ECG—should be stressed. Cope connected a photoelectric gauge amplifier to the pacemaker cardiac monitor for auditory and visual display of digital pulse. There are commercially available pulsometers that may be connected to pacemaker monitors.

The ability to achieve pulse monitoring at the nasal septum has occurred with the development of a rhinoplethysmography device. This monitoring system uses a rhinotransducer containing photoelectric components in two curved aluminum shafts that fit into the nares, extending above the level of the inferior turbinates. The light beam passes through the septum and, with each heartbeat, senses density changes in the terminal branches of the anterior ethmoidal artery. This nosepiece monitoring system receives its signals primarily from the internal carotid arterial system. It can be positioned quickly and easily.

Pulse monitoring at the nasal septum has been studied by Groveman and associates as a means of reflecting the cerebral blood flow. It was Groveman's belief that monitoring at the nasal septum above the level of the inferior turbinates reflects a constant picture of the internal carotid circulation. In at least three instances of cardiac arrest, the rhinoplethysmography pulse monitoring device was used to monitor the patient during cardiac massage. The efficacy of the massage apparently was reflected in the amplitude and configuration of pulse waves. It was noted that as the compression efforts lagged, there was an evident decrease, and the relieving operator's efforts were reflected in an increase in the amplitude of the waves (see Fig. 8-2).

RESPIRATORY MONITORING IN INFANTS

An apnea alarm system has been devised (see Fig. 8-3) that sounds an alarm and flashes a light when breathing stops in infants. The device is so simple that there are no electrodes or connections to the infant.

Recognition of cardiac arrest

The appearance of a sudden bradycardia and subsequent drop in blood pressure may provide a few seconds of warning that ventricular asystole is close at hand. Ventricular arrhythmias, especially ventricular tachycardia, may signal the onset of ventricular fibrillation.

Ziegler calls attention to the frequency of cardiac arrests in operations upon patients with cyanotic heart disease and states that in 80% of 175 patients some type of arrhythmia occurred. Nine of the patients died from cardiac arrest that was first manifested as a persistent bradycardia.

DeCamp says cardiac arrest almost never occurs without warning signs. He lists these signs as cyanosis, bradycardia, hypotension, changes in respiration, downward displacement of the pacemaker, repetitive ectopic beats, change in atrioventricular or interventricular conduction, and unexplained changes in the level of anesthesia. Harken and co-workers indicate that in their experience almost all instances of ventricular fibrillation occurring during cardiac surgery were preceded by a period of ventricular

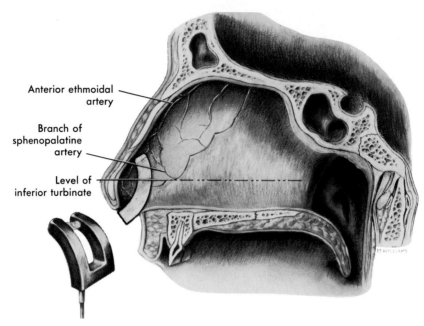

Anterior ethmoidal
artery

Branch of
sphenopalatine
artery

Level of
inferior turbinate

Fig. 8-2. Rhinoplethysmography pulse monitoring at the nasal septum. Rhinoplethysmography allows monitoring of branches of the internal carotid artery by means of a photoelectric plethysmograph placed at the nasal septum. Efficacy of cardiac massage may be indicated by the amplitude of the pulse waves recorded. (From Groveman, J., and others: Anesth. Analg. 45:63-68, 1966; Courtesy Corbin-Farnsworth Division of Smith, Kline & French Instruments, Inc., Palo Alto, Calif.)

tachycardia. Blades relies on ECG changes as reliable signs of impending ventricular fibrillation in patients under hypothermic anesthesia.

Greenberg analyzes events preceding arrest in a group of twenty infants and reports one or more signs of respiratory embarrassment in most cases. Laryngeal spasm, excessive tracheobranchial secretions, tracheal rales and rhonchi, tachypnea, and cyanosis are the usual signs of respiratory distress.

With an acidotic state, the ventricular fibrillation threshold may be so lowered that the usual premonitory arrhythmias, such as extrasystoles, may be absent and ventricular fibrillation may occur without warning.

Mazel and associates consider the most common changes preceding cardiac arrest during surgery to be hypotension (a 10- to 20-mm. drop without apparent cause), sudden bradycardia or tachycardia, cyanosis, and

unexplained changes in the level of anesthesia and changes in respiration.

PALPATION

If a surgeon is operating in the vicinity of a large vessel, then palpation of that vessel should offer an immediate appraisal as to whether a satisfactory cardiac output is being maintained and if there is pulse. The carotid, femoral, and brachial arteries are usually easily accessible.

AUSCULTATION

Prolonged auscultation with a stethoscope should be warned against. Not only can it be time consuming but also it seldom provides reliable evidence of the action of the heart when the blood pressure and pulse no longer are present.

How much reliance can be placed on the absence of heart sounds? The probable

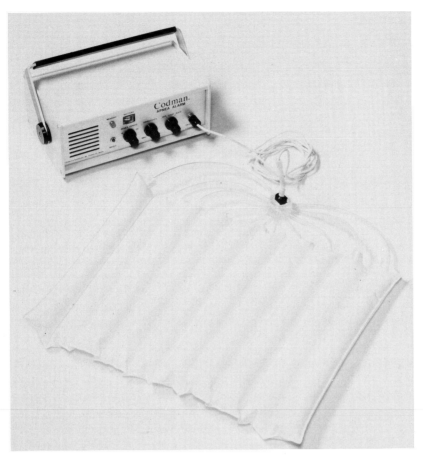

Fig. 8-3. Apnea Alarm mattress. (Courtesy Codman & Shurtleff, Inc., Randolph, Mass.)

answer to this is that, for the most part, a great deal of reliance can be placed upon the presence or absence of heart sounds and the relationship to an adequate circulation. In dogs all heart sounds cease at a systolic pressure of 50 mm. Hg (Swan). Therefore if no sounds can be heard it is likely that circulation has probably failed. Swan believes that, in man, heart sounds presumably fail at about the same pressure; hence, the absence of heart sounds in man following anoxic accidents probably means that the circulation has also failed. Therefore, if there is not too much extraneous noise and if the patient's chest is not too bulky, the absence of heart sounds will usually be indicative of inade-

quate cardiac output, although not necessarily complete cardiac standstill.

Table 8-2 provides helpful differential aids in the diagnosing of cardiac arrhythmias.

HICCUPS

The significance of the hiccup as an indication of poor ventilation and oxygenation with a high frequency of association with cardiac arrest is stressed by White (as quoted by Stiles). This well-known Seattle surgeon reports a high incidence of both hiccup and cardiac arrest in patients with biliary-pancreatic disease or recurrent ulcers, often with accompanying pulmonary problems. He recommends that a celiac-ganglion block be used

Table 8-2. The heart rate as a valuable clue in diagnosis of certain cardiac arrhythmias*

Arrhythmia	Rhythm	Ventricular rate (beats per minute)	Comments
Sinus tachycardia	Regular	100 to 180	May exceed 200 in children; slight variation in rate over period of hours is common
Paroxysmal atrial tachycardia	Regular	140 to 240	Rhythm usually perfectly regular over period of time
Atrial flutter	Regular	150, 100, 75	Conduction usually 2:1, 3:1, 4:1, etc.; not irregular
Atrial fibrillation	Grossly irregular	140 to 200	Usually in range of 140 to 170 in untreated case
A-V nodal tachycardia	Regular	100 to 180	Behaves like PAT
Ventricular tachycardia	Regular or slightly irregular	100 to 180	Sometimes slightly irregular; usually not affected by carotid sinus pressure
Sinus bradycardia	Regular	40 to 60	Normal P-R relationships
A-V nodal rhythm (escape)	Regular	40 to 60	May be associated with A-V dissociation; look for capture beats
Idioventricular rhythm	Regular	30 to 40	Associated with complete heart block

*From Hurst, J. W., and Myerburg, R. J.: Cardiovascular arrhythmias: evolving concepts (1), Mod. Concepts Cardiovasc. Dis. **37**:73, 1968.

in patients who have hiccup at the time of surgery. Ritalin (10 mg. four times a day) is effective in stopping hiccups occurring postoperatively.

CESSATION OF RESPIRATIONS

There may often be a discussion as to whether respiratory arrest preceded or followed cessation of cardiac action. Sudden and complete anoxia may be characterized initially by hyperventilation and convulsive action and eventually by agonal, gasping respiratory activity. Initially, tachycardia is seen. The blood pressure usually rises temporarily, only to fall precipitously. Thus abrupt cardiopulmonary failure may not always have its origin on a cardiac basis but may simply be a respiratory arrest with subsequent cardiac collapse. It may occur after various instances of airway obstruction, near drowning, drug overdose, electrical shock, and a variety of other causes.

Often, within a matter of several seconds after the circulatory system breaks down with complete absence of cardiac output, the respiratory center will likewise cease func-

tioning. Following resuscitation of the heart, the respiratory center responds in a variety of ways, and there is no set pattern indicating the point at which it will return. Occasionally, weak voluntary respirations will continue for several minutes after cardiac output is absent. Unfortunately, cessation of respirations is sometimes the first thing noted, when actual circulatory arrest may have been present for some time. Frequently a few agonal respiratory efforts will follow sudden cessation of heart action. The mechanism of these agonal movements has been well discussed by Negovskii.

In some patients, cessation of respiration may be difficult to ascertain quickly, even though one carefully observes for respiratory motion or listens for breath sounds. In such instances it will be wise to assume that ventilation is inadequate, regardless of the cause.

OPHTHALMOLOGIC EVIDENCE OF CARDIAC ARREST

The pupillary findings under conditions of severe anoxia must be differentiated from those seen with complete circulatory arrest.

Jordanov and Ruben considered the reliability of pupillary changes as a clinical sign of anoxia and concluded that patients in respiratory failure who had clinical signs of severe anoxia and extremely low oxygen tension levels did not display any increase in pupillary size. Pupillary size cannot, according to their studies, be used as a reliable sign of anoxia, even when the anoxia ·is severe. Pupillary diameter does increase to marked dilatation when circulatory arrest occurs. In hundreds of dogs arrested with electrical fibrillation, full pupillary dilatation was a regularly observed response; I cannot recall a single instance in which pupillary dilatation failed to occur. The importance of the size of the pupil as a critical monitor of survivability during the use of expired air ventilation and closed-chest massage is emphasized by Lee and associates. They found that small pupils nearly always predict survival in dogs being resuscitated with expired air.

Some dispute continues as to the value of the size of the pupils as a reliable sign of cerebral anoxia. There is the occasional case in which pupils remain contracted in spite of unsuccessful external cardiac massage.

Rather large dilated pupils may be encountered under conditions of both light and very deep anesthesia. Bilaterally fixed pupils may occasionally be seen in patients with epidural hematomas and if resuscitative efforts are prompt, the patients may survive.

It has been suggested that pupillary dilatation (because of the ease with which it can be observed) affords a satisfactory means of diagnosing cardiac arrest, especially if one is not adept at feeling large vessel pulsations. Since there is an appreciable lag between cessation of cardiac output and full dilatation, it is most desirable that resuscitation be started before such dilatation occurs.

As a rule, pupils begin dilating within 20 seconds after complete circulatory arrest and reach full dilatation by 45 seconds. Similarly, the pupils represent a reliable index of return of cerebral perfusion, either by manual or artificial means, or as an indication of return of spontaneous cardiac output.

Gilston has pointed out that pupils may remain small even after death of the patient, particularly in patients having been administered morphine sulfate or other opiates. On the other hand, dilated pupils do not

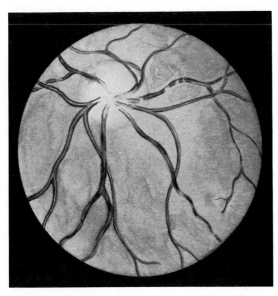

Fig. 8-4. Segmentation of blood flow as seen upon funduscopic examination.

always mean circulatory arrest. Patients under varying degrees of hypothermia may exhibit widely dilated pupils, as will patients who have recently received atropine, quinidine, or epinephrine. Halothane anesthesia and ganglion-blocking drugs also dilate the pupils.

Pupils are not a reliable index of respiratory insufficiency and anoxia. Jordanov's studies point out that, during anoxic episodes, pupils often either contract or fail to change in size.

Retinal changes indicative of insufficient cardiac output have been known for many years. Segmentation of retinal venous columns and disappearance of the retinal arterial pattern are noted within a minute or so after cardiac output ceases (Fig. 8-4). Unquestionably, such findings are of considerable diagnostic value if there is a serious question as to whether or not cardiac arrest has occurred. It does appear, however, that the value of the funduscopic examination as a diagnostic tool in cardiac arrest is limited. Other physical findings are more easily available at an earlier stage. The question of availability of an ophthalmoscope, the extra delay necessitated by its use, and the questionable interpretation of the findings tend to dampen my enthusiasm for this diagnostic procedure.

There are times, however, when ophthalmoscopic determination of cardiac arrest may be of distinct value. Failure to visualize segmentation of retinal venous vessels would raise a question as to whether cardiac arrest has occurred. A good review of the ophthalmoscopic findings following circulatory arrest has been provided by Kevorkian.

A most significant observation on the circulation of the retinal vessels during exsanguinating hemorrhage is recorded by Farmati (Kirimli and others). Ophthalmoscopy and retinal photography were performed during the experiments.

It is important to realize that fixed, dilated pupils are not always a sign of irreversible brain damage. In a case reported by Shocket and Rosenblum, dilated pupils were present for 45 minutes during cardiac resuscitation techniques without any neurologic sequelae. Two years later the patient, a stockbroker, was functioning effectively. The observation that pupils are widely dilated and fixed does not constitute reason to abandon resuscitation efforts because it has repeatedly been observed that unresponsive pupils during the period of resuscitation does not in itself demonstrate conclusively that irreversible brain injury has occurred or that further efforts at resuscitation are futile.

ELECTROENCEPHALOGRAPHY

It is significant to note that flattening of the EEG waves occurs rather suddenly in dogs after about 20 seconds of circulatory arrest and within another 5 to 10 seconds thereafter, the EEG becomes isoelectric. Sealy and his group have shown that at this point (20 seconds) the cerebral synthesis of its primary source of chemical energy, ATP, is reduced 10%. In dogs this occurs within an average of 3.1 seconds.

Electroencephalography provides an excellent means of determining cessation of circulation. EEG tracings will reveal absence of alpha, gamma, and beta waves after about 20 seconds of total anoxia of the brain—even before respiratory arrest may be noted or before the ECG tracings show cessation of cardiac electrical activity (Fig. 8-5).

The practicality of obtaining constant EEG tracings has become a reality with the introduction of relatively low-cost machines. The value of the electroencephalogram lies not only in its diagnostic ability but also in its usefulness as an index of the expected prognosis.

CAPILLARY REFILL

Capillary refill cannot be depended upon since it is often observed for 20 to 30 minutes after the heart has stopped.

INTRACARDIAC NEEDLE INJECTION

Formerly it was a common practice, upon making the diagnosis of cardiac arrest, to

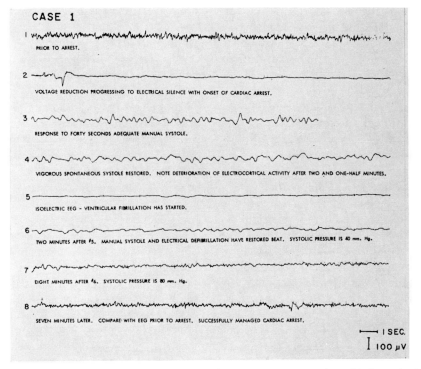

Fig. 8-5. Serial EEG pattern in patient with cardiac arrest. (From Brechner, V. L., and others: Anesth. Analg. **40**:1, 1961.)

insert a needle into the heart through the intact chest wall and to inject epinephrine hydrochloride. It is true that stimulation of the heart through the intact chest wall by needle will occasionally revive spontaneous beating in some hearts, particularly those in which a sudden vagovagal arrest has occurred. As far as I am able to determine, however, this practice is to be partially condemned. The time needed for making this observation and finding and preparing the needle often eliminates the possibility of being able to do anything else if this measure is ineffective. The time lag has already been too great. Successful cases probably result from the mechanical stimulation of a needle on the pericardium and on the myocardium. If the heart is in complete standstill, the injection of a drug can be of little value since it will only pool in the lumen of the portion of the heart into which it has been injected. This procedure is to be condemned not only

for the above reasons but also because, first, it will occupy a valuable portion of the time necessary before irreversible damage will occur and, second, by injecting drugs into the heart, one obscures the true diagnosis of the condition of the arrest. Cardiac standstill may be present; however, the possibility of ventricular fibrillation should not be overlooked, for in such a patient recovery will seldom occur without the use of manual systole and attempts at defibrillation.

VENOUS PULSE

Occasionally, because of atrial activity, a venous pulse may be temporarily visible in the neck. Auricular contractions do not, of course, necessarily cease with the onset of ventricular fibrillation.

CYANOSIS

If one relies upon the clinical manifestations of anoxemia as indicated by cyanosis, particularly of the lips, lobules of the ear, and the face, then one may occasionally fail to suspect anoxia because it has not become clinically apparent. Five grams of reduced hemoglobin is necessary before cyanosis is evident.

Dwyer and Gunner encountered a 28-year-old nurse with phenacetin cyanosis who, at laparotomy for recurrent intestinal obstruction, experienced cardiac arrest. The preoperative cyanosis from phenacetin overdose presented an interesting complication.

Cyanosis may not be an obvious feature of arrested cardiac output of several minutes duration, especially if the patient has been breathing air with a high oxygen concentration. Dark-skinned individuals pose an additional problem in this regard.

DIASTOLE OR SYSTOLE?

Cessation of the heart in a tetanic-like spasm or in systole is extremely rare in my experience. Cessation in diastole is much more common. Although cessation in systole is an extremely rare occurrence, DeCamp suggests it would be wise to apply 5 to 10 ml. of a 1% procaine solution to the surface of the heart and to inject 5 to 10 ml. into the left ventricle. Massage should be continued in the hope that the myocardium will relax.

Several cases of cardiac arrest have been observed in patients following severe exsanguinating hemorrhage from an ectopic pregnancy. The hearts of these patients have been noted to be small and contracted before massage was begun.

ASYSTOLE, VENTRICULAR FIBRILLATION, OR PROFOUND CARDIOVASCULAR COLLAPSE?

These three clinical conditions, asystole, ventricular fibrillation, and profound cardiovascular collapse, have a common denominator—inadequate cardiac output. All lead within a few minutes to irreversible cerebral cortical damage. At the onset, the precise state of the heart is an almost academic consideration because cardiopulmonary assist is urgent and the initial steps in resuscitation are similar. If respiratory arrest is not already present, failure of respiration will follow within seconds.

The relative frequency of asystole and ventricular fibrillation is discussed in another section. Since resuscitative efforts now involve large groups of myocardial infarct cases, ventricular fibrillation is encountered much more frequently and has become a prominent feature in cardiopulmonary resuscitation.

With the sudden occurrence of cardiac arrest, a differentiation between cardiac standstill and ventricular fibrillation is all but impossible on physical examination. On several occasions I have witnessed the inability of physicians to diagnose ventricular fibrillation, even with the chest open, particularly if it is through the intact pericardial sac. In these instances when the pericardium is not open, the fibrillary action of the myocardium may be so weak that a diagnosis is not readily made. It is also true that some physicians simply are unaware of what a fibrillating ventricle looks like.

Although of questionable diagnostic value, it should be mentioned that a venous pulse may often be present in ventricular fibrillation for a period of time. This is due to auricular activity, which seldom ceases with the onset of ventricular fibrillation.

Certain situations that may occur should suggest the possibility of ventricular fibrillation. Accidental electrocution is perhaps the outstanding example of this. Cardiac arrest following the rapid administration of digitalis sometimes may be assumed to consist of ventricular fibrillation. If an electrocardiograph is connected to the patient at the time of the arrest, then the diagnosis of ventricular fibrillation can be made almost with certainty. If the chest has been opened, ventricular fibrillation can be diagnosed as readily by palpation as by visualization. Holding the heart in the palm of the hand, one notes the sensation of a fluttering, undulating convulsiveness of a wormlike nature. This is caused by various blocks of myocardial tissue contracting with different degrees of strength at different rates and rhythms. Various descriptions have been given to this sensation. Grudel described it as a wormlike movement of the ventricular muscle; Wiggers described it as a fluttering, undulating, convulsive sensation; and McWilliam called it an arrhythmic oscillation of the ventricular walls.

DIAGNOSIS OF VENTRICULAR FIBRILLATION

Attacks of ventricular fibrillation are most frequently initiated by an acceleration of the basic ventricular rhythm, by premature beats, or by short runs of irregular ventricular oscillations.

If ventricular fibrillation persists 3 seconds or more, a sensation of faintness is experienced. After 10 to 20 seconds, syncope occurs. If the arrhythmia persists for 40 seconds, convulsions, apnea, and often incontinence will occur.

Patients dying suddenly from an acute myocardial infarct or following accidental electrocution are frequently described as having suddenly cried out in pain and anguish. Children dying suddenly with anomalous coronary artery disease have been described in the same way. This observation may be of diagnostic value in ventricular fibrillation, since anginal pain and fibrillation theoretically may relate to the same altered physiology, that is, localized anoxia of the myocardium. Generalized anoxic myocardium, however, seldom seems to associate itself with anginal pain.

In several instances the diagnosis of ventricular fibrillation has been made by the insertion of a spinal needle through the chest wall. In such cases, the needle has been noted to have a fine, oscillating movement interpreted as ventricular fibrillation. Medford states that in several instances he has confirmed the transthoracic needle technique by simultaneous ECG.

DIAGNOSIS OF RUPTURED VENTRICLE

Much of the picture of an acute cardiac arrest may present itself with the rupture of a ventricle. Robinson, in a personal communication with Wynn, reports a successful resuscitation with a 3-week survival using internal cardiac massage and surgical repair of the ruptured ventricle.

A cardiac rupture may be suspected when the arrest occurs in a patient several days after a myocardial infarct. If the patient is being monitored, the ECG may continue to reveal a sinus rhythm with normal QRS complexes.

ATRIAL STANDSTILL

Persistent atrial arrest is extremely rare. In a review of world literature, Bloomfield and Sinclair-Smith were able to find only thirty-three reports of atrial arrest in the presence of beating ventricles. They did, however, describe a patient who experienced persistent atrial standstill. For such a diagnosis, the following criteria are suggested:

1. Absence of P wave activity in any lead of the ECG
2. Absence of A wave in the neck veins
3. Regular rhythm, the ventricular complex of ECG being the usual supraventricular type
4. No evidence of P wave activity with intracardiac ECG
5. No evidence of A wave component in intra-atrial pressures
6. Immobility of the atrium as shown by fluoroscopy and cineangiocardiography

The rate of their patient's heart increased from 38 to 64 beats per minute on atropine sulfate, and he was subsequently managed on a maintenance dose of atropine sulfate.

CARDIAC TAMPONADE

As pointed out elsewhere in this book, the diagnosis of cardiac arrest resulting from tamponade may be suspected in some instances because of the nature of the trauma or the history preceding the arrest. Pericardiocentesis is of questionable diagnostic value since the bleeding into the pericardium tends to clot if the blood loss has been rapid. The agitation of the blood by action of the heart and lungs, in instances of rapid bleeding, is not adequate to defibrinogenate the blood. Defibrinogenation is more likely to occur with relatively slow bleeding.

The ECG cannot be relied upon for diagnosis of pericardial tamponade since it may be unchanged except for a decreased amplitude. It should be noted that positive pressure artificial respiration will increase the intrathoracic pressure, which in turn aggravates the degree of cardiac tamponade and further reduces the blood pressure.

CARDIAC ARREST CAUSED BY AIR EMBOLISM

Air in the right side of the heart or in the pulmonary circulation characteristically produces what is termed a "washboard" type of sound (also, the murmur is often described as a "water-wheel," "mill-wheel" [bruit de moulin], or "washing-machine" sound). The pathognomonic sound heard with air emboli to the right side of the heart results from the churning and splashing of the blood and air mixture in the heart. Often there will be a preliminary episode of chest pain and dyspnea. If air or gaseous mixtures enter the left side of the heart or arterial circulation, cerebral manifestations may be present in addition to cardiac manifestations. Air bubbles may even be seen passing along in the retinal circulation. "Air bleeding" sometimes may be noted from open vessels.

The continuous "mill-wheel" murmur was audible in three of eleven documented cases of air embolism. An elevation of venous pressure, a decrease in arterial blood pressure, and a cardiac arrhythmia are all suggestive of obstructed flow in the right side of the heart.

Since direct aspiration of air from the heart has not always been successful, Michenfelder and co-workers report the successful aspiration of air by a percutaneous central venous monitoring catheter.

THORACOTOMY AS A DIAGNOSTIC PROCEDURE

With present monitoring equipment, the indications for doing a diagnostic thoracot-

omy when cardiac arrest is suspected seem less urgent. Our general plan is to use closed-chest compression and mouth-to-mouth respiration until an ECG can give the precise condition of the cardiac activity. If an electrocardiograph is not available, an open thoracotomy will sometimes be a wise action. In such situations the words of Johnson and Kirby regarding a thoracotomy still hold:

> This may seem like an unnecessary, aggressive policy to those who are not familiar with this catastrophe because of the possibilities that the heart may be beating so feebly that signs of effective circulation are lacking. It is true that this possibility does exist, but we believe that this risk must be accepted.*

They state that they have found the heart to be beating feebly only once, and that patient survived. I have seen one chest opened under a similar situation when apparently the stimulatory effect from the thoracotomy was sufficient to provoke nodal rhythm of the heart. In the three cases of cardiac arrest in our registry in which the chest was opened and the heart was found beating, even though feebly, there was no fatality.

Summary

It should be pointed out that some monitoring devices fail to signal the presence of ventricular fibrillation, particularly because the ventricular fibrillary waves are of sufficient potential to be sensed as an impulse by the monitoring device. It is important to have a device that will trigger tachycardia or ventricular fibrillation.

Despite a large number of monitoring devices, the advantages and reliability of the "finger-on-the-pulse" method of following cardiac activity during surgery are, indeed, still obvious. Knowledge of limitations and drawbacks of mechanical devices is, likewise, obviously advantageous.

Even with direct vision of the heart, mis-

---

*From Johnson, J., and Kirby, C. K.: Cardiac standstill and ventricular fibrillation, Am. Pract. Digest Treat. 5:264-269, 1954.

takes in diagnosis are not uncommon. A vigorously fibrillating myocardium has been mistaken for ventricular tachycardia. More commonly, however, a weakly fibrillating ventricle can appear, through the unopened pericardial sac, to be in asystole.

During an abdominal or thoracic procedure, the diagnosis of cardiac arrest should present little difficulty. I have, however, seen at least two cases in which the heart had stopped during an intrathoracic operation and the attention of the surgeon was directed to the heart action by the anesthetist. Either visualization of the heart itself or palpation of the aorta or one of the larger vessels should quickly reveal whether or not any cardiac output is present. If, for example, the patient is undergoing anesthesia induction, then the absence of any blood pressure or pulse should be regarded as most significant.

In spite of the possibility that a rare instance may occur when cardiac standstill is not actually complete, it would seem logical to place the burden of proof on the individual who insists that the output of the heart is sufficient to maintain adequate cerebral circulation. Since the 4-minute period during which reversible changes may occur passes so rapidly, I have little patience with those who would urge needless diagnostic procedures to confirm what is already obvious.

During a 1-year period at the Toronto General Hospital, 184 arrests were analyzed. In 60% of the cases the initial recognition of the arrest was made by the nurse and in 33% by the physician. The diagnosis was made by a monitoring device in only 15% of the instances. The clinical findings of no pulse, respiration, or a combination of both constituted the first sign of the arrest in the remaining cases.

The delay in making a diagnosis of cardiac arrest (with its subsequent delay in instituting treatment) is responsible for the bulk of the failures of resuscitation. Until the simplicity of making a diagnosis of cardiac arrest is understood, it is likely that the appalling mortality from episodes of sudden failure of the heart will continue. The best rule of thumb is that if there is no palpable pulse and no obtainable blood pressure, both of which have disappeared suddenly, then the diagnosis of cardiac arrest can be made with every reasonable degree of assurance. Let those who disagree assume the burden of proof that under such situations the cardiac activity is sufficient for life. Again, more patients lose their chance for recovery during this crucial period between arrest and diagnosis than from any other aspect of the resuscitative procedure. The time factor represents the crux of successful resuscitation. Few patients can survive after a delay of more than 4 minutes before artificial circulatory activity is maintained by manual systole. Since the period of reversibility is almost always present in cardiac arrest, it is tragic to allow this period to pass in following time-consuming diagnostic procedures such as searching frantically for a stethoscope or trying to obtain consultation from others. The patient's chance for survival rests with the personnel who are with the patient at the time of arrest.

PART THREE

MECHANISM
OF CARDIAC ARREST

Chapter 9

PATHOPHYSIOLOGY OF CARDIAC ARREST

In the more than 25 years since work began on this book, there has been an increased understanding of the mechanisms involved in sudden arrest of the heart's functioning ability. Many isolated and recorded clinical observations along with research efforts in related fields have served to further complete the picture. Less controversy over interpretation of information exists. Even so, this chapter has been written with the intent to present a range of viewpoints since the final scheme is still ahead. Through a better understanding of the pathophysiology of cardiac arrest will inevitably come more effective therapy.

In any consideration of cardiac arrest, we almost always refer to a sudden acute stoppage of the heart and not to the gradual cessation of cardiac contractions.

The role of the vagus nerve in production of cardiac arrest

To paraphrase a famous reply a reporter over 80 years ago made to a little friend's inquiry about Santa Claus, Yes, Virginia, there *is* a vagovagal reflex. The role of the vagus nerves as significant factors in the causation of cardiac arrest has been a source of dispute over the years. In 1953, when I reported on the first 1,200 cases of cardiac arrest in the Cardiac Arrest Registry, I concluded there was suggestive evidence of significant vagovagal effect as a major factor in the etiology of almost 25% of the cases. Even so, numerous authors continue to omit vagal nerve reflex action in their discussions of the etiologic aspects of cardiac asystole or ventricular fibrillation. One intent of this chapter is to reemphasize the significant role played by the tenth cranial nerves in their relationship to the heart. By collating some

of the varied clinical relationships we may more nearly define the action of the vagi on the neuromuscular control of the heart. Furthermore, it is increasingly apparent that significant preventive measures are available that need to be used in a wider variety of clinical situations.

While our knowledge of vagal reflex actions may still be in its infancy, the last two decades have seen a considerable unfolding of the various sensory, motor, and secretory relationships of the vagus nerve. Witness the remarkable strides toward a clinical understanding of the vagus in gastric functions and peptic ulcer disease. Changes in pancreatic secretory function and biliary stasis have been observed as by-products of vagus section for duodenal ulcer. It is obvious that most medical specialties are involved in the neurovisceral aspects of this, the longest cranial nerve.

More recently, vagal inhibition has been purposefully applied in a variety of ways. For example, knowledge of the vagal effect from the carotid sinus reflex is reported by Braunwald and co-workers for the treatment of intractable angina pectoris. By augmenting the frequency of efferent vagal stimuli and reducing the frequency of sympathetic efferent impulses distributed to the heart by stimulation of the carotid sinus nerves, the oxygen requirements of the myocardium are decreased. As a result of a slowing of the heart rate there is a decrease in myocardial contractility and a fall in arterial pressure.

Also noting that oxygen consumption by the left ventricle appears to decrease and cardiac efficiency appears to increase during vagal stimulation, Bilgutay and co-workers utilized vagal tuning to slow heart rate and preserve sinus rhythm. Progressive slowing of the P-R interval, leading to atrial ventricular block and nodal rhythm, occurred as the voltage level increased.

The vagomimetic action of anoxia on the myocardium has more clearly come into focus with the realization that a large percentage of myocardial infarctions are associated with marked vagotonia including nausea, vomiting, tenesmus, and sinoatrial bradycardia. Atrial bradycardia is estimated to be as frequent as once in every five myocardial infarctions. Particularly is this likely to occur when the area of the right atrium is affected from an inadequate right coronary artery blood supply. Adequate amounts of atropine often may be lifesaving. Pantridge found bradyarrhythmias in 44% of 1,150 patients with acute myocardial infarction managed by a mobile coronary care unit. He stresses the importance of treating bradyarrhythmia in order to protect against ventricular fibrillation, especially if associated with a lower blood pressure or ventricular ectopic beats. Other pathophysiologic states occur that are now recognized as examples of increased vagal tone. The characteristic sinus bradycardia and hypotension, responding to treatment with atropine, is a cardiogenic reflex activated in patients with acute posterior myocardial infarction and is often referred to as the Bezold-Jarisch reflex.

Although Reid centered attention on the relationship of the vagus nerve to reflex inhibition of the heart and cardiac arrest, the term "vagovagal reflex" was credited to Bayliss by Newman in 1923. Bayliss used the term quite broadly in speaking of the homeostatic mechanisms of the circulatory system. A more specific modification was suggested by Weiss and Ferris, who used the term to describe those cases of heart block produced by vagal inhibition resulting from reflexes set up by stimulation of efferent vagal fibers in the pharynx, esophagus, or respiratory tract. In their classic experiment in 1940, Reid and Brace demonstrated that mechanical irritation of the pharynx and larynx

during anesthesia can produce atrioventricular blocks, atrial premature systoles, and even ventricular premature systoles.

As early as 1889 McWilliam called attention to those cases in which cardiac failure assumed the form of an inhibition of the heartbeat by impulses reaching the organ along the vagus nerve. He accurately prophesied: "In certain forms of cardiac arrest, there appears to be the possibility of restoring by artificial means the rhythmic beat, and tiding over a sudden and temporary danger."

What happens when the cardioinhibitory nerve (vagal nerve) is stimulated in the human heart? Most commonly observed effects on the cardiac conduction mechanism involve depression of the sinus node; depression of the A-V node; and impairment of the A-V conduction, resulting in auricular or ventricular slowing or standstill in all degrees of A-V block (Capps).

Because of the "conduction mechanism" of the human heart, a study of the reflex pathways affecting the heart is of importance. As stated by Reid, the pathway by which a reflex can travel to the heart from those areas of our present interest, such as the respiratory passages and the gastrointestinal mucosa, involves three routes: first, by the vagal network to the vagal center and from there by an efferent path to the heart; second, by an axon reflex in the vagal system where there is passing from one branch to another without going centrally; and third, by irradiation of vagal impulses in which the stimulus originates at vagal nerve endings and passes to a ganglion, where it transfers to a branch of the sympathetic system and then to the heart. These pathways take on added significance when one contemplates the many examples of mechanical irritation to the mucosa of the respiratory or gastrointestinal tracts that occur in present-day medicine. The widespread use of endotracheal tubes and catheters and the frequency of bronchoscopy, gastroscopy, and esophagoscopy are all examples of such mechanisms. Stimuli can originate at any area where there are vagal nerve endings. Two such areas are as follows:

1. *Bronchial group.* This includes the treachea and nasal pharynx. The trigger stimulus appears most commonly to be an endotracheal tube, inflation of an intratracheal tube cuff, or insertion of a bronchoscope.

2. *Vascular group.* The trigger stimulus here seems to be the stretching of the vessel wall by the presence of an embolus—for example, the so-called pulmocoronary reflex described by Scherf. The ligation of either the right or left pulmonary artery is not a serious procedure in the course of an operation. However, the occlusion of a small vessel with a foreign body embolus is frequently accompanied by dyspnea and even bronchial spasm. These effects disappear immediately on vagal section.

A certain percentage of cases of pulmonary emboli in which ECG changes are observed depends, in part at least, on the fact that the vagal control of the coronary circulation is not very efficient.

In considering reflex action from the vagus nerve, it is vital to realize that the type of stimulus is the factor that determines the effector organ. A stimulus of an electrical nature applied to the vagus in the neck, if of a certain frequency, will result in bradycardia, whereas another frequency will produce minimal gastric secretion and little bronchial spasm. When the frequency is again changed, a large amount of gastric secretion, high in acid and rich in enzymes, will be observed—with only minimal cardiac slowing. Severe bronchial spasm can be seen following still another change in frequency of the stimulation current.

Morton and associates, in a study of thirty patients, conclude that the relative infrequency of cardiac change secondary to vagal stimulation suggests that, under satisfactory anesthesia, cardiac arrest caused by vagovagal reflex is less common than previously supposed. They suggest anoxia as probably the most important factor in the pathogenesis

of such cardiac derangement. These associates have performed several vagotomies as palliative measures in alleviating discomfort in patients with bronchogenic carcinoma and intractable asthma.

By traction on the vagus nerve in the lower portion of the thorax between the hilus of the lung and the diaphragm, by electrical stimulation with current obtained from an induction coil, by cutting, or by crushing in clamping, Chester and associates came to several conclusions after a group of fifteen dogs had been studied. They were unable to note any relationship between the type of anesthesia and the type of vagal response elicited. A combination of traction and electrical stimulation seemed to be the optimum method of obtaining the most pronounced amount of stimulation. They were able to abolish, by local infiltration of the intrathoracic vagus with procaine hydrochloride, any cardiovascular response that seemed to be produced by the electrical stimulation. Procaine did not abolish the effect of traction. Atropine sulfate appeared to be of no value, although dibenzyl-beta-chlorethylamine (Dibenamine) completely abolished any cardiovascular response to vagal stimulation in this area.

Using dogs, Young and associates found that the effects on the heart following vagal stimulation are greatly enhanced by hypercapnia. As the degree of carbon dioxide accumulation increases and the arterial blood pH falls, the degree and duration of cardiac asystole during vagal stimulation increases. In several animals atropine sulfate was given, and, even though the pH was below 7.0, the effect of vagal stimulation was abolished. In 1924 Andrus and Carter demonstrated that vagal stimulation of the perfused turtle's heart shows an increased sensitivity in an acid medium. As early as 1934, Heymans noted similar responses, as did Young and associates. Young, Sealy, Harris, and Botwin concluded from their studies that hypoxia appears to decrease instead of increase the effect of vagal stimulation. On the other hand, Sloan arrived at an opposite conclusion.

The studies of Ebert and co-workers attempt to define the mechanisms of cardiac arrest during hypoxia. In order to determine whether cardiac arrest under an hypoxic condition is initiated by neural stimulus or by the direct effect of oxygen deficit on the heart (as well as to investigate the relative effects on the heart of slowly and rapidly induced hypoxia), Ebert perfused dog hearts with fully oxygenated blood. Hypoxia was acutely produced in the systemic circulation. He notes that with acute systemic hypoxia a severe bradycardia occurred within 3 minutes in all animals and that cardiac arrest supervened in two of them. With gradual systemic hypoxia and normal cardiac oxygenation, mild bradycardia occurred during the initial 5 minutes; in two of these four animals, severe bradycardia and "vagal escape" were produced after 8 minutes. With cardiac hypoxia for 10 minutes during normal systemic oxygenation, dogs with either normal hearts or denervated hearts showed no significant changes in rate or rhythm. When, however, cardiac hypoxia and systemic hypoxia were both acutely produced, four of five dogs had cardiac arrest after 1 minute. This arrest was preceded by arrhythmia, bradycardia, and "vagal escape." Gradual systemic hypoxia, induced during cardiac hypoxia, resulted in a less pronounced response; but arrest did occur in one of four dogs after 3 minutes.

Vagal section abolished the effect of systemic hypoxia on the heart. Blood pH studies did not indicate a significant change during these brief periods. Ebert and associates conclude that neurogenic stimuli originating in peripheral receptors are responsible for the cardiac effect of systemic hypoxia. These effects are more profound when systemic unsaturation is suddenly induced, and they are more deleterious when the heart is also hypoxic.

Jensen studied two patients who were undergoing thoracic surgery. The arterial pH of each patient was studied closely during the entire operation; in one patient the pH went down to 6.98, and in the other to 6.82. Because of the remarkably low pH, surgery was discontinued in each patient and the chest was closed rapidly. Both patients went into cardiac arrest when they began to blow off the retained carbon dioxide. Both cases of cardiac arrest occurred in spite of arterial oxygen saturation which had failed to show any evidence of hypoxia. In spite of the ability to maintain high concentrations of oxygen to keep the arterial blood level at normal oxygen saturation, the patient had been unable to adequately remove the carbon dioxide excess.

Undoubtedly, the breathing tension of carbon dioxide results in an increased concentration of potassium in the plasma. This concentration in the plasma will continue to rise even for a period after the patient again begins to breathe room air. During hyperventilation, the blood potassium level will decrease in the serum.

In summary, it is important to realize that a vagal reflex will not produce a cardiac arrest in a normal healthy individual. For cardiac arrest to occur, three essential mechanisms are necessary (Reid and associates): (1) there must be disease of the ventricular specific tissue; (2) there must be depression of the ventricular specific tissue that still remains functioning, by drugs or anesthetic agents; and (3) there must be suppression of stimulus formation in the auricles.

CARDIAC ARREST IN THE JAUNDICED PATIENT (AND WITH SURGERY OF THE BILIARY SYSTEM)

Clinically and for many years, the patient with obstructive jaundice has been associated with an increased vagal tone manifested by sinus bradycardia. It was not surprising that the most common clinical entity associated with cardiac arrest in our first 1,200 cases studied was that of obstructive jaundice. There were thirty-two cases of obstructive jaundice with sudden failure of the heart.

These patients were noted to have been clinically jaundiced at the time of the cardiac arrest. Sixteen cases were associated with carcinoma of the pancreas, others with carcinoma of the gallbladder, carcinoma of the common bile duct, congenital atresia of the bile ducts, and, in one case, with carcinoma of the duodenum.

Waltman Walters of the Mayo Clinic stated that in 28 years of surgery he had witnessed only two cases of cardiac arrest. Both cases were associated with obstructive jaundice. Both patients were being explored for common bile duct obstruction. He called attention to a third patient who was jaundiced from the obstructive effects of a carcinoma of the head of the pancreas. Although cardiac arrest did not occur, an abrupt drop in systemic blood pressure did occur.

As long ago as 1928, Buckbinder reported irregularities in the pacemaker in dogs noted 10 days after the induction of jaundice. Two years later, Ivy and associates noted that jaundice produced in dogs regularly causes a bradycardia, an evidence of increased vagal tone.

Crittenden and associates observed in 1932 that preexisting icterus increases the occurrence of cardiac irregularities associated with nausea, retching, vomiting, and pain produced by distension of the biliary passages. They noted that dogs made icteric by obstruction of the biliary passages develop a bradycardia. The degree of the arrhythmia or irregularities of the cardiac rhythm is not constant; this depends upon the degree of icterus. They did note, however, that the changes caused by distension of the biliary system parallels the degree of icterus. It was their conclusion that jaundice definitely sensitizes the cardiovagal mechanisms. Crittenden produced these irregularities in the cardiac rhythm of animals that were not anesthetized, and he was able to produce such irregularities as heart block, cardiac arrest, and ventricular and atrial ectopic beats. He found that these irregularities are most likely to occur during retching. Owen showed that cardiac irregu-

larities could be produced in dogs by stimulation of hollow abdominal viscera if jaundice was present; this could not be duplicated in nonjaundiced dogs. Johnstone reported the presence of bradycardia and partial A-V block during induction of anesthesia with ether a jaundiced patient. I believe that clinical evidence supports this view.

Over 30 years ago, Reid called attention to the importance of the vagovagal reflex in the etiology of cardiac arrest. Clinically, the patient with obstructive jaundice has been associated with an increased vagal tone for many years. The relative bradycardia that occurs is one of the more pronounced associations. The most widely accepted factor responsible for this hypervagotonic state is ascribed to the deposition of bile salts in the tissues of the body. Therefore it is not surprising that one might encounter an increased number of cases of cardiac arrest in patients with obstructive jaundice which has in turn produced a hypervagotonic environment for the patient. Particularly might this have been expected had there been greater awareness of some of the laboratory data recorded over 25 years ago.

The work of Engel is significant. He cites twenty-three patients with acute symptomatology arising from the biliary tract. Eighteen, or 78%, of these patients showed cardiac standstill of 3 seconds or more after massage of the carotid sinus. Postoperative examinations were made on ten of these eighteen patients, and carotid sinus hypersensitivity had disappeared in seven. Draper interprets this evidence as showing a summation of afferent impulses arising from the end organs in the biliary tract that had reached the threshold of reaction of vagal centers in the medulla.

Patterson reported his experience with patients with coexistent biliary tract disease (gallstones) and heart disease. He was impressed with the unusual frequency with which angina-like pain disappeared following removal of the gallbladder. Other patients with electrocardiographic evidence of myocardial disease seemed to show marked improvement following removal of gallstones. He cites the work of Ravdin, who demonstrated the decreased coronary blood flow that follows stimulation from the biliary tract. Gilbert was able to show almost the same thing following distension of the stomach in dogs. These effects could be abolished after atropine administration or vagal section. An excellent review of the association of gallstones and heart disease is provided by Patterson.

So closely related is Adams-Stokes disease to biliary tract disease and gallstones that Levine has declared that he routinely orders a gallbladder study on every patient with Adams-Stokes attacks. In about 50% he found evidence of gallstones, and an operation was performed. Multiple episodes of cardiac arrest invariably occur during the operative procedure and may sometimes be controlled by use of the cardiac electrical pacemaker. In one patient, over seven different periods of cardiac standstill occurred prior to completion of the surgery. Seven of fourteen patients were completely relieved of syncopal attacks following surgery (Levine).

In a study of over 1,700 cases presented in the first edition of this book, there was but one case of cardiac arrest in a patient with nonobstructive jaundice. This was in a 10-month-old white male upon whom a splenectomy was being performed. Cyclopropane and ether were administered. Cardiac arrest occurred at the time of extubation of the endotracheal tube. An intracardiac injection of drugs through the intact chest was unsuccessful. The patient died.

On August 23, 1954, a 75-year-old white woman was taken to the operating room, and an abdominal exploration was performed under spinal anesthesia supplemented by 5 ml. of 2.5% Pentothal. Forty-seven minutes after the anesthetic was begun, sudden cessation of cardiac activity was noted just as the common duct was being palpated. The chest was quickly opened, and within 2 minutes after the arrest occurred intermittent cardiac compression was being accomplished at the rate of 50 to 60 times per minute. The heart was in asystole. Artificial respiration was accomplished by means of endotracheally administered oxygen by compression of the rebreathing bag. The heart was restored to a normal spontaneous rhythm. Cardiac resuscitation was indeed quite prompt. It was decided to leave the chest open for the remainder of the procedure, and, accordingly, the surgeon returned to the abdominal exploration. Again, just as the area about the common duct was manipulated, a marked slowing of the heart occurred. The stimulation and the wound retractors were quickly removed; the heart rate increased and the blood pressure came up. This was noted on a second occasion. Atropine sulfate, 0.4 mg., was administered intravenously, and the abdomen and chest were closed. The patient did not return to consciousness but remained in a semicomatose state and had a convulsion on the fourth postoperative day. In addition, lower nephron nephrosis was diagnosed. (Reported by Dr. Irvin C. Shaffer.)

During an exploratory laparotomy for obstructive jaundice under Pentothal, nitrous oxide, oxygen, and ether, a 68-year-old white man suddenly developed cardiac arrest approximately 12 minutes after the start of the anesthesia and just as the operative incision was begun. The heart, on thoracotomy, was found to be in diastole and required only a short period of massage before normal rhythm returned. The patient was awake and out of bed that afternoon. (Author's own case.)

A middle-aged woman, an inmate of a mental institution, was operated upon for disease of the biliary system. The operation was performed under spinal anesthesia without an unusual amount of trauma or loss of blood. Suddenly during the course of the operation, the anesthetist noted a fall of the blood pressure to zero and could not feel any peripheral vessel pulsation. The surgeon was unable to feel cardiac pulsation through the diaphragm. By means of subdiaphragmatic massage for approximately 10 minutes, the rhythm was restored to its spontaneous rate, and the patient made a subsequent recovery. The patient was discharged from the mental institution, and her family reports that since discharge she seems to be mentally improved and is much more cooperative. (Courtesy Dr. Wadley Glenn.)

A 76-year-old man was operated upon for an obstruction of the common duct. Four hours after the preoperative atropine sulfate (gr. 1/200) had been given, at the time the patient was lifted upon the operating table for insertion of the x-ray box for dye visualization of the common duct, sudden cardiac arrest occurred. Cardiac massage was instituted and was almost immediately successful in restoring the normal cardiac rhythm. The patient survived the procedure. (Courtesy Dr. K. Anderson.)

Just as the endotracheal tube was inserted, the heart stopped in a 78-year-old male who was markedly jaundiced. The left leaf of the diaphragm was opened, and the heart was massaged at the rate of 60 per minute. In spite of severe hypertensive heart disease, cardiac rhythm was restored and the patient made an uneventful recovery. (Courtesy Dr. Henry Faxon.)

It is now generally agreed that adequate doses of atropine sulphate are especially indicated in patients being operated upon for jaundice with marked deposition of bile salts in body tissues.

ADAMS-STOKES DISEASE AND
VAGAL STIMULATION

The effect of chronic or long-term disease on vagal stimulation is noteworthy. Dr. Samuel Levine, for example, observed over 20 years ago that some patients with Adams-Stokes syncope were completely relieved after a diseased gallbladder had been removed. In addition, two well-documented cases of Adams-Stokes syncope unexpectedly "cured" by vagotomy for peptic ulcer disease are reported (Obel and Marchand). Frequent and disabling episodes of syncope with electrocardiographic evidence of asystole have not recurred in 3 and 7 years respectively. Cerebral vagal center stimulation from afferent vagal impulses is believed to stimulate efferent vagal fibers suppressing impulse formation and transmission in the S-A and A-V nodes and in the automatic cardiac cells. Episodes of idiopathic Adams-Stokes disease have been successfully treated by right vagotomy (Greenwood). Truncal vagotomy below the level of cardiac innervation interrupts the afferent fibers of this visceral reflex arc.

That such reflexes do occur is supported by the interesting observation of Gallivan and co-workers who note a high incidence of electrocardiographic abnormalities after infracardiac truncal vagotomy, which they believe result from retrograde conduction and central autonomic stimulation.

REFLEX CARDIOVASCULAR REACTIONS
DURING ABDOMINAL SURGERY

Reflex cardiovascular patterns of a vagal nature are generally well known to most surgeons. An excellent appraisal of cardiovascular reactions occurring during abdominal surgery is presented by Folkow and co-workers. There are numerous regions from which reflex cardiovascular reactions can be elicited. Surgeons are particularly aware of those that occur during simple exploration of the upper abdominal viscera, downward displacement of the stomach, traction on the gallbladder, mobilization of the duodenum, traction of the mesentery and/or greater omentum, and distension of the common duct. Folkow was able to show that bradycardia and a falling blood pressure could also be provoked by pulling the broad ligament of the ovary.

This work calls attention to the reflex cardiovascular pattern, first, as being one that manifests itself as a bradycardia from vagal inhibition of the sinus node with escaped beats elicited from the atrioventricular node. This portion of the reflex pattern, the bradycardia, can regularly be counteracted by the intravenous injection of 0.5 mg. atropine. Intravenous administration of atropine does not, however, exert an effect upon the second aspect of the reflex pattern, that is, a fall in blood pressure associated with reduction in pulse pressure. Folkow and co-workers state:

> Decreased pulse amplitude, indicating a reduced stroke volume of the heart, however, can well be due to reflex inhibition of tonic sympathetic activity. Reflex sympathetic inhibition can cause a decrease of stroke volume both by decreasing positive inotropic sympathetic effect on the ventricles and by reflex inhibition of constrictor fiber influence on the venous side, with a consequent pooling of blood within the capacitance vessels.

The investigators show that forearm volume generally increases simultaneously with reflex decreases of pulse pressure. Peripheral resistance and the venous return to the heart decrease. The generalized inhibition of tonic sympathetic activity produces a relaxation or a dilatation of both the arterioles and the veins. All contribute to the sudden fall of mean arteriolar blood pressure.

What nerve pathways are used? Folkow and co-workers agree that afferent fibers from specific visceral mechanoreceptors within the thoracic and abdominal cavities run within the vagal nerves. Pain fibers from the visceral organs, however, proceed in a different fashion, reaching the spinal medulla mainly by sympathetic nerve channels. This explains why electrical stimulation of vagal nerve endings at the abdominal level does not evoke reflex cardiovascular changes. This, indeed, is an important consideration to keep in mind regarding the vagus nerve.

The causal relationship between cardiac arrest and certain types of procedures employing traction on abdominal viscera continues to have a considerable clinical implication. Kihn notes that cardiac arrest occurred twice during one operation when downward traction on the stomach was exerted in order that ligation of the left gastric artery could be performed. Following each incidence, open-chest cardiac massage was employed. The patient was successfully resuscitated. An endotracheal tube was in place throughout the sequence of events, and it was felt that the patient was being adequately oxygenated. Kihn raises the question of whether anoxia is necessary for the effect of a traction reflex.

CARDIAC ARREST FOLLOWING VAGOTOMY

Transabdominal truncal vagotomy was performed on 106 patients at the Connecticut Health Center during a 17-month period. Gallivan and co-workers report on ischemic electrocardiographic changes in 9% of the truncal vagotomies. The ECG abnormalities were primarily noted 1 day after vagotomy, lasted one to several weeks, and were not accompanied by correlative clinical or serum enzymolysis. They suggest that all patients undergoing vagotomy should have preoperative and postoperative electrocardiogram studies.

Their work further supports the work of Manning (1937) who showed that prolonged stimulation of the vagal nerves seems to produce myocardial damage, with the presence of negative T waves. He was able to prevent these changes by administration of atropine. Gallivan speculates that retrograde induction along the vagus may produce a central vagosympathetic reflex. The cardiac and the pulmonary plexus have considerable intermingling of vagal and sympathetic innervation to both atria and ventricles. The initial parasympathetic overreaction may be balanced by increased sympathetic tone or by the release of catecholamines.

A total gastrectomy was being performed on a 69-year-old man under cyclopropane-oxygen-ether anesthesia. One hour and 15 minutes after induction, the blood pressure was 140 systolic and 90 diastolic. The pulse rate was 72. At this point the surgeon informed the anesthesiologist that he was to cut the left vagus nerve. Fifteen seconds or less after the nerve was cut, blood pressure readings could not be obtained. Since the procedure was under a thoracoabdominal approach, the heart was promptly examined and was in complete standstill. After a period of massage for 11 minutes, the heart was returned to its normal rhythm, and the operation completed. Postoperatively the patient did well, and the followup 3 years later failed to reveal any obvious mental changes in the patient. (Courtesy Dr. J. Bonica.)

Alvarez calls attention to one patient who died after a ligature was placed about one of the vagus nerves and to another patient who died while a vagus nerve was being mobilized.

TRACTION OF VAGUS NERVE IN THE CHEST

Lindskog and Liebow, in their book on thoracic surgery, mention the danger from traction on the pulmonary hilum with mechanical stimulation of the vagus nerve in the mediastinum as an etiologic factor in cardiac arrest. They call attention to the frequency of cardiac arrest during light anesthesia when procedures such as endotracheal intubation or extubation, bronchoscopy, or endotracheal catheter suction are employed. I noted fourteen cases that occurred during dissection about the pulmonary hilus.

VALSALVA MANEUVER

Disturbances in heart rhythm induced by the Valsalva maneuver are well known. It is usually after the strain that the "overshoot" in blood pressure occurs, accompanied by marked vagal stimulation and slowing of the heart rate. Berant and Gassner believe that extraordinary expiratory effort during an asthmatic attack in the presence of anoxemia and sympathetic overactivity may induce severe cardiac arrhythmia and cardiac arrest. In reporting such a case they ascribe the arrest to excessive vagal tone.

HYPERVENTILATION AND CARDIAC ARREST

Excessive vagal stimulation following full inspiration has repeatedly been the basis for sinus arrest in a 51-year-old male over a 20-year period, with arrest periods lasting almost 3 seconds. These episodes of sinus arrest with inspiration are illustrated in Fig.

9-1. As might be expected, these episodes are modified by the sublingual administration of 0.6 mg. atropine sulfate. In discussing this case, Adams attributes the physiologic mechanism to vagal stimulation from stetch reflexes occurring at the time of full inspiration of the lung. These reflexes are transmitted by way of the carotid sinus to the cardioinhibitory center in the medulla oblongata. From the medulla oblongata center, located in the dorsal nucleus of the vagus in the floor of the fourth ventricle, efferent impulses pass by way of the right vagus nerve to the sinoatrial node. These impulses are inhibitory and result in slowing or arrest of sinoatrial impulse transmission. Interestingly enough, the patient would seem to be an individual in whom parasympathetic influence appears to be predominant. The patient has hyperchlorhydria and bradycardia and has had vagotomy for a perforated peptic ulcer.

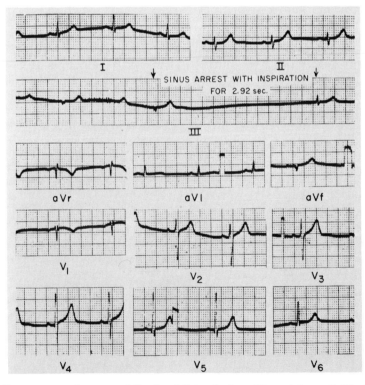

Fig. 9-1. Sinus arrest and syncope following full inspiration. (From Adams, C. W.: Dis. Chest 45:546, 1964.)

The vagal reflex response mediated during the surgical repair of an arteriovenous fistula has been noted on several occasions; it may be caused by a sudden increased pressure in the carotid sinus and aortic arch. The effect of hypotension could be prevented by intravenous injection of 5 mg. methantheline bromide (Stephen and co-workers).

Branham's bradycardiac sign, produced by temporarily occluding an arteriovenous communication, is a well-known diagnostic measure. By increasing the arterial tree blood flow, the resulting rise in systemic blood pressure stimulates the carotid sinus mechanism and the aortic depressor nerve, producing vagal inhibition of the heart.

TIC DOULOUREUX, THE VAGOVAGAL REFLEX,
AND CARDIAC ARREST

One of the most interesting conditions associated with a reflex inhibition of the heart is that occurring in association with glossopharyngeal neuralgia. This observation has been made by different physicians for several years.

A well-documented case of glossopharyngeal tic douloureux associated with cardiac arrest is reported by Kjellin and associates. Their patient was a 50-year-old man who for 4 years had experienced attacks of facial pain accompanied by loss of consciousness. Along with the attacks, hypersecretion from the ipsilateral parotid gland was observed. Swallowing, more than any other activity, brought on the attacks of syncope, preceded by bradycardia. Lemon was especially likely to provoke an attack, as were other foods with a strong, bitter, salty, or acid taste. Sweet foods had no effect. Yawning also precipitated the attacks.

In 1942 Riley and co-workers called attention to such a case. Ray and Stewart reported a similar case in 1948. Glossopharyngeal neuralgia (an entity somewhat similar to trigeminal neuralgia, or tic douloureux as it is commonly called) is associated with symptoms producing pain in the region of one ear and one side of the throat. The pain occurs at brief intervals and is of short duration. It is accompanied by a bradycardia, at times resulting in an attack of syncope and convulsions. Richburg and Kern, in discussing this condition, point out its relatively rare incidence. Its incidence is about one fortieth as common as trigeminal neuralgia. It is generally assumed to be completely cured by intracranial section of the ninth or glossopharyngeal nerve.

Richburg and Kern, in explaining the mechanism of syncope with glossopharyngeal neuralgia, state:

It is our assumption that, during the attacks of neuralgic pain, the glossopharyngeal nerve and its central pathways, which are presumably the principal pathways over which carotid sinus impulses are carried, are bombarded with an intense overload of afferent impulses. These travel to the autonomic centers of the brain and find their way to the vagus, which mediates the increased "vagal effect" with cardiac slowing and blood pressure fall, to the point where cerebral ischemia occurs. This results in syncope and convulsions exactly like that seen in the carotid sinus syndrome. We have demonstrated that atropine will abolish the vagal response even though neuralgic pain is unaffected.

The patient was a 36-year-old man who had many of the typical symptoms and complaints of glossopharyngeal neuralgia, including intense pain of a burning, lancinating character occurring at brief intervals and lasting only a short while, starting deep within the left ear and spreading to the deep structures of the upper portion of the throat on the left side. These attacks were precipitated by swallowing, particularly if cold liquids were taken. Simply clearing the throat or talking would produce such attacks and accordingly the patient refused to swallow and carried a cup into which he could drool. In spite of this, periods of sudden unconsciousness would occur during which he would fall and occasionally injure himself. His past history was essentially negative and he had been well until a cold had developed several months prior to the attack. As many as twenty or thirty attacks might occur within a 24-hour period.

Complete neurologic examination was entirely negative. Gag reflex was hyperactive; there were no cardiac abnormalities on physical examination and the ECG was within normal limits as was the EEG. Extensive x-ray examinations were negative, and repeated tests for carotid sinus hyperactivity were negative. Finally, after all efforts had failed, the patient was operated upon and the left glossopharyngeal nerve and the upper two filaments of the vagus nerve were sectioned through the usual left suboccipital craniotomy. Following the operation the patient made a rapid recovery and there were no recurrences of his previous symptoms.*

CAROTID SINUS REFLEX

Much attention has been given to the carotid sinus reflex and its relationship to the vagus nerve. It will be recalled that the afferent fibers of the carotid sinus reflex arc are found in the sinus nerve of Herring, a branch of the glossopharyngeal nerve. Although terminating in pressure-sensor organs in the adventitia of the sinus wall, these fibers make central connections with the cardio-inhibitory and vasomotor centers, the efferent limb of the reflex being the vagus nerve. The reflex can generally be adequately blocked by atropine, as pointed out by Hendrickson who reports marked hypertension and bradycardia in 47% of patients being operated for radical neck dissections.

CARDIAC ARREST FOLLOWING CAROTID SINUS PRESSURE

The accepted criterion for diagnosis of hypersensitive carotid sinus syncope is a post-carotid stimulation period of asystole greater than 3 seconds duration or a systolic or diastolic decrease in blood pressure of at least 50 mm. Hg. Diabetes mellitus, ischemic heart disease, and hypertension are often associated with the hypersensitive carotid sinus syndrome.

The hazards of indiscriminate use of carotid sinus pressure in various cardiac arrhythmias is not always well recognized. Numerous well-documented cases illustrate this danger. Ventricular fibrillation or ventricular asystole is not an uncommon result of carotid sinus pressure.

---

*From Richburg, P. L., and Kern, C. E.: Glossopharyngeal neuralgia with syncope and convulsions, J.A.M.A. **152**:703-704, 1953.

Pressure or massage of the carotid sinus is a valuable diagnostic tool in paroxysmal atrial and nodal tachycardia. Serious ventricular arrhythmias, although rare, do occur following pressure. Transient ventricular fibrillation has been reported as a latent manifestation of digitalis intoxication.

Periods of sudden slowing of the heart, unconsciousness, and, occasionally, convulsions have been noted for many years to be associated with pressure in the region of the carotid sinus. The carotid sinus syndrome is differentiated from the hyperactive carotid sinus reflex in that the former is associated with syncope whereas the latter is not. The carotid sinus syndrome is characterized by episodes of unconsciousness occurring suddenly and is sometimes preceded by a period of dizziness, weakness, ringing in the ears, or epigastric distress. The attack may last as long as 20 minutes but usually involves only a period of 1 to 4 minutes.

Why the carotid sinus becomes hyperactive in one patient but not in another is still a mystery, although we do know that predisposing factors such as age, sex, emotional state, organic disease that increases vagal tone, and vascular disease as well as cerebral and cardiac medication seem to play a part. Classically the carotid sinus syndrome is found in men in at east eight out of ten cases. The average age of the patient is usually in the fifth or sixth decade. Reviews of several series indicate that a history suggestive of a carotid sinus syndrome is found in the patient's family in as high as 50% of all cases.

Selvin and co-workers describe five different characteristics of carotid sinus reflexes:

1. Bradycardia alone
2. Hypotension alone
3. Hypotension and bradycardia
4. Hypotension and tachycardia
5. Hypotension, bradycardia, and apnea

The carotid sinus syndrome can be manifested in three different ways: (1) the vagal type, with cardiac slowing or asystole; (2) the vasodepressor type, which is associated with a fall in blood pressure but is not related to bradycardia; (3) the cerebral type in which there is loss of consciousness without significant cardiac or blood pressure effect. There can be combinations of all three. The vagal type, associated with cardiac asystole, or slowing, is the primary concern in this chapter. This occurs in at least one third to one half of all the cases.

A fatality resulting from a carotid sinus reflex is relatively rare. Heart action usually is resumed in 30 to 40 seconds after removal of the carotid sinus reflex stimulation. It is seldom that resuscitative measures will have begun before this time period expires.

Capps states that he has observed cases of hyperactive carotid sinus syndrome in which complete ventricular standstill following carotid sinus pressure was recorded on the ECG for more than 30 seconds. Further pressure was not deemed wise and was discontinued, but it was believed that the asystole could have been further prolonged. He also indicated that, in addition to this mechanism, there is the possibility that ventricular fibrillation may occur during a period of increased vagal tone. According to Hoff and Nahum, this arrhythmia can be produced by epinephrine acting on an irritable myocardium that is under the influence of at least a moderate degree of vagal tone. If, as seems reasonable, coronary or arteriosclerotic heart disease can cause an irritable myocardium, then the condition suitable for ventricular fibrillation must frequently be present.

The treatment of a sensitive carotid sinus manifested during surgery is not difficult. It can best be treated by the infiltration of the carotid sinus with a 1% solution of procaine hydrochloride. This can be done by introducing the solution under the adventitia of the vessel and allowing it to diffuse between the layers of the carotid artery. Approximately 3 to 7 ml. is usually necessary. Atropine sulfate should be injected intravenously, and the head of the patient should be placed in a low position by tilting the table into a Trendelenburg position.

Greeley has reported favorable response to radiation therapy of the carotid sinus in the patient with this syndrome, whether it be of vagal, depressor, cerebral, or mixed type. His experience, as reported, was limited to thirteen cases; twelve of the patients had been free from syncope for 6 months to 6 years. The technique of Greeley was similar to that of Stevenson, who used three roentgen exposures in 1 week, using 200 to 220 kv., 2 mm. of copper and 1 mm. of aluminum filters, 50 cm. T.S.D., 200 R. with a 10 cm. round portable. Occasionally one or two similar exposures are added to this routine. In an emergency, epinephrine and ephedrine are used to reduce the risk of asystole by rendering the cardiac muscles more irritable and less liable to vagal stimulation. Surgical denervation of the carotid sinus is seldom resorted to. Predisposing factors such as the quick motion of the neck, pressure on the neck, straining, bending, and lifting may sometimes serve as a trigger mechanism to bring on the attack. Morphine, digitalis, nitrites, dessicated thyroid, and methacholine (Mecholyl) are preoperative drugs that should be avoided. These drugs accentuate the vagal type of hypersensitivity in the carotid sinuses. Caffeine, calcium gluconate, and niacin may also be added to this list.

A carotid sinus syndrome attack can be abolished within a matter of several minutes by the intravenous injection of atropine sulfate, which acts to paralyze the vagal endings and thus prevents reflex cardiac slowing. Five tenths of a milliliter of a solution of epinephrine, 1:1,000, administered subcutaneously, prevents the attacks through its local stimulating effect on the ventricles. In addition to atropine and epinephrine, belladonna, alcohol, and quinidine diminish or abolish the vagal type of hypersensitivity.

An interesting case has been reported by Prinzmetal and Kennamer. A 65-year-old woman suffered from severely incapacitating effects of frequent syncopal attacks due to ventricular asystole produced by the slightest stimulus. Swallowing or slight external pressure on the carotid sinus would provoke a temporary cardiac arrest. The various drugs such as atropine, epinephrine, and hydroxy-amphetamine were used without benefit. When all other measures had failed, the patient was placed on thyroid hormone in doses sufficient to produce a mild hyperthyroidism and tachycardia. The episodes of asystole and syncope ceased. She was kept on this dosage for several months, during which time the attacks did not occur, nor did they recur after the drug was discontinued.

Hehre and co-workers report on a patient who, they believe, exhibits the common criteria of carotid sinus syndrome, namely, a male over 50 years of age with evidence of arteriosclerotic heart disease manifested by posteroinferior myocardial infarction and angina pectoris. He suffered an episode of carotid sinus hypotension and bradycardia, followed by a second episode of carotid sinus asystole during the removal of a parotid tumor while a surgical retractor was in place in the retromandibular space. Closed-chest massage and ephedrine were effective.

Master and others call attention to the case of a young Midwestern preacher who experienced periods of syncope while wearing tight collars. On examination, carotid sinus pressure repeatedly induced asystole and syncope. The attacks were eliminated when the patient stopped wearing tight collars.

The authors state that a diagnosis of syncope due to carotid sinus hypersensitivity should be made only if the following criteria are satisfied. (1) The attacks must occur without the premonitory signs usually seen in other forms of vasodepressor syncope, for example, those associated with fright or the sight of blood. (2) The attacks should be reproducible by sinus stimulation. (3) The attacks should not occur after the administration of adequate doses of atropine or ephedrine, that is, doses large enough to prevent bradycardia on manual carotid sinus stimulation.

For prolonged therapy, Master and associates recommend ephedrine sulfate (25 mg. three times a day) or atropine (0.3 mg. three

times a day). Hydroxyamphetamine (Paredrine), 60 mg. three times a day, or phenylephrine hydrochloride (Neo-Synephrine), in oral doses of 20 to 25 mg. three times a day, will occasionally be successful when other medication fails. They further suggest that small doses of sedatives (barbiturates) may be indicated to prevent any untoward effects such as insomnia or excessive nervousness.

Von Maur and co-workers treated a 43-year-old male patient with a 2-month history of episodic dizziness, mental confusion, and syncope. He had been treated unsuccessfully with administration of belladonna, orally, and atropine, intravenously. Xylocaine, injected percutaneously to block the right glossopharyngeal nerve prevented syncope and asystole during right carotid sinus compression. The patient responded to the use of a temporary, transvenous, fixed-rate cardiac pacemaker electrode positioned in the right ventricle. A permanent, demand-type cardiac pacemaker was then employed. Subsequently, carotid sinus compression was accompanied by immediate pacemaker-triggered systole with only a transient and slight reduction in arterial blood pressure. Voss and Magnin have reported an additional successful case with demand pacing for carotid syncope.

VAGOVAGAL REFLEX AND CARDIAC ARREST UPON SWALLOWING (DILATATION OF ESOPHAGEAL STRUCTURE AND DISTENDING ESOPHAGEAL DIVERTICULUM)

Profound bradycardia and, occasionally, syncope have been reported during swallowing. There has been no paucity of reports of cardiac arrest occurring after swallowing a large bolus of food (Sigler, Brown, Prinzmetal, and Reiniger). In one patient the syncope produced by swallowing food could also be provoked by distending the patient's esophageal diverticulum with a rubber balloon. At the American Surgical Association meeting in 1961, Haight called attention to a sudden cardiac arrest provoked by dilatation of an esophageal stricture 20 months after repair of a tracheoesophageal fistula in an infant.

Stretching of the esophagus with subsequent traction on the right vagus nerve regularly caused disappearance of P waves and a marked slowing of the QRS in a 4-year-old child who had had a tracheoesophageal fistula repaired at birth (Kenigsberg and others). It is believed that manipulation of the vagus nerve during repair of the tracheoesophageal fistula may cause adhesions between the nerve and the esophagus and may be the cause of unexplained postoperative death in patients with tracheoesophageal fistula repair.

In the case mentioned above, it was noted that the cardiac reaction to swallowing was first blocked by atropine and later, at an operation in which the vagus nerve was found to be firmly bound by adhesions, the reflex reaction was abolished by right vagotomy, including division of the inferior cardiac branches. Syncope when swallowing carbonated beverages, with subsequent distension of the esophagus by carbon dioxide, was reported. Stretching of the esophagus results in bradycardia and atrioventricular disassociation by stimulation of the afferent limb of a vagovagal reflex.

Sigler in 1941 called attention to possibility of cardiac arrest during swallowing, and reported a patient Starling had observed in 1921. The patient had had recurring attacks of unconsciousness attributed to asystole of the heart that was induced by swallowing. These could be abolished by the administration of atropine sulfate. When the patient finally expired, gross pathologic changes in the conduction apparatus appeared evident; Starling attributed the attacks to vagal impulses that played on a "highly diseased structure and yielded an unphysiologic response." Brown described a case in which syncopal attacks occurred in a middle-aged woman whenever large amounts of food were swallowed. Prinzmetal and Kennamer reported a 65-year-old woman who suffered innumerable syncopal attacks caused by ventricular asystole from such a stimulus as swallowing. In Reiniger's remarkable case, cauterization of a discrete area in the larynx of a 64-year-old man prevented further episodes of asystole occasioned by swallowing.

The subject of vagovagal syncope is discussed by Kopald and co-workers. This group, working at the Western Reserve University School of Medicine, was prompted to investigate the problem after they encountered a 48-year-old dental technician who had frequent "fainting spells" associated with the ingestion of food. Repeated episodes of unconsciousness occurred when the patient drank carbonated beverages. A bilateral splanchnic nerve block (using 2% lidocaine) was of no benefit. The attacks could be abolished, however, by large doses of atropine (2 mg.) given intravenously. Swallowing the carbonated beverage resulted in a prolonged elevation of intraesophageal pressure, possibly because of continued release of carbon dioxide. The authors believe that, with the rise in intraluminal pressure, esophageal muscle spasm occurs and is accompanied by stimulation of vagal nerve fibers. The efferent pathway of the reflex responsible for the arrhythmia appears to be vagal since splanchnic nerve block did not prevent the arrhythmia, whereas large doses of atropine did so.

Other cases have been reported in which vagovagal syncope was associated with esophageal disease. Weiss and co-workers and James (1964) reported patients with esophageal diverticulae in whom syncope occurred during the swallowing of water or a bolus of food. Attacks were potentiated by the administration of digitalis.

The vagovagal syncope is not to be confused with vasovagal syncope. In the latter, there is a sharp decline in blood pressure secondary to a loss of vasomotor tone resulting from a variety of stimuli such as postural changes, sight, pain, and so on. Vasovagal syncope is often associated with some degree of tachycardia. Vagovagal syncope, on the other hand, is accompanied by cardiac slowing or standstill.

CARDIAC ARREST AND REMOVAL OF PHARYNGEAL OR TONSILLAR PACK

The probable cause of a cardiac arrest in a young woman, following a dental clearance, was believed to be a vagovagal reflex instigated by the removal of the pharyngeal pack under light anesthesia (Keep). It is now my practice to give 1.2 mg. atropine sulfate intravenously with the administration of a general anesthetic and repeat this injection if the operation outlasts the tachycardia it produces.

A significant number of cardiac arrest cases are associated with tonsillectomies. One of the most dramatic examples of a reflex mechanism occurring in this area is the following case:

An adenoidectomy was performed with some difficulty on a 6-year-old boy. Considerable bleeding occurred. This necessitated that a nasopharyngeal pack be placed snugly against the nasopharynx. During the packing of the area, cardiac arrest occurred. Intracardiac injection of epinephrine was carried out without any result, and the thorax was subsequently opened and massage of the heart was soon instituted. Cardiac massage was successful in restoring the heart to a normal rhythm and at this point it was decided that the child would be returned to his room. Before this was done the nasopharynx was inspected and the pack was moved in such a fashion as to place it more securely against the breathing surface. At this point cardiac arrest again occurred, and only with great difficulty was the heart again restored to a normal rhythm.

The next morning the child was again taken to the operating room for removal of the pack. It was noted, however, that any mechanical stimulation to the nasopharynx gave rise to a very slow pulse and even actual transient cardiac arrest. Since the cardiac disturbance occurred only during nasopharyngeal stimulation, it was decided to again return the patient to his room.

On the third day, however, after considerable discussion, it was decided that the child should be given atropine just before the nasopharynx was disturbed. On taking the patient to the operating room, the pack was removed and no unusual activity of the heart occurred. Prior to the original surgery, the patient had been examined by his family physician and was found to have a heart murmur, although other findings were normal. (Courtesy Dr. L. Corsan Reid.)

GASTROSCOPY, ESOPHAGOSCOPY AND VAGOVAGAL RESPONSE

Definite changes in the electrocardiographic pattern were noted in 37% of a group of 49 patients during upper gastrointestinal endoscopy (Ewan-Alvarado and co-workers). Sixty percent of these patients showed electrocardiographic changes if there was any preexisting cardiovascular disorder. Ninety percent of the changes occurred after the stomach had been distended with air. The incidence was higher with the fiberscope than with the other scopes. It is interesting to note that Crittenden and Ivy, almost 40 years ago, intubated 92 students with a gastric tube. In those who showed gagging and vomiting, ectopic ventricular contractions were seen in five, A-V block in three, auricular extrasystoles in two, ventricular extrasystoles in one, and cardiac arrest in one.

REGURGITATION AND CARDIAC ARREST

Reflexes initiated under anesthesia following aspiration of regurgitated gastric contents or during vomiting have been associated with cardiac arrest in a sizable number of cases. Aspiration of regurgitated gastric contents can occur during anesthesia even though signs of vomiting have not been obvious.

Crittenden produced obstructive jaundice in dogs and then, by producing nausea, retching, and vomiting with the injection of apomorphine hydrochloride, he was able to produce cardiac irregularities. By the intravenous injection of atropine sulfate, he was able to inhibit almost completely the previously produced cardiac irregularities.

He noted the correlation between pH and cardioinhibition in the hyperventilated dogs that were given acetylcholine. There was no correlation between pH and acetylcholine or acetylcholine-inhibition of the heart following sodium bicarbonate. A possible factor in this apparent discrepancy was an alteration in the ratio of sodium to potassium in the cardiac nodal tissue during acetylcholine administration.

ENDOTRACHEAL INTUBATION AND
CARDIAC ARREST

There seems little question that there is an increase in arrhythmias in intubated patients. Kuner and Goldman noted a 72% incidence among 97 intubated patients. Bertrand and co-workers noted an incidence of 84%. In a group of 90 patients, 47 arrhythmias occurred at the time of intubation and 17 at the time of extubation.

There also seems to be little question that the procedure of endotracheal intubation represents an episode in the handling of the patient during which time the likelihood of cardiac arrest is increased. Among the 1,710 cases analyzed in the first edition of this book, a significant number of arrests occurred at the time the endotracheal tube was inserted. Shumacker has written an excellent report on this aspect.

Although many associate the aberrations in blood pressure and pulse and the cardiac arrhythmias that occur during tracheal intubation with anoxia and possibly with carbon dioxide retention, these factors were ruled out in a study originating at the University of Pennsylvania by King and associates. In a series of a considerable number of patients, laryngoscopy was completed less than 15 seconds after ventilation was discontinued. They were unable to note any circulatory responses that appeared to be dependent upon the anesthetic agent used. They believed that the results were more frequently due to the depth of anesthesia, and they advised discretion in performing tracheal intubation during very light anesthesia. In patients allowed to remain apneic for periods longer than usually required for tracheal intubation, they failed to note the typical responses seen in the controlled experiments.

BRONCHOSCOPY AND
CARDIORESPIRATORY REFLEXES

Cardiac arrest during bronchoscopy is uncommon. However, Burman and Gibson showed that 36% of fifty-nine patients developed arrhythmias at the time of bronchoscopy, especially when the bronchoscope touched the trachea, carina, and mainstem bronchi. They were unable to abolish these responses with usually employed doses of atropine.

SUDDEN DEATH FOLLOWING TRACHEOTOMY
AND TRACHEAL SUCTIONING

It is increasingly recognized that cardiac arrest may follow successful completion of an emergency tracheotomy. I have experienced this unexpected complication on at least three occasions. The most plausible explanation is that these patients represent examples of long-standing carbon dioxide retention. Sudden hyperventilation, with relief of hypoxia and carbon dioxide retention, removes an effective respiratory stimulus and compensatory hypertension. The resultant apnea and hypotension precede the cardiac arrest.

In some instances, intratracheal suctioning may provoke either a vagovagal arrest or ventricular fibrillation. In addition, the prolonged apnea following an uncomplicated tracheotomy may be caused by the vasodilator effect on the peripheral circulation when metabolic acidosis is suddenly reversed.

There is experimental evidence (Oppenheimer and Quinn) that the posthypercapneic ECG, resembling that seen with potassium intoxication, is actually associated with a marked increase in the serum potassium. This increase is added to the already high potassium associated with asphyxia.

Green discusses five deaths attributed to tracheotomy (rather than to the condition for which tracheotomy was performed). He cites other reports attempting to explain this untoward reaction after apparently successful tracheotomy. He believes the most probable explanation of this phenomenon is related to the rapid alteration in pulmonary ventilation produced by the tracheotomy—the improved pulmonary ventilation resulting in a rapid reversal of preexisting respiratory acidosis.

The pathogenesis of circulatory and respiratory collapse after an emergency tracheotomy is believed to involve the sudden removal of the tremendous sympathetic response provoked by hypoxia and hypercapnia secondary to airway obstruction (Bendixen and associates).

Because of a reduction in the normal coronary-sinus pressure gradient during cardiac massage, it is likely that coronary filling is further reduced during cardiac massage· accompanied by tracheal suction. The respiratory unit at the Massachusetts General Hospital has a rule that tracheal aspiration must be preceded by a period of maximum oxygenation and must never last more than 15 seconds at a time. Formulation of this rule was prompted by frequent episodes of cardiac arrest during tracheal suctioning. In discussing this in their book *Respiratory Care,* Bendixen and associates mention a 22-year-old man who required intermittent positive pressure respiration after a crush injury of the chest. Three days after the injury, while a nurse was aspirating bloody secretions from the trachea, the heart stopped. External cardiac massage restarted the heart, but, over the course of the next 2 days, the patient suffered cardiac arrest twice, each time responding to external massage. In each instance the cardiac arrests were associated with prolonged tracheal aspiration.

ECG ALTERATIONS DURING RECTAL
EXAMINATION, PROSTATIC MASSAGE, AND
BARIUM ENEMA

Sudden cardiac asystole has appeared at the time of rectal examination. Bilbro documents episodes of either frank syncope or marked faintness associated with bradycardia as slow as 36 beats per minute in a group of soldiers during prostatic manipulation. Changes in the electrocardiogram can be documented during sygmoidoscopic procedures. It is generally believed that there are reflex changes in the coronary circulation and cardiac-nerve tone mediated to the vagus nerves. Eastwood documents electrocardiographic abnormalities associated with the

barium enema in a group of 95 patients. Forty-six percent of the group showed ECG changes, over a third of which were thought to be potentially serious. The ECG changes have been noted by a number of authors to be more common in the aging individual and in persons with a heart disease.

An interesting report of an Adams-Stokes attack produced by rectal stimulation is reported by Scott and Sancetta. The patient was a 62-year-old white woman. During the patient's hospital stay, it was observed that her attacks occurred while using the bedpan. ECG tracings showed an almost complete atrioventricular block prior to the attacks of unconsciousness and absence of pulse. The attacks could be initiated by digital examination of the rectum. The ECG revealed transient ventricular standstill on several occasions. On one occasion, the ECG first revealed a high ventricular tachycardia that later became a coarse ventricular fibrillation with a ventricular rate over 300 per minute. The patient subsequently died during her hospital stay and an autopsy examination, interestingly enough, revealed only slight coronary arterial sclerosis. No areas of fibrosis were seen. There were slight atrophy, fibrosis, vacuolation of the myocardial cells, and moderate arteriolar sclerosis; the latter was commensurate with similar arteriolar changes in other organs.

POSTMICTURITION SYNCOPE

The exact mechanism of postmicturition syncope is not clear, but it is true that atropine administration can prevent the sinus arrest demonstrated on electrocardiograms, which indicates that viscerocardiac reflexes with vagal connections are present.

VAGAL ARREST PROVOKED BY OPERATIONS
ON THE EYE

Early in our Cardiac Arrest Registry study it became evident there were a disproportionately large number of cardiac arrests during eye operations, especially in children. Arrhythmias during mobilization of the rectus muscles during strabismus surgery are a good example. Bradycardia from pressure on the eyeball has been known for almost 80 years. The afferent arc of the oculocardiac reflex is the trigeminal nerve. The efferent limb of the reflex arc consists of the vagus nerve. Varying degrees of sinus depression occur, particularly that which affects the upper regions of the sinoauricular node in patients with known cardiac disease.

There is a real danger of cardiac arrest during eye operations. A glance at current programs of ophthalmologic societies indicates a considerable interest in and emphasis on this problem by ophthalmologists. As noted elsewhere in this book, numerous examples of cardiac arrest occurring during ophthalmologic procedures have been cited— to an extent that would appear out of proportion to the expected incidence. Kirsch and associates have demonstrated that the vagal relationship is a real one in the etiology of cardiac arrest during eye surgery (particularly surgery involving the muscle groups). A marked bradycardia, in some instances profound, can be produced by muscle traction. It will disappear upon release of the muscle and subsequently recur after repeated traction. ECG tracings can also demonstrate an occasional conversion from sinus rhythm to nodal rhythm.

Enucleation procedures have been associated with cardiac arrest (Bailey, 1935; Vialard, 1935; Merigot de Treigny, 1940). In each instance the patient developed a marked bradycardia following enucleation of an eye, and subsequent cardiac asystole occurred.

Sorenson and Gilmore, in an excellent presentation, established that various types of arrhythmias occur with mobilization of the rectus muscles during strabismus surgery. Since manipulation of the recti is an integral part of the squint operation, it is difficult to avoid tension on these muscles. Apparently even very slight unilateral tension on the medial or lateral rectus oculi will consistently result in a minor degree of bradycardia.

These authors note varying degrees of bradycardia, sometimes combined with extrasystoles, in all seventeen cases for which careful ECG monitoring was present. In one case ventricular fibrillation occurred, and in a second case cardiac arrest occurred. The latter case was a 3-year-old girl whose operative pulse rate was 120 per minute until tension was exerted on the medial rectus, at which time the pulse fell to 20. With further tension on the muscle, cardiac arrest occurred. Thumping on the anterior chest wall resulted in restoration of the former heart rate of 120 per minute. Stretching of the rectus muscle again produced a marked bradycardia.

In 1908 it was demonstrated by Aschner that pressure on the eyeball results in a slowing of the radial pulse. Aschner's further work establishes that the efferent limb of the reflex arc consists of the vagus nerve, whereas the trigeminal nerve constitutes the afferent limb. It now seems possible that the oculocardiac reflex results from the stimulation of the first division of the trigeminal nerve (ophthalmic nerve). Various manipulative efforts have demonstrated the validity of this reflex clinically. Subconjunctival hematoma may elicit an oculocardiac reflex (Stortebecker).

In his paper on oculocardiac reflexes, Berler states that pressure on the globe and the extraocular muscle stretch are the most dependable stimuli that produce ECG changes. ECG abnormalities are especially produced by traction on the medial rectus nerve.

An excellent study of ECG effects of eyeball compression was done by Shamroth. Of 148 patients, 102 with cardiac disease, considerable emphasis is given the role of the vagus nerve in the production of various cardiac arrhythmias. The role of vagal action in cardiac rhythm was studied by means of eyeball compression (Aschner-Dagnini reflex). The afferent arc of the oculocardiac reflex is the trigeminal nerve which, when stimulated by eyeball compression, causes an increase in vagal tone. Almost invariably, this reflex produces a varying degree of sinus depression, particularly affecting the upper regions of the sinoauricular node. Arrhythmias were exceedingly rare in normal patients used as controls, but were inevitably present in patients with known cardiac disease. Shamroth speculates that an abnormal myocardial focus is a necessary condition for this occurrence.

The eyeball compression reflex is elicited by manual pressure exerted simultaneously on both eyes for 3 to 20 seconds. The degree of pressure is sufficient to cause some slight pain. Eyeball compression produces changes that include sinus depression, shift in the site of the primary pacemaker, auricular ventricular dissociation, precipitation of ventricular ectopic beats with fixed couplings, abolition of coupled ventricular ectopic beats, transient lengthenings of the coupling interval with intermittent parasystole, variation in the duration of the P-R intervals, prolonged P-R intervals at higher degrees of atrioventricular block, transient atrial and ventricular tachycardia, and nodal and ventricular escape. A significantly greater precipitation of ectopic rhythms is present in patients receiving digitalis. This is in agreement with experimental work on animals showing that vagal stimulation will produce a more likely effect on the heartbeat if it is combined with certain drugs such as thiobarbiturates, digitalis, and aconitine.

Magoon and Norton strongly recommend that some kind of audible or visual monitoring system be used for recording pulse or blood pressure during operations upon the eye. Much ophthalmologic surgery is done under local anesthesia and with the patient completely draped so that only the eye is visible. The presence or absence of bleeding is seldom significant. Magoon and Norton suggest that there have been cases in which cardiac arrest occurred during eye surgery under local anesthesia and that the patient's condition was not diagnosed until the operation had been completed.

As noted, the oculocardiac reflex is especially common in children. It is, as a matter of fact, seldom obtained after 40 years of age. This is not surprising since vagal tone is maximal in young people. As a matter of fact, if one excludes cardiac arrest in those patients with known coronary artery disease, the most common decade for cardiac arrest is the first decade of life. Of the initial 1,700 cases studied in our Cardiac Arrest Registry, 24.3% were encountered in the first decade. Numerous other studies have confirmed the high incidence of cardiac arrest in the young age group. Reid believes that this may partially be explained by the fact that children have highly sensitive reflexes as demonstrated, for instance, by the response of the sinus node to respiration and its influence upon cardiac rhythm. With increasing age this sensitivity gradually decreases.

Strictly speaking, the oculocardiac reflex is not a vagovagal reflex since the afferent pathway is via the trigeminal nerve.

FRIGHT AND DEJECTION

Wolf has repeatedly called attention to the striking bradycardia that may be seen under situations provoking extreme dejection or sudden fright. He compares the pathophysiologic influences produced to the profound bradycardia regularly occurring in man and animals during diving.

There is even some evidence to indicate that the rare episodes of sinus arrest of a volitional nature are caused by vagotonia.

James is quite convinced that the layman's term of "being frightened to death" or "dying of a broken heart" does, in fact, have some scientific support. The many neural responses that influence the electrical stability of the heart are undoubtedly influenced by emotions generated from fear, pain, apprehension, and grief.

SUBARACHNOID HEMORRHAGE AND VAGAL STIMULATION

Vagal tone increased at the cortical level has clinical significance. For example, electrocardiographic changes attributed to vagal stimulation secondary to subarachnoid hemorrhage are strongly suspected—particularly when there is involvement of area 13 of the brain, which contains the chief cortical representation of the vagus nerve. Shuster abolished S-T segment depression associated with subarachnoid hemorrhage by the use of atropine administered intravenously.

The frequency of cardiac arrest in patients with epidural hematomas is revealed by Verdura. He presents three classic cases of epidural hematomas that exhibited cardio-respiratory arrest. Two of the patients had decerebrate rigidity and bilateral dilated pupils, yet all three survived without neurologic sequelae after cardiac resuscitation and removal of the hematoma.

CARDIAC ARREST IN THE PSYCHIATRIC PATIENT RECEIVING ELECTROSHOCK THERAPY

The incidence of cardiac arrest in patients receiving electroshock therapy (ECT) was originally thought to be low. More recently, however, it appears that this is not altogether true. In fact, the list of causes of death during ECT is headed by cardiac arrest. Arneson and Butler note that the incidence of cardiac arrest among psychiatric patients receiving ECT appears to be more common in good risk patients than in poor risk patients. They cite the work of Richardson, who was able to demonstrate cardiac arrhythmias of vagal origin in 30% of patients receiving ECT under anesthesia. Atropine in doses of 2.4 mg. or $\frac{1}{25}$ grain could prevent this fatality.

The grand mal seizure following the electrical stimulation of the brain is accompanied by a marked vagal discharge that can be observed in about 30% of all patients receiving ECT (Richardson and co-workers).

After studying one hundred successively admitted psychiatric patients and comparing them with one hundred patients admitted to the general hospital for general care, Bernreiter notes a distinct difference in the comparative A-V conduction times of the psychi-

atric patients and those of the general hospital population. Of the patients admitted to the psychiatric department, 20% showed an accelerated A-V conduction rate, as compared with only 5% in the second group. The short P-R interval indicates that the A-V node permits an unusually fast conduction rate that could be differentiated from the Wolff-Parkinson-White syndrome, in which an accessory bundle is responsible for the P-R interval. In the psychiatric patients studied, a normal QRS conduction time was present, whereas a widened QRS conduction complex was present in the patients with Wolff-Parkinson-White syndrome.

Since two patients died following arrhythmias that developed after ECT, Bernreiter cautions that patients with accelerated A-V conduction rates should receive prophylactic treatment such as quinidine, procainamide (Pronestyl), or digitalis prior to ECT. Fifty percent of the patients receiving ECT developed paroxysmal tachycardia. The second patient died after paroxysmal auricular tachycardia that could not be controlled. The explanation for the increased conduction rate across the A-V node in psychiatric patients is not clear. Sympathetic stimulation resulting from drugs or hypothalamic stimulation may be related to the shortening of the P-R interval. In addition, Bernreiter speculates that variations in the vagosympathetic tone may play a part.

In discussing the cause of cardiac arrest in a 29-year-old woman receiving ECT, Tropper and Hughes consider that repeated shock, such as that received by this patient, accentuates the vagal stimulation to the point that it is a most potent factor in the causation of the cardiac arrest.

An additional case of cardiac arrest following ECT, in this case successfully managed, is reported by McNichol and Seale. Their article reviews the growing list of documented cases of cardiac arrest under ECT.

History of a previous cardiac arrest does not appear to contraindicate administration of ECT. Wilson and Mayfield have, in fact, reported successful use of ECT in a patient with previous history of cardiac arrest.

A short period of asystole occurred almost every time that ECT was used in dogs (Dobkin and Olszewski). The arrest is the result of stimuli that reach the heart through vagal nerves, and the arrest is effectively prevented either by the administration of atropine or by the cutting or freezing of the vagi.

Barrett used a unique method of external cardiac massage to successfully resuscitate a patient who had cardiac arrest under ECT. He observed that the patient had a very thin abdominal wall, and cardiac massage was attempted by pushing the hand well up under the left costal margin and rhythmically pushing and squeezing. After a few such maneuvers, the patient's heartbeat was restored, and she eventually recovered with no signs of increased organic impairment. Barrett believes that this method is particularly applicable to people with weak abdominal walls.

VAGAL STIMULATION, HYPERPOTASSEMIA, AND HYPERCAPNIA

Augmentation, or an increase in the sensitivity of the heart to a vagal stimulation, may be possible in the *hypercapnic* state. Hoff and Winkler showed that the sensitivity of the heart to vagal stimulation is increased in hyperpotassemia. Young and associates point out that the effects of vagal stimulation on the heart are increased in hypercapnia, even before there is a rise in serum potassium.

After reviewing the problem, Casten and Bardenstein support the idea that hypercapnia and respiratory acidosis reinforce vagal bradycardia and prevent vagal escape.

Casten and Bardenstein, referring to the work of Dripps and co-workers, emphasize the importance of hypercapnia, or respiratory acidosis, as a potent factor in the production of cardiac arrest. They mention that of seven patients, six died just as the operation was nearing completion, that is, after anesthetic agents had been discontinued. They state:

Most all anesthetic agents are associated with some degree of stagnation of pulmonary ventilation and an increase in alveolar carbon dioxide tension. Since compensatory renal mechanisms are largely inoperative during the stress phase of surgery, this increased alveolar carbon dioxide tension causes a true, uncompensated respiratory acidosis and a decrease in blood pH. This situation not only potentiates vagal reflexes, but also, more significantly, lays the foundation for the so-called posthypercapnic phenomenon. This phenomenon refers to the development of severe cardiac arrhythmias, ventricular fibrillation or cardiac arrest in the immediate recovery phase from anesthesia; the phase in which the patient is suddenly "washed out" with oxygen after termination of the anesthesia.*

Electrocardiographic tracings of the dog heart illustrating that CO_2 accumulation augments the cardioinhibitory effect of vagal stimulation are shown in Fig. 9-2.

VAGOMIMETIC ACTION OF MORPHINE

Many house staff officers and other physicians are, in my experience, unaware of the marked vagomimetic action of morphine. I have often encountered a marked bradycardia in a patient receiving morphine sulfate. In postoperative patients I have employed 0.6 mg. atropine sulfate intravenously, given over a 5-minute period, to effectively relieve the bradycardia and in such instances have switched to Demerol or other medications for the control of pain.

ASYSTOLE FOLLOWING NEOSTIGMINE ADMINISTRATION

Before neostigmine (Prostigmin) is administered, it should be recognized that its vagal stimulatory effects are quite real, often with extreme bradycardia. A number of sudden deaths have been attributed to the use of neostigmine given during anesthesia to neutralize any remaining relaxant (for example, d-tubocurarine) at the close of an operative procedure. It is sometimes considered satis-

---

*From Casten, D. F., and Bardenstein, M.: Cardiac arrest in children, Bull. Hosp. Joint Dis. **16:** 13-21, 1955.

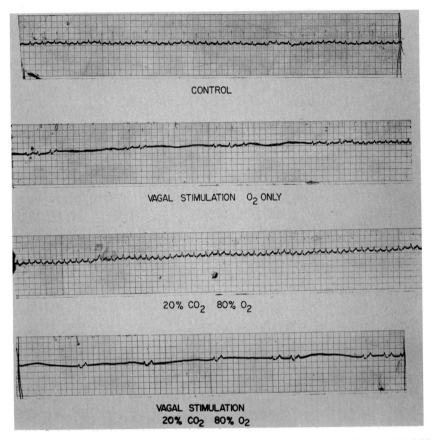

Fig. 9-2. ECG illustrating failure of carbon dioxide accumulation to potentiate vagal inhibitory effect on the heart.

factory to give neostigmine simultaneously with an antagonizing dose of atropine. This procedure, however, appears unwise. The atropine should be given at least 2 to 3 minutes preceding the neostigmine. A good review of this subject has been presented by Lawson. Usually, a sudden transition occurs; a patient with normal vital signs develops sudden cardiovascular collapse, dilated pupils, and absent respiration. As with most vagal-type arrests, these patients seem to respond well to resuscitative attempts.

Pohlmann reports a patient experiencing respiratory arrest following the intravenous administration of polymyxin B sulfate. Hiscox notes a cardiac arrest occurring in a patient on echothiophate iodide, an anticholinesterase somewhat like neostigmine. The drug

was being used for chronic open-angle glaucoma.

Ten patients with cardiac arrest following the administration of neostigmine are reported by Dinnick. It is his opinion that in each instance there was evidence of underventilation. He emphasizes the importance of maintaining adequate ventilation, of restoring the circulatory blood volume, and of correcting any acid-base disturbance.

CARDIAC ARREST WITH PENTYLENETETRAZOL

Sinus arrest has been reported while pentylenetetrazol (Metrazol) was being administered intravenously as an activating agent during an EEG examination (Ferriss and Hackett). Two additional cases are also noted. Recovery occurred in all instances. In systemic lupus erythematosus, cardiac electrical mechanisms may be interfered with as a result of structural damage to the cardiac conduction system.

RESPIRATORY ARREST WITH NEOMYCIN

Neomycin may be absorbed in considerable amounts from damaged intestinal mucosa and in cases of large bowel obstruction. Infants appear to be particularly sensitive to the neuromuscular-blocking effect of neomycin. Neomycin in the pleural cavity may produce respiratory arrest.

CARDIOPULMONARY ARREST WITH INTRAVENOUS KANAMYCIN

Kanamycin may produce cessation of cardiopulmonary function when administered intravenously (Ream). In addition, kanamycin, polymyxin, and neomycin are also capable of producing neuromuscular block of the nondepolarizing type identical to that produced by dimethyl tubocurarine. In contradistinction to the foregoing discussion, neostigmine may prove to be life-saving in this situation. In reversing the neuromuscular, curare-like block, its effect may be dramatic. In Ream's case, 0.25 mg. neostigmine was administered intravenously every 30 minutes. The muscarinic effects of the drug were kept at a minimum. Atropine was not necessary.

CARDIAC ARREST WITH ANTICHOLINESTERASE DRUGS

Lycoramine derivatives, used in the management of myasthenia gravis, have been responsible for cardiac arrest in several instances. A transient period of cardiac asystole followed the administration of lycoramine methiodide, an extremely short-acting anticholinesterase.

Three cases of cardiac arrest have been reported to me by Somers, all which have immediately followed the use of edrophonium chloride (Tensilon). Fortunately, two of the three patients were successfully resuscitated. In each case edrophonium chloride was being used for its anticholinesterase effect. In fact the Tensilon test is widely used in diagnosing myasthenia gravis. Moss and Alecort have evaluated edrophonium chloride for the treatment of certain cardiac arrhythmias. Because of their transient effect upon the heart, lycoramine derivatives should be used with caution.

RIGHT VAGUS VERSUS LEFT VAGUS

It is generally considered that there is some difference between the right and left vagus nerves as they affect the heart. Stimulation of the left vagus nerve exerts its effects more commonly on the atrioventricular node (A-V), whereas stimulation of the right vagus nerve predominately affects the sinoatrial (S-A) node, suppressing impulse formation at this node.

It is apparent that the right vagus, in particular, is capable of retarding the intrinsic rate and rhythm of the heart and may block conduction of the pacemaker center. There undoubtedly must be considerable fiber crossover from one side to the other.

ARE THERE VAGAL FIBERS IN THE HUMAN VENTRICLE?

Although there are occasional articles to the contrary, it is generally conceded that there are no vagal fibers in the mammalian ventricle. The ventricles, however, have the capacity to form stimuli independently and automatically. This capacity for automaticity in the ventricles results from the outstanding feature of what is known as the ventricular specific tissue. Since reliable, anatomically distinguishing features of ventricular specific tissue are not available, other criteria must be used for differentiation. The criterion for the differentiation of this specific tissue lies in its capacity to form stimuli independently. It is here that one must mention the law of auxomeric conduction, which states: "As long as there is one healthy fiber present, then conduction will be normal." Ventricular specific tissue is the body's most resistant tissue and can function for long periods without oxygen or even blood supply. This point is of crucial importance in a discussion of the role of anoxia. Ventricular specific tissue is capable of revival as long as 72 hours after death.

A point emphasized by Reid, and one worth remembering, is that the heart is composed of two types of tissue that are dissimilar phylogenetically, morphologically, and functionally, but which operate as a unit. It is composed of a specific tissue, of which every single unit or fiber has the capacity to originate stimuli, and the common myocardium, which does the mechanical work but which is unable to originate stimuli.

There are no vagal fibers in the human ventricle, according to most authorities. The vagal inhibition is restricted to the auricles and the junctional tissue. That this is true can be illustrated by failure of atropine sulfate to produce an effect on the ventricles in the presence of experimental heart block. Schwartz has shown, however, that in experimentally produced atrioventricular disassociation, stimulation of the vagus nerves may yield an inhibitory action on the centers that regulate the idioventricular pacemaker of the heart and thus slow the ventricles. This slowing may occur, presumably, through the vagus itself, or through factors that may influence the vagus reflexes by way of the carotid sinus.

Waggoner encountered a most interesting case. A young boy was being operated on for ligation of a patent ductus arteriosus. An anomalous left vagus nerve was encountered and was accidentally clamped, at which time cardiac activity suddenly ceased. Resuscitation was successful in restoring heart action, whereupon traction on the vagus again took place. Resuscitation was not successful. At the postmortem examination, the vagal fibers were seen entering the left ventricle. This is the only such case of which I am aware. Vagal tone is thought to be at a maximum during adolescence and early childhood. During infancy, vagal tone is at a minimum.

Under normal conditions, regardless of periods of reflex inhibition of the atria, the ventricles are able to originate a contraction spontaneously. The ventricular specific tissue, indistinguishable anatomically in the ventricle, has this unique physiologic feature of being capable of initiating stimuli independently. It is not surprising that in analyzing several hundred cases of cardiac arrest one sees such a high incidence of sudden cardiac standstill immediately following a probable reflex action on the heart. If there is disease of the specific tissue and vagal stimulation depresses stimulus formation in the auricles, sudden and complete stoppage of cardiac contractions may occur. As Reid states: "A heart under anesthesia is as vulnerable to vagal stimulation as a heart with diffuse organic lesions would be without anesthesia." A probable vagovagal reflex action was found likely in approximately one fourth of all cases studied. These included instances in which cardiac arrest occurred immediately after insertion of the endotracheal tube, during tracheal suction through the endotracheal tube, at the time of extubation, at the exact time of cutting the vagus nerve in the chest, during the dissection about the hilus of the lung, during downward traction on the stomach, during bronchoscopy at the end of operation, during traction on the mesentery, while stripping the periosteum, during positional changes of the patient, and during passage of a Levin tube. Several cases have been reported in which cardiac arrest recurred on subsequent occasions following the repetition of an identical stimulus, such as during reinsertion of the endotracheal tube.

Turk and Glenn believe that in many cases listed as unknown or uncertain, cardiac arrest was secondary to vagal reflexes. In their group of forty-two cases reported from the Grace–New Haven Hospital, they felt that at least five were directly caused by vagovagal inhibition.

If there are no vagal fibers in the ventricle, one might well ask: "How can one get cardiac arrest from vagal stimulation?" The point that should be brought out is that no healthy, normal heart can ever stop from vagal stimulation in the sense that serious symptoms will arise. One will never see a carotid sinus syndrome in a healthy heart. If there are widespread areas of destruction from disease in the specific tissue of the ventricles and if under these conditions vagal stimulation depresses the stimulus formation in the atria, the automaticity of the specific tissue in the ventricles will have been abolished and a contraction does not occur, or it occurs with insufficient rapidity to provide an adequate circulation. It is here that anesthetic agents have a similar action on the functional response of the specific tissue, giving the same result as if there were widespread areas of nonfunctioning tissue. To quote Reid again, "A heart under anesthesia is as vulnerable to vagal stimulation as a heart with profuse organic lesions would be without anesthesia."

Levy and his associate question the assumption that the parasympathetic division of the autonomic nervous system fails to directly affect the ventricles—at least in the dog. Their studies indicate that the vagus nerves mediate a significant fraction of the reflex depression of ventricular performance induced by carotid sinus baroreceptor stimulation. In fact, an appreciable elevation of left ventricular systolic pressure was produced by atropine and vagal cooling after blockage of sympathetic junctions. They conclude that this enhancement of ventricular performance is an indication of a negative inotropic influence of the vagus nerves upon the ventricular myocardium.

Additional evidence of vagal innervation of the ventricles (in the dog) is reported by Hirsch, Kaiser, and Cooper. The nerve distribution in the septal tissues and in other myocardial tissues was identified by noting retrogressive changes in the morphology of the intrinsic cardiac nerves and of their terminals after bilateral cervical vagotomy, bilateral thoracic sympathectomy, or total extrinsic denervation in the canine heart. They believe that nerve-ganglion relationships of cardiac nerves imply vagal characteristics.

Eliakim and Bellet and co-workers studied the effect of vagal stimulation and acetylcholine on the ventricle of dogs. Electrical vagal stimulation caused slowing of the ventricular rate in nine of twenty-three animals with experimental complete A-V block. Acetylcholine produced various degrees of bradycardia. The cardioinhibitory effects were enhanced by neostigmine and were abolished by atropine. They conclude that vagal influences may possibly play a role in the regulation of the spontaneous changes of ventricular rate in patients with complete A-V block.

Knowledge is becoming more plentiful regarding events triggered by an increase in vagal tone. By abolishing the normal sympathetic balance, high spinal anesthesia may increase vagal tone, as will overdistension of the lungs during controlled respiration or administration of neostigmine or suxamethonium as parasympathetic stimulants.

Chapter 10

ROLE OF ANOXIA AND HYPOXIA IN ETIOLOGY OF CARDIAC ARREST

B. G. B. Lucas

Death of the body, or a part, is always the result of anoxia. Irrespective of the original mechanism precipitating cardiac arrest, once the arrest has occurred, there is a state of acute anoxia that may result in permanent damage to parts of the body, even if death does not occur. To many, oxygen lack is associated only with cyanosis or a diminished oxygen saturation in the blood. This is not necessarily true. Anoxia has a multitude of causes and, for this reason, there is much confusion about the condition. Barcroft (1920) was the first to clarify the term. He defined oxygen lack as a failure of oxygen to reach the tissues, and from this he was able to classify anoxia into three groups: (1) *anoxic,* in which oxygen cannot gain access to the bloodstream; (2) *anemic,* in which the blood is incapable of carrying a sufficient quantity of oxygen for the tissues; and (3) *stagnant,* when, for some reason, the circulation fails. Later, a fourth group, *histotoxic,* was added (Peters and Van Slyke, 1931); in the histotoxic form, the cell is poisoned in some way so that oxygen, although freely available in the bloodstream, cannot be utilized by the tissues.

It has become convenient to define anoxia as failure of a cell to metabolize efficiently. There are still the same four standard groups, but histotoxic anoxia can be further clarified and broken down into four subdivisions according to the way in which the metabolism is affected:

1. Extracellular histotoxic anoxia—the tissue oxygen enzyme systems of the body are poisoned. The classic example is cyanide poisoning, in which the cytochrome enzyme system is destroyed, resulting in immediate death of the cell. The action of most hypnotic and anesthetic drugs is also included in this group, since they depress enzyme activity and have been shown to inhibit cellular respiration in the brain (Quastel and Wheatley).

2. Pericellular histotoxic anoxia—oxygen cannot gain access to the cell because of a decrease in cell membrane permeability, such as occurs with lipoid-soluble anesthetic agents such as chloroform and ether.

3. Substrate histotoxic anoxia—there is insufficient foodstuff for efficient metabolism.

4. Metabolite histotoxic anoxia—the end products of cellular respiration cannot be removed, thereby preventing further metabolism, as in uremia or carbon dioxide poisoning.

Anoxic states therefore arise from a variety of causes, but what is not always appreciated is that the effect on the cell is the same whatever the cause and that combinations of types summate their individual effects (Fig. 10-1) so that minor degrees of several types occurring at the same time may produce severe anoxia in a cell. It is seldom that the body suffers from one type of anoxia alone. For example, with cardiac arrest a combination of types occurs: stagnant, because the circulation has failed; metabolite, because waste products will accumulate; and probably extracellular histotoxic, because this condition

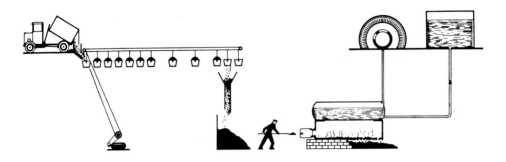

ANOXIC	STAGNANT	ANAEMIC	H I S T O T O X I C			
			EXTRACELLULAR	PERICELLULAR	METABOLITE	SUBSTRATE
(No coal)	(Breakdown of motor)	(Not enough buckets)	(Failure of stoker)	(Furnace door shut)	(Failure to remove ashes)	(No water)
High altitudes	Shock	Anaemia	Hypnotics	Aether	Carbon dioxide	Hypoglycaemia
Asphyxia	Cardiac failure	Carbon monoxide	Barbiturates	Chloroform	Uraemia	
Drowning			Opiates	Cyclopropane		
Lung diseases			Cyanide	Trilene		
Pulmonary oedema						
Nitrous oxide -				Nitrous oxide		
Cerebral ischaemia -				Cerebral ischaemia-Cerebral ischaemia		

U.C.H.M.S. 818/236-53.   V.K.ASTA.

Fig. 10-1. In this diagram, coal, representing oxygen, is transported to a furnace, representing a cell. Atmosphere is portrayed by the lorry and the energy produced in the cell by the turbine. Circulation and heart are shown by the bucket conveyor system and motor. Tissue respiration is represented by both the stoker (extracellular) and by the furnace door (pericellular). Cell substrate is depicted by water in the boiler, and end products of metabolism are represented by ashes from the furnace. The transportation of coal may fail at any point, and several minor defects at different stages will have a major effect upon the steam pressure. Clinically, more than one type of anoxia often occurs at the same time. For example, in a patient with acute cerebral ischemia, the brain will suffer from stagnant anoxia caused by failure of oxygenated blood to reach the head; also, there will be no substrate for the brain to metabolize because of the absent circulation, nor can the metabolites be removed. In cerebral ischemia caused by cardiac arrest occurring during surgery, there is the added factor of the anesthetic agent. (From Lucas, B. G. B.: Asphyxia [anoxia]. In Camps, F. E., and Purchase, W. B.: Practical forensic medicine, London, 1956, Hutchinson & Co., Ltd.)

is usually associated with or occurs during anesthesia.

To many physicians, anesthesia is not associated with anoxia, and it has even been suggested that drugs increase resistance to anoxia. This is because the oxygen consumption of a cell measured while the patient is under the influence of hypnotic or anesthetic drugs is found to be reduced; however, it is erroneous to conclude that a cell will tolerate an increased degree of anoxia. Actually, the drug poisons the cell, so preventing full oxidation that the cell suffers from oxygen want (in this instance, histotoxic anoxia) and will die more easily than a cell not so drugged. This concept is of fundamental importance in the etiology and treatment of cardiac arrest from the point of view of both the heart and the brain. In other words, the heart and brain already poisoned are more likely to fail. It is obvious that if the heart is already suffering from a state of oxygen lack, cardiac arrest is more likely and successful resuscitation less likely.

Cardiac arrest may occur in three ways: (1) by pure asphyxial action on the heart muscle, which, having to beat under anoxic conditions, progressively builds up a larger and larger oxygen debt and ultimately stops; (2) reflexly, as a result of vagal stimulation; or (3) as a result of an overdose of anesthetic agents.

The first response of the heart and circulation to anoxia is attempted compensation. The heart increases its output, and at the same time there is peripheral vasoconstriction, resulting in raised blood pressure and increased coronary flow. After a period, however, the anoxia has a direct effect on both the conducting mechanism and the heart muscle itself, with profound and rapid results. The effect on the conducting mechanism is to cause ectopic rhythm, particularly ventricular extrasystoles. These are dangerous because the ectopic beat, although using up cardiac energy, has a much reduced stroke-volume so that during these beats there is a marked reduction in cardiac output and

a fall in blood pressure. This hypotension results in a diminished coronary flow, which in an already anoxic myocardium may lead to arrest. Alternatively, a run of ventricular ectopic beats leads to ventricular tachycardia and subsequently to ventricular fibrillation. Such a sequence of events occurs occasionally during cardiac surgery when manipulation of the heart causes ventricular extrasystoles that lead to ventricular tachycardia and fibrillation (Fig. 10-2).

The direct effect of anoxia on the heart is a slowing and finally a stoppage of the heartbeat. Although capable of working for short periods under anaerobic conditions, the heart muscle fails to function as soon as its store of glycogen becomes exhausted. Under such circumstances it stops and becomes completely inert; it will not fibrillate.

The heart may stop suddenly as a result of vagal overactivity. Sloan (1950) has shown experimentally that, if the vagi are stimulated in the presence of anoxia, sudden asystole rather than the normal vagal slowing of the heart occurs. Vagal stimulation per se is unlikely to occur spontaneously when the circulation is anoxic, but respiratory irritation causing bronchial spasm results in both vagal overactivity and anoxia. The fact that bronchial spasm causes a rapid fall in blood oxygenation is easily demonstrable. If a relaxant technique is used to induce anesthesia, a period of apnea will cause a fall in oxygenation to about 80% in 1 minute, but if a state of bronchial spasm is induced, either deliberately or inadvertently, very rapid suboxygenation occurs. Also, the social experience of laryngeal spasm induced by "something going down the wrong way" results in rapid cyanosis. The explanation must be that, with bronchial and laryngeal spasm, small bronchi and bronchioles shut and prevent further supplies of oxygen from reaching the alveoli. The pulmonary vein blood then remains unsaturated and myocardial anoxia occurs. This anoxia, in the presence of cardiac vagal stimulation, can produce asystole. Such a cardiac arrest fits well into the category of the forensic

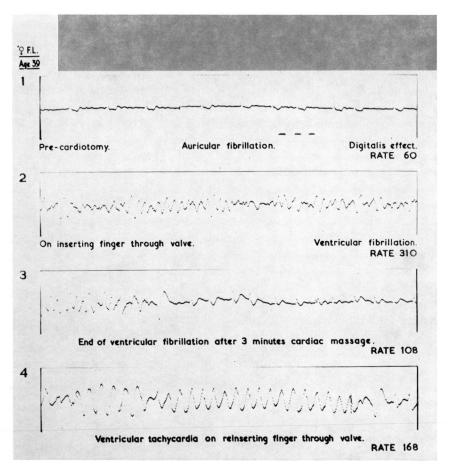

♀ F.L.
Age 39

1

Pre-cardiotomy.   Auricular fibrillation.   Digitalis effect.
RATE 60

2

On inserting finger through valve.   Ventricular fibrillation.
RATE 310

3

End of ventricular fibrillation after 3 minutes cardiac massage.
RATE 108

4

Ventricular tachycardia on reinserting finger through valve.
RATE 168

Fig. 10-2. Mitral stenosis. ECG tracings during mitral valvulotomy. Lead II.

pathologist's status of thymolymphaticus, and it has been postulated that patients suffering from a natural overactivity of the parasympathetic system are more likely to have such a reflex arrest. It has been shown that the use of decamethonium compounds as relaxants, which have marked autonomic activity, is associated with an increase in this type of arrest, particularly in patients suffering from burns (Bush and others, 1962).

Cardiac arrest may also be caused by overdosage of anesthetic agents. An overdose of anesthetic is usually associated with respiratory depression. (Absolute information about the effect of anesthetic agents on the heart itself can be obtained only from isolated heart preparations or from the intact ani-

mal.) Since the introduction of extracorporeal circulation, however, it has been possible to ascertain the effect of anesthetic drugs on the heart and circulation separately.

In general, all anesthetic drugs, with the possible exception of nitrous oxide, are poisons and have a depressant action on the heart and the whole cardiovascular system. This action varies with individual drugs but, in general, the more potent the agent, the greater its depressant effect. At the same time many anesthetic agents cause an increase in catecholamines, which, in the early stages of anesthesia, may mask the direct depressant effect of the drug itself (Kelman, 1971). For example, during light anesthesia with ether or cyclopropane the cardiac output is usually raised and does not fall unless anesthesia is deepened or has been maintained for some while. Halothane, on the other hand, does not cause an increase in catecholamines, and with deep anesthesia there is a most marked reduction in cardiac output.

The intravenous barbiturates have a somewhat similar effect to halothane. Moreover, by virtue of their route of administration, rapid induction has an almost catastrophic effect on the heart, which in someone whose output is already reduced may be lethal. Patients with severe aortic stenosis or constrictive pericarditis are likely to die suddenly when induction of anesthesia with these agents is too rapid.

As far as can be ascertained, nitrous oxide given with an increased concentration of oxygen has little action on heart muscle, but without oxygen it has effects similar to ordinary anoxic anoxia.

The physical state of anesthesia itself causes changes in acid base balance, which also have an effect on the cardiovascular system. For example, a respiratory acidosis, which often accompanies anesthesia because of the depressant action of the agent on respiration, produces similar effects to those of cyclopropane anesthesia, that is, an increase in cardiovascular function in the early stages, followed by a depression if the acidosis is prolonged.

Overdosage of anesthesia, therefore, can be due either to a true poisoning effect over a period of time or to a too rapid induction.

There is a third effect of anesthetic agents on the heart, that of producing changes in cardiac rhythm. Agents that are particularly likely to do this are the halogenous compounds, chloroform, Fluothane, and trichlorethylene, as well as cyclopropane. With all these drugs, the presence of epinephrine may increase the incidence of arrhythmias and, under certain circumstances, may induce ventricular tachycardia and fibrillation. I have discussed the mode by which arrhythmias cause cardiac arrest by producing a fall in coronary blood flow.

Apart from the reflex cardiac arrest associated with vagal overactivity, the essential feature of arrest is defective myocardial metabolism caused either by a failure of substrate to reach the myocardium or by a failure of the substrate to be oxidized due to poisoning of the enzyme systems or lack of circulating oxygen; in short, defective coronary flow.

Once fibrillation has started there is no output whatever from the heart; therefore myocardial anoxia increases. Fibrillation is, in fact, worse than an anoxic heart in asystole because the energy requirement of the fibrillating heart is greater than that of a heart that is in asystole. Thus ventricular fibrillation is more damaging to heart muscle than asystole, and it is for this reason that it is more difficult to restart a heart in fibrillation than one in arrest.

In summary, once the heart has contracted a large oxygen debt and has used up its intrinsic supply of glycogen, it cannot be restarted in the absence of myocardial oxygenation. If the heart has accumulated sufficient anoxic metabolites or has been severely poisoned by drugs, including anesthetic agents, then coronary perfusion by massage or by other means may have to continue until the metabolites or poisons are washed out before the heart will restart. Practically speaking, elimination of poisons and provision for coronary oxygenation will restore the tone of the heart. The heart without tone cannot beat.

Objective evidence to indicate factors responsible for the cardiac effect of systemic hypoxia has been contributed by Ebert and his colleagues. It is their conclusion that vagal stimulation, originating in peripheral receptors, is responsible for these deleterious effects. By using the cardiopulmonary bypass, dog hearts were kept oxygenated but the systemic circulation was allowed to become hypoxic. With either acute or gradual systemic hypoxia, bradycardia and eventual "vagal escape" did occur. When the reverse situation was presented—a normal systemic oxygenation but a hypoxic heart—no appreciable changes in cardiac rhythm occurred. When the heart and the systemic circulation were both allowed to become hypoxic, 80% of the dogs had cardiac arrest after 1 minute. Blood pH changes were insignificant during the periods of hypoxia studied. These studies support the use of atropine prophylactically when systemic deoxygenation appears as a predictable hazard.

The effect of anoxia on the isolated rabbit atrium is to decrease excitability (Torchiana and Angelakos). Anoxia can not be implicated as a contributing factor in increasing myocardial irritability in this instance.

It is true that anoxia produces an added work load on the heart. It is thought (G. R. Graham) that anoxia may release catecholamines, which sensitize the myocardium. In this fashion, the fibrillary threshold may be lowered. An additional comment regarding hypoxia and its influences on the myocardium relates to the reaction of the heart to differential oxygenation. With generalized hypoxia, a lowering of the fibrillary threshold may be particularly prone to occur with a diseased myocardium. Beck and his co-workers have discussed this important aspect in detail.

Few problems concerning cardiac arrest are of a more controversial nature than that concerning the precise role of anoxemia and hypoxia in the etiologic mechanism of cardiac arrest. Johnson and Kirby state:

We have been impressed, in reviewing our experience, that the etiologic factor of greatest importance is hypoxia. Partial obstruction of the airway or inadequate ventilation of the lungs has been present in most of our patients. Preexisting arteriosclerotic or valvular heart disease may increase the susceptibility to anoxemia.*

This statement sums up the beliefs expressed by perhaps a majority of the anesthesiologists and by many of the surgeons writing on the subject.

---

*Johnson, J., and Kirby, C. K.: Cardiac arrest during pulmonary resection, etiologic factors and management, Am. J. Surg. **89:**56-63, 1955.

Gerbode, Lee, and Herrod state: "Anoxia is probably responsible for more cardiac difficulties during surgery than any other toxic influence."

Even though many authors attach great importance to anoxia or hypoxia as the primary factor responsible for sudden cardiac stoppage, Reid has questioned this concept for some years, and the clinical data that have been gathered from a study of 1,710 cases of cardiac arrest as well as from animal experimentation make me support his doubts and question this concept even more.

It is true that adequate oxygenation is essential for enzymatic destruction of all drugs in anesthetic agents and therefore in its absence their depressant action is prolonged. Anoxia, although it alone cannot cause a vagovagal reflex, nevertheless potentiates the action of the anesthetic agent so that the net result is a further decrease in the capacity of the specific tissue to form stimuli. In a high percentage of dogs, vagovagal reflexes can be elicited by mechanical irritation in the trachea or esophagus when the animal is breathing 100% pure oxygen. Sloan, however, reports that he was unable to produce cardiac arrest in dogs with vagovagal reflexes unless anoxia or hypoxia was present.

Experiments have been performed by Reid and associates (1954) in which the tracheas of dogs were completely ligated. Fig. 10-3 illustrates by means of ECG tracings that the cardiac activity was maintained for 53 minutes after oxygen to the lungs was completely interrupted.

The failure of the heart results ultimately from lack of sufficient oxygen to the common myocardium, and it is due to failure of formation of stimuli in the specific tissue. A movie made in the animal laboratory by Reid and his co-workers showed at one point the dog's heart beating for 9 minutes when completely separated from the body and completely without blood within its chambers. This experiment was believed to demonstrate that anoxia per se does not cause sudden failure of the heart. In this instance, it eventually failed because the common myocardium did not respond to stimuli received from the specific tissue.

Clark and associates studied the role of hypoxia in relation to cardiac arrhythmias and the cardiac conduction bundle. Of fifteen dogs that underwent total replacement of the mitral valve, twelve had postoperative arrhythmias and conduction bundle hemorrhage. They died 3 to 10 days after surgery. Of seventy-five surgical cardiac deaths, 48% were found to be associated with hemorrhage in the cardiac conduction bundle. This compared with 6% of fifty-two unselected cadavers.

From a study of 300 fatal cases of cardiac arrest associated with surgical procedures occurring in various South African public hospitals, it was concluded (Kok and Kitay) that "hypoxia alone very seldom led to a sudden cessation of cardiac function."

The effect of vagal stimulation of the heart under conditions of hypoxia and hypercapnia was studied by Sealy and his colleagues at Duke University by stimulating the right vagus nerve until "a vagal escape" occurred. By increasing the content of carbon dioxide, they noted that the duration of cardiac asystole markedly increases. In fact, they believe that the duration of asystole varies directly with the degree of hypercapnia. Mixtures of 30% to 40% carbon dioxide were used.

Sealy and his co-workers found in their experiments that an acute hypoxia actually *decreases* the period of asystole produced by vagal stimulation. Sealy reports on thirty-six cases of cardiac arrest studied at Duke University and concludes that few instances of arrest were due to hypoxia. These are usually the result of long-standing, diminished circulation to the airway.

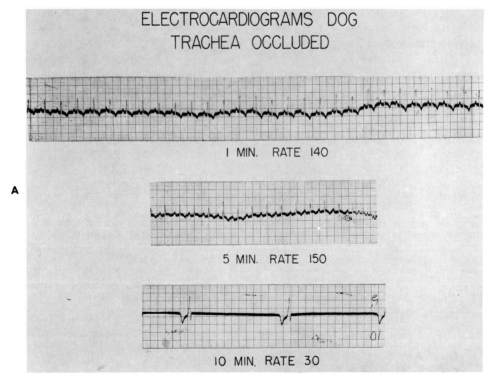

Fig. 10-3. A, B, and C, ECG revealing cardiac activity after total occlusion of the trachea in the dog. In spite of complete anoxia, rhythmic activity of the heart continues for a considerable period of time.

In considering anoxia and/or hypoxia, one should keep in mind factors other than simply that of obstruction of the airway. These would include anemia, congenital cardiovascular disease, acute blood loss, excessive preoperative sedation, and overdose of the anesthetic agent.

One of the major contributions to our knowledge of the events taking place during circulatory, respiratory, and cerebral failure and death has been made by Swann, who found that, in dogs, fulminating anoxia causes respiratory failure, which always precedes circulatory failure. This time lapse averaged 84 seconds. A relationship between the two could not be demonstrated by examining the various components of the breathing pattern.

Reid, in discussing this point at the 1954 meeting of the American Surgical Association, stated:

> If anoxia is a significant factor in the cause of cardiac arrest, why does it not occur in asphyxia; in hypoglycemia; in hibernation; in cerebral accidents with respiratory suppression when the cardia goes on; in people removed from submersion in

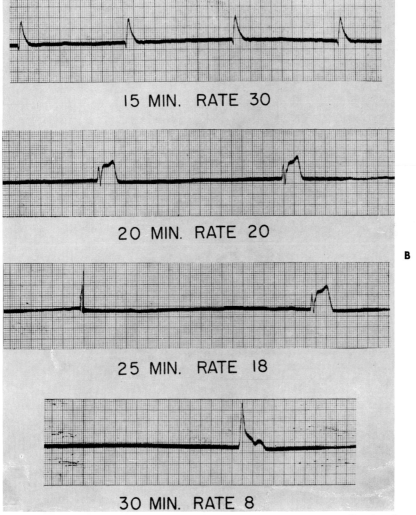

15 MIN. RATE 30

20 MIN. RATE 20

25 MIN. RATE 18

30 MIN. RATE 8

B

Continued.

Fig. 10-3, cont'd. For legend see opposite page.

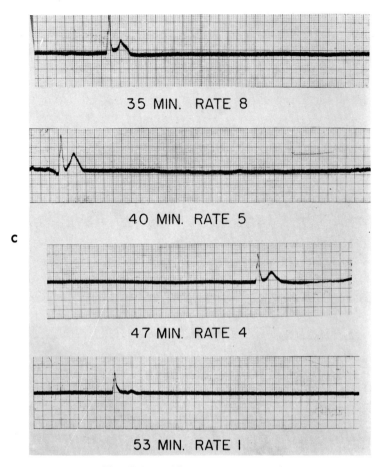

C

Fig. 10-3, cont'd. For legend see p. 172.

whom the respiration fails with long periods of cardiac activity; when an animal is subjected to tracheal occlusion and the heart goes on for long periods? Why is it never reported in congestive failure, in emphysema, and in asthma? Why is it not seen in the newborn infant in the delivery room, which would seem to be a place where anoxia frequently occurs?*

*From Reid, L. C.: (Discussion of West, J. P.) Cardiac arrest during anesthesia and surgery; analysis of thirty cases, Ann. Surg. **140:**623-629, 1954.

Again, it must be emphasized that the myocardium is relatively resistant to hypoxia and to anoxic states as compared, for example, with the cerebral cortex. Irreversible changes in the central nervous system can easily occur prior to any effect anoxia may have on the myocardium. It is because of this differential in the ability to withstand anoxic states that we have, at the same time, both a fortunate and an unfortunate circumstance.

Chapter 11

ANESTHETIC AGENTS AND THEIR RELATIONSHIP TO CARDIAC ARREST

Since the death of 15-year-old Hannah Greene on January 28, 1848, in Newcastle, England, while having a toenail removed under chloroform anesthesia, a direct relationship between cardiac arrest and anesthesia has been the source of much discussion. The specialty of anesthesia has contributed significantly to our present-day knowledge of cardiac arrest and resuscitation and has quite naturally provided much effective leadership. Since the area of primary concern with cardiac arrest has moved out of the operating arena with the advent of practical resuscitative efforts available throughout the hospital, less attention has been directed, perhaps, to anesthesia and its etiologic role in the production of ventricular fibrillation or cardiac asystole.

The relative frequency of cardiac arrest under anesthesia is discussed elsewhere in the book. The relative safety of anesthesia is illustrated in a study reported by Memery. It involves anesthesia mortality experienced from a total of 114,866 anesthetics administered over a 10-year period (1955 to 1964) by a seven-man group of anesthesiologists in private practice. The overall hospital mortality was 1.4% (43,045 anesthetics were obstetrical). A total of twenty-two cardiac arrests occurred (an incidence of 1:3,149 anesthetics). Forty-one percent of the cardiac arrest patients were successfully resuscitated and released from the hospital. More recently, McClure and associates at Emory University reported an incidence of twenty-four episodes of cardiac arrest in 76,556 administrations of general anesthetics and 6,115 administrations of spinal anesthetics over a 7-year period.

In 1964 Dinnick reported to the Association of Anesthetists in England on 600 deaths based on confidential case reports received by the association. Regurgitation of stomach contents, underventilation, overdosage, anoxia, respiratory obstruction, and circulatory collapse caused by sympathetic blockade or intravenous barbiturates were listed among the major hazards of anesthesia. Hypovolemia was identified as a major factor contributing to death in over a third of the patients. In thirty-nine patients adequate spontaneous respirations could not be restored after the use of relaxants. In these cases of "neostigmine-resistant curarization," there was invariably clear evidence either of severe underventilation or of gross fluid depletion and, in a majority, both factors could be identified. Bronchoscopy was associated with twenty-five deaths.

Pierce has provided an interesting study of cardiac arrest associated with anesthesia in a 540-bed, teaching, community hospital where seven certified staff anesthesiologists work. In 1957 there were eight episodes of cardiac arrest from a group of 8,227 patients receiving anesthesia (a cardiac arrest rate of 1:1,025). During a 2-year period between April 1, 1963, and March 31, 1965, there were 18,062 anesthetics administered with twenty-two cardiac arrests. This represents an increased rate of cardiac arrest (1:821), despite recent advances in anesthesia, including the more sophisticated means of monitoring patients in order not only to diagnose cardiac arrest instantly but also to allow for a detection of early warning signs. Pierce attributes a great deal of the higher incidence of cardiac arrest to an acceptance

175

Table 11-1. Cardiac arrests associated with anesthesia*

	1957	April 1, 1963 to April 1, 1965
Total anesthesias	8,227	18,062
Cardiac arrests	8	22
Cardiac arrest rate	1 : 1025	1 : 821
Patients expiring in operating room	2 (25%)	11 (50%)
Patients surviving in operating room	6 (75%)	11 (50%)
Patients surviving in operating room but subsequently expiring in hospital	3 (37%) 50% of O.R. survivors	3 (14%) 27% of O.R. survivors
Patients discharged from hospital	3 (37%) 50% of O.R. survivors	8 (36%) 73% of O.R. survivors

*From Pierce, J. A.: Cardiac arrests and deaths associated with anesthesia, Anesth. Analg. (Cleve.) **45**: 407-413, 1966.

of poor risk patients for anesthesia and surgery.

A comparison of cardiac resuscitative efforts in the 1963 to 1965 period with the 1957 series is of some interest. In the 1957 series all successful resuscitations occurred by the open-chest means of cardiac compression. In the more recent group of cases, it was also noted that all successes required eventual thoracotomy and direct cardiac compression. There was not a single case of permanently successful external cardiac massage.

The precise relation of any specific anesthetic agent to the etiology of cardiac arrest is a particularly difficult matter to document. It is my impression that the advances in anesthesiology have contributed so significantly toward diminishing the patient's operative risk that it is difficult to talk critically in specific terms about any particular agent.

At the annual meeting of the American Medical Association in 1961, a discussion of the role of anesthesia in surgical mortality was led by Dripps and Eckenhoff. The records of 33,224 patients were analyzed in an effort to determine the degree and nature of the contribution of anesthesia to death in this group of surgical patients who received either spinal or general anesthesia and a relaxant. Spinal anesthesia was received by 18,737 of these patients. In this group there were twelve patients whose deaths were believed to be definitely related to the anesthetic—a mortality of 1:1,560; twelve others

died, and anesthesia may possibly have contributed to the deaths—a mortality of 1:780. Of 14,487 patients receiving general anesthesia supplemented with a muscle relaxant, twenty-seven died from causes directly related to the anesthesia—a mortality of 1:536. An additional twenty-nine patients died from a possible anesthetic contribution —a mortality of 1:259. In contrast to the study of Beecher and Todd, Dripps and Eckenhoff failed to note any evidence of toxicity of the muscle relaxants.

The interpretation of data is not easy because of the multiplicity of agents used and the degree of the variables that may enter into any one case. Since the introduction of ether, the armamentarium of the well-trained anesthesiologist has enlarged from a single agent to a wide choice of agents.

The first fifty cases of cardiac arrest reviewed in the literature by Green shortly after the turn of the century were found to include thirty-seven cases in which chloroform had been the anesthetic agent. The file of cardiac arrest cases now contains those which were associated with almost every available agent, including chloroform, ether, cyclopropane, ethyl chloride, ethylene, halothane nitrous oxide, intravenous barbiturates (Pentothal and Surital), vinyl ether (Vinethene), tribromoethanol (Avertin), trichloroethylene (Trilene), alcohol, curare, cocaine, and many others. Almost all routes of administration have been associated with cardiac arrest, including local and regional blocks, intravenously administered agents, open-drop ether, spinal anesthesia, topical and rectal anesthesia with hypothermia.

Oktawiec, speaking before the New York State Anesthesiology Assembly, reported a case of acute circulatory failure in the operating room during a 6-year period at the University of Kansas Medical Center. She concluded that, in reviewing the causes of acute circulatory collapse in the present series of seventy-three cases, two things were apparent: first, that the incidence of cardiac arrest far exceeded that of peripheral circulatory failure, and, second, that unfortunately anesthesia was to be blamed in the majority of cases. In the latter group she placed fifty-two of the cases. These, she stated, were due to (1) errors in technique and judgment, (2) anesthetic overdosage, (3) aspiration of vomitus, and (4) anesthetic management. Of twenty-six cases, 50% of the cardiac standstills occurred during the first hour of anesthesia.

In our study of cardiac arrest cases presented in the first edition of this book, over 60% of all cases had at least two different agents employed at one time or another. A large number had as many as five different agents. Those with spinal anesthesia were supplemented in almost one half the instances with another agent, usually thiopental sodium (Pentothal), with or without oxygen.

Probably most would be in agreement, especially in view of the recent work of Morrow, that all anesthetics may decrease the performance ability of the ventricles and that this reduction is influenced significantly by the size of the dose administered. Increasing scrutiny is being directed to this ability of anesthetic agents to modify the myocardial capacity to propel blood.

Cardiac arrhythmias occurring during anesthesia

The frequency of cardiac arrhythmias occurring during anesthesia and surgical procedures has been a source of investigation by many persons. Of particular note is the recent

Table 11-2. Incidence of arrhythmias related to age and sex*

	Number of patients in series		Patients with arrhythmias		
	Male	Fe-male	Male	Fe-male	Per-cent
Under 10	18	8	9	8	65.4
Under 20	7	3	4	2	60.0
Under 30	6	8	5	3	57.1
Under 40	1	15	1	8	56.2
Under 50	8	19	3	14	63.0
Under 60	8	11	7	6	68.4
Under 70	4	11	8	7	55.6
Over 70	4	11	3	7	66.7
Total	56	86	40	55	61.7

*From Kuner, J., and others: Cardiac arrhythmias during anesthesia, Dis. Chest **52**:580, 1967.

study by Kuner and associates. The validity of their findings is augmented by their method of identifying the arrhythmias. A Holter monitoring system was used. This system continuously records the ECG signal on a magnetic tape for prolonged periods of time. The recordings can be rapidly analyzed by data-reduction systems and any portion can be printed out.

The tracings taken by Kuner and associates were studied by the electroscanner computer. One hundred fifty-four consecutive patients were observed from before induction of anesthesia to the conclusion of surgery. Fifty-six males and eighty-six females, ranging in age from 6 weeks to 86 years, were involved. Table 11-2 relates the incidence of arrhythmias to age and sex. None of the patients was operated on specifically for cardiac problems. Anesthesia usually consisted of thiopental sodium, halothane, nitrous oxide, ether, or cyclopropane, either alone or in combination. The most frequent combination was thiopental sodium and halothane. Forty-four patients received regional block anesthesia, either epidural or spinal. Two patients received local anesthesia. Tracheal intubation was used in ninety-seven instances, forty-eight of which were associated with succinylcholine.

About 62% of the patients were found to have a cardiac arrhythmia. Of these ninety-five patients, a total of 195 arrhythmias were seen. Interestingly enough, the incidence of arrhythmias in patients with preexisting cardiac disease was no higher than in patients without known cardiac disease. Sinus tachycardia was not included as an arrhythmia. The types and frequency of arrhythmias are listed in Table 11-3. The most frequently encountered arrhythmias were wandering pacemaker, isorhythmic A-V disassociation nodal rhythm, and premature ventricular systoles. A number of precipitating factors are suggested. These include types of anesthetic, duration of surgery, intubation, and hyperventilation. Interestingly enough, atropine was believed to be responsible for producing several cases of A-V disassociation during anesthesia.

Wheeler, Corwin, and Martt of the University of Missouri Medical Center studied cardiac rhythm disorders during anesthesia in a random group of forty patients coming to surgery (Table 11-4). The ECG was continuously recorded in each patient prior to and during induction of general anesthesia. Of significance is the fact that 90% of the patients developed some type of cardiac arrhythmia. One half of the patients developed ventricular arrhythmias, most of which occurred during laryngoscopy or endotracheal intubation, or within 3 minutes following intubation. The majority of the ventricular arrhythmias consisted of a premature ventricular contraction that was occasionally of multifocal origin.

Once again, it seems that the frequency of cardiac arrhythmias developing during induction of general anesthesia is sufficiently high to justify routine cardiac monitoring in order to detect and identify these arrhythmias that may be of sufficient severity to predispose to asystole or fibrillation of the ventricles.

Cardiac arrhythmias associated with hyperventilation

A high incidence of ectopic arrhythmias is noted in association with hyperventilation during anesthesia. Several explanations are given. Kuner and associates explain that

Table 11-3. Arrhythmias occurring during anesthesia and surgery (excluding sinus tachycardia)*

Type of arrhythmia	Number of patients
Wandering pacemaker	43
Isorhythmic A-V disassociation	34
Nodal rhythm	29
Premature ventricular systoles	28
Sinus bradycardia	22
Premature supraventricular systoles	19
Paroxysmal supraventricular tachycardia	5
Paroxysmal ventricular tachycardia	5
Others (including atrial flutter and fibrillation, idioventricular rhythm, ventricular standstill, and blocks)	10
Total arrhythmias	195

*From Kuner, J., and others: Cardiac arrhythmias during anesthesia, Dis. Chest 52:580, 1967.

Table 11-4. Cardiac rhythm disorders in forty patients monitored prior to and during induction of general anesthesia*

	Number of cases	Percent of cases
Number with cardiac arrhythmia	36	90
Ventricular arrhythmia	21	53
a. Bigeminy	14	
b. Ventricular tachycardia	4	
c. Isolated premature ventricular contractions	3	
Wandering atrial pacemaker	18	45
Sinus tachycardia	17	43
ST-T wave abnormalities	15	38
Sinus bradycardia	10	25
Supraventricular tachycardia	4	10
S-A block with nodal escape	1	3

*From Wheeler, J., and others: Cardiac rhythm disorders during anesthesia, Mo. Med. 62:680, 1965.

hyperventilation may produce arrhythmias by changing intrathoracic pressure and thereby stimulating stretch-receptors in the visceral pleura or parietal parenchyma. A vagal reflex can also be induced by venous filling of the heart or by alteration in blood gases. It is noted, as a matter of fact, that prolonged respiratory alkalosis causes a migration of potassium across the cell membrane and increases the irritability of the heart because of the alteration of cellular membrane potentials.

Cardiac arrest associated with chloroform

Since chloroform is used so seldom today, it will be considered only briefly. Certainly, for many years chloroform was the center of much controversy. Its association with sudden deaths was common.

Considerable evidence exists that epinephrine hydrochloride and chloroform represent a dangerous combination—one conducive to ventricular fibrillation. In 1911 Levy and Lewis observed that small intravenous injections of epinephrine hydrochloride produces a high incidence of ventricular fibrillation under chloroform administration.

Ventricular fibrillation was produced experimentally in cats during chloroform anesthesia by Levy in 1913; he noted that ventricular fibrillation could be produced by allowing the animal to struggle under induction, by intermittent administration of the anesthetic, or by suddenly increasing the chloroform concentration. Beecher has stated that he believes the same effect occurs in man.

As early as 1847 John Snow wrote a monograph on the sudden deaths occurring during ether and chloroform anesthesia. In this monograph he carefully distinguished between asphyxial deaths and the sudden chloroform deaths. He insisted that chloroform death was associated with a sudden failure of the heart, in that respiration stopped only after cardiac arrest, whereas in asphyxia cardiac activity continued long after respiratory

paralysis. Still more than 100 years later there are those who fail to distinguish between asphyxial death and a primary cardiac death.

One of the outstanding facts in the chloroform deaths was the minute quantity of chloroform that produced cardiac arrest even though the anesthesia produced was extremely light. There is a famous case of Mrs. Crie, a Boston victim of chloroform, whose last words were: "The only fault I find with Dr. Eastman is that he never gives me enough." In Chelsea a sailor at the Marine Hospital was able to reach unaided for a sponge of chloroform and take the fatal breath. Such cases made physicians question that the cardiac arrest was caused by overdosage, although such beliefs persisted for over 50 years. Even as late as 1908 the Commission of Anesthesia of the American Medical Association still persisted in the notion of overdosage.

Deaths continued despite the low concentrations administered, and another complete study was made that was financed by the Nizan of Hyderabad. His physician, Edward Lorarie, had investigated the matter and believed that asphyxia alone was the cause of chloroform deaths. The report of this committee, which was appointed by the British Medical Society, was that asphyxia alone caused the sudden death.

Sansom made a rather complete study of patients dying under anesthesias and it was, his conclusion that the vigorous healthy individual was more likely to succumb to chloroform than the ill or feeble patient. Furthermore, as the number of deaths steadily increased under chloroform, it became apparent that the agent was itself a direct cause of deaths.

Cardiac arrest associated with cyclopropane

An adverse effect by cyclopropane anesthesia on the cardiac "conduction mechanism" has been the subject of many reports since the advent of its use.

Eiseman and associates reported the incidence of cardiac arrhythmias during 334 major surgical procedures in which electrocardiograms were taken on all patients. An incidence of 62% of some type of arrhythmia was noted when cyclopropane was administered to seventy of 113 patients. When compared with Pentothal–nitrous oxide–ether anesthesia, a striking contrast was noted in that only 9% of the latter evidenced any signs of cardiac arrhythmias (twenty-one of 221 patients)! Of the various types of cardiac arrhythmias, the incidence of ventricular arrhythmias was noticeably higher in patients under cyclopropane anesthesia.

Light, Livingstone, and Adams, in reporting on anesthesia for operation on the heart and great vessels, state that they have not found cyclopropane satisfactory for such procedures:

> . . . because of the cardiac irregularities which this agent may in itself produce or render the heart most sensitive to under other conditions which are apt to be present during operations of the heart. The further tendencies of cyclopropane to slow the pulse, depress the respiration, and accentuate the vagal reactions have made us hesitate to use this drug.*

Cyclopropane was used in combination with ether in thirty of a total of sixty-six patients with cardiac arrest reported from the Los Angeles Children's Hospital.

It has been stated that cyclopropane is responsible for vagal stimulation. Cyclopropane does not stimulate the vagus but is itself a drug or agent whose action mimics that of acetylcholine, the mediator of vagal nerve action. To quote Reid and associates:

> Recent work with acetylcholine clarifies some paradoxical reactions which characterize the action of this substance. A few remarks along this line will illuminate for the surgeon the almost labyrinthine complexity underlying the results of vagal stimulation. There is excellent evidence to suggest that the myocardium produces acetylcholine and that a certain level or concentration is essential

for its normal activity. Under certain conditions acetylcholine depresses and under others it stimulates. Bulbring and Burn have shown that if a heart is perfused with Tyrode's solution and oxygen, it will gradually stop beating at the end of twenty-four to thirty-six hours; if acetylcholine is then added to the bath, the heart immediately starts to beat, and if a little more is added, it will beat still more vigorously. After the beat is well established, the addition of acetylcholine then inhibits it. If acetylcholine is added to the newly beating heart, it causes inhibition. The same is true of extracts made from these hearts in their ability to synthesize acetylcholine.*

Beecher and Todd cite the use of cyclopropane in hyperthyroidism as a serious error in the choice of agents and one likely to produce cardiac arrest.

As with chloroform and ethyl chloride, cyclopropane has been repeatedly linked with the likelihood of an increased occurrence of ventricular fibrillation, especially when used in conjunction with epinephrine.

Because of an alarming incidence of cardiac arrest (three in 2 weeks) on one surgical service during the 1950s at Bellevue Hospital in New York City, it was decided to discontinue cyclopropane as an anesthetic. Cyclopropane was the predominant agent being used at this time. Although not of statistical significance, no additional cases of cardiac arrest occurred on this service for a full year. Other surgical services continued to encounter their usual number of cases of cardiac arrest.

Cardiac arrest associated with curare and curare-like drugs

Beecher has repeatedly called attention to the high incidence of anesthetic deaths associated with curare. He has not stated the number representing cardiac arrests; but Beecher and Todd studied anesthetic deaths in 599,548 anesthesias and found that an anesthetic death occurred once in every 370 cases in which curare was used. All of the

---

*From Light, G. A., Livingstone, H. M., and Adams, W. E.: Anesthesia for operations on the heart and great vessels, Arch. Surg. **60:**42-54, 1950.

*From Reid, L. C., Stephenson, H. E., Jr., and Hinton, J. W.: Cardiac arrest, Arch. Surg. **64:**409-420, 1952.

various muscle relaxants were included under curare. An anesthetic death was six times as common under curare as with the general anesthetic death rates of 1:2,100. Death during induction of anesthesia occurred thirty-five times in 555,548 cases, a ratio of 1:15,500, when no muscle relaxants were used; and twenty-one times in 44,090 cases, a ratio of 1:2,000, when muscle relaxants were used.

In addition, these data indicated that death with curare is just as common in the good-risk patient as in the poor-risk patient. Of particular significance is their observation that many of these patients died of a circulatory collapse that had previously not been recognized. They caution especially against the combination of ether and curare. There were thirty-two deaths in 2,000 cases, an incidence of 1:62. There were sixteen deaths in 1,600 cases with cyclopropane and ether.

In the initial 1,710 cases of cardiac arrest studied by us, curare or one of the muscle relaxants was used 102 times. Curare was associated with an arrest once in every sixteen cases, about 6% of the 1,710 cases. The survival rate in curare cases was only 16%, almost half of the overall survival rate.

Cardiac arrest associated with halothane

The potential danger of liquid halothane delivered to the circle system of an anesthetic machine has been pointed out by Kopriva and Lowenstein. They describe a 50-year-old woman whose heart stopped suddenly under halothane anesthesia but who was subsequently resuscitated. Inspection of the anesthetic machine after the incident revealed that the flowmeter bobbin moved the entire range of the halothane flowmeter when the control knob was turned a quarter turn. When the control knob was turned further, liquid halothane flowed briskly from the delivery tube. Examination of the flowmeter needle-valve assembly revealed a damaged needle set, which was responsible for

the exchange altered sensitivity of the flowmeter control. I have observed a sudden case of cardiac arrest during an inadvertent delivery of an excessive amount of halothane during a thyroidectomy procedure. This patient also made a subsequent recovery. Obviously, if inadvertent delivery of liquid halothane occurs, the patient should immediately be disconnected from the anesthetic machine and ventilated and oxygenated by other means. It is important that valves limit flow through the vaporizer to 900 ml. per minute and prevent inflow of pressure high enough to force the liquid anesthetic agent into the delivery tube.

Cardiac arrests associated with halothane anesthesia have been the subject of numerous reports. Forbes studied 100 patients under halothane anesthesia in an effort to document arrhythmias, especially those related to the addition of epinephrine. Thirteen percent showed cardiac arrhythmias related to halothane; and an additional 11% developed arrhythmias after epinephrine had been injected. Most of the former patients showed a nodal rhythm that was attributed to the vagotonic action of halothane in depressing conduction both at the sinoatrial node and in conduction tissue generally—thus allowing ectopic centers to discharge. Atropine (0.6 mg., administered intramuscularly) did not abolish these spontaneous arrhythmias.

Premature systoles are more likely to be observed during halothane anesthesia in the presence of acidosis or after catecholamine administration. One explanation is that halothane inhalation enhances vagal tone and causes bradycardia, a diminished cardiac output, and arterial hypotension. The reflex effects of hyperventilation are accentuated in the presence of halothane as well as in thiopental sodium anesthesia.

The hazards of tipping the vaporizer during halothane administration are pointed out by Munson. In one instance, a Fluotec vaporizer had been momentarily dislodged to the floor. Cardiac arrest occurred shortly thereafter. It was thought that the patient suffered some unusually severe depression from the anesthetic agent as the halothane may still have been vaporizing within the tubing during the period of "100%" oxygen administration.

Repeated episodes of cardiac arrest under halothane anesthesia are described by Skyes. The administration of halothane in low concentration resulted in heart block and cardiac arrest on two successive occasions in a 3-year-old girl.

Propanidid

As an induction agent, propanidid, which has been felt desirable because of its quinidine-like action on the cardiac conductive tissue, exerts a protective antiarrhythmic action on the heart. Certain untoward reactions to its use have been reported, however. These have been reviewed by Johns. He adds a case of cardiac arrest in an 8-year-old boy. The event occurred following induction with propanidid and he attributes this to a massive histamine release.

Cardiac arrest associated with ethyl chloride (isopropyl chloride)

Because of its rather pronounced effect on the heart, isopropyl chloride has not been used extensively for anesthesia, in spite of its obvious advantages, that is, nonirritation of the respiratory tract and rapid recovery of consciousness following its use. Definite toxic effects on the heart, as shown by cardiac arrhythmias, have been demonstrated. These appear to occur at a lighter plane of anesthesia than those seen under cyclopropane or chloroform, and as Cope mentions:

> They develop at a level which coincides with maintenance of light anesthesia, at which death's strong reflexes (e.g., those moving the head of an intubated patient) are not completely abolished, and the combination of this stimulus on an already sensitized heart may initiate ventricular fibrillation and cardiac arrest. For this reason I have discontinued the use of isopropyl chloride anesthesia.*

*From Cope, D. H. P.: Isopropyl chloride as anaesthetic, Br. Med. J. 2:1116-1117, 1950.

Only in three instances of 30,788 anesthetics was ethyl chloride used at the Mayo Clinic. It was not even given consideration in the report by Beecher and Todd.

In the first statistical study, I was surprised to find that ethyl chloride had been associated with cardiac arrest in fifty-eight cases of the total of 1,710.

Cardiac arrest associated with procainamide (Pronestyl)

A report of a case of cardiac arrest following intravenous administration of procainamide has been made by Weingarten and co-workers. The patient was a 30-year-old black man with pulmonary tuberculosis upon whom a right upper lobectomy was to be performed. Following premedication with morphine sulfate and scopolamine hydrobromine as well as secobarbital (Seconal), anesthesia was induced with ether oxygen and continued with cyclopropane and oxygen. During the operation an ECG revealed multiple premature ventricular contractions and ventricular tachycardia. Procainamide hydrochloride, 250 mg., was given intravenously followed by widening of QRS complexes within 1 minute. An additional dose of 150 mg. of procainamide was given 10 minutes later, and an additional 200 mg. was repeated in 5 minutes. At 5-minute intervals an additional 500 mg. was given, and cardiac arrest occurred. Cardiac massage was successful in restoring rhythm to the heart. The patient had an uneventful recovery, and follow-up ECG studies were negative.

Epstein encountered three cases of ventricular standstill during intravenous administration of procainamide for ventricular tachycardia. Even though procainamide is used to correct various conduction defects in the heart, it may, as has been demonstrated, precipitate even more severe irregularities than those which it is intended to treat, such as ventricular fibrillation or cardiac arrest. This paradox has been observed in animal experimentation.

Other authors have reported sudden death

following the administration of procainamide (Kayden and associates; Berry and associates; and Schwartz and co-workers). Kayden calls attention to a case of ventricular fibrillation developing after too rapid administration of the drug. It appears that procainamide often fails to abolish or prevent ectopic beats produced during cardiac catheterization and some mechanical stimuli may be too great to be inhibited by the drug.

A number of cases have been reported in which sudden ventricular fibrillation has followed the injection of procainamide. The improper use of procainamide for arrhythmias caused by overdosage of digitalis must be noted. Ventricular flutter and/or fibrillation have been reported. In a study of the action of procainamide on the heart, Wedd and co-workers conclude that the drug may be particularly dangerous when there is disease of the junctional tissue. It was suggested by Denny and his colleagues that when procainamide is given, a widening of the QRS wave during the administration of the drug may represent a precursor to ventricular fibrillation and is an indication for a discontinuance of the use of the drug.

Procainamide hydrochloride, like procaine hydrochloride, depresses the irritability of the ventricular muscle. The action of procainamide is more prolonged, and procainamide is tolerated in larger intravenous doses than is procaine. It is about one half to two thirds less toxic than procaine.

Cardiac arrest after stellate ganglion block

Moore, in his writings on the stellate ganglion block, mentions cardiac arrest as a possible complication. Adriani and co-workers, in discussing fatalities and complications after attempts at stellate ganglion blocks, mention cardiac arrest as a possible complication.

Although a number of possibilities can be advanced as to etiologic mechanisms, they suggest that reactions to the drug caused by rapid absorption, intravascular injection, or intolerance represent the most likely cause.

Cardiac arrest from analgesic agents

As previously pointed out, cardiac arrest cases have occurred during all types of anesthesia, local and general. Cases appear under various forms of analgesia. Analgesic agents administered by means of special inhalers have received a certain amount of popularity within the last several years, in most instances during obstetric and minor surgical procedures. Trilene and Trimar are trade names for the agent most frequently used, namely, trichloroethylene. Ostlere reports twenty cases of sudden death under the agent. The exact nature of these deaths is not specifically known.

A case of cardiac arrest under trichloroethylene anesthesia was reported by Burstein. The case was that of a 19-year-old soldier injured with multiple missile wounds of both legs and feet and requiring frequent dressings. Trichloroethylene analgesia was elected for these procedures. The agent was administered by means of a Cyprane inhaler (the most commonly used in this country are the Cyprane and the Duke inhalers). Failing to get adequate analgesia, the dial on the inhaler was moved from its original reading of 5 up to 7, and the patient suddenly became flaccid; gasping respiratory movements appeared, and a sudden absence of pulse occurred.

An interesting case of cardiac arrest under trichloroethylene analgesia is that of a 20-year-old white woman was administering trichloroethylene analgesia to herself at the time of artificial rupture of the membranes for a 34-week pregnancy. Intermittent manual compression of the heart was successful in restoring a normal rhythm, but the patient died 5 hours later, having remained comatose.

Cardiac arrest under spinal anesthesia

Six cases of cardiac arrest occurred in 11,136 consecutive peridural anesthetics reported by Lund (Table 11-5). Two-thirds were resuscitated by the open-chest technique.

Table 11-5. Cardiac arrest during peridural anesthesia (11,136 cases) *†

Number	1	2	3	4	5	6
Age and sex	70 M.	70 M.	66 F.	55 M.	56 F.	37 F.
Physical status‡	V	VI	II‖	VII	II‖	I
Preoperative diagnosis§	Arteriosclerosis; perforated ulcer	Heart failure; bundle branch block; strangulated hernia	Hypertension; arteriosclerosis; incisional hernia	Moribund; heart failure; acute obstruction	Hypertension; serum amylase 622	Cystocele; rectocele
Operation	Closure ulcer; thoracotomy	Herniorrhaphy; thoracotomy	Herniorrhaphy; thoracotomy	Exploratory lap.; thoracotomy	Thoracotomy	Thoracotomy
Anesthetic agent and site	Xylocaine 2% 30 cc. at L2	Xylocaine 2% 30 cc. at L3	Chloroprocaine 3% 30 cc. at L1 (cath)	Xylocaine 2% 25 cc. at L2	Xylocaine 2% 30 cc. at L1	Xylocaine 2% 30 cc. at L2
Anesthesia course	Precipitous hypotension	Uneventful to arrest during manipulation	Uneventful until 10 cc. via catheter	Uneventful to arrest during surgery	Cardiovascular and respiratory collapse	Cardiovascular collapse
Precipitating factors	Massive spinal block; hypotension	Stimulation; celiac plexus; reflex (neurogenic)	Reflex or spinal block hypotension	Reflex or chemical	Toxic reaction; hypotension	Anoxia (induct); toxic reaction; hypotension
Postoperative course and result	Recovery; no sequelae	Recovery; no sequelae	Cardiovascular failure secondary to anoxia	Cardiovascular decompression anoxia	Recovery; no sequelae	Recovery; no sequelae

*From Lund, P. C.: Peridural anesthesia—current concepts, Western J. Surg. 72:150-156, 1964.
†One unverified case with complete recovery.
‡A.S.A. code.
§Most significant factors only.
‖Marked obesity.

In a comprehensive study of over 599,544 anesthesias gathered from ten institutions over a 5-year period, Beecher and Todd studied the deaths that were associated with anesthesia and surgery. From this group they noted 58,840 spinal anesthetics. Roughly, spinal anesthetics represented 10% of all types of anesthetics administered. For the group of over 58,000 patients there were thirty-three deaths, an incidence of 1:1,780. These of course were not regarded as being only cardiac arrest deaths.

There are a number of independent reports on successful cases of cardiac resuscitation by cardiac massage carried out on patients under spinal anesthesia. MacLeod and Schnipelsky described such a successful case in 1942. A period of 3½ minutes elapsed before cardiac massage was instituted; subsequently, the patient had a 48-hour period of cerebral edema but recovered satisfactorily. Graham and Brown, in 1939, reported five fatal cases of cardiac arrest, all of which occurred during abdominal surgery. Beecher speculated that sudden collapse after spinal anesthesia is perhaps caused by a sensitivity of certain patients to the drug rather than the effect of an overdose. After investigating experimentally the mechanism of death from spinal anesthesia, Waters reports that an initial decrease in peripheral resistance to blood flow by skeletal muscle paralysis and vasomotor nerves is the first event during high spinal block. This is followed by a decrease in minute volume respiration accompanying intercostal nerve paralysis and then by inadequately oxygenated blood. There is a diminished minute volume of blood flow. As a result of the oxygen deprivation, there comes a progressive loss of vascular tone over the entire body and an acute cardiac incompetence. Next, as the nutrient blood flow becomes inadequate, the medullary respiratory mechanism fails. Oxygenation can still revive the heart during this latter event.

Hebert and colleagues studied complications of spinal anesthesia and listed sudden blood pressure fall that was severe enough to produce signs of cerebral hypoxia in 11.2% of their cases. In 4.2% there was a decided cerebral hypoxia evident. Of the complications studied by Hebert and associates, 5.7% were those due to high spinal anesthesia in which death occurred from vascular and respiratory failure. Lorhan and Merriam made a rather extensive analysis of the causes of death in the fatalities among 580 patients in 1,716 successive spinal anesthesias over an 18-month period. In this group there were twenty-six deaths from all causes, an overall mortality of 3.63%.

There were fifty-nine cases of death under spinal anesthesia reported by the Anesthesia Study Commission of the Philadelphia County Medical Society from a group of 307 deaths under anesthesia. Of the deaths from the single-dose method of spinal anesthesia, 73% were listed as preventable.

Cardiac arrest under spinal anesthesia was associated with other agents that had been used to supplement the spinal anesthesia in almost one-half of all the cases. It would appear that perhaps supplemental or complemental anesthesia increases the hazard of cardiac arrest in patients under spinal anesthesia.

Of course, one of the great dangers in spinal anesthesia is that the spinal block will reach too high a level and in too great a concentration. The motor routes of the thoracic nerves will be paralyzed, causing an intercostal paralysis. Along the phrenic route the second, third, and fourth cervical nerves will be paralyzed, resulting in cessation of movements from the diaphragm. Respiration ceases, and anoxia occurs. Before anoxia effects the circulatory mechanism, however, a marked slowing of the heart results from blocking of the cardiac accelerator fibers originating from the upper five thoracic segments.

Cardiac arrest during induced hypotension

Elective hypotension as an adjunct to certain surgical procedures has not experienced widespread acceptance, although there are still those who are enthusiastic about its use on specially indicated cases. Vandewater has called attention to an incidence of cardiac arrest with induced hypotension of 1.3% in his own experience. This calculated risk, he emphasizes, should be carefully weighed in the light of the nature of the operation and the benefit of the hypotension to the patient. Trimethaphan camphorsulfonate (Arfonad) and hexamethonium bromide are two agents commonly used for inducing hypotension.

Cardiac arrest associated with hypothermia

As the use of hypothermia becomes more widespread and its indications increase, it is imperative that the physician acquaint himself with the dangers and complications resulting from a marked lowering of the patient's body temperature. Already a large number of deaths have occurred under hypothermic anesthesia. Perhaps 90% have been caused by cardiac arrest and particularly by ventricular fibrillation. Bigelow and associates believe that, since ventricular fibrillation and cardiac standstill are not uncommon complications in hypothermia and since one or the other invariably occurs if the body temperature is reduced to a low enough level, a knowledge of cardiac resuscitation is imperative.

Beattie and others, in studying the effect of refrigeration in experimental surgery of the aorta, found that one of the major complications in their study was the production of cardiac arrest or ventricular fibrillation. Of ten dogs dying during refrigeration experiments, seven died from cardiac arrest or ventricular fibrillation. They noted that rectal temperatures below 25° C. are particularly prone to cause cardiac arrest or ventricular fibrillation.

The problem of cardiac arrest in association with hypothermia is so vital and so large in magnitude that it is the principal barrier toward a more widespread application of the principles of reduced body oxygen requirements as produced by general hypothermia.

Da Costa, Ratcliffe, and Gerbode state: "The linear decrease in oxygen consumption found in mammalian species has been reported extensively in the literature and constitutes the basis for the application of hypothermia to surgery." At 20° C. (68° F.) oxygen consumption is approximately 15% of normal. A greater tolerance to decreased temperature levels appears to be noted in the infant.

During cooling, the pulse rate declines, there is a gradual fall of blood pressure, and venous pressure rises somewhat. Physiologic responses have been measured by the ECG tracing and the EEG changes. As mentioned elsewhere, the electrical potentials noted after EEG studies give evidence of a marked decrease in cortical activity. At 20° C. (68° F.) a total absence of cortical activity can be noted in the monkey. These are entirely normal on rewarming.

Bigelow states that in his experience most of the danger from hypothermia may be expectetd when the temperature falls to between 20° C. (68° F.) and 24° C. (75° F.). In the pioneer work of Bigelow and associates, it was demonstrated experimentally that by lowering the temperature of dogs from 38° C. (100° F.) to 20° C. (68° F.) oxygen demand in metabolic activity was reduced to 18% of normal, and survivals could be accomplished when great vessels were occluded over an extended period of time.

Mortality figures on patients subjected to hypothermic anesthesia have not been low. It must be considered, however, that many of these patients are extremely poor risk patients who under ordinary circumstances would not be subjected to operative procedures. Bailey stated in 1954 that so far he had completely interrupted the circulation in more than twenty patients under hypothermia. A mortality rate of 66% was incurred. Deterling, at the same time, stated that of a total of eight patients placed under hypothermic conditions and operated upon by his group a mortality of 30% occurred.

The use of general hypothermia as an aid in operations to correct intracardial defects appears to have had its stimulus primarily from the inability to occlude the inflow and outflow tracts of the heart for an appreciable period of time which would allow for satisfactory opportunity to repair the intracardial defect. Swan states that total inflow tract occlusion associated with open cardiotomy in the normal dog at normal body temperature can be tolerated for $1\frac{1}{2}$ minutes with essentially no deaths, but the risk becomes extremely high if the inflow tract is occluded more than 4 minutes. Death is usually caused by ventricular fibrillation.

Hacker reports an instance of survival of a dog in whom the outflow tract was occluded for a period of 10 minutes. Hypothermia received its chief stimulus from the desire to increase the time period for working in the heart.

A report by Swan calls attention to sixteen patients upon whom open-heart surgery has been carried out under hypothermia. In describing his method of producing hypothermia, Swan seems to feel that rapid cooling and warming reduced the hazards of hypothermia. He notes that the lower the temperature that is achieved under hypothermia, the greater the risk of cardiac arrhythmias. It is also true that the lower the temperature, the longer circulatory arrest may be prolonged without danger of central nervous tissue damage.

Biochemical determinations were made during general hypothermia by Swan and his group in Colorado and have been confirmed by others. Their findings revealed that serum sodium levels remain constant and that serum chloride shows a slight but consistent rise during general hypothermia. The blood volume tends to decrease.

The pH of blood as determined during hypothermia on dogs (Fleming) dropped on an average from 7.35 to 7.03. There was evidence of carbon dioxide retention, which is due to diminished respirations occurring during hypothermia and the increased solubility of carbon dioxide in blood at lowered body temperatures. Few changes were observed by Fleming in the cation or anion concentrations, and he concluded that the acid-base balance changes that occur at reduced body temperatures are those of an uncompensated acidosis, which is mainly gaseous in origin because of either inadequate pulmonary ventilation, cardiopulmonary pathology, or carbonic anhydrase inhibition due to lowered temperature.

Experimentally, the acidosis was corrected by administering base in the form of sodium bicarbonate or by increasing pulmonary ventilation. The mortality rate and the frequency of cardiac irregularities were not altered much by the addition of sodium bicarbonate. The most effective way to combat cardiac standstill in ventricular fibrillation under hypothermia seems to be by increasing the degree of pulmonary ventilation. This can be done by increasing the respiratory rate, the flow of oxygen, and the duration of positive pressure with each breath. In this way the blood pH and the carbon dioxide content can be maintained as a constant.

Schimert and Cowley discuss their experience with forty resuscitations in dogs at temperatures ranging from 15° to 29° C. Their evidence considerably substantiates previous impressions that proper concentrations of sodium, potassium, and calcium ions are essential for the production of a normal heartbeat. First, the body temperature was lowered to hypothermic levels (15° to 29° C.); second, ventricular fibrillation was induced; and finally, the heartbeat was restored by massage and the administration of electrolytes. The latter consisted of an injection of 3 ml. of a 15% solution of potassium chloride to stop the ventricular fibrillation, followed by 15% sodium lactate into the left ventricle, and immediate cardiac massage. Within about 30 seconds, contractions of the heart could be felt. Ringer's lactate solution, with all of the necessary electrolytes for heart action, was then administered. Again it was confirmed that (1) calcium increases myocardial contractility and when present in excessive amounts will stop the heart in systole; and (2) potassium reduces contractility of the heart and when present in excessive amounts will stop the heart in diastole. The action of sodium seems to be that of maintaining myocardial excitability and contractility.

Ventricular fibrillation is one of the main deterrents to the use of hypothermia. The exact mechanism of the onset of ventricular fibrillation under hypothermia is probably caused by a variety of factors. Of particular importance is the tendency toward development of accelerating discharges from ectopic centers in the ventricles coupled with prolongation and variations in the relatively refractive periods produced by the lowered temperature (Badeer). Ventricular ectopic discharges are favored by changes in blood pH, disturbed myocardial calcium-potassium balance, mechanical stimuli, increased activity of cardiac sympathetics, increased amounts of circulating catecholamines, interference with coronary artery flow, and the use of certain drugs.

Attention has centered on the role of the cardiac sympathetic nerves as representing an important factor in the spontaneous development of ventricular fibrillation under hypothermia. Nielsen and Owman's study suggests that hypothermia activates the sympathetic system through a central mechanism producing ventricular fibrillation under deep hypothermia. Using cats as an experimental medium and subjecting them to cardiac sympathectomy, only two out of seventeen denervated animals died in ventricular fibrillation while all seventeen unoperated, controlled animals subjected in the same way to hypothermia developed ventricular fibrillation.

Ventricular fibrillation during neurosurgery in patient under profound hypothermia

The advantages in operating upon the brain during periods of profound hypothermia have appealed to many neurosurgeons. Dissection and excision can be achieved in a relatively bloodless field and without risk of exsanguinating hemorrhage. Anatomic planes are more clearly delineated. The tissues and areas of the brain are more readily explored.

The perimeters of neurosurgical procedures under hypothermic conditions await further expansion following greater security from the likelihood of ventricular fibrillation. Certain protective measures, however, do seem to be already available. The likelihood of ventricular fibrillation occurring will be diminished with gradual cooling and warming, using 100% oxygen and relatively deep anesthesia. The heart will be more likely to tolerate temperature changes if the changes are not encountered abruptly. Galindo and Baldwin point to considerable protection against ventricular fibrillation under such circumstances by a combination of an epidural block and quinidine gluconate. Spontaneous ventricular fibrillation appears, in addition, to be less likely under deep halothane anesthesia. In fact, the diminished cardiovascular excitability afforded by halothane anesthesia may reduce the necessary quinidine gluconate dose level by one third. Shoemaker and others have demonstrated protection against ventricular fibrillation by a sympathectomy. The beneficial effect afforded by the epidural block cannot be entirely explained, but Galindo and Baldwin speculate that such a block may provide a reduction in catecholamine secretion. This secretion is thought to be a sequel to cold stimulation of the sympathetic system with the subsequent production of catecholamine and an increase in cardiac excitability.

Using moderate general hypothermia and profound preferential cerebral hypothermia of 3° C., ventricular fibrillation and respiratory arrest were tolerated by monkeys for periods of 30 to 60 minutes without supportive cardiopulmonary bypass and all of the animals were successfully resuscitated without neurologic damage. Mechanical external cardiac massage (using the Nachlas-Siedband "iron heart") maintained circulation during the early phases of recovery and was considered a major adjunct in the success of the procedure. Despite prolonged precordial compression, visceral and skeletal trauma from excessive thrust were not apparent. In some instances, 2 hours of effective automatic external cardiac massage was continued (Tyers and Wolfson). The efficacy of automatic external cardiac massage as an adjunct to recovery from prolonged hypothermic cardiopulmonary arrest with selective cerebral hypothermia as carried out with laboratory animals would seem to be an attractive procedure for use in certain neurosurgical and vascular surgical procedures and perhaps could be applied to selected trauma situations. Tyers and Wolfson, in an excellent discussion on the use of hypothermia, caution that recovery must be monitored most carefully during the middle phase of rewarming when cardiac output is highest, the greatest amount of peripheral metabolic waste is mobilized, and severe acidosis and fibrillation are most likely to develop.

Ventricular fibrillation in hibernating animals

Although ventricular fibrillation is not an infrequent complication of induced deep hypothermia in man and most animals, Nielsen authoritatively states that it has never been observed in hibernating animals. He attributes this to a fundamental difference between nonhibernators and hibernators such as bats, thirteen-lined ground squirrels, and hedgehogs. For example, he found that in the nonhibernators, the adrenergic nerves in the ventricle are distributed both to the vascular system and to the myocardium proper, while in the hibernators, the myocardial muscle cells receive only a few, if any, adrenergic nerve terminals. He notes that kittens are remarkably tolerant to hypothermia and, significantly, kittens have a poorly developed cardiac sympathetic innervation. Experimentally, Nielsen was able to control hypothermic ventricular fibrillation

by cardiac sympathetic denervation by bilateral incision of the cervical sympathetic chains between and including the superior cervical and stellate ganglia. The superior cervical ganglia contribute approximately 25% to the adrenergic innervation of the heart by way of axons, most of which run down in the vagal trunks. In addition to surgical ablation, adrenergic mechanisms important in the mechanism of ventricular fibrillation during hypothermia can be controlled by depletion of the adrenergic nerves of their noradrenalin with drugs such as prenylamine reserpine. By blockade of the transmitter release from the adrenergic neurons by bretylium, the same effect can be achieved.

Malignant hyperpyrexia

Death under anesthesia caused by a sudden unexplained hyperthermia is receiving increasing attention. While the problem remains one of cardiopulmonary resuscitation, a brief mention here would seem appropriate. A significant feature in many of these cases, along with laryngeal spasms and cyanosis, is the tonic contraction of the skeletal muscle. Massive water and electrolyte shifts and metabolic acidosis develop rapidly. Apparently the susceptibility to development of extreme temperature elevations is genetically determined and chromosomally dominant. Wyant lists halothane, succinylcholine, atropine, monoaminooxidase inhibitors, and chlorpromazine and other phenothiazines as agents that are particularly likely to trigger malignant hyperpyrexia in susceptible individuals. Instead of the expected relaxation following succinylcholine administration, muscle rigidity, along with tachycardia, tachypnea, and cyanosis, develops rapidly. There is occasionally a history of an unexplained operative death in the family; and there is a possibility that susceptible individuals have a high creatine phosphokinase blood level. At any rate, most of the reported cases seem to be occurring in generally healthy adults and adolescents. Byrd reports two cases; one in the recovery room and one occurring 9 hours after induction.

Gatz theorizes that the hyperthermia is caused by the uncoupling (in the mitochondria) of oxidative phosphorylation, the process by which energy liberated in respiration is conserved by the cell in the form of adenosine triphosphate (ATP). When this uncoupling occurs, it is suspected that the cell cannot make ATP. Heat is produced instead.

Unless there is routine monitoring of body temperature, early recognition of hyperthermia may be delayed. Obviously, upon recognition, most vigorous efforts to cool the patient should be immediately instituted and should include gastric or peritoneal lavage if possible as well as external cooling with ice and thermal blankets. Large doses of sodium bicarbonate will combat the severe metabolic acidosis. Pulmonary ventilation should be aggressive, and fluid replacement should be given particular attention. Byrd advocates intravenous calcium and hydrocortisone as well.

Succinylcholine-induced hyperkalemia

It is now apparent that multiple cardiac arrests caused by serum potassium following the administration of succinylcholine are by no means rare—particularly in the patient suffering from a severe burn. This may be also true in the patient suffering from other moderate to severe trauma. The potassium elevation is thought to be caused by the alteration of the muscle-cell membrane and appears to come from injured as well as noninjured areas of the body. The magnitude of serum potassium rise does seem, however, to depend upon the severity and duration of the illness. Lowenstein has demonstrated that maximal succinylcholine "sensitivity" is greatest about the third week of injury. This is important because the uneventful use of succinylcholine repeatedly before this period does not preclude the subsequent possible occurrence of severe acute hyperkalemia and cardiac arrest.

Mazze and co-workers have demonstrated

that the "vulnerable" period seems to vary from 7 to 70 days. Krupp has suggested that serious cardiac complications under these circumstances may be avoided if the patient is pretreated with d-tubocurarine or gallamine triethiodide.

Everett and Allen stress the potential hazard of multiple injections of succinylcholine and caution that atropine in clinically used doses cannot be relied upon to totally eliminate the hazard.

Serum potassium levels may be markedly elevated within seconds preceding the cardiac arrest and may reach levels of even 8 to 13 mEq. per liter. The serum potassium, fortunately, falls rapidly. Successful resuscitation is probably as frequent in this group of patients as in any specific etiologic group since these hearts respond very promptly to adequate techniques.

It is most important to understand that there is an excessive liberation of potassium from the muscle cell membrane in the patient under the influence of muscle relaxants. The bradycardia following intravenous administration of succinylcholine in infants and children is well known and has prompted Gravenstein at Case Western Reserve University School of Medicine to insist that the omission of atropine constitutes an error in management if not given to a child under halothane anesthesia who is to be given succinylcholine in preparation for orotracheal intubation. The effect upon the cardiac rate, cardiac rhythm, and arterial blood pressure may lead to cardiac standstill or fibrillation.

Gravenstein suggests that atropine be given intravenously immediately before the induction of anesthesia to ensure a high atropine effect when it is most needed—namely, during induction of anesthesia. In addition, the anesthesiologist is provided with an opportunity to observe the patient's response to the atropine. Reasonably large doses rather than conservative small doses are urged, and Gravenstein recommends for the normal newborn, 0.1 mg., and for the average adult, 0.6 or 0.7 mg. atropine sulfate intramuscularly for premedication. When the drug is given intravenously, 75% of this dose can be injected rapidly with safety in all patients who are candidates for atropine medication.

The danger of prolonged cardiac asystole subsequent to bradycardia when successive intravenous doses of succinylcholine are administered is much greater in those patients receiving cyclopropane and halothane than with patients being given thiopental or ether.

In the fully digitalized patient, the danger of producing serious ventricular arrhythmias is particularly great (Dowdy and Fabian).

Paraplegic patients being anesthetized with succinylcholine are subject to cardiac arrest because of the significant hyperkalemia that develops, probably from the paralyzed muscle distal to the level of the spinal cord injury (Tobey).

Chapter 12

EFFECT OF ANOXIA ON MYOCARDIAL CONTRACTILITY

Although it has been known for a long time that anoxia will severely damage the myocardial cell and will affect the contractility of the muscle, a more precise explanation of how these detrimental effects are elicited is gradually becoming clearer. Following periods of anoxia, irreversible damage occurs to the mitochondria.

Since the mitochondria contain all the enzymes necessary to catalyze the reactions in the Kreb's citric acid cycle, fatty acid oxidation, electron transport system, and oxidative phosphorylation, the "powerhouse" of the cell can be knocked out. Failure in free energy release may occur as a result of anoxia. Since, in the final analysis, it appears that energy metabolism in the myocardium revolves around the synthesis and utilization of ATP and other like substances, any disturbance in the release of ATP will seriously affect the contractility of the muscle cell.

Anatomically, the changes from anoxia seem to be associated with fragmentation, swelling, and distortion of the normal ultra-structure of the myocardial sarcosomes. It has been demonstrated that the decline in work capacity associated with anoxia is roughly proportional to the decline of possible phosphocreatine contents, and subsequently proportional to a fall in ATP concentration. Fortunately, many of the anoxic changes in the cell are reversible, providing that the anoxia has not been too prolonged.

Action potentials after periods of anoxia have been studied. Using intracellular electrodes on isolated, electrically stimulated, anoxic rat atrial tissue, the height of the action potential fell within 4 minutes after the onset of anoxia. Muscle contractility, on the other hand, was seen to diminish within 1 to 2 minutes; within 15 to 20 minutes complete cessation of activity occurred.

Bing and his group note that the action potential shortens after a brief period of anoxia, but the membrane resting potential diminishes only slightly. After 17 minutes, no action potentials could be elicited. When using papillary muscle and muscle from the dog ventricle and when subjecting muscle to lower oxygen tension, they found that the duration of the action potential shortened rapidly, followed by a diminution in the amplitude.

The amplitude of the transmembrane resting potential fell to an average of 65% of the control value at the time of complete cessation of electrical activity. Bing speculates that the findings are compatible with a more rapid passive transfer of potassium ions outward across the concentration gradient. The diminution of the amplitude of the transmembrane resting potential during anoxia may result from an increased uptake of sodium and a consequent loss of potassium by the cell during recovery. The fall in the amplitude of the action potential can be related to the effects of the lowered resting potential. Alterations induced by anoxia in the ionic transfer across the cell membrane are closely related to the high-energy phosphate concentration within the cell.

Even though the transmembrane potentials may be changed and even eliminated by anoxia, the contractile proteins of the heart seem to be extremely resistant to anoxia. The actomyosin bands do not appear shortened, even 6 hours after death. As pointed out, the high-energy phosphate compound ATP seems to show the fastest disappearance rate. With anoxia, there is an increase in inorganic phosphate, which is the result of breakdown of ATP and phosphocreatine. Glycogen also disappears rapidly from the anoxic heart's muscle cell activity.

When coronary flow is insufficient to meet myocardial oxygen demands, there are profound alterations in metabolism, structure, function, and chemical composition of the myocardial cell. Aerobic metabolic systems are compromised and are unable to maintain myocardial ATP stores. A compensatory acceleration of the glycolysis ensues; glucose extraction is enhanced and glycogen stores are depleted. Although glycolysis is increased, it cannot compensate adequately, and neither transmembrane potential nor normal contractility is maintained.

Chapter 13

ACID-BASE AND ELECTROLYTE IMBALANCE

Herbert L. McDonald

The important role of the concentration of potassium on myocardial function was first described by Ringer in 1882 and 1883. This classic work demonstrated that high extracellular potassium concentration caused cardiac arrest in diastole. d'Halluin (1904), Hooker (1929), and Wiggers (1930) further demonstrated that potassium infusion converts ventricular fibrillation to standstill. In 1955 Melrose and associates described a simple technique for the utilization of these principles in open-heart surgery. Cardioplegia modeled after his method was used extensively. Kolff and Effler and Lam and their co-workers led the implementation of the technique in this country. Despite the fact that potassium citrate cardioplegia has since been generally abandoned, the experience gained by its use, coupled with the basic concepts of Ringer, has furnished the stimulus for the increasing interest in the relation of potassium alterations to the etiology of clinical cardiac arrest. The purpose of this discussion is to present the salient features concerning that relationship.

The changes in the ECG caused by serious fluctuations in serum potassium are now well documented (Fig. 13-1). These changes correlate roughly with the serum potassium concentration. Levels of 3 mEq. per liter or below will usually be reflected in the ECG by the alterations shown. In hyperkalemia, the depicted T wave disturbances, increased P-R interval, and other changes occur when serum potassium reaches 6.5 mEq. per liter or greater. At levels of 8 mEq. per liter, absence of these changes would be very unusual. In the vicinity of 8 to 10 mEq. per

liter, a biphasic curve is followed by ventricular standstill or fibrillation in the majority of instances. Darrow states that the following sequence of changes accompanies increasing concentrations of potassium in serum: appearance of high-peaked T waves, increased duration of the the P-R interval leading to atrial standstill, a biphasic curve with progressive delay in ventricular conduction, and, finally, total arrhythmia leading to cardiac arrest.

In hypokalemia, the resting membrane potential is slightly increased and the duration of the action potential is considerably increased. Therefore repolarization is progressively lengthened. If not corrected in a reasonable time period, hypokalemia may delay repolarization enough that the myocardial cell is depolarized by the following stimulus before it has been completely repolarized. One may then speak of a lower excitability threshold. This state of affairs will be reflected in the ECG by a negative S-T displacement with lengthening of Q-T interval, inversion of the T wave, lengthening of Q-T, and, frequently, the presence of a U wave. The lengthened Q-T is caused by the great duration of T, especially its ascending limb. A prolonged P-R interval may also occur with any of the above patterns. These changes quickly disappear with correction of the serum potassium levels.

In hyperkalemia, the resting membrane potential is decreased and the action potential is shortened. Up-stroke velocity of the action potential is decreased. Intraventricular conduction is slowed and the QRS duration is increased. Repolarization changes precede

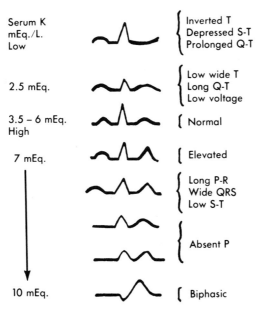

Serum K mEq./L. Low		Inverted T Depressed S-T Prolonged Q-T
2.5 mEq.		Low wide T Long Q-T Low voltage
3.5 – 6 mEq. High		Normal
7 mEq.		Elevated
		Long P-R Wide QRS Low S-T
		Absent P
10 mEq.		Biphasic

Fig. 13-1. ECG changes produced by alterations in serum potassium (K) concentrations. The spreading of the QRS and lengthened Q-T interval in hypokalemia has been attributed to hypocalcemia rather than the hypokalemia. (Redrawn from Darrow and Pratt; from Statland, H.: Fluids and electrolytes in practice, Philadelphia, 1954, J. B. Lippincott Co.)

an appreciable decrease in velocity. This explains why the earliest manifestation of hyperkalemia in the ECG is a peaking of the T wave.

In hyperkalemia, the alterations of the ECG are augmented when serum sodium is normal. A similar relationship has been established with serum calcium levels. In hypokalemic alkalosis, decrease of the calcium level contributes to the abnormal pattern, but this effect is less than that of lower potassium. It should be stressed that the presence of all these ions in appropriate concentrations is necessary for normal cardiac excitability and contraction. The ionic systems involved are extremely complex, and one must constantly keep in mind that the relationships of these ions to one another is the best and only course by which a given clinical situation may be understood. However, the extracellular and intracellular concentrations of potassium seem to play the central role.

The frequently expressed opinion that the ECG is the result of forces operating across the surface membrane of cardiac cells stems from Bernstein's theory of opposing electrical charges at this interface. The membrane separates a layer of anions on its inner side from a layer of cations on its outer side, thus creating an electrical potential across it. Permeability is increased and ionic redistribution occurs with depolarization. This theory was originally proposed for nerve fibers but has since been applied to myocardial cells as well. Actually, the ionic transport at this interface is much more complex, but in principle the theory is useful. The magnitude of the membrane potential at rest is determined chiefly by the ratio of the intracellular to the extracellular concentrations of potassium. In the pacemaker fibers, the transmembrane potential is brought to a critical level by spontaneous slow diastolic depolarization. At this level, depolarization becomes rapid and gives rise to a new action potential. In the nonpacemaker fibers of the atria and ventricles, the resting potential remains steady until the fiber is ·depolarized by the spread of excitation.

This "ionic hypothesis" has received support from the work of Hodgkin and Huxley utilizing the axon of the giant squid. In the resting state, intracellular potassium concentration is relatively high. With deloparization, efflux of intracellular potassium and influx of sodium occurs. After a short plateau, the membrane potential returns to its resting level by a slower process of repolarization, during which potassium influx and sodium efflux take place, restoring both the electrical and chemical equilibrium of the cell membrane.

Ionic transport through the cell membrane is also influenced by cell enzyme systems. Equilibrium after depolarization is attained by a biologic mechanism often termed the "sodium-potassium pump." The ionic redistribution occurring with depolarization— egress of potassium and ingress of sodium— is reverted during repolarization. To effect this latter process, cellular work is required to "pump" sodium from the cell. The energy for this process is supplied by the action of adenosinetriphosphatase on adenosine triphosphate. Potassium ions presumably increase adenosinetriphosphatase activity. Reentry of potassium during diastole is apparently necessary for reestablishment of mechanical as well as ionic equilibrium of membrane potential. The description of ischemic contracture of the heart or "stone heart" by Cooley and associates and a following editorial on the subject by Katz and Tada implicate the depletion of adenosinetriphosphatase in this interesting form of cardiac arrest. The possibility that decreased extracellular myocardial potassium is part of this complex problem is alluded to.

Aberrations in the ratio of potassium ions on either side of this still poorly understood membrane were considered to be an important cause of ventricular fibrillation by Kehar and Hooker in 1935. It has been observed that rapid perfusion of potassium results in immediate ventricular fibrillation, whereas slower perfusion with the same extracellular potassium concentration causes decreased conduction, but fibrillation does not ensue. Many contemporary writers and investigators have stressed the importance of the ratio of intracellular potassium to extracellular potassium rather than the absolute values of either. The same can be said for the relationship of potassium to sodium and potassium to calcium.

From the foregoing discussion, it is hoped that the reader has been logically lead to the understanding that the key to maintenance of normal cardiac excitability lies in the ratios of these important ions at the cellular interface. Their transport may be altered by hemorrhagic shock, trauma, drugs, blood pH changes, various disease processes, and hormones, especially the catecholamines. The manner by which these phenomena influence the intracellular-extracellular potassium ratio will be discussed in an attempt to correlate body potassium variations and their possible role in the etiology of cardiac arrest.

The studies of Swann and Spafford concerning ventricular fibrillation resulting from freshwater drowning implicate potassium. They attribute the increase in potassium to anoxemia and to hemolysis, with subsequent release of intracellular potassium. Even though the extracellular potassium concentrations were not extremely high, the ratio of potassium to the other extracellular ions was greatly increased. They term this the "fibrillating ratio" and attribute much importance to it, noting that in seawater drowning the serum potassium may even be doubled and often is much higher than in freshwater drowning. Fibrillation does not occur because the "fibrillating ratio" is not exceeded.

The association of cardiac arrest with abrupt changes in extracellular potassium concentration caused by clinical misadventure receives considerable impetus when such events cause death. Elman and associates say this of their experience with too rapid infusion of potassium salts:

Cardiac standstill immediately followed with all the appearance of death, but fortunately three minutes later action started again with the dramatic return of all the vital signs to normal.*

High serum potassium levels leading to potassium intoxication are not rare. Adrenal insufficiency, diabetic acidosis, severe burns, shock, and renal insufficiency are clinical states that may be frequently associated with hyperkalemia. The latter is probably the most apparent cause of cardiac arrest due to potassium toxicity.

Finch and his co-workers note the frequency with which uremic patients exhibit ECG's indicative of potassium intoxication. Hypertonic sodium chloride and glucose are effective in temporary amelioration of these tracings. Both agents promote the transgression of extracellular potassium to the intracellular space. The sequence of events in experimental hyperkalemia is well duplicated in experimental anuria. Here, the concentration of serum potassium rises progressively because of cellular damage, inability to store potassium, and poor excretion of this ion. Enselberg's observations that ECG records in the agonal state are similar to those of hyperkalemic dogs lends considerable credence to the idea that serum potassium excess is very frequently associated with the end stages of life, regardless of the basic disease process.

Potassium variation associated with concomitant blood pH changes, especially acidosis, is an important facet in the consideration of potassium-induced cardiac arrest. Casten and Bardenstein point out that the ECG tracings in experimental animals and in patients during the *posthypercapnic phase* (such as may occur near the termination of an anesthetic agent) may closely resemble those observed in hyperkalemia. They state:

Several factors may be responsible for this similarity. First, the stress and trauma of surgery may mobilize intracellular potassium into the plasma. Secondly, respiratory acidosis, by diminishing blood pH, may further cause an increase in circulating potassium, in an attempt at compensation. Finally, the posthypercapnic phase, in which the most marked electrocardiographic changes are observed may also sensitize the myocardium to slight increases in circulating potassium. It is usually in this phase that arrest occurs, and it is also at this time that the highest potassium level has been found.*

The significance of electrolyte changes is particularly great in infants and children who, because of their increased percentage of body water, are more sensitive to changes in electrolyte concentration.

Brown and Miller showed that rapid correction of severe hypercapnic acidosis is followed by ventricular fibrillation in the experimental animal. Young and colleagues analyzed the effect of electrolyte metabolism during and immediately following acute hypercapnia. These changes correlate closely with ECG abnormalities that occur with hyperkalemia. It is not known precisely from where the potassium is mobilized. The liver, skeletal muscles, and bones represent likely sources.

Increased hydrogen ion concentration is thought to interfere with the transport of potassium at the cell membrane. It is known to be a strong stimulus to liberation of epinephrine, which in turn causes mobilization of potassium from the liver. Increased potassium levels in serum also result as a compensatory effort of the kidneys in metabolic acidosis. The report of Stewart and associates supports the concept that acidosis and potassium toxicity are closely related to maintenance of normal cardiac excitability with equilibrium at the cell interface. Resuscitation of their patient was not satisfactory until alkali was infused, despite peritoneal dialysis, administration of insulin and glucose, and the use of calcium gluconate. The pH was

---

*From Elman, R., and others: Intracellular and extracellular potassium deficits in surgical patients, Ann. Surg. 136:111-131, 1952.

*From Casten, D. F., and Bardenstein, M.: Cardiac arrest in children, Bull. Hosp. Joint Dis. 16:13-21, 1955.

7.08 and the potassium was 8.6 mEq. per liter when correction of the acidosis was begun.

The reverse side of the coin, hypokalemia, is usually associated with alkalotic states. This situation has generally been considered to be less alarming than hyperkalemic states. However, the increased use of controlled ventilatory support in the postoperative period, especially following cardiac surgery, has frequently been associated with decreased serum potassium levels. Controlled ventilation is associated with hyperventilation more often than not and, despite theoretic consideration to the contrary, is considered to be reasonably well tolerated. These patients are often ones who have been using diuretics preoperatively. Many are taking digitalis which further complicates the matter. The report of Verska emphasizes the profound levels of hypokalemia, which may occur rapidly and without warning. To control ventricular arrhythmias in his patient it was necessary to give 120 mEq. of potassium chloride in a 2½-hour period.

In an excellent clinical study by Flemma and Young, the importance of this problem is pointed out. Serious ventricular arrhythmias occurred in some of their patients. Correction of the arrhythmia was accomplished by infusions of rather small doses of potassium. Selmonosky and Flege report on seven patients who developed serious ventricular arrhythmias following open-heart surgery. Five of these patients had been receiving long-term diuretic therapy with thiazide drugs, and all seven had been maintained on digitalis therapy. Following rapid administration of small doses of potassium chloride, the arrhythmias ceased. In two patients the arrhythmia recurred within a few minutes, but repeated small doses of potassium corrected the situation. Ebert, Sampson and Anderson, and Lown and co-workers have all called attention to the probability that patients treated with these drugs will develop serious arrhythmias when hypokalemia is allowed to occur. The plea of

Flemma and Young that more careful consideration be given to respiratory alkalosis and accompanying hypokalemia in such patients is strongly endorsed here.

Extensive study of potassium decreases following cardiac surgery has been reported by many observers. Breckenridge and others have shown the efficacy of infusing potassium solutions at the time of such surgery and have given guidelines for expected losses. These vary widely in individual cases. Potassium salts, usually potassium chloride, may be given rapidly when indicated. Doses of 1 mEq. per minute are satisfactory and relatively safe. ECG monitoring and several K^+ serum determinations are essential. Yikoyarna and associates, Dieter and co-workers, and others have also studied this problem. It is transient in nature and if potassium stores are normal the body tolerates the insult well. Often, these patients are those most likely to have decreased total body potassium so that preoperative and postoperative vigilance by the clinician is mandatory.

Roebuck and co-workers have demonstrated the beneficial effect of hypertonic saline solution in hypercapnic dogs with elevated serum potassium and decreased serum sodium. They conclude that a sodium-potassium ratio of less than 12 results in ventricular fibrillation in hypercapnic dogs. Bellett has repeatedly emphasized the deleterious nature of low pH and high potassium on cardiac function. Ledingham and Norman have shown experimentally that metabolic acidosis accompanying respiratory acidosis may be an important variant in cardiac arrest. Malamos and associates have emphasized that metabolic disorders accompanying acidosis are probably the cause of ventricular fibrillation in hypothermic dogs.

The beneficial effect of hypertonic saline solution in potassium toxicity referred to previously has been substantiated in human beings by Garcia-Palmieri. Decrease in serum potassium and improvement of heart action as monitored by the electrocardiogram were observed. He assumes, as have others, that increased serum sodium causes the cellular influx of potassium. An experimental study by Danielson and co-workers further corroborates the salutory effect of dextrose and potassium salts on the cardiac rhythm after myocardial infarcts. The relation of potassium concentration to that of sodium and calcium is treated in more detail elsewhere in this book.

Leveen and co-workers have called attention to the increased incidence of cardiac arrest in patients with hemorrhagic shock treated by massive transfusion with bank blood. Several factors in hemorrhagic shock compound the dangers of using such blood. The increased circulating epinephrine in patients with shock results in glycogenolysis by the liver with release of potassium stored there. This potassium ascends directly to the heart before it can reach the tissues where equilibration occurs, as when blood is transfused intravenously. The warming of bank blood substantially restores the normal extracellular-intracellular potassium ratio. Transfusion of cold blood should be avoided. The papers of Boyan and Howland further discuss this subject.

Taylor and co-workers, Pew, and others report on cardiac arrest during exchange transfusion in the newborn infant. Increased potassium levels have often been present, but no direct correlation is drawn. Taylor stresses that acidosis appears to be a common denominator in his cases.

The "antagonistic" nature of digitalis to the adverse effects of hyperkalemia on cardiac conduction is well accepted. Use of potassium, conversely, is an important adjunct in treatment of digitalis intoxication. It is usually considered that digitalis prevents the influx of potassium, thereby helping preserve the equilibrium of extracellular and intracellular potassium at the cell interfaces. This beneficial effect may be reversed when toxic levels are reached. Fisch and colleagues administered relatively small doses of potassium to dogs receiving toxic amounts of digitalis, thereby producing serious ventricular arrhythmias. Potassium should be used discretely in the treatment of digitalis intoxication, especially in those patients with A-V conduction defects.

Quinidine decreases myocardial excitability by a direct action. It has been postulated that this action is mediated by the ability of quinidine to stablize membrane permeability, resulting in decreased potassium efflux and sodium influx.

The bearing of various sugars, buffers, and ions on the transport of potassium has been the subject of recent reports (Kaplan and Fisher; O'Brien and Guest). The ionic ratios at cell interfaces are shown to be influenced quite definitely by perfusion of carbohydrate solutions. Extracellular potassium is reduced by the use of these sugars, especially 10% glucose and fructose in normal saline solutions. In the latter instance, impressive increases of myocardial potassium were noted in dogs subjected to ventricular fibrillation by potassium chloride infusion.

The association of hypothermia and ventricular fibrillation is well known. In 1947 Elliot and Crimson noted that serum potassium and calcium levels rise in rats under hypothermia. Swan has commented that potassium levels (in hypothermia) are among the most marked aberrations from normal physiology that he has observed. He notes that the blood potassium falls to as low as 40% of control values in dogs subjected to hypothermia and hypoventilation. With inflow occlusion, it appears that potassium accumulates in the tissue spaces to the extent that, after circulation is resumed, the serum concentration rises to levels considerably higher than before. More potassium leaves the extracellular space during hypothermia than is excreted in the urine. With warming, the excreted potassium is commensurate with the decreased serum level noted.

Varying degrees of metabolic acidosis occur in hypothermia, depending on the degree and length of cooling. Bigelow states that most of the aberrations of hypothermia occur at temperatures between 20° and 24° C.

Taylor has suggested that hypothermia alters myocardial electrolyte equilibrium by permitting potassium influx and sodium efflux.

This discussion has been largely concerned with phenomena thought to occur in instances of elevated levels of extracellular potassium, since this is the most important aspect regarding this ion's role in the cause of cardiac arrest. Severe hypokalemia, however, is known to result in systolic standstill. This is attributed to the unmitigated effect of extracellular calcium.

Pathologic changes in potassium-depleted rats have been studied by Molnar and associates. Earliest abnormalities noted were cytoplasmic changes in myocytes with preservation of mitochondria and nuclei, indicative of altered membrane permeability induced by electrolyte imbalance.

Surawicz and Gettes have demonstrated two types of arrest caused by potassium. First, the usual changes of hyperkalemic asystole were noted in rabbits, as recorded by measuring several parameters of myocardial function, including membrane potentials and conduction time. In a second group, perfused with hypokalemic solutions (0.8 mEq. per liter) for 3 to 15 minutes then suddenly with normokalemic solutions (4.8 mEq. per liter), arrest occurred. However, the arrest was different from that caused by high levels of potassium (12 mEq. per liter). These differences were manifested as dissimilar findings in resting potentials, among others. Surawicz and Gettes concluded that such arrest may or may not occur in situ. It is caused by depression of pacemaker fibers, probably by inhibition of the diastolic repolarization, and not by the depression of atrial and ventricular excitability and conduction that characterizes the action of high potassium levels.

Another intriguing clinical setting for critical changes in potassium ratios at the myocardial level has been associated with the use of succinylcholine during surgery. Cardiac arrest and serious ventricular arrhythmias caused by succinylcholine used during sur-

gery were reported by Roth and Wuthrich in 1969. Since then, numerous reports have followed showing that very large amounts of potassium are liberated in several disease states and trauma. Extracellular potassium is increased resulting in cardiac arrhythmias. The mechanism of this release is not precisely known. A recent review of this phenomenon as well as other causes of hyperkalemia during anesthesia has been made by Robbins and co-workers.

Ascribing to potassium a singular role in the etiology of cardiac arrest would be unrealistic except in those instances when such striking laboratory and clinical findings exist to make this etiologic diagnosis secure. This is the exception, not the rule. The probability that potassium changes play a dominant role is supported by a preponderance of clinical and experimental evidence.

Cardiac arrest in the burn patient

As mentioned elsewhere in this book, repeated episodes of cardiac asystole in the burn patient may be associated with succinylcholine-induced hyperkalemia. Even though normal serum potassium levels are recorded prior to anesthesia, a rapid rise in serum potassium concentration following the injection of succinylcholine may occur. The rise in serum potassium concentration following the injection of succinylcholine is especially likely to occur in the patient with moderate to severe trauma, including particularly those patients with burns and upper motor neuron lesions. Succinylcholine-induced hyperkalemia also has been reported in patients with diffuse lower motor neuron disease and spinal cord trauma. It should be noted that there may be a perfectly normal serum potassium prior to the injection of succinylcholine. Following injection of the succinylcholine, a marked peaking of the T wave and sinus bradycardia may be noted.

Attention has previously been called to the apparent increased frequency of cardiac arrest in patients being anesthetized for the treatment of burns. Finer and Nylen, Upsala,

Sweden, have also been impressed with the relative frequency of cardiac arrest in the burn patient and have reported on their experiences. Their reported incidence of cardiac arrest during anesthesia for burns is 1:209. This can be compared with an incidence of only 1:2,744 during anesthesia for other plastic procedures. Of the cardiac arrest cases occurring on the plastic surgery service at the University of Upsala, 75% occurred in patients with burns. Many authors have commented on this particular problem (Moncrief and co-workers).

In summarizing the experience of cardiac arrest occurring in burn patients, Finer and Nylen point out that all the cases reported in medical literature have been examples of burns that were of a severity not usually thought to be fatal. In every reported case, they state that the cardiac arrest occurred during operations between 21 and 50 days following the burn.

Anuria and cardiac arrest

Sudden death in the anuric patient is not rare. Stock has reported sudden death in three of twenty-two anuric patients. In all of these, death was attributed to potassium intoxication. Suppression of urinary excretion is one of the most important factors in potassium intoxication. Even in severe renal disease, potassium clearance remains remarkably constant. Apparently the limiting factor is the amount of urine excreted. In discussing the clinical syndrome of potassium intoxication, Finch and co-workers note the frequency with which these ECG abnormalities occur in uremic patients and believe that they are due to the hyperpotassemia resulting from the uremia. Hypertonic sodium chloride and glucose temporarily correct these ECG abnormalities due to the hyperpotassemia.

Hardy, in his book *Fluid Therapy,* states:

In uremia, potassium is liberated from the cells and may so increase the extracellular level as to stop the heart. Potassium intoxication due to an abnormally elevated concentration of this ion in the extracellular fluid may be observed in states of renal insufficiency in which potassium is not excreted normally, in diabetic acidosis, and following trauma or severe burns, where large amounts of nitrogen and potassium are mobilized in the presence of a reduced output. In such patients the plasma potassium may rise to dangerously high levels and cardiac arrest may supervene.*

As with other clinical states associated with elevated serum potassium levels (extreme dehydration, diabetic ketosis, massive tissue injury, sudden release of circulatory obstruction in an ischemic limb, and administration of large amounts of cooled stored blood), digitalis may help thwart the untoward effect on the heart. Glucose, insulin, ion exchange resin, and, ultimately, dialysis may be needed to lower the serum potassium levels.

Relationship between ventricular fibrillation and potassium and calcium

Swan shows at least two definite relationships between potassium and ventricular fibrillation: (1) ventricular fibrillation produces a marked extravasation of potassium into the coronary circulation and (2) if the coronary vessels of a heart in ventricular fibrillation are perfused with potassium chloride, the fibrillation will cease. Also, a possible relationship between acetylcholine, the cholinesterases, and the distribution of potassium in the heart was pointed out. Acetylcholine or an anticholinesterase produces a pronounced change in the tendency of the heart to fibrillate when certain stimuli are applied, and, too, there is a definite change in the disposition of the potassium.

Grumbach and colleagues studied the effect of injections of calcium and potassium-free perfusion media on the isolated perfused heart. Calcium chloride injected into the perfusion stream was observed to initiate ventricular fibrillation, whereas perfusion with a potassium-free perfusion medium also produced ventricular fibrillation. The latter did not occur if calcium had also been re-

---

*From Hardy, J. D.: Fluid therapy, Philadelphia, 1954, Lea & Febiger, p. 21.

moved from the perfusion medium. Calcium produced ventricular fibrillation with increasing ease as the potassium concentration of the tissue fluid was lowered. They concluded that the removal of the potassium from the tissue fluid leads to a failure of the heart to resist the stimulating action of the potassium present in normal Krebs solution, with the result that the tissues begin to discharge impulses spontaneously if the potassium concentration falls below a certain level.

The mechanism of ventricular fibrillation in 246 dogs was studied by Gordon and Jones. They rapidly injected high levels of potassium into the femoral vein. Of animals that received 20 mg. per kilogram body weight, 90% went into ventricular fibrillation. They cite a definite time-dose response as the serum potassium level falls rapidly. In addition, they conclude from their experiments that anoxia, hypercapnia, hemorrhage, stress, various drugs, and anesthetic agents all are capable of producing a significant elevation in the serum potassium. In referring to the work of Houssay, they indicate the liver as the source of this potassium, with the sympathetic nervous system acting to release the potassium–hexosephosphate complex from the liver.

The electrical potential across the myocardial cell membrane is affected by the extracellular concentration of potassium. With high concentration, it is possible that the myocardium is suddenly depolarized.

Magnesium and cardiac arrest

Next to potassium, magnesium is the major intracellular cation. Its precise measurement in the various body components has not been readily accomplished. Some generalizations, however, now appear warranted (Seller and Moyer). With excessive administration, intraventricular conduction is delayed and the spontaneous rhythm of the heart is depressed. Presumably this may be caused by a decreased loss of intracellular potassium resulting from a magnesium-induced decrease in permeability of the cell membrane to potassium. Potassium is known to activate adenosine triphosphate. ATP is essential for membrane activity allowing active transport of cations across the cell membrane which maintains transmembranous cationic gradients including the high intracellular concentration of potassium.

On the other hand, when there is a diminution in the level of magnesium there may be a secondary loss of intracellular potassium that is related to an uncoupling of oxidative phosphorylation, the latter being necessary to maintain intracellular potassium concentration. Low magnesium levels may be observed in patients with such problems as hyperparathyroidism, primary aldosteronism, diabetic acidosis, hepatic cirrhosis, chronic alcoholism, malabsorption syndrome, and situations with prolonged and excessive loss of body fluids. In addition, many diuretic drugs not only produce hypokalemia but also hypomagnesemia. Seller emphasizes that not only the level of potassium but also the cell level of magnesium may need to be elevated when arrhythmias caused by toxicity follow the administration of digitalis preparations. The predisposition of hypomagnesemia to digitalis toxicity should, in many instances, prompt the physician to administer a slow intravenous infusion (1 ml. per minute) of 10 to 20 ml. of 20% magnesium sulfate. The electrocardiographic activity should be monitored at the same time.

The effect of magnesium on cardiac arrhythmias has been studied by Enselberg. He failed to note changes of a significant nature following doses of 10% to 20% magnesium sulfate given intravenously, injecting 10 to 20 ml. at a time. The only consistent effect of the injection was the subjective observation by the patient of the flushing action and a feeling of intense heat in the throat radiating downward through the body and accompanied by visible blushing. In animals, the intravenous infusion of magnesium chloride or magnesium sulfate causes distinct cardiac effects such as increasing the P-R interval and slowing of the heart rate for a short while. Following large doses, the fall in the heart rate may progress to actual cardiac standstill, which then may be followed by spontaneous resumption of the heartbeat (Hoff, Smith, Winkler, and Miller and associates). The depressant action of magnesium apparently is not affected by prior administration of atropine sulfate and is therefore presumed to be due to a direct effect on the myocardium. If concentrations of magnesium sulfate are increased beyond 20%, cardiac arrest may result. The cardiac arrest that occurs consistently when the magnesium concentration is elevated high enough is difficult to explain as a result of the depression of conduction since, in most instances, the last beat showed a well-defined and vigorous systole. Szekely, in looking for an accurate explanation of the arrest, thought it necessary to assume a more direct toxic action of magnesium on the myocardium itself. Magnesium sulfate has been suggested for the intravenous administration and use in the treatment of paroxysmal tachycardia. Magnesium salts may protect against ventricular fibrillation in the posthypercapnic period by neutralizing the elevated serum potassium level.

Some of the information regarding the effect of the magnesium ion on the heart is derived from the work of Sealy and Merritt and co-workers in their cardioplegic experimentation. Excess magnesium ion apparently does not influence the diastolic length of the myocardial fibers (as does potassium) but shortens the extent of contraction. It is a synergistic action from potassium administration that arrests heart action. The magnesium ion is thought to inhibit the energy transfer mechanism in the heart muscle, in contrast to potassium, which acts at the cell membrane and blocks the polarization of the cell. Magnesium stops the heart in diastole.

Magnesium sulfate given parenterally or orally may have a beneficial effect upon some patients with cardiac arrhythmias. Chadda and associates were able to abort supraventricular tachycardia with magnesium sulfate administered intravenously and subsequently maintain a normal sinus rhythm. In the patients who benefited from magnesium, it was usual for hypokalemia to be present also but potassium replacement therapy alone was unsuccessful in controlling the arrhythmias. They are presently measuring serum magnesium routinely in patients suspected of having hypokalemia and believe that this will bring to light a relationship between hypomagnesemia and refractory cardiac arrhythmias. The patients with low serum magnesium levels were in the range of 0.4 to 0.7 mg. per 100 ml. The normal serum magnesium level is 1.4 to 2.7 mg. per 100 ml.

The potential cardioplegic effect of magnesium ion may possibly play a part in the morbidity from seawater drowning since the magnesium content of aspirated seawater is considerable. Seawater is said to contain 100 mEq. of magnesium or about 50 times the plasma concentration (Malm).

Sudden death following intravenous injection of calcium chloride

Although calcium chloride has been used extensively in cardiac resuscitation it should be noted that intravenous injection of calcium chloride has been responsible for sudden death. Stimulation as well as inhibition of ectopic impulse formation with calcium chloride has been reported repeatedly (Sherf). I have observed ventricular fibrillation in dogs in the laboratory on numerous occasions after the injection of calcium chloride solution into the heart.

Calcium gluconate in a 10 ml. injection of a 20% solution is a commonly used drug. Lloyd observed sinus arrests of the heart after an intravenous injection of 4 ml. of a 10% solution of calcium chloride. Sherf cites two cases reported by Bower and Mengle in which sudden death occurred immediately after the intravenous injection of calcium. The patients had both been given digitalis previously. In both cases cardiac arrest was diagnosed within a 2-minute period. These authors believed that the effect of calcium gluconate on impulse formation is similar to that of calcium chloride, Sherf reported a case of cardiac arrest following an intravenous injection of 10 ml. of a 10% solution of calcium chloride. Fortunately, cardiac contractions started again after severe blows to the precordium. I have heard verbal reports of at least three other cases of cardiac arrest following the intravenous injection of a calcium solution.

Sodium chloride and ventricular fibrillation

In 1932 Hooker called attention to his experiments dealing with the sodium chloride content of isolated dog hearts. His conclusions were that, if the content of sodium chloride is high (1.58%), the heart appears to be relaxed, to beat slowly, and to be less irritable to electrical stimulation. If the content is below normal (0.45%), the heart rate is greatly increased. If the content of the perfused mixture of sodium chloride is still further reduced (such as to a level of below 0.23%), ventricular fibrillation occurs.

Further experiments by Hooker show that an increase of sodium bicarbonate or an increase of calcium chloride in the perfusate prepared for use in the isolated dog heart will produce ventricular fibrillation. If the two drugs are both increased in the same solution, the effect is even more pronounced. He regards these results as supporting the hypothesis originally advanced by Gotch, who indicates that ventricular fibrillation, whether produced by electrical stimulation or otherwise, may be caused by a disassociation of some protein-salt molecule, as previously conceived by Loeb, such that an abnormal chemical state exists in or surrounds the muscle fibers, with a consequent change in their behavior.

Sudden death during parathyroid crisis

Serum calcium levels over 17 mg.% are not rare. Hewson has reviewed this aspect of parathyroid crisis and reports the case of a 38-year-old man who died suddenly with a serum calcium of 18.9 mg.%. The heart is thought to have stopped in systole.

Role of carbon dioxide in etiology of cardiac arrest

Hypercapnia itself has apparently no direct effect on the myocardium, but, since hypercapnia does lead to a fall in blood pH and an associated rise in potassium concentration of the blood, it produces a potentially hazardous situation. In addition, Graham observed that hypercapnia may sensitize the heart to the effects of the catecholamines and may thus lower the threshold to fibrillation.

Perhaps the greatest danger with the hypercapnic state is related to the sudden return to the carbon dioxide level in the blood to normal. This occurrence, often referred to as posthypercapnic phenomenon, is frequently associated with various types of atrial and ventricular arrhythmias and with ventricular fibrillation.

One should remember, however, that the role of carbon dioxide is to delay conduction in the specific tissue, but it does not suppress stimulus formation in the ventricle. Therefore failure of the heart results from inadequate oxygenation of the common myocardium, and this is never sudden.

Young and associates pointed to the augmentation of respiratory acidosis on the effects of vagal stimulation to the heart. An additional aspect of the problem has been studied further by Young's group. They analyzed the effect of electrolyte metabolism on the ensuing cardiac abnormalities. Their work was designed to study the effects of acute, severe respiratory acidosis on intracellular and extracellular electrolyte composition and to correlate, if possible, associated ECG changes. By working with rats and dogs, definite conclusions were reached. These consisted of finding pronounced changes in the potassium metabolism during and immediately following acute hypercapnia. These changes were closely correlated with ECG abnormalities that occur with hyperpotassemia. Others have confirmed the finding of a rise in serum potassium following prolonged exposure to high concentrations of carbon dioxide. Such increases are well known in asphyxia. It is not known precisely from where the potassium is mobilized. The liver, skeletal muscles, and bones represent likely sources. One should note, however, that heart muscle, in contrast to skeletal muscle, shows a definite increase in potassium concentration during and after hypercapnia.

In recent years, much emphasis has been placed upon the effect and importance of hypercapnia in cardiac irregularities and in cardiac standstill. Wiggers realized that the carbon dioxide level may rise dangerously high in patients under anesthesia, and that the level of carbon dioxide concentration in the alveolar air and the blood bears no constant relationship to the oxygen concentration in the blood, and that it does occur even in the presence of normal blood oxygenation. He showed that when the blood pH is significantly lowered with a concentration of carbon dioxide, a prolongation of the conduction time of the heart may be produced. Wiggers was able to produce this condition by lowering the blood pH to 7.0.

The blood pH can shift to 7.2 or even as low as 7.0. During a long operation under a closed system with poor absorption of carbon dioxide by the apparatus, if the carbon dioxide is allowed to rise to high levels in the alveoli, then high carbonic acid levels are produced. Indirectly, this leads to many of the cardiac irregularities and even arrests that may occur.

Other observations have been made that refer to this as the posthypercapnic phenomenon. This phenomenon refers to a sudden return of an elevated carbon dioxide level to normal in the blood. This is frequently associated with ventricular fibrillation. Some would classify "cyclopropane shock" under a similar category as a posthypercapnic phenomenon.

Just as anoxia will potentiate the effect of the vagovagal reflex, likewise hypercapnia appears to do the same thing. Experimentally,

in dogs, stimulation of the vagus nerve in the neck or the introduction of acetylcholine into the right atrium results in a longer period of cardiac asystole and more bradycardia when the blood pH is lowered (Campbell). This increased vagal effect accompanies carbon dioxide ventilation or intravenous injection of dilute hydrochloric acid. Therefore it would appear that no condition should be allowed to precipitate an acidotic condition such as arises from the accumulation of carbon dioxide.

An analysis of 300 South African cardiac arrest cases, all of which were fatal, led Kok and Kitay to the assumption that 70 of the 300 cases were precipitated by hypercapnia. Chronic pulmonary or cardiac disease was present in a majority of these patients who were elderly.

Snyder and his co-workers suggest the possibility for a marked increase in cardiac arrest at the Los Angeles Children's Hospital to be in some way associated with the use of anesthetic machines employing the use of the closed-cycle carbon dioxide absorption technique of administering anesthetics, whereas in previous periods the simple open-drop ether method had been used. They suggest that the dead space and respiratory resistance in the tubes leading from the mask could be a factor in producing hypoxia or hypercapnia.

Working with dogs, Reid failed to note any appreciable effect of carbon dioxide accumulation on the potentiation of the vagal inhibitory effect on the heart. One such ECG tracing is shown in Fig. 10-3.

Since the work of Brown and Miller over a decade ago called attention to the ventricular fibrillation that follows a rapid fall in alveolar carbon dioxide concentration, considerable attention has been directed to this phenomenon. Hyperventilating the experimental animal with 100% oxygen to rapidly correct severe hypercapnic acidosis produces ventricular fibrillation in a high percentage of instances. Other methods of correcting the acidosis of severe hypercapnia have been employed; Epstein and his co-workers did so with the administration of THAM (tris-[hydroxymethyl]-aminomethane). Instead of ventricular fibrillation, cardiac asystole occurred in every instance. In attempting to explain the mechanism of the cardiac arrest, they note that a high plasma potassium is invariably accompanied by a low plasma sodium. When the sodium-potassium ratio drops below 12, asystole generally occurs. Invariably, the asystole or arrhythmias can be prevented by the administration of sodium, which can be in the form of sodium chloride. The administration of calcium ion will accomplish the same result.

Because of the cerebral vasodilating properties of an increased carbon dioxide tension of the blood, with a concomitant increase in blood flow to the brain, there has been wide employment of increased carbon dioxide tension during carotid artery surgery and occlusion. With an increase in the arterial carbon dioxide tension to 55 to 60 mm. Hg, ventricular rhythm disturbances in the form of ventricular extrasystole or alternate nodal or ventricular beats are common (White and Allarde). These disturbances are corrected promptly when the carbon dioxide concentration of the inspired mixture is decreased somewhat.

Cardiac arrest and acidosis

Gerst and co-workers determined that there is an increased susceptibility of the heart to ventricular fibrillation during metabolic acidosis. Experimentally they were able to note a definite decrease in the ventricular fibrillation threshold value. During metabolic acidosis, the threshold to ventricular fibrillation increased. It is interesting that in these studies, variations in pH because of respiratory acidosis and alkalosis did not affect the ventricular fibrillation threshold. Hyperventilation in dogs with metabolic acidosis, even though resulting in alkaline arterial blood pH, does not protect the dogs from the increased susceptibility to ventricular fibrillation that exists as long as the base deficit is present. Thus, respiratory acidosis and alka-

losis not associated with other alterations in acid-base balance may not necessarily have an influence on the vulnerability of the heart to fibrillation. These studies reinforce the clinical observations that attempts to resuscitate the fibrillating human heart in the presence of severe metabolic acidosis may not be successful unless the latter can be corrected. Variations in gradients of hydrogen ions across the membrane of the myocardial cell can be altered by a number of clinical situations. Ventricular fibrillation may occur after removal of occluding aortic clamps or when reversing venous inflow occlusion after restoration of blood flow to large masses of hypoxic tissue. The promptness with which cardiac arrest may occur after the heart is first perfused with blood-carrying, acidic end products of anaerobic metabolism from hypoxic cells has been clinically noted for at least 20 years and was discussed in the first edition of this book.

Although the work of Leveen indicates that the turtle heart is resistant to acidosis, there is some doubt whether this information can be transferred to the human being. The frog heart, likewise, is remarkably resistant to changes in the acidity of its perfusate. These studies have been made with perfusate as acid as pH 5.5 and as alkaline as pH 10.0.

Leveen and colleagues studied the effect of various hydrogen ion concentrations on the perfused and isolated turtle heart with two concentrations of potassium. They concluded that acidosis does not affect, to any great degree, the contractility of the isolated turtle myocardium. In addition, they suspect that cardiac arrest during acidosis (in experimental animals) is secondary to other causes, possibly hepatic potassium release.

The heart in severe acidosis is generally thought to arrest in extreme diastole, with the conductivity of the heart suddenly abolished. The effect on intraventricular conduction is minimal, and the heart rate may be maintained almost up to the time of the sudden arrest.

Chapter 14

TOXIC RESPONSE AND CARDIAC ARREST

Sudden sniffing death

The sudden and unexpected deaths occurring among teenagers who sniffed volatile hydrocarbons reached epidemic proportions within the last 10 years, but hopefully the rate is leveling off at the present time.

Bass, in reporting on 110 sudden sniffing deaths in American youths during the 1960s, emphasizes that the deaths were almost instantaneous as noted by observers and are probably best explained on the basis of a sudden ventricular arrhythmia resulting from light plane anesthesia and often intensified by hypercapnia or stressful activity. The volatile hydrocarbons most frequently involved in sniffing deaths are trichlorofluoromethane and dichlorodifluoromethane. These nonaqueous, soluble, pressurized fluorinated refrigerants serve as agents for propelling the liquid ingredients out of the aerosol can.

Although not as popular as it was a few years ago, the practice of sniffing airplane glue, aerosol sprays, and fumes of certain solvents continues in young people. Flowers has pointed to the mechanism that is triggered by the gas used to propel the sprays. The most common propellant is Freon, which is the gas usually added to various glues and solvents to speed up evaporation and drying. The effect of Freon on the electrical conduction system of the heart is to slow the heart rate and eventually produce cardiac asystole. In a series of dogs studied, eight died from one to nine whiffs of Freon-propelled aerosol.

Sudden death (ventricular fibrillation) following intravenous injection of mercurial diuretics

Over 50 years ago Salant and Kleitman (1922) observed that ventricular fibrillation in dogs frequently follows intravenous administration of inorganic mercurial salts. This was further substantiated by Jackson 4 years later when he reported that he was regularly able to produce death by ventricular fibrillation in normal dogs under ether anesthesia 3 to 5 minutes after intravenous injection of various mercurial components.

Volini reported three patients who died suddenly after intravenous injection of mercurial diuretics. Each had received standard doses of the drug given; two had received prior injections of the mercurial diuretics before the fatal episode. ECG studies were available on two patients with tracings shortly before and during the reactions. Both patients showed the development of ventricular fibrillation following administration of the drug. Speculating on the mechanism of death following the injection of mercurial diuretics, Volini pointed to clinical and experimental evidence indicating that the action results from the direct effect on the heart by the mercury ion.

Cardiac arrest due to digitalis intoxication

Either ventricular fibrillation or ventricular asystole may result from digitalis intoxication in patients with atrial fibrillation or even with partial heart block. Asystole may occur because of a depression of impulse formation and thus a prevention of conduction through the atrioventricular bundle. Ventricular action may cease temporarily after either paroxysmal or nonparoxysmal tachycardia. Increased refractoriness from rapid beating of the ventricles may stop the whole heart or it may stop only the ventricles.

207

Arrhythmias are estimated to occur in approximately 80% of cases of digitalis intoxication. Ventricular fibrillation is a not uncommonly encountered arrhythmia. In 1966, McLaughlin and associates were able to find only one instance of successful resuscitation in a patient with ventricular fibrillation following digitalis intoxication. They report, however, the successful management of digitalis intoxication and ventricular fibrillation in a 25-year-old woman. Over a period of 60 hours the patient received approximately 150 electric countershocks for ventricular fibrillation during ninety-nine episodes. Under careful monitoring, sternal compression was often unnecessary because of the rapid resumption of effective myocardial contraction after defibrillation.

Cases of digitalis-induced ventricular fibrillation were recorded electrocardiographically by Castellanos and co-workers. In the first two patients, fibrillation evolved from a rapidly progressing, bidirectional, ventricular tachycardia. In the second case, ventricular fibrillation appeared suddenly when a ventricular extrasystole fell in the vulnerable phase of the preceding contraction after the intravenous administration of digoxin to a patient with an undiagnosed digitalis-induced arrhythmia.

It should be emphasized that, while ventricular fibrillation from digitalis intoxication is a reversible situation, repeated electric countershock may be necessary to reverse ventricular fibrillation until the arrhythmic effects of the drug have ceased. In addition to the usual attention to prevention of metabolic and respiratory acidosis, intravenous potassium should be given in an effort to decrease the digitalis effect.

Pierce states that acidosis itself hinders restoration of normal circulation for the following reasons:

1. Myocardial contractility, followed by cardiac function, are both reduced.
2. The effect of catecholamines, which the body elaborates to enhance the efficiency of existing circulation, is impaired.
3. There is depression of the central nervous system, inhibiting respiration.
4. The same degree of respiratory effort produces less compensation in profound acidosis than it does when the metabolic state is more nearly normal.
5. The affinity of hemoglobin for oxygen is less in acidosis, hence hypoxia is increased.*

In the presence of a low pH, cardiac output and venous return are diminished. In acidotic conditions the response to pressor drug injections is diminished.

Twenty years ago Finch and Marchand reported ventricular fibrillation relating to existing hyperpotassemia in a digitalized patient. It is also known that the potassium-depleting effect of thiazides can precipitate cardiac arrest due to the resultant digitalis sensitization and toxicity.

Arsenic poisoning

Although arsenic poisoning is not common, it continues to be seen in urban areas where rodenticides containing arsenic are being used. Sprays containing arsenic are used extensively as pesticides, particularly in rural areas. St. Petery and Victorica report on a 3-year-old white female admitted to the hospital with acute arsenic poisoning. She experienced repeated episodes of ventricular flutter-fibrillation requiring frequent cardioversion using an external defibrillator set at 25 watt-seconds. Lidocaine (1 mg. per kilogram every 15 minutes) and procainamide hydrochloride (75 mg. intramuscularly) could not control the arrhythmia. It was not until a transvenous bipolar electrode catheter was inserted into the apex of right ventricle by way of the right saphenous vein that the ventricular rhythm was captured at a rate of 150 per minute. The pacemaker was discontinued after 72 hours and the patient eventually recovered. The mechanism involved in the cardiovascular effect of arsenic is not generally agreed upon. In human

---

*From Pierce, J. A.: Cardiac arrests associated with anesthesia, Anesth. Analg. (Cleve.) 45:407-413, 1966.

arsenic poisoning, however, electrocardiographic changes have often been noted that include nonspecific S-T segment changes, T wave inversion, and Q-T interval prolongation. St. Petery and Victorica suggest that patients with a history of acute arsenic poisoning, because of the tendency to develop dysrhythmias, be monitored continuously with an electrocardiogram.

Excess oxygen as a factor in cardiac arrest

The implication of overoxygenation or oxygen intoxication has been made on several occasions in conjunction with cardiac irregularities. S. E. Stephenson, Jr., was able to produce cardiac arrest in animals receiving 40% oxygen in the inspired air, and he speculates that the associated fall of pH and elevation of carbon dioxide tension that may occur with overoxygenation may be a precipitating factor in cases of cardiac arrest of unknown etiology. He was able to show that animals subjected to pneumonectomy displayed no cardiac irregularities with arterial oxygen saturations of 86% to 92% accompanied by normal carbon dioxide tension and normal pH. If the same procedure is performed in such a way that animals breathing 30% to 40% oxygen are subjected to simple hyperventilation, a considerable number of arrhythmias occur, particularly with manipulations about the hilus of the lungs.

It will be interesting to follow cardiac evaluations of patients subjected to prolonged hyperbaric conditions.

Cardiac arrest from topically applied agents

The observation has been made that hydrogen peroxide in 3% mixture applied directly to the myocardium produces ECG abnormalities in 100% of the instances when used experimentally on dogs. A case of cardiac arrest is reported by Sellers following irrigation of a chest wound infection with 3% hydrogen peroxide. There was communication of the chest wound with the pericardium. Although the cardiac arrest occurred outside the operating room and recovery room, mouth-to-mouth rescuscitation and open-chest cardiac massage were carried out with subsequent recovery of the patient. Seven days prior to the arrest, the patient had undergone a simple fainting episode during the irrigation procedure with 3% hydrogen peroxide.

Sellers and co-workers speculate on possible mechanisms by which hydrogen peroxide produces this effect upon the myocardium and upon cardiac activity. They conclude that the effect probably results from the direct action of the hydrogen peroxide on the myocardium, perhaps through the mechanism of differential oxygen tensions in adjacent areas of the myocardium or by the release of nascent oxygen. Since the arrest occurs as an asystolic episode rather than fibrillation and since bradycardia is seen in animal experimentation, the possibility of a vagovagal reflex action was investigated but seems unlikely. The possibility of action of the peroxide on the coronary circulation cannot be excluded.

Cardiac arrest after triple-strength plasma infusions

Sudden cardiac asystole may occur if triple-strength plasma is rapidly infused. In 1962 Marshall described a case of cardiac arrest attributed to triple-strength plasma. Three years later, Zorab and associates encountered a sudden cardiac arrest in a 37-year-old woman who was admitted to the hospital as an emergency patient after an antepartum hemorrhage. Following the rapid administration of 400 ml. of prepared triple-strength plasma, cardiac asystole occurred.

Both authors believe that their cases represent potassium arrest from the rapid infusion of triple-strength plasma. They note that, where multiple transfusions of blood and plasma have been given, the citrate will produce low serum levels of ionized calcium, making the heart even more sensitive to potassium than is normally the case.

Whitehouse describes a third case of cardiac arrest after triple-strength plasma had been rapidly infused under positive pressure. The patient was successfully resuscitated.

Cardiac arrest during exchange transfusions

A number of instances of sudden cardiac arrest have been reported in newborn infants receiving exchange transfusions for hemolytic disease. In a case reported by Glassford and Motamedy, the blood from the donor was neither refrigerated nor subsequently warmed. One milliliter of 10% calcium gluconate had been slowly injected after each 100 ml. of replacement. Taylor and co-workers have also reported on exchange transfusions in infants. No clear-cut explanation has been offered relative to the etiology other than that suggesting such factors as hyperpotassemia, cooling of the heart, hypocalcemia, and acidosis.

Continued monitoring during exchange transfusions is indicated.

Phenothiazine derivatives and sudden death

Antipsychotic drugs were believed to be the cause of death in six patients reported by Hollister and Kosek. These were all previously healthy patients being treated with phenothiazine derivatives (chlorpromazine, prochlorperazine, trifluoperazine, and thioridazine). Although ventricular fibrillation was documented in one instance, it is not known whether asystole or fibrillation was present in the other five patients. In each instance the attacks began as an abrupt syncopal or seizure-like attack (resembling a fatal Adams-Stokes attack), followed immediately by death.

Sudden death during disulfiram-alcohol reaction

A review of the occasional danger of disulfiram (Antabuse) is provided by Amador and Gasdar. They point to autopsy studies following sudden death in heavy alcoholics taking disulfiram. Autopsy findings showed both coronary arteries and the myocardium to be normal.

Sudden death from anaphylactic reactions

The whole gamut of severe constitutional reactions, including sudden death, occur in allergic emergencies. Severe reactions from penicillin, foreign serum used as antitoxin, hyposensitization treatments with allergenic materials, insect stings (bee, wasp, or yellow jacket), and rupture of the hydatid cyst all provide good examples. Sudden unexpected cessation of the heart occurred as a fatal anaphylactic reaction to triphenylmethane dye (Alphazurine 2G) in a 44-year-old man. The dye was being given to determine the depth of a burn he had received (Hepps and Dollinger). Although sudden death is not the rule, cardiac resuscitative measures may be necessary since collapse may occur immediately. Immediate treatment may forestall cardiovascular collapse and will vary somewhat with the injected antigen. When a person is stung by a bee, for example, the stinger should immediately be scraped off with the fingernail, since contraction of the stinging apparatus may continue to inject venom. Oral administration of antihistamines or sublingual administration of isoproterenol hydrochloride may be effective. Certainly, injectable epinephrine will be more effective. A tourniquet should be placed above the site of the injection if it is on an extremity. Adrenocortical steroids are not rapid-acting anaphylactic agents, but may be partially effective. If ventricular fibrillation occurs, the usual resuscitative procedures should, of course, be followed.

Sudden death following the injection of penicillin (thirty reported penicillin deaths occurred in New York City from 1952 to 1957) and other sudden anaphylactic responses have been reported, including those caused by various types of sera, local anesthetic agents, almond extracts, vaccines, and even ACTH.

Allergic reactions to penicillin now account for approximately 10% of all reported adverse drug reactions in the United States and are the most common type of anaphylactic shock (Westerman and co-workers). It is estimated that 300 persons a year die from this reaction. A need for a safe and reliable test to determine the likelihood of the penicillin reaction is obvious. Apparently the most promising new technique is the penicilloyl polylysine (PPL) skin test. Its use is suggested by the finding that one of the metabolic products of penicillin, penicilloyl, is capable of conjugating with body protein to form potent antigens that provide the major stimulus for penicillin hypersensitivity. When penicilloyl haptenes are combined with a lysine polymer in the test tube and then injected subcutaneously, they do not stimulate antibody production but elicit a typical wheal-and-flare response in patients with circulating antipenicillin antibodies.

Simultaneously administered antihistaminics do not decrease the incidence of penicillin reactions as compared with a control group. Seiple came to this conclusion after using antihistaminics simultaneously with penicillin in a series of 4,537 patients. The overall penicillin reaction rate in this series was 4.8 per 1,000.

The exact mechanism of death following a penicillin injection is not clear. Some evidence exists that the heart muscle itself participates in tissue sensitization. Bernreiter lends encouragement to this concept by a demonstration of the serial ECG tracings in a 74-year-old man following an injection of 600,000 units of penicillin. Respiratory distress and cardiovascular collapse occurred rapidly. Although the patient was not in cardiac arrest, auricular fibrillation plus intraventricular conduction disturbances and evidence of severe coronary insufficiency with marked injury to the posterior wall of the left ventricle were thought to be present. Within less than 1 hour, however, ECG indications had rturned to normal. Bernreiter suggests that the cardiac muscle with its

coronary circulation is capable of participating directly in an anaphylactic response.

Of interest is the study of Booth and Patterson in which they record electrocardiographic changes during anaphylaxis in humans. In a group of twenty-three instances of anaphylaxis, a variety of significant electrocardiographic changes were noted. Although they can only speculate on the etiology of the electrocardiographic changes in human anaphylaxis, the following possibilities are considered: (1) a direct antigen-antibody-myocardial reaction, (2) a pharmacologic effect of mediators released during anaphylaxis, (3) the effects of agents such as epinephrine used for treatment, (4) anoxia, (5) preexisting heart disease, and (6) other unknown factors or a combination of several factors. It would seem likely, however, that cardiac abnormalities play a decisive role in influencing the morbidity and mortality of patients with anaphylaxis. Autopsy data concerning human anaphylaxis are limited. The study by Booth and Patterson would tend to emphasize the advisability of cardiac monitoring to detect potentially fatal arrhythmias at an early stage.

James and Austin studied the clinical and postmortem findings in six cases of fatal systemic anaphylaxis and conclude that the "shock organ" was the respiratory system in five patients. Four of these patients had obstructing edema of the upper respiratory tract (two with obstructing pharyngeal edema), and the fifth patient had respiratory symptoms demonstrating gross acute pulmonary emphysema.

At first it was thought by some that perhaps procaine penicillin was responsible for the fatal reactions and that the sensitivity was due to the procaine. On the other hand, penicillin reactions have occurred with crystalline penicillin as well as with procaine penicillin and penicillin in beeswax and oil. It is true, however, that the absorption of antigens when penicillin is given in beeswax and oil is much slower, so that the chances of a sudden severe anaphylactic reaction are much less. The full picture of penicillin re-actions has probably not been revealed as yet.

Boger and associates have reported severe convulsions resulting from the direct injection of 50,000 units of penicillin intrathecally. From 1946 to 1951 there was one fatality reported following penicillin injection. However, during 1953, four fatal reactions from penicillin were reported in the New York area alone. Crystalline penicillin and/or aqueous suspension of procaine penicillin were used in these instances. I was present at the autopsy of a middle-aged black woman who had been given an injection of procaine penicillin in her hip for a Bartholin's abscess. Almost immediately following the injection of penicillin, the patient collapsed and died. A thoracotomy was performed for massage of the heart, but the thoracotomy incision was entirely unsatisfactory and massage of the heart was not adequate. At autopsy, no demonstrable lesions could be noted as having caused the death of the patient.

Therefore it would seem that, regardless of whether or not a sudden reaction to penicillin with sudden death can be classified as a true case of cardiac arrest, attempts at cardiac resuscitation may prove lifesaving, as in cases of procaine sensitivity. If the circulation can be artificially maintained until the response to the penicillin is over, recovery should follow. A rather typical picture of what one might encounter occurred with the sudden collapse of a young nurse who experienced an anaphylactic reaction to cocaine. Following massage of the heart the patient appeared to have been resuscitated, but after the circulation was maintained for a few seconds, additional cocaine was recirculated and the patient went into a second sudden anaphylactic reaction requiring further massage. (The patient lived.) It is well to keep in mind that the indications for cardiac resuscitation may not always exactly parallel the true definition that one may have for cardiac arrest.

It is the physician's responsibility to always inquire with respect to any previous sensitivity to penicillin. Patients with hives, asthma, hay fever, eczema, and evidence of other allergies appear particularly likely to have anaphylactic reactions to penicillin. Skin tests are generally unreliable and give both false positives and false negatives.

The treatment of an acute penicillin reaction should include the use of a tourniquet proximal to the injection site whenever possible as a means of preventing more systemic absorption. Epinephrine hydrochloride, 0.3 to 1. ml. of 1:1,000 solution, should be given rapidly by subcutaneous or intramuscular injection. This may be repeated every 5 to 10 minutes to control symptoms. One hundred milligrams of intravenously administered hydrocortisone may then be given. Antihistamines (chlorpheniramine maleate, 5 to 10 mg.) are next indicated. Large doses of penicillinase (Neutrapen)—800 units intravenously, followed by the similar amount intramuscularly—should be given and repeated in 1 to 4 hours.

Fatal reactions following subcutaneous and intramuscular injections of antitetanus serum have been documented many times. A fatality following the injection of a therapeutic dose of tetanus antitoxin is estimated to occur approximately once in every 1,000,000 administrations.

Epinephrine and ventricular fibrillation

One of the early observations related the administration of epinephrine to ventricular fibrillation when associated with chloroform, ethyl chloride, or cyclopropane anesthesia, particularly with the patient under light anesthesia. The obscure mechanism of fibrillation in such instances has not been clarified. Fauteux speculated that general anesthetics have, at a certain moment, a depressive action on the conductive system and that in such a condition cardiac stimulation provoked by epinephrine is sufficient to create heterotropic centers leading to fibrillation.

Many others have confirmed the relationship between epinephrine and ventricular fibrillation and have related it to instances of sudden death during excessive fear and fright. Caution is still urged in the use of epinephrine with cyclopropane anesthesia.

There are numerous instances of cardiac standstill reverting to ventricular fibrillation after epinephrine was given.

Papaverine hydrochloride and ventricular fibrillation

Papaverine hydrochloride raises the fibrillation threshold significantly and for a considerable period of time. Papaverine, like quinidine, if administered too rapidly or in excessive doses, may induce fibrillation of a very coarse type (Wegria and associates).

Quinidine intoxication and ventricular fibrillation

Quinidine syncope or sudden death associated with ventricular arrhythmia in patients receiving quinidine is well documented (Selzer; Rubeiz). In most of the reported cases there seems to be no relation in the dosage of quinidine to the etiology of the heart disease or to cardiac surgery. The tendency of the heart to revert to the basic rhythm spontaneously has frequently characterized this problem. A most dramatic case of quinidine syncope or quinidine-induced recurrent ventricular fibrillation is reported by Miller and Blount. A 28-year-old woman was given quinidine sulfate for atrial fibrillation following mitral valve surgery at an initial dosage of 200 mg. orally every 6 hours. On the second day after four doses, ventricular fibrillation occurred. After a sudden episode of apnea and loss of consciousness, the patient responded quickly to external cardiac massage and assisted ventilation and regained consciousness. Within a few minutes and while the cardiac rhythm was being monitored, ventricular fibrillation reappeared but reverted to atrial fibrillation on closed chest compression. There was evidence of prolongation of the Q-T interval with multifocal premature ventricular contractions, with R-on-T patterns. All of this prompted

the diagnosis of quinidine cardiotoxicity. Amazingly enough the patient had 200 separate bouts of recurrent ventricular fibrillation within the next 11 hours. Half of these episodes spontaneously reverted to the basic rhythm and ninety-five separate episodes of fibrillation were successfully treated by D.C. defibrillation using 70 watt-seconds. Despite a number of different attempts at medical therapy to control the recurrent ventricular fibrillation, no success was achieved until blind passage of a pacemaker electrode catheter to the heart at the bedside, and then not until the pacemaker rate was increased to 120 per minute, a rate rapid enough to suppress irritable ectopic foci. Initially 88 mEq. of sodium bicarbonate and 10 mg. of dexamethasone sodium sulfate were used without any benefit. This was followed by 500 ml. of 1/6 molar sodium lactate, which acts predominantly by lowering serum potassium, but in this case it failed to produce any beneficial effects. Lidocaine, 50 mg. intravenously, was given twice with an actual increase in the frequency of the arrhythmias. No benefit was obtained from intravenously administered atropine.

Isoproterenol, through its stimulation of beta receptors, increases the heart rate, which may suppress ventricular arrhythmia in some cases of quinidine syncope. There is some experimental evidence that tromethamine (THAM) may be of benefit in that it changes the intracellular pH more rapidly than the slower-acting sodium buffers and the diuretic effect of tromethamine enhances urinary potassium excretion.

With widespread use of quinidine, particularly over a prolonged period of time, a number of cases of quinidine intoxication have been reported. Many have terminated in ventricular fibrillation. Quinidine is, of course, used therapeutically in a variety of situations, for example, as a prophylactic against arrhythmias following myocardial infarction, for patients with hypersensitive carotid sinus syndromes, Wolff-Parkinson-White syndrome, and atrial arrhythmias.

Quinidine-induced cardiotoxicity is more commonly associated with ventricular fibrillation but seldom with asystole.

Quinidine-induced ventricular fibrillation is discussed by Ranier-Pope and associates, among others. Rokseth and Storstein report twenty-seven cases of quinidine syncope due to transient episodes of ventricular fibrillation. Selzer considers the rare instance of ventricular fibrillation in patients taking quinidine to be dose related and also, in some instances, to be due to an idiosyncratic reaction in susceptible individuals who are taking low doses of the drug. Quinidine syncope is more likely to occur in patients with diseased hearts than in those with normal hearts and is more apt to develop during the early phases of quinidine therapy than in patients who have been treated by this drug over a long period.

Aconitine and ventricular fibrillation

The classic work of Scherf should be cited. He studied the cardiac arrhythmias produced by an intensely poisonous alkaloid from *Aconitum napellus*. By the application of aconitine crystals to an area of the ventricular surface, he was able to produce various types of ventricular flutter that often changed into ventricular fibrillation. Whenever the site of application of aconitine was cooled, ventricular tachycardia could be arrested. Cooling at the site of aconitine application did not influence the course of ventricular fibrillation; however, it is from this study that Scherf concludes: "The primary disturbance in ventricular fibrillation is the rapid impulse formation in several ectopic centers." He also concludes that the local reentries and interference between such contractions are caused by the rapid impulse formation in several centers, but are not a circus movement.

Diphenylhydantoin and ventricular fibrillation

The effect of diphenylhydantoin (Dilantin) on the cardiovascular system is discussed elsewhere in this book. It has a direct myocardial depressive effect as well as a peripheral vascular effect that results in vasodilatation. It is well recognized for its value in the treatment of arrhythmias of varying etiologies. Experimentally, diphenylhydantoin prevents aconitine-induced ventricular tachycardias in dogs from progressing to ventricular fibrillation, even when the ventricular pulse rate rises to 500 beats per minute (Scherf). The primary toxic changes of diphenylhydantoin as reflected on the ECG are widening of the QRS complex and prolongation of the P-R interval. Gellerman and Martinez report a patient who developed ventricular fibrillation almost immediately after receiving 150 mg. of diphenylhydantoin intravenously (3 mg. per kilogram body weight) over a 3-minute period. This episode was not preceded by extrasystoles.

Cardiac arrest occurring in two patients following the intravenous injection of diphenylhydantoin sodium (Dilantin sodium) have been reported (Unger and Sklaroff). In both instances the drug was given for atrial flutter. Scherf earlier caused cardiac asystole in dogs by giving large doses of diphenylhydantoin.

Voigt reports a patient who died suddenly after receiving intravenous Dilantin. Progressive AV nodal block and ventricular asystole occurred. After reviewing six other such reported deaths he concludes that Dilantin depresses impulse formation and prolongs AV nodal conduction. The drug may also impair myocardial contractility and decrease peripheral vascular resistance. Atropine may correct Dilantin-induced bradycardia and AV nodal block, but a vasopressor acting directly on peripheral vessels is probably best given for the hypotension.

Chapter 15

SPECIFIC MEDICAL RELATIONSHIPS TO CARDIAC ARREST

Deaf-mutism, ECG abnormalities, and sudden deaths

Although syncopal attacks and sudden deaths associated with a prolongation of the Q-T interval are now known to be present in at least 1% of all infants born with congenital deafness, the delayed ventricular repolarization represented by the prolongation of the Q-T interval is seen clinically in a number of other situations also in which the duration of the vulnerable period is increased with an accompanying greater susceptibility to ventricular fibrillation. Digitalis, quinidine, diuretics, hypocalcemia, and hypokalemia are all well known in the etiology of Q-T prolongation (James). In addition, James called attention to certain phenothiazine drugs associated with Q-T prolongation and subsequent ventricular dysrhythmias and syncope. A Q-T prolongation may occur also with the administration of certain hydrocarbons and catecholamines and the simple aliphatic aldehydes.

There is always the danger that an electronic pacing signal, by falling randomly among spontaneously generated cardiac beats with long Q-T intervals, may increase the chance of a fatal arrhythmia.

Jervell and Lange-Nielsen have called attention to the unusual relationship of deaf-mutism, ECG abnormalities, and sudden death. Levine and Woodward have further documented their observation. Others have subsequently contributed to our knowledge of this syndrome and to the possible explanation for the sudden cause of death (Fraser, Froggatt, and James; James, 1967).

Of particular importance is the distinctive ECG finding of a considerably prolonged Q-T interval. Since this represents the period of increased vulnerability in the cardiac cycle, critically timed premature beats may produce a paroxysm of ventricular arrhythmias, including ventricular fibrillation. Cardiac conduction system defects have been noted at autopsy in some of the patients. James indicates that cardiac arrhythmias become less frequent in these patients as they grow older.

Not all members of a family with the cardio-auditory syndrome will have the expected congenital high-frequency deafness despite a prolonged Q-T interval (Mathews and co-workers). Perhaps the auditory and cardiac defects are inherited separately. In a summary of all cases from the world literature, Mathews and his colleagues conclude that the syncopal attacks that accompany the arrhythmias may be mild with loss of consciousness or, on the other hand, may be associated with complete loss of consciousness, grand mal seizures and residual disorientation, and other signs of neurologic damage. Apparently both kinds of attacks vary in frequency and are often precipitated by emotional or physical exertion. They may begin in early infancy. Pathologic changes of the coronary artery have been notably absent. Episodes of documented transient ventricular fibrillation are recorded.

In addition to their excellent review of the subject, Mathews and co-workers report, for the first time, on a family in which some members (with or without mild congenital high-frequency perceptive deafness) are af-

215

fected by Q-T interval prolongation and syncope. The exact mechanism of the genesis of the arrhythmias and the etiology of the prolongation of myocardial repolarization is still not well understood. They emphasize that management must be directed at preventing or controlling precipitating factors that may induce an arrhythmia and the use of drugs that are effective in preventing arrhythmias, particularly propranolol (because of its beta-adrenergic blockade and quinidine-like effect) and diphenylhydantoin, which slightly reduces the Q-T interval.

Since the last edition of this book was published there has been a considerable resurgence of interest in the pathogenesis of sudden death as it relates to instances of familial occurrence. Sudden death in patients without congenital deaf mutism or Q-T interval prolongation has been observed in families both with and without delayed ventricular repolarization. Alternating bidirectional tachycardia leading to death during attempted suppressive therapy was observed in a 16-year-old girl without prior clinical evidence of cardiac disease and reported by Gault and co-workers. Fatty and mononuclear cell infiltration in the atrioventricular conduction system and the main left bundle branch were thought to be significant. It is their belief that the origin of the arrhythmias lies in the degenerative change of the conduction system and has a genetic base. Their patient died of continuing unsuppressed reentry phenomena and uncontrollable ventricular fibrillation. A variety of local anomalies of the heart have been identified at autopsies in or near the sino-atrial node and Purkinje system.

Contrary to the belief of some, the survival rate in complete congenital heart block is excellent, particularly in contrast with acquired complete heart block. This excellent prognosis prevails only if there is no associated congenital structural heart disease, the QRS complexes are supraventricular in configuration, and the condition is not familial. Corne and Mathewson, for example, present a 25-year follow-up of one patient who has progressed in excellent fashion.

Sudden unexpected death in several members of a family has been noted by numerous authors. Of interest is the report by Green and associates who document ten instances of sudden unexpected death in three generations of one family. One instance involved the sudden death of a 15-year-old boy just as he had completed a 100-yard dash. When his 14-year-old sister learned of her brother's death, she suddenly developed ventricular fibrillation and efforts by her physician to resuscitate her were unsuccessful. One year previously, their 10-year-old sister died suddenly and unexpectedly while playing on a beach. Efforts to elucidate a common defect in the cardiac conduction system have not proved successful.

Green and associates also studied the medical records of eight generations (127 members) of a family. Twenty-one cases of unexpected death—the average age at the time of death was 17—were uncovered in the 127 family members. Syncope following psychic trauma preceded the deaths in most instances. Green and his group conclude that a non-sex-linked gene had produced anatomic defects of the conduction system in members of the family, predisposing them to ventricular arrhythmias and death precipitated by environment. In both of the children mentioned, they found a defect in the conduction bundle. In one instance the left bundle failed to contact the rest of the conduction system, and in the other the bundle of His was exceedingly small. Wilson and Reese tell of two 32-year-old women, both hospitalized for schizophrenia, who died suddenly and unexpectedly within 1 hour of each other.

Treatment continues to be a problem. An effort to prevent the arrhythmias is usually made by the prophylactic use of propranolol or diphenylhydantoin. The former is used for its beta-adrenergic blockade properties and its quinidine-like effects. Diphenylhydantoin acts to shorten the Q-T interval. Neither seems to work in all patients. An intracardiac ventricular pacemaker has been used in an effort to capture the rhythm and prevent ventricular disturbances but this, too, has been ineffective.

The reader who is interested in a discussion of familial heart block and sinus bradycardia should refer to the paper of Sarachek and Leonard.

Dystrophia myotonica and cardiac arrest

This familial hereditary disease is briefly mentioned to call attention to an apparently increased sensitivity to thiopental sodium anesthesia (Pentothal). Pachomov and Caughey have reviewed the subject in detail. They observed a 12-year-old girl whose heart stopped shortly after an operation for ptosis of the left eyelid and on whom cardiac resuscitative efforts were to no avail. Diffuse adipose infiltrations and fibrosis of the left ventricular wall and focal fibrosis of the interventricular septum were found at autopsy. Not only is there a damaged myocardium in patients with this disease but also, as these authors pointed out, there is thought to be a possible interrelationship of the metabolism of thiopental sodium with certain enzyme deficiencies in dystrophia myotonica. They believe that thiopental sodium detoxification in the body depends largely on the presence of certain enzymes such as cytochrome C, adenosine triphosphate, nicotinamide, and a substrate: citrate, ketoglutarate, formate, or malonate. In addition, they indicate that inhibition of the phosphocreatine synthesis by 2-4 dinitrophenol decreases the thiopental sodium metabolism by 30%, which suggests that other oxygenative processes are involved in metabolism of thiopental sodium.

Sudden death associated with fear and apprehension

Episodes of fright and syncopal attacks have often been associated and a satisfactory explanation has not always been forthcoming except in a small percentage of clinical situations. For example, individuals with congenital deafness and a prolonged Q-T interval are particularly prone to syncopal attacks and sudden death during episodes of excitement and fright. James considers the possibility that nervous impulses coming from the central nervous system act as stimuli to produce either premature beats or transient further prolongation of the Q-T interval.

The frequent association of sudden death with an unusual degree of apprehension and fear has been noted for a long time. The presence of excessive amounts of endogenous secreted epinephrine has never been substantiated, but the possibilities must be considered. A case cited by Dillon illustrates this point:

The operation was to be done with ligation of the patent ductus arteriosus. As far as could be determined, the patient was in good condition physically. However, it was ascertained later that he had in all seriousness told his friends and the nurses on the ward that he was going to die. Neither the surgeon nor the anesthesiologist was informed of this statement. The course of this patient during induction in the first part of the operation was entirely uneventful. Cardiac arrest occurred without warning.*

The observation has long been made that a patient unduly fearful of the operative procedure when brought to the operating room represents a distinct hazard from an anesthetic standpoint. Adequate premedication has contributed a great deal in this regard.

Cases of cardiac arrest in which the patient expressed a tremendous amount of terror at the onset of induction have been noted frequently in our survey. Speculation on how fear and apprehension play an undesirable role in such cases has been made, and many have associated this with an undue amount of epinephrine being secreted which, on occasion, has thrown the patient into ventricular fibrillation. The observation has

---

*From Dillon, J. B.: A consideration of some of the factors causing death in the operating room, Calif. Med. **71:**353, 1949.

been made that ventricular fibrillation is more prone to occur with cyclopropane after the addition of epinephrine in a local anesthetic agent. That this could occur through the body's own mechanism seems also likely.

One patient in the series was described by his physician as being extremely apprehensive and as displaying violent shivering, cringing, and drawing back in alarm when approached by doctor, nurse, or corpsman. (This patient was a prisoner of war and spoke no English.) Cardiac arrest occurred during a relatively minor operative procedure. I believe that such patients should have their surgery canceled or postponed until their apprehension has been relieved. Much of this problem may be obviated by preoperative sedation.

Wolf has often called attention to the diminution of regulatory inhibitions by the autonomic nervous system in situations that are interpreted as overwhelming and without hope. It is well known that many deaths have been noted in presumably healthy individuals under circumstances of intense fright or profound dejection. The possibility that such a mechanism might explain the fatal arrhythmias or cardiac arrest associated with voodoo is discussed by Wolf. Death occurring at times of bereavement in patients with coronary disease suggests to him that the damping action of the autonomic inhibition may have lost its effectiveness in the face of the massive assault on the nervous system by an overwhelming event.

Cardiac arrest through volition

The ability of a patient through his own volition to slow his heartbeat, even to the point of complete arrest, has been questioned. However, McClure verified this phenomenon several times over a 5-year period in a 44-year-old aircraft mechanic. The patient could "sit quietly, relax completely, and allow everything to stop." On several occasions when the radial pulse was observed to the point at which it could not be felt, the patient would become ashen gray and partial loss of consciousness would occur. Electrocardiographic evidence is shown in Fig. 15-1. The sinus rate slowed to the point of sinus arrest for a period of 5 seconds.

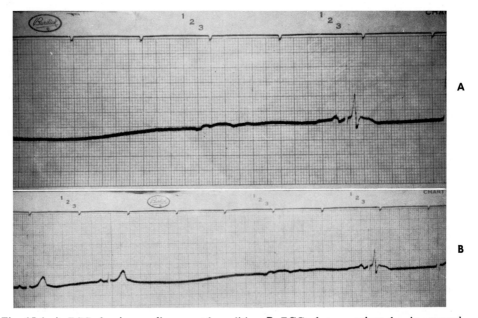

Fig. 15-1. A, ECG showing cardiac arrest by volition. B, ECG of same patient showing normal tracing. (From McClure, C. M.: Calif. Med. **90:**440, 1959.)

Occasional atrioventricular nodal beats were observed. The ECG would always be normal following one of these episodes. Atropine and a number of other drugs could not abolish this effect. The dose of atropine is not mentioned. Of interest is the mention that the patient had suffered rheumatic fever at age 7. McClure feels that the bradycardia and cardiac arrest represent exaggerated vagotonia. The production of vagotonia was not clear. No breath-holding or Valsalva maneuver was performed. McClure speculates that perhaps the patient abolished all sympathetic tone by complete mental and physical relaxation.

In the practice of yoga one finds evidence supporting the possibility of voluntary control of the autonomic nervous system. Engel has reported extensively upon the operant conditioning of heart rate slowing. And Pavlovian techniques have been applied to cardiovascular conditioning (Hnatiow).

Cardiac arrest subsequent to cardiac trauma

Although the effect of penetrating wounds on the heart is well known, that of non-penetrating injuries from a blow or blunt trauma to a chest wall is less well understood. Particularly common today is the myocardial injury following a steering wheel compression. Many medicolegal considerations have been raised in such cases and the claim has often been made that the heart was not normal prior to the accident. Usually it is difficult to identify the possible causal relationships of cardiac disease or to attribute them to the presence or absence of associated myocardial trauma when adequate autopsy findings are not present. Commonly the suspected mechanism of death is dysrhythmia. Dreifus reports on observed periods of S-A arrest alternating with intractable supraventricular tachycardia. Heart trauma is found in about 15% of all fatal thoracic injuries (DeMuth and co-workers). One of the three mechanisms is usually responsible: ventricular fibrillation, myocardial rupture, or myocardial failure. It is believed that the area of injury in the heart muscle appears to possess an electrical potential differing from that of the surrounding myocardium. A so-called electrical death ensues. Patients with a history suggesting possible cardiac contusion should be observed carefully. The ECG is the most reliable diagnostic aid. In some instances, these patients should be monitored for a period of several days in the coronary care unit.

Grand mal seizures and cardiac arrest

The neurologic clinic of the University Hospital, Utrecht (The Netherlands), has documented a remarkable case of "flicker-induced cardiac arrest" in a patient with epilepsy. Using a conventional electronic stroboscope for photic stimulation, EEG and ECG recordings were made in a 34-year-old male with a history of frequent episodes of unexplained unconsciousness. Ossentyuk, in reporting the case, believed the patient to be suffering from two problems: epileptic seizures and increased vagal excitability—both provoked by photic stimulation. One episode of cardiac arrest lasted for 40 seconds before spontaneous rhythm returned. After an 8-month period, the patient seemed to be under satisfactory control with a cholinergic blocking agent and phenobarbital.

It has been observed that certain types of epilepsy, particularly temporal lobe epilepsy, are associated with mild disorders of cardiac rhythm. Phizackerley and associates described a case of cardiac arrest during a grand mal seizure which they believe indicates temporal lobe firing into vagal autonomic pathways to produce cardiac arrest. Glossopharyngeal neuralgia may sometimes need to be differentiated from grand mal seizures if the glossopharyngeal neuralgia is associated with loss of consciousness caused by cardiac asystole.

Hosler and co-workers speculate on the possibility of sudden death in certain grand mal seizures. The attacks, they speculate, are caused by cardiac standstill or ventricular fibrillation. They point out that autopsy on these patients often fails to reveal the cause of death.

Sudden and unexpected death in young adults and children

It is estimated that sudden, unexpected infant death in the United States is between 10,000 and 25,000 per year (Beckwith and co-workers). An epidemiologic study in the greater Cleveland area over a 10-year period has been reported by Strimer and co-workers, which reported 1,134 sudden unexpected infant deaths. These were deaths in apparently healthy infants that occurred within a matter of a few seconds or minutes and were generally unexplained. Autopsy findings were of little value. A few common denominators in Strimer and associates' epidemiologic study include greater frequency among non-whites, among male infants, in infants less than 25 weeks of age, and in infants during cold months. They reemphasize the fact that the etiology is still unknown in the sudden unexpected death in infancy often referred to as "cot-death," "crib-death," or "sudden death syndrome."

The sudden deaths that occur after parents put an allegedly well child to bed were studied by Segard and Koneman from autopsy material at the Billings Deaconess Hospital in Montana. From their view, the majority of crib deaths are caused by laryngotracheo-bronchitis. Histologically a characteristic inflammatory infiltrate is found beneath the mucosa of the trachea and was a consistent finding in 35 of 54 children studied.

The sudden and unexpected death of young adults has been the source of much mystery and conjecture. Kuller and colleagues report an epidemiologic study of sudden and unexpected nontraumatic deaths among Baltimore, Maryland, residents over a 1-year period. One third of the sudden, unexpected deaths were attributed directly to alcoholism. Surprisingly, almost 22% of the sudden and unexpected deaths were due to arteriosclerotic heart disease.

Nakamura and Natas have studied sixty-one children with complete heart block. In an excellent review of the subject, they discuss the incidence of associated heart disease, the natural history, and indicated therapy. It is interesting to note that 10% had familial conduction disturbances. In seven patients the duration of the QRS complex was 0.10 second or longer. In over 50% it was assumed with relative certainty that the conduction disturbance was congenital in origin. In contrast to other studies stressing the benign prognosis of congenital heart block, this study presents a mortality of 21.3%.

Some cite the incidence of 10% to 15% as representative of all natural deaths occurring suddenly and unexpectedly. No cause of death could be determined at autopsy in 14% of 1,000 cases of sudden, unexpected death in military personnel from 18 to 40 years of age, in whom the only sign or symptom was syncope.

Death of a child who was thought to be in good health, or whose terminal illness appeared to be so mild that the possibility of a fatal outcome was not anticipated, indicates to Adelson a case of cardiac arrest in the infant. Morrison is of the opinion that the cause of the great majority of sudden deaths can be determined accurately and investigation would include most careful pathologic studies such as cultures of blood from the heart, nose and throat cultures, and lumbar punctures. In Morrison's series, the majority of deaths were caused by meningitis and septicemia. Three of the seventeen deaths were thought to be due to endocardial fibroelastosis. From this study, it would appear that efforts at cardiac resuscitation might be limited and unrewarding.

Occasionally when sudden death occurs from an apparently insignificant cause such as during a minor operation or under light anesthesia, autopsy will not reveal the cause of death, and the pathologist will be unable to account for the death other than by an enlargement of the thymus, the spleen, and certain lymph nodes. A special committee appointed by the Medical Research Council and the Pathological Society of Great Britain and Ireland reported as long ago as 1921. Their report doubted the justification in assigning status thymicolymphaticus as a satisfactory cause of sudden death. Elaborate data were assembled by this committee, comparing the weight of the thymus in health and disease and its proportionate size to the spleen and lymph glands. Instances of sudden death were carefully studied for the circumstances surrounding the event. In spite of their efforts, they were completely at a loss to explain satisfactorily how hypertrophy of lymphoid tissue could cause sudden death or even predispose to it.

It is now generally agreed by most investigators that status thymicolymphaticus or an abnormality of the thymus of such a nature as to be responsible for sudden death is a remote possibility. The size of the thymus normally varies greatly, particularly in regard to body weight. Autopsies on infants dying suddenly, even when large thymus glands are present, have seldom been preceded by symptoms referable to thymic enlargements that might suggest pressure on other organs. For a long time the question of this condition was debated and articles continued to appear describing it. The *Quarterly Cumulative Index Medicus*, however, has discontinued this heading since 1942.

Other causes of sudden death

Sudden unexpected death in the Pickwickian syndrome is well documented (MacGregor and co-workers).

Sudden cardiac arrest is reported in a patient with pseudoxanthoma elasticum. Huang discusses the role of pseudoxanthoma elasticum in the heart in the genesis of cardiac failure and arrythmias.

POLIOMYELITIS

Patients with poliomyelitis, both in the acute stage and for some months afterward, represent potential candidates for cardiac arrest. Thomas illustrates this point in his report on a 38-year-old woman who was successfully resuscitated from cardiac arrest during the recovery period of the disease.

The occurrence of sudden failure of the cardiac "conduction mechanism" is noted by Steigman, who reports twelve such cases. In each of the twelve patients an immediate emergency thoracotomy was performed. One patient, a 2-year-old boy, lived 4½ days following the thoracotomy and was restored to normal consciousness. An additional patient survived 2½ days, but the other patients died. Steigman believes that better methods for the instantaneous detection and correction of abrupt cardiac arrest and for artificially maintaining circulation by other means are needed. He further speculates that artificial maintenance of ventilation and circulation in poliomyelitis has not yet reached a maximum period of development.

GRANULOMATOUS (FIELDER'S) MYOCARDITIS

Inflammatory reactions of the myocardium are not rare. They may be associated with infectious, toxic, or granulomatous states. Cases of granulomatous myocarditis have been reported—nearly all of which end in sudden death (Long). Fielder's isolated myocarditis may be a diffuse, inflammatory infiltration of the heart muscle or a granulomatous process with firm gray plaques noted in the myocardium, chiefly of the septum and left ventricle. A diffuse infiltration of lymphocytes and mononuclear cells with some neutrophils is seen. The disease is generally fatal within a matter of weeks and is seldom diagnosed prior to autopsy. Most cases of granulomatous myocarditis may be suspected by rather rapid onset associated with fainting spells and frequent dizzy spells.

SICKLE CELL ANEMIA

Jones and co-workers suggest that sickle cell crisis be considered in a differential diagnosis after sudden death of any black person despite his previous state of health. They document four sudden deaths attributable to sickle cell crisis.

GOUT

Brief mention should be given the fact that gouty involvement of the heart does occur and that total heart block attributed to urate deposits in the conduction system have been observed at an autopsy (Virtanen and Halonen).

SUDDEN DEATH DURING EXERCISE

Rarely does even the most strenuous exercise cause death in subjects with normal hearts. While unexpected, sudden death of athletes is an unusual event, invariably it is due to an asymptomatic heart disease. Most frequent postmortem findings are those of coronary arteriosclerosis and degenerative changes in the myocardium. Myocarditis, cardiac tumors, and obstructive cardiomyopathy, more rarely, will be found.

With increasing interest in jogging and exercise programs, an occasional case of sudden death from exercise is reported. From the Seattle area, Bruce and Kluge report seven patients who developed exertional cardiac arrest manifested by ventricular fibrillation. In two instances the arrest occurred during exercise testing and in five during exercise training of coronary patients. Fortunately, however, because of immediate availability of both a physician and a defibrillator, all were successfully treated. In each instance a single shock with a defibrillator restored normal sinus rhythm and return of consciousness. Only one of the seven patients exhibited any clinical or ECG manifestations of a possible acute myocardial in-farction. All but one were discharged from the hospital within 1 week and encouraged to continue physical activity including deliberate physical training. Bruce and Kluge urge that physicians should not encourage high-risk coronary patients to undertake physical training exercises that are strenuous in relation to their limited capacity without providing appropriate facilities and supervision. This would include the immediate availability of a defibrillator as well as other resuscitation equipment.

It is estimated that only 2% to 5% of all sudden coronary deaths are preceded by strenuous physical exercise. Around 10% occur while the victim is at work. On the other hand, at least 50% of coronary victims are at home when they encounter their attack and most often in bed.

THE SMALLEST TUMOR THAT CAUSES SUDDEN DEATH

On rare occasions, heart block in a young person may be caused by a small tumor of the atrioventricular node. At least twenty of these tumors have been reported and often represent an autopsy finding in younger persons with a history of Adams-Stokes attacks or complete heart block. Lewman and coworkers describe a 19-year-old girl who had had frequent blackout spells characterized by loss of consciousness and convulsions since the age of 3. In spite of a permanent demand pacemaker implanted in the right ventricular apex, the patient died suddenly at her home. Autopsy findings included a poorly circumscribed light yellowish-brown nodule in the region of the A-V node. Twenty similar lesions are reported by Morris and Johnson.

Chapter 16

SURGICAL AND DIAGNOSTIC PROCEDURES RELATED TO CARDIAC ARREST

Cardiac arrest during cardiac surgery

Within the past several years, physicians performing cardiac surgery have had opportunities to acquire considerable experience in cardiac resuscitation. One of the major obstacles toward further developments in cardiac surgery has been within the realm of cardiac arrest and resuscitation. Various authors have commented upon the nature of this problem. Hanlon states that one of the great stumbling blocks to the successful performance of aortic valvotomy had been the notorious tendency of the patient to go into ventricular fibrillation. Now with employment of coronary perfusion, selective hypothermia, or induced ventricular fibrillation, the nature of the problem has changed. An even greater depth of knowledge and understanding of cardiac resuscitation is required.

In a discussion of the dangers and difficulties likely to be met during surgical correction of interventricular septal defects, Bailey and associates list first the dangers of functional disturbance of the cardiac mechanism while the heart is being manipulated or subsequent to its manipulation. These include ventricular fibrillation and cardiac arrest. Paine and Varco commented upon the frequency of cardiac irregularities and cardiac arrest in patients undergoing surgery for pulmonic stenosis. In reporting their impressions relative to the frequency of ventricular fibrillation in patients with aortic stenosis on whom valvotomy is being performed, Cooley and DeBakey stated that ventricular fibrillation

is very prone to occur in the myocardium of patients with severe left ventricular hypertrophy. In their experience, the manipulation required to insert the valvulotome tends to develop fibrillation even if depressants are employed. Therefore it is their belief that such patients with acquired aortic stenosis should be operated upon before advanced stages of deterioration in myocardial decompensation.

Hypothermia as a means of reducing body oxygen requirements during cardiac surgery is being employed with some frequency. Ventricular fibrillation and cardiac arrest represent the major difficulties encountered under hypothermia. This has been discussed previously.

Cardiac arrest from pericardial tamponade

A tamponade of the heart may be produced in a variety of ways: (1) traumatic penetrating wounds of the heart from stabbing or from gunshot, (2) contusion of the heart from accidents such as steering wheel injuries, (3) rupture of the heart itself, or (4) an aneurysm of the ventricle. Cardiac tamponade is a not infrequent complication of both open- and closed-cardiac surgery. Iatrogenic cardiac tamponade has been produced in a number of instances by the diagnostic catheterization of the various chambers of the heart. The physiologic aspects of cardiac tamponade have been the subject of research by many investigators. Martin and Schenk record alterations in pericardial pressure, arterial pressure, venous pressure, and left ventricular output as the volume of fluid in the pericardial sac is acutely altered. They experimentally confirmed the observation that arterial blood pressure is in reality a poor index of cardiac output in the early phases of tamponade. Despite a considerable fall in cardiac output, peripheral resistance in vasoconstriction serves to maintain the arterial blood pressure. Cardiac output falls in a linear fashion as the interpericardial pressure is increased. Venous pressure rises in the same fashion.

Galenko and associates demonstrate that the pulsus paradoxus characteristic of acute pericardial tamponade is caused by a gradient between the pulmonary venous and left atrial pressures. Actual reversal of flow, back into the pulmonary veins, can be shown during inspiration.

Myocardial irritability

It is my impression, following clinical experience, that certain clinical entities appear to be associated with a decreased amount of cardiac irritability as observed in the operating room. Patients with constrictive pericarditis in particular may have surprisingly few rhythm abnormalities despite the considerable manipulation and myocardial trauma associated with pericardiectomy. Others have commented upon the somewhat unexpected finding that the same is true with patients undergoing resection of a left ventricular aneurysm. In such patients, the pericardium is usually firmly adherent to the myocardium about the site of the aneurysm. Despite the fact that the etiology of most of the aneurysms involves postmyocardial infarction and the fact that coronary atherosclerosis is present, few arrhythmias of any seriousness are encountered.

Cardiac arrest associated with declamping shock

Cardiac arrest is occasionally associated with an operation for correction of a co-

arctation of the aorta, frequently at the time of the removal of the clamps following the anastomosis. In 1948 Porter and co-workers called attention to the marked hypotension that often develops when the aortic clamps are removed at the completion of the anastomosis or following the resection of the coarctated segment of the aorta. The peripheral resistance is decreased because the heart has not only a well-developed collateral bed but also a normal aortic channel in which to empty; therefore the blood pressure falls sharply until the various vasomotor mechanisms can be brought into action or until death supervenes. As treatment, they suggest centripetal arterial transfusion. Most cardiovascular surgeons, however, find that they can avoid this complication if the clamps are removed slowly.

Blood transfusions administered in the usual manner are generally contraindicated because of the hazard of overtransfusion since the hypotension is not caused by decreased blood volume.

Crafoord, disagreeing with this concept, has commented upon the rapid fall of blood pressure caused by the sudden release of the aortic clamps. In his experiences with seventy cases of coarctation and patent ductus, he has never had a significant blood pressure fall connected with the removal of the clamps, even though he has taken no precaution to remove them slowly. He reports that in patent ductus cases where there is no collateral circulation, the blood pressure sometimes rises to 200 mm. Hg or more when the aortic clamps are applied. When these clamps are removed, these elevations return to their previous levels. Crafoord does not agree with the explanation given by Gross that releasing the clamps is responsible for the fall in blood pressure. He is convinced that some other mechanism is responsible, such as unsatisfactory ventilation during anasthesia, since, to his knowledge, these patients were not under controlled respiration at the time. Therefore he believes that with the use of adequate ventilation the heart would not be affected by the small additional stress caused by removal of the aortic clamps.

Strandness and colleagues believe that the problem represents a simple redistribution phenomenon. In a large number of animal experiments, they note that mean aortic pressure decreases 23% after aortic clamps are released in animals with aortic occlusion of 1 hour without significant blood loss. A subsequent decrease in cardiac output averages 21%. As an indication that the declamping shock is not related to the time factor, almost identical decreases in aortic pressure and cardiac output are recorded after aortic occlusions of 1 to 2 minutes and 15 minutes, respectively.

It should be noted that vasopressor drugs administered systemically prior to the release of the aortic clamp exert an undesirable effect. The increased systemic blood pressure speeds the rate of flow into the distal bed, resulting in sequestration of blood in the lower extremities of a great magnitude (Deterling).

Fry and co-workers used 1 to 1.5 mg. of phenylephrine hydrochloride injected directly into the iliac arteries prior to release of the aortic clamp. In a series of fifteen patients the average fall in blood pressure upon the release of the aortic clamp was 15 mm. Hg; in contrast, in twenty unselected patients undergoing aortic resection, the blood pressure fell an average of 110 mm. Hg following release of the aortic clamp.

The problem of aortic declamping is one that usually refers to patients undergoing resection of aortic aneurysms. Patients undergoing arterial reconstruction for insufficiency in the lower extremities do not, as a rule, experience an appreciable hypotension following declamping. This would lend support to the explanation offered by Fry and associates that the hypotension that follows release of the aortic clamp is due to reactive hyperemia and intravascular sequestration of a significant proportion

of the total circulating blood volume into the lower extremities. This sequestration of blood into the lower extremities promotes a decreased venous return to the heart, a reduced cardiac output, and an associated fall in systemic blood pressure.

Schneiweiss and co-workers found that they could alleviate aortic declamping hypotension in dogs by a dextran infusion into the iliac artery. They attribute the beneficial effects to the increased intravascular volume produced by the dextran which in turn aids in maintaining the normal tone of the small vessels.

Bowey and McClerkin gave dogs the amine buffer THAM to combat acidosis, but they were not able to prevent declamping hypotension.

It has been demonstrated that there is a considerable accumulation of acid metabolites distal to the cross-clamped aorta (Mansberger and others). For example, a significant drop in venous pH is noted during occlusion as well as significant elevations in the absolute values of lactate and pyruvate. The venous carbon dioxide and venous oxygen saturation suffer a profound fall. Mansberger and associates decided that, particularly following resections of ruptured aortic aneurysms, there is a triple mechanism at work in producing large quantities of acid metabolites: massive transfusion, hypotension, and cross-clamping. For this reason they recommend the infusion of commercial dextran above the aortic clamp at the rate of 2.5 ml. per kilogram of body weight per hour to reduce the anaerobic metabolism during the period of occlusion. In addition, they suggest that sodium bicarbonate also be employed routinely—particularly in resection of ruptured aortic aneurysms.

Levarterenol injected distal to the aortic clamp immediately prior to declamping is the most effective method of preventing the pressure drop. The gradient of pressure across the aortic clamp at the time of release is a major factor in determining the magnitude of the blood volume shift and resultant drop in pressure.

Fry's group noted experimentally that a marked drop in blood pressure occurs after clamping the aorta of dogs for only 10 seconds. This suggested to them that the rapid onset of vasodilatation points more to a reflex and mechanical phenomenon than to decreased vasomotor tonus and pooling of blood on the basis of an accumulation of acid metabolites.

Engler and associates approach the problem of declamping shock following release of the aortic clamp by providing for a small arterial shunt. They were able to eliminate the hypotension in dogs, and they speculate that metabolic acidosis, hypoxia, and vascular pooling are decreased.

In summary, declamping shock or hypotension is usually attributed to at least three major factors: profound metabolic acidosis, expansion of the vascular space in the lower extremities, and, occasionally, considerable blood loss through the interstices of the graft. In addition, Brant demonstrated the presence of a vasopressor substance in the effluent blood from dogs' lower extremities following a resection of a segment of the aorta and placement of a Teflon sleeve graft.

Relationship of cardiac arrest to operative procedure

Because of the significance of various phases of the operative procedure, cardiac arrest has been implicated in all periods of the operation. In 35% of the cases in my 1958 statistical study, cardiac arrest was experienced before surgery was begun or at the beginning. In 40% of the cases cardiac arrest occurred during the middle of the operative procedure. In 18% it was at the end of the procedure. In only 5% of the cases did cardiac arrest occur in the postoperative period.

Cardiac arrest associated with bone cement

Use of cold-curing acrylic cement to anchor the components of artificial joints to bones has become widespread. Numerous authors have referred to the fall in blood pressure shortly after use of this cement. Phillips and co-workers carried out clinical observations to study the cardiovascular effects of implanted acrylic bone cement and concluded that there is often, but not invariably, a fall in systemic arterial blood pressure after implantation. They theorize that the observed hypotension may be explained by the toxic effect of methylmethacrylate monomer or additives such as dimethylparatoluidine absorbed into the circulation. While others have speculated that the hypotensive effect may be due to the occurence of fat embolism, Phillips and associates failed to observe any of the clinical features of fat embolism in patients during or after operations. The effects of cement temperature, air embolism, and sensitivity to the acrylic warrant further investigation.

At least six cases of sudden cardiac arrest have been reported with the use of bone cement during orthopedic procedures (Powell and co-workers). Absorption of the cement monomer has produced sudden fall in blood pressure as well as pronounced vasodilation in experimental animals.

Cardiac catheterization and cardiac arrest

With the advent of cardiac catheterization as a diagnostic tool, it was not long before cases of cardiac arrest began to appear as a result of such a procedure. Episcoto reported a series of forty catheterizations of the heart under electrocardiographic observation. These were patients who had congenital heart disease, rheumatic heart disease with mitral stenosis, and/or aortic regurgitation. Three of the patients had auricular fibrillation prior to cardiac catheterization and all the others had a sinus rhythm. Thirty-eight, or 95%, of the forty catheterizations resulted in disturbances of cardiac rhythm. The location of the tip of the catheter was associated with a particular type of arrhythmia in most cases. Points of particular danger appeared to be when the catheter was passed through the tricuspid valve, when the tip of the catheter lay against the interventricular septum and the ventricular walls, and when it penetrated into the lumen of the pulmonary artery. One 9-year-old patient with congenital heart disease experienced a marked arrhythmia when the catheter was passed into the left median basilic vein. Although there were no cardiac arrests, the severe arrhythmias included one case of supraventricular tachycardia and one case of atrial fibrillation which persisted. Cardiac arrhythmias of a permanent nature may be produced in a small percentage of cases. A direct-writing ECG observation should be used routinely.

In general, the danger is greater with an increase in the degree of pathology present in the heart. Ravin indicates that the low incidence of fatalities in cardiac catheterization speaks highly for the ability of the heart to withstand mechanical stimulation. Catheterization is so valuable a diagnostic tool that it is important to keep the mortality rate at the lowest possible figure to avoid putting the procedure in disrepute. As more people with little experience participate in the procedure, it is possible that the number of fatalities may rise. It is therefore important that every precaution possible be taken to avoid mishap. If the catheter is being monitored by electrocardiographic observation, it is possible to withdraw the catheter when the arrhythmias become alarming. On the other hand, it is also true that often one must push past the area giving the arrhythmia to get the catheter into the pulmonary artery. The safest place for the catheter tip is in the pulmonary artery. If the catheter must be left in place more than a few seconds and especially if the patient is to be exercised or moved, the catheter should, if possible, be passed into the pulmonary artery. Dimond and co-workers report a case of temporary standstill with recovery in one patient out of a total of 130 catheterizations of the right side of the heart.

A case of cardiac arrest occurred during cardiac catheterization in a 46-year-old patient with congestive heart failure on the medical service at the Grace–New Haven Hospital and, at the time of massage, ventricular fibrillation was present. Electrical defibrillation occurred, but the patient survived only 20 hours. A second case at the same institution occurred in a 1-year-old child with cyanotic congenital heart disease. Resuscitation occurred but was not permanent, and the patient died within 6 hours. Asystole was present in this patient.

Angiocardiography and cardiac arrest

The association of angiocardiographic studies with the sudden cessation of the cardiac "conduction mechanism" has become increasingly well known with the publication of case reports from time to time. The autonomic nervous system effect from the injection of dyes is such that a strong vagal cardiac impulse is listed in a sizable number of cases. Stevens and associates demonstrate the vagovagal effect from injection of dye during arteriograms. This effect, they point out, is alleviated by the intravenous injection of atropine (0.2 mg.).

In twenty-five of twenty-six deaths during angiocardiography, out of a total of 6,824 diagnostic procedures collected from 182 hospitals by Dotter and Jackson, iodopyracet (Diodrast, Diodone, or Pyelosil) was the drug used. The frequency of death associated with angiocardiography from this large series was 0.38%. Dimond and Gonlubol report a sudden death following iodopyracet injection during angiocardiography, although the patient had reacted negatively to skin sensitivity tests. Sixty milliliters of 70% concentrated iodopyracet was injected intravenously, and within a second or so after the dye was given, the patient suddenly become cyanotic and complained of a warm sensation and headache. Artificial respiration was given; heart sounds suddenly stopped; the patient failed to respond to nikethamide (Coramine). Preparatory medication consisted of 0.4 gm. of quinidine 5 hours and 2 hours before the procedure and 100 mg. of cortisone 2 hours before angiocardiography. Autopsy findings revealed pulmonary veins from the right side entering the right atrium. A widely patent foramen ovale was present, and there was stenosis of the mitral valve.

Cournand and associates note twenty-six sudden deaths in a group of 6,224 patients having angiocardiographic examinations. Koszewski and co-workers record a sudden death in a 68-year-old white man on whom a translumbar aortography procedure was carried out. It is believed that this represents a hypersensitivity reaction.

A case occurred in 1952 in which iodomethamate sodium (Neo-Iopax) was injected intravenously (20 ml. of a 75% solution). A skin test had been negative. Cardiac arrest occurred 45 seconds after the injection. Normal rhythm was restored after intracardiac instillation of epinephrine, but this provoked ventricular fibrillation. The chest was opened and massage instituted. Electrical defibrillation was attempted three times but without success. Procainamide was also given. Massage was continued for 3 hours without effect. The patient had previously had a cardiac catherization that was uneventful for which the preparatory medication consisted of 0.2 gm. of quinidine and 0.1 gm. of pentobarbital (Nembutal) given 3 hours before angiocardiography. A continuous record of the heart action was obtained by the ECG, which varied from atrioventricular dissociation to ventricular tachycardia and then to ventricular fibrillation.

Evidence relative to the nature of the contrast medium, the number of injections, and the type of premedication or anesthesia was not of apparent significance in influencing a death from angiocardiography. There was a higher incidence of death among those patients receiving larger doses and in those examined in the horizontal position. The incidence of death was higher in children.

Although widely used for other indications, Renografin-76 (meglumine diatrizoate and sodium diatrizoate injection) should not be used for selective coronary arteriography because of a significant incidence of ventricular fibrillation associated with the drug. In a letter to physicians dated April 17, 1970, E. R. Squibb & Sons advised against the use of this preparation for purposes of coronary arteriography.

Arrhythmias in the denervated transplanted human heart

In a review of the electrocardiograms of forty-three cardiac transplant patients at Stanford University it is concluded by Schroeder and associates that innervation is not necessary for production of cardiac arrhythmias in the transplanted heart. Atrial arrhythmias occurred in 50% of the patients and usually were associated with acute rejection episodes. Sinus arrest occurred in two, necessitating permanent pacemaking. In sixteen of the patients, ventricular premature beats were detected and were usually associated with either acute rejection or ischemia secondary to accelerated coronary atherosclerosis. Two acute rejection episodes were associated with ventricular fibrillation.

Chapter 17

EMBOLIC MECHANISMS

Amniotic fluid embolism

An excellent description of the hemodynamic effects of amniotic fluid embolism is provided by Reis and co-workers. They have reviewed the arguments incriminating an anaphylactic response to fetal epithelial material, mechanical pulmonary vascular obstruction, or intravascular thrombosis. The physiologic responses observed after injection of amniotic fluid into the circulation of ewes include marked systemic vasodilatation and profound pulmonary vasoconstriction. The circulatory effects of amniotic fluid were not altered by filtering the fluid or by injecting it into the left atrium. The suspicion persists that it is a humoral material in amniotic fluid that produces a marked decrease in systemic vascular resistance and a profound and prolonged increase in the pulmonary vascular resistance following its introduction into circulation.

A diagnosis of amniotic fluid embolism should be considered in any obstetric patient when sudden syncope develops during or after labor. Particularly is this likely to occur in association with placenta accreta, cesarean section, rupture of the uterus, partial retention of the placenta, or premature marginal separation of the placenta. If death occurs suddenly, pulmonary embolism by amniotic fluid should be strongly considered and the appropriate treatment for resuscitation should be instituted. In spite of the gaps in knowledge concerning the mechanism of death with pulmonary embolism from amniotic fluid, it is appropriate that we consider this problem in a book on cardiac arrest and resuscitation, since the problem resolves itself around cardiopulmonary resuscitation and should be amenable to an approach embodying the principles as stressed throughout this book. The controversial nature of the role of amniotic fluid in such cases is to be remembered.

Amniotic fluid emboli to the pulmonary circulation occur most frequently in multiparas of the older age group. Violent uterine contractions followed by dyspnea, cyanosis, and shock may lead to a suspicion of this diagnosis. Steiner and Lushbaugh believe that deaths from amniotic fluid range in the neighborhood of 1 in 8,000 deliveries.

Sublethal episodes of embolization must occur considerably more often. It is not intended that a detailed consideration of amniotic fluid embolism be considered in this book; excellent discussions of this problem are available (Nickerson; Fowler and Goode). It does appear likely, however, that a small percentage of these patients may be candidates for cardiac resuscitative efforts in addition to the usual therapy, which includes the use of oxygen, vasopressors, blood or plasma replacement, and the administration of fibrinogen to combat the afibrinogenemia that is so often associated with the embolism.

The incidence of pulmonary embolism by amniotic fluid has been estimated by various authors to vary from as frequent as 4 cases in 1,000 obstetric deaths in North Carolina (Sluder and Lock) to an incidence of 1 in 8,000 deliveries or more. Gross and Benz reported three cases that occurred within a general hospital averaging 1,300 deliveries annually and represented the only maternal deaths within that period. May and Winter were unable to find any such deaths after reviewing the deliveries in Charity Hospital, New Orleans, over a 10-year period. The first such report was that of Steiner in 1941. This was a case of sudden obstetric death in which the embolism occurred without warning and which resulted in instant death of the patient.

Since Steiner's report first appeared in the literature, there is still considerable doubt in many obstetric areas that amniotic emboli do actually exist and cause sudden death. Tunis wrote that he had never been quite convinced, first, that there was an amniotic embolus, second, that the amniotic embolus was the cause of the fatal outcome, and finally, that there were not other factors operating to cause the death.

During the first 2,400 deliveries at Chicago Lying-In Hospital of the University of Chicago, there were three cases of amniotic fluid embolism with death. Eames reports a case of sudden death that he believes was a fatal pulmonary embolism from amniotic fluid. Sluder and Lock conclude from their observations that amniotic fluid embolism has been demonstrated in a sufficient number of instances to establish this condition as a cause of sudden death during labor or in the early puerperium.

Deaths occurring during or shortly after labor have been reported with increasing frequency since Steiner and Lushbaugh first described in 1941 eight patients in whom autopsies showed widespread embolism of the small pulmonary arterioles and capillaries by the particulate matter found in the amniotic fluid and meconium. The mechanism of such deaths might well be explained by the so-called pulmocoronary reflex described by Scherf in 1937. Reid has attributed the mechanism of this reflex to the stimulation that occurs following the stretching of vessel walls by the presence of an embolism and the inadequate clearing of accumulated metabolites and to the metabolites acting on local nerve endings setting up an impulse. Whether the theory of this reflex is correct or not, the existence of the reflex seems well established, and it is well known that the simple occlusion of the pulmonary vessel is a harmless affair except for the subsequent local changes. As Reid has pointed out, the occlusion of very small vessels in animals with foreign body emboli is frequently accompanied by dyspnea and sometimes bronchial spasm. This effect cannot be produced if vagal section has occurred previously. The effects of the reflex may be manifested in the coronary circulation.

Uterine tetany, unusually strong uterine contractions, intrauterine death of the fetus, an oversized baby, multiparity, and advancing age of the mother have been listed as predisposing factors. An editorial in the *Journal of the American Medical Association* noted that embolism had been reproduced in animals by injecting human amniotic fluid and meconium into the intravenous system.

The exact mechanism of the entrance of the amniotic fluid into the maternal circulation is thought to be by way of the uterine or placental vessels that have been opened abnormally, such as might occur in premature marginal separation of the placenta, partial retention of the placenta, placenta accreta, or a rupture of the uterus. Others believe that, instead of a mechanical and reflex mechanism, the cause of death is an anaphylactoid reaction.

Although not of practical significance from the standpoint of instituting treatment, a diagnosis of amniotic embolism (when an autopsy cannot be performed) may be suggested by the methods described by Gross and Benz. They found that blood aspirated from the right ventricle or from the inferior vena cava, when centrifuged, shows a characteristic third flocculent stratum above the layer of leukocytic cream. If the material from this layer is smeared or sections are taken, constituents of amniotic fluid and meconium can de demonstrated.

Fowler and Goode report the case of a

40-year-old woman who died suddenly following rupture of fetal membranes. In this case, the lower uterine segment showed a detached chorionic membrane and an exposed, ruptured venous sinus containing a mixture of blood and vernix. Death was attributed to pulmonary circulatory obstruction by amniotic debris.

The diagnosis may be made if formed elements of amniotic fluid are found in the pulmonary arterioles and alveolar capillaries.

Air and gas embolism

Sudden death following introduction of air or other gases into the arterial or systemic venous systems is a mechanism that has become increasingly clear. The occurrence of cardiac arrest or serious impairment of cardiac output depends upon several factors such as the amount of air introduced, the solubility of the gas, the condition of the heart at the time it receives the insult, and the location of the gas as well as the position of the patient.

Air embolism as a lethal complication of subclavian venapuncture with the usual clinical findings of the immediate development of tachypnea and a "mill-wheel" murmur heard over the precordium presents very much the same picture as air embolism from any other transvenous source (Flanagan and co-workers).

There are many examples of situations leading to fatal embolism. For example, air embolism may occur when air enters or is sucked into a collapsing vein as it is torn and cut in the neck. The fascia of the neck sends out fibers that invest the large veins of the neck and, when cut, instead of allowing for closure of the cut into the vein, the fascial fibers attached to the circumference of the vein pull the vein wider apart at its cut end, allowing air to be sucked in. A fatal amount of air may enter the circulation quickly, and death may occur.

Other sources of air embolization may include diagnostic or therapeutic air injection such as during pneumoperitoneum, vaginal insufflation, perineal air insufflation, postpartum following knee-chest exercise, introduction of air into the urinary bladder, maxillary antrum lavage, encephalography, angiocardiography, during the production of an artificial pneumothorax, and associated with a therapeutic abortion.

A fatal case of air embolism occurred in a 16-year-old girl following voluntary mouth-to-mouth yoga breathing exercises with a teenage boy. At autopsy, massive extension of the right ventricle and atrium of the heart and of the carotid vessels of the superior mediastinum was present. Corrigan states that the case represents the fatal sequela of acute transient respiratory obstruction as produced by human-to-human, mouth-to-mouth air exchange, with air embolization at the level of the small nondissectible vessels and the subsequent embolization of the coronary vessels.

Another source of air embolization is bubbles flowing in the blood-flow line from the kidney to the patient during renal hemodialysis. Kolff, in discussing air embolization during hemodialysis, cautions that air emboli may originate by being sucked into the system whenever a pump is used. Its origin may be an artificial kidney that is not properly flushed. Occasionally air is used to displace blood during removal of blood from a Kiil or a coil kidney.

Residual coronary air embolus after heart-lung bypass may occasionally be the reason for poor myocardial contractility and low cardiac output. In a report on dog experiments before the Society of Thoracic Surgeons, Justice emphasizes that small amounts of air produced an additive effect with more depression and a slower recovery after each injection. By far the most effective method of removing air from the coronaries and improving contractility of the myocardium is through increasing the perfusion flow rate for 1 minute to one and a half to two times normal. Hearts intractable to electrical defibrillation become pink when exposed to such increased flow rates and respond to a single countershock.

It has been pointed out that the transdiaphragmatic approach for production of a pneumoperitoneum can be the source of serious air emboli. Higgins and Batchelder describe two cases of right-sided cardiac air embolization following an upper right lobectomy. It is believed that in each instance air was inadventently injected into the liver. Both cases recovered uneventfully after the pericardium was opened and air was aspirated from the right side of the heart. To substantiate their suspicion, they were able to show that air injected into the parenchyma of the dog's liver quickly appears as bubbles in the inferior vena cava and subsequently in the right side of the heart.

The mechanism by which air emboli will prove fatal can be by any one of several ways. Air entering through veins to the right side of the heart may act as a large bolus in the right atrium, preventing blood from entering the right ventricle. Air entering the left side of the heart by means of an intra-arterial transfusion or during open cardiac surgery may proceed to the cerebral circulation or to the coronary circulation and act like a small thrombus, causing myocardial ischemia and subsequent death.

Lindskog discusses the danger of an air embolism during a therapeutic pneumothorax for treatment of tuberculosis. He points out that the embolism can occur when the needle point enters or tears a blood vessel in an adhesion or a branch of the pulmonary vein in the lung, or simply when an adhesion is torn. In the past, sudden death following a therapeutic pneumothorax was often attributed to "pleural shock." Most writers at the present time believe that such instances actually are unrecognized examples of air embolism. An air embolism may occur during thoracentesis. Rossle suggests that fatal air emboli may occur in fliers and in victims of explosions in the air or under water because of the sudden changes in the atmospheric and intra-alveolar pressures with a subsequent rupture of the pulmonary capillaries. Air enters into the pulmonary capillaries or veins and from there goes to the left side of the heart and, subsequently, to the coronary arteries.

Shires and O'Banion describe the case of a 49-year-old man who was receiving emergency care following a gunshot wound. Blood was being administered rapidly by intravenous route with the use of an air-bulb for pressure. The transfusion bottle had been inadvertently emptied and large quantities of air under pressure had entered the patient's venous system. A thoracotomy was immediately performed and the heart was "tremendously dilated." No contractile activity could be noted under manual compression. Air under pressure was removed by inserting a needle into the right ventricle; in fact, the air was under such pressure that the plunger was rapidly pushed out of the end of the syringe. The patient subsequently made an uneventful recovery. It is estimated that the patient received in excess of 300 ml. of air within a few seconds.

Unless methods are used to prevent the entrance of air into the coronary vessels during surgery on the left side of the heart, the results are likely to be unsuccessful. As already mentioned, the clinical picture of air in the left side of the heart is of much greater significance than that on the right side. Air injected intravenously into dogs at the rate of 25 ml. per minute until the amount of 76 ml. per kilogram is reached fails to provoke death in dogs, whereas no more than 1.5 ml. per kilogram can be injected into pulmonary veins before death results (Van Allen). Only small amounts of air in the left side of the heart, however, are required to produce death unless means are taken to reverse this procedure. Geoghegan and Lam speculated on the cause of death from air in the left side of the heart and concluded that the sudden death is caused by filling of the coronary arteries with air. Their experimetal data fail to indicate that air in the cavity of the left ventricle greatly impairs the function of the heart, and air in the cerebral arteries does not result in immediate death. Severe brain damage does result if sufficient air is present in the coronary arteries.

Air in the coronary arteries is not necessarily an irreversible situation. Massage of the heart can create sufficiently high pressure in the coronary arteries to force the air through the venous side and restore the heart to a normal rhythm. To increase the pressure in the coronary vessels, it has been recommended that the aorta be clamped beyond the great vessels either by use of a rubber-shod clamp or with the fingers.

The diagnosis of air embolism may occasionally be overlooked in sudden death. If the air enters by means of a sudden sucking of air into the veins, the surgeon may become conscious of hearing the noise produced by such suction. Air in the right side of the heart characteristically produces what is described as a "washboard" type of sound and may be suspected when such a sound is heard. On palpation and inspection, the heart will appear dilated. If closer inspection is carried out, columns of air can be seen moving back and forth in the coronary vessels during massage or when the heart has been restored to a sinus rhythm.

The position of the patient during the operation has direct relationship to the likelihood of development of an air embolus. Hamby and Carry particularly call attention to this danger during neurosurgery since the sitting position is often used. A diagnosis of an air embolus can often be made when the patient is shifted to the supine position, for, in this case, a to-and-fro, swishing, "mill-wheel" murmur can be heard.

Tisovec and Hamilton report an incidence of 2.6% to 15% in venous air embolism during posterior fossa craniectomies done with patients in the sitting position. In this position, venous pressure in the head and neck may be less than atmospheric; therefore an opening into a venous channel affords a portal of entry for air.

During neurosurgical procedures, the danger of air embolism appears to be greatest in the patient upon whom surgery is being performed on the posterior cranial fossa. Of 2,002 neurosurgical procedures with the patient in a sitting position, thirty-nine of forty episodes of air embolism occurred during surgery on the posterior cranial fossa. Routine placement of the catheter, ideally in the right atrium, in all patients scheduled for suboccipital craniectomy in the sitting position is suggested by Michenfelder and associates at the Mayo clinic. The sudden appearance of a heart murmur was the first feature to suggest the diagnosis in all but four of the episodes. Confirmation was by aspiration of air from the right atrium. The murmur was generally not the classic "mill-wheel" murmur but was characterized by a "sloshy" quality. In cases where a central venous pressure was being monitored, the pressure elevation occurred when air entered the heart.

Once the diagnosis has been made, further entry of air may be discouraged by increasing the venous pressure in the head by bilateral compression of the internal jugular veins. Vasopressors not only improve the perfusion pressure but also aid the heart in ejecting the intracardiac air into the pulmonary circulation. Aspiration of the air may be accomplished if there is a catheter present in the right atrium or superior vena cava. In one instance, as much as 400 ml. of air was aspirated. It seems likely that in most instances air was aspirated by noncollapsible venous channels (diploic veins or dural sinuses). While a sitting position favors the development of air embolism by permitting the central venous pressure to be markedly lower than the intracranial venous pressure when the system is open under surgical conditions, air embolism may also occur with the patient in the prone position in cases explored intracranially with mechanically controlled respiration.

In summary, a central venous catheter in the right atrium and constant monitoring with an esophageal stethoscope are indicated in patients subjected to increased risk from air embolism. Pump/oxygenators used during the course of open-heart surgery are a major source of air emboli. Simmons and Lichte at the University of Missouri have demonstrated that these air bubbles can be detected by the use of the ultrasonic flowmeter in the carotid and temporal arteries during open-heart surgery.

After the heart has been closed following open-heart surgery, most of the air can be removed from the aorta by puncturing the aorta at its highest point. If air is seen in the coronary artery during open-heart surgery, high perfusion pressures will eventually push the air through the coronary arteries.

Air can enter any vein under the proper circumstances and will do so spontaneously if negative pressure exists, as in the case of an open jugular vein in the neck. I recall seeing a cardiac arrest result from an air embolus taking place during a cystectomy. Only after a lengthy period of cardiac massage was a diagnosis of air embolism made when inspection of the coronary vessels revealed columns of air moving to-and-fro within their walls. Hearts that are opened following air emboli will reveal a right ventricle and pulmonary artery filled with a foamlike material that has prevented adequate emptying of the right side of the heart. Ventricular fibrillation may follow an air embolism. In the experimental laboratory I have witnessed dog hearts thrown into ventricular fibrillation following injection of 50 to 100 ml. of air into the femoral vein.

Geoghegan and Lam speculate on the possibility that deaths occurring during pneumothorax treatments (so-called pleural shock deaths) are actually due to air being injected into the venous side of the pulmonary vascular bed. These authors consider three possible mechanisms responsible for death when air enters the left heart: (1) air entering and occluding the coronary arteries; (2) the bolus of air in the ventricles, itself resulting in a failure of the cardiac pumping action; (3) cerebral air embolism. In regard to the third mechanism, they note that in twelve animals in which large amounts of air were injected into the left common carotid artery, death did not ensue nor was cardiac action impaired. However, when more than 0.25 ml. of air was given, there was evidence of marked neurologic damage, and the damage seemed, in general, proportional to the amounts of air injected and resembled effects produced by increasing periods of cerebral anemia. Relative to the second mechanism, they attempted to simulate conditions by placing a balloon in the apical regions of the left ventricle through an ingenious maneuver. In all of the cases, there was very little alteration noted in the aortic pressure, as the ventricle apparently was able to compensate satisfactorily to the alteration in volume. Thus the likelihood of a compressible bolus of gas in the left ventricle causing mechanical pump failure in the absence of air in the coronary arteries seemed less likely. In 1949 Kulka demonstrated a device with which he could collect the gas bubble in the heart and also save it for further examination.

Air entering the systemic circulation in association with open-heart surgery is a well-recognized complication. Steps to prevent air entrapment and subsequent embolization include several techniques. Induced elective fibrillary arrest, extensively utilized by Glenn, provides an excellent means of controlling air entrapment. Prior to restoration of a beating heart, the cardiac chambers may be allowed to fill and air venting may be allowed to take place. I have been satisfied with induced fibrillary arrest, particularly with regard to surgery on the left side of the heart.

Starr calls attention to the particular likelihood of air embolization during correction of a congenital cleft mitral valve. Air may be trapped in the left ventricle during operations for correction of acquired mitral disease while the patient is in the left lateral decubitus position. In such a position, the right pulmonary veins may serve as an additional source of trapped air. Air introduced into the left atrium while the patient is in the supine position can gravitate into the left ventricle. Starr recommends the use of a left ventricular vent (Fig. 17-1) as a means of avoiding air emboli in such situations.

Carbon dioxide flooding of the operative field has been utilized as a preventive measure against air embolization in the belief that it will displace the oxygen and, in ad-

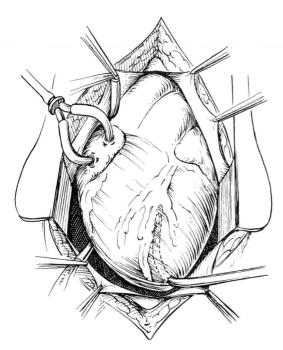

Fig. 17-1. Method used for decompression of left ventricle as well as for removal of retained air in ventricle. (Modified from Starr, A.: J. Thorac. Cardiovasc. Surg. **39**:808, 1960.)

dition, will be readily diffusible. Carbon dioxide is over twenty times as soluble as air at normal body temperatures. This type of displacement is not widely used at present.

Impressed by the fact that air embolism may occasionally occur despite the use of ventricular vents, aspiration of the ascending aorta, or elective fibrillation, Taber advocates the use of a combined cardiotomy suction and intracardiac aspiration system. This allows for multiple aspiration of the left heart and aortic areas before the heart is defibrillated. A crystalloid solution may be injected through a left atrial catheter to help fill the heart, and the heart may subsequently be compressed to displace bubbles of air into the apex. Taber suggests that aspiration be performed sequentially, beginning in the atrial appendage, then the ventricular apex, and finally the ascending aorta.

Although experimental studies have shown that the dog heartbeat can be maintained for considerable periods of time by perfusion of oxygen alone into the coronaries, one must not fail to appreciate the fact that oxygen embolism has much the same effect as that resulting from air. A paradoxic air or gas embolism may explain the devastating effect of a relatively small amount of air or gas. When it is recalled that as little as 0.5 to 1 ml. of air admitted to the left side of the heart in dogs can be fatal, as compared with as much as one hundred times that amount on the right side, then one realizes the potential danger of air entering the systemic venous system in patients with such lesions as ventricular septal defect or trilogy of Fallot.

Treatment of massive air emboli

Once cardiac arrest due to air emboli is suspected, resuscitative efforts should include the following (Nicholson):

1. Obviously, the source of the air emboli should be discontinued if it is known.
2. Steps should be employed to prevent the air emboli from entering the cere-

bral circulation by lowering the head of the patient.

3. The patient should be placed in the left lateral position in order to encourage a release of "air lock" in the right side of the heart and into the right uppermost pulmonary arterial bed. Gradual absorption of the air entrapped in the right lung will occur.

4. Needle aspiration of the right side of the heart, in case of right-sided emboli, is indicated if large amounts of air have accumulated. Needling of the left side of the heart for air emboli is of little value.

From preliminary animal observations, there is serious doubt that closed-chest compression is the most effective method of treating right-sided or venous air embolism. The large bolus of air in the right side of the heart is not readily dissipated.

Fat emboli

Although cases of sudden death in young adults with fatty livers, fatal fat emboli in diabetic patients, and pulmonary fat emboli following trauma have been described, each as a cause of sudden death, adequate documentation of these cases has been infrequent. Holler and co-workers studied fourteen patients who died suddenly with massive fatty infiltration of the liver, but these authors are not impressed with the evidence suggesting that fat embolism was the cause of death.

Pulmonary embolism

In discussing pulmonary emboli, Crafoord reported that all of the twenty-three patients with pulmonary emboli upon which he has operated have had periods of cardiac arrest. Among resuscitative measures used were procaine hydrochloride (Novocain) in the pericardium itself, vigorous massage, and epinephrine (1:1,000) intracardially. In about 50% of these cases he was able to restore function of the heart.

As early as 1937 Beck and Mautz suggested that the method of resuscitation of the heart in cardiac arrest may also apply to pulmonary embolus. They stated: "The obstacle to success in pulmonary embolectomy is not so much the removal of the embolus and suture of the pulmonary artery as the revival of the heartbeat." Pulmonary emboli, of course, are more commonly due to a blood clot, but in a few cases gas or fat may be responsible. Occasionally, pieces of tumor tissue and pieces of normal organ tissue torn off by trauma, or even amniotic fluid, may be the cause of pulmonary emboli. Bile embolism has even been reported in jaundiced patients after needle biopsy of the liver. These emboli will be discussed further.

Considerable evidence indicates that cardiac changes occurring after a pulmonary embolism are reflex in nature. The work of Byrne and Cahill (1958) fails to substantiate that this occurs in rabbits. They conclude that the cardiac changes found in pulmonary embolism are caused by increased intraventricular pressure secondary to the pulmonary embolism and associated vascular constriction but are not related to a reflex coronary spasm.

A massive pulmonary embolism occurring under general anesthesia may present diagnostic problems. I encountered such a case in a patient on whom a lumbar sympathectomy was being performed under spinal anesthesia. During the course of the dissection, hypotension occurred and became progressively more severe. The hypotension was associated with marked distension of the patient's neck veins, and it was felt by the anesthesia service that the patient was in cardiac decompensation. An attempt was made to digitalize the patient. The blood pressure was maintained at around 80 mm. Hg systolic. The procedure was promptly completed and, while the bandage was being applied, all heart action ceased. Closed-chest cardiac resuscitation was begun almost immediately. Since closed-chest resuscitation did not seem to be effective, after 2 or 3 minutes a decision was made to open the chest at the fourth intercostal space. This was done, and manual cardiac compression was carried out for well over 1 hour. Pupil constriction could be maintained at a satisfactory level, but resuscitative efforts appeared generally inadequate. The neck veins remained distended, and the right side of the heart was enlarged. Repeated attempts at defibrillation were only temporarily successful. The patient responded poorly to epinephrine and calcium chloride. After approximately 1½ hours of resuscitative efforts, attempts were abandoned. At autopsy, a large pulmonary embolus was found at the bifurcation of the pulmonary artery and extending into the main pulmonary artery.

The use of a surgical approach to pulmonary embolism has waxed and waned during much of this century since the first pulmonary embolectomy was performed at the University of Leipzig by Trendelenburg in 1908. The procedure, which bears his name, has been modified considerably since Sharp, Cooley, and others reported their successful efforts in removing pulmonary emboli with the assistance of the heart-lung bypass apparatus. The addition of extracorporeal support not only provides mechanical aid for the failing circulation prior to and during the embolectomy but it allows for a more deliberate and thorough extraction of the clot by providing added time for the surgeon to work in a nearly bloodless field.

The indications for a pulmonary embolectomy have tended to narrow rather than broaden. Thrombolytic agents and the administration of anticoagulants as well as an increased awareness of the natural potential for spontaneous lysis have decreased the frequency of the procedure. In addition, the reports of the operative results have not always been glowing.

What we are concerned with in this particular section on pulmonary embolism in a book on cardiac arrest and resuscitation is the patient who suddenly throws a massive embolism to obstruct the right side of the heart and the pulmonary circulation. We will not concern ourselves with the many considerations revolving around the diagnosis and technical approach to the semielective removal of a pulmonary embolism, although it is true that a number of these patients will also develop cardiac arrest during the procedure and will require active resuscitative efforts. It is estimated that perhaps only about 5% of all patients with major pulmonary embolism require surgery on a real emergency basis. These patients, however, are faced with a highly critical situation with the clock rapidly running out. The obstruction is such that the right ventricle fails to empty, acute right-sided heart failure occurs, and inadequate pulmonary ventilation and cyanosis quickly follow as well as a moribund state. Fig. 17-2 attests to this situation and represents a patient of ours whom we saw some years ago and who died within a matter of 20 to 30 minutes while on the ward. The massive size of the clot is obvious and dramatically demonstrates the need for an embolectomy. These are truly individuals with whom a last ditch effort must be attempted—and generally within a matter of minutes.

In the face of acute cor pulmonale, marked reduction in cardiac output, cyanosis, and shock, the clinical features concomitant to smaller embolization are not seen. For example, pleuritic pain is not a common feature. Since no infarction has occurred, no hemoptysis is seen, and no area of infarction is visible on the roentgenograms. In fact, the decreased vascularity of the lungs may show an increased radiolucency. Enzyme studies will not be of great value, again because of the absence of an infarct. Alerting one to the possibility of a massive pulmonary embolism is a sudden onset of dyspnea, with or without cyanosis or chest pain, syncope, and frequently convulsions caused by inadequate cerebral circulation. Unexplained hypotension occurs.

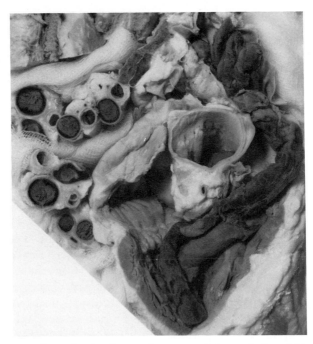

Fig. 17-2. Autopsy specimen showing huge pulmonary embolus occluding right ventricle, pulmonary outflow tract, and pulmonary arteries.

If the obstruction is not complete, pressure agents may help maintain the patient for a short time. Even though the electrocardiogram in a massive pulmonary embolism may be confused with that of an acute inferior myocardial infarction, one should, if possible, obtain an ECG. Obviously emergency angiographic studies will be confirmatory. At the same time, right pulmonary artery and right ventricular pressure studies will help define the hemodynamic alterations.

In the meantime, an emergency partial cardiopulmonary bypass should be done at the bedside with a femoral vein–femoral artery connection and a portable oxygenator. A pulmonary lung scan is not generally indicated in this particular situation as it is with the more semielective problem.

Attention should be called to the emergency thoracotomy, which can expose the pulmonary artery within a minimum of time. This procedure allows removal of the clot without extracorporeal circulation. Basically

it is a modified Trendelenburg procedure. In describing the technique, Borja and Lansing suggest a posterior-lateral incision on the left side with entrance to the chest through the fourth intercostal space. The left main pulmonary artery is palpated. The pericardium is opened to gain access to the main pulmonary and right pulmonary arteries (Fig. 17-3, A and B). The left main pulmonary artery is dissected free and an umbilical tape is passed around the vessel both proximally and distally. After the arterotomy is performed as pictured, a Fogarty catheter is passed for clot extraction. Subsequently, suction is applied to the bifurcation of the main pulmonary and to the right pulmonary arteries. A Fogarty catheter can be passed in these directions also. The lung should be compressed gently to further mobilize emboli that are in the smaller branches of the pulmonary artery and the Fogarty catheter again inserted to remove any residual clots. The ideal patient for this procedure, of

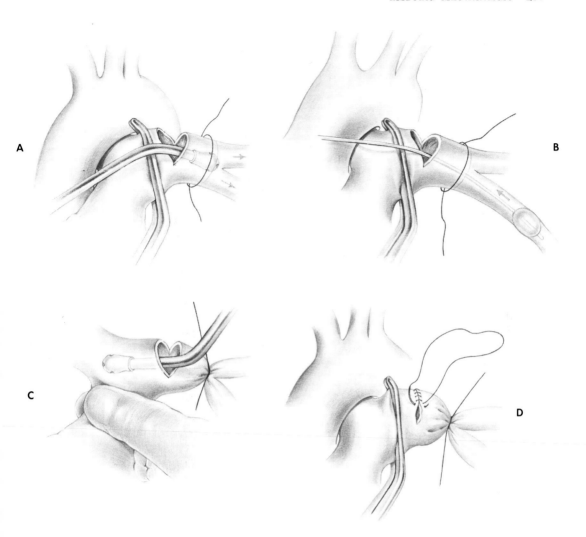

Fig. 17-3. A, Arteriotomy is performed at anterosuperior aspect of left main pulmonary artery after occlusion at its origin in order to selectively remove pulmonary embolism without the use of a cardiopulmonary bypass. **B,** For extraction of distal clots, the Fogarty catheter is passed into the branches of pulmonary artery. **C,** With fingers compressing main pulmonary artery, suction catheter and/or Fogarty catheter is passed to bifurcation in main pulmonary artery and into right pulmonary artery. **D,** A continuous arterial suture is used to repair the arteriotomy site after embolectomy is completed. (From Borja, A. R., and Lansing, A. M.: Surg. Gynecol. Obstet. **130:**1073-1076, 1970; by permission of Surgery, Gynecology & Obstetrics.)

course, would be one in whom the embolism is obstructing the pulmonary artery on just one side. If an arteriographic study indicates the embolus to be in the right pulmonary artery, the embolectomy can be performed using a right-sided thoracotomy or with a midsternotomy approach. An anterior thoracotomy in the third interspace is also an appropriate incision for pulmonary artery exploration. Once the right ventricular obstruction has been removed usually the heart can be resuscitated.

Chapter 18

VENTRICULAR FIBRILLATION

When the fibrillar contraction is excited by stimulation (e.g., faradisation of the surface of the ventricles) there appears to be a condition of violent excitement set up in the muscular tissue. The excitation of the muscular fibres travels peristaltically, producing the characteristic movement; the incoordinated contraction of the various fibres may be most distinctly realised when the ventricles are held between the forefinger and thumb; there is a sort of wriggling sensation to be felt as the individual muscular bundles become hard and wiry while the contraction is passing over them in succession. The co-ordinating arrangements of the ventricles are powerless to regulate and guide the contractions; those co-ordinating arrangements are very possibly not paralysed nor rendered incapable of action, but they are temporarily superseded and rendered inoperative by the excessive state of excitement which pervades the muscular fibres—just as the cerebrospinal co-ordinating mechanism might be rendered impotent by strong local stimulation of the skeletal muscles. When the fibrillar movement, having become less rapid, has at length stopped—its duration depending on the excitability of the muscle—there ensues a pause. . . .*

One of the great advances in the last half-century and particularly within the last 25 years is associated with the problem of ventricular fibrillation. No longer does this malignant arrhythmia of the human ventricle necessarily carry with it an irreversible and fatal prognosis. The advances in surgery, particularly those for correction of developmental defects of the heart, have been extended because ventricular fibrillation need no longer be feared to the extent that it was previously; instead, it can be looked upon as an unfortunate complication which, in the majority of instances, can be coped with successfully. Even so, our knowledge of ventricular fibrillation still leaves much to be desired. In this discussion I will attempt to present the current status of ventricular fibrillation.

Over the years, ventricular fibrillation has been given many different names in an effort to describe what was occurring. Some of the names applied to this fibrillary action are: delirium cordis (Ludwig); intervermiform movement (Mills); fibrillary twitching, contraction fibrillaire, tremulations, tremulatories and movement fibrillaire, tremblotements musculaires, undulatory movements (Gaskill); undulation (Wuhlen and Wagen); flimmern (Hoffa and Ludwig); herzzittern (Einbrodt, Kronecker); circulatory rhythm (Mines); and circus contractions (Garrey). As a practicing British surgeon in 1842, Erichsen described the visible phenomena of ventricular fibrillation. The ectopic focus theory of ventricular fibrillation was introduced by Rothberger and Winterberg in 1914.

The classic work of Prevost and Battelli in 1899 opened up a new frontier in the treatment of ventricular fibrillation. From their original article appearing the next year, I have translated material dealing with some of the effects of electrical discharges on the heart of mammals. It would be worthwhile to quote the conclusions made by these authors after they had reviewed their experimental data:

Today we are reviewing experiments done in the physiological laboratory of the University of Geneva with the same technique, except that one

---

*From McWilliam, J. A.: Fibrillar contraction of the heart, J. Physiol. 8:296-310, 1887. As cited by Willius, F. A., and Keys, T. E.: Cardiac classics, vol. 2, New York, 1961, Dover Publications, Inc., p. 677.

of the electrodes was placed directly upon the bared heart. This electrode consisted of one or several metallic discs covered with wet cloth which was applied to the anterior wall of the ventricles. These experiments were done with mammals (dogs, cats, rabbits) curarized or anesthetized with chloroform, chloral, morphine, or ether. In a previous note (March 13, 1899) we have shown that fibrillary tremulations produced in the dog, where they are definite, can be arrested under certain conditions, the heart beating normally again when the animal is subjected to the passage of an alternating current of high voltage.

By means of electrical discharges made directly on the heart, we have arrived at analogous results, which we review in the following conclusions:

1. Whatever the cause of fibrillary tremulations in the dog or adult cat, they can be abolished and replaced by true rhythmical cardiac contractions with restoration of arterial pressure when one applies to the heart an appropriate electrical discharge (neither too weak nor too strong); that is, if not more than fifteen seconds have elapsed.

2. When more than fifteen seconds have passed since the appearance of fibrillary tremulations, it is necessary to resort to a more or less prolonged massage of the heart, in order to apply the discharge in an effective manner and obtain the cessation of tremulations and the reestablishment of rhythmical beating of the heart. The discharge usually stops the heart momentarily in diastole, then the ventricles revert to effective contractions.

3. Induced currents applied to the region of the heart which has received a strong electrical discharge no longer produced fibrillary tremulations. These tremulations may, however, be produced if one electrifies a point other than the one which has received the discharge.

4. The inhibition of the area which has received the discharge can be more or less intense, according to the energy of the discharge; this area could be completely inhibited or its reactions might simply be weakened.

5. The inhibition of the area which has received the discharge does not proceed to a profound anatomical lesion.

6. With discharges of moderate energy, applied to the area of the discharge, acceleration of the heart is often produced.*

Thus Prevost and Battelli worked out what has proved to be a fundamental contribution, little of which has been improved upon during the ensuing 75 years.

As late as 1951, Johnson and Kirby reported that they could find only five cases of successful recovery from ventricular fibrillation in the literature. Today, with a proper understanding of the procedure of defibrillation of the ventricles of the heart, few instances will occur among surgical patients in which ventricular fibrillation need be regarded as irreversible. However, this discussion will not limit itself to those cases of ventricular fibrillation that occur under the controlled environment of the operating room, but will deal also with ventricular fibrillation as a sequel of cardiac conduction abnormalities that may be encountered under a variety of circumstances.

When we speak of ventricular fibrillation, we refer to an irregular, uncoordinated activity of the ventricles of the heart or to a quivering-like motion resulting in an almost complete absence of any cardiac output. Death will result from ventricular fibrillation (using the period necessary for irreversible brain damage to occur as a standard) in almost the same length of time as that resulting from cardiac asystole.

McWilliam emphasized that in ordinary circumstances sudden cardiac failure does not usually take the form of a simple ventricular standstill in diastole, but in many instances the terminal event is actually ventricular fibrillation. His description of ventricular fibrillation is worth repeating.

. . . A sudden, unexpected, and irretrievable cardiac failure may, even in the absense of any prominent, exciting cause, present itself in the form of an abrupt onset of fibrillar contractions (ventricular delirium). The cardiac pump is thrown out of gear, and the last of its vital energy is dissipated into a violent and prolonged turmoil of fruitless activity in the ventricular wall.*

*From Prevost, J. L., and Battelli, F.: Quelques effects des décharges électriques sur le coeur des mammiféres, J. Physiol. 2:40-52, 1900.

*From McWilliam, J. A.: On the effects of increased arterial pressure on the mammalian heart, Proc. Roy. Soc. 44:287-292, 1888.

Pathophysiology of ventricular fibrillation

Wegria defines ventricular fibrillation as follows:

Ventricular fibrillation is a cardiac mechanism in which, because of the lack of coordination in the activity of the ventricular fibers, no blood is expelled from the heart and this results in generalized anoxia and death.*

No detailed effort has been made in this book to review the evidence in support of the various theories and hypotheses regarding the mechanism of ventricular fibrillation, a number of which have been advanced. At present there is still some disagreement as to exactly what takes place. The ectopic focus theory of fibrillation envisages that a single ectopic focus discharges repeatedly and acts as a pacemaker. The circus movement theory explains fibrillation by reentry of an impulse into a portion of the heart that has just responded to the same stimulus or excitation wave. Holland and Cline are of the opinion that the mechanism of ventricular fibrillation may not be caused by a single agency and that two different forms may be present.

In support of the multiple reentry theory, it can be demonstrated that electrical stimulation to one portion of a ventricle does not always institute fibrillation, whereas if two points of the ventricle are stimulated, ventricular fibrillation more often results. Iwamoto and co-workers state:

With regard to the difference of each refractory period and excitability, it is clear that the refractory period caused by the stimulation in one point intercepts the excitation provoked in other points, and consequently the excitation is spread only over the receptive parts and soon resumes its original place which has recovered its excitability. The above complicated alterations of excitability and refractory period are named multiple reentry. This multiple reentry will easily explain the superiority of two-point stimulation. Now, if we attach the primary importance to multiple reentry, repeated stimulation by current having square waveform or the stimulation by more than two electrodes ought to provoke the fibrillation more easily.*

Few individuals have so thoroughly studied the problem of ventricular fibrillation as did Wiggers. Some of his understanding of the pathologic physiology occurring during ventricular fibrillation resulted from his study of the heart by means of a recording ECG and simultaneous moving pictures of the cardiac activity. Intraventricular pressure curves were optically recorded. His conclusions by such means were the following:

1. Fibrillation induced by faradic stimulation continues naturally for fifteen to fifty minutes and may be divided into four stages, on the basis of surface changes, electrocardiographic deflections and intraventricular pressure variations.
2. The initial stage of tachysystole lasts less than one second and is characterized by the spread of rapidly recurring but coordinated contraction waves, by large electrocardiographic deflections with steep gradients and by definite if small intraventricular pressure variations.
3. The second stage of convulsive incoordination ordinarily lasts fifteen to forty seconds and is characterized by rapid irregular localized contractions which spread short and variable distances over the heart. They are accompanied by large electrial deflections, 600 or more per minute, which vary considerably in size, amplitude, and contour.
4. Third stage of tremulous incoordination ordinarily continues two or three minutes and is characterized by multitudes of irregular yet forceful shivering or trembling motions, each spreading very short distances and with highly variable frequencies over different surface regions. They give rise to small irregular electrocardiographic oscillations having frequencies between 1100 and 1700 per minute, and are capable of increasing the intraventricular pressure level slightly.
5. The fourth stage of atonic incoordination is characterized by feeble wavelets of contrac-

*From Wegria, R.: Ventricular fibrillation, Bull. Am. Assoc. Nurse Anaesthetists 10:14, 1942.

*From Iwamoto, K., Matsubara, Y., Machiyama, S., and Iwabuchi, K.: Study on ventricular fibrillation, Bull. Heart Inst. Jap. 1:71-84, 1957.

tion spreading irregularly and at slow rates over small areas until more and more areas become quiescent, and finally the very slightest movements remain in a few areas only. The electrical deflections perhaps become slightly more regular in contour and spacing, but their amplitude becomes progressively smaller, and their frequency is gradually reduced to 400 per minute or less.

6. Potassium chloride injected into both ventricular cavities does not modify the stages through which fibrillation naturally passes; it merely hastens the process so that fibrillation stops within an average period of 2.4 minutes.

7. Intraventricular injections of CaCl₂ after potassium inhibition combined with massage, first inaugurate a coordinated idioventricular rhythm, characterized by slow waves of contraction sweeping over the two ventricles asynchronously but in coordinated fashion. After a short interval, a supraventricular rhythm is reestablished, the electrocardiogram regaining all its normal characteristics.*

It is significant that these stages of fibrillation described by Wiggers do not follow if myocardial anoxia is prevented by coronary perfusion of the fibrillating heart as seen during cardiopulmonary perfusions. The rate and strength of the uncoordinated contractions are related to the degree of myocardial anoxia.

In their excellent book, *Extrasystoles and Allied Arrhythmias†*, Scherf and Schott summarize some of their thoughts about ventricular fibrillation by saying: "Evidence is discussed in support of the views that, in ventricular fibrillation, the primary factor is the simultaneous activity at a high rate of several ectopic centers of impulse formation, resulting in local areas of depressed conductivity and local reentries, but is not a circus movement."

Omura has made a significant contribu-

tion in determining the minimum number of cardiac cells required for the induction of ventricular fibrillation. He studied fibrillation induced by local administration of toxic doses of digitalis to tissue-cultured, spontaneously beating, cardiac cell masses. He found that typical fibrillation can be induced in a minimum of four to ten cardiac cells forming a beating mass; these cells must be in mutual close contact and not lined up in a series in order to fibrillate. Omura also noted that a fibrillating cell group and a regularly contracting cell group can coexist within the same cell mass having a diameter of less than 200μ.

The rapid, nonsynchronized, and ineffective contraction resulting from many isolated groups of contracting muscle units presents a picture that we know as fibrillation. The induction of ventricular fibrillation is the result of many separate or combined factors such as the duration of the refractory period, the length of conduction pathways, conduction velocity, and the permeability of cell membranes. Oxygen levels, pH values, temperature, and concentration of ions such as potassium, sodium, calcium, and magnesium—all seem to play a part.

Surawicz believes that at least three conditions must be present in order for ventricular fibrillation to be initiated and maintained: (1) a certain critical mass of myocardium is needed to maintain the fractionated activity, (2) an excitable stimulus to initiate the disorder is needed, (3) the conduction velocity and duration of the refractory period in the entire myocardium must maintain a certain critical relationship in order to produce and maintain this disorganized activity.

Oxygen consumption of the fibrillating heart

Oxygen consumption in the fibrillating ventricle is less than that in the normally beating heart. As the fibrillating heart distends, a considerable increase in oxygen

*From Wiggers, C. J.: Monophasic and deformed ventricular complexes resulting from surface applications of potassium salts, Am. Heart J. **5:** 346-365, 1930.
†From Scherf, D., and Schott, A.: Extrasystoles and allied arrhythmias, New York, 1953, Grune & Stratton, Inc.

consumption occurs. The volume and pressure of the ventricular chamber can be increased during cardioplegia without any change in oxygen consumption. Beyond a certain point, pressure and volume increases in the fibrillating ventricle cease to be associated with an increase in oxygen consumption. At this critical point, coronary flow is decreased. Studies by Monroe and French indicate that injections of epinephrine increase both the intraventricular pressure and coronary flow during ventricular fibrillation.

The vulnerable phase of systole

Wiggers and Wegria demonstrated unequivocally that the local application of very short condenser shocks to a spot on the ventricle induce fibrillation when the shocks fall during late systole but never at any other phase of the heart cycle. Sixteen years earlier Garrey noted that a single electrical shock or mechanical stimulus would often produce fibrillation when timed to fall immediately after the refractive phase of a preceding contraction. De Boer called attention to this in 1920. Garrey believed that this condition was far from necessary since, given the physiologic conditions for fibrillation, any single stimulus to a resting muscle will cause fibrillation. Wiggers and Wegia believed that the danger of fibrillation induced from a needle puncture of the heart is a temporal, not a topographic, matter since late systole constitutes the period when the ventricle is especially vulnerable to stimuli.

Over 35 years later, Lown used the knowledge of the vulnerable phase of systole to avoid induced ventricular fibrillation during treatment of atrial fibrillation or ventricular tachycardia with direct current. He utilized an electronic synchronizer to trigger the discharge during the R wave of the ECG. Discharges outside the T wave avoided ventricular fibrillation in over 3,500 synchronized shocks. Of shocks delivered during the T wave, 35% produced ventricular fibrillation. It was the interval within the 30 msec. preceding the apex of the T wave that represented the precise point of susceptibility.

The R-on-T phenomenon has been a source of increasing interest to cardiologists for the last several years. Apparently it is by no means uncommon, and may be seen in association with a number of clinical situations such as myocardial infarction, ischemic heart disease, hypertensive heart disease, and several distinct myocardiopathies. Smirk and Palmer, Otago University Medical School, Dunedin, New Zealand, report eighty cases of a well-defined myocardial syndrome, an important feature of which is the interruption of T waves by premature QRS complexes. In addition, other features of the syndrome are multiform premature ventricular complexes, aberration in the form of ventricular complexes of supraventricular origin, variation in the interval between each successive ectopic complex and its preceding sinus complex, and ectopic complexes in runs of two or more.

Smirk and Palmer suggest that the phenomenon may be suspected clinically when premature beats are noted on auscultation and that it is frequently found in ECGs recording such arrhythmias as multiform ventricular systoles, ventricular tachycardia, flutter and fibrillation, auricular paroxysmal tachycardia, and auricular fibrillation. Because the syndrome is so often associated with sudden death, they recommend prophylactic administration of quinidine as a therapeutic measure in treatment of the underlying lesion.

Rabbino and associates report two instances of fatal ventricular fibrillation occurring 30 to 120 seconds after D.C. countershock for paroxysmal atrial tachycardia. The fact that a delay of $\frac{1}{2}$ to 2 minutes followed each shock before onset of ventricular fibrillation would indicate, perhaps, that factors were responsible other than the "vulnerable phase of systole."

Low-energy capacitor discharges are more likely to produce ventricular fibrillation than high-energy discharges. This fact is also true for A.C. shocks.

In Gutierrez and co-workers' study of 166 patients in a coronary care unit, twelve exhibited the R-on-T phenomenon on twenty-six separate occasions in thirty-two incidences of ventricular tachyarrhythmia. Two ventricular tachycardias and one ventricular fibrillation were present. There were six episodes of ventricular standstill, and in only one instance did it occur without an antecedent ventricular arrhythmia. The ECG of this patient revealed many multifocal, multiform premature beats showing isolated T wave introductions before death. Existence of the T wave was determined by interruption. At a point in which an intact T wave immediately preceded an interrupted T wave, the Q-T interval of the cardiac cycle was measured and then the Q-R interval from the the beginning of the cycle with the interrupted T wave to the beginning of QRS complex of a premature beat was measured. The R-on-T phenomenon is considered to be present when the Q-R:Q-T ratio is less than one, and when the Q-R is shorter than the Q-T. Again it is most important to realize that ischemic heart ectopic foci falling on the descending of the T wave may initiate ventricular fibrillation. The inherent danger of numerous premature systoles in acute myocardial infarction is well recognized as a forerunner of ventricular fibrillation. In a group of 851 patients with proved myocardial infarction, twenty developed primary ventricular fibrillation. In sixteen, ventricular ectopic beats falling in the vulnerable phase of systole constituted the mechanism of onset of the ventricular fibrillation. In the other four patients, ventricular tachycardia progressed to ventricular fibrillation (Dhurandhar and co-workers).

Patients who exhibit ventricular arrhythmias preceding ventricular fibrillation invariably show ventricular premature beats during the vulnerable period of systole. The appearance of ventricular premature beats interrupting T waves in the early hours after acute myocardial infarction should be regarded as a forewarning of possible impending ventricular fibrillation (Dhurandhar and co-workers).

Particular attention to the R-on-T phenomenon is, of course, given to patients in coronary care units where even a few premature beats falling on the T wave of the preceding complex suggest the need for vigorous treatment with antiarrhythmic drugs. Gutierrez and associates treat the R-on-T phenomenon with lidocaine 1 mg. per kilogram administered intravenously followed by continuous dose of 2 to 4 mg. per minute for the next several days. If this therapy does not control the extrasystoles, then quinidine is given, 200 to 400 mg. every 6 hours, or propranolol hydrochloride, 10 mg. four times a day orally or 1 to 5 mg. intravenously in 1 mg. increments each 5 minutes as necessary.

An impulse discharge during the vulnerable phase of systole must pursue a rather tortuous pathway, thereby predisposing to reentrant and self-sustained activity. It is the vulnerable period that exhibits the greatest disparity in the degree of recovery from the refractory period (Lown). If it is true that ventricular fibrillation is initiated by reentrant depolarization, then it is not surprising that it is much more frequent during pathophysiologic states increasing the myocardial excitability and refractoriness.

Ventricular fibrillation threshold

The fibrillation threshold has generally been determined by applying a single square-wave shock through the heart during the vulnerable phase of the cardiac cycle or by applying alternating current of 60 cycles per second. Sugimoto and associates studied factors determining vulnerability to ventricular fibrillation induced by 60 cycles per second alternating current. They confirm that the onset of fibrillation induced by a single shock of alternating current is preceded by ventricular tachysystole that lasts for sereval beats. The fall in fibrillation threshold during an accelerating tachysystole may help to explain the observation that a leak of very weak current from improperly grounded equipment may cause ventricular fibrillation. Similarly, with the pacemaker, if the pulse supplied by a pacemaker should fall during the vulnerable period after one or more spontaneous premature ventricular beats, the fibrillation threshold may be lower than the output of the generator and fibrillation may result.

Much attention has been directed toward a determination of the factors likely to influence the threshold of ventricular fibrillation. Obviously much of this work has been on an experimental basis in the animal laboratory, and perhaps not all of the data can be transferred to the human patient. Nevertheless, a multitude of factors is thought to be important. Certainly, high on the list would be the effects of acidosis and alkalosis on the ventricular fibrillation threshold. It is known that this threshold falls as the patient becomes more acidotic. A markedly alkalotic heart is more difficult to fibrillate and maintains a marked tendency to resume a synchronous beat (Dong and associates). With the maintenance of an alkalotic state, there is a greater tendency for ectopic rhythms to extinguish themselves.

One of the areas of the heart particularly vulnerable to fibrillation is that near the lower, apical end of the anterior coronary sulcus. Stimulation is prone to produce ventricular fibrillation.

The relatively long refractory period of cardiac muscle (150 to 300 msec.) has a tendency to protect the heart from ventricular fibrillation. (The refractory period of skeletal muscle is 2 to 3 msec.)

Fibrillation thresholds of the ventricle were studied by Sakakibara and associates on myocardial infarctions produced in dogs by coronary artery ligation. Although the fibrillatory threshold fell markedly with the production of the infarcted area, the threshold returned to an almost normal level after surgical resection of the infarcted myocardium. These physicians believe that these findings lend support to the ectopic focus theory of Prinzmetal regarding the mechanism of ventricular fibrillation. In addition, the findings would seem to support the work of Brofman, Leighninger, and Beck, who report that either ligation of a major coronary artery or multiple ligation of all smaller arteries to a given myocardial area produces a "trigger" area susceptible to ventricular fibrillation. They express the relationship of current of oxygen difference and the fibrillation threshold as the fibrillation index:

$$\text{Fibrillation index} = \frac{\text{Current of oxygen difference}}{\text{Fibrillation threshold}}$$

Pifarré, Wilson, and Hufnagel studied the effect of oxygen and helium upon ventricular fibrillation after acute myocardial infarction in thirty dogs. A significant reduction in the incidence of ventricular fibrillation was noted with a mixture of 75% air and 25% oxygen. On the other hand, when 20% helium was added along with a combination of 50% air and 30% oxygen, ventricular fibrillation was completely prevented in fifteen dogs in which the left circumflex coronary artery had been occluded. The mechanism of the elevation of ventricular fibrillatory threshold with the use of helium is still a matter of conjecture.

Pifarré and his associates have subsequently done additional studies on the effect of oxygen and helium mixtures on ventricular fibrillation and have concluded that there is a faster development of collateral circulation, which results in an increased blood flow throughout the ischemic area of the heart. A significant increase in the coronary sinus blood flow is noted and experimentally there is a reduction in the size of the infarcted area. The incidence of ventricular fibrillation is reduced from 54% in the control group to 11% in the helium group. A mixture containing 20% helium and 40% total oxygen appears to be ideal.

Many different experimental models have

been established to more nearly delineate ventricular fibrillation thresholds in experimental animals. By producing myocardial infarcts of a specific size, Myers and Cherry show that all infarcts that included over 15.6% of the epicardial ventricular surface lead to ventricular fibrillation. Ventricular fibrillation is a consistent finding if a certain amount of the myocardium is rendered totally avascular.

These studies show that the presence of a junctional zone in dogs is not enough to produce ventricular fibrillation; a definite size factor exists. The critical mass in pigs is shown to be different than in dogs.

Experimentally, cesium chloride will prevent the fibrillation produced by coronary ligation in 63% of cases (Prasad and co-workers). This effect of cesium in raising the fibrillatory threshold may be related to its effect on the rate of rise of action potential and the action potential duration in the cardiac muscle (it lengthens the action potential duration and decreases the rate of rise of action potential). Cesium chloride, which is known to stimulate the membrane adenosinetriphosphatase in cardiac muscles, has an effect on the transmembrane potential similar to potassium and other antiarrhythmic drugs. Unlike many antiarrhythmic agents, it does not greatly depress the myocardium and may actually increase the force of contraction after a brief initial decrease.

In the work of Han, ventricular vulnerability to fibrillation is estimated by measuring the fibrillation threshold, that is, the least intensity of an electrical stimulus applied to the ventricle to initiate fibrillation. The vulnerability is inversely related to the fibrillation threshold. Han delivered gated pulses to the ventricle during the vulnerable period. He found the fibrillation thresholds, as determined by applying test stimuli at an identical site unaffected by coronary occlusion, to be consistently lower after creation of an ischemic area. These observations could not be explained on the basis of any electrophysiologic changes at the site of application of test stimuli since no such changes

are expected at the site. The ventricle with an ischemic area responds differently to premature impulses initiated at the stimulated site. Changes in the behavior of the conduction of these premature impulses through the ischemic area account for the increased vulnerability. A strong pulse delivered during the vulnerable period may induce fibrillation by its ability to set up a focus that will fire repetitive impulses at an accelerating rate. Excitability and conduction velocity are irregularly depressed. The repetitive impulses that are initiated during the relative refractory period may travel rapidly through areas in a more excitable state, propagate slowly through less excitable segments, and fail to excite some refractory areas. Han concludes that irregular excitability and conduction are the conditions that favor development of reentrant activity, fractionation of wave fronts of excitation, and total disorganization of impulse propagation; this is, of course, fibrillation. The increased incidence of premature ventricular beats in patients with myocardial infarction may be a result of enhanced automaticity of Purkinje fibers or development of reentrant activity at the boundary between intact and ischemic areas (Harris and Matlock). Because of this, a premature beat with its relatively long coupling interval is more likely to induce ventricular fibrillation in patients with myocardial infarction.

At the Heart Institute of the Tokyo Women's Medical College, Sakakibara and co-workers performed infarctectomies on dogs after regional myocardial infarctions were induced on the left ventricular wall by the coronary artery ligations. They were impressed with the elevation of the ventricular fibrillatory threshold after resection of the infarcted myocardium. The ventricular fibrillatory threshold decreased markedly after the ligation of the coronary artery but returned to an almost normal level after surgical resection.

Because of the increased incidence of sudden death observed in coronary subjects who are heavy cigaret smokers, Bellet and co-workers studied the effect of cigaret smoke inhalation on the ventricular fibrillation threshold in dogs. Their results showed rather significant decreases in the ventricular fibrillation threshold in dogs from a controlled value of 1.02 watt-seconds to as low as 0.67 watt-second in the dogs inhaling cigaret smoke.

STEROIDS AND VENTRICULAR FIBRILLATION THRESHOLD

In commenting on asthmatic deaths in England that might be considered related to the use of a pressurized aerosol nebulizer containing highly concentrated isoproterenol, Lehr believes that there is circumstantial evidence that drug-drug interaction may be involved in the isoproterenol-induced cardiac death, related to the interaction of corticosteroids and pressurized isoproterenol inhalers. In rats treated with desoxycorticosterone acetate–saline, ventricular fibrillation occurred within 20 minutes after injection of an otherwise almost innocuous dosage of isoproterenol, an extraordinary potential of toxicity.

Transient ventricular fibrillation (spontaneous defibrillation)

It is now apparent that spontaneous defibrillation occurs clinically more often than was suspected. For example, Miller and associates report an incidence of ventricular fibrillation following a myocardial infarction in which the fibrillation was converted by external cardiac massage without countershock. With coronary care units now a recognized necessity for any modern hospital, monitoring of the patient with the acute coronary occlusion will aid in rapidly diagnosing the arrhythmia. It seems likely that spontaneous defibrillation may be expected with a much higher frequency when effective cardiac massage is started early.

Fleming reports that a heart was found in ventricular fibrillation twice in 1 week during two episodes of cardiac arrest in a 6-year-old girl being anesthetized for skin grafting following burns. In each instance, the heart reverted to a normal sinus rhythm following a period of massage, and subsequent recovery was uneventful.

Ventricular fibrillation spontaneously reverted to ventricular tachycardia as the pericardium was being incised to allow direct manual massage in a case reported by Gurewich and his colleagues. The patient had previously experienced a 30-minute period of closed-chest compression.

The first case of spontaneous reversion of ventricular fibrillation to normal cardiac rhythm occurring under closed-chest cardiac massage was reported by Wetherill and Nixon. The patient was a 12-year-old girl being treated for chronic renal insufficiency. Following hemodialysis, the serum potassium level fell to 2.4 mEq. per liter. She was started on potassium citrate, and 4 hours after the third dose, the cardiac arrest occurred. During the cardiac arrest, a blood sample revealed the serum potassium to be 8.6 mEq. per liter. Peaston observed another such case of spontaneous reversion in a woman with a myocardial infarction.

Wiggers was unable to note a single case of spontaneous defibrillation in dogs. As one goes down the scale phylogenetically, one observes an increasing tendency toward spontaneous defibrillation. Spontaneous recovery after induced ventricular fibrillation is said to be frequent in the rat, cat, mouse, hedgehog, rabbit, monkey, guinea pig, hen, pigeon, and blackbird. In the dog, however, once fibrillation has begun, it responds much as does the human heart. Sheep and goats are also difficult to defibrillate. On the other hand, ventricular fibrillation is difficult to induce in the frog and turtle and probably does not occur spontaneously in these species (Gregg). In the several-weeks-old puppy, spontaneous defibrillation is the rule rather than the exception. I have worked with the hedgehog. Spontaneous defibrillation did occur but was the exception rather than the rule.

Swan described a case of spontaneous defibrillation before the American Surgical Association in 1951. While arteriography was being performed in the x-ray room, cardiac arrest occurred at the moment the needle was placed in the aorta. The chest was opened quickly and ventricular fibrillation was noted. Massage was begun. Unfortunately, no defibrillation instrument was available. In spite of a probable failure, therapy was continued for 65 minutes. At this point, spontaneous respirations appeared, and after 82 minutes the heart suddenly began beating under its own power. The only medication was procainamide given intravenously. One month later the patient appeared "quite well."

It is well known that ventricular fibrillation may occur with episodes of Adams-Stokes attack. In one well-documented case of Adams-Stokes seizures (Sacolick and others), a total of ninety-three attacks was recorded—all associated with ventricular fibrillation. Seventy-two of the paroxysms terminated spontaneously. Twenty-one of the attacks required electrical defibrillation (applied externally) because the duration of the fibrillation seemed excessively long.

Transient attacks of ventricular fibrillation simulating those of Adams-Stokes syndrome have been recorded (Robinson and Bredeck). Others have made ECG recordings of hearts that spontaneously reverted from ventricular fibrillation to normal contractions (Smith and Hoffman). Schwartz reported ECGs obtained from a patient showing transient ventricular fibrillation with auriculoventricular disassociation and recurrent syncopal attacks.

Transient fibrillation has been observed after carotid sinus massage for diagnostic purposes. Frequently, digitalis intoxication is an associated feature.

Dock (1929) recorded his view as follows: The most rapid ventricular fibrillation ever recorded in man terminated abruptly and the patient recovered (Kerr), while in 37 moribund patients studied by various groups, only 5 showed transient fibrillation

and 2 terminal fibrillation. I think that we must conclude from this that ventricular fibrillation is not easily established or maintained in man.*

In the case of ventricular fibrillation in a 58-year-old infarction patient, all efforts with electrical countershock were unsuccessful (Harden and others). When, however, 20 ml. of an 8.4% solution of sodium bicarbonate (1 mEq. per milliliter) was administered into the external jugular vein, spontaneous reversion to sinus rhythm was noted on the ECG within 2 minutes. It is for this reason that Harden and co-workers recommend that 200 mEq. of sodium bicarbonate be administered empirically as soon as possible after cardiac arrest. If ventricular fibrillation is present, it will be more easily corrected with electrical countershock, and left ventricular function will improve.

In an excellent experimental study on ventricular fibrillation thresholds in respiratory acidosis and alkalosis, Dong, Stinson, and Shumway not only note a marked elevation of the ventricular fibrillation threshold in alkalosis but also note a marked tendency for the alkalotic heart to resume a synchronous beat. In fact, spontaneous defibrillation is frequently seen in alkalotic hearts. In contrast, the acidotic heart seldom participates in spontaneous defibrillation.

Repeated episodes of external defibrillation were attempted in a 58-year-old engineer shortly after admission for an acute myocardial infarction. Within 2 minutes after the administration of 20 mEq. of an 8.4% solution of sodium bicarbonate into the left external jugular vein, spontaneous defibrillation occurred and there was a reversion to sinus rhythm. The radial pulse immediately became palpable, and the blood pressure rose to 100/60 mm. Hg.

Spontaneous defibrillation, even after 10

---

*From Dock, W.: Transitory ventricular fibrillation as a cause of syncope and its prevention by quinidine sulphate, with case report and discussion of diagnostic criteria for ventricular fibrillation, Am. Heart J. 4:709-714, 1929.

to 20 seconds of fibrillation, is frequently seen after bretylium tosylate administration in the dog. In fact, the heart protected by bretylium tosylate may have fibrillation induced, but the heart spontaneously reverts to a sinus rhythm within a fraction of a second—or even as long as 20 seconds—after the electrodes are removed. In the search for an agent that will suppress the vulnerability of the heart to ventricular fibrillation, Bacaner suggests bretylium tosylate. A remarkable influence on the myocardium is apparent in dogs. The vulnerability of the normal dog heart to ventricular fibrillation is drastically reduced with the use of bretylium tosylate. Even after coronary ligation, bretylium tosylate protects the heart against fibrillatory stimuli. It was found that the period during which the fibrillatory stimulus can be tolerated without inducing fibrillation is prolonged three to several hundred times. Spontaneous defibrillation is the rule rather than the exception after induced fibrillation. The action of bretylium tosylate, according to Bacaner, may be considered to be roughly that of a chemical sympathectomy. The drug is thought to depress adrenergic transmitter release, probably by lowering the excitability of the adrenergic nerve endings.

Semple witnessed spontaneous reversion of ventricular defibrillation in five patients during external cardiac compression. Hebert and co-workers record the case of a 25-year-old patient being operated upon for removal of the left lung. The patient had pulmonary tuberculosis. Cardiac arrest occurred during ligation of the pulmonary artery and, following a period of cardiac massage, it was decided to inject epinephrine into the left ventricle. Within 2 minutes after the injection of epinephrine, ventricular fibrillation occurred and, following continued cardiac massage, spontaneously reverted to a normal rhythm in about 10 minutes.

Lampson and associates report ECG evidence of spontaneous defibrillation by the use of procaine hydrochloride. The patient was a 7-year-old boy in whom cardiac arrest occurred in the operating room during suture of lacerations of the foot. Anesthesia had been maintained by open-drop ether induced with cyclopropane. The arrest occurred at the close of the operation after anesthesia had been discontinued and while preparations were made to apply a plaster boot. Within a period of 3 minutes a thoracotomy was performed and visual examination of the heart revealed "fine ripples of ventricular fibrillation passing aimlessly across the left ventricle beneath the pericardium." Cardiac massage was started and continued for a period of 15 minutes, after which an intravenous injection of 3 ml. of a solution of 1% procaine hydrochloride was given. Approximately 6 minutes later a second dose of procaine hydrochloride was given, and 30 seconds following this, the tone of the heart changed to the extent that it was felt to stiffen beneath the massaging fingers and to assume, 27 minutes following the initial arrest, spontaneous contractions.

Although the patient had evidence of severe cerebral anoxia following the arrest, including periods of unconsciousness, impaired vision, and confusion, he improved to the extent that on the fourth day he was alert, calm, oriented, and in good rapport. He was discharged on the twenty-sixth postoperative day. Five months after the operation his visual acuity was normal. He obtained a score of 108 in the Form A, Otis Quick Scoring Mental Ability Test.

Fell had a patient with a severe tear of the left atrial wall during a commissurotomy procedure. Hemorrhage was controlled by occlusion of the tear with the fingers. Cardiac arrest occurred abruptly and then the large tear was closed in approximately 3 minutes. The heart was manually compressed at once, and shortly afterward ventricular fibrillation was noted. This continued for about 5 minutes, but the heart spontaneously reverted to normal sinus rhythm as attempts at electrical defibrillation were begun.

In 1965 Marcuson was able to find only twelve reported cases of spontaneous defibrillation in patients without a previous heart block. In adding a twelfth case, Marcuson documents (see Fig. 18-1) ventricular fibrillation occurring in a 72-year-old woman admitted to the Central Middlesex Hospital of London following an acute myocardial infarction. Neither external cardiac massage nor mouth-to-mouth breathing was employed during a period of ventricular fibrillation which was known to have lasted 3 minutes. Marcuson speculates that the heart and brain in this patient were better able to stand the period of anoxia because of the reduced demands for oxygen by the tissues since the patient was suffering from myxedema.

Under cardiopulmonary bypass, twelve instances of spontaneous reversion of ventricular fibrillation to a normal rhythm were observed among fifty-two cases by Marchanz in Johannesburg, South Africa. Four cases of spontaneous defibrillation occurred during cases of ventricular fibrillation that complicated mitral valvulotomies.

SPONTANEOUS DEFIBRILLATION AFTER ELECTIVE VENTRICULAR FIBRILLATION

Elective ventricular fibrillation has been employed with increasing frequency as a means of elective cardioplegia (see Wada's discussion of elective arrest). Levy reports approximately 70% spontaneous defibrillation of the hearts on which this technique has been employed during correction of congenital heart defects with the cardiopulmonary bypass. Apparently it is not common to note spontaneous defibrillation in cardiopulmonary bypass procedures employed on the quiet heart.

Glenn, Yale University School of Medicine, has had extensive experience with induced fibrillary arrest in open-heart surgery and in one discussion notes a 40% incidence of spontaneous defibrillation. Interestingly

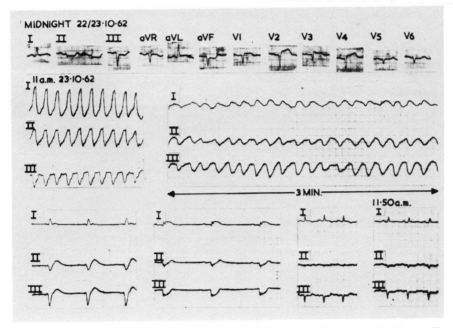

Fig. 18-1. ECG tracings showing spontaneous defibrillation. (From Marcuson, R. W.: Br. Heart J. 27:456, 1965.)

enough, all of his cases of spontaneous defibrillation were associated with congenital heart defects.

Although procainamide has been found useful in the abolition of various forms of premature beats of the ventricles and in the control of ventricular tachycardia, its beneficial effect on various forms of ventricular acceleration and ventricular fibrillation, such as those that may form the basis of Adams-Stokes seizures during heart block, has not been well known. It has been understood (Mautz) that procaine applied to the heart locally may make it somewhat more difficult to induce ventricular fibrillation. Schwartz and others studied the effect of procainamide on three patients with transient ventricular fibrillation during established A-V disassociation. A variable action was noted from patient to patient and in the same patient from day to day. Its early effect seemed to be that of a transitory depressant of the sinoauricular node, since it slowed the atrial rate even in the well-atropinized patient. They concluded that procainamide is contraindicated in patients with the various forms of ventricular acceleration leading to ventricular fibrillation during established A-V disassociation. The drug favors the development of ectopic beats of the ventricles resulting in various forms of ventricular acceleration and ending in a series of ventricular fibrillations, all of which appear earlier and last longer when the drug is given in the presence of interventricular conduction disturbance, premature beats of the ventricles, or when recurring seizures of ventricular fibrillation are present. Procainamide is also contraindicated when quinidine sulfate has been administered.

EFFECT OF AGE

Experiments by Wiggers over a 10-year period, during which time observations were made on ventricular fibrillation in 208 dogs, failed to reveal a single instance of spontaneous recovery. It was therefore his assumption, based on this statistical evidence, that spontaneous recovery does not occur in the normal adult dog's heart. Hooker recalls, however, that he was able to repeatedly induce ventricular fibrillation in a young female puppy for short periods of time, but each time the ventricles were converted spontaneously to a normal rhythm after remaining in fibrillation for about 1 minute. I have also noted repeatedly that the heart of the puppy is more likely to revert spontaneously than the heart of the adult dog.

PART FOUR

TECHNIQUES OF CARDIOPULMONARY RESUSCITATION

Chapter 19

THE TECHNIQUE OF RESUSCITATION: GENERAL CONSIDERATIONS

The immediate goal in cardiac resuscitation is to reverse the sudden deprivation of essential oxygen necessary for survival and continued function of vital organs.

The successful management of any case of cardiac arrest revolves first and foremost around a proper realization of the importance of the *time factor* (see Fig. 66-1). Efforts are doomed to failure in all but a negligible percentage of cases unless the proper treatment is instituted 3 to 4 minutes after cessation of circulatory activity. Few unexpected emergencies in medicine will so tax the speed and efficiency of the physician as will that of cardiac arrest. The very nature of its unexpectedness may so disrupt the inexperienced that efficient management of the case will be delayed.

The term cardiac resuscitation applies to that action taken to save the life of a patient whose heart has suddenly ceased to beat, when there is reasonable expectation that with prompt treatment his normal cardiac and cerebral function can be restored for an indefinite period.*

This definition offered by Turk and Glenn expresses my sentiment.

The management of the usual case of cardiac arrest is essentially a simple procedure. Often, however, unless the pathophysiology of the heart is understood, attempts at resuscitation may fail. Various adjuncts in therapy now available may be neglected.

Once cardiac arrest occurs, therapy should be instituted with the efficiency that characterizes other procedures in medicine. Unless the individual physician has his own plan of action worked out, this necessary speed and efficiency will be lacking once a case of cardiac arrest is encountered. Likewise, it is absolutely essential that a hospital should have its own general plan of action for handling cases of cardiac arrest.

Finally, all steps in the resuscitative procedure must be kept in the proper perspective. First things must come first. Swann, from Galveston, Texas, believes that the desired reversal of the process of death is accomplished solely by reoxygenation, and therefore measures of resuscitation should be directed at the first function to fail. In other words, oxygenated blood must be artificially propelled to the central nervous system. This is the first order of business.

Once cardiac arrest has been diagnosed, the competent physician will immediately have his own plan of action to put into use. He will be careful to place each aspect of the resuscitative procedure in its proper perspective and will employ each adjunct at the proper time. Even during the period when cardiac arrest is suspected, efforts should be initiated to facilitate cardiac resuscitation. The following discussions describe steps in the resuscitation procedure as well as the rationale for their use. These procedures, as described, are those I have found most valuable in my own efforts.

Tenaciousness of the myocardium

The amazing resistance revealed by the human heart, or the heart of animals, is

*From Turk, L. H., III, and Glenn, W. W. L.: Cardiac arrest: results of attempted cardiac resuscitation in forty-two cases, N. Engl. J. Med. **251:** 795-803, 1954.

sometimes surprising to those unfamiliar with cardiac physiology. Lee and Downs summarize this well by stating:

The functions of irritability and contractility are intimately characteristic of the myocardium. They begin to be manifested in earliest embryonic life, when the heart of the chicken, and doubtless of other embryos, begins rhythmic contractions almost before the mesenchyme has become differentiated to muscular tissue about the primitive heart tube, and they continue without interruption for many years in man and other long-lived animals. The greatest mechanical imperfections of the heart, the greatest changes in its histology, in its nutrition, or in its innervation are not sufficient to destroy its irritability or its contractility until the myocardium is too exhausted to respond or until it has used up all of its stored nutrients.*

Kountz's work on the revival of human hearts after death emphasizes the fundamental ability of the heart to contract rhythmically and effectively under most adverse conditions. His classic work (1936)

_____
*From Lee, W. E., and Downs, T. M.: Resuscitation by direct massage of the heart in cardiac arrest, Ann. Surg. 80:555-561, 1924.

laid much of the groundwork for our present-day optimism about the practicability of cardiac resuscitation and, indeed, many aspects of cardiac surgery. Kountz developed a method of perfusion of the heart that would permit the development of different pressures in the ventricle and in the coronary arteries. Cannulae were inserted into the coronary arteries through the aorta. A large cannula was then introduced over the coronary ones through the aorta and past the aortic valves. He was able to revive sixty-five of 127 hearts to the point of ventricular contraction. Of the sixty-five hearts, forty-eight developed regular cardiac mechanisms and beat for a period of at least 2 hours. He observed that the time after death and the nature of the disease causing the death had definite influence upon the viability of the heart. The sooner the heart was obtained after death, the more readily it could be revived. Particularly was this true of patients who were in good health when they died of acute heart disease but not so true of persons with chronic disease.

Chapter 20

ARTIFICIAL RESPIRATION AND RESUSCITATION

In my experience, one of the most difficult aspects of training personnel for cardiopulmonary resuscitation has revolved around the establishment of a patent airway and adequate ventilation. I have, for example, been impressed with the difficulty experienced by many physicians in establishing "ventilation" even on the Resusci-Anne manikin!

The fundamental objectives of artificial respiration must always be kept in mind. The words of Coryllos are appropriate. He states:

> Life is continued as long as exchanges of oxygen and carbon dioxide in the tissues are carried on in a normal way. Gas exchanges depend upon and are regulated by their respective positive pressures.*

It is the aim of pulmonary ventilation to maintain these pressures precisely at constant levels, whatever may be the metabolic needs of the different tissues. Since the supply of oxygen and the removal of carbon dioxide are accomplished by the circulating blood, circulation is but a part of respiration.

The whole problem of artificial respiration and cardiopulmonary resuscitation has been generally neglected in medical school education. Little training is given in the practical demonstration of pulmonary resuscitation and, subsequently, it is of little surprise to see grossly ineffective maneuvers

---

*From Coryllos, P. N.: Mechanical resuscitation in advanced forms of asphyxia: a clinical and experimental study in different methods of resuscitation, Surg. Gynecol. Obstet. **66:**698-722, 1938.

being carried on in the anoxic patient. In several cases of cardiac arrest where resuscitation of the heart could not be achieved, it was noted that an adequate exchange of air in the lungs was not occurring. *One of the most common errors rests with a failure to maintain an open airway.* The base of the tongue may have shifted posteriorly to occlude the airway by pressure against the posterior pharyngeal wall. The neck may be markedly flexed on the anterior chest wall.

Mouth-to-mouth artificial respiration ("expired air" resuscitation)

Karpius calls attention to the widespread interest in and employment of mouth-to-mouth respiration between 1740 and 1800. In 1767 a Society for the Revival of Persons Apparently Dead by Drowning was formed in Amsterdam. Among the methods recommended was mouth-to-mouth respiration. It is interesting to note that, in order to avoid the entry of air into the stomach, one was advised to press the larynx against the spine. Expired air was not considered to be of great value and was even thought to be of possible harm. Bellows were constructed for the use of fresh air, and sometimes even oxygen was used for artificial respiration.

Mouth-to-mouth respiration as a satisfactory method of artificial respiration is well documented and is to be strongly encouraged. Some have questioned whether the exhaled air of an individual contains a sufficient amount of oxygen to maintain another's life. Exhaled air contains 15.5% oxygen and is therefore more than adequate to maintain life. (The normal inspired air is 20.94 vol.%.) The expired air of the rescuer also contains 4 vol.% of carbon dioxide, as compared with the normal inspired air of .04%, which is less than 7% to 10% carbogen used for resuscitation by some. (The use of carbogen for artificial respiration is not advised.) In addition, the mouth-to-mouth procedure gives an adequate amount of tidal air, which is more than many manual methods of artificial respiration can claim. The advantages of mouth-to-mouth respiration, if physiologically sound, are great. In desperate situations in which a respirator is not at hand or when an anesthesiologist is not present to insert an endotracheal tube, mouth-to-mouth respiration can be readily employed.

Although the most effective methods of artificial respiration are provided by the various mechanical breathing machines, the physician should not forget that he is personally equipped with an efficient "breathing machine."

The average normal adult in the resting stage inhales about 500 ml. of fresh air with each breath. When applying mouth-to-mouth respiration, the rescuer almost always breathes more deeply than usual and converts his expired air to gas containing as much as 18% oxygen and only about 2% carbon dioxide. The rescuer can provide the patient with as much as 1,000 to 1,250 ml. of expired air with each inflation. Pulmonary oxygen concentration may be restored to almost normal within 20 seconds by performing mouth-to-mouth resuscitation consisting of only four to five inflations. The previously popular Schafer and Holder-Neilsen manual methods of artificial respiration are unable to adequately supply an asphyxiated victim's oxygen need. In addition, these techniques have the disadvantage of requiring a position of the victim's body that precludes cardiac resuscitation.

The work of Lee and associates at the University of Manchester in England supports the use of expired air ventilation along with external cardiac massage, particularly when 100% oxygen is not available. Their results indicate satisfactory oxygenation during expired air resuscitation in dogs and lead them to conclude that in previously healthy individuals expired air resuscitation in conjunction with external cardiac massage is as likely to provide satisfactory oxygenation as is ventilation with oxygen. Prolonged resuscitation by expired air ventilation should not be abandoned because oxygen is not available.

Whittenberger's excellent monograph on artificial respiration is suggested for a detailed summary on respiratory resuscitation.

PROCEDURE

During mouth-to-mouth respiration, the nose should be compressed with one hand; the other hand should be used to make pressure over the patient's upper abdomen and epigastrium to prevent distension of the stomach by air. The mouth of the patient may be covered by several thin layers of gauze, a handkerchief, or even a thin towel. Prior to expiration, the operator should take a deep inspiration and then immediately apply his widely opened mouth over the mouth of the patient and make a forcible exhalation. The uninitiated will be surprised at the degree of inflation produced by this method. The patient's chest will be observed to expand as the air is blown into his mouth, and when the operator raises his mouth from that of the patient, a rush of air will be heard coming from the patient's lungs. This latter aspect can be improved by forcible pressure on the patient's chest. As in all other methods of artificial respiration, the tongue must be brought forward, since it may occlude the oral pharynx. Again it should be pointed out that one may have confidence in his ability to perform mouth-to-mouth respiration when it is recalled that 16 mm. Hg pressure is the level of oxygen pressure developed by most of the positive-negative pulmonary resuscitators. Men, according to Swann, can exhale with a force of 50 mm.

Hg and this figure may even reach 100 mm. Hg. A rate of at least twelve times a minute is suggested. One should exhale twice his normal resting tidal volume (about 1,000 ml.). Inadequate oxygenation is often the result of exhalations that are too slow.

Elam, Brown, and Elder concluded that mouth-to-mouth insufflation is the ideal method for artificial ventilation for the following reasons:

1. The patient's alveolar oxygen pressure can be elevated more quickly than by any other known method.
2. No equipment is necessary.
3. The operator knows immediately whether or not the patient is being ventilated.
4. Sufficient inflating pressure is exerted to deliver an adequate volume, as the operator continuously compensates for changes in airway resistance and in lung compliance.*

Attention should be called to several precautions and pitfalls in this procedure. Because of the limited endurance of the individual performing mouth-to-mouth respiration, the question of physical fatigue for the operator has been considered. I doubt that this should be much of a limiting factor. It is true that the operator may experience a degree of hypocapnia from his prolonged efforts and may therefore experience some vertigo. If additional personnel are available to take over the procedure, the decrease in the carbon dioxide concentration of the blood will not be sufficient to cause the operator any discomfort. Brown and Elam, in their special report to the Chemical Corps Medical Laboratories, describe a method that would eliminate this objection. They added a 300 ml. tube to be connected to the mask in which mouth-to-mouth respiration is being carried out. The mouth-to-tube device ensures that adequate volume of sufficient gas composition is delivered to the patient. Brown and Elam

---

*From Elam, J. O., Brown, E. S., and Elder, J. D., Jr.: Artificial respiration by mouth-to-mask method, N. Engl. J. Med. **250**:749-754, 1954.

point out that, unlike other forms of artificial respiration, the mouth-to-tube method does not depend upon the operator's observation and judgement to determine whether ventilation of the patient is adequate. The mouth-to-mask or mouth-to-tube methods have advantages over the simple mouth-to-mouth procedure in that both hands of the operator are available to maintain patency of the upper airway. The operator is able to sense any increase in pulmonary resistance by the amount of exertion it takes for the deflation of his own lungs. From a study of nine patients temporarily paralyzed by succinylcholine, Brown and Elam find that normal respiratory gas exchange can be consistently achieved by intermittent inflation of the patient's lungs with the expired air of the operator. Oxygen saturation studies all gave results above 90%. In addition, the mouth-to-tube method of respiration has several points in its favor besides that of prevention of hypocapnia in the operator. These include the prevention of cross-contamination between the operator and the patient if a disposable filter is placed in the breathing tube. The method can be continued for long periods of time, and no special position of the patient is required by the operator. The equipment is of minimal expense and adequate ventilation is ensured in spite of abnormalities in airway resistance and in lung compliance.

Another drawback to the mouth-to-mouth procedure is that in some instances, particularly in large city hospitals, the operator may be in danger of exposure to patients with pulmonary tuberculosis or other infectious diseases. Patients with anaerobic suppuration of the lungs and with an associated foul odor make the problem increasingly difficult. In addition, the rescuer may be reluctant to contact the lips of a dying patient. Prevention of cross-contamination can be implemented by the use of a handkerchief. The mouth-to-tube method will also obviate this objection. The danger of gastric dilatation can be mitigated to some degree if the operator places his hand upon the epigastrium of the subject to prevent the gastric dilatation from occurring. The possibility of lung rupture is present, particularly if the operator applies too much effort, as in the case of infants. Elam suggests that the operator will be more efficient in his efforts if he hyperventilates while executing mouth-to-mouth insufflation. In order to ensure an adequate airway, a backward tilt of the head and overextension of the neck are required (Fig. 20-1). Pillows may be placed beneath the shoulders. The mandible may be brought forward and an endotracheal tube can be passed through the mouth. We have seldom found it necessary to do a cricothyroid membrane puncture or a tracheotomy as an emergency procedure associated with cardiac resuscitation.

Mouth-to-mouth breathing can be quite effective in infants and should not be delayed until a breathing machine is available. Caution should be exerted lest the pressure of the exhaled air be such that it will rupture the alveoli of the infant.

An unusual case of artificial respiration concerned a 19-year-old lifeguard who was trapped under 9 feet of water in a municipal swimming pool. For 8 minutes, other lifeguards took turns surfacing, inhaling large breaths of air, diving down again, and forcing the air into the victim's mouth. After the victim was finally freed from the underwater entrapment, mouth-to-mouth respiration was continued for a short while and the patient regained consciousness. Certainly, this instance of mouth-to-mouth respiration with the victim underwater is an unusual example of successful artificial respiration.

PREVENTION OF AIR ENTERING ESOPHAGUS

If one uses excessively high inflation pressures during artificial ventilation, some of the

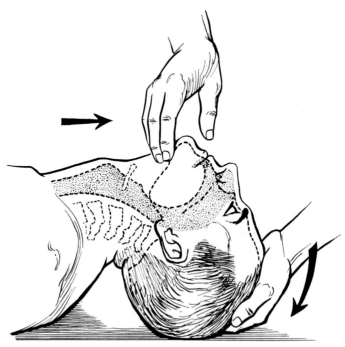

Fig. 20-1. Overflexion of head on the neck is usually necessary to maintain an open airway. Note elevation of chin. In addition, support beneath the back and shoulders may be helpful.

air will be forced into the stomach by means of an open esophagus. Don Michael, concerned about the inflation of the stomach that occurs in the course of routine mouth-to-mouth respiration, has developed an airway that can be easily introduced into the esophagus and can be manipulated so that the balloon obliterates this orifice.

During mouth-to-mouth respiration, especially in infants, one may readily force air into the esophagus and stomach. In addition, pressure on the sternum may provoke regurgitation of stomach contents into the upper airway. Both active and passive regurgitation in air-venting into the esophagus can be prevented by esophageal compression from the cricoid cartilage displaced posteriorly, as illustrated in Fig. 20-2. Brown suggests that this be done by applying posterior pressure to the skin over the anterior surface of the cricoid and by compressing the esophagus between it and the anterior surface of the cervical vertebrae. With moderate pressure, air can be prevented from entering the esophagus, and gastric contents can be kept from regurgitating through it. As shown in Fig. 20-2, the

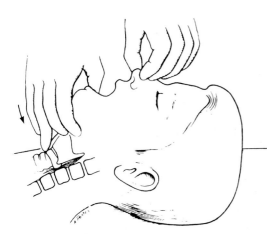

Fig. 20-2. Prevention of air-venting into the stomach or regurgitation into the upper airway by compression of the esophagus by posterior displacement of cricoid cartilage with ring finger. (From Brown, B. R., Jr.: J.A.M.A. **203:**156, 1968.)

ring finger and little finger of the hand supporting the chin and tongue are free to displace the cricoid backward with sufficient strength to occlude the esophagus. One must be sure to place pressure on the cricoid cartilage and not on the thyroid cartilage.

Mouth-to-nose respiration

Artificial respiration may be best applied by the mouth-to-nose technique in several instances. For example, the individual applying artificial respiration may be unable to completely seal his mouth around the patient's mouth. If transient rigidity, trismus, or convulsions are present, mouth-to-nose respiration should be used. A patient with a broken jaw may have his teeth wired. Even so, blowing between the teeth has been successful.

Airways

Although mouth-to-mouth resuscitation will usually be instituted without the advantage of an airway, at least three types of airways are available (Fig. 20-3).

LABIODENTAL AIRWAYS

These airways simply provide a channel through the victim's lips and teeth. They usually incorporate a mouth guard to provide a seal and a short blow tube for the rescuer. Unfortunately, they do not overcome any obstruction in the front of the mouth due to opposition of the tongue against the palate.

ORAL AIRWAYS

Oral airways are of a medium length, long enough to ensure the passage of air through the victim's lips, teeth, and front of the mouth. Obstruction by the tongue in the throat is prevented by correct hyperextension of the victim's head and, in the case of the Brook airway (Fig. 20-4), a nylon bite-block maintains a channel between the teeth. A mouth guard provides the seal. A flexible extension is available.

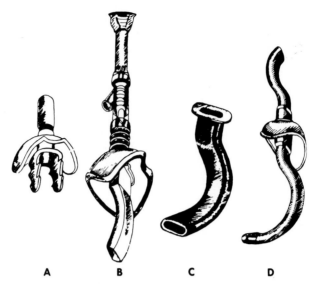

Fig. 20-3. Examples of airways used for emergency resuscitation: **A**, Rescue breather; **B**, Brook airway; **C**, Guedel airway; and **D**, Safar airway.

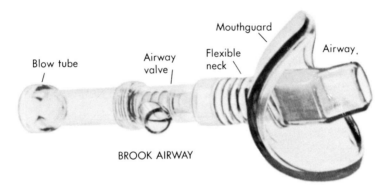

Fig. 20-4. Brook airway, a simple oral airway with a nonbreathing blow tube. (Courtesy Dr. Joseph Brook.)

It facilitates resuscitation when the victim cannot be ideally positioned. The extension is connected to a nonreturn valve that diverts the victim's expired air from the rescuer's mouthpiece. The Brook airway minimizes the danger of cross-contamination.

PHARYNGEAL AIRWAYS

Pharyngeal airways are full-length airways that traverse the victim's mouth and reach the back of the throat. Safar's resuscitube contains a large mouthpiece to provide a seal. Because of their length,

retching, vomiting, and aspiration of stomach contents may be induced when the victim is not deeply unconscious. An oversized pharyngeal airway may occasionally impact the epiglottis and obstruct the larynx.

Face masks

A great deal of time is spent in teaching endotracheal intubation, which is no doubt justified, but the proper use of the face mask deserves equal attention. Sabel makes a plea for the use of the face mask during

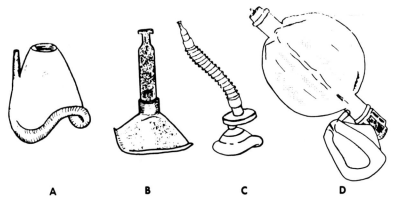

Fig. 20-5. Face masks for emergency resuscitation: **A,** oronasal mask; **B,** Ventibreather; **C,** Emerson resuscitator; and **D,** AMBU resuscitator.

the early stages of cardiac resuscitation, reserving endotracheal intubation for the later stages when prolonged maintenance is required and when the tube can be inserted in relative leisure in an already oxygenated patient. As we have stressed repeatedly, valuable time should not be expended in passing an endotracheal tube during the early stages of resuscitation when simple mouth-to-mouth or face-mask and bag techniques can more quickly ventilate the patient.

As pictured in Fig. 20-5, several designs of face masks are available for emergency resuscitation. These include the simple oronasal mask, the oronasal mask with mouthpiece, and the oronasal mask with bag or bellows. The oronasal mask, while satisfactorily used by most physicians, is not easily used by the inexperienced: mask leakage is often a problem. Inspiration may occur through the nose, and expiration may be blocked by a valving action of the soft palate.

The *AMBU* (Air-Mask-Bag-Unit) bag, pictured in Fig. 20-6, provides a satisfactory method of artificial respiration using manual compression of the bag. The AMBU bag may be attached to an endotracheal tube.

Comparative features of respirator bags

Realizing that self-inflating respirator bags achieve quite adequate ventilation when used with a tight-fitting face mask (or when connected directly to an endotracheal or a tracheostomy tube) and realizing their particular application to cardiopulmonary resuscitation, Carden and Bernstein (1970) compared some of the features of nine most commonly used resuscitative bags. Without detailing all of the aspects of their testing, the conclusion of their results was that all of these bags gave an increased concentration of oxygen with an increase in oxygen flow but none gave 100% oxygen when the oxygen flow was twice the minute ventilation. For intermittent positive-pressure respiration, the AMBU and the AMBU compact bags with E-2 valves or the Air-Viva bag seem most suitable. The latter appears easier to clean and sterilize, the former delivers a slightly higher percentage of oxygen. With oxygen input of greater than 5 liters per minute, the Ruben valve with the AMBU bag has a tendency to jam. Carden and Bernstein do not believe that the AMBU, Air Shields, Inc. (similar in appearance to the AMBU bag with Ruben valve but with a different option inflow), performed as well as the Danish-made AMBU bag and was far less comfortable to use.

The advantages of the Laerdal bag consist of its extreme portability and ease of use. It can be packed in a first aid kit. Since the bag and mask are transparent, any regurgitation can be seen immediately. The

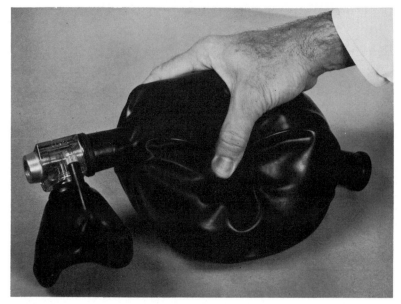

Fig. 20-6. AMBU bag.

bag is easy to clean. The valve tends to jam in the inspiratory position but this is not a drawback with the use of a face mask. For a patient being transported from one area to another, the AGA bag or the AMBU bag with an optional extension tube fitted between the bag and inflating valve appears to work quite well. They report that the HOPE, Puritan PMR, and Pulmonator bags deliver low quantities of oxygen at all flow rates and that some oxygen is blown past the air-inlet valve.

Mask-tube-mask resuscitator

As a result of the threat of chemical warfare employing the anticholinesterase compounds, the U.S. Army has developed a mask-tube-mask respirator that allows the rescuer's face and lungs to be protected while applying artificial respiration to the victim.

Portable ventilator

A simple portable ventilator for emergency resuscitation (Carden and Bernstein) allows ventilation of the patient automatically with 100% oxygen at any rate volume, is small enough to be carried in a pocket, and works effectively enough to be connected to either wall oxygen or any oxygen cylinder. In addition, it can be adapted for spontaneous respiration (see Fig. 20-7). The ventilator has an optimal-pressure-ventilating valve attached to the patient connector of the respirator.

Effect of artificial respiration on circulation

For many years, considerable disagreement existed as to the amount of circulation or movement in the vascular channels that occurred from the mechanical process of artificial respiration. In spite of several reports to the contrary, it is my belief at the present time that this augmentation of circulation is essentially zero and need hardly be considered in the total picture. The general consensus is that artificial respiration, at best, promotes a minimal degree of movement in the vascular channels of the body.

Although the final chapter on this story does not appear to have been written, it is my opinion that there is some degree of cir-

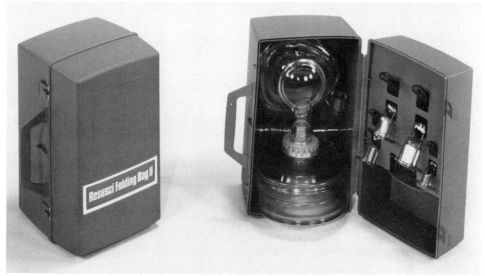

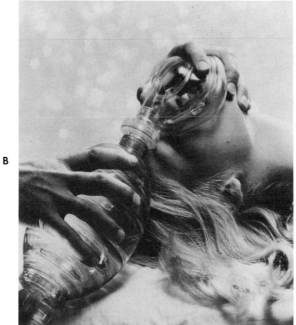

Fig. 20-7. Portable ventilator for emergency resuscitation. **A,** Can be carried in a pocket or connected to either wall oxygen or any oxygen cylinder. **B,** Can be adapted for spontaneous respiration.

culation, obviously quite small, provoked by positive pressure respiration. Safar and associates have shown that inflation of the lungs with positive pressure simultaneously with closed-chest massage produces a blood flow rate and an arterial pressure that are somewhat higher than when only one of the techniques is employed.

Degree of pulmonary pressure that should be maintained

In 1951 Taylor and Gerbode added much to our knowledge of the effect of high intrapulmonary pressures given to patients in the unconscious state. They considered relatively high intrapulmonary pressures as those having a range of 15 to 50 mm. Hg. With high intrapulmonary pressures, a rather uniform and persistent drop in cardiac output and evidence of circulatory depression occur. The mechanism of this reduction in systemic arterial pressure has not been clearly defined. Taylor and Gerbode believe that the autonomic reflex pathway can be excluded, since denervation of the possible reflex pathways did not significantly alter the circulatory response to pulmonary inflation with high pressures. The most logical explanation seems to be that the elevated pulmonary pressures (with unusual degrees of inflation of the lungs) exert an obstructive effect on the pulmonary circulation. Although the tamponade factor cannot be excluded, circulatory depression will still occur in spite of its presence. The obstruction of the pulmonary circulation acts directly on the pulmonary capillary bed with production of strain on the right ventricle. This, of course, causes a decrease in the left ventricular pressure. Taylor and Gerbode state:

In addition the decline in left ventricular pressure and the rise in right ventricular pressure during acute pulmonary inflation tend to reverse the normal gradient of the coronary circulation and might lead to myocardial embarrassment. This may afford an explanation for certain instances of circulatory collapse or cardiac arrest occurring during operations upon the heart or great vessels. The

heart and circulatory system already heavily burdened by congenital or acquired disease may not tolerate slight increases in peripheral resistance in the pulmonary circulation.*

During coughing or shouting, the intratracheal pressure in the adult may rise to above 50 mm. Hg with no ill effects.

The Council on Physical Medicine of the American Medical Association has recommended that automatic positive-negative resuscitators be set at pressures in the neighborhood of 14 mm. Hg in the positive phase alternating with 9 mm. Hg in the negative phase, the total excursion of 23 mm. being achieved.

In the use of the mobile cardiac resuscitation unit at Bellevue Hospital, however, it was noted that these pressures failed to maintain adequate inflation of the lungs when the chest was open, and adequate oxygenation could not be maintained. Therefore, the pressure in the positive phase was increased by several millimeters. Although the Council on Physical Medicine of the American Medical Association recommended that the pressure as set by them had proved safe and satisfactory for infants as well as adults, I have had better results clinically in cardiac resuscitation using the open chest with a positive-negative pulmonary resuscitator with which the alveolar pressures of infants could be reduced. In the usual type of artificial respiration with the closed chest, the small air passages of the infant lung safely withstand the same pressures that are employed for adults, since the pressures are not maintained. The pressure peaks are reached only momentarily and cannot hold continuously, even with moderate pressures employed. However, with the amount of pressure used for the adult chest, the degree of inflation in the infant lung would be too

---

*From Taylor, G., and Gerbode, F.: Observations on the circulatory effects of short duration positive pressure pulmonary inflation, Surgery 30:56-74, 1951.

large. The degree of positive pressure or the degree to which the anesthetist may be allowed to use rhythmic compression of the breathing bag may depend upon the cardiac status of the patient. If the patient has an already depressed cardiac output, then a dangerous situation may be provoked by an unsuspectedly high alveolar pressure being maintained by pressure on the breathing bag.

Should an oxygen–carbon dioxide mixture be used in resuscitation?

During the initial phase of respiratory resuscitation, the patient will be receiving only expired air. If the AMBU bag is used, he will receive room air. Ideally, one should strive to administer 100% oxygen as soon as possible. There would seem to be little justification for using anything other than 100% oxygen during the early phase of cardiac resuscitation. Little excuse will exist for the use of carbon dioxide mixture, in spite of the vasodilatation effect of a 7% to 10% carbon dioxide mixture or a mixture of helium and oxygen. As complete a saturation with oxygen as possible is desirable. When total anoxia is present, there need be no additional stimulus to the respiratory center from either carbon dioxide or helium.

Should 100% oxygen be given?

During the initial period of resuscitation, 100% oxygen should be given. However, because of the possible complications of prolonged high oxygen concentrations such as intra-alveolar hemorrhage, fibrosis, and inhibition of the mucociliary apparatus, lower oxygen concentrations should be used after the initial period of resuscitation.

Should an endotracheal tube be passed?

The importance of maintaining adequate ventilation and utilizing endotracheal intubation in prolonged cardiopulmonary resuscitation is emphasized by the work of Fillmore and co-workers, who carefully studied blood gas and lactate levels serially during cardiopulmonary resuscitation in fifteen patients. They point out that preintubation samples of mean Pa_{CO_2} fell from 66 to 41 mm. Hg following intubation. The sooner the endotracheal tube was in place, the sooner the pH was normalized and the more easily it could be controlled with bicarbonate. In the patients not subjected to endotracheal intubation, lactate rose to a mean of 128 mg. per liter by 20 minutes but was only 80 mg. per liter in the group with endotracheal tube.

In general, it is desirable to have an endotracheal tube in place when administering artificial respiration. As a rule, however, passage of the endotracheal tube during the early and critical period of resuscitation means delay at a time when every second counts. Applying the mask directly to the mouth (provided steps are taken to be sure the airway is open) will be adequate at the onset. Should the stomach be inflated, pressure applied to the epigastrium at intervals will correct this complication. Elam, in listing the indications for endotracheal intubation during resuscitation, includes a full stomach, excessive gastric inflation, gastric hemorrhage, regurgitation and imminent pulmonary aspiration, and the need for prolonged ventilation with oxygen.

In summary, although it is true that an endotracheal tube provides the best assurance that the airway is patent, it should only be employed when it does not contribute to any delay. The endotracheal tube can usually be inserted with ease, often by the inexperienced, since the vocal cords will be relaxed and a sizeable aperture evident.

May I again stress that *under no circumstances should cardiopulmonary resuscitation be delayed by waiting for an anesthetist or an endotracheal tube.* If the condition of the patient makes intubation possible, so much the better, but no undue risk should be taken. (The mobile cardiac resuscitation unit should always be equipped with endotracheal tubes of various sizes.)

Regurgitation during resuscitation

It is not infrequent that a patient will regurgitate at some time during the period of resuscitation. Obviously, the resulting chemical irritation to the tracheobronchial tree compounds the problem of respiratory resuscitation. Precautions should be taken either to prevent vomiting or, if present, to allow for effective clearing of pharyngeal secretions. Ambulances, coronary care units, and all areas likely to encounter this problem should have suction catheters readily available. If suction is not available, one must resort to mechanical cleansing of the pharynx by proper positioning of the patient and by clearing the secretions from the mouth and pharynx with the use of gauze, a handkerchief, or whatever may be available. Once the endotracheal tube has been inserted, the problem of tracheal aspiration is largely solved. Occasionally, it may be necessary to pass the bronchoscope quickly in order to remove pieces of aspirated food particles. This problem is dealt with more specifically in a section devoted to the neonate. If other aspects of resuscitative procedure are under control, a Levin tube may be passed into the stomach to allow adequate emptying. In some patients, the maneuver of closed-chest compression will provoke gastric regurgitation, as discussed in the section on the closed chest.

Emergency airway via cricothyroid membrane puncture

Cardiac arrest may be associated with a number of respiratory difficulties that respond poorly to the usual method of artificial respiration. Acute obstructive laryngeal edema from an allergic reaction to penicillin, hemorrhage into neck tissue planes, epiglottitis, and lodgement of particulate matter such as food in the larynx provide such examples. If an inability to inflate or de-

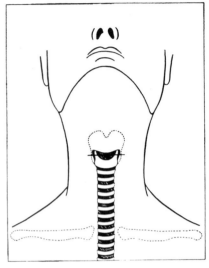

Fig. 20-8. Anatomic relationships of cricothyroid membrane. (Redrawn from Nicholas, T. H., and Rumer, G. F.: J.A.M.A. 174:1934, 1963.)

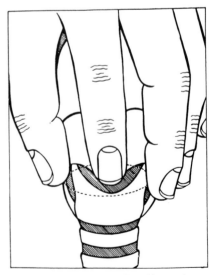

Fig. 20-9. Location of cricothyroid membrane and position of hand in stabilizing larynx prior to puncture of cricothyroid membrane. (Redrawn from Nicholas, T. H., and Rumer, G. F.: J.A.M.A. 174:1934, 1963.)

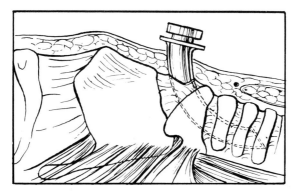

Fig. 20-10. Position of cannula after insertion through cricothyroid membrane. (Not to be left in place for more than 24 hours.) (Courtesy Drs. D. S. Ruhe, G. O. Proud, and G. V. Williams, and Pfizer Laboratories.)

flate the lungs is noted upon mouth-to-mouth respiration, obstructions of this nature can be suspected. High insufflation pressures may partially relieve the obstruction; further extension of the neck may be indicated, as may be further pushing of the mandible forward to prevent obstruction of the pharynx by the tongue. If ventilation is still inadequate, then a puncture of the cricothyroid membrane is the quickest, simplest, and safest means of establishing an airway (Fig. 20-8).

Entry through this relatively avascular membrane offers several advantages over a conventional tracheotomy. It is easily reached due to its superficial position and adjacent cartilagenous landmarks. The cricothyroid space is quite large and can accept fairly large tubes. Posterior perforation is unlikely, due to the heavy posterior projection of the cricoid cartilage. An elective tracheotomy can be done at a later date, if necessary. The cricothyroid membrane approach should not be utilized for much over 24 hours.

To perform a cricothyroid membrane puncture, the physician stabilizes the larynx between left thumb and middle finger (Fig. 20-9). The skin is incised by scissors or knife over the cricothyroid space. The scissors or knife is then guided down the index finger to puncture the membrane.

Fig. 20-10 shows the tracheotomy tube in position.

Mini-tracheotomy

Two British anesthesiologists, Davies and Belam, suggest that a standard intravenous transfusion needle be inserted into the trachea through the cricothyroid membrane in instances of airway obstruction where anesthetic apparatus is unavailable. The volume of air that can be drawn through the needle (at pressures reached during obstructed inspiration) is believed to be sufficient to prevent asphyxia and to enable the patient to make forced expiratory efforts.

In evaluating the clinical applications of a needle tracheotomy, Hughes and Williamson conclude from their ventilation experiments in dogs that a No. 13 needle tracheotomy may temporarily restore an adequate airway to the irfant but not to the child or adult with acute obstruction of the upper airway. Those who have used percutaneous insertion of size-13 needles into the trachea of infants state that it is not always a technically easy procedure to accomplish.

Indications for tracheotomy

A tracheotomy is seldom indicated in the immediate phase of cardiac resuscitation. Other and more effective means are available to supply oxygen to the lungs. The time required to perform a tracheotomy is usually excessive.

If a cricothyroid membrane puncture is not elected, one may perform a tracheotomy using essentially the same indications. Over a 25-year period, I have, as mentioned, infrequently used emergency tracheotomy during the immediate or early cardiopulmonary resuscitation period. In some instances of multiple facial fractures and injuries about the nose and mouth with considerable bleeding, a tracheotomy may prove to be a prophylactic measure. Further discussion of the use of the tracheotomy in varied clinical situations is found in the section on postresuscitative care.

When tracheotomy is performed electively, it must be done under a well-controlled situation, preferably in the operating room with the patient well oxygenated. A change of the airway from an endotracheal tube to a tracheostomy tube should be considered after about 72 hours (Safar). This time lag need not be as long if it is obvious that the patient will need an artificial tracheal airway for a prolonged period of time because of a severe crushing injury of the chest or a head injury. Better cuff design shows promise of markedly reducing injury to tracheal mucosa, which could produce tracheal stenosis.

Although tracheotomy will often be necessary and even lifesaving, one should be aware of its complications. Almost a 10% incidence of complications was noted in an analysis of 688 patients undergoing tracheotomy for a variety of indications and conditions (Rogers). There were three deaths from massive tracheal hemorrhage. Patients with tracheostomies require continuous observation by experienced personnel. While severe endotracheitis is the most common complication, numerous others such as pneumothorax, an improperly positioned cannula, aspiration, delayed arterial bleeding, atelectasis, diminution of the tracheal lumen, mediastinitis, and wound infections may be encountered.

Toy and Weinstein described a technique of rapid percutaneous tracheotomy performed within 1 minute (by carefully inserting a No. 13 needle into the tracheal lumen between the second and third tracheal wings in the midline of the suprasternal area, a small polyethylene catheter about 14 cm. long can be then passed through the needle and the needle withdrawn, leaving the tube as a guide). Following removal of the needle, a tracheostomy tube (No. 5) is slipped into a specially made bougie and secured to the bougie. The entire assembly is lubricated and inserted percutaneously until the tracheostomy tube is in place. The removal of the bougie and attached catheter completes the procedure.

How to cope with airway obstruction

It takes only a period of between 5 and 10 minutes for complete airway obstruction to cause death. The hypoxia as well as hypercarbia or hypercapnia (accumulation of carbon dioxide) obviously represents an emergency of almost the same time proportions as sudden cessation of cardiac output. Under conditions of asphyxia the heart may continue to beat for several minutes but all available oxygen stores are rapidly depleted. Cardiac output becomes ineffective and ventricular fibrillation may be initiated.

Aspirated foreign bodies are responsible for an inordinately large percentage of accidental deaths in the young child. In the adult there is a condition that is termed the "cafe coronary." This refers to the clinical observation suggesting an apparent sudden heart attack when in actuality it represents the inadvertent swallowing of too large a bolus of food with resultant airway obstruction and often death.

It may seem that airway obstruction would be readily recognized. Such, however, is not always the case. In the unconscious patient with head and neck muscles relaxed and the patient's neck in a partially flexed position the tongue may be relaxed so as to press against the posterior pharyngeal wall. Not all victims become cyanotic. In some there may actually be a vasodilation set off by the hypoxemia that is present. An appraisal of the color of the nail beds, conjunctiva, or mucous membranes may be misleading, particularly in dark-skinned individuals. In some patients there may be no airway obstruction but respiratory movements of the chest or abdomen cannot be detected. Under such a profound state of hypoventilation as may be found in patients somnolent from hypercarbia or suffering the effects of massive drug overdose, one may need to hold a wisp of cotton in front of the patient's mouth or nose to detect any air current.

There are, of course, already implied various degrees of partial airway obstruction. Depending on the degree of obstruction, intrathoracic pressure fluctuations are increased along with the efforts of breathing. Gradually the respiratory center becomes less sensitive to the usual stimulus from a buildup of carbon dioxide.

Marked activity of the accessory muscles of respiration in the neck, supraclavicular, and intercostal areas should alert one to the presence of severe or even complete airway obstruction. If the airway obstruction is complete, one will hear no airflow; if it is incomplete, various degrees of noise intensity may be provoked, depending upon the degree of obstruction. Snoring is probably the best known example of partial airway obstruction and is simply produced by hypopharyngeal obstruction by the tongue. The wheezing effect of the asthmatic from partial bronchial obstruction is well known. Laryngospasm produces a characteristic crowing sound. Foreign matter obstructing the airway may occasionally produce a gurgling noise.

Safar has repeatedly stressed the principles in the recognition and management of space airway obstruction. He recommends that a sequence of activities be followed until one is satisfied that an open airway exists:

1. The unconscious patient should be properly *positioned*. He should be supine with the head tilted back. Do not place the unconscious patient in the prone position for a number of reasons. Not only is the face inaccessible for mouth-to-mouth respiration but such a position may further promote mechanical obstruction.

2. Perhaps the most effective step to take in promoting an open airway in the unconscious patient is to simply *tilt the head backward* by placing one hand under the patient's neck and the other at the patient's forehead. This maneuver stretches the tissues between the larynx and the mandible and lifts the base of the tongue from the posterior pharyngeal wall. In some instances elevation of the patient's shoulders may further facilitate the tilting of the patient's head. The patient's mouth will usually open when the head is tilted back and this may, indeed, be advantageous particularly when there is partial or complete nasal obstruction.

3. Apply mouth-to-mouth or mouth-to-nose respiration by exhaling into the patient's air passages. The *positive airway pressure* may help overcome obstruction by increasing the pressure gradient for airflow and by dilating the air passages.

4. In approximately one out of five patients the above steps will still not result in an open airway and an additional maneuver should be performed, namely the *forward displacement of the mandible*. This can be done simply by lifting the mandible with your hands at the ascending rami or placing your thumb in the mouth and pulling the mandible forward. If the mouth does open with the backward tilting of the head then the patient's lips and teeth should be separated in the event that an expiratory nasal obstruction is present.

5. The airway may still not be open. *A foreign body may be in the back of the pharynx and can be quickly removed by turning the patient's head to the side, forcing the mouth open and wiping the pharynx and*

mouth clean with the fingers or, if available, by the use of suction. Obviously you must not risk further spinal cord damage by twisting the cervical spine in cases of possible fracture of that area.

6. *Artificial oral airways* may be necessary to hold the base of the tongue forward and maintain the lips and teeth in an open position. The nasopharyngeal tube, if available, may be particularly valuable in the patient with trismus (spasm of the jaw muscles preventing easy opening of the mouth). The familiar S-shaped oral pharyngeal airway may be used as may the simple comma-shaped airway, often referred to as the Guedel airway. If a nasopharyngeal tube is not available, the mouth may be forced open by sliding the index finger backward between the cheek and the teeth and then wedging the tip of the index finger behind the last molars. If the jaws are not clenched, the oral pharyngeal tube may be inserted by forcing the mouth open with the thumb and index finger crossed and inserting the tube over the tongue and twisting it into position. The Brook airway is an oral airway with which hyperextension of the victim's head prevents any throat obstruction by the tongue. Unlike the oropharyngeal airways, it is not likely to stimulate vomiting and cause aspiration of the gastric contents in the partially comatose patient. Occasionally an oral airway may even reach beyond the pharynx and obstruct the air passage by impacting the epiglottis.

Every individual can serve as an effective pulmonary resuscitation unit. The air we breathe contains over 20% oxygen and 0.04% carbon dioxide. Our exhaled air contains 16% oxygen and 4% carbon dioxide. Instinctively a person will breathe more deeply when applying mouth-to-mouth resuscitation, thereby enhancing the quantity and quality of his expired air and the victim will subsequently receive twice his normal tidal volume of air containing as much as 18% oxygen and 2% carbon dioxide. Generally speaking, after about 15 seconds or

five deep inflations, the victim's lungs will contain near normal amounts of oxygen and carbon dioxide.

7. *Tracheal intubation:* When it is imperative that the tracheobronchial tree be rapidly suctioned, when gastric contents have been aspirated, and when the above steps have not been sufficient to maintain adequate oxygenation, a rapid insertion of the endotracheal tube is indicated. Obviously the endotracheal tube may not be available in many emergency situations but it should be a part of the equipment on every ambulance. The endotracheal tube will not be tolerated easily by the conscious or partially conscious patient.

Should automatic ventilators be used in resuscitation?

Mechanical respirators have many obvious advantages. However, their inability to alert the physician to increased airway resistance prompts me to use either airway-to-mouth or bag breathing until I am reasonably sure that an adequate airway exists.

A number of pulmonary resuscitators have been advocated for maintenance of ventilation during cardiac arrest. Several disadvantages inherent in these resuscitators have been pointed out by Safar and co-workers.

1. Airway obstruction is difficult to detect and difficult to treat because of a lack of pressure reserve.
2. Mask leakage, which is common during emergency artificial ventilation, leads to failure in cycling of the apparatus.
3. The rate, pressure, volume, and flow for each inflation cannot be changed according to the resistances encountered in the patient.
4. Lung-thorax compliance and airway resistance vary greatly from patient to patient, and within each patient during the course of resuscitation.*

With these considerations in mind, Safar and associates conclude that exhaled air

*From Safar, P., Brown, T. C., and Holtey, W. J.: Failure of closed chest cardiac massage to produce ventilation, Dis. Chest **43:**6, 1962.

resuscitation and the use of hand-operated equipment such as bags or bellows provide the best methods of positive-pressure ventilation necessary for both closed and open cardiac resuscitation.

Moreover, external cardiac compression does not lend itself effectively to a combination with positive-pressure-cycled automatic ventilators since airway pressure increases with each compression of the chest causing premature termination of the inflation cycle and insufficient ventilation.

Electrophrenic respiration

On the original mobile cardiac resuscitation cart at Bellevue Hospital (1951), there was an electrophrenic stimulator for providing artificial respiration either by direct application to the phrenic nerve in the neck or by application of current over the appropriate cutaneous area.

Although I do not have extensive clinical experience with electrophrenic respiration, it does appear that it would be helpful to the patient experiencing prolonged inadequate spontaneous respiration or to the patient in whom a delayed return to spontaneous respirations occurs. (I can testify to the efficacy of electrophrenic stimulation after experiencing this form of artificial respiration during a visit to Sarnoff Laboratory in Boston in the early 1950s.)

Interest in electrophrenic stimulation has been rather dormant during the last 25 years. Daggett and co-workers revived interest in the procedure by their report on intracaval electrophrenic stimulation. As shown in Fig. 20-11, they observe that placement of catheter electrodes in either the superior or inferior vena cava in the dog makes possible the rhythmic contraction of the diaphragm by intermittently applied

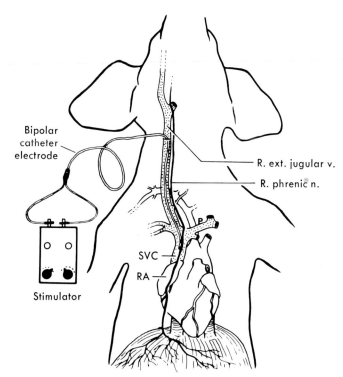

Fig. 20-11. Daggett's method of intracaval electrophrenic stimulation. *SVC,* superior vena cava; *RA,* right atrium. (From Daggett, W. M., and others: J. Thorac. Cardiovasc. Surg. **51:** 677, 1966.)

electric stimuli. They attribute this reaction to the close proximity of the right phrenic nerve to the vena cava.

Daggett and his colleagues compare intracaval electrostimulation with positive-negative pressure breathing under a number of different conditions. They find, for example, that under barbiturate intoxication intracaval electrophrenic stimulation is a more effective method of ventilatory support than is positive-negative pressure (see Table 20-1). Cardiac output consistently appears to be higher and ventilation is more physiologic as measured by the carbon dioxide tension and pH. Cardiac arrhythmias were not noted.

There are several apparent advantages of electrophrenic stimulation. A better maintenance of circulation, at least in dogs, can be achieved than with positive-negative pressure ventilation. A number of studies have shown that, in shock, positive pressure breathing depresses cardiac output and arterial pressure. Active contraction of the diaphragm by phrenic nerve stimulation prevents disuse atrophy of respiratory musculature, which is thought to occur during prolonged periods of ventilatory support by a positive pressure respirator. With phrenic nerve stimulation, apnea occurs as mediated through the vagus nerve. There is therefore no effort of spontaneous respiratory activity to counter artificial efforts. In addition, negative pressure breathing, which takes place during electrophrenic stimulation, promotes

increased venous return to the heart. It should be noted that adequate ventilation of the contralateral lung during direct stimulation of the right phrenic nerve has been previously demonstrated by Sarnoff.

Although electrical stimulation by radio-frequency induction has been applied to many clinical conditions including bladder paralysis, hypoventilation, intractable pain, anal and urethral incontinence, hypertension, and angina pectoris, this apparently is the first example of its use for stimulation of the phrenic nerve. It appears that electrical stimulation of one phrenic nerve to effect maximum contraction of the diaphragm is attended by fatigue after 12 to 18 hours. For this reason the phrenic nerves are stimulated in alternating periods of 12 hours each. After stimulation is discontinued, recovery of the nerve is rapid and apparently complete in a few hours.

If necessary, long-term electrophrenic respiration is practical. Glenn and co-workers report on a patient with respiratory paralysis from injury of the cervical cord. He received ventilatory support for his quadriplegic condition with radiofrequency electrophrenic respiration over a 14-month period. He was unable to support adequate ventilation by voluntary effort, alone, for more than a few minutes.

More recently Bilgutay and associates at St. Mary's Hospital in Minneapolis have developed a synchronous phrenic nerve stimulator that has been used clinically (Fig. 20-12, *A* and *B*). The advantage of syn-

Table 20-1. Physiologic variables in artificial respiration*

Measured variables	Intracaval electro-phrenic respiration	Positive-negative pressure respiration	Spontaneous respiration
Arterial pressure (mm. Hg)	130.0	105.0	160.0
Heart rate (beats/minute)	145.0	150.0	165.0
Arterial pO_2 (mm. Hg)	500.0	260.0	350.0
Arterial pCO_2 (mm. Hg)	43.0	27.0	95.0
Arterial pH	7.4	7.6	7.1
Cardiac output (L./min.)	1.9	1.6	1.5

*From Daggett, W. M., and others: Intravenous electrical stimulation of the phrenic nerve: a new technique of artificial respiration, Surg. Forum **16**:177-179, 1965.

chronous stimulation is that it provides for an automatic control of stimulation, utilizing the patient's own servomechanism. In tachypnea it slows and regulates ventilation and it maintains cyclic ventilation in apnea.

Bilgutay has not observed paradoxical motion of the diaphragm or difficulty with swallowing or phonation in patients with synchronous phrenic nerve stimulation.

Transmission of electrical stimuli to the

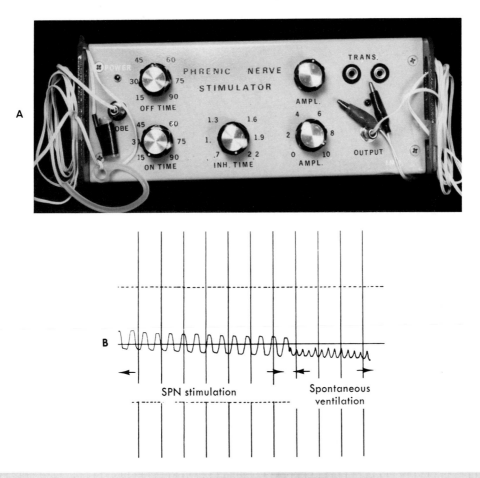

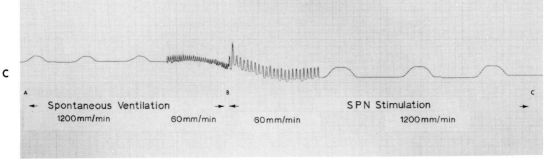

Fig. 20-12. A, Synchronous phrenic nerve stimulator. B and C, The advantage of synchronous phrenic nerve stimulation is that it provides for an automatic control of stimulation. (From Bilgutay, A. M., and others: Trans. Am. Soc. Artif. Intern. Organs 16:213-219, 1970.)

phrenic nerve by radiofrequency induction is reported by Glenn and his associates at Yale. In six patients with hypoventilation of central origin, it was applied for up to 22 months. Long-term phrenic stimulation often leads to fatigue. The cause of this electrophrenic respiration–induced fatigue (Sato and co-workers) does not lie in either the nerve or the diaphragm as the site of the fatigue but is caused by interference with the transmission of impulses across the neuromuscular junction. When the pulse interval is adjusted to the lowest possible frequency for greater contraction, significantly prolonged respiration results without diaphragm fatigue. Stimulating with alterating bidirectional current also greatly prolongs effective diaphragmatic contracture. Reinforcement of ventilation with electrophenic pacing of the paralyzed diaphragm is reported by Johnson and Eiseman.

Return of spontaneous respiration after cardiac arrest

In my own clinical experience with cardiac arrest and in studying the experience of others, I have been impressed with the variability of the response with which return of spontaneous respiration occurs following cessation of the heartbeat and respiration.

If cardiac compression and augmentation of circulation are begun at once, it is frequently noted that spontaneous respirations will resume within a matter of seconds. These spontaneous respirations occur within 5 to 10 minutes after apparent cardiac resuscitation has been effected; however, they may not return for a period of 20 to 30 minutes, and therefore patience in awaiting the return of respiratory center activity is mandatory.

In individuals who have suffered severe cerebral damage from anoxia during the arrest, the respiratory center will usually survive, even though the patient remains a decerebrate. This was not the case, however, in a recent cardiac arrest that involved a 4-year-old girl who was operated upon for strabismus of the eye. It was necessary to maintain artificial respirations for 36 hours, despite the fact that the heart had been resuscitated. Spontaneous respiratory action did not return and the patient died.

Swan mentions a case of ventricular fibrillation in which massage was carried out for 65 minutes before spontaneous respirations returned. A spontaneous heartbeat did not occur until after 82 minutes had elapsed.

Obviously, return of spontaneous respiration may be considerably delayed if respiratory arrest is caused by drug or chemical overdose, CNS depression, or conditions causing neuromuscular paralysis.

Chapter 21

ARTIFICIAL MAINTENANCE OF CIRCULATION: PRECORDIAL PERCUSSION AND CLOSED-CHEST RESUSCITATION

Precordial thumping

As is illustrated in Fig. 21-1, a thump to the chest can revert ventricular tachycardia in a patient with ischemic heart disease. Lown and associates were led to believe that a low-energy source such as provided by a chest thump might be effective in human ventricular tachycardia, after they had induced prefibrillatory arrhythmias in dogs with acute myocardial infarction and had terminated the arrhythmias with transthoracic shocks of less than 1 watt-second. They believe that precordial concussion or chest thump is indicated as an emergency procedure in cases of cardiac asystole and that it may prove lifesaving when the mechanism is prefibrillatory ventricular tachycardia. Obviously, use of low-energy cardioversion, being more predictable and less traumatic, is preferable with the patient who is tolerating the ventricular tachycardia.

The important contribution of Pennington, Taylor, and Lown in more closely defining cardioversion energy requirements for various arrhythmias is noteworthy. Whereas atrial fibrillation conversion to sinus rhythm requires energy of only about 100 watt-seconds, we know that ventricular defibrillation requires much greater energy. On the other hand, cardioversion of atrial flutter needs only a low-energy discharge. These workers speculate that all of these arrhythmias are caused by reentrant mechanisms sustained by the continuous traverse of a depolarization wave front over fixed single or multiple and variable pathways and that

at any one instance part of the circuit is refractory and part recovered. The arrhythmia is abolished when premature depolarization of the recovered portion blocks conduction of the circulating wave front. When depolarization of multiple pathways at differing stages of recovery is required, a larger electrical discharge is necessary for terminating the reentrant mechanisms. Only low energies are necessary for depolarizing the heart when the arrhythmia is sustained by conduction over a single circuit. It is believed that the chest thump serves as an external pacemaker to produce ectopic depolarizations of a fraction of the reentrant circuitry with subsequent termination of the arrhythmia. The blow to the chest induces focal excitation, which propagates as a single ectopic systole.

Scherf has pointed out that the increasingly hypoxic arrested heart may develop ventricular fibrillation following thumping of the precordium because the blow may activate groups of bizarre complexes. Don Michael was able to maintain an effective heartbeat for 90 minutes by repetitive precordial concussion. In this instance the arrest was due to asystole. Lown and his associates speculate that the wide acceptance of precordial thumping for cardiac resuscitation stems from its effectiveness in the termination of prefibrillatory ventricular tachycardia rather than asystole.

Don Michael has considered, in several publications, the question of precordial percussion in cardiac resuscitation. In one

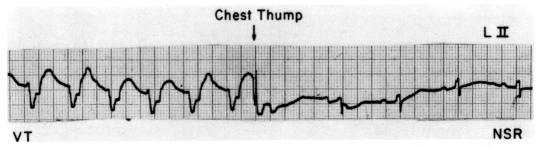

Fig. 21-1. A single sharp blow delivered to lower sternum terminates ventricular tachycardia. (From Pennington, J. E., Taylor, J., and Lown, B.: N. Engl. J. Med. 283:1192-1195, 1970.)

instance, he was able to maintain intermittent pacing of the heart by precordial percussion for 1½ hours, with eventual recovery of the patient. The patient was electrocardiographically monitored during the entire period. Don Michael observes that a sharp blow delivered with the ulnar border of the hand activates the heart, producing one or more ventricular complexes. He also notes that a palpable pulse and recordable blood pressure coincide with the mechanical stimulus. It should be realized, of course, that the activation of an ECG complex is not synonymous with a palpable pulse and recordable blood pressure. Don Michael proposes that precordial percussion should be tried before external cardiac massage in all cases of cardiac arrest. Fig. 21-2 shows ventricular complexes that coincided with the precordial percussion.

Several years ago I had an opportunity to observe the effectiveness of precordial chest wall blows in initiating cardiac activity. The patient apparently went into cardiac arrest from an elevated potassium level while being monitored by an electrocardiogram. Shortly after the arrest, the anesthesiologist pounded on the left chest wall over the precordium. With each such fist percussion, an ECG complex was evident—a forceful contraction of the heart took place. Crum and Harris report a 51-year-old man who had a cardiac arrest following a myocardial infarction. A pulse

rate of 68/80 beats per second was maintained simply with forced fist percussion to the precordium. The chest was subsequently entered and the heart was found to be in asystole. Transient ventricular fibrillation occurred but reverted to a sinus rhythm after approximately 20 minutes' massage.

Roberts and co-workers found that an apparent case of cardiac arrest with multiple episodes responded twice in a period of several days to a strong blow on the precordium. They urge that such a procedure be carried out in all cases before any incision is made. They state:

The speed and ease with which the precordium may be struck certainly justifies the trial of this procedure in many cases of cardiac arrest before cardiac massage is undertaken.*

On more than one occasion, a heart in cardiac arrest has resumed normal nodal rhythm following a rather severe precordial concussion. As a general rule, precordial concussion refers to a sharp or abrupt blow with the folded fist upon the lower portion of the sternum or precordium.

In Brandenburg's case, three quick, heavy blows were struck on the left chest with the clenched fist during simultaneous palpation of the radial pulse. After the

*From Roberts, B., Schnabel, T. G., Jr., and Ravdin, I. S.: Multiple episodes of cardiac arrest, J.A.M.A. 154:581-584, 1954.

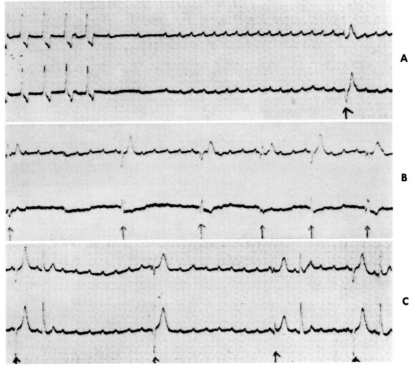

Fig. 21-2. Effect of precordial concussion on cardiac asystole. **A,** ECG showing epinephrine-induced ventricular tachycardia giving place to asystole, terminated by thumping the chest. **B,** ECG showing ventricular complexes coinciding with precordial percussion. **C,** ECG showing activation of spontaneous ventricular complexes following those produced by precordial percussion. (From Don Michael, T. A., and Stanford, R. L.: Lancet 1:699, 1963.)

third blow, a sustained pulse could be felt and the patient regained consciousness. A similar case was reported by McLachlan, with survival of the patient for 7 months.

In eleven patients, Scherf documents the effect of precordial thumping in evoking ectopic beats that give way to regular idioventricular rhythm. He credits Schott (1920) with first describing this type of mechanical stimulation to the heart. Surprisingly enough, several instances of ventricular fibrillation are said to have reverted with this technique. Therefore precordial thumping, pounding, or percussion is worthy of trial in the first few seconds after arrest. It is apparent that the effectiveness of this technique is too little known.

Continuous rhythmical chest pounding can successfully maintain the heart rhythm for a considerable period of time. Wild and Grover report three such instances in which ventricular asystole successfully responded to precordial concussion. In one instance it was successful for more than 40 minutes. Meanwhile a transvenous pacemaker was introduced to pace the heart. With each blow on the chest, ventricular depolarization and asystole occurred, but with no metabolic acidosis. Fig. 21-3 shows the electrocardiogram tracings in a 77-year-old man who experienced syncopal episodes in the coronary care unit. QRS complexes with each blow were followed by strong pulses.

Paroxysmal ventricular tachycardia abolished by a blow to the precordium is reported

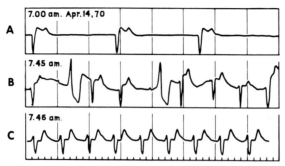

Fig. 21-3. **A,** Ventricular complexes occurring every 2 to 6 seconds; **B,** tracing recorded during early moments of chest pounding; **C,** tracing recorded during chest pounding 1 minute after **B.** Figure was traced from monitoring electrocardiogram. Long vertical lines are at 1-second intervals. (From Wild, J. B., and Grover, J. D.: Lancet 2:436-437, 1970.)

by Bornemann and Scherf, but they point out that mechanical stimulation during ventricular tachycardia is hazardous as it may unpredictably induce ventricular fibrillation. The negative after-potential may be increased, leading to firing off of impulses at a rate sufficiently rapid to cause the fibrillation. Thus it would appear that precordial thumps are not without hazard and it should be reasonably certain that one is dealing with cardiac asystole or ventricular fibrillation before attempting them.

Semple and co-workers have reported on the effect of "thumping" the precordium in a patient with complete heart block with standstill on over twenty occasions within the space of an hour while preparations were being made for transvenous pacing. Pennington and co-workers report that a precordial blow to the chest successfully terminated twelve episodes of ventricular tachycardia in five patients. They suggest that the precordial thump provides a low-energy current capable of depolarizing a reentry pathway through electromechanical transduction. Repeated efforts with cardioversions to convert ventricular tachycardia are generally successful with energy ranging from 50 to 300 watt-seconds. Lown and his group at Harvard recently subjected to cardioversion fourteen patients who exhibited thirty-two episodes of ventricular tachycardia. In twenty-seven episodes of eleven patients, the initial energy employed was only 10 watt-seconds or less. Thus in 93% of episodes of ventricular tachycardia, 10 watt-seconds or less was the effective energy.

In one case reported by Wild and Grover, chest pounding was continued for more than 40 minutes with each blow on the chest being followed by ventricular depolarization and systole.

Instances of the conversion of a ventricular fibrillation to normal sinus rhythm by a thump on the chest have been reported (Fig. 21-4). An interesting corollary is the "endocardial thump" instituted by Kwast. While placing an intravenous pacing catheter into the right ventricle of a patient with complete heart block, ventricular fibrillation occurred. Defibrillatory efforts were unsuccessful owing to a broken wire at the base of one of the paddles. In desperation, Kwast gave two or three rapid and forceful jolts to the distal end of the catheter with subsequent conversion to normal sinus rhythm. Unfortunately, within several minutes complete heart block again occurred.

Technique of closed-chest cardiac massage

Jude and his associates have emphasized the importance of placing the patient on a firm, rigid surface to most effectively in-

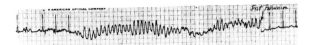

Fig. 21-4. A vigorous thump to patient's chest converts ventricular fibrillation to normal sinus rhythm. (From Barrett, J. S.: N. Engl. J. Med. 284:392-393, 1971.)

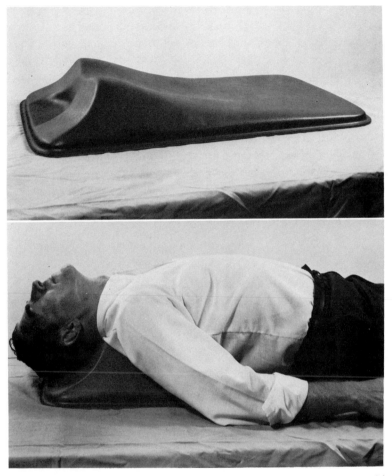

Fig. 21-5. Special cardiopulmonary resuscitation support that allows for proper positioning of head, neck, and thorax. (Courtesy Cordis Corp., Miami.)

itiate external cardiac massage. Most hospital wards now have special resuscitation boards that can be easily slipped under the patient. Ideally, these boards should support the entire length of the body rather than just the chest. The operating room table is of satisfactory firmness, but the usual hospital bed does not provide adequate support to allow maximal effectiveness for compressing the space between the lower end of the sternum and the vertebral column. To facilitate the venous return to the heart, it is my usual custom to elevate the legs as much as 30 to 40 degrees. Often it is not practical to delay resuscitation in order to place the patient on a rigid surface. For example, the resuscitator may be the only individual present. In such instance, closed-chest resuscitation should be carried out as effectively as possible until help is available either to insert the bed board or to place the patient on the floor or on a table.

In order to effectively compress the space between the lower end of the sternum and the vertebral column, pressure should be delivered over a relatively localized area of the sternum (see Fig. 21-5). In adults, this involves the lower two sternebrae. One places the heel of the palm at the lower end of the body of the sternum, with the other hand placed upon the back of the first to provide additional pressure directed to the forearms from the back and shoulders (Fig. 21-6). The arms should be maintained in a generally straight position. It may be most effective to stand on a chair or stool if the patient is on the operating table or in a hospital bed. In instances where the patient is on the floor, one may kneel beside the abdomen or occasionally kneel beside the head and face the feet. In any event, a rate of between 60 and 80 compressions per minute will generally provide cardiac output compatible with the maintenance of cerebral function.

In any consideration of closed-chest cardiac resuscitation, the reader should refer to the well-written and beautifully illustrated book by Jude and Elam. These authors recommend that the adult sternum be depressed by the heel of the hand (the thenar and hypothenar eminences) for a distance of 1½ to 2 inches. The downward thrust, which is a rather rapid thrust held for approximately half a second, should be at right angles to the vertebrae. With an instant release of the hand, the patient's chest wall will recoil, producing negative intrathoracic pressure that aids in the venous return to the heart. (The reader is referred to the sections on infant resuscitation for variations of the technique as applied to this age group.)

As pointed out elsewhere, artificial respiration is maintained at approximately twelve ventilations per minute. These ventilatory efforts are interposed between every fifth external cardiac compression effort.

Again it is emphasized that the use of manikins appears to be a relatively reliable practice method for closed-chest resuscitative techniques and should be resorted to frequently in the training of house staff physicians and students. Cardiac resuscita-

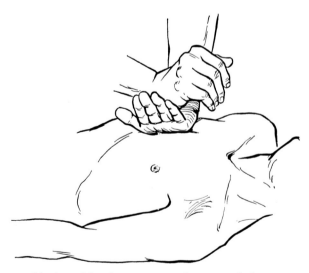

Fig. 21-6. Proper positioning of hands on sternum for external chest compression. Note that procedure is basically a sternal compression effort.

tion in the animal laboratory is best combined with open-chest approaches. Experimentally, it is well recognized that the dog is seldom an ideal experimental control upon which to study closed-chest cardiac compression. Because of the very mobile mediastinum, long thoracic cage, narrow sternum, and high-positioned liver, closed-chest resuscitation is less than ideal. Boxers and basset hounds, perhaps, are an exception.

The necessary depression of the sternum will vary in certain instances. In large, emphysematous chests, it may be necessary to eventually depress the chest more than the usual 1½ to 2 inches. The mobility of the sternum revolves essentially around the body of the sternum and the xiphoid. The manubrium is relatively fixed during closed-chest compression. In an unconscious adult or a fresh cadaver, the sternum can easily be depressed 3 to 4 cm. (Iung and Wade). It has also been demonstrated that the maximum lateral shift of the heart with depression of the sternum averages about 0.5 cm.

A number of relatively minor variations in the technique described by Jude and Kouwenhoven have been suggested. For example, Dr. James Thomson of Cape Town, South Africa, suggests that the closed fist may be used to give a more localized depression of the lower third of the sternum. With this method, the ulnar aspect of the closed fist of the left hand is placed over the lower third of the

sternum just above the xiphoid process. The right hand is placed on top of it, and the sternum is depressed 1½ to 2 inches. Because of the more localized area of pressure, cardiac compression may be more efficient, while fractures and visceral lacerations may be less common.

Because of the pulmonary and circulatory disturbances with cardiopulmonary resuscitation, deterioration may progressively increase as longer resuscitative efforts are attempted. Metabolic acidosis increases. Myocardial contractility decreases. For this reason, Orkin suggests that closed-chest resuscitation be abandoned and open-chest resuscitation be tried if evidence of adequate circulation—normal pupillary size, return of consciousness, normal color, and capillary refill—is not rapidly produced.

Closed-chest resuscitation in infants and children

Closed-chest resuscitation seems ideally suited to the infant and certainly would seem desirable as compared with the thoracotomy approach. The possibility of neurologic sequelae in resuscitation of the newborn infant has been raised, but to date no evidence is available to contraindicate prompt institution of resuscitative measures if the above requisites are met.

Jude points out that only moderate pressure by the fingertips on the middle third of the sternum should be employed in infants. One hand only may be all that is required to give adequate pressure to the

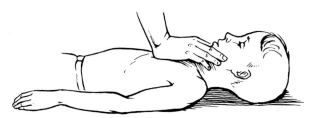

Fig. 21-7. Closed-chest resuscitation of young child. Gentle pressure is sufficient. With infants, compression by pressure with thumb over sternum is adequate. Pressure on xiphoid is avoided, as is simultaneous pressure over abdomen and chest.

flexible thoracic cage of patients from infancy up to 9 or 10 years of age. Fig. 21-7 illustrates the position of the hand for closed-chest massage in the young child.

Because of the frequency of rupture or tear of the liver during external cardiac compression in infants, Thaler recommends that the site of thoracic compression be moved away from the xiphoid end of the sternum to a point near the midsternum. In infants, the ventricle lies behind the midsternum, whereas the lower sternum extends over the liver. The liver is particularly likely to be injured when the thorax and upper abdomen are compressed simultaneously. Thaler suggests that external cardiac compression in infants and young children should consist of compressing the midsternum with superimposed thumbs. This point is found halfway between the sternal notch and the xiphosternal junction. The operator's fingers are linked behind the infant's back for additional support, and the head is held toward the operator.

Considerable interest has been shown in the application of closed-chest cardiac massage technique in the newborn infant. One of the first such reported cases, using the closed-chest approach, was by Surks. Moya, in 1961, reported the first successful closed-chest resuscitation of a newborn infant. Surks lists four requisites for cardiorespiratory resuscitation in newborn infants:

1. A trained staff and proper equipment must be on hand in the delivery room.
2. A rapid examination must show the infant to be mature with no evidence of major birth trauma or congenital anomalies.
3. There should be no background of prolonged intrauterine asphyxia or severe systemic disease.
4. Good fetal heart sounds must be heard in the five-to-ten–minute period preceding the delivery.*

---

*From Surks, S. N.: Closed-chest massage of stillborn infants, Obstet. Gynecol. 18:182-186, 1961.

Various methods of closed-chest massage in infants are illustrated in Figs. 21-8 to 21-10.

In general, cardiac resuscitation guidelines can be applied uniformly to patients of all ages. Certain comments should be

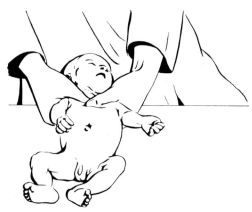

Fig. 21-8. Closed-chest cardiac compression in the infant. Physician stands behind the infant, with his hands cradling the infant's back and his fingers locked behind the scapulae. Thumbs extend up over either shoulder and then rest one upon the other on the midsternum. The rate of 90 to 100 compressions per minute is carried out. (From Wolcott, M. W.: Med. Times **94:**645, 1966.)

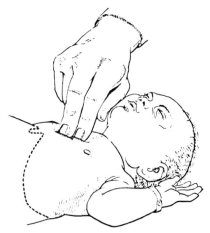

Fig. 21-9. Location of fingers for sternal compression in cardiac massage in the newborn infant. (From Moya, F., and others: Anesthesiology **22:** 1961.)

made, however. External cardiac massage, or closed-chest resuscitation, seems to be especially effective in the child, particularly since the chest wall is more easily compressed. Spencer and Bahnson recommend that the rate of compression should be 80 to 100 times per minute for children. Although two hands are often required for external cardiac massage in the adult, it is seldom necessary to use but one hand with the infant and young child.

In 1957 Rainer and Bullough described a method of closed-chest cardiac massage and augmentation of the venous return with elevation of the lower extremities. They successfully resuscitated all eight children described in their first report. In their description of the method used, they outlined the steps as follows:

1. Any blankets, towels, instruments, or other impediments close to the patient have been quickly discarded,

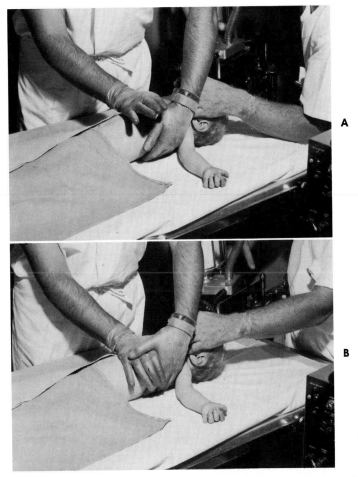

Fig. 21-10. Method of closed-chest cardiac resuscitation in the infant. **A,** Position of left hand for elevating, extending, and supporting left thoracic cage. Thenar and hypothenar eminences of right hand are placed on sternum immediately above xiphosternum. **B,** Position of both hands during massage, with compression of sternum, costocartilages, and ribs produced by alternate flexion and extension of right hand at wrist. (From Dawson, B., and others: Circulation **25:**976, 1962.)

the table is lowered to approximately 10 degrees Trendelenburg by the anesthetist, while the surgeon positions himself at the patient's right side.

2. A nurse is instructed to check the time and call each minute.

3. Having made sure the airway is clear, the anesthetist rhythmically inflates the lungs with 100% oxygen. Unless an endotracheal tube is already in position or can be inserted immediately, no time is wasted over intubation at this stage. The lungs can be adequately ventilated through a facepiece and reservoir bag connected to a Boyle's machine.

4. Meanwhile, the surgeon places his right forearm under the patient's knees and his left forearm behind the patient's neck.

5. The patient's bent knees are raised and the hips fully flexed, forcing the thighs against the upper abdomen and chest, the spine being flexed at the same time. When full flexion is reached, the surgeon compresses the patient's chest with the bent knee, using some of his own weight judiciously to add to the pressure.

6. He then lowers the patient's legs, fully extending them on the operating table. At this point, the anesthetist inflates the lungs.

The maneuver is repeated twelve to fifteen times per minute. If there is no response after 1 to 1½ minutes, the chest is opened and direct cardiac massage is begun.

With widespread application of closed-chest massage for maintaining artificial circulation, adequate opportunities have been provided to evaluate this technique in the infant and young child. There seems little doubt that this technique readily lends itself to this age group, particularly since the chest wall is easily compressed, as pointed out elsewhere. Overenthusiastic use of this method with application of too much pressure can, however, easily result in complications, including rupture of the liver or spleen and fracture of the ribs.

Resuscitation of the elderly patient

Although the likelihood of fracture is increased in the relatively rigid rib cage of the elderly patient, cases of successful closed-chest massage in older persons are encountered almost daily. Iung and Wade report a 9-month follow-up on an 87-year-old man who was successfully resuscitated following cardiac arrest during surgery and on whom closed-chest massage was carried out.

Hemodynamics of closed-chest resuscitation

Systemic arterial pressure, central venous pressure, cardiac output, and arterial pressure were monitored during three cases of closed-chest cardiac massage at the University of Edinburgh (MacKenzie and others). Clinically, adequate "systolic" peak pressures were recorded during cardiac compression. In two of the patients, this systolic impulse was accompanied by a reasonable forward stroke output, but in the third patient (with a no less adequate systolic peak pressure), forward flow was negligible. The right arterial pressure tracings showed a wave-form pattern essentially similar to that recorded from the aorta. Although the mean atrial pressures were only slightly increased during thoracic compression, peak pressures of 116 and 88 mm. Hg were recorded from the atria during the phase of cardaic compression. The work of MacKenzie supports the fallacy of accepting systolic pressure pulses as indicative of proportionate forward blood flow. Table 21-1 shows the systolic peak in one patient to be six times greater during cardiac compression than during spontaneous activity, although the stroke volume and total cardiac output were reduced more than half by cardiac massage. MacKenzie questions the efficiency of external cardiac compression as demonstrated by

Table 21-1. Circulatory changes during spontaneous heart activity and external cardiac compression*

Patient	Circulatory state	Systemic arterial pressure (mm. Hg)			Cardiac output (litres per min. per sq.m.)	Heart-rate (per min.)	Stroke volume (ml. per sq.m.)	Right atrial pressure (mm. Hg)			Systemic vascular resistance (dyne sec. cm.-5 sq.m.)	Mean transit time (sec.)	Cardio-pulmonary blood volume (ml. per sq.m.)
		Sys-tolic	Dia-stolic	Mean				Max.	Min.	Mean			
A. B. Woman, age 71; height 1.67 m.; weight 62.5 kg.; surface area 1.69 sq.m.	Normal sinus rhythm	155	70	92	2.095	88	24	30	14	21	2709	32.2	1124
	External cardiac compression	143	46	57	1.300	53	25	116	11	26	1906	36.4	790
C. D. Man, age 49; height 1.75 m.; weight 74 kg.; surface area 1.88 sq.m.	Normal sinus rhythm	62	48	53	2.583	98	26	26	10	15	1176	20.5	883
	External cardiac compression	115	35	42	1.039	48	22	88	7	19	1769	82.8	1432
E. F. Woman, age 66; height 1.57 m.; weight 59 kg.; surface area 1.58 sq.m.	Normal sinus rhythm	34	21	25	0.883	68	13	†	—	19	543	36.8	541
	External cardiac compression	102	2	10	0.405	68	6	†	—	10	0	81.1	551

*From MacKenzie, G. J., and others: Haemodynamic effects of external cardiac compression, Lancet 1:1242-1245, 1964.
†Owing to over-damping of the venous catheter system, phasic pressures were not available.

cardiac output figures. Compression of the anterior thoracic cage results, he believes, in a generalized increase in intrathoracic pressure that would be expected to expel blood into the great veins outside the thorax as well as into the aorta. Large elevations in venous pressure have been demonstrated during cardiac massage. Not only is blood expelled into the great veins outside the thorax, but it is expelled from the left atrium into the thin-walled pulmonary veins. Pulmonary edema is found in some postresuscitation cases and may well be a result of vascular damage from increased pressure in a low-pressure venous system.

External cardiac massage produced systolic pressures of between 80 and 100 mm. Hg in eight cardiac arrest cases studied by Safar. On the other hand, Safar states that he has observed five patients who had no artificial pulse produced by the external compression method but who had the chest subsequently opened. Four of the five patients had an artificial pulse provoked by internal cardiac compression.

Larka and Sawyer have demonstrated in an 8-year-old boy with cardiac arrest that closed-chest cardiac compression can maintain a circulation in the Kolff twin-coil kidney. The resulting flow through the coil was sufficient to provide an adequate dialysis for at least a 2-hour period. Although the patient died, it is believed that the feasibility of adequate hemodialysis during external cardiac massage may be of value in such conditions as acute barbiturate intoxication.

CAROTID BLOOD FLOW

Cozine resuscitated ten dogs after 20 minutes of closed-chest compression in spite of the finding that carotid blood flows during the period of massage reach only 7% to 19% of the control value.

ARTERIAL PRESSURE

Nachlas and his colleagues conclude that, experimentally, arterial pressures appear to be good indicators of effective perfusion. When these exceeded values of 75/25 mm. Hg, the results were often good; when they used pressures below 50/25 mm. Hg, no animal was resuscitated.

Nachlas and associates find that when pure oxygen is delivered through an endotracheal tube, interruption of sternal compression for pulmonary ventilation is unnecessary in the dog (diffusion respiration or apneic oxygenation).

In an effort to further define the hemodynamic effects of closed-chest cardiac massage or intravascular pressure changes, Tomsen, Stenlund, and Rowe measured intracardiac pressures of the left side of the heart and systemic arterial pressures during cardiac arrest and closed-chest cardiac massage in human subjects. Values were recorded via pressure transducers on an oscillographic recording system. Mean pressures were determined by fluid dampening of the galvanometers. In their group of twelve cases of cardiac arrest, an average peak systolic pressure was 91 mm. Hg as registered in the left atrium and in the femoral artery. The average left atrial mean pressure was 55 mm. Hg, and the average femoral artery mean pressure was 60 mm. Hg. All of their cases of cardiac arrest were seen in the cardiovascular research laboratory.

In seven patients, cardiac arrest followed the injection of contrast material into the central aorta. In two patients, arrests occurred with the injection of the contrast material into the left atrium, and in two it occurred when the injection was into the left ventricle. Ventricular fibrillation occurred in one patient while a catheter was being passed from the right ventricle into the pulmonary artery. It is interesting to note that, in six patients, the heart spontaneously reverted to the prearrest arrhythmia. These workers conclude that the elevations of left arterial pressure, when transmitted to the pulmonary capillaries, contribute to the development of pulmonary edema as a relatively common complication following prolonged closed-chest massage. They further believe that, during open-chest cardiac massage, pressures can be more selectively applied to the ventricles so that pressure relationships between the atria and ventricles more closely approximate normal. This, they believe, may explain why open-chest cardiac massage is frequently found to be more effective than closed-chest massage in producing a forward blood flow.

Falsetti and Greene believe that the mean arterial pressure must be higher than 25 mm. Hg for flow to occur during cardiac resuscitation if cardiac output is to follow traditional pressure-flow relationships (flow = pressure/resistance). Their criticism of closed-chest methods is concerned with the very slight elevation in mean blood pressure associated with the brief systolic ejection spike. They find that the pulse contour is considerably different during direct cardiac massage and most nearly approaches the normal pulse wave. Falsetti and Greene are of the opinion that a satisfactory mean pressure may be obtained by a prolongation of sternal depression that prolongs the systolic phase of the pulse wave and thereby increases the mean pressure. Their data indicate that the sternum should be depressed 0.4 to 0.5 seconds.

CEREBRAL VENOUS OXYGENATION

An opportunity to study the oxygen saturation of jugular venous blood during external cardiac massage was provided in the case of a 41-year-old man who was undergoing a carotid endarterectomy. Ventricular fibrillation suddenly occurred without arrhythmias being recognized prior to the onset of fibrillation, even though the patient was being constantly monitored. Oxygen saturation of the jugular venous blood remained in excess of 80% prior to the arrest. Within less than 1 minute after the arrest, the oxygen saturation in the lateral sinus blood fell to 61%, but rose to 66% as soon as massage was started. When

massage was interrupted for attempted D.C. defibrillation, the venous oxygen saturation fell precipitously to as low as 20%. It also fell consistently when there was a change of operators. During a 6-minute period of massage, the cerebral venous saturation was maintained at 76%. The patient was never successfully defibrillated. In commenting on the case, White and Allarde estimate that neurologic deficit is unlikely if saturation of venous blood from the brain is maintained at 60% or higher. They emphasize that there is a rapid fall in cerebral venous oxygen if the massage is not consistent.

Effectiveness of closed-chest massage on cerebral circulation

The effectiveness of closed-chest massage in maintaining adequate cerebral oxygenation has been repeatedly documented. Although a report from Peter Bent Brigham Hospital in Boston recorded only eight instances of return of consciousness in sixty-five attempts at closed-chest resuscitation, Nixon recorded pressure tracings of the pulse during closed-chest massage and found that it was not difficult to produce arterial pressure pulses reaching more than 100 mm. Hg. Bernier reports a 63-year-old man with a history of repeated Adams-Stokes attacks. While in the hospital, the patient suddenly cried out and became unresponsive, pulseless, and cyanotic. Closed-chest massage was instituted and the patient soon began to move his extremities and shortly was able to answer questions. Ventricular fibrillation was present as recorded on the ECG. Closed-chest massage was continued for 35 minutes until a decision was made to do a thoracotomy for defibrillation since no closed-chest defibrillator was available. This was done under local procaine (Novocain) infiltration and successful defibrillation of the heart was achieved with a 100-volt shock. The chest was closed under local anesthesia, and throughout the procedure the patient remained conscious. One year after the cardiac arrest, the patient was working at a part-time job; no repeat episodes of Adams-Stokes attack had been experienced.

Effect of closed-chest cardiac massage on pulmonary ventilation

There is some debate as to an accurate assessment of the value of rhythmic sternal compression on artificial respiration. Most generally, it is believed to be of rather minimal value. Safar and associates at Baltimore City Hospital attempted to evaluate this feature under several different conditions. In thirty curarized patients with natural airways, no respiratory tidal exchange was produced by using closed-chest compression. The head was unsupported and probable upper airway obstruction was present. If the airway was improved with elevation of the shoulder and backward tilting of the head, some improvement in the respiratory tidal exchange occurred but was minimal. If an artificial airway was introduced, tidal volume was recorded as high as 390 ml. The faster the chest compression, the lower the tidal volume registered.

The tidal exchange was also studied in twelve patients with cardiac arrest on whom resuscitative attempts had been started with closed-chest massage and an endotracheal tube in place. Basically, no tidal exchange was detectable. Therefore it would seem that closed-chest compression should not be relied upon to produce much tidal exchange. It does seem, however, that an occasional patient has benefited in this fashion. It is possible that an adult with a more rigid chest receives less benefit than a young person.

When to start closed-chest massage

If a patient is adequately monitored and the systolic arterial pressure falls to less than 50 mm. Hg (40 mm. Hg in infants), adequate cerebral oxygenation may be questioned and closed-chest augmentation of the circulation is probably indicated.

A historical note

From a historical point of view, it is interesting to cite the work of Crile. Discussing the indirect approach to cardiac resuscitation, he divides the indirect method into (1) compression of the chest wall, (2) electrical applications to the chest wall and massage of the heart itself, and (3) the use of infusions. In discussing all of these methods, he emphasizes the necessity of continuous artificial respiration.

In discussing the first item, he states:

In dogs, the forcible rhythmic compression of the thorax over the heart by compressing the heart itself and the great vascular trunks, raises the blood-pressure to a certain extent and then thus aids its action. A mere stimulation of the first few compressions has a tendency to make the heart resume automatic action, and a feeble circulation may be maintained by the continuation of the rhythmic pressure upon the chest. If the capacity of the medullary centers be early increased by the subsequent diminution in their relative anemia, the resumption of heart activity is much more apt to be permanent. Success will be in inverse ratio to the feebleness of the heartbeat, if present, and to the duration of its inactivity, if absent.

In adults, and especially in children, something can doubtless be accomplished by forcibly activating the elastic chest wall.

With the child flat on his back, pressure should be applied at the rate of about 30 to 40 times a minute. This will also afford efficient expiration as, in the Schafer method, elasticity of the thorax will take the place of the inspiratory efforts. Care should be taken not to use too much force, although the action should be firm and vigorous. The application should continue for at least twenty minutes, or for as much longer as necessary (if a stethoscope is not at hand) so that the lack of heart action can be determined with accuracy. If no action can be detected with the stethoscope at the end of twenty minutes, there is little or no hope that the heart action will be established and, in all probability, the higher cerebral centers will long have passed any hope of recovery.

. . . even while the heart is inactive, the blood may be artificially circulated through the brain by rhythmic compression of the thorax and abdomen. This pressure is doubtless beneficient; it simultaneously produces artificial respiration and artificial circulation. It serves to supply to the brain enough oxygen to keep the slender thread of life from breaking. In artificial respiration, by the

Schafer method especially, an artificial circulation of no mean value is simultaneously produced.

It must be borne in mind that when any part of the body, but especially the chest and the abdomen, is subjected to pressure, the valves of the heart and the veins inevitably cause the blood of the veins to flow toward the heart, and the blood in the arteries to flow toward the periphery. Now this is precisely what the heart does. If, instead of a single local pressure, a series of rhythmic pressures upon the thorax and abdomen are made, the entire blood stream may be energized and moved, that is to say, the person who makes the rhythmic pressure furnishes an external pseudo-cardiac action. The author has personally been able to effect a complete circulation in a recently dead subject producing a radial pulse and bleeding of peripheral vessels, and even to make a blood pressure of measurable tension (registered by a sphygmomanometer) by the combined effort of a tightly inflated rubber suit covering the lower extremities and the abdomen and strong rhythmic pressure from the broadly extended hands applied upon each side of the chest. Indeed, the face could be made to flush and fade appreciably at will. Undoubtedly, such an excellent method as Schafer's for producing artificial respiration owes its effectiveness as much to the factor of artificial circulation as to artificial respiration. This point seems to have been missed.*

Dr. Crile first demonstrated his method of "rhythmic pressure on the chest as a means of resuscitation" before the Cleveland Medical Society at Western Reserve University Medical College.

Professor Crile cites three cases, all eventually unsuccessful, in which cardiac action was restored after closed-chest compression of the heart had been carried out. In each of these cases, epinephrine had been injected into the axillary artery during the closed-chest compression of the heart as a part of the process of artificial respiration. These cases, all encountered before 1914, represent some of the earliest recorded examples of intentional closed-chest cardiac compression.

*From Crile, G. W.: Anemia and resuscitation, New York, 1914, D. Appleton and Co., pp. 229-232. (The author is grateful to Dr. Charles S. White, Washington, D. C., for supplying a copy of this book.)

As mentioned earlier, in 1957 Rainer and Bullough first described a method of closed-chest cardiac massage and venous return augmentation in the *British Medical Journal.* Their method concerns itself primarily with the pediatric patient, and in their report they show 100% survival in eight cases of cardiac arrest. Fig. 21-11 illustrates the tech-

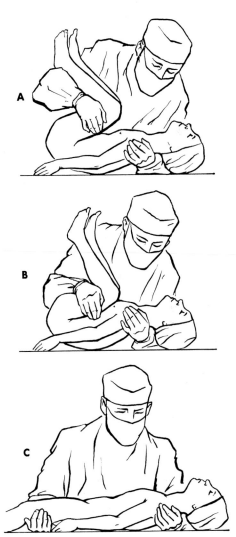

Fig. 21-11. Method of infant resuscitation suggested by Rainer and Bullough. Provides assistance to venous return, chest compression, and opportunity for rhythmic pulmonary ventilation. (From Rainer, E. H., and Bullough, J.: Br. Med. J. **2:** 1024, 1957.)

nique used. The physician places his right forearm under the patient's knee and the left forearm behind the patient's neck. The patient's flexed knees are raised and the hip fully flexed, forcing the thigh against the upper abdomen and chest. The spine is flexed at this time, also. When full flexion is reached, the bent knees are used to compress the patient's chest with the additional added pressure from the weight of the physician. Their explanation of the beneficial effect from this method consists of the following points:

1. Raising the legs causes venous blood to gravitate toward the abdomen.
2. Flexing the knees and hips squeezes venous blood out of the legs into the abdomen.
3. Pressure of the thighs on the abdomen forces blood from the abdomen into the chest, where it reaches the heart.
4. Pressure of the thighs on the chest squeezes the blood out of the chest into the periphery, the brain especially receiving some blood, being lower than the heart.
5. When the chest reexpands, release of external pressure and negative intrathoracic pressure will initiate entry of blood into the chest.

The same authors mention that their technique is not really new since Byrd described a somewhat similar method of resuscitation in asphyxia neonatorum in 1870. With this method, the obstetrician holds the supine infant in the crooks of his arms and, by compressing his whole body like a concertina and then stretching it, he actively deflates the child's lungs (and incidentally, at the same time, stimulates the circulation) before allowing the elastic recoil of the chest wall to take in air.

In the same year, both Rainer and Bullough, and Stout, at the University of Oklahoma School of Medicine, wrote on "Cardiac arrest—massage without incision." The latter technique is very much the same as the previously mentioned method. Stout recommended placing the right arm under the patient's knees, and jack-knifing the patient, thereby thrusting the knees up into the

epigastrium and onto the lower chest, actually rocking the hips off the table, with the buttocks higher than the heart. In this fashion, he believed that he would thrust a column of blood from the leg veins up through the inferior vena cava into the right auricle of the heart where the sinus node is located, stretching the right auricle and forcing blood into the right ventricle through the tricuspid valve. By using a knee-pumping action, pressing the knees together and the thigh muscles against the abdomen and lower chest, and then relaxing the knees to horizontal position, one can continue the knee-pumping action at a rate of sixty or more times per minute.

Barrett, a psychiatrist, describes an alternate method of external cardiac massage that he believes to be a simple method applicable to persons with weak abdominal walls. The patient had experienced a cardiac arrest following electroshock therapy. It was observed that the patient had a very thin abdominal wall and "cardiac massage" was attempted by pushing the hand well up under the left costal margin and rhythmically pushing and squeezing. The heartbeat returned after a few such maneuvers, and the patient recovered uneventfully.

It is said that the Japanese samurai, centuries ago, developed rather refined resuscitative techniques for posttraumatic syncope. This method, Kuatsu or "life technique," was passed down from teacher to student by word of mouth. It involves precordial compression, indirect pressure via the epigastric transdiaphragmatic route, and dorsal percussion.

Cardiopulmonary resuscitation by a single individual

When cardiac arrest occurs outside the hospital, emergency ventilation of the victim as well as closed-chest compression will need to be carried out simultaneously (Fig. 21-12). Adequate, although not ideal, resuscitation may be possible. In such in-

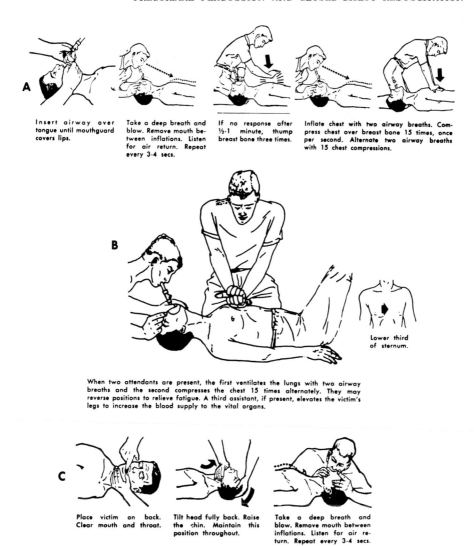

A, **Insert airway over tongue until mouthguard covers lips.** **Take a deep breath and blow. Remove mouth between inflations. Listen for air return. Repeat every 3-4 secs.** **If no response after ½-1 minute, thump breast bone three times.** **Inflate chest with two airway breaths. Compress chest over breast bone 15 times, once per second. Alternate two airway breaths with 15 chest compressions.**

B, Lower third of sternum.

When two attendants are present, the first ventilates the lungs with two airway breaths and the second compresses the chest 15 times alternately. They may reverse positions to relieve fatigue. A third assistant, if present, elevates the victim's legs to increase the blood supply to the vital organs.

C, **Place victim on back. Clear mouth and throat.** **Tilt head fully back. Raise the chin. Maintain this position throughout.** **Take a deep breath and blow. Remove mouth between inflations. Listen for air return. Repeat every 3-4 secs.**

Fig. 21-12. **A,** Artificial respiration and artificial circulation by trained rescuer; **B,** emergency resuscitation when two or more attendants are present; **C,** artificial respiration by the chance rescuer. (From Brook, J., and others: Can. Med. Assoc. J. **93:**387, 1965.)

stances, attention should first be directed to respiratory ventilation by either mouth-to-mouth or mouth-to-nose techniques. After an initial period of rapid hyperventilation for three or four excursions, the resuscitator should execute fifteen chest compressions followed by two full lung inflations. Chest compression should be at the rate of eighty per minute.

If an airway such as an S tube is available, the operator will find it considerably easier to switch rapidly from ventilatory efforts to those of cardiac compression.

Fig. 21-13, *A,* illustrates a method for providing artificial respiration and at the same time having one's hands free to aid in transportation of the patient. Greene and co-workers, in describing the expired air ventilator, state that it may be used with an oronasal mask, tracheal tube, or tracheotomy. Expired air ventilation consists of using a simple mouthpiece and a special

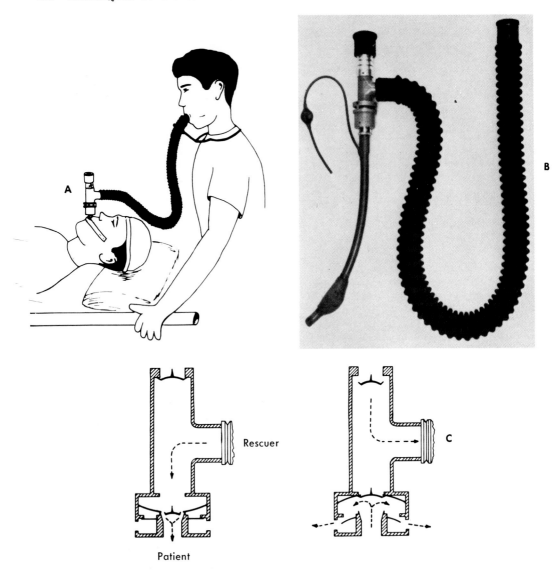

Fig. 21-13. **A**, Expired air ventilator that facilitates resuscitation by single operator and transportation of patient by ambulance, elevator, or hospital cart; **B**, expired air ventilator connected to an endotracheal tube; **C**, diagram of the valve assemblies: left, inflation; right, passive expiration. (From Greene, D. G., and others: Am. J. Surg. **97**:407, 1959.)

three-way valve connected by a flexible tube of about 300 ml. volume (Fig. 21-13, *B*). The use of a 300 ml. dead space in the apparatus helps to provide excellent gas exchange. One of the physicians at the University of Missouri Medical Center (Dyer) has been interested in the use of an

expired air ventilator for situations requiring both closed-chest resuscitation and ventilation by a single operator.

Effectiveness of resuscitation efforts

If one is not successful in providing enough cerebral oxygenation to constrict the

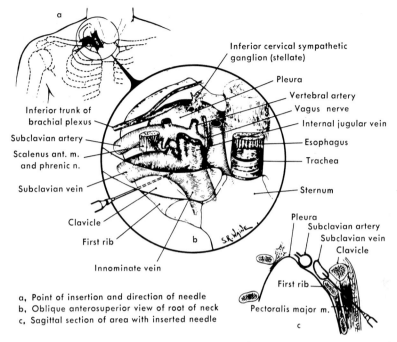

a, Point of insertion and direction of needle
b, Oblique anterosuperior view of root of neck
c, Sagittal section of area with inserted needle

Fig. 21-14. Technique for subclavian venipuncture. Patient lies flat on his back, with the head facing forward. Needle is inserted immediately below clavicle at the junction of its middle and medial thirds (*a* and *b*). Needle is directed backward, inward, and slightly upward to a point where subclavian, internal jugular, and innominate veins join (*c*). Negative pressure is applied through syringe attached to the needle until free flow of venous blood occurs. After blood return occurs, syringe is disengaged and a sterile plastic cannula is passed through the needle into the vein. Needle is then withdrawn. (From Davidson, D., and others: Lancet 2:1139, 1963.)

dilated pupils, it is doubtful that cardiopulmonary resuscitative efforts are adequate. Even if readily palpated with each sternal compression, presence of a femoral, radial, or carotid pulse may be misleading in that it may represent transmitted pulsation rather than effective circulation. Should spontaneous respirations return during resuscitative efforts, one can be encouraged that one's efforts are probably adequate. Occasionally, of course, the patient will regain consciousness and speak, even though spontaneous cardiac activity has not returned.

Establishment of an intravenous route

The usual site for inserting a needle or catheter into a vein during cardiopulmonary resuscitation is at a cutdown in the greater saphenous vein just anterior to the medial malleolus of the ankle. Ideally, a catheter should be introduced directly into the vein and anchored securely.

A cutdown on an ankle vein is a satisfactory manner of obtaining an intravenous route for immediate delivery of drugs to the heart and body tissues. Venotomy does require valuable time; and, because external cardiac massage produces a poor blood flow at best, a more rapid route for drug injection may sometimes be needed. A peripheral venipuncture with a sufficiently large needle is not usually possible, because of the collapse of the patient's veins. The intracardiac injection rate interferes with closed-chest resuscitation, and it is difficult to perform repeatedly over a short period of time.

SUBCLAVIAN CATHETERS

Bergman and Aazon advocate the use of subclavian catheter insertions in all cardiac arrests. In a series of twenty-two cardiac arrest patients, twelve were resuscitated with nine eventually being discharged from the hospital. In all twenty-two patients subclavian catheter was used. Bergman and Aazon believe that the catheter insertion via the infraclavicular route can be accomplished in nearly all cases within 1 to 2 minutes without interruption of closed-chest cardiac compression or artificial resuscitation measures. They suspect that on several occasions the catheter may have directly stimulated the myocardium and was thus a factor in establishing a sinus rhythm. In addition, any lag in effect of cardiotonic drugs because of peripheral flow deficit from cardiogenic shock is eliminated by the subclavian catheter route. Their technique is as follows: a patient is placed in a slightly head-down position with the head inverted. A 1 ml. tuberculin syringe is connected to a 14-gauge needle and is inserted approximately at the midclavicular line. The needle is advanced immediately, slightly cephalad in the direction of the suprasternal notch at a 15 to 20 degree angle to the long axis of the clavicle. Then the needle is advanced to a point beneath the posterior head of the clavicle, maintaining a position close to the chest wall while slightly negative pressure is maintained within the syringe. When venous blood is obtained, the catheter is rapidly advanced and the needle can then be removed.

Intracardiac puncture

Intracardiac puncture through the unopened chest has been a common practice in cases of suspected cardiac arrest, and beneficial results have been attributed to the procedure. Although there may be cases of helpful mechanical stimulus caused by the needle prick, injected drugs are likely to be ineffectually pooled within the lumen of the injected chamber unless adequate closed-chest massage is used.

Preferably, intracardiac injections should be avoided if there is any alternative. Intracardiac needling is, at best, a blind technique. Laceration of a coronary vessel or a tear of the myocardium, while not common, may result. In addition, closed-chest massage must be discontinued while intracardiac needling is taking place. Nevertheless, this approach remains the quickest way to administer epinephrine if a venous approach is not available.

Chapter 22

ADJUNCTS FOR CIRCULATORY ASSISTANCE

Substernal cardiac massage and assistance

In 1968 Johnson, Prisk, and Whitney published a description of their technique for a substernal method of cardiac massage and assistance. They considered their technique a closed method of cardiac massage and assistance, except that the physical forces required are not exerted externally but substernally. As illustrated in Fig. 22-1, a small, 1-inch stab wound is made at the tip of the xiphoid into the peritoneal cavity. A specially designed, curved, substernal trocar is introduced into the wound and is manipulated beneath the sternum into the anterior mediastinum or into the pericardial space. The obturator from the trocar is subsequently removed, and a conical-shaped, plastic balloon on a catheter is passed into the lumen of the trocar and on into the anterior mediastinum or directly into the pericardial sac. The trocar is then removed, and the plastic balloon-catheter massager and assister is then connected directly to a cyclic pneumatic pulsator. (The pulsator consists of an air compressor, a volume regulating device, and a special solenoid operated spool valve. The spool valve is operated by an electronic control unit. See Fig. 22-2.) The pulsator controls the rate and duration of the massaging and synchronizes the massaging with the systolic contraction of the heart by keying with a QRS complex of the patient's ECG should the heart alone be needing assistance. These authors state that they can insert the device and begin the massaging within 1 minute.

In the experimental animal, mean arterial pressures of 45 to 60 mm. Hg were recorded.

The device was tested on sixty cadavers in the necropsy room. This experience indicated that the trocar could be inserted directly into the anterior mediastinum without injury to the surrounding anatomic structures or directly into the pericardial sac without injury to the heart. Circulation pressures higher than 200 mm. Hg were recorded with flow rates of more than 6 liters per minute.

So far, only limited clinical experience has been recorded. After conventional methods of cardiac resuscitation had failed, three of the seven patients in cardiac arrest tested were converted to sinus rhythm. In one patient, assistance of the failing heart was maintained for 31 hours.

Johnson and co-workers list four indications for the use of their device:

1. Unresponsive resuscitation efforts after 5 minutes of external cardiac massage
2. Prophylactic placement in the pericardial sac following open-heart surgery
3. In the assistance of the heart in patients with acute myocardial infarction who develop arrhythmias and subsequent failure with no response to drug therapy
4. Immediately after death to preserve organs for transplant

Value of the Trendelenburg position

During cardiac arrest, it is extremely important that all residual oxygen in the blood be available to the vital centers, particularly the brain. For this reason, I recommend that the patient be placed in a head-down position immediately upon diagnosis of cardiac arrest. Gaghon and Telmosse state that, in their experimental work, the Trendelenburg position (10 to 15 degrees) is the op-

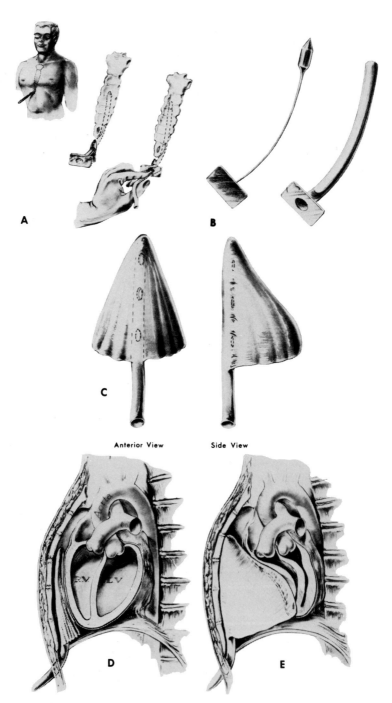

Fig. 22-1. Technique for substernal cardiac massage and assistance. **A,** Technique for insertion of balloon. **B,** Insertion instruments (trocar and cannula). **C,** Massaging balloon. **D,** Balloon deflating while heart is filling. **E,** Balloon inflated, forcing blood from heart. (From Johnson, Prisk, and Whitney, and General Motors Research Laboratories, Warren, Mich.)

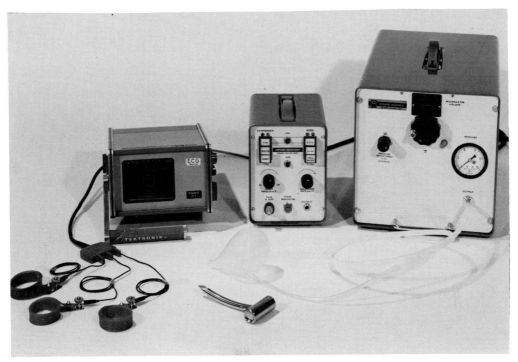

Fig. 22-2. Equipment for substernal cardiac massage and assistance. (Courtesy General Motors Research Laboratories, Warren, Mich.)

timal position at the onset of cardiac arrest. It may be that this measure is effective only for a relatively short time.

Brierley emphasizes that postural hypotension may contribute to brain damage under general as well as local anesthesia. The normal cerebral blood flow is reduced to a critical level when the blood pressure falls below 50 mm. Hg systolic, particularly if this is a sudden and prolonged occurrence. Elevating the head of the patient increases the likelihood of brain damage during episodes of severe hypotension, that is, during cardiopulmonary resuscitation.

Cole reported on his work relative to the beneficial effect of the Trendelenburg position. He believed the restorative action of head lowering results, in part at least, from an actual, significant, rapid, demonstrable, and consistent increase in the blood pressure in the upper extremities and, undoubtedly, in the brain. From this study he concluded that increased oxygenation of the vital

centers, including the brain, is accomplished in the presence of low arterial pressure, when gravity is allowed to aid rather than hinder the work of the heart.

According to Engel, a period of 4 to 8 seconds of asystole will produce coma when patients with Adams-Stokes syndrome are in the erect position. If the patient is recumbent at the time of the attack, 12 to 15 seconds are required before coma develops.

Therefore, to stretch that delicate period between reversibility and irreversibility of cerebral cortical activity, I feel that the Trendelenburg procedure should be employed as a worthwhile adjunct.

Even while the patient is being placed in Trendelenburg position and during efforts at effective artificial respiration, preparations should be under way for artificially maintaining the circulation by intermittent manual compression of the heart, either by the closed-chest or open-chest approach.

One advantage of the Trendelenburg

position, particularly as it applies to the closed-chest resuscitation technique, is that it tends to prevent aspiration of vomitus and gastric contents following pressure on the sternum and, in some instances, on the epigastrium.

The argument against the Trendelenburg position has been seriously considered by Guntheroth, a pediatric cardiologist at the University of Washington in Seattle. In a personal communication, he stated his belief that the common error in thinking about cerebral blood flow has been the assumption that gravity could assist in perfusion. Since the cerebral circulation is essentially a rigid V tube, Guntheroth believes any additional pressure added on the input must be substracted on the output side, and the net driving force across the cerebral vascular bed would be unchanged by position.

Guntheroth further emphasizes that the theoretical advantage of increased venous return from the lower part of the body is obviously nullified by other factors. The slight increase in arterial blood pressure may be secondary to interference with the respiratory pump, or it may be due to the carotid baroreceptors "interrupting" the total intravascular pressure at that site as representative of the general *vis a tergo*.

Pulmonary ventilation is adversely affected by an increased workload of ventilation, decreased vital capacity, and uneven ventilation. In addition, a definite, although slight, vasodilatation results in a decreased mean aortic pressure and a very slight decrease in cerebral blood flow. A study done by Weil at the Los Angeles County Hospital revealed a lower survival rate in a group of rats kept in a head-down position following severe hemorrhage than in a group kept in a horizontal position. Weil questions the value of the Trendelenburg position for treatment of hypotension resulting from bacterial infection, endotoxin, hypersensitivity, or depression of neural control.

Milstein, in his excellent monograph on cardiac arrest, makes a plea for the recumbent position for any patient with any condition of a hypotension state. It is the decreased venous return to the heart that may prevent recovery from an otherwise relatively benign episode of syncope. Otherwise, cardiac output may be so altered that a progressive and fatal sequence will follow. Elderly patients are sometimes found dead strapped into their wheelchairs. It is thought that some of these cases originally represent a simple fainting episode. Cardiac arrest has been reported on the myelographic tilt table (Cooper). Patients with poor muscular tone react poorly to a sudden upright position. MacLean voiced the belief 20 years ago that the margin between adequacy and incompetence is so narrow that, when man stands erect without moving, he hovers on the verge of circulatory collapse.

The value of a 10 to 15 degree head-down position, used either when an arrested circulation is suspected or in the immediate resuscitation period, must not be confused with the apparent failure of the Trendelenburg position to improve circulation during clinical shock when the head-down position is maintained for protracted periods.

One of the advantages of the Trendelenburg position, admittedly a rare one, is in cases of suspected air emboli (left-sided air emboli).

Taylor and Weil emphasize other potential complications of the head-down position as a routine use in shock patients. In addition to the increased impingement against the diaphragm by the viscera and subsequent reduction in vital capacity, the risk of increased cerebral edema should be mentioned. At Duke University, studies were done to determine the effect of a head-down position during hypotension in ten male baboons. Tindall and associates, in reporting this work, conclude that tilting the primates to a 10 degree head-down position produces a significant increase in internal carotid artery blood flow, as well as an increase in mean arterial pressure, presumably due to increased cardiac output. When norepinephrine was intravenously administered to the hypotensive, hypovolemic baboons, there was a substantial increase in the internal carotid artery blood flow in the head-down position. They conclude that the 10 degree head-down position is a useful adjunct to the treatment of hypovolemic hypotension and should not be abandoned.

Venous filling of the heart and the "Woodward maneuver"

In a consideration of cardiac resuscitation, concern with the venous return to the heart has usually been assigned a rather secondary role. However, it is frequently noted that the filling of the heart appears quite inadequate, even in resuscitative attempts on patients whose circulating blood volume has not been appreciably depleted. If cardiac arrest has been present for more than a few minutes, considerable cooling takes place, and marked peripheral dilatation will have occurred. Both may have taken place even prior to the arrest. In such instances, the output from the heart, with manual intermittent compression or with the closed-chest approach, is inadequate, and a cycle is set up that perpetuates this inadequacy. Unfortunately, the closed-chest method of massage does not allow as adequate an appraisal of the venous filling of the heart as does the direct approach. In general, however, it may be assumed that the venous filling is not normal.

Woodward, in Australia, has repeatedly emphasized the beneficial effect on the venous return to the heart caused by elevation of the patient's lower extremities. Compression of the lower extremities by Esmarch bandages applied from the feet to the groin may accomplish the same purpose, although there is always the disadvantage of the time required for bandaging. The effectiveness of simple elevation of the limbs into the vertical position has been demonstrated on several occasions. Wood-

ward has observed four instances of cardiac pulsations returning in the arrested heart after elevation of the extremities. In all four cases, the heart was being observed directly through the opened thorax.

The mechanism allowing this desired effect is somewhat speculative. Woodward suggests that the rush of blood into the large veins depresses vagal tone by a Bainbridge-like reflex that will allow the inhibited heart to escape the vagus. Furthermore, he suggests that this sudden augmentation of venous refilling of the heart may produce its desired effect by stretching the cardiac fibers. While this is an adjunct for venous refill of the heart, an important contribution is also apparently made by recoil of the chest wall after manual compression, thus increasing negative pressure within the thorax. Venous pressure itself probably accounts for the bulk of the venous return.

Woodward, in 1952, encountered a case of cardiac arrest in a 4-year-old boy. The patient was being operated upon for reduction of multiple fractures of the left hand. During intermittent compression of the heart, Woodward was unable to restore normal cardiac rhythm successfully, and he attributed part of his failure to the fact that the heart felt small and empty. However, when the patient's legs were held vertically and Esmarch bandages were applied from the toes to the trunk, the heart was immediately felt to enlarge twice its previous volume or more. He noted that as soon as it filled, the heart began to beat. He also applied Esmarch bandages to the arm from the fingers to the shoulders and again noted some increased filling of the heart. I have used this method both in the animal laboratory and clinically. I agree that this adjunct may be particularly beneficial when cardiac refill seems grossly inadequate. Woodward has continued his interest in the beneficial effect achieved by elevation of the limbs in cardiac arrest. He suggests that elevation of the unbandaged extremities be carried out immediately upon recognition of cardiac arrest.

With elevation of the legs, venous return is increased by making as much as 1,000 ml. of additional blood available. The stretching effect of distending the right atrium or right ventricle may, in itself, provoke a heartbeat on the basis of Starling's law of contractility of the heart.

Negovskii estimates that about one fifth of the blood volume may be mobilized by raising the legs in man. Silber showed an increase in the volume of the circulating blood by 500 to 1,000 ml. by raising the legs of anesthesized adult subjects.

In addition to the procedures just mentioned, the venous return to the circulation may be improved if generalized vasoconstrictors are administered. Fowler emphasizes the futility of cardiac massage in those instances when venous return to the heart is clearly inadequate. He observes a dramatic response to the use of Esmarch bandages applied to the lower extremities in such a case.

Sjostrand, in 1953, demonstrated that more than 600 ml. of blood can be added

to the venous return of the heart in the adult by placing the patient in a leg-up position. Maass describes the application of rubber bandages to both legs in one of his cases of cardiac arrest successfully treated in December, 1891.

In many cases of cardiac arrest, one may find it to advantage to wrap the extremities with elastic bandages. This assumes, of course, that adequate personnel are available. Pike and his co-workers had commented as early as 1908 on the beneficial effect of bandaging the limbs and the abdomen when the venous return was too low for satisfactory filling of the heart.

Cardiac arrest and pulmonary edema

The combination of pulmonary edema complicated by cardiac arrest should not be considered a contraindication to resuscitative procedure; successful resuscitation is possible. Stannard and Rigo have reviewed resuscitation attempts in patients with acute pulmonary edema and strongly recommend that resuscitation should be attempted in such instances. In addition to the usual methods of resuscitation, venesection and

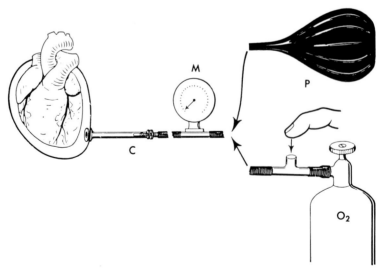

Fig. 22-3. Cannula used for pneumomassage in position and ready for use. (From Bencini, A., and Parola, P. L.: Surgery **39**:375, 1956.)

the use of rotating tourniquets may be of great help.

Mechanical devices for direct and indirect cardiac massage

In spite of the ease with which cardiac massage can be carried out without the use of special instruments and in spite of its application to all types of circulatory arrest, a number of approaches to the problem of artificial maintenance of the blood flow through the vascular system have been considered. At Western Reserve University, "suction" cup applicators have been available for use for some time as a means of compressing the cardiac musculature. Bencini and Parola have experimented with a method that they term "pneumomassage." This method embodies the rhythmic insufflation of gas into the pericardial cavity, taking advantage of the relative inelasticity of the pericardial sac. Compression of the heart occurs as a result of the increased pressure in the pericardial cavity. They find that the pressure necessary to compress the heart is considerably less than needed to rupture the pericardial sac.

Their apparatus consists of a cannula that is introduced via a small hole in the pericardium and held in place by a screw device (Fig. 22-3). By means of an elastic rubber ball or an oxygen tank with a double outflow tract, intermittent compression can be accomplished. The endopericardial pressure is allowed to vary between 0 and 140 to 160 mm. Hg. They find that higher pressures do not result in further increases of the maximal blood pressure as usually maintained by an endopericardial blood pressure of 100 mm. Hg. They do not feel that reflux into the vena cava is alarming or that the coronary circulation is impaired.

Additional work embodying the principle of pneumomassage of the heart has been done in the Department of Surgery at the University of Chicago (Jones and co-workers). By maintaining a positive pres-

sure phase within the pericardial sac of 120 mm. Hg. at 60 to 70 cycles per minute, adequate systemic pressures can be maintained in the dog. The average systolic systemic pressure is 64 mm. Hg. Pressures in the inferior vena cava average 14/2 to 50/5, which is considerably elevated over the normal range. In addition, Jones and associates employ mechanical heart compression by intermittent inflation of a balloon placed behind the left ventricle and within the pericardial sac. Air pressure is intermittently delivered to the balloon at around 250 mm. Hg. at 60 cycles per minute, which means systolic systemic pressures near 80 mm. Hg. A similar technique is employed using a mantled balloon placed behind the left ventricle, with pressures in the balloon ranging from 450 to 500 mm. Hg. Similar systemic artery pressures are recorded. In all instances the systemic pressure is higher than that which can be produced with manual cardiac compression (Fig. 22-4).

Although compression of the heart by pneumomassage through the open chest is not considered particularly practical at present, certain desirable features are, nevertheless, provided. Adams and his group at Chicago point out that mechanical compression of the heart does allow a constant pressure in the systemic circulation that is in contrast with a rather variable pressure with manual massage. In addition, these methods appear to be less traumatic to the myocardium and thus they allow a prolonged period of compression and may give possible assistance, if needed, after cardiac resuscitation.

A mechanical heart massager designed by Wolcott and Wherry utilizes a rather simple pneumatic cuff that can be applied to the heart and with which alternate negative and positive pressures allow the heart to be alternately compressed and expanded. Vineberg describes a mechanical heart massager with a somewhat similar, though more intricate, construction.

A closed-chest heart-lung machine has

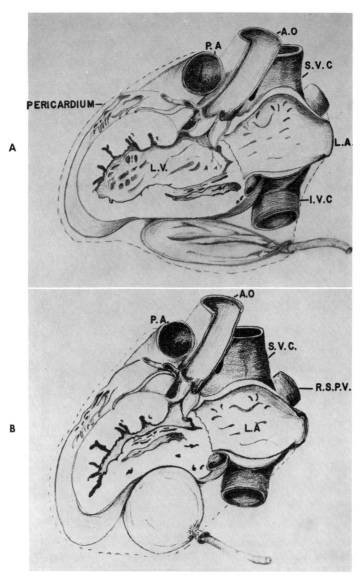

Fig. 22-4. Mechanical means of producing artificial systole using intrapericardial balloon. **A,** Mantled balloon in diastolic phase behind left ventricle within pericardial sac. **B,** Mantled balloon in systolic phase (inflated) behind left ventricle within pericardial sac. Note selective compression of left ventricle. *L.A.,* Left auricle; *L.V.,* left ventricle; *A.O.,* aorta; *P.A.,* pulmonary artery. (From Jones, G. A., and others: Dis. Chest **39**:207, 1961.)

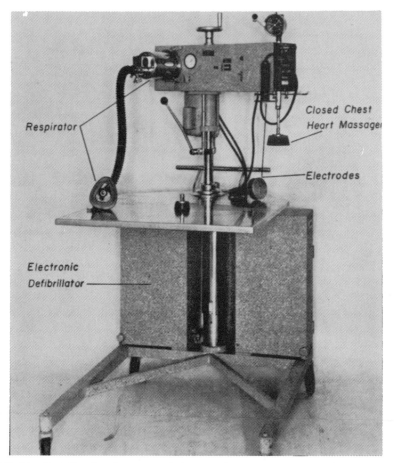

Fig. 22-5. The Beck-Rand unit for closed-chest cardiopulmonary resuscitation. (From Hosler, R. M.: Biochem. Clin. 1:327, 1963.)

been introduced by Beck and Rand (Fig. 22-5). It compresses the heart by rhythmically applying pressure of a selected amount upon the proper area of the sternum. A synchronizing mechanism operates a device that forces air into the trachea at the correct time.

A further refinement in the mechanization of massage has been introduced by Harkins and Bramson. It is an apparatus that can be used for imposed systole but also may assist the failing heart by synchronization in such a way that it automatically follows in and out of the weak systole. Assisted circulation is further discussed in other parts of this book.

The CardiO$_2$ external cardiac compressor (Fig. 22-6) can duplicate the best manual technique, and, unlike the physician, it is not subject to fatigue or varied effectiveness. The compressor is cycled at 60 compressions per minute. The pressure-limited ventilator is automatically synchronized to deliver full volume ventilation during every fifth diastolic cycle of the compressor. The unit features simplified controls and has many built-in safety features. Other types of mechanical heart-lung resuscitators are shown in Figs. 22-7 and 22-8. A portable hand pump is shown in Fig. 22-9.

The effectiveness of various machines for

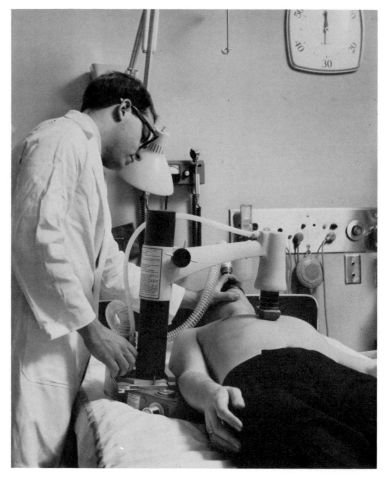

Fig. 22-6. CardiO₂ external cardiac compressor. (Courtesy Corbin-Farnsworth Division of Smith, Kline & French Instruments, Inc., Palo Alto, Calif.)

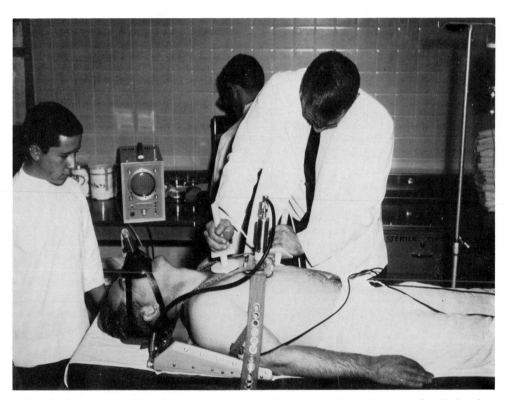

Fig. 22-7. Example of heart-lung resuscitator applied to a patient. Note that debrillation is being carried out with an external D.C. debrillator. (Courtesy Travenol Laboratories, Morton Grove, Ill.)

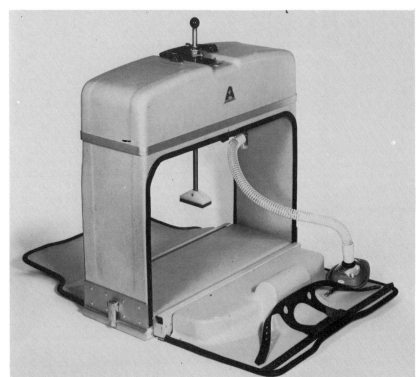

Fig. 22-8

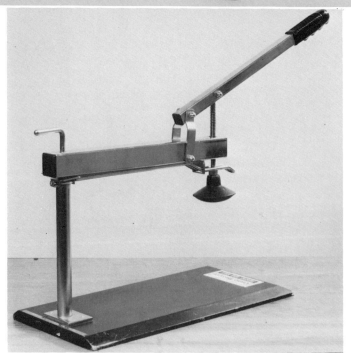

Fig. 22-9

Fig. 22-8. Heart Reactivator. (Courtesy American Safety Equipment Corp., New York.)
Fig. 22-9. Portable hand pump for external cardiac massage designed by Dr. James J. Lally. The plunger can be adjusted according to size of the individual.

external heart massage has not been universally accepted. Wolcott was able to achieve 100% survival in dogs using such a device after 30 minutes of ventricular fibrillation. Using this device, cardiac output was only one third of normal, and pulmonary edema was the main cause of death in dogs massaged for 1 to 2 hours (due to selective right over left heart emptying). No evidence of pulmonary congestion, however, was encountered in seven human patients massaged from 1 to 8 hours.

Although such mechanical devices may not receive widespread utilization, they do provide certain inherent advantages. Greater uniformity of compression is provided than will be experienced among different physicians in their varying ability to massage the heart. Structural damage to the heart may be decreased. The exhausting effort by the operator can be avoided. The operator can be free for attention to other aspects of resuscitation. Last, the advantages of coordinated assist to the heart may be considerable.

Chapter 23

ARTIFICIAL MAINTENANCE OF CIRCULATION: OPEN-CHEST RESUSCITATION

Although several approaches can be used, the thoracic approach for cardiac massage is the method of choice. The advantages of the thoracotomy exposure include the following:

1. Direct visualization of the heart is possible with a more accurate estimation of the heart's activity.
2. The thoracic exposure allows easy application of the electrodes for electrical defibrillation.
3. Drugs need not be injected blindly but can be accurately injected into the lumen for which they are intended, thereby avoiding the coronary vessels.
4. The pericardial sac, which may need to be opened, can be easily approached. The phrenic nerve is less likely to be severed.
5. Manual massage through a thoracotomy incision allows for a more adequate cardiac output and subsequently less likelihood of irreversible cerebral damage. Clinical experience as well as repeated work on dogs has convinced us that proper massage should maintain a circulation only slightly below the normal level.
6. The aorta can be pinched off, with the fingers or with the rubber-shod clamp, just beyond the origin of the great vessels, and thus more blood will be shunted into the cerebral and coronary circulations.
7. The procedure can be accomplished within a matter of seconds.

Subdiaphragmatic route

As late as 1948 the subdiaphragmatic route for massage of a heart in asystole was still recommended by many authors. That this method has been effective in the past is true; nevertheless, with the stakes so high, it is imperative that the method most likely to succeed in supplying adequate oxygen for an anoxic brain be used. Clinical and laboratory data heavily support this thoracic route.

Some years ago Bost suggested that the heart be approached through the diaphragm by separation of the diaphragm from its insertion to the ribs by a 2-inch transverse incision. The hand is then placed into the left thoracic cavity and the heart massaged through the intact pericardium. He believed this method opens up an easier route of access to the heart and that the hand, in plugging the diaphragmatic opening, usually will prevent pneumothorax.

In summary, there are few instances when direct cardiac resuscitation is elected that the thoracic approach to the heart will not be superior to others. It is possible that in cases of pulmonary tuberculosis there would be some advantage in massage by the subdiaphragmatic route.

A subcostal approach to the heart

In 1964 Fitzgerald, department of anatomy, University College, Cork, Ireland, gave added encouragement to use of the subcostal approach to the heart in cardiac arrest. As he emphasizes, the procedure requires no more than a sharp knife and knowledge of the appropriate anatomy. Fitzgerald's approach takes advantage of the heretofore poorly realized knowledge that there is an actual continuity between the anterior portions of the transversalis layer and the sternal costal portion of the diaphragm. In the dissecting room it can be demonstrated that the anterior sheath of

310

the rectus as well as the rectus muscle can be detached from its costal cartilage at the insertion, leaving the posterior sheath intact. Two fingers can be pushed upward along the posterior rectus sheath under the costal margin and onto the thoracic surface of the diaphragm without causing a break in continuity between the sheath of the rectus and the diaphragm itself.

Therefore, to reach the heart rapidly, the left rectus can be incised transversally along the costal margin until the posterior rectus sheath is reached. Two fingers can then be inserted between the xiphosternum and the left costal margin and the posterior layer of the rectus, and the diaphragm can be pushed backward from the sternal and costal margins. The fingers then slide readily onto the thoracic surface of the diaphragm from which the heart can be approached easily.

Approach during abdominal operation

The question is often asked: "If I am operating in the abdomen at the time of cardiac arrest, should I try the subdia-phragmatic route?" My answer is that the surgeon should first place his hand under the diaphragm beneath the heart and try massage. Occasionally just the mechanical stimulus (as may occur with a sudden, forceful precordial blow) will be sufficient to restore heart action. In the meantime, the assistant should make a thoracic incision as described and prepare for exposure via the transthoracic approach. Closed-chest compression is preferred by some at this point. Survival figures are not yet conclusive.

The incision

Individual variations will occur, but in the majority of cases the fourth intercostal space on the left side offers the most satisfactory approach for manual massage of the heart (Fig. 23-1, *A*). Time need not be taken, however, to count the rib spaces, since an incision just beneath the nipple in the male or along the lower margin of the breast in the female will be satisfactory. Beginning near the midline just to the left of the sternum, the incision should sweep

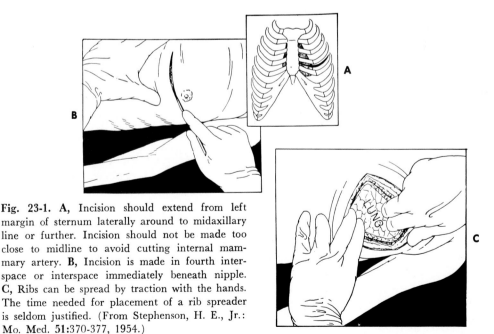

Fig. 23-1. **A,** Incision should extend from left margin of sternum laterally around to midaxillary line or further. Incision should not be made too close to midline to avoid cutting internal mammary artery. **B,** Incision is made in fourth interspace or interspace immediately beneath nipple. **C,** Ribs can be spread by traction with the hands. The time needed for placement of a rib spreader is seldom justified. (From Stephenson, H. E., Jr.: Mo. Med. **51:**370-377, 1954.)

laterally in the interspace and should penetrate the skin and subcutaneous tissue on the first sweep. Laterally the incision should extend liberally, going as far as the midaxillary line. Within the next several seconds, the hand can be on the heart and artificial maintenance of circulation begun.

To allow manual massage, the interspace must be spread. This can be done easily, as noted in Fig. 23-1, *C*. In an elderly person there is more rigidity of the rib cage and the adjacent ribs occasionally may be fractured. If a rib cutter is available, the distal rib can be severed. This latter step should wait till the actual massage has been instituted, however. Massage through an interspace in an infant or child is relatively simple because of the elasticity of the rib cage. Due precaution is indicated to prevent rib fracture since such damage may contribute to a laceration of the lung or even a laceration of the myocardium during either manual massage or electrical defibrillation of the heart.

RIGHT-SIDED CHEST INCISION

Although the heart can obviously be approached through the left intercostal incision in the fourth interspace, there will be occasions when an incision in the right chest may be elected. Tuberculosis involving the left lung or extensive left-sided pleural disease, for example, would influence one toward an incision on the right side, and, if properly carried out, it is likely that cardiac massage would be successful. However, I have had no clinical experience with the right chest incision. Maurer states that, due to the previously mentioned circumstances, he has been forced to enter the right side of the chest for cardiac resuscitation and has found it adequate, although the left ventricle is not as readily accessible.

Opening the pericardium

If closed-chest resuscitation is not elected and the transthoracic approach is used for cardiac resuscitation, the question of whether to open the pericardial sac arises. In general, the following policy has been carried out. I do not routinely open the pericardial sac. To open the pericardium at the onset is to delay the beginning of cardiac compression by several seconds and thus increase the risk of irreversible cerebral damage at this most critical stage. Physicians who are not familiar with the anatomy of the pericardial sac will often delay considerably before entrance has been gained. In a majority of cases the myocardium can be visualized and its status evaluated through the intact pericardium.

Once cardiac arrest has been diagnosed and the chest incision made, artificial circulation should be attempted immediately by compression of the heart through the intact pericardium. Opening the pericardium only increases the risk of added complications, especially if the physician is inexperienced. The myocardium or a coronary vessel may be injured, the left phrenic nerve may be cut by mistake, and, if there has been previous disease of the pericardium, adhesions may be present.

In my opinion, the pericardium should be opened under the following conditions:

1. When a diagnosis of ventricular fibrillation is made, the pericardial sac should be incised to allow direct application of electrodes for electrical defibrillation. It is true that defibrillation is possible through the intact pericardial sac. I have successfully accomplished defibrillation on several occasions without opening the pericardial sac, but at present I still believe that it is desirable to open the pericardium and apply the electrodes directly to the epicardium.
2. The pericardial sac should be opened in all cases in which ventricular fibrillation is suspected but cannot be definitely diagnosed because of inability to visualize the myocardium through the intact pericardium. In elderly patients the pericardium may often be thickened sufficiently to prevent visualization. Previous pericardial disease will present a similar situation.
3. In young infants I have found it necessary to open the pericardial sac in most cases.

This is necessitated by the diaphragmatic attachments of the pericardial sac which make adequate compression of the heart difficult.

4. Should rupture of the heart occur, then it will be necessary, of course, to open the pericardium if an attempt is to be made to repair the myocardial tear. (Fig. 23-2 illustrates the correct procedure.)

There are several advantages to leaving the pericardial sac unopened, some of which are as follows:

1. Within the pericardial sac there will usually be about 15 ml. of pericardial fluid. This acts as a lubricant during compression of the heart and minimizes the degree of trauma to the myocardium.

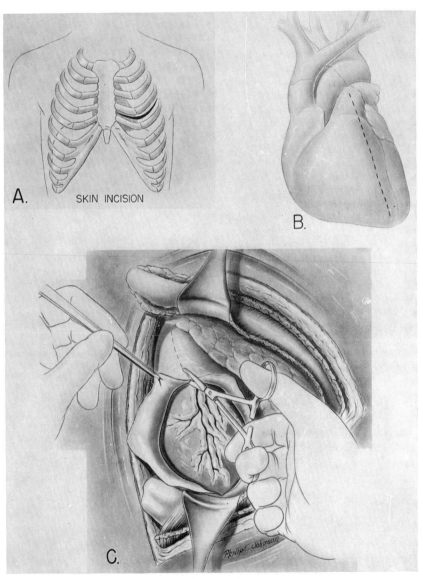

Fig. 23-2. In opening the pericardium, care should be taken to avoid left phrenic nerve. Coronary vessels can also be easily damaged unless caution is observed. **A,** Skin incision. **B,** Dotted line indicates where pericardium should be incised. **C,** Retractors placed and incision made. (From Stephenson, H. E., Jr., Reid, L. C., and Hinton, J. W.: Arch. Surg. 69:37, 1954.)

2. The incidence of traumatic rupture of the right ventricle by prolonged pressure with the compressing fingers is much greater when the pericardial sac is opened. I am aware of at least ten cases of traumatic rupture of the heart from cardiac massage when the pericardial sac was opened. With the intact pericardium and pericardial fluid, the compressing finger seldom remains in one spot for a prolonged period.

3. Following successful resuscitation, the problem of adequately closing the pericardial sac arises. This is associated with several complications that are not encountered when the pericardium is left intact throughout the resuscitative procedure. If the pericardial sac is tightly closed, a tamponade effect may very likely be caused by an accumulation of serosanguineous material. In several cases a pericardial tap has been necessary in order to relieve the cardiac tamponade. If the pericardial sac is not closed adequately, an occasional herniation of the heart will occur, with a resultant tamponade effect on the heart. This can usually be diagnosed by x-ray examination. I am aware of at least three cases of herniation of the heart through an opening in the pericardial sac. Should one elect to open the pericardial sac, the correct method of closure is by loose approximation of the sac at approximately three or four places. Some surgeons prefer closing the original opening in the pericardial sac in a tight fashion and then making a small pericardiotomy at a second site in order to allow drainage of any fluid accumulation.

On a subsequent opening of the chest several weeks or months after cardiac arrest has been encountered and cardiac compression carried out, an examination of the pericardium has failed to show any appreciable evidence of pericardial disease or thickening. On a number of experimental animals opened 14 weeks after cardiac compression, no pericardial adhesions to the myocardium were noted.

Manual compression technique

What is the correct method for manual compression of the heart? *The inability to compress the heart properly in cardiac arrest is second only to a delay in its compression as a major factor in the failures of cardiac resuscitation.* In most instances, when competent surgeons massage a heart for the first time, it is exceedingly disappointing to note the relative ineffectiveness of their first attempts at manual compression. All too often the frequently used term "cardiac massage" is taken literally, and actual compression of the walls of the heart fails to occur; subsequently, the amount of blood being pumped into the systemic circulation is inadequate.

There are several different ways by which one may compress the heart adequately, depending on the individual surgeon, the size of the heart, the type of approach to the heart, and a variety of other circumstances. Regardless of the method used, the correct procedure for cardiac compression is one by which the operator is able to maintain an adequate artificial circulation that will force an optimal amount of blood through the cerebral and coronary arteries. Again disregarding the method used, pulse in the peripheral arteries should be easily palpable, the color of the patient should be maintained in an oxygenated-appearing state, and, in the ideal situation, the pupils should be contracted.

Fig. 23-3 demonstrates the method that we have found most effective in approximately 250 cases of cardiac arrest. Through an incision in the left fourth or fifth anterior interspace, the *left* hand, as indicated by the illustration, is inserted after the ribs have been spread. As much of the hand as possible is clasped around the heart. Compression correctly applied should develop an even pressure, the apex of the heart being well up in the palm of the hand, with the fingers extending outward toward the base. Fingertip pressure should *at all times* be avoided. As discussed in a subsequent chapter, rupture of the myocardium can easily occur if constant and active pressure is applied by the thumb on the thin portion of the upper part of the right ventricle. This particularly is

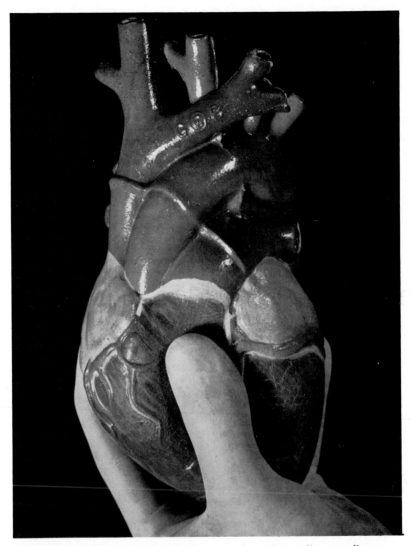

Fig. 23-3. Effective method of holding the heart for intermittent direct cardiac compression. Rupture of right ventricle may occasionally occur if continual and undue pressure is applied with left thumb.

likely to occur if the pericardium is opened and if there is much coronary artery disease. For this reason, the position of the hand should be changed slightly from time to time to avoid excessive pressure over any particular portion of the heart and also to avoid occlusion of any of the coronary vessels.

As I have repeatedly emphasized, proper cardiac compression can seldom be carried out by a physician encountering his first case—unless he has obtained some degree of effectiveness through practice elsewhere. It is for this reason that cardiac compression should be practiced in the animal laboratory. Whenever cases of cardiac arrest occur in the hospital, we endeavor to have house staff members attempt manual compression of the heart for brief periods of time. *This, of course, must be done under careful supervision.* Fig. 23-4 illustrates a model which we have used for teaching purposes and which we find relatively successful. The heart is of normal size and made of a rubber-like material. It is of the same approximate weight as the average human heart and requires a similar type and force of compression as that required by the living heart. When adequately compressed, the amount of pressure exerted through channels placed in the heart is great enough to light an electric bulb. If compression is inadequate the light will not illuminate.

I find it most advantageous to massage with the left hand, to stand on the left side of the patient, and to face the patient's head. Some physicians encounter an equal degree of success by standing on the right side of the patient and massaging with the right hand in the chest. The two-handed method of compression of the heart has not proved effective for me. Neither have I been as successful with the method of compression in which the heart is held against the sternum. In these latter two methods, I have been unable to obtain a femoral blood pressure consistent with that

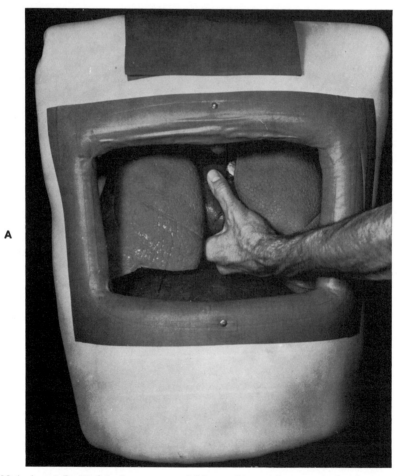

A

Fig. 23-4. **A** and **B**, Models shown are useful in teaching students methods of adequate direct massage of heart. **A** illustrates method that I find effective, although **B** is considered superior by others.

achieved by compression with only one hand. In the animal laboratory, Johnson and Kirby demonstrated the two-handed method and the method of compression of the heart against the sternum, but neither developed a level of cardiac output comparable to that developed by the single-handed method.

The foregoing statements apply to the average-sized human heart. In the infant heart and in the dilated heart, some modification of this standard method of compression may be necessary. Effective cardiac compression, of course, is limited to the compression of the ventricles, particularly the left ventricle.

Closure of the pericardial sac after direct cardiac resuscitation

In many instances it is necessary to open the pericardial sac for indications previously discussed. Closure of the pericardial sac should entail no particular problem in the usual instance if certain precautions are observed. In the majority of cases the pericardial sac should not be closed tightly. When sutures are placed too close together, an effective filling of the pericardial sac

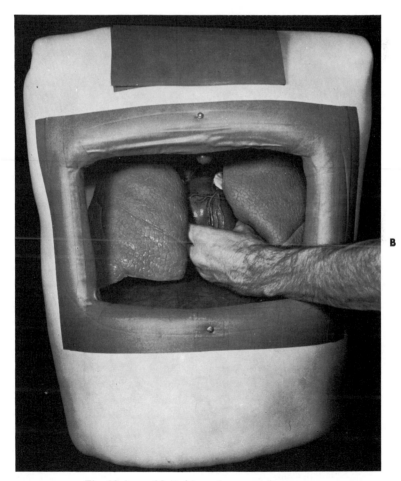

B

Fig. 23-4, cont'd. For legend see opposite page.

will occur, and it is possible that the collection of serosanguineous fluid within the pericardial sac will be such that an effective cardiac tamponade will occur. As mentioned elsewhere, herniation of the heart also occasionally may be seen in those instances where the pericardial sac has not been closed tightly enough. In such instances a portion of the apex of the heart may protrude through the open edges of the pericardium and a tamponade-effect may be the result.

When closing the pericardial sac, Harken often closes the original incision tightly and then makes an additional small incision anteriorly and inferiorly in order to allow for drainage of any accumulated pericardial fluid. This would seem to be a logical procedure.

Ideally, the heart should function best when enclosed in the intact pericardial sac. However, in several cases of cardiac resuscitation, particularly following open-heart surgery, I have removed the entire anterior pericardial sac. It is my opinion that one seldom is aware of any harmful effects from the absence of a large portion of the pericardium, although it should be recognized that it undoubtedly serves a most useful purpose in providing a lubricating effect to eliminate friction. It is also recognized that an intact pericardium tends to prevent anatomic displacement of the great vessels as well as the superior and inferior venae cavae. The pericardium provides a barrier against the extension of infection from neighboring anatomic structures. Its supporting action on the heart seems to be a most desirable feature. Overdistension of the heart in diastole is limited by the pericardium.

Closure of the chest following direct cardiac massage

How long should one wait to close the chest after the heart has been restarted? There is a general rule that one may wait 5 to 8 minutes following resuscitation of the heart. If at the end of that time cardiac activity seems adequate, then closure of the chest may be accomplished. In some instances, however, one may elect to wait for a longer period of time. This is particularly true if epinephrine hydrochloride has been given and the heart appears to be showing the maximal response to the stimulating effect of the drug. One should wait until the drug action has worn off to see if cardiac activity continues in an adequate state. Occasionally, cardiac output will be inadequate once the effect of epinephrine has worn off. This is especially true when an overdose of the drug has been administered.

One surgeon states that he approximates the edges of the thoracotomy incision with towel clips for a period of several minutes. In this way the heart may be followed before the final closure of the chest incision is carried out. If an abdominal procedure or any other extrapleural operation is being performed, time may be allowed for its completion before proceeding to closure of the chest.

Following electrical defibrillation and the resumption of a regular heartbeat, one need not always wait longer than 5 minutes. If the heart is going to revert to ventricular fibrillation, it will generally do so before then.

In some instances when an operation is already in progress, the chest is left open so that the heart can be observed while the operation is completed. Shaffer reported the case of a 75-year-old white woman who was being operated upon for obstructive jaundice. Cardiac arrest occurred as the common bile duct was being palpated. Resuscitation was prompt and effective after a left thoracotomy was performed. It was decided to leave the chest open until the operation could be completed, but as soon as the abdominal retractor was replaced in the abdominal wound, a marked slowing of the heart rate occurred which almost resulted in standstill. When the retractor was removed, the heart rate increased and the blood pressure went up. This was repeated at least twice with the heart under direct vision.

If one is familiar with chest surgery, of course, closure of the chest following cardiac resuscitation would be of little note here. For one not familiar with chest surgery, several points should be mentioned. After one is certain that the lungs are expanding satisfactorily, at least one and preferably two chest tubes may be placed in the left chest and brought out through stab wounds one or two intercostal spaces below the incision. One chest tube should be placed near the apex of the chest and the other just above the diaphragm.

Because the chest has been opened under septic conditions in all likelihood, I employ catgut sutures throughout the closure, approximating the ribs above and below the incision with No. 0 chromic catgut, the sutures encircling the two ribs. These retention sutures facilitate the remainder of the closure considerably. The rest of the procedure is completed with continuous or interrupted No. 00 chromic catgut. Prior to the closure I always check once again to be certain that I have not incised the internal mammary artery at the time of incision. If so, and if it has not been ligated, profuse bleeding may occur. It will particularly do so after the blood pressure begins to rise. I know of four patients who have subsequently bled to death from an unrecognized cut in the internal mammary artery. The intercostal arteries do not usually present a problem. The catheters that have been brought out through a stab wound are anchored to the skin with sutures and then, with a 50 ml. syringe attached, are used to suction all remaining free air in the left hemithorax. Often this will amount to 200 to 300 ml. or more. In order to facilitate drainage and relieve any potential pneumothorax, the catheters are attached to an underwater drainage bottle or suitable thoracic pump. With each respiratory excursion, the column of fluid rising out of the bottle will be seen to move. Within about 12 to 36 hours this column will cease moving and may indicate that no more free air exists in the left chest and that the chest tube may be removed with safety. This is done by placing a piece of petrolatum gauze around the stab wound at the exact moment of removal of the catheter in order to prevent any suctioning of air back into the chest. If the chest was entered under septic conditions, it is preferable that the lower chest tube remain in place several additional days.

Postponing or continuing the operation after cardiac massage

If cardiac arrest occurs during an operative procedure, it may reappear at a later point in the operation in a certain number of cases. It is for this reason that the operation may best be postponed when it is of an elective nature. I have seen cardiac arrest occur, for example, halfway through a subtotal gastrectomy. In such instances it is imperative that the procedure be completed. In operations upon the heart, especially for mitral stenosis, it seems wise to complete the intended procedure. Sometimes the outcome will not be successful. The following is an example.

A 65-year-old white man had been brought to the operating room for removal of a tumor of the left lung. As the patient was turned to a right lateral position, cardiac arrest occurred. The chest was opened immediately and massage was started within 1½ minutes. Excellent return of function followed within 30 seconds. The left pneumonectomy was then performed and cardiac arrest again occurred suddenly at the time of the closure of the wound. Resuscitation measures at this second episode were unsuccessful. Autopsy showed the lesion to be secondary to a small asymptomatic clear cell cancer of the kidney. Severe sclerosis of the coronary arteries was also reported. (Courtesy Dr. Mark H. Williams.)

A patient who has experienced a cardiac arrest under surgery usually tolerates a subsequent operation satisfactorily. Hanks and Papper point to fifty-seven operations performed on forty-two patients following cardiac resuscitation. In this group there was one death caused by exsanguination during a partial hepatectomy.

Rate of cardiac compression

Difference of opinion exists as to the optimal rate at which the heart should be compressed in treating a case of cardiac arrest. The late Dr. Frank Lahey advocated that the heart should be directly massaged at a rate of about 40 to 50 compressions per minute in order for the heart to refill. Others have supported his view, including Dr. Alfred Blalock of Johns Hopkins. I agree with Dr. Blalock's impression that most surgeons are likely to be too timid in their compression of the heart and his recommendation for more vigorous compression if irreversible brain damage is to be prevented. I am not in complete agreement, however, with his suggestion that the heart be compressed at the rate of 40 to 50 times a minute.

As long ago as 1915, Gunn and coworkers argued for compression of the heart at a very slow rate. They reasoned that in the normally beating heart, the ventricles fill by active propulsion of blood from the auricles and that the circulation is aided by other factors that are no longer present during cardiac arrest. In the case of massage of the arrested heart, the filling is effected by a suction process resulting from the elasticity of the ventricles, such a process taking longer than in the normal heart.

If one views an exposed heart during a period of vagal nerve stimulation and witnesses atrial arrest and origination of the stimulus formation in the ventricles, one will be impressed by the ability of the right ventricle to fill in spite of complete inactivity of the right atrium. The degree of filling of the right ventricle by gravity as well as by the "suction" effect is considerable. I believe that cardiac compres-sion, by either the direct or the closed-chest approach, should be maintained at a rate between 55 and 70 per minute. There are variables that may alter this rate, for example, the size of the heart.

In addition, Gunn and associates believed that compression should be done gradually to avoid injury to the heart. Conversely, they believed that the massaging hand should relax in an abrupt and jerking fashion so that the maximal pressure drop in the ventricles would occur in the shortest possible time. I have not found these maneuvers especially worthwhile.

The rate at which the heart should be compressed will vary to a certain extent according to the individual performing the operation. In our hands, a rapid rate (between 65 and 80 per minute) has given the best result. In the animal laboratory, massage of the dog heart at a rapid rate produces a more vigorous rise in the arterial pressure than does a relatively slow rate. In the human heart, the pulse in the femoral and other peripheral arteries is stronger, the patient's color is better, and the constriction of the pupils is more easily maintained when a rapid rate of compression is employed.

Johnson and Kirby demonstrate by means of the Dumke bubble meter that a greater output of the heart can be maintained by means of rapid compression. This work has been the basis for some of our support of rapid cardiac compressions. They suggest that even a rate as high as *120 times per minute* might be the optimal rate. It is true that a rapid rate is perhaps more traumatic to the heart than a slower rate, but in dogs as well as in human beings we have been able to maintain a better blood pressure with the rapid rate of compression and justify our opinion on this basis. *Clinically, it is not necessary to consciously allow filling of the heart.* I have not been impressed with the argument that the rapid rate of massage should be avoided because of fatigue to the operator. A rate of 70 to 80 per minute can be maintained for a number of minutes. Very rarely is the operator alone in the resuscitative procedure, an assistant being at hand to give relief in the great majority of instances.

The work of Lape and Maison should be mentioned. They attempted to confirm the studies of Johnson and Kirby, who had previously indicated better cardiac output when a faster rate of massage was maintained. Lape and Maison came to the opposite conclusion. Their work showed that the mean arterial pressure was not increased by increasing the rate of massage; however, the difference was not great. Lape found that the increased output was in favor of a slower rate. This has not been in accordance with my own observation in human beings or in dogs. The simple procedure of inserting a needle in the femoral artery is a very convincing means by which to demonstrate that a much higher head of pressure occurs with a rapid rate of massage than when a slower rate is used. Lape and Maison produced cardiac arrest by large doses of magnesium sulfate, the cessation probably resulting from abolishment of all vasoconstrictor tone.

In summary, it should be mentioned that, although the value of manual intermittent compression of the heart is universally accepted as a means of artificially maintaining circulation and preventing irreversible brain damage, the prevalence of various misconceptions on the part of many practicing physicians is surprising. Schiff, as early as 1874, demonstrated the reality of the value of intermittent cardiac compression or massage in artificially establishing adequate circulation. In addition there are many who fail to realize that intermittent compression of the heart is necessary in both cardiac asystole and in ventricular fibrillation. The misconception also occasionally exists that massage in ventricular fibrillation may perpetuate the arrhythmia. It must not be forgotten that the function

of massage is that of maintaining adequate circulation while other therapeutic measures are being readied. Deuchar and Venner recorded intra-arterial blood pressure determinations by means of an electric condenser manometer and a thin plastic catheter introduced into a peripheral artery. With the pericardium intact they recorded systemic blood pressure levels of 75/30 and 55/20. Every physician should feel confident that he can apply intermittent cardiac compression in a manner that will sustain life and make successful resuscitation possible.

Intracoronary artery pressure with cardiac massage

How effective is manual massage of the heart in supplying adequate pressure in the coronary artery circulation, and what effect on the coronary arterial pressure occurs following compression of the aorta, elevation of the foot of the table, and intra-arterial and intravenous transfusions? These questions are answered to a large extent by Veal and associates in the department of surgery, Georgetown University School of Medicine. Prompt elevation of the coronary artery pressure almost to a hypertensive state is noted on occlusion of the thoracic and abdominal aorta, even in states of mild shock. They caution against the danger of overloading the heart by intracarotid transfusions when the aorta is occluded. Similarly, a change in the position of the animal from a supine to the Trendelenburg position (30 degree elevation of the foot of the table) causes mild to severe states of hypertension and a definite shifting of blood with a rise in the coronary pressure, but the rise in pressure is only a fraction as great as that caused by occlusion of the thoracic aorta.

A marked change in the appearance of the heart should be noted routinely after massage has begun. The degree of flaccidity grows less, the coronary vessels gradually begin to distend, and the myocardium takes on its characteristic pink color once again.

Open-chest cardiac massage in the infant

In the very young, the operator will have difficulty in massaging the heart in an effective manner if he applies the same method used in the adult patient. In the infant or very young pediatric patient I have found it necessary to open the pericardial sac in order to massage the infant's heart in an effective manner because of the diaphragmatic attachment of the pericardial sac. In those cases it is difficult to get one's hand about the apex. The problem is similar to that found in the dog, and, in general, it seems that a one-handed method of intermittent manual compression lends itself to the most satisfactory results.

Useful adjuncts during cardiac compression

Along with manual intermittent compression of the heart, to artificially maintain adequate circulation to the brain, myocardium, and vital organs, one should be aware of certain additional measures that may be employed as adjuncts in a most effective manner.

Ripstein mentions the use of the tilt-table as an effective method of aiding circulation.

AORTIC ARTERY (THORACIC) COMPRESSION

At the beginning of cardiac massage the return circulation to the heart is sometimes inadequate and cardiac output likewise is reduced. Therefore it would seem logical for as much as possible of the oxygenated blood to be sent to the cerebral circulation and through the coronary vessels to the myocardium. In order to shunt more blood to these vital centers, it is worthwhile, on occasion, to clamp the aorta at a point distal to the exit of the last great vessel to the neck (the left subclavian artery). This can be done by pressing the aorta

between the fingers or by use of a rubber-shod clamp. In some instances the aorta may be constricted by compressing it against the vertebral column with the fingers. The effectiveness of this procedure is often dramatic. Although Schiff provides us with the first recorded suggestion of this sort (he applied this method on dogs in 1874), others (Carter, Wiggers, Harken, Guthrie, and Pike) report using a similar procedure. The clamp or fingers should be relieved at intervals of every 5 to 10 minutes.

INTERMITTENT PRESSURE ON THE ABDOMINAL AORTA

Because of the beneficial results noted in the animal laboratory on the increase of venous return to the heart due to intermittent manual compression of the abdomen, the above-mentioned men felt justified to use it on a patient. Although only very general means were available for observation, it was the impression of the operating team that the cardiac output was greater as measured through the peripheral pulse and blood pressure. If cardiac arrest occurs during an abdominal procedure, then I would suggest that the aorta be compressed either between the fingers or posteriorly against the vertebral column. In thin persons this may prove to be an effective maneuver even though the abdomen is unopened. I have tried this procedure in the animal laboratory and am satisfied of its merit.

In a thin patient some degree of abdominal aortic artery compression can be maintained along with closed-chest resuscitation.

ATRIAL ASSISTANCE

The concept of atrial assistance as an aid to cardiac massage is discussed by Das of the Moti Lal Nehru Medical College in India. In a series of experiments, he notes that atrial assistance (by compressing and releasing the right atrium alternately) not only prevents atrial distension and atrial inactivity but also contributes significantly to proper filling of the ventricles.

In normal subjects, atrial systole apparently contributes very little to cardiac function. Its role in the closure of the A-V valves has been disputed from time to time although Braunwald and co-workers have concluded from a study of forty-three patients that properly timed contraction of the atria is not always essential for effective closure of the mitral valve. In an abnormal heart, however, it is a different story. Benchimol and co-workers have demonstrated considerable increase in cardiac output with the use of atrial pacing techniques in diseased hearts. Therefore, it seems there is definitely some enhancement of ventricular cardiac output by effective contraction in the abnormal heart.

Permanent atrial standstill may be compatible with normal activity. Messinger and Mirkinson were able to document permanent atrial standstill over at least an 8-year period in a 47-year-old man. The atrial standstill fulfilled all of the requirements for such a diagnosis by the absence of P waves in all the electrocardiographic leads, no A waves in the neck veins, and regular rhythm with the QRS of the usual supraventricular type. In addition, there was no evidence of mobility of the atrium on fluoroscopy. Although uncommon, atrial standstill may be seen in cases of digitalis and quinidine intoxication.

Induction of atrial fibrillation by alternating current stimulation of the right atrium is still another mode of atrial stimulation that is therapeutically effective. There are disadvantages to induction of atrial fibrillation in patients with underlying heart disease since these patients benefit from the atrial contribution to ventricular contraction and induction of atrial fibrillation would eliminate this mechanism.

Chapter 24

CLOSED-CHEST MASSAGE VERSUS DIRECT MANUAL COMPRESSION OF THE HEART

It seems unfortunate that the training of physicians in the techniques of open, direct cardiac compression has considerably diminished with the advent of closed-chest compression techniques. Every physician, particularly the surgeon, should have the ability to effectively open the chest and adequately maintain circulation artificially by compressing the heart.

In addition to the indications for open-chest cardiac compression cited in this section, there are obvious general advantages:

(1) From the standpoint of most parameters studied, the hemodynamics of open-chest massage is superior to that of closed-chest massage. (2) A knowledgeable physician may more likely determine the optimum drug indicated by a careful observation not only of the volume of the heart and its rhythm (Foley), but by the character of the cardiac contractions and by the tone of the cardiac muscle. (3) After the drug has been given, its effectiveness can be more nearly ascertained. (4) Augmentation of the heart's own contraction by manual compression is often indicated, and its need can be monitored carefully by direct vision. (5) Stroking the interventricular septum for its pacemaker effect has often been of considerable aid in our resuscitative efforts. (6) Epicardial pacemaker wires can be placed if necessary. (7) If deterioration of the heart after defibrillation appears to be present, efforts can often be successful in avoiding a recurrent episode of ventricular fibrillation.

Again, as Foley emphasizes, the physician has a great asset in being able to see and feel the heart rather than make judgements based on secondary evidence.

Blood flow and arterial pressure levels consistently less than 50% of base line can be expected with either open- or closed-chest cardiac massage.

Although many authors state that the mortality rate is significantly greater with open-chest or direct cardiac massage than with external cardiac compression (Grossman and Rubin), overall comparative figures do not necessarily substantiate this conclusion. In some ways, it is like comparing apples with oranges in that different groups of patients have been used for the direct method. The success rate with external cardiac compression has yet to approximate that obtained in the operating room using the open-chest approach. Obviously the open-chest technique does not lend itself to the delay inherent in an arrest occurring outside the operating room, to the added trauma and complications of a thoracotomy outside the operating room, and to the inadequate training of personnel. Each approach has its place, its indications, and its aspects of superiority.

A substantial number of follow-up studies are now available to lend a note of encouragement to the long-term prognosis of patients successfully resuscitated and discharged from the hospital. Many of these long-term follow-ups concern patients resuscitated during episodes of ventricular fibrillation in a coronary care unit after a myocardial infarction. Workers at the Royal Victoria Hospital in Belfast report on 173 patients with ventricular fibrillation who were resuscitated during a 5-year period from 1964 through 1969. As in most of these studies, there was a preponderance of male patients. All had received direct current countershock. Forty-one had repeated episodes of cardiac arrest and two of the survivors had more than 100 separate episodes of fibrillation that were successfully treated. A "separate episode" was considered as a recurrence of the dysrhythmia half an hour or more after an earlier successful restoration. Sixty percent of the long-term survivors were those who had fibrillation within 24 hours of the onset of symptoms. The survival rate of patients who have ventricular fibrillation less than 4 hours after the onset of symptoms is better than that of patients who fibrillate later.

Generally speaking, ventricular fibrillation associated with clinically mild coronary attacks carries a prognosis not unlike that of an episode unassociated with ventricular fibrillation. Among twenty-nine survivors who had ventricular fibrillation within the first hour of the onset of symptoms, twenty suffered the arrest while outside the hospital.

In the group of 173 survivors, 15 subsequently died a sudden and unexpected death. In Dupont's series, nearly 25% subsequently died suddenly; but there was only one sudden death among fifty-three survivors in the Lawrie series, and no sudden death among twenty survivors in Stannard's group.

Sixty-eight percent of the survivors eligible to work were at work in occupations similar to those they had had prior to the myocardial infarction.

One of the first large surveys to indicate the effectiveness of closed-chest massage was made by Cotlar at Charity Hospital of New Orleans. A progressive improvement in survival from cardiac arrest was demonstrated since the introduction of external cardiac massage at Charity Hospital; from June, 1960, through March, 1962, seventy-three patients were treated for cardiac arrest. These excluded patients on whom cardiac or pulmonary operations were being performed. Nineteen of the cases occurred outside the operating room. Of the seventy-three patients, an overall survival rate of 42% was achieved during this period. With closed-chest massage, however, a survival rate of 80% in twenty-five cases was recorded. Only three patients of the nineteen survived outside the operating room, regardless of the method employed. Of particular significance was the fact that no permanent residual brain damage occurred in any of the twenty-eight patients on whom successful resuscitation was employed in the operating room. Irreversible brain damage was present, however, in five patients who died in the postresuscitative period of from 6 hours to 4 days.

Working at Saint Bartholomew's Hospital in London, Weale and Rothwell-Jackson made several interesting observations relative to the efficiency of closed-chest cardiac massage versus internal or direct compression of the heart. This comparison was presented to the English Surgical Research Society (1962). In a series of nineteen dogs, arterial and venous pressure tracing readings were taken after ventricular fibrillation was induced. Atrioventricular valve incompetence, as measured by a rise in venous pressure readings, could be produced by both internal and external compression. However, and perhaps significantly, internal cardiac compression resulted in a higher mean arterial and a lower mean venous pressure than when external or closed-chest compression was applied. It was emphasized that pulses as high as 60 mm. Hg in the venous system can hardly avoid producing cerebral damage when these pressures are transmitted peripherally to the capillaries of the brain. Increased neurologic sequelae may be a result of closed-chest compression techniques involving higher venous pressure readings; however, these pressures can be partially relieved if epinephrine is given. Weale and Rothwell-Jackson would tend to cast doubt on the generalization that closed-chest compression is superior to the internal approach because of an enhanced venous return to the heart when the chest is unopened. Little attention has been paid to the importance of venous pressure elevations in the past. Almost certainly, a considerable amount of back flow through the tricuspid valve occurs with closed-chest massage. Weale and Rothwell-Jackson believe the high venous pressure pulses illustrate the fallaciousness of regarding a pressure pulse as good evidence of forward flow. In concluding their remarks on the comparison of the two methods of cardiac massage, these authors emphasize that the ease of performance with the closed-chest technique (and the reluctance of physicians to be involved in an emergency surgical procedure) should not obscure the fact that the internal cardiac massage technique has allowed a success rate of as high as 75% in some series. Even in resuscitation of patients with myocardial infarct, the direct approach has been equally as effective among reported cases.

It is, of course, almost impossible to selectively apply compression to the heart without other structures within the chest being partially or equally affected. Dissipation of pressure effects to noncardiac structures would seem to be considerably less with the direct thoracotomy or internal compression techniques. Leighninger has recorded higher flow rates in the carotid artery in dogs during the open method as compared with the closed-chest method.

Redding and Cozine studied carotid flow rates in dogs with both closed-chest and open-chest massage. The average of over fifty determinations with each technique indicates that the direct or open method of manual massage of the heart is superior to the closed-chest technique. Nevertheless, it would seem that many advantages can be attributed to the closed-chest technique. Not only is it simple and easily applied, but also it is perhaps less fatiguing to the operator. Since no skin incision is required, the danger of infection and localized or generalized sepsis is absent. Artificial ventilation without an open thorax is perhaps easier and more effective. Damage to the heart itself is probably decreased. Myocardial burns are unlikely. Perhaps of most importance is its wide applicability under so many variable situations.

On the other hand, certain additional disadvantages would seem to be inherent in the closed-chest technique. It is sometimes desirable to closely inspect the heart, as has been discussed elsewhere. Complications, as with the open-chest approach, do occur and have been discussed in some detail. The closed-chest approach may not be applicable if the patient is unable to assume a supine position. Severe emphysema does not lend itself as readily to closed-chest techniques in the experience of some. Likewise, the obstetric patient near term is probably not an ideal candidate for the closed-chest technique. Drugs cannot be injected as accurately and their pharmacologic effect cannot be assessed as readily. Also, the closed-chest technique does not allow selective diversion of more blood to the brain by pinching off the aorta. The closed-chest method of cardiac massage, although obviously effective, does allow for considerable ventriculoatrial reflux. This reflux can be reduced by left ventricular compression as it is employed in the one-hand method following a thoracotomy.

Bizzarri and co-workers report a 15-year-old patient whose cardiac arrest occurred during spinal anesthesia for a forceps delivery. She did not respond to external cardiac massage, but did respond to internal cardiac massage. The patient was transferred to the recovery room and hypothermia was begun because of cerebral irritation. Eight hours later, the endotracheal tube became obstructed and another cardiac arrest occurred. Again, external cardiac massage was ineffectual; a normal sinus rhythm was restored after the chest was opened and direct cardiac massage was applied. The patient subsequently made a complete recovery after being maintained at 92° to 94° F. for 5 days.

Some have suggested that loss of elasticity of the chest wall in advanced age may represent a relative contraindication to closed-chest resuscitation. Many exceptions to this concern would indicate that it is probably unwarranted. For example, Egerton and associates report the successful resuscitation of an 85-year-old man upon whom external cardiac compression was continued for 15 minutes.

It is rather widely accepted that cardiac output with open-chest cardiac compression is almost double that with closed-chest compression. The disappointingly low cardiac output with closed-chest compression may further compound certain aspects of the problem. For one thing, stagnant anoxia results along with progressive metabolic acidosis, which in turn not only increases the likelihood of ventricular fibrillation, but also sustains cardiac asystole by a reduction in myocardial contractility. This further reduces cardiac output with a worsening of the cycle.

The high arterial peaks with cardiac compression do not necessarily indicate adequate forward flow of blood. Mean arterial pressure may continue to be low—especially with closed-chest resuscitation. Therefore one must remember that palpable peripheral pulses are not conclusive of a satisfactory cardiac output.

Seventy-five minutes of closed-chest massage were used on a 32-year-old patient in ventricular fibrillation after a colectomy. Eight attempts at conversion with D.C. electroshock had only transient effects. External pacing was attempted, but was unsuccessful. Levophed, sodium bicarbonate, and calcium gluconate were given at intervals. Finally, in desperation, the chest was opened, and, in spite of a now flat ECG tracing, the heart was subtly fibrillating, although greatly dilated and flabby. The patient's heart action was restored with open-chest massage, and recovery followed, despite a period of pulmonary edema in the postresuscitative period.

The feasibility of treating venous air embolism and subsequent cardiac arrest with closed-chest resuscitation has been demonstrated in the seven patients treated by Ericsson and associates. All were patients selected for elective craniotomy in the head-up position. In four patients the air-

embolism occurred as the skull was being opened with a nitrogen-driven drill. The other three patients suffered air emboli 1 to 2 hours after the beginning of the procedure. The diagnosis of air embolism was made in each case by the typical "mill-wheel" murmur heard over the precordium. Closed-chest massage was begun in five of the seven patients, with effective restoration of circulation.

In describing a case of cardiac arrest in a 29-year-old female at the time of a ruptured uterus, Paul and associates comment that the soft foam pad on the operating table made closed-chest resuscitation relatively ineffective. Following a thoracotomy, the heart was resuscitated and the patient survived.

The contribution of Jude, Kouwenhoven, and Knickerbocker in advocating closed-chest resuscitation is, undoubtedly, one of the real major advances in resuscitation. Because of their efforts, large groups of patients are now candidates for closed-chest resuscitation where resuscitative efforts may not have been practical in the past. The technique of closed-chest resuscitation can be utilized by physicians in all types of specialties; its use is, of course, even applicable to groups of laymen having received special training in resuscitation. Many of the complications of open-chest resuscitation are avoided, such as intrathoracic infection, rupture of the heart, and postresuscitative bleeding. Artificial respiration is more easily applied and, most importantly, resuscitative techniques need not be limited to the confines of the hospital. Closed-chest resuscitation allows almost immediate efforts to be directed toward improving the cardiopulmonary function, and elaborate equipment need not be required.

It is my belief that the two techniques of closed-chest and open-chest cardiac massage are not in themselves competitive but that there are situations in which one technique may be preferable to the other. For example, pulmonary emboli have responded poorly to closed-chest resuscitation. I encountered such a massive pulmonary embolism while operating upon a 70-year-old man under spinal anesthesia. Closed-chest resuscitation seemed to be wholly inadequate, and the left chest was finally opened after 2 or 3 minutes of closed-chest compression. This was prompted by failure to achieve any appreciable cardiac output and by marked stasis of the neck veins. In spite of more than 30 minutes of open-chest resuscitation and repeated attempts at ventricular defibrillation, the heart could not be restarted. The possibility of a massive pulmonary embolism was overlooked and therefore attempts to remove the clots were not made. Had the diagnosis been recognized, their successful removal may well have occurred.

There are now numerous instances on record illustrating the beneficial effects of open-chest, or direct, massage when the closed-chest technique proved to be unsuccessful. Shocket and Rosenblum encountered cardiac arrest in a 32-year-old male following a colectomy for ulcerative colitis at the Mount Sinai Hospital in Miami Beach, Florida. Closed-chest massage was carried out promptly following the arrest, which occurred in the recovery room. Despite vigorous efforts with closed-chest massage augmented by adequate ventilatory efforts and repeated injections of sodium bicarbonate, calcium gluconate, and levarterenol, the patient showed no response. The pupils were fixed and dilated. Because of the youthfulness of the patient, the decision was made to open the chest and apply direct massage. Within seconds of manual cardiac compression, the heart returned to a spontaneous sinus rhythm. Spontaneous defibrillation had occurred.

Using open-chest techniques, Sykes and Ahmed were able to successfully resuscitate over 12% of thirty-five patients who failed to resuscitate with closed-chest massage.

The open-chest, or direct, approach may be indicated for patients with myocardial infarction who do not respond to closed-chest techniques and in whom a ventricular rupture may be suspected. Several successful applications of open-chest massage under such circumstances have been reported.

I believe the closed-chest cardiac resuscitation is contraindicated and that the open-chest technique is generally more likely to be successful in the following situations:

1. The patient with a pectus excavatum or a marked pectus carinatum
2. Massive air embolism
3. Cardiac tamponade
4. The patient with a bilateral pneumothorax
5. Lack of availability of an external defibrillator in the presence of ventricular fibrillation
6. A failure to respond adequately to closed-chest compression (should the patient be in the operating room under a well-controlled situation, one should open the chest in 2 to 3 minutes)
7. In some instances of severe mitral stenosis (commissurotomy may be the emergency procedure of choice)
8. Pregnancy (third trimester)
9. Flail chest
10. Massive pulmonary embolism
11. Evidence of intrathoracic hemorrhage or severe trauma to the chest
12. Known or suspected tension pneumothorax
13. Penetrating thoracic injuries
14. Ventricular herniation after cardiac surgery
15. When the heart's anatomic position is not in the midline
16. When one desires visual monitoring of the heart
17. With other causes of intracardiac obstructions, such as a left atrial myxoma
18. When the chest is already opened
19. For management of the tetanic (stone) heart
20. Myocardial laceration
21. Refractory ventricular fibrillation
22. Ventricular aneurysm

The presence of a mitral or aortic valve prosthesis should prompt open-chest resuscitation if closed-chest defibrillation and massage are not immediately successful. There is a high incidence of complications from the pressure effect of the valve being compressed between the sternum and the vertebral bodies.

Although probably not of major overall significance, some protective effect may be provided by the relative hypothermia that occurs when the thorax is opened. Isselhard, at the Second International Symposium on Emergency Resuscitation, indicated that the temperature of the heart with an open thorax will drop to about 30° or 28° C. if the room temperature is about 20° C. He believes that the degree of ischemia tolerated by the heart can be extended from a period of 20 to 25 minutes at normothermia, up to 40 or 50 minutes at hypothermia.

A detailed study of sixteen cases of cardiac arrest is reported from the department of surgery of Istanbul Medical School and the surgical unit of the 1,000-bed Istanbul Army Hospital (Degerli). It is significant that ten of the sixteen patients had severe respiratory difficulties. Three had broncho-spasm and seven had insufficient ventilation or dyspnea. Cardiac standstill was the mechanism of arrest in thirteen patients and ventricular fibrillation in three; but a history of coronary insufficiency was present in only two patients. The need for flexibility in one's approach to the problem of cardiac arrest is well illustrated in Degerli's report (1972). Open-chest massage was resorted to in eight of the sixteen patients. In six patients external cardiac massage was entirely satisfactory for restoration of cardiopulmonary function; but external massage failed to restore an effective heartbeat in the former group. In fourteen of the sixteen patients cardiovascular function was restored; but in two instances of ventricular fibrillation, defibrillation was not achieved. Seventy-eight percent of the patients survived (eleven of sixteen).

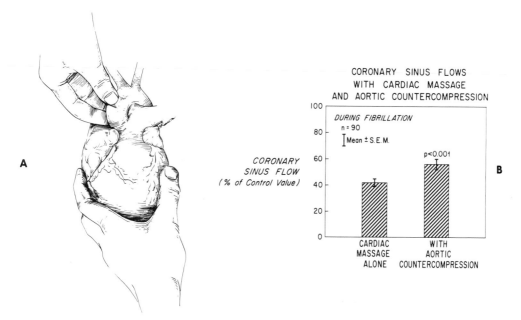

Fig. 24-1. A, Improved coronary blood flow can be achieved by alternately compressing the heart and proximal aorta as shown. Fingers of the left hand are positioned over posterior wall of the ventricles with the ventricular apex in the palm and the thumb over anterior wall of the left ventricle. The right hand is placed so that index and middle fingers are positioned transversely across posterior wall of the ascending aorta approximately 7 cm. above the level of aortic valve with right thumb across anterior wall of the vessel. B, Mean coronary sinus blood flow measured during conventional cardiac massage and massage with aortic countercompression. (From Molokhia, F. A., and others: Chest 62:610-613, 1972.)

Special adjuncts available with open-chest cardiac massage

A method of augmenting coronary perfusion during direct manual compression of the heart is reported by Molokhia and associates from Boston City Hospital. As shown in Fig. 24-1, the method involves alternate manual compression of the heart and of the ascending aorta as a means of selective diastolic augmentation to increase coronary flow during direct cardiac massage. Experimental models confirm that coronary sinus blood flow is significantly greater during massage and aortic countercompression than during massage alone. In fact, sequenced ventriculo-aortic countercompression is able to produce coronary sinus flows that average 32% greater than those achieved by the usual and conventional methods. Arterial pressures continue to be maintained at their same levels without decreased peripheral blood flow and its associated contribution to anaerobic metabolism.

Resuscitation in association with thoracoabdominal injury

In the active emergency room frequent instances of cardiovascular collapse requiring cardiopulmonary resuscitation in association with severe thoracoabdominal injuries are encountered. It is estimated that over half the trauma patients who are alive on arrival at the hospital but who succumb within 24 hours have severe chest injuries. Frequently external cardiac massage is contraindicated because of a severe chest injury and the chest should be opened for direct cardiac compression. Lahdensuu and Rokkanen report the successful resuscitation of a 32-year-old man who required 6 hours of intrathoracic cardiac compression, drug therapy, and ventricular defibrillation before success was achieved. He was eventually discharged.

Pulmonary embolism

While the results are quite poor in the management of pulmonary embolism by means of closed-chest cardiac massage, occasional successful cases are reported. In Sandoe's series, there is one success in eight individuals who had cardiac arrest caused by pulmonary embolism.

Further indication for open-chest massage

Cardiac arrest that has followed unrecognized exsanguinating hemorrhage will receive only minimal and temporary benefits from closed-heart massage. It is not always easy, in postoperative circumstances, to be entirely certain that hemorrhage has not occurred. For this reason, I have employed closed-chest resuscitation long enough to get the patient to the operating room for a thoracotomy on several occasions when hemorrhage was suspected. Even though underwater chest-tube drainage is employed, a completely adequate reflection of intrathoracic bleeding may not occur.

If there is suspicion of cardiac tamponade, it is my opinion that efforts at cardiac resuscitation by closed-chest compression methods are to be avoided unless the environmental conditions make a thoracotomy impractical. An additional contraindication applies to the patient with cardiac arrest that resulted from ventricular herniation through a portion of the pericardial sac. Several such cases have been reported and are mentioned elsewhere in this book. If massive intrathoracic bleeding is suspected, closed-chest resuscitation is contraindicated. Although any herniation of the left ventricle will usually occur relatively soon after cardiac surgery, one case did not become manifest until 62 hours later. Roentgenograms may provide some clue to the diagnosis of such herniation by showing the heart lying in a more transverse position. Unfortunately, however, this would have no practical application if sudden cardiac arrest occurred.

If a massive air embolism is suspected, the usual methods employed in closed-chest compression may need to be altered. The head of the patient should be lowered to prevent embolization to the cerebral circulation. If large quantities of air are accumulated in the right side of the heart, it will probably be best to directly visualize the heart and aspirate as much of the air from the right atrium or right ventricle as is possible. Correction of the marked distension should be employed as promptly as possible.

Cardiac resuscitation in obstetric patients

Once cardiac arrest has been diagnosed at the time of delivery, efforts should first be made to resuscitate the mother by taking steps to ensure adequate pulmonary ventilation. Closed-chest compression has been used on obstetric patients at term. Because of the marked elevation of the diaphragm by full-term pregnancy, my own vote, however, would be in favor of a thoracotomy for direct massage of the heart—particularly if the patient were in the delivery or operating room.

Thomas reports a successful cesarean section on a 22-year-old woman whose heart stopped for 3 minutes after the administration of 10 mg. of tetracaine (Pontocaine) for spinal anesthesia. The baby was delivered and breathed spontaneously, but the mother was not resuscitated.

Jain and Pandey (Banaras Hindu University, Varanasi) showed that external cardiac compression can be successfully applied, even if associated with a full-term pregnancy. Cardiac arrest occurred in a 21-year-old primigravida being prepared for a cesarean section. A full, pounding pulse appeared after 5 minutes of external cardiac massage and a healthy baby was subsequently delivered.

Hemodynamic effects of closed- and open-chest massage

Attention to the hemodynamics of closed- and open-chest massage seems to indicate that the bulk of the evidence is in favor of a higher perfusing arterial pressure with open-chest cardiac massage.

Without question, both approaches to the artificial maintenance of circulation, combined with adequate artificial respiration and augmented with other aids when indicated, combine to successfully restore cardiopulmonary function. If any doubt exists about the value or adequacy of cardiac massage in maintaining blood flow, one should be reminded of the numerous patients who regain consciousness during cardiac massage. I have had several patients who have regained consciousness during open-chest compression and who have required general anesthesia before completion of the efforts.

Is lateral displacement of the heart a significant factor in closed-chest resuscitative techniques? In attempting to answer this question, Pryor of Christchurch, New Zealand, placed water-filled balloons inside the pericardium of cadavers from which the heart had been removed. The volume displaced with each compression was measured during external cardiac massage and radiographs were taken. These studies show that lateral displacement of the "heart" does not occur. In other words, it is apparent that the pericardium does prevent any significant degree of lateral displacement of the heart.

Therefore it behooves the physician to be well versed in the techniques of both open-chest and closed-chest cardiac compression, as there will be times when each technique will be lifesaving. While the apparent simplicity of closed-chest resuscitation is appealing, cardiac resuscitation continues to be an effort that requires rather sophisticated knowledge. If the percentage of successful resuscitation (that is, patients discharged from the hospital) is to rise significantly over the 15% or 16% level, it will require improved efforts on the part of the medical profession.

Complications of either closed-chest or open-chest resuscitation are, to be sure, of relative insignificance when compared with a dead patient. Nevertheless, an awareness of these complications and knowledge of their avoidance is necessary. Closed-chest resuscitation, if improperly applied, may result in severe laceration to the pulmonary parenchyma, ventricular rupture, rupture of the inferior vena cava near its junction at the right atrium or rupture of internal mammary vessels, relaxation of costochondral junctions, myocardial damage of varying degrees, fat emboli to the pulmonary parenchyma and to the brain, rupture of the liver, spleen, transverse colon, or stomach, multiple rib and sternal fractures, and aspiration from gastric regurgitation. A discussion of these complications is presented elsewhere in this book.

Successful resuscitative efforts have not been limited to human beings. Williamson reports resuscitation of a circus lion! Because of ventricular fibrillation, the chest was opened and, after direct massage, successful electrical defibrillation occurred.

COMPARATIVE HEMODYNAMIC EFFECTS

Considerable data are now available concerning the various cardiorespiratory parameters in cardiac resuscitation using either the closed-chest or the open-chest approach (Del Guercio and co-workers; Weiser and co-workers; Leighninger; Pappelbaum and co-workers; Cohn and associates).

It is unfair to transfer data in their entirety from dog resuscitative techniques to the human. Closed-chest resuscitation is hampered in the dog because of anatomic characteristics. Smaller dogs have more favorable chest contours; therefore, with less exaggerated anterior-posterior dimensions, better massage can be accomplished. Because earlier investigators justify the human clinical application of data from closed resuscitative techniques obtained from dogs, Weiser and associates conducted a comparative study of closed-chest resuscitation techniques versus open-chest techniques. They note that, despite seemingly comparable systolic pressures with either the open or closed technique, the cardiac outputs and mean pressures are consider-

ably less with the closed-chest technique. In their opinion, the high systolic pressures recorded during closed-chest compression are related to direct mechanical transmission of pressures applied to the closed thorax and to catheter freeing—both without significant increase in blood flow. As noted elsewhere, carotid artery flows and aortic pressures (Redding and Cozine) are higher with an open-chest technique. A summary of Weiser's experiments indicates that the open-chest method provides greater cardiac output (average 61% of control values) and greater aortic systolic, diastolic, and mean pressures (48% of control mean aortic pressure) than the closed-chest technique (20% and 21% respectively). Systolic ejection period and stroke volume are considerably diminished with the closed-chest technique and therefore a rapid rate of compression is more effective than slower rates. With either the closed-chest or open-chest technique, administration of epinephrine during massage results in increased values of the systolic, diastolic, and mean aortic pressures.

In contrast, Pappelbaum and associates studied closed- and open-cardiac resuscitative techniques in dogs, paying particular attention to cerebral arterial oxygen saturation levels. They conclude that there is no significant difference in the quantity of blood delivered to the brain by the left common carotid artery per minute, or per heart compression, during either open or closed techniques. Both closed- and open-chest resuscitation provide satisfactory cerebral tissue perfusion. Among the first to document hemodynamic parameters during closed- and open-chest techniques were Del Guercio and co-workers (1963).

In an effort to determine how much blood flow can actually be produced by compression of the human heart between the sternum and the vertebral column, they used serial indicator-dilution curves and calculated cardiac output, mean transit time, and central blood volume. They used closed-chest cardiac compression on three patients. Their indicator-dilution curve suggests inefficient stroke output and valvular incompetence during external cardiac massage and a cardiac index less than one half of normal. Arterial pressures, determined by direct cannulation or sphygmomanometry, correlated poorly with flows being produced by resuscitative efforts. The brief systolic ejection spike, no matter how high, produced very little elevation in mean blood pressure. Two years later, Del Guercio reported cardiorespiratory variables measured during resuscitation attempts on eleven patients. In three patients, both open- and closed-chest techniques were used. In their experience, a direct method of massage with the open chest produced significantly more physiologic blood flow than did compression of the heart through the intact chest. During internal massage, the cardiac index was twice that achieved by external massage. Stroke index and mean circulation times were significantly better with the open technique. In all three instances, the open-chest resuscitations were performed after the closed-chest technique had been previously used and, even so, produced significantly

greater total blood flow. With direct cardiac massage, the best flow rates were produced by pulse rates between 70 and 120 strokes per minute. The best flows during external cardiac massage occurred at lower pulse rates. These workers make a plea that one not delay too long in using direct cardiac massage in instances where closed-chest techniques are ineffective.

In a 1966 communication, Cohn and Del Guercio report on eighteen patients studied by means of a mobile cardiac catheterization laboratory prior to cardiac arrest and during resuscitative attempts. In six of the patients, the cardiac index was measured during both direct and external cardiac massage. Much higher blood flows were noted during open-chest massage. Although stroke index was not a great deal higher, elevated stroke rates were effective in producing a higher output with a shorter circulation time. (See Table 24-1.)

Again, it needs to be reemphasized that the physician should assume an obligation to maintain his ability with both external cardiac compression and open or direct heart massage. While the latter has obvious disadvantages, the open-chest approach does

Table 24-1. Cardiorespiratory parameters in cardiac resuscitation*

	Data prior to arrest: 10 patients	Both external and internal massage in 6 patients		Postresuscitation data: 12 patients	
		External	Internal	C.I. < 2.0	C.I. > 2.0
Cardiac index (L./min./M²)	1.91	0.56†	1.28	0.93†	3.09
Stroke index (cc./M²)	20.2	10.6	14.2	14.9†	32.2
Pulse rate (beats/min.)	110	57†	90	75†	101
Mean circulation time (sec.)	42.0	106.8†	46.3	51.8†	15.6
"Central blood volume" (L.)	1.31	1.77	1.64	1.05†	1.44
B.P.:S./D.	93/49	55/12	67/22	55/34	55/31
Mean (mm. Hg)	62	25	33	40	38
Peripheral resistance (dyne-sec./cm.⁻⁵)	2461	2291†	1210	2205†	558
Central venous pressure (cm. H_2O)	9	22	20	17	19
Arterial blood					
pH	7.24	7.21	7.25	7.24†	7.23
P_{CO_2} (mm. Hg)	43.2	62.3	56.9	49.5†	70.9
Buffer base (mEq./L.)	38	39	42	39	48
O_2 (% saturation)	89.0	73.1	89.4	85.1	91.3

*Adapted from Cohn, J. D. et al.: Department of Surgery, Albert Einstein College of Medicine, New York.
†Indicates chance probability less than 0.05.

produce a higher cardiac output and there is a lower mean circulation time. The survival rate using the open-chest approach in trained hands, overall, is probably higher than with the external cardiac compression technique, particularly with regard to selective groups of cases.

Effect of prolonged massage

The limit of prolonged cardiac compression that is compatible with successful resuscitation is not known. I examined a heart that had been massaged for a period of 2 hours, and there were no gross indications of any epicardial hemorrhages or other signs of trauma. The pericardial sac had not been opened.

In other instances, however, prolonged massage is associated with many of the complications that have been discussed in a previous chapter. Prolonged massage, especially with the pericardium open, has frequently provided enough pressure on a given point to allow the compressing finger to push through the wall of the ventricle. In other instances coronary vessels have been damaged by prolonged massage and epicardial hemorrhages and hematomas have been produced.

Instances of successful resuscitation following prolonged massage are not infrequent. I have seen an individual in whom the normal cardiac rhythm was restored after a period of 2 hours. There are a number of recorded cases of continual cardiac compression periods of between 40 minutes and 2 hours. Touroff and Adelman recorded an uneventful recovery following 40 minutes of cardiac massage. No neurologic sequelae were noted in a 63-year-old man upon whom intermittent cardiac compression was carried out by Carter for over 25 minutes.

Cardiopulmonary resuscitation in patients with prosthetic heart valves

The problems posed by cardiac resuscitation in the patient with a mitral or aortic

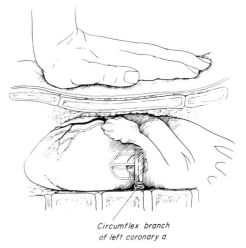

Circumflex branch of left coronary a.

Fig. 24-2. The circumflex coronary artery is in an excellent anatomical position to be injured during external cardiac compression in the presence of a mitral valve prosthesis. (From Burnside, J., Daggett, W. M., and Austen, W. G.: Ann. Thorac. Surg. 9:267-271, © 1970, Little, Brown and Co.)

valve prosthesis are several. The metallic ring of the prosthesis is anchored on a plane opposite that of the sternum and vertebral bodies. With the use of closed-chest external cardiac compression, the unyielding ring is in excellent position to apply damaging pressure in the region of the posterior A-V groove (between the mitral prosthetic ring and the vertebral bodies). It may exert pressure on the myocardium causing myocardial hematoma. Disruption of the ventricle, rupture of a coronary artery or intractable conduction disturbances may result. Burnside and co-workers (see Fig. 24-2) report an instance of rupture of the circumflex branch of the left coronary artery at the time of closed-chest compression for cardiac arrest. The patient had a Starr-Edwards mitral valve prosthesis. They believe that the hematoma found at autopsy was due to pressure necrosis caused by the prosthetic valve ring during the brief period of external cardiac massage. Thomas reports one patient with extensive biventricular and septal hematoma extending as much as 3 cm. in thickness and obstructing the ventricular chambers. In addition, two patients had lacerated atrioventricular grooves in addition to perforation of the posterior left ventricular wall. Two of the patients had ball valve prostheses with the metallic cage; the third had a disc valve prosthesis. All three of these were in the mitral position.

Although successful resuscitations of patients with heart valve prosthesis subjected to prolonged external cardiac resuscitation are well known (Stein), the presence of the valve does present an inherent complication, which prompts Burnside to urge electrical defibrillation as the first maneuver in patients requiring resuscitation after prosthetic valve replacement, ventricular asystole being relatively rare. If the patient does not respond quickly to defibrillation and a short period of closed-chest compression, then the situation may well constitute an indication for open-chest cardiac compression to avoid the effect of compressing the valve between the sternum and the vertebral bodies.

Ventricular defibrillation in obese individuals

In an effort to determine the electrical energy and current requirements for external closed-chest ventricular defibrillation, Geddes and associates at Baylor report that the minimal electrical requirement for defibrillation at all weights is 1 ampere (peak current) per kilogram body weight with electrodes applied over the manubrium and apex beat of the heart. Energy is not the best criterion for specification of electrical parameters required. For adequate defibrillation of a subject weighing greater than 100 kilograms, the electrical dose is greater than that supplied by currently available defibrillators. Their study would imply that in such individuals one might need to resort to open-chest defibrillation.

Chapter 25

VENTRICULAR DEFIBRILLATION: GENERAL CONSIDERATIONS

Un coeur qui tremule n'est pas un coeur mort (a quivering heart is not dead).

d'Halluin

Ventricular defibrillation by electrical countershock has not long been the widely accepted and prognostically favorable technique that it now is. The historic contributions of Prevost and Batelli in 1900, followed by the work of Hooker and associates in 1933, are particularly noteworthy and are presented in greater detail elsewhere in this book. However, it has only been 27 years since the first successful case of ventricular defibrillation by electrical countershock—an accomplishment that we are likely to consider remote when contrasted with today's almost routine presence of the electrical cardiac defibrillator throughout most hospitals.

Wiggers lists the following four general requirements (still relevant after four decades) that must be fulfilled if successful defibrillation is to occur:

1. Fibrillation must cease completely in every fraction of the myocardium. If even a vestige of fibrillating muscle remains, coordinate contractions never develop.
2. Adequate pacemakers must survive to initiate impulses with an excitatory value sufficient to inaugurate coordinated contraction.
3. Not too many pacemakers should be present —preferably one—to dominate the reexcitement of the defibrillated ventricle. If there are too many, they cause reversion to fibrillation.
4. The muscle fractions that are so excited must be capable of responding with reasonably vigorous contractions; otherwise weak, incoordinated beats result, and the heart dies in a hypodynamic state or reverts to fibrillation.

Electrical countershock is clearly the most effective means of defibrillating the human heart. Regular sinus rhythm may resume almost immediately following electrical countershock, sometimes, however, being preceded by an episode of atrial fibrillation or other arrhythmias induced by the countershock.

Mechanism of defibrillation

For electrical ventricular defibrillation to be successful, it would seem that the split-second electrical contact received by the ventricular myocardium must result in abrupt and complete contraction of all muscle fibers. By eliminating all uncoordinated ectopic foci of activity and converging them into one single contractile effort, followed by complete refraction of the muscle mass of the ventricles, a coordinated effort by individual muscle fibers is subsequently encouraged.

Since increasing interest has been centering on the mechanism of production and the treatment of ventricular fibrillation, knowledge has increased considerably.

Factors in the development of closed-chest defibrillation

Although this topic is dealt with in detail in other chapters, some generalities will be mentioned here.

Unquestionably, the successful application of closed-chest defibrillation tech-

336

niques (Figs. 25-1 and 25-2) has greatly enhanced and altered cardiac resuscitative techniques.

Ventricular defibrillation can be satisfactorily accomplished in some instances, even though no artificial ventilation has taken place. Such a situation is possible if electrical defibrillation is applied within 45 to 50 seconds after the arrest occurs. If longer periods of time do ensue, Hosler has shown that defibrillation attempts alone will not be successful.

At the sixth conference on Electronic Instrumentation and Nucleonics in Medicine (1952), MacKay presented a paper in which he discussed the problem of electrical defibrillation without applying the electrodes directly to the heart itself. With closed-chest defibrillation, the momentary current of many amperes at several thousand volts can be supplied by the sudden discharge of a condenser that has slowly stored this energy. MacKay found in his experiments on dogs that condensers, from 2 to 12 μf. charged to from 500 to 4,000 volts, can be discharged through the chest without producing ill effects aside from trivial burns. A current of this amplitude discharged through the spine did not produce paraplegia. A typical value of the peak current was noted to be 55 amperes, indicating a body resistance of 75 ohms. He found that these intense discharges did stop fibrillation. Guyton and Satterfield suggested that 440 volts would be more than adequate for defibrillation of the human heart through the unopened chest. The use of electrodes 20 cm. in diameter or larger would necessitate as much as 30 to 60 amperes of current flow.

With A.C. defibrillators (now largely replaced by D.C. defibrillators), three to four hundred volts by the closed-chest approach are known to be adequate to defibrillate the average ventricle. I have, however, felt it necessary to apply over 750 volts on occa-

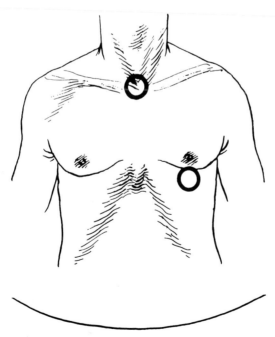

Fig. 25-1. Optimum position for placement of electrodes for closed-chest defibrillation. Electrode paste should be liberally applied.

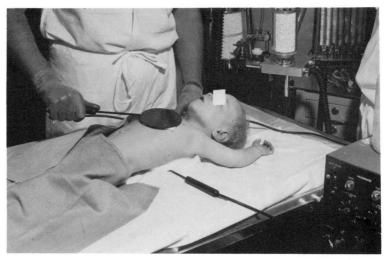

Fig. 25-2. Closed-chest defibrillation in the infant. Saline-soaked sponges are employed for good electrical contact. (From Dawson, B., and others: Circulation **25:**976, 1962.)

sion. Two patients had aortic stenosis, and repeated attempts with a smaller voltage were unsuccessful. The first attempt with the large voltage, however, was successful. For a child, 250 volts is usually adequate.

Guyton and Satterfield attempted to determine optimal conditions for electrical defibrillation of the heart through the unopened chest. They believe that the use of electrodes lodged in the heart itself promote the greatest density of current flow at the lowest possible voltage and that small electrodes may require several times as much voltage as do large electrodes to achieve the same results. Hooker and his co-workers and Ferris and associates, in the early 1930s, demonstrated that defibrillation can be accomplished by applying electricity through the thorax with external electrodes, but that a relatively low frequency of success can be anticipated. High voltage requirements are necessary when applied through the unopened chest. In order for a single stimulus to defibrillate a heart, it is necessary that a large condenser charged to several thousand volts originate the stimulus. Yet, as pointed out by Guyton and Satterfield, a short train of sinusoidal stimuli of only 50

volts is capable of stopping fibrillation. A single stimulus delivered from a condenser charged to 2,000 volts will not accomplish the same effect. They conclude that a train of stimuli can stop fibrillation without causing complete refractoriness of the ventricular muscle; it can, instead, act by simply blocking the pathway of the fibrillary impulses as they momentarily arrive within the effective field of the defibrillary stimulus. It appears that prolonged stimuli are essentially no better than shorter ones. The important factor in defibrillation is the density of current flow through the heart.

Direct versus alternating current for ventricular defibrillation*

During a visit to Negovskii's laboratory in Moscow in the summer of 1962, I was able to observe repeated use of direct current for ventricular defibrillation through the unopened chest. It was the opinion then

---

*As used in this chapter, the term "A.C. defibrillation" refers to defibrillation with a 60 c.p.s. bidirectional shock of relatively long duration, while the term "D.C. defibrillation" refers to defibrillation with a much shorter and typically higher amplitude unidirectional shock.

of Negovskii and Gurvich that direct current offers certain advantages over alternating current.

The relative merits of D.C. and A.C. defibrillation have been more clearly defined within recent years. Several large clinics report clinical impressions to the effect that D.C. defibrillation is advantageous. Lefemine and his co-workers from Harvard Medical School reported to the Surgical Forum of the American College of Surgeons on their comparative studies. Using a D.C. defibrillator constructed by the American Optical Company of Buffalo, New York, and described by Lown and associates, Lefemine was convinced that the defibrillation is consistently more effective across the intact chest of normothermic animals. In addition, fewer undesirable side effects are noted. In this study, 172 attempts at defibrillation with D.C. are compared with 137 attempts with A.C. Failure is generally defined as inability to defibrillate after three rapidly repeated shocks. D.C. was unsuccessful in two attempts on one animal. On the other hand, A.C. failed to defibrillate a heart in twenty instances; and in each of these episodes, D.C. countershock returned the heart to a normal sinus rhythm. Most of the A.C. failures occurred during the hypothermic state at approximately 20° C.

Russian workers have shown interest in the D.C. defibrillator for some time. At the 1956 session of the Scientific Research Institute for Experimental Surgical Apparatus and Instruments, Nevotonova reported on experiences with a defibrillator. External defibrillation was being used at that time. The defibrillator described was capable of developing a potential of from 100 to 6,000 volts that can be discharged through the patient's body for 5 to 10 msec. It was believed that defibrillation can be more quickly and easily accomplished by a high-tension discharge than by other methods. One clinical trial with the apparatus involved a patient who developed ventricular fibrillation while

undergoing cardiac surgery. Interestingly enough, one electrode was connected by placing it beneath the patient's spine and the other was placed directly on the heart. After 5,000 volts were applied, defibrillation occurred.

Myocardial burns have been reported by the pathologist after unsuccessful efforts at defibrillation, and they have been observed clinically. Obviously, this is an undesirable feature of electrical ventricular defibrillation, although its relative importance as a complicating factor may be somewhat exaggerated. At any rate, D.C. shock appears to cause less temperature elevation than A.C. Burns do occur, however, and have been reported following D.C. shocks with 50 watt-seconds during internal or direct application. Most patients require only 30 watt-seconds or less when the electrodes are applied directly to the myocardial surface.

Lefemine and Harken, in reporting on experience at the Peter Bent Brigham Hospital, state that successful defibrillation at low body temperatures can be routinely accomplished with D.C. In several instances, a single shock of 30 watt-seconds was successful, although repeated alternating current shocks at 250 volts failed.

The advantages of successfully defibrillating the hypothermic heart following elective cardioplegia are several. A reduction in total bypass time may be accomplished. If present, heart block can be noted early.

After prolonged massage and repeated efforts at defibrillation, multiple cardiac arrhythmias may be experienced following successful defibrillation. These may include ventricular tachycardia, complete heart block, and ventricular asystole. Most comparative studies indicate that the D.C. application appears to provoke fewer post-defibrillation arrhythmias than does the A.C. defibrillator. Fewer ECG changes indicative of myocardial damage are likewise claimed.

Advocates of D.C. defibrillation stress

certain advantages over the use of A.C. Some of the advantages are:

1. D.C. defibrillation can deliver an electrical discharge of an extremely brief duration, measured in milliseconds. Theoretically, less injury to the heart muscle may occur.

2. The D.C. defibrillators can be plugged into any electrical outlet since the current drain is equivalent to that of a 100-watt lamp. An additional advantage is that the apparatus can be used at any place where a 12-volt battery is present, such as in an ambulance.

3. Since the D.C. defibrillator should not be affected by line voltage variations, the accuracy in calibration of countershock intensity is greater.

4. Since the D.C. defibrillator can deliver only the amount of energy stored in the capacitor, it is unlikely that a voltage drop and fuse burnout or a line overload will affect the energy delivered by the unit.

5. Experimentally and clinically, the D.C. countershock appears to have greater success in difficult defibrillation efforts than the A.C. countershock.

6. Evidence of acute myocardial infarction, as demonstrated by ECG changes, is observed more commonly following A.C. countershocks than with D.C. countershock.

7. Cardiac arrhythmias, which frequently occur following A.C. defibrillation, are less frequent after D.C. countershock.

8. There is a potential reduction of the hazard to the operator by the nonrepetitive nature of the D.C. pulse and its short duration.

An added advantage in favor of D.C. defibrillation is that there is a marked decrease in the total body response of striated muscle at the time of the shock because of the shorter duration of shock. This convulsive-like motion can be most disconcerting. For example, intravenous needles may be displaced from the vein.

An important feature of D.C. is its relative inability to throw the normal heart into ventricular fibrillation should it receive an accidental shock. Even though shock is applied in the T wave phase of the cardiac cycle as well as during the other phases of the cycle, Jude and colleagues were unable to induce ventricular fibrillation in 314 tests performed on forty dogs. There are certain disadvantages, however. Since the capacitors need recharging after each shock, it is impossible to deliver serial countershocks at intervals of less than 5 seconds. It is possible that this undesirable feature can be corrected. In addition, the capacitor discharge defibrillator may be somewhat more dangerous because of the high voltages employed.

As the A.C. defibrillator does not require charge-up time, repetitive shocks may be administered. "Serial shocking," as first described by Wiggers, may prove helpful in the refractory case of persistent fibrillation.

The effect of A.C. and D.C. countershock on ventricular function was studied by Yarbrough and colleagues, regarding heart rate, left ventricular and diastolic pressure, mean aortic pressure, and peak ventricular pressure. Both A.C. and D.C. were effective and well tolerated in dogs, but it was evident that the D.C. shock produced significantly fewer changes in the above variables than did A.C. For example, in the A.C. series, there is a greater rise in heart rate and a greater decrease in both aortic and ventricular pressures. In two instances, D.C. countershock was effective in terminating episodes of ventricular fibrillation refractory to repeated A.C. shocks.

Empirical defibrillation

The few questionable disadvantages of "blind" electrical countershock seem outweighed by the potential benefit to the patient even if an exact electrocardiographic rhythm diagnosis has not yet been attained. Hubbell estimates that 60 to 80 seconds are consumed in applying electrolyte jelly, securing electrode leads, and taking an ECG rhythm strip. Since the majority of patients with cardiac arrest are fibrillating, since time is of the essence, and since some of the complications of closed-chest resuscitation can be avoided, empirical "blind" defibrillation is indicated in special instances.

Whenever possible, I attempt defibrillation even before artificial ventilation and closed-chest massage. Ideal situations arise infrequently unless the patient is being carefully monitored. Experiences during cardiac catheterization and coronary arteriography, particularly, attest to the value of this approach.

With the realization that successful resuscitation rather closely parallels the rapidity with which the heart is restored to a regular effective rhythm; that relatively minimal damage is done to a patient with cardiac arrest who is electrically shocked even though the heart is in asystole; and that a preponderance of patients with acute myocardial infarction needing cardiopulmonary resuscitation are, as a matter of fact, patients with ventricular fibrillation, it is apparent that electrical shocking can be accomplished in the emergency situation, regardless of whether or not fibrillation has been confirmed by electrocardiography.

There seems little doubt today that the treatment of choice for ventricular fibrillation under such ideal conditions as in the cardiac care unit is immediate defibrillation. Many of the patients will not lose consciousness.

Portable ventricular defibrillator

With the possibility for successful cardiac defibrillation outside the operating

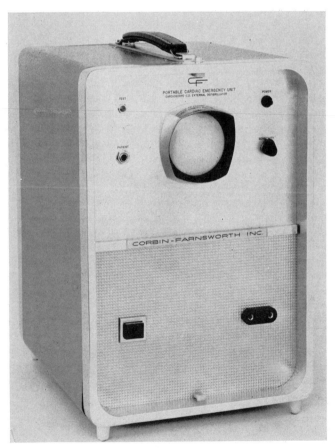

Fig. 25-3. Portable machine for ventricular defibrillation. (Courtesy Corbin-Farnsworth, Inc., Palo Alto, Calif.)

room and, indeed, occasionally outside the hospital, the development of a practical and inexpensive portable electrical difibrillator unit represents a desirable addition to the equipment for cardiac resuscitation. Undoubtedly, additional improvements will be made on existing portable units—a few of which are now available. Such a unit (Fig. 25-3) is available complete with internal and external electrodes. Desirable features include the absence of a warm-up period. For external defibrillation, only two settings are available: a 440-volt setting for an adult and a 330-volt setting for a child. A shock duration of 0.18 second is the only duration allowed. Unfortunately, voltage and duration of shock requirements are empirical features and may vary from one individual to the next; nevertheless, the simplicity of set voltage and time requirement may, in some instances, represent desirable features.

The development of a portable electrical defibrillator was reported to the American Institute of Electrical Engineers by Kouwenhoven and Knickerbocker; Jude reported on this portable defibrillator before the Surgical Forum of the American College of Surgeons. The advantages of the portable defibrillator are obvious. Not only can the capacitor-discharge external defibrillator be charged from 115 volts A.C. but also from 6- to 12-volt batteries. This voltage is increased to 2,200 volts by the use of converters and a power pack and is stored in two 25 μf. capacitors. During 196 defibrillation attempts on seventy-seven animals, ventricular defibrillation was successful in all but one instance. In about 90% of the cases, only one countershock was required.

To what extent are defibrillators being used in office practice? Because of the realization that the earliest possible defibrillation attempt leads to more probable success in resuscitation, an increasingly large number of medical clinics and private physicians' offices are being equipped with electrical defibrillators.

Defibrillation and the pressor response

The clinical observation of a sudden rise in blood pressure immediately after cardiac resuscitation has been made by us on numerous occasions. Crowell and co-workers warn that experiments in dogs indicate the wisdom of allowing the pressor response to run its course in those cases needing defibrillation since ease of defibrillation is facilitated. Usually, catecholamines are liberated by the vasoconstriction and by sympathetic discharges from tissue anoxia. These catecholamines are suddenly thrown into the circulation, but with massage they can be dissipated in about 5 minutes.

Asystole as a primary result of countershock defibrillation

Even though ventricular defibrillation is often reported to result in cardiac asystole, in actual practice, once an actively fibrillating ventricle is defibrillated with countershock, ordinarily it will spontaneously resume its normal contraction. This is particularly true in the dog. Only in rare instances will asystole result, which, of course, demands cardiac assist. Often, massage may be helpful during the first few feeble beats that occur immediately following defibrillation.

Arrhythmias following ventricular defibrillation

A variety of disturbances may be observed after ventricular defibrillation, including 2:1 A-V block, complete A-V block, and frequent premature ventricular contractions.

The incidence of arrhythmias is apparently higher in the patient who is digitalized. An induced arrhythmia is a complication of electroshock using the cardioversion technique, and it may lead to ventricular fibrillation or cardiac standstill. Schuder has, over a period of 15 years, conducted a systematic experimental study involving over 50,000 fibrillation-defibrillation episodes in dogs. Along with Stoeckle, he is currently studying arrhythmias induced by directional shock in digitalized dogs. In contrast to unidirectional shock, a bidirectional wave form has zero net electrical charge transport associated with it. It is the impression of Schuder and Stoeckle that fewer arrhythmias are associated with the bidirectional shock.

Failure to defibrillate

If one is unable to successfully achieve defibrillation, one should use another defibrillator. As emphasized by Edmark and his colleagues, there is a relatively high incidence of D.C. defibrillator failure—more than may be suspected. They note three types of defibrillator output failures in nine instruments tested. They emphasize that skeletal muscle jerk occurring at the time of defibrillator discharge is no indication of proper defibrillator function. Among other problems, breaks in the wires to the defibrillator paddles were occasionally seen. Edmark describes a simple bolometer-type dependent defibrillator tester.

Summary of factors conducive to successful ventricular defibrillation

If a high degree of success in defibrillation is to be achieved, the following conditions should usually be satisfied:

1. Adequate coronary artery flow
2. Good ventricular muscle tone
3. Adequate decompression of the left side of the heart
4. Normothermia

5. Vigorous ventricular fibrillary action
6. Unobstructed outflow tract
7. Adequate pulmonary ventilation
8. Provision of pacemaker activity—either normally or by an electric pacemaker
9. Correction of metabolic acidosis
10. Correction of abnormal ion ratios

Effects on fetus after electrical defibrillation of mother's heart

Can electrical countershock be applied for ventricular defibrillation in the pregnant patient without producing iatrogenic fetal arrhythmias or initiating uterine contractions? Curry and Quintana have helped answer this question by successfully defibrillating a 29-year-old woman with a 6-month uterine pregnancy who developed ventricular fibrillation while in the coronary care unit. The ventricular fibrillation was preceded by a premature ventricular beat, followed by a normal sinus beat, and then a rapid run of five premature ventricular beats with progressively diminishing amplitudes ending in ventricular fibrillation. A D.C. shock of 300 watt-seconds was delivered across the precordium. Fortunately fetal electrocardiographic monitoring was carried out throughout the procedure and revealed a regular ventricular rate of 150 beats a minute not affected by the countershock.

No fetal distress has been noted in at least four other instances in which D.C. countershock has been used to correct either ventricular fibrillation or atrial flutter in the mother.

Chapter 26

CARDIAC DEFIBRILLATION

Juro Wada

Possibly, a working picture of defibrillation might consist of general depolarization of the heart by a sufficiently strong current that abolishes multifocal incoordinate and ineffectual contractions, which is followed by the resumption of normal rhythm.

The present use of electrical defibrillation is one of the modern developments in cardiac surgery. To obtain more effective defibrillation, several defibrillators were developed and tested with approximately 7,000 discharges in laboratory animals.

Comparison of D.C. and A.C. defibrillation

It was found that each dog had the same threshold for fibrillation and defibrillation. Within the value of the defibrillatory threshold, the failure rate of defibrillation with D.C. was 0.8% (two out of 257) and with A.C., 7.8% (eighteen out of 204).

Repeated application of D.C. defibrillation showed little change of SGOT or ECG. Occasionally after A.C. defibrillation, hypotension persisted that required vasopresser drugs and cardiac massage. This circulatory influence after D.C. defibrillation is less common. It suggests that D.C. defibrillation is superior to A.C.

In order to determine the most satisfactory methods of D.C. defibrillation, various investigations with dogs have been carried out in our laboratory.

D.C. defibrillator apparatus

WAVE FORM

Effectiveness of defibrillation varies with the wave form of the discharge. The wave form itself can be varied by different combinations of inductance and capacitance and it can also be varied from single to multiimpulse. We found that the single-peaked wave form used externally was most effective. However, the double-peaked wave form, when used for internal defibrillation, is safer and less myocardial damage results.

INDUCTANCE

A single-peaked wave form with 1 msec. total energy discharge time is less effective than one of 3 to 10 msec. discharge time, using a 32 μf. condenser with a 100 to 200 mh. choke coil. If inductance is over 300 mh., effectiveness of defibrillation becomes unstable and poor in result. Moreover, if the inductance approaches 500 mh., there is increased myocardial damage and generally unreliable effectiveness.

CAPACITANCE

At present, there is some discussion over which is more important: the joule or the volt. A change in capacitance influences the duration of discharge. Under varying capacitances, the minimal threshold of defibrillation was measured. With a capacitance below 32 μf., effective defibrillation depends upon joules rather than upon volts

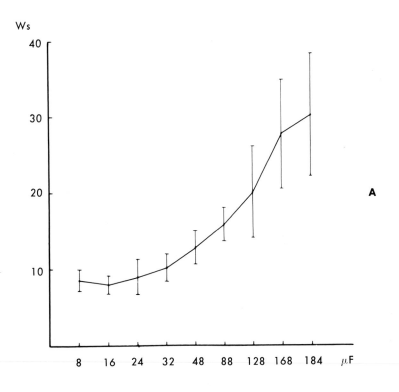

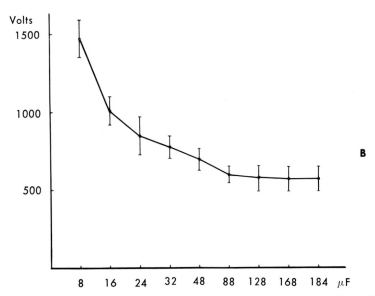

Fig. 26-1. A, Defibrillation threshold in relation to joules watt-seconds. **B,** Defibrillation threshold in relation to volts.

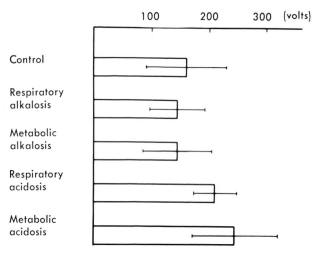

Fig. 26-2. Influence of alkalosis and acidosis for threshold of defibrillation.

(Fig. 26-1). There is less stability when values exceed 50 μf. Upon prolongation of discharge time into the vulnerable period with a 50 μf. condenser, defibrillation is increasingly less effective. In clinical cases, we use a 16 to 32 μf. condenser; in this range of capacitance, effective defibrillation is dependent on joules.

Influence on the myocardium of D.C. defibrillation

Arrhythmias frequently appear soon after shock of 3 kv., and abnormal finding of ECG continues for several days. With a shock of 4 kv., these findings appear more frequently and occasionally A-V block develops. If the voltage is over 5 kv., these changes are irreversible, and the heart occasionally goes into fibrillatory arrest without relation to vulnerable period. Myocardial necrosis is often observed microscopically. The defibrillation threshold of the dog was 8 to 32 watt-seconds (700 to 1,400 volts), and there was practically no harmful high energy required.

Influence of alkalosis and acidosis on threshold of defibrillation

The threshold of defibrillation was constant in each dog and was similar to that used to induce fibrillation. The measurement of the threshold of defibrillation was made during both acidosis and alkalosis. In both respiratory and metabolic alkalosis, the threshold was decreased by 9.4%. However, the threshold was increased by 31% in respiratory acidosis and by 59% in metabolic acidosis (Fig. 26-2). These experimental findings correspond well to clinical experiences that defibrillation is difficult in patients with acidosis.

Clinical application of D.C. defibrillation

One hundred and seventy-five patients were treated with external application of the D.C. defibrillator 403 times for various arrhythmias. During open-heart surgery, approximately 400 patients received direct application of D.C. defibrillation.

ATRIAL FIBRILLATION AND FLUTTER

Atrial fibrillation and flutter were treated most frequently in the clinical setting. The effectiveness of converting to sinus rhythm was not related to the duration or origin of arrhythmias or to the patient's sex or age. Occasionally, patients who had suffered from atrial fibrillation for over 20 years were successfully defibrillated. Long-term follow-up studies of these patients after

Table 26-1. Conversion of arrhythmias using D.C. defibrillator (external use)

	Number of cases treated	Effective conversion	
		Immediate (cases)	Long-term (cases)
Atrial fibrillation	144	128	57
Atrial flutter	17	16	9
Tachycardia	22	19	11
Extrasystole	21	17	4
Ventricular fibrillation	18	13	7
Total	222	188 (84.7%)	88 (39.6%)

defibrillation indicate recurrence of atrial fibrillation or arrhythmias to be similar to that reported in world medical literature. The appearance rate of arrhythmias is greater in the group of hypertensive cardiovascular disease patients than in postoperative patients, particularly following the replacement of cardiac valves (Table 26-1).

Eight patients with paroxysmal tachycardia after open-heart surgery were satisfactorily treated by D.C. fibrillation. Twenty-one patients with extrasystoles were treated with D.C. fibrillation with partial success. Extrasystoles of bigeminal or trigeminal type had less recurrence after treatment. Perhaps the explanation is that, with D.C. defibrillation, depolarization occurred simultaneously, even in ectopic foci of contraction (Table 26-1).

Eight cases of ventricular fibrillation that developed on the ward were satisfactorily converted to sinus rhythm following application of D.C. defibrillation. One patient, however, who had severe cardiac lesions and congestive heart failure, did not survive. One of the eight patients had a mitral valve replacement and, in the first 12 postoperative hours, developed fifty-three episodes of ventricular fibrillation. On each occasion, D.C. defibrillation was successfully applied, and she had a satisfactory recovery. Follow-up ECG revealed only a slight S-T depression. In conclusion, we feel that D.C. defibrillation is safe in clinical use.

Chapter 27

OPEN-CHEST ELECTRICAL CARDIAC DEFIBRILLATION

As mentioned in the chapter on prognosis, the chances of successful ventricular defibrillation are quite good, regardless of whether open- or closed-chest defibrillation is used. In certain instances, it is easier to attempt to resuscitate a heart that is fibrillating than one that is in complete standstill.

The physician must remember that all the principles of cardiopulmonary resuscitation apply to ventricular fibrillation up to the application of the electrodes. *After a diagnosis of cardiac arrest is made, cardiac compression should be started at once regardless of whether asystole or fibrillation is the cause of arrest.* After about 4 or 5 minutes of massage, electrical defibrillation can then be attempted. An exception can be made in the case of almost instantaneous recognition of ventricular fibrillation in areas such as the coronary care unit. *Immediate* electrical defibrillation without closed-chest massage will often suffice.

Electrical internal cardiac defibrillator unit

The constructing of an instrument capable of delivering an appropriate shocking current to the human heart is not difficult. The earlier cardiac electrical defibrillators satisfied several basic considerations:

1. They were capable of delivering an adequate amount of current.
2. They were safe. Precautions could be taken for protection against any injury to the patient or to the operator.
3. They were reliable.
4. Their cost was not prohibitive.

Fig. 27-1 shows an internal defibrillator

designed by us in 1948, complete with electrodes and foot switch. The new D.C. defibrillators are considerably more sophisticated in design.

THE ELECTRODES

In order to have optimal electrode contact, various sizes of electrodes should be available for various size hearts. Although I have on occasion used unsterile electrodes without a resulting infection following large doses of antibiotics, it is urged, of course, that this not be done and that the electrodes as well as their extensions be sterilized for 15 minutes at 250° F. Some electrodes do not withstand sterilization well. Electrodes having a back covering of nonconductive plastic are desirable, as are electrodes padded and soaked with saline prior to use.

It is apparent that there is considerable merit in the use of relatively large electrode paddles to achieve maximal depolarization with minimal voltage requirement. Thermal damage may thus be minimized. McLean's studies indicate that a heart-shaped defibrillator of about 8 by 12 cm. is ideal. It should be backed with insulating polyvinyl plastic and should have a silver conducting surface. Before shocks are given, it is important to caution all personnel to avoid touching the patient or items in contact with the patient.

For direct defibrillation, electrodes are chosen that most nearly correspond to the size of the particular heart. The electrodes are then applied directly to the myocardium. The metal should be moistened or

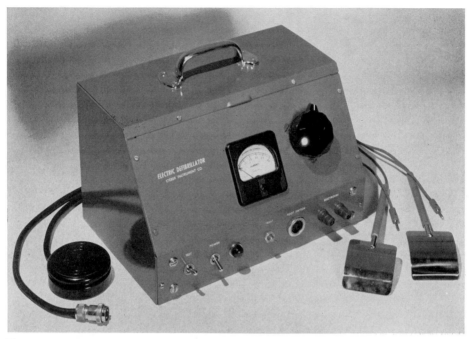

Fig. 27-1. Relatively simple and inexpensive electrical defibrillator that has repeatedly proved its value in defibrillation of the human ventricle. A more satisfactory electrode is described in the text. (Courtesy Steber Instrument Co., St. Louis, Mo.)

wrapped in gauze soaked in saline solution to increase conductivity and to avoid localized burns of the myocardium. It is advisable to compress the heart somewhat between the electrodes, as this considerably lowers the amount of voltage required for defibrillation (Guyton and Satterfield). The electrodes should be placed so that as much of the heart musculature as possible is placed between the two electrodes (Fig. 27-2). Rivkin, in fact, strongly advocates that electrode padding with moistened polyvinyl sponge be used to increase electrode contact and decreased incidence of burns.

If the electrodes are to be applied outside the chest they should be applied as shown in Fig. 25-1. Rivkin advises against wrapping the electrode with gauze; he suggests instead the polyvinyl sponge because it gives a much better contour effect and overcomes the mismatch between the curvature of the electrode and the actual shape of the heart.

Dr. Albert Star, in a motion picture illustrating placement of an artificial mitral valve, demonstrates a technique that has been effective in the occasional case of ventricular fibrillation when it is difficult to place both electrodes in an adequate fashion about the heart. In the heart requiring a repeated surgical effort, mediastinal and intrathoracic adhesions may be dense. Because of the desire to avoid annoying bleeding from the dissection of the adhesions, they are left undisturbed. Should such a heart develop ventricular fibrillation, defibrillation may be accomplished by placing one electrode within the open heart and the other on the outside of the heart.

Probably the most desirable location of the two electrodes during open-heart defibrillation is one electrode over the apex of the left ventricle and the other over the right atrium. Lung tissue or mediastinal fat should, of course, not be incorporated between the electrodes.

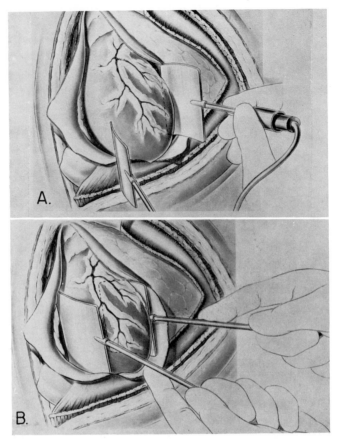

Fig. 27-2. Method for introducing metal electrodes for electrical defibrillation of heart in ventricular fibrillation. **A,** Electrodes should be moistened and held snugly against the heart. **B,** Electrodes that most nearly correspond to the contour and size of the heart should be used. (From Stephenson, H. E., Jr.: Mo. Med. 51:370-377, 1954.)

Electrical resistance of the heart

Since Ohm's law states that the current flow is dependent upon both the voltage and the resistance, it is helpful to know the electrical resistance of the human heart. Blades and co-workers studied the problem on dog hearts, living and dead, and human hearts at autopsy. They determined the total resistance of the average living dog heart to be approximately 50 ohms. If a potential difference of 110 volts was applied to the average dog heart, the current flow would equal 2.2 amperes. The average resistance of nine dead dog hearts was 97 ohms. Twenty human hearts were studied at autopsy, and a wide range from 32 to 135 ohms was noted.

The size and composition of the electrodes as well as the surface area of the heart and the contents of the fluid (Hufnagel) in the chambers of the heart must all be taken into consideration.

Regulation of current flow

Once the electrodes have been placed (as soon after massage has been discontinued as possible), the operator is ready to apply the current. This may be done by stepping on the foot switch or by pressure on a band switch, if available. The operator can thus regulate the duration of current flow as he desires.

An interval timer can be incorporated which automatically regulates current application to various fractions of a second (with A.C. defibrillators). For direct defibrillation, I no longer use the timer but prefer to regulate the time myself. The duration of current flow seems to be an empirical factor and will need to be altered from one patient to another, or even from one shock to another in the same heart.

Various combinations of time and intensity of current may be necessary for successful defibrillation. With closed-chest defibrillation, these factors are generally fixed at established levels.

"Serial" defibrillation

The electrical countershock method of ventricular defibrillation was modified somewhat by Wegria and Wiggers in 1939 by using what they termed "serial defibrillation." Wiggers explained this modification by stating:

> [It] consists in applying to the ventricles, through padded electrodes, not one, but a series, of brief and weaker alternating current shocks. Each shock lasts less than one second and has a strength of approximately 1 ampere; one or two seconds elapse between the shocks. As a rule, from three to seven such shocks suffice.*

The rationale of such a maneuver appears to be in the tendency of each successive A.C. shock to merge smaller fibrillating areas into larger ones until a convulsive state involving larger blocks of tissue is redeveloped. A final shock then stops the fibrillation and allows coordinated beating to be initiated by natural pacemakers (Wiggers). By this method, it seems likely that the interventricular septum in the deeper myocardium could be defibrillated more frequently. Atrial

---

*From Wiggers, C. J.: The physiologic basis for cardiac resuscitation from ventricular fibrillation—method for serial defibrillation, Am. Heart J. **20:** 413-422, 1940.

fibrillation, often produced by a single, strong electrical countershock, is less likely to be induced by the method of serial defibrillation.

Energy requirements for open-chest defibrillation

It is advisable to have a ventricular defibrillator with a variable voltage, or watt-seconds in the case of a D.C. defibrillator. The resistance of the child's heart is low. A voltage of from 80 to 120 volts will often revert a fibrillating child's heart to normal rhythm. In the adult heart, I have found a voltage of around 100 to 150 volts to be adequate. A voltage requirement of 220 or more has been needed in the patient with the large, hypertrophied left ventricle. With D.C. fibrillators, shock varying from 20 to 100 watt-seconds (joules) may be required. Sakakibara and co-workers have suggested rather precise positions for the placement of electrodes for the most effective method of defibrillation. Iwamoto and associates discuss this aspect and demonstrate that application to the longitudinal axis is always able to stop ventricular fibrillation with a lower voltage than if the horizontal axis is used. Reference to the longitudinal axis indicates line A-B as illustrated in Fig. 27-3. Interestingly, also, these same workers show that the threshold for defibrillation of the ventricle is lowest at the apex of the left ventricle (Fig. 27-4). The threshold rises as one goes more cranially from the apex. The interventricular septum does not represent a low threshold for defibrillation. There is no entirely clear explanation for the adequate "longitudinal" defibrillation being more effective than "horizontal." The longitudinal axis has, likewise, been a recommended plan for employment during external cardiac defibrillation (Kouwenhoven, Knickerbocker, and Jude). The work of the previously mentioned Japanese investigators fails to indicate that the impulse conducting system plays a major part, but that the difference between the length and breadth of the

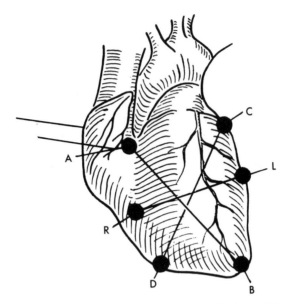

Fig. 27-3. Electrode position in bipolar stimulation of defibrillation. *A-B* represents most satisfactory position. (From Iwamoto, K., and others: Bull. Heart Inst. Jap. **1**:71, 1957.)

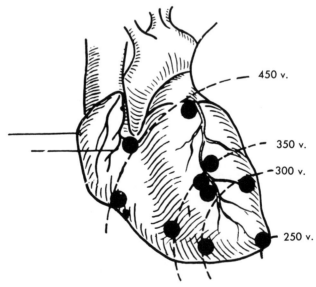

Fig. 27-4. Thresholds of defibrillation. (From Iwamoto, K., and others: Bull. Heart Inst. Jap. **1**:71, 1957.)

ventricle is the factor that makes longitudinal stimulation effective. In other words, the impulse conducting system apparently has no relationship to the efficiency of defibrillation.

Ventricular defibrillation where hazards of explosion exist

I am unaware of any explosion having occurred during elective ventricular defibrillation. The hazard is, however, real if ven-

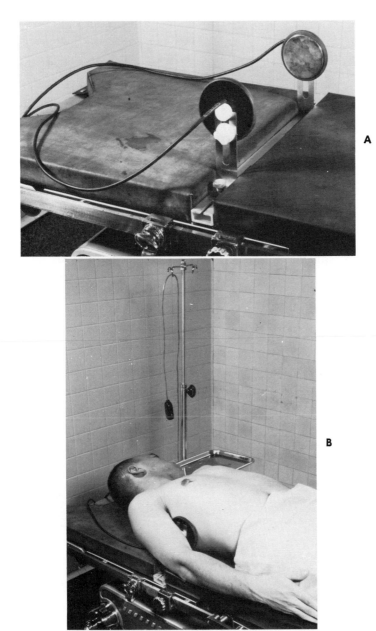

Fig. 27-5. A, External defibrillation with the chest open by means of electrodes mounted on adjustable set in which transverse bar is recessed in slot in mattress. B, Position of external electrodes on the chest (median sternotomy to be used). (From Rastelli, G. C., and others: J. Thorac. Cardiovasc. Surg. 55:116, 1968.)

tricular fibrillation is carried out in the presence of explosive gases. Under conditions of hyperbaric oxygenation, the hazard of explosion from electrical spark is increased. Under conditions likely to expose the patient and the physician to the possibility of explosion, ventricular fibrillation may require reversion by potassium.

Cardiac arrest following an explosion in the operating room is reported by Chandra. The operation was taking place in India and occurred at the time diathermy was started in connection with a resection of the maxilla for a carcinoma in a 30-year-old male. A considerable explosion occurred, but other than the cardiac arrest the patient suffered only superficial burns on the face and no other apparent injuries were noted. He made an uneventful recovery.

External defibrillation with the thorax open

An alternative approach to ventricular fibrillation in the operating room is by means of electrodes applied externally with the chest open. Rastelli and associates at the Mayo Clinic have evaluated this technique in more than fifty patients, using electrodes positioned as shown in Fig. 27-5. There are several advantages of this technique. Defibrillation may be accomplished at any moment during the operation by positioning the electrodes before the procedure begins. The promptness with which ventricular defibrillation thus occurs may add considerably to the survival rate.

In instances of multiple pleural or pericardial adhesions, one often experiences difficulty in placing the electrodes about the heart. Rastelli and his co-workers, have consistently demonstrated that external defibrillation can be applied effectively and safely in patients undergoing cardiovascular surgery through a median sternotomy. Both Rivkin and Kortz have also suggested external defibrillation even though the chest is open.

External-internal defibrillation

Most cardiac surgeons have occasionally encountered the patient with an obliterated

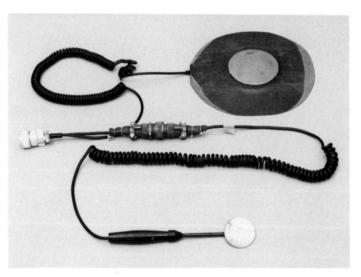

Fig. 27-6. The flat metal plate imbedded in a round, rubber pad whose thickness is tapered around the periphery is placed under the patient's left lower scapula. Attached to an interchangeable connector is a standard internal panel with a button switch allowing for internal-external defibrillation. (From Roe, B. B.: Ann. Thorac. Surg. **13:**189, © 1972, Little, Brown and Co.)

pericardial space either from a previous operation or from some prior inflammatory condition. Obviously the pericardial symphysis poses some problems if ventricular defibrillation should be necessary. If the operative approach is from the right side, application of electrodes may be all but impossible.

In coping with this problem, Benson Roe supports the use of an external-internal defibrillator for just such occasions (Fig. 27-6). It consists of a smooth, flat electrode mounted on a rubber pad, which is placed under the patient's left chest prior to the start of the procedure and before draping. A single standard internal electrode paddle is connected by wire from the external plate and can be applied to any surgically exposed surface of the heart. The energy requirements have varied from 60 watt-seconds to 200 watt-seconds.

There are a number of advantages to the external-internal defibrillation technique. It has been extensively studied by Borman and associates at the Hadassah University Hospital in Jerusalem on both an experimental basis and a clinical basis in more than eighty patients undergoing open-heart surgery. Their work was stimulated, to some extent, by their inability to reproduce the defibrillation results obtained by Rastelli using external defibrillation, even with the chest open.

The technique involves the use of a 12 by 12 cm. stainless steel rectangular plate on a sponge-rubber base as the external electrode; it is placed under the back in order to lie posterior to the heart. The patient's chest is opened by a midline sternotomy incision. One must ensure good conduction by liberal application of conductive paste and by making certain that the patient's back actually rests on the electrode. The internal electrode is a slightly concave, circular paddle, 8 cm. in diameter for adults or less for children. The stainless steel paddle is well padded to prevent contact thermal burns. It may also be used as an external

electrode when necessary. Defibrillation is usually successful with the D.C. defibrillator set for 20 to 30 watt-seconds, although occasionally up to 45 watt-seconds may be required. The internal electrode is pressed firmly against the anterior surface of the heart for adequate conduction purposes.

It appears that the external-internal defibrillation technique provides a more homogeneous current distribution to the heart with a lessened possibility of thermal damage, particularly when increased energy levels are applied to hearts resistant to defibrillation. Borman believes that the most striking benefit from the external-internal defibrillation technique is that it avoids freeing dense vascular adhesions that may remain between the heart and pericardium as a result of previous surgery, which may provoke considerable blood loss if removed especially following heparinization and cardiopulmonary bypass.

Braimbridge and co-workers reported on the use of external D.C. defibrillation during open-heart surgery at St. Thomas Hospital in London. They found the technique of Rastelli to be most effective except in the grossly hypertrophied ventricle of aortic valve disease, in which case internal D.C. defibrillation is usually more effective. External defibrillation is particularly valuable in second operations in which only the aorta and right and left atria need to be dissected and the ventricles may be left entirely undisturbed. With this technique there is less chance of encountering a low cardiac output induced by mobilization of the left ventricle prior to going on the bypass; and the chance of hemorrhage, following bypass, is reduced. They find that external defibrillation has also prevented the occasional recurrence of ventricular fibrillation when internal defibrillator plates are removed from the pericardium. In addition, the likelihood of myocardial damage from the heat of defibrillation is reduced. Altogether they treated sixty patients with external defibrillation using the method of Rastelli.

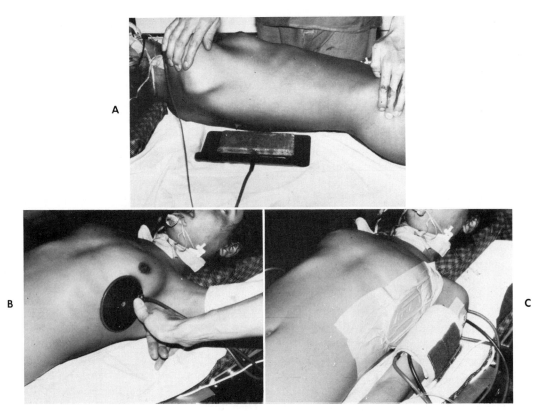

Fig. 27-7. A, The posterior defibrillation plate is placed behind the right hemithorax. **B,** A low profile plate is placed over the apex. **C,** Low profile plate is fixed in position with adhesive tape. (From Braimbridge, M. V., and others: Thorax 26:455-456, 1971.)

In Fig. 27-7 the D.C. defibrillator plate is shown being placed behind the right hemithorax. The patient's weight is allowed to rest on the plate. The anterior plate is a specially developed, low-profile plate that is attached over the apex of the heart and fixed in position with adhesive tape and is then covered with a sterile plastic sheet. Using this method, thirty-five of the sixty patients were converted to a sustained, co-ordinated beat by a single D.C. shock. Only three patients needed three or more shocks. Twelve of the patients could not be returned to a coordinated beat with external defibrillation; this is thought to be because of the grossly hypertrophied left ventricle attributed to aortic valve disease. In several cases, however, the plates were positioned too far posteriorly.

Chapter 28

THE DIFFICULT RESUSCITATION: RECURRENT EPISODES OF VENTRICULAR FIBRILLATION

The patient who experiences repeated periods of ventricular asystole or fibrillation presents a considerable challenge in management. To successfully restore a heart to its normal rhythm, only to have a short-lived period of success, taxes one's ingenuity. McLaughlin and associates were able to successfully resuscitate a 25-year-old woman despite ninety-nine separate episodes of ventricular fibrillation requiring over 150 indirect current shocks over a period of 60 hours. Cases have been reported in which over eighty separate episodes of Adams-Stokes attacks occurred during a period of several days. I encountered a 35-year-old woman who experienced thirty separate episodes of ventricular asystole over a 9-hour period. The patient was 4 days postpartum, with generalized peritonitis following retraction of an ileostomy. Final efforts were unsuccessful.

Questions in recurrent fibrillation

In such instances, one might pose the following questions:

1. By reestablishing circulation, is one providing for recirculation of a noxious agent? Numerous drug sensitivities have been manifested by a cardiotoxic effect. I recall a nurse who experienced ventricular fibrillation shortly after cocaine was applied to the mucous membrane of the nose. Although cardiac resuscitation was easily accomplished, repeated episodes of ventricular fibrillation occurred until the cocaine had been metabolized. Similar encounters with penicillin sensitivities, for example, have been experienced. In a patient reported by McLaughlin a digitalis intoxication was suspected. It is necessary to repeatedly use electrical countershock to reverse the ventricular fibrillation until the arrhythmic effects of the drug have subsided.

Digitalis intoxication is a good example of a reversible disorder that may require multiple efforts at defibrillation until the toxic effects of the drug have dissipated. In the meantime, any possible measures to decrease the effect of the specific toxicity should be taken. In the case of digitalis, use of intravenous potassium is indicated.

Episodes of cardiac arrest may recur from the reinfusion of blood carrying end products of anaerobic metabolism from hypoxic cells when occluding aortic clamps are removed or when venous inflow occlusion is reversed. The restoration of blood flow to large masses of hypoxic tissue will shortly perfuse the heart with blood likely to precipitate asystole or, more likely, ventricular fibrillation.

Most hearts can be defibrillated even if metabolic acidosis is present—but not always without recurrence. Gerst, Fleming, and Malm suggest that gradients of hydrogen or other as yet undetermined ions across the myocardial cell membranes may be responsible for important changes in cardiac physiology—as evidenced by the promptness with which the arrhythmia occurs after the heart is perfused with acidotic blood and the rapid improvement in cardiac function following correction of metabolic acidosis by infusion of alkalis or buffer solutions.

Recurrent bouts of fibrillation are common in hypokalemic states and may be precipitated by any factor that decreases the refractory period of the heart. Obviously, ventricular premature beats occurring in the vulnerable 30 milliseconds of the upstroke and at the peak of the T wave are prone to precipitate ventricular fibrillation, as is anything that shortens electrical systole.

Mechanical cardiac massage with a Brunswick heart-lung resuscitator was done for 3 hours during peritoneal dialysis in an effort to correct the biochemical effects produced by salicylate poisoning. The patient was a 49-year-old woman who had attempted suicide and whose heart subsequently stopped.

2. Is a cholinergic-blocking agent indicated? By interfering with the action of acetylcholine on the patterned cell receptor, atropine prevents the vagovagal reflexes from taking effect. Well-documented examples of the value of atropine have established this drug's effectiveness in an occasional cardiac arrest case. For example, the vagovagal effect produced by the oculocardiac reflex can be prevented with atropine. Trigger zones producing cardiac arrest in instances of glossopharyngeal tic douloureux may be controlled with atropine. I know of several repetitious instances in which traction of abdominal viscera produced cardiac asystole that finally responded to the administration of atropine sulfate.

Studies by Pansetrau and Abboud on the hemodynamic effects of ventricular fibrillation support the rationale for the use of atropine in the treatment of ventricular fibrillation, particularly when fibrillation recurs spontaneously after countershock. They conclude from their study that ventricular fibrillation is associated with two major hemodynamic responses; one is a negative chronotropic response that appears to be mediated through a cholinergic mechanism, and the other is a positive inotropic response that is related to adrenergic mechanisms. The former response is illustrated by sinus bradycardia and sinus node arrest. Although sinus node arrest may last only 10 to 20 seconds after ventricular defibrillation, sinus bradycardia may be maintained for up to 10 minutes after conversion; its magnitude seems related to the duration of fibrillation. Also associated with bradycardia are frequent premature ventricular beats. If atropine is given or if the vagi are sectioned, sinus tachycardia is reduced and the premature ventricular beats are abolished. With cholinergic blockade by atropine the incidence of spontaneous recurrence of ventricular fibrillation was reduced from 43% to 13% in the experimental animal. Just how the cholinergic pathway is activated is not clear, but it may originate from the coronary vessels, myocardial stretch receptors, baroreceptors, or chemoreceptors. It is even speculated that the response may result from cerebral ischemia.

3. Will open-chest cardiac massage provide additional support? Although closed-chest resuscitation is now a well-established technique for resuscitation, there are times when an open-chest approach may be indicated. Shocket and Rosenblum maintained closed-chest massage for 75 minutes in a 32-year-old male following a total colectomy for ulcerative colitis. In spite of repeated attempts at conversion with D.C. electrical shock, it was not until the chest was finally opened and open-chest defibrillation attempted that the heart was successfully defibrillated. Despite a period with fixed, dilated pupils and loss of spontaneous respiration, the patient made an eventual recovery. Because of the reflux of blood into the pulmonary veins during closed-chest massage, pulmonary edema— otherwise unexplained—may provide a major complication. In a case that I observed, the resultant storage shift to the alveoli was of massive proportions. An increased likelihood of pulmonary edema with closed-chest resuscitation may be explained on the basis of these theoretical factors: Resistance to ve-

nous return may be less with a closed chest. With the open-chest approach, massage is usually more or less in the nature of ventricular compression rather than an involvement of the entire heart. Compression of the chest wall over a prolonged period of time may mechanically traumatize the pulmonary parenchyma.

4. What effect does bone marrow and fat embolization have on the pulmonary circulation? Jackson and Greendyke found pulmonary fat emboli in forty-six of fifty-seven patients on whom closed-chest resuscitation was used. Of these, 81% showed emboli in the alveolar capillaries and occasionally in the larger vessels as well. Lee and Merkel report finding these emboli in twelve of sixteen patients on whom external cardiac massage had been carried out. It appears that the effect on the vascular bed may be considerable.

A decision to open the chest may be prompted by suspicion of a massive pulmonary or coronary embolus. Occasionally a large right-sided air embolus, requiring aspiration, may be diagnosed. An unrecognized cardiac tamponade may be contributing to the failure of resuscitation. An unrecognized pneumothorax may be discovered.

5. Should the cardiac pacemaker be used? Obviously, it should be used if there is an A-V conduction block. Ideally, a standby pacemaker should be available when there is suspicion of A-V conduction block.

Left atrial pacing with a permanently implanted, transvenous pacemaker for the management of recurrent ventricular fibrillation complicating acute myocardial infarction was first reported by Moss and associates. In their patient, a 67-year-old male with an acute myocardial infarction, twelve episodes of defibrillation occurred before there was a stabilization of the patient's cardiac situation. The usual methods of controlling recurrent ventricular arrhythmias were used, including the combined use of atropine, lidocaine, and pro-

cainamide. Right atrial pacemaking and left ventricular pacing were used but did not prevent the recurrent episodes of ventricular fibrillation. It was not until the transvenous catheter was passed into the left atrium, probably through the intra-atrial septum (foramen ovale), that the episodes of recurrent ventricular fibrillation were prevented. A rapid supraventricular pacing at the rate of 110 per minute proved most advantageous. This represents the first successful use of left atrial pacing with a permanently implanted transvenous pacemaker for the management of recurrent ventricular fibrillation complicating acute myocardial infarction. Moss reviews the hemodynamic effects of atrial pacing, which apparently are proving to be slightly superior to those of ventricular pacing, in the absence of atrioventricular block. For one thing, the production of ventricular irritable rhythms by mechanical impact of the catheter against the ventricular wall is eliminated. Pick and co-workers have documented the mechanism by which rapid pacing suppresses ventricular irritability.

In spite of the fact that the patient's skin was mottled, no blood pressure could be obtained during external cardiac compression with an external cardiac compressor machine, and that resuscitation efforts had continued for almost 2 hours, the resuscitation team at Lower Bucks County Hospital in Bristol, Pennsylvania, was encouraged to persist in resuscitation efforts because the patient's pupils still remained constricted. In addition, the patient was suffering from acute myocardial infarction. After eight countershocks, an attempt at external cardiac pacing, and various pharmacologic assists, the patient was successfully resuscitated (Quan). Lillehei reports a successful resuscitation with closed-chest massage lasting 3 hours. Others have reported prolonged resuscitation with eventual success (Stept and Russell).

6. Ventricular defibrillation of the hypothermic patient often presents serious difficulties. When the patient is in a controlled environment within the operating room,

these can often be handled promptly. A patient admitted to the emergency room with profound accidental hypothermia presents a more challenging situation. Towne and his associates encountered such a patient in a 58-year-old alcoholic admitted comatose, hypotensive, and with a bradycardia. His rectal temperature was 25° C. Ventricular pacing was attempted but induced ventricular fibrillation, presumably because of the lowered fibrillation threshold associated with hypothermia. Prolonged efforts at cardiac massage and assisted ventilation along with external defibrillation were unsuccessful. Sodium bicarbonate, lidocaine, and potassium were administered intravenously. Thirty minutes later the patient's pupils were beginning to dilate and become nonreactive to light but his rectal temperature was still 25° C. At this point the patient was placed on partial cardiopulmonary bypass with the use of the left femoral vein and artery and the blood was warmed to 37.8° C. Two hours after the onset of ventricular fibrillation the patient's temperature reached 34.4° C., and at this point the heart responded to a single shock of 350 watt-seconds. The externally applied defibrillator restored the patient's sinus rhythm and the blood pressure returned to a near normal level. After a somewhat stormy postoperative course, the patient was finally discharged. Fell reported a somewhat similar case of a patient whose temperature was 22.2° C. Fibrillation could not be corrected until the patient was rapidly rewarmed by the use of partial cardiopulmonary bypass via the femoral artery and the vein and internal defibrillation was successfully applied when the patient's temperature had reached 30° C.

7. When should hypothermia be instituted? The patient being subjected to repetitive episodes of cerebral anoxia will receive some protection from a lowered metabolic rate provided by moderate hypothermia. The patient suspected of having a cerebral insult from anoxia should be placed on the cooling blanket. Obviously, the patient's state of oxygenation should be carefully reviewed.

8. In patients with recurrent episodes of cardiac arrest, when should resuscitative efforts cease? Successes in the resuscitation of such patients are being reported with a frequency sufficient to lend encouragement to persistent efforts. Resuscitative efforts are justifiable as long as there is any reasonable expectation of functional cerebral activity. This is particularly true in the patient with no major underlying irreversible disease process or terminal malignancy. Most hearts can be defibrillated. Most hearts can be restored to a regular rhythm. To maintain this activity, however, taxes the ingenuity of the physician.

9. At what point does life end? Is it when the heart stops while the brain still has the ability to function or is it when the brain dies but the heart still beats? The answer to the question is, of course, predicated upon several considerations. For example, how does one determine brain "death"? The electroencephalogram has been used increasingly to help this determination. In spite of its reliability, however, its interpretation must be made with caution in some instances. For example, in barbiturate intoxication, recovery after as long as 72 hours of "flat" EEG tracings has been known. The American Electroencephalographic Society suggests that serial tracings 24 hours apart should be utilized with both tracings being absolutely flat at maximal gain. The tracings should be made with high-quality, 8-channel equipment and with no electronic resuscitation equipment or monitoring devices in operation during the period of recording (which ideally should last 20 to 30 minutes). To be sure there is no machine error, the electrodes should also be placed on the head of the technician.

• • •

Various cardiac augmentation systems are being used on experimental animals and a few have been tried in clinical situations. It would seem that such efforts are a logical extension of present efforts toward a solution of this problem, that is, tiding the failing heart over a variety of pharmacologically, mechanically, or disease-induced hurdles.

Although there has been only limited clinical experience with the Anstadt cup, a biventricular mechanical assister, numerous experimental studies have indicated its potential usefulness. With the Anstadt cup, nine of eleven animals had a restoration of cardiac function following 2 hours of mechanical massage. In a group of control animals, cardiac function could not be restored in a single instance (Massion and associates). It is the conclusion of Massion and co-workers that direct mechanical ventricular massage may be the method of choice in supporting circulation in cases in which the heart can be expected to resume near normal function only after assistance. If successful and prolonged cardiac massage can be promoted, then a cardiotoxic agent such as digitalis or carbon tetrachloride may have time to be metabolized.

Skinner and co-workers make a strong case for mechanical ventricular assistance using the Anstadt, Schiff, and Baue cup. As it requires no more than 2 minutes to apply, it lends itself to emergency situations and, in addition, does not require heparin administration since no vascular cannulations are needed. The control console for regulating rate and pressure is portable. Although there is some cardiac damage from the device, it is hoped that as the technical aspects are improved this can be significantly reduced. Skinner and associates from their experiments with laboratory animals speculate that mechanical ventricular assistance provided by this method may enable the human brain to survive longer periods of arrest because of the improved hemodynamics.

There are reports of the intra-aortic balloon's effectiveness in helping defibrillate the heart in resistant cases.

In one patient reported by Okel, fifty-six electrical shocks were required within a 10-hour period before a stable rhythm could be obtained. All shocks used direct current and were applied to the chest wall. Lidocaine (120 mg. intravenously in divided doses) decreased the frequency of fibrillatory episodes, but it was only after 4 gm. of procainamide hydrochloride was given intravenously in a 6-hour period that electrical countershock was successful. The patient was a 48-year-old male suffering from an acute myocardial infarction.

If, after ventricular defibrillation, the ECG reveals ventricular tachycardia, one must be alert for the return of ventricular fibrillation. As mentioned elsewhere, use of lidocaine hydrochloride, quinidine gluconate, or procainamide hydrochloride may be indicated in such cases.

Over 300 episodes of ventricular fibrillation requiring external countershock are reported by Zoll in a 68-year-old man being treated for Stokes-Adams attack. At autopsy there was no evidence of damage from the electrical shock, either to the chest wall or to the heart.

Guyton and Satterfield set some sort of a record when they successfully resuscitated one dog by external countershocks after 130 episodes of electrically induced ventricular fibrillation. Rivkin successfully resuscitated a patient who required cardiac massage and defibrillation over 100 times during a 5-day period.

There seems little question that the human heart can withstand repeated shock of therapeutic intensity from either D.C. or A.C. over a prolonged period with little evidence of anatomic or physiologic damage. Flynn and co-workers, after a study of seventeen cases requiring twenty or more electric countershocks, conclude that the damage is minimal. Although no obvious gross muscle necrosis or inflammation was noted, electron microscopy showed disruption of sarcolemma, clumping of sarcoplasm, necrosis of individual myofibrils, some nuclear proliferation, and some increase of fibroadipose tissue. These authors say that the frequency of recurrent ventricular arrhythmias can be decreased with the vigorous but carefully monitored use of cardiosuppressant drugs such as quinidine, lidocaine, and procainamide.

Ventricular fibrillation requiring 179 separate episodes of defibrillation over a period of 60 hours is reported by Milliken. Sudden syncope began just after quinidine gluconate was started. As in the case previously cited there was apparently a complete recovery. In each instance, fibrillation recurred after a sequence of ventricular premature beats, bigeminal rhythm, and ventricular tachycardia. Unger successfully treated a patient who received over 200 D.C. shocks. Hubbell reports a successful discharge of a patient who had been defibrillated fifty-six times in a 10-hour period. In May, 1969, Kubik and Gupta successfully treated a 56-year-old man with a myocardial infarction, who required ventricular defibrillation on 195 occasions plus three episodes of complete cardiac standstill. He, too, eventually left the hospital in a satisfactory state.

Although the pharmacology of resuscitation will be discussed in more detail later in this book, some brief repetition is appropriate in this section. A patient with recurrent ventricular fibrillation should be considered a candidate for bretylium tosylate because of its apparent antifibrillatory qualities; in fact, ventricular fibrillation may even revert to a sinus rhythm if the drug is given within 70 seconds of the onset. Bacaner has given bretylium tosylate intravenously or intramuscularly in doses of 2.5 to 5.0 mg. per kilogram of body weight. Ventricular fibrillation was successfully reverted in nine patients who were resistant to the usual treatment. The effect of bretylium tosylate is prolonged for 12 to 20 hours after a single dose. The patient should remain in bed after taking bretylium tosylate because of its orthostatic hypotensive qualities.

Theoretically, there would seem to be an occasional use for hyperbaric oxygen if it is easily available.

Despite repeated episodes of ventricular fibrillation over an 18-month period during which she was treated with diphenylhydantoin, bretylium, atropine, and phenobarbital, a 40-year-old woman without any personal or family history of heart disease had an idiopathic Q-T interval prolongation (Q-T equals 0.64 second). It was suspected by Moss and McDonald that an imbalance of a right-left sympathetic cardiac nerve activity contributed to the Q-T interval prolongation. Within 6 minutes following a left stellate ganglion block with local lidocaine infiltration, the Q-T interval shortened to 0.42 second. A right stellate ganglion block produced a Q-T interval prolongation to 0.72 second. The Q-T interval remained normal after a left stellate ganglionectomy was performed.

Working at the Palmerston North Hospital in New Zealand, Parkinson and Dickson were faced with a posterior myocardial infarction in a 62-year-old man. Ventricular fibrillation, with no premonitory ectopic beats, developed while the patient was in the coronary care unit even though he was receiving intravenous lignocaine at a rate of 2 mg. per minute. Defibrillation with 150 watt-second shock was successful within a minute and a half of onset; but ventricular fibrillation recurred 8 minutes later even though 400 mg. of procainamide was used intravenously. During the next 48 hours the patient required 201 separate episodes of ventricular defibrillation. He was conscious between attacks. Numerous attempts were made to prevent the repeated episodes of fibrillation, including quinidine sulfate 300 mg. intravenously and a potassium-glucose-insulin infusion. Transvenous pacing was not effective, nor was propranolol 5 mg. intravenously. Magnesium sulfate 20% intravenously (40 ml.) produced remissions lasting up to 1 hour on three occasions. Finally, dexamethasone 4 mg. given intravenously was followed by complete cessation of attacks of ventricular fibrillation. Despite the repeated ventricular fibrillations, metabolic acidosis was not a problem. The patient made an eventual recovery and returned to work with no evidence of a physical or mental defect.

Episodes of recurrent ventricular fibrillation associated with quinidine cardiotoxicity not necessarily related to the dose of quinidine is discussed elsewhere. In managing such a case all efforts should be directed toward sustaining life long enough for the quinidine to be metabolized and the cardiotoxic effect to be dissipated. Several hundred episodes of ventricular fibrillation within a matter of several hours have been reported in such patients. It is not infrequent for some of the episodes of ventricular fibrillation to self-terminate and revert to the previous basic rhythm of the heart. Temporary transvenous electrical pacing of the heart has been successful provided the pacemaker rate was rapid enough to suppress irritable ectopic foci.

Thirty-four paroxysms of ventricular fibrillation were encountered in a 64-year-old man with an acute myocardial infarction. Despite a 100 mg. bolus of lidocaine injected intravenously in a total dosage of 1.5 gm. of procainamide hydrochloride in a 2-hour period, the recurrent bouts of ventricular fibrillation continued. It was not until propranolol hydrochloride (5 mg.) was administered by intravenous drip that sinus rhythm was restored by a D.C. electric shock. The action of propranolol is not completely understood, but it does produce a decrease in the automaticity of the sino-atrial and ectopic pacemakers and an increase in the refractory period at the sino-atrial and atrioventricular junctions. In addition, it has a nonspecific depressant action upon the heart similar to that of procainamide and quinidine sulfate. As mentioned elsewhere, its use has been demonstrated to prevent ouabain-induced ventricular fibrillation in guinea pigs. Because there are adverse effects on the myocardial function,

including hypotension and profound bradycardia (which occurs as the result of the negative inotropic and chronotropic properties), Rothfeld and co-workers recommend the use of propranolol in such cases of resistant fibrillation only after other antiarrhythmic drugs have failed. Propranolol, as a beta-adrenergic blocking agent, has been successful when other drugs fail. A maximum dose of 10 mg. is recommended. The drug should be injected slowly and in the smallest possible dose, preferably less than 10 mg.

Unexplained myocardial failure from the residual effect of propranolol during cardiac surgery may present an unexpected problem. Viljoen and associates recommend that propranolol be withheld for 2 weeks prior to surgery. If, however, problems arise during surgery on a patient when propranolol has not been withdrawn, they recommend the following plan of action:

1. Atropine sulfate in a 1 mg. intravenous dosage should be given if bradycardia is present and if the bradycardia persists along with a low mean arterial pressure or high central venous pressure, and isoproterenol infusion (0.8 mg. per 250 ml.) should be started.
2. Because of the positive inotropic effect of calcium, especially in patients who have a beta blockage, calcium chloride salts should be administered.
3. Rapid intravenous digitalization should be accomplished if resistant cardiac failure continues.
4. If digitalization does not help, then a rapid injection of epinephrine, followed by an infusion (2 mg. per 250 ml.), should be given.
5. Intravenous glucagon (15 to 20 mg. in repeated doses), although admittedly of questionable value, should be given if myocardial irritability ensues and if a cardiotonic drug is required.
6. Along with the above measures, massive doses of intravenous steroids (2 gr. of hydrocortisone) should be included.

The possibility of blood flow from the ventricle to the myocardium is challenged by experimental work of Pifarré and co-workers. They note that during systole the pressure in the intramural segment of an implanted venous graft is greater than in the aorta and in the ventricle. During diastole it is lower than in the aorta but, at all times, greater than in the left ventricular cavity.

Successful defibrillation

Although it is recognized that the risk of mortality increases with each subsequent episode of ventricular fibrillation associated with a myocardial infarction, it should be noted that successful defibrillation can, on occasion, be achieved. Miller, Mower, and Nachlas report two such instances. In one patient, a 64-year-old man who developed a large myocardial infarction, ventricular fibrillations on the fifteenth, twenty-ninth, and thirty-second hospital days were successfully treated by external countershock. The patient subsequently died from neurologic sequelae. The second patient was a 59-year-old woman who had suffered a severe and extensive myocardial infarction 11 months earlier. Because of a second infarction and congestive heart failure, she was readmitted to the hospital. Successive episodes of ventricular fibrillation developed at 16, 28½, and 29¾ hours after arrival at the hospital. She was subsequently discharged from the hospital and was well 22 months later, at the time of the report.

Following a myocardial infarction with subsequent ventricular fibrillation and defibrillation, a recurrence of ventricular fibrillation is to be expected if cardiac function is inadequate. These patients are generally refractory to defibrillation. It is in this group of patients that the possible benefits of an emergency infarctectomy (to remove the focus of electrical irritability) may prove practical. As Heimbecker points out, marginal zones of nutrition may be further depressed by metabolic acidosis arising in the infarcted area.

Almost any clinician dealing with an occasional episode of ventricular fibrillation has been faced with the problem of successful defibrillation in the heart that is refractory to repeated electrical shocks. The

effectiveness of left ventricular drainage in permitting defibrillation after prolonged, refractory ventricular fibrillation in experimental acute myocardial infarction is reported by Kuhn and associates. Prolonged ventricular fibrillation without circulatory support was continued up to 48 minutes with subsequent unsuccessful electrical defibrillation regardless of the amount of direct current applied. When, however, left ventricular drainage by means of transaortic or transatrial cannulation was used, the defibrillation was successful in each instance.

It has been my impression for many years that the heart is much more difficult to defibrillate when it is distended. Kuhn and his co-workers now demonstrate that successful defibrillation appears related to a reduction of the volume of the distended, fibrillating left ventricle and that the size of the left ventricle is of particular importance in permitting and maintaining the development

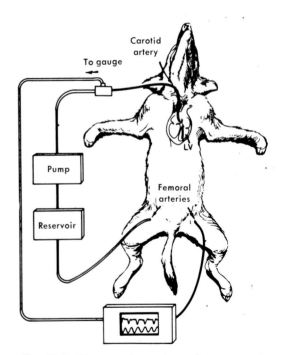

Fig. 28-1. Diagram of experimental arrangement. (From Kuhn, L. A., and others: Am. J. Cardiol. **30**:248-251, 1972.)

of ventricular fibrillation. They suggest that perhaps large hearts provide more reentrant pathways for perpetuation of fibrillatory "circus" rhythms than do smaller hearts in which refractory tissue may be present, thus allowing the rhythm to terminate. In addition, reduction of myocardial oxygen requirements and increment of coronary flow as by-products of left ventricular drainage are considered as facilitating mechanisms for defibrillation. In view of this experimental work it would seem likely that transarterial left ventricular drainage through a closed chest may have clinical indications, particularly in the patient who is refractory to defibrillation and who otherwise would seem to have reversible pathology (see Fig. 28-1). Although not always possible in the human, prolonged and refractory ventricular fibrillation may be successfully reversed in dogs if left ventricular drainage via transaortic or transatrial cannulation is carried out. Acute reduction of left ventricular volume permits defibrillation in refractory instances both in normal animals and in those with acute myocardial infarction. Adequate reduction of left ventricular volume deserves increased clinical application.

Chapter 29

RELATIONSHIP BETWEEN WAVE FORM AND EFFECTIVENESS IN TRANSTHORACIC COUNTERSHOCK FOR TERMINATION OF VENTRICULAR FIBRILLATION

John C. Schuder

In most commercially available D.C. defibrillators, the energy is stored in a capacitor. To deliver a defibrillatory shock, the capacitor discharges through the chest via a series inductor. A modification of this arrangement involves storing the energy in the capacitors of a lumped delay line. This yields a quasi-rectangular defibrillatory pulse. Earlier A.C. defibrillators supplied 60 hertz sinusoidal shocks. Lown and associates (1962), Balagot and co-workers (1964), and Kouwenhoven and his colleagues (1957) have discussed the various arrangements. In addition, Peleška (1963, 1965, 1966) has reported detailed studies in which the size of the energy storage capacitor and of the inductor were varied. These systems do not lend themselves to convenient and independent adjustment of the various parameters of the defibrillatory shock, even though the amplitude of the shock is under the control of the operator.

This section of the book is in the nature of a review of a long-term study, involving over 53,000 fibrillation-defibrillation episodes, in which the parameters of the wave form could be conveniently and independently adjusted. Most of the material was initially reported by Schuder and co-work-

ers (1963, 1964, 1966, 1967, 1970, 1971, 1972), Rahmoeller and colleagues (1966), and Stoeckle and associates (1967, 1968).

Special apparatus

Much of the apparatus employed in the investigations is shown in Fig. 29-1. The center and left-hand relay racks, together with a very large capacitor bank (which is not shown), comprise a 24,000 watt vacuum tube linear amplifier capable of supplying transthoracic shocks of almost any desired wave form at peak current levels up to 10 amperes for bidirectional shocks and up to 20 amperes for unidirectional shocks. The right-hand relay rack houses a 600,000 watt hydrogen Thyratron defibrillator that can supply unidirectional rectangular shocks of up to 100 amperes. Provisions are made for the convenient induction of fibrillation and for the monitoring of the wave form of the applied shock and of the ECG.

Procedure

Each wave form was evaluated on the basis of 120 fibrillation-defibrillation procedures and involved six or more dogs. A given animal was anesthetized and 9 cm. diameter electrodes were taped or

366

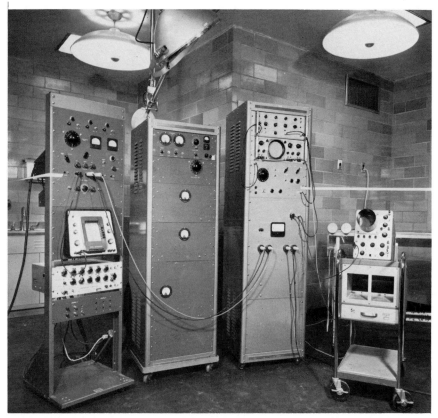

Fig. 29-1. Arrangement of apparatus for experimental fibrillation-defibrillation procedure. (From Schuder, J. C., and others: Institute of Electrical and Electronics Engineers, Inc., International Convention Record **14**(9):32, 1966.)

held on the anterior portion of the chest. The left electrode was located approximately over the apex of the heart, and the right electrode was placed slightly to the left of midline and higher on the chest. Fibrillation was induced with a low-current shock, and unassisted fibrillation was allowed to continue for 30 seconds. At the end of 30 seconds, the wave form being investigated was applied to the chest of the animal. If defibrillation and an effective beat were not realized on the initial attempt, the episode was recorded as a failure, and a shock of known high effectiveness was used to save the animal. A given animal was used in not more than twenty episodes in the evaluation of any given wave form.

Results and comments

Figs. 29-2 and 29-3 illustrate the results of a series of investigations involving unidirectional rectangular wave shocks with durations of 40 μsec. through 200 msec. and at amplitudes of from 5 to 100 amperes. From the curves of Fig. 29-2, it is evident that the effectiveness of shocks of a fixed amplitude tends to increase, reach a peak, and then decrease with increasing duration of the shock. At a fixed duration, an increase in the amplitude of the shock may, for the longer durations, actually yield a less effective shock. Figs. 29-2 and 29-3 show that unidirectional rectangular shocks of suitable duration can be highly effective over a current range of 10 through 100 amperes. The

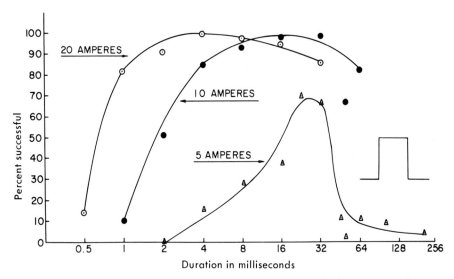

Fig. 29-2. Relation between percent success of ventricular defibrillation and duration of unidirectional rectangular shocks. (From Schuder, J. C., Stoeckle, H., and Dolan, A. M.: Circ. Res. 15:258, 1964.)

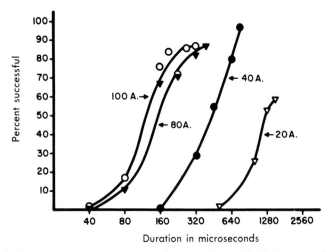

Fig. 29-3. Relation between percent success of ventricular defibrillation and duration of unidirectional rectangular shocks. (From Schuder, J. C., and others: J. Appl. Physiol. 22:1110, 1967.)

100 ampere curve of Fig. 29-3 indicates that an occasional defibrillation is realized with shocks of only 40 μsec. duration—a shock so short that 25,000 could be contained in 1 second. Although not immediately apparent from the curves, the 40, 80, and 100 ampere shocks tend to require progressively more energy for a given level of success than do the 10 and 20 ampere shocks.

While transthoracic electrical shocks can

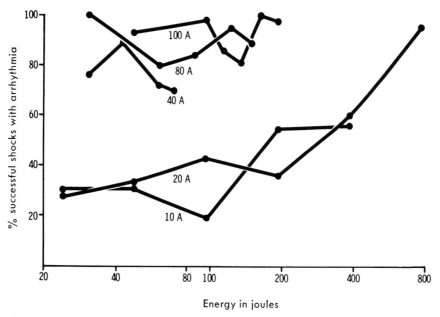

Fig. 29-4. Relation between percent of successful shocks that induce one or more arrhythmias and energy content of unidirectional rectangular shocks. (From Stoeckle, H., Nellis, S. H., and Schuder, J. C.: Circ. Res. 23:343, 1968.)

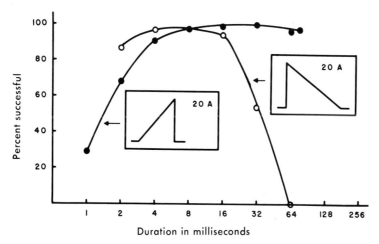

Fig. 29-5. Relation between percent success of ventricular defibrillation and duration of 20-ampere triangular shocks. (From Schuder, J. C., Rahmoeller, G. A., and Stoeckle, H.: Circ. Res. 19:689, 1966.)

terminate ventricular fibrillation, they may also induce a variety of other arrhythmias. Often, more than one type of arrhythmia will be observed in the ECG taken immediately following a defibrillatory shock. In

Fig. 29-4, the results of a study of induced arrhythmias for unidirectional rectangular waves are plotted. For this illustration, the horizontal axis is in terms of the energy content of the shock, while the vertical axis represents the percent of successful shocks that yield one or more types of arrhythmias. Of particular interest is the comparatively low incidence of arrhythmias with the 10 and 20 ampere shocks as compared with the 40, 80, and 100 ampere shocks. However, at the lower current levels, there is a definite trend toward a higher incidence of arrhythmias with increasing duration or energy content of shock.

Fig. 29-5 illustrates the results of a study involving triangular wave forms. One case involves a wave form in which the current starts at zero, increases linearly with time to 20 amperes, and then decreases abruptly to zero. In the other case, the current jumps abruptly to 20 amperes and then decreases linearly with time. For any given duration, the energy content of the two types of wave forms is identical. At a duration in the neighborhood of 8 msec., both wave forms are nearly 100% effective. For longer durations, the increasing ramp wave form continues to be very effective, while the decreasing ramp wave form decreases rapidly in effectiveness and is completely ineffective at 64 msec. duration. It is postulated that the leading portion of the descending ramp

wave form successfully defibrillates the heart, while the lagging edge or tail of the wave form refibrillates as it sweeps through low-current values. When the 64 msec. descending ramp wave form is modified by merely cutting off the last 32 msec. and thereby making it into a trapezoidal wave, the effectiveness increases to over 90%.

Some of the results of a study involving defibrillation in large 24 through 32 kilogram dogs with truncated and untruncated exponential stimuli of the general type sketched in Fig. 29-6 are illustrated in Fig. 29-7. There is currently (1972) considerable interest in the possibility of using such wave forms in commercial defibrillators because of the ease with which they can be generated with solid-state electronic switching devices. In Fig. 29-7, untruncated exponential wave forms have final current values that approach zero; truncated wave forms have nonzero values for final current. Of particular interest is the very low effectiveness of the untruncated wave forms, which have an initial current of 20 amperes, as compared with their optimally truncated counterparts. As with the descending ramp triangular wave forms, it is postulated that the low

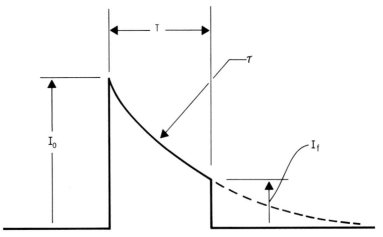

Fig. 29-6. Truncated wave forms. In the untruncated decay, current is not abruptly terminated but allowed to approach zero in an asymptotic fashion as suggested by the dashed curve. The symbol τ denotes the time constant of decay. (From Schuder, J. C., and others: IEEE Trans. Biomed. Eng. BME-18:410, 1971.)

effectiveness of the untruncated wave forms is due to a refibrillation phenomenon. Additional studies indicate that the effectiveness of defibrillation with untruncated exponential stimuli of a given energy content can be increased by using a higher value of initial current and a shorter time constant of decay.

The results for unidirectional rectangular shocks are compared with those for the corresponding bidirectional shocks in Fig. 29-8. For any given duration, the energy content of the two types of shocks is the same. In contrast to the unidirectional shock, the bidirectional shock involves zero net charge transport. An important finding

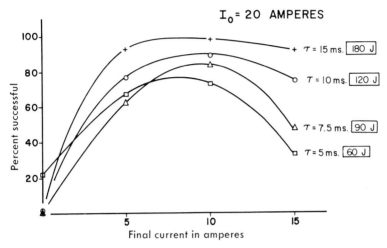

Fig. 29-7. Relation between percent success of ventricular defibrillation and final current of exponential stimuli with initial current of 20 amperes. Numbers within the boxes denote energy content in joules of the untruncated wave form associated with each of the curves. (From Schuder, J. C., and others: IEEE Trans. Biomed. Eng. **BME-18**:410, 1971.)

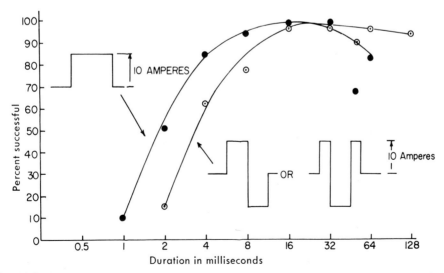

Fig. 29-8. Relation between percent success of ventricular defibrillation and duration of 10-ampere unidirectional and bidirectional rectangular shocks. (From Schuder, J. C., Stoeckle, H., and Dolan, A. M.: Circ. Res. **15**:258, 1964.)

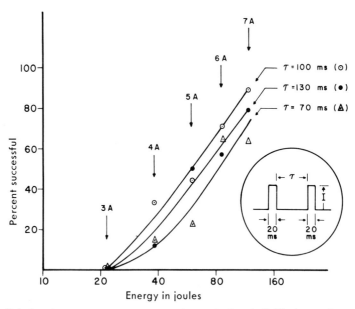

Fig. 29-9. Relation between percent success of ventricular defibrillation and energy content of unidirectional rectangular double pulse shocks in which the pulse duration is fixed at 20 milliseconds. The symbol τ denotes pulse separation. (From Schuder, J. C., and others: Cardiovasc. Res. 4:497, 1970.)

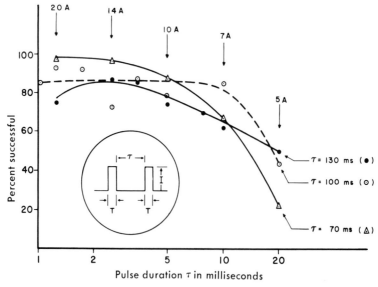

Fig. 29-10. Relation between percent success of ventricular defibrillation and pulse duration of unidirectional rectangular double pulse shocks in which energy content is fixed at 60 joules. (From Schuder, J. C., and others: Cardiovasc. Res. 4:497, 1970.)

is that bidirectional shocks appear to continue to be quite effective at the longer durations of shock, whereas unidirectional shocks have a noticably reduced effectiveness. A study of 5 ampere shocks (not shown) reveals similar results.

Kugelberg (1966, 1967), and Resnekov and colleagues (1968) have suggested that open-chest defibrillation of the heart can be achieved at reduced energy levels by the use of suitably spaced double pulses. However, the results of extensive studies, as summarized in Figs. 29-9 and 29-10, fail to support a corresponding superiority of double pulse shocks over single pulse shocks for transthoracic defibrillation.

An abrupt jump in current on the leading edge of a defibrillatory shock, which is present, for example, in a straight capacitor discharge, has been suggested as a possible cause of low effectiveness and a high incidence of induced arrhythmias in such shocks. However, in a carefully controlled series of experiments in which 1 msec. 20 ampere unidirectional rectangular shocks were alternately supplied with very short rise times (approximately 3 μsec.) and relatively long rise times (approximately 200 μsec.), no significant difference in either effectiveness of shock or the incidence of induced arrhythmias could be demonstrated.

The energy required for transthoracic defibrillation when neither cardiac massage nor assisted respiration is used is a function of the duration of fibrillation. In a detailed study of this relationship, unidirectional rectangular shocks were employed and episodes in which attempts to defibrillate after 5 seconds of fibrillation were alternated with episodes in which defibrillation was attempted after 30 seconds of fibrillation. The results demonstrated that a given level of effectiveness after 5 seconds of fibrillation could be achieved with approximately 75 per cent of the energy required to achieve the same level of defibrillation effectiveness after 30 seconds of fibrillation.

Conclusion

Although the probable effectiveness and the incidence of induced arrhythmias in ventricular defibrillation procedures are dependent upon certain detailed features in the wave form of the applied shock, there are a wide variety of types of countershocks suitable for defibrillation. In general, the wave form specifications for such shocks are not critical.

Chapter 30

TOTALLY IMPLANTED STANDBY VENTRICULAR DEFIBRILLATION SYSTEMS

John C. Schuder

Ventricular fibrillation is presumably an important cause of sudden death in patients who suffer a coronary occlusion. Although highly trained ambulance crews prepared to initiate cardiac massage and defibrillation procedures and sophisticated coronary care units with extensive monitoring and resuscitation capabilities are helping to reduce the mortality from ventricular fibrillation, they are of little value to the patient who develops ventricular fibrillation in the absence of trained medical personnel.

The mortality from ventricular fibrillation might be further reduced by the availability of standby automatic defibrillation systems that could be implanted on a prophylactic basis in selected patients. This chapter constitutes a review of recent experimental work in the area of implantable automatic defibrillation systems.

A block diagram of the first completely implantable defibrillation system to be successfully used in animals is shown in Fig. 30-1 (Schuder and co-workers, 1970). In this system, the electrocardiographic electrodes are placed in the musculature of the chest wall so as to yield a signal with a high amplitude R wave. The electrodes through which the defibrillatory shock is delivered are 7.5 cm in diameter and are implanted between the pectoralis muscle and the rib cage with one electrode over the apex of the heart and the other electrode higher on the chest and slightly to the right of midline. The remaining apparatus,

weighing about 1 kilogram, is implanted subcutaneously in the abdominal region.

As long as R waves are present in the electrocardiogram, the fibrillation detector shown in Fig. 30-1 does not deliver a turn-on signal to the D.C.-to-D.C. converter and the system remains in its quiescent state. The absence of R waves for a period of 5 seconds triggers the solid-state D.C.-to-D.C. converter via the fibrillation detector and this, in turn, initiates the process of charging the 600 microfarad (μf.) capacitor bank from the 19.5 volt alkaline battery pack. When the capacitor bank potential reaches 500 volts, typically in about 12 seconds, the solid-state pulse generator is activated and delivers a quasi-trapezoidal shock to the chest via the implanted electrodes. A signal from the pulse generator also deactivates the D.C.-to-D.C. converter which, in turn, reactivates the fibrillation detector and places the system in a position to once again sense the presence or absence of an R wave in the electrocardiogram. If an R wave is present, the system will then remain in a quiescent state. If no R wave is present, the events described above will be repeated and another shock delivered to the chest.

Mirowski and colleagues (1970) suggested an alternative approach to the development of an implantable standby automatic defibrillator. In their original paper, they proposed an electrode system with one electrode at the tip of a catheter and positioned within the right ventricle and with the other elec-

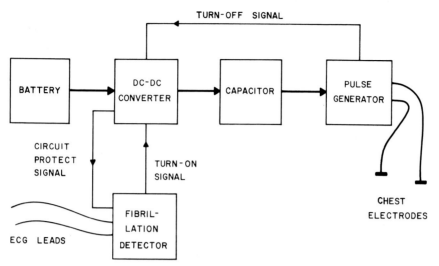

Fig. 30-1. Block diagram of completely implantable standby automatic defibrillation system. (From Schuder, J. C., and others: Trans. Am. Soc. Artif. Intern. Organs 16:207, 1970.)

trode positioned under the skin of the anterior chest wall. Fibrillation was detected by a pressure transducer that was an integral part of the intracardiac catheter and that sensed the absence of a pulsatile right ventricular pressure. After fibrillation was detected, a capacitor bank was charged and then discharged by means of a solid-state switch to furnish an untruncated exponential wave form to the heart and chest. Although their original apparatus was too large for implantation, it was visualized that with engineering improvements implantation might be possible.

Mirowski and co-workers (1971) and Denniston and colleagues (1971) have suggested the concept of ventricular defibrillation via a single intravascular catheter having one electrode in the apex of the right ventricle and the other electrode in the superior vena cava. Such an arrangement is potentially attractive because the same catheter could also be conveniently utilized for cardiac pacing. Thus, one might visualize an implanted system with both pacing and standby defibrillation capabilities. Schuder and colleagues (1971) in cooperation with Denniston have studied the effective-

ness of one type of bielectrode catheter in the defibrillation of large dogs. In this study, a Silastic catheter of the type shown in Fig. 30-2 was inserted through the jugular vein and the tip positioned under fluoroscopy in six anasthetized animals weighing 24 through 30 kilograms. The effectiveness of truncated exponential shocks in reversing fibrillation of 30 seconds duration was studied on the day of catheter insertion, one week postinsertion, and two weeks postinsertion. In 144 fibrillation-defibrillation episodes with a truncated exponential shock having an initial current of 10 amperes, a final current of 5 amperes, a pulse duration of 6.9 milliseconds, and an energy content of 37 joules, successful defibrillation was achieved 98% of the time. Truncated exponential shocks with an energy content of 18.5 joules and 10 amperes initial current or with an energy content of 37 joules and 7 amperes initial current were appreciably less effective in achieving defibrillation.

Mirowski and colleagues (1972), working with Gott, have used catheter defibrillation in patients undergoing bypass grafting for coronary artery disease. In evaluating an arrangement in which one electrode was

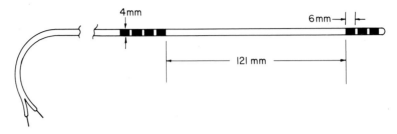

Fig. 30-2. Catheter used in experimental defibrillation studies. The three platinum sleeves that constitute the ventricular electrode are connected together electrically as are the four sleeves that constitute the vena cava electrode.

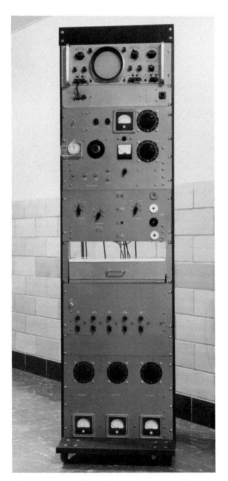

Fig. 30-3. Multielectrode–time sequential laboratory defibrillator.

placed in the apex of the right ventricle by means of a catheter inserted through an atriotomy and the other electrode consisted of a saline-soaked sponge placed upon the superior vena cava near its junction with the right atrium, successful defibrillation was achieved at the 5 joule level in two patients, at the 10 joule level in two patients, and at the 15 joule level in an additional two patients.

It is anticipated that the level of acceptance of implantable defibrillation systems by physicians and their patients will be, in part, a function of the size and weight of the system. Since the size and weight of an implantable defibrillator is directly related to the energy that must be delivered in the defibrillatory pulse, there is current interest in finding the most effective implantable electrode system. A multielectrode–time sequential laboratory defibrillator for the convenient study of implanted electrode systems has been developed and described by Schuder and co-workers (1972). It is shown in Fig. 30-3. The instrument consists of three isolated pulse generators. Each generator has a 1,350 volt, 450 μf. capacitor bank from which truncated exponential discharges are initiated by firing a hydrogen thyratron and terminated by firing shunt silicon controlled rectifiers. Pulse widths can be varied from 100 microseconds to more than 45 milliseconds. Pulse separations are adjustable from 100 microseconds to 1 second. Depending upon the wishes of the operator, up to three pulses can be delivered in time sequence to any two of the four available output terminals or, alternatively, all four terminals may be utilized and individual pulses delivered to different terminal pairs. We have employed this and other apparatus in studying the relationship between electrode geometry and effectiveness of defibrillation with a 7-lead experimental catheter in which the geometrical composition of the electrode within the right ventricle and of the electrode within the superior vena cava could be effectively controlled by switching leads external to the animal. The study served to emphasize the necessity of having the tip of the distal electrode well positioned in the apex of the right ventricle and to suggest that the effectiveness of a catheter of the general type shown in Fig. 30-2 could be appreciably increased by using greater surface area for the vena cava electrode.

The results of the studies described in this chapter suggest that the prospects are reasonably favorable for the development of implanted standby defibrillation systems for clinical application. In the early stages of clinical evaluation, the use of systems in which pacing and standby defibrillation capabilities are incorporated into a single device may facilitate the problem of patient selection.

Chapter 31

RESUSCITATION OF THE NEAR-DROWNING VICTIM

Imburg and Hartney estimate that in the United States more persons under the age of 24 die from drowning than from any other cause. Of an estimated 6,000 persons dying from drowning each year, most are young and in good health.

In the 20-year period between 1947 and 1967, over 110,000 people died from drowning. With increasing interest in skin diving and the use of scuba diving equipment, water skiing, and other types of water sports, the need for adequate management of the near-drowning victim becomes increasingly relevant.

Every year in France there are 3,000 to 4,000 cases of drowning. Because of this there is a resuscitation training center in Paris where lifeguards are specifically trained in mouth-to-mouth respiration and external cardiac massage.

Modell divides the near-drowning victims into two groups: "near drown without aspiration" and "near drown with aspiration." In both groups, acute asphyxia is the major consideration. Fluid and electrolyte changes taking place in the victim will depend particularly on the quantity and composition of the fluid being aspirated. The chances of eventual recovery of the victim are considerably decreased if large quantities of either freshwater or seawater are aspirated.

If there is much freshwater aspirated, in the experimental animal, ventricular fibrillation occurs shortly after onset of immersion. In addition, there is rapid hypervolemia along with a marked lowering in serum sodium and chloride concentrations, an increase in serum potassium, hemolysis,

hypoxia, hypercapnia, and acidosis. Modell and Moya show that 80% of dogs that aspirate at least 44 ml. of freshwater per kilogram body weight will fibrillate. Dogs aspirating less than 22 ml. per kilogram generally will not fibrillate.

The difficulty of reinflation is compounded by atelectasis of the pulmonary alveoli and by the destruction or alteration of normal surfactant activity that occurs after freshwater aspiration.

The concentration of serum sodium, chloride, potassium, and calcium is increased in experimental seawater drowning. Also, plasma is removed from the circulating blood volume.

As more data become available, it is evident that earlier concepts relating to significant features of near drowning need to be altered. Much of our earlier experimental information was based on the assumption that death from drowning resulted from exposure to large quantities of aspirated water—a feature that is apparently lacking in most instances. For this reason, there is less concern with the composition of water aspirated, be it saltwater or freshwater. However, the common denominator is more nearly a matter of acute asphyxia with arterial hypoxemia and acidosis. Significant electrolyte changes in near-drowning victims have not been documented (Modell and co-workers). Some investigators originally believed that victims of immersion in freshwater experienced a rapid onset of hypervolemia, hyponatremia, hypochloremia, hyperkalemia, and significant hemolysis, with rapid progression to ventricular fibrillation

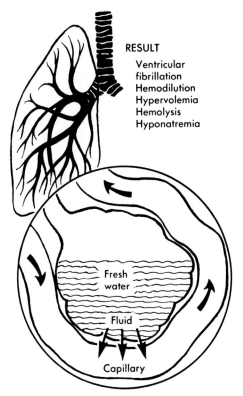

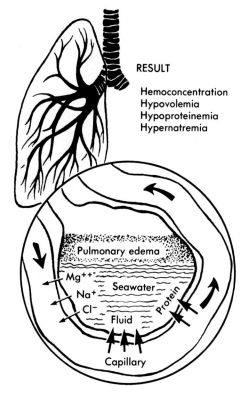

Fig. 31-1. Schematic diagram of events associated with freshwater drowning. (Modified from Redding, J. S., and others: J.A.M.A. **178:**1136, 1961.)

Fig. 31-2. Events taking place during saltwater drowning. (Modified from Redding, J. S., and others: J.A.M.A. **178:**1137, 1961.)

(Fig. 31-1). Saltwater drowning was thought to be associated with hypovolemia and a marked increase in concentration of serum electrolytes (Fig. 31-2). Although both mechanisms do occur, it seems unlikely that they are active in the majority of near drownings (Fuller).

Mouth-to-mouth ventilation should be initiated, if possible, even before the patient is removed from the water. Many workers agree that any attempt to drain water from the lungs in freshwater drowning is a waste of time because it is so rapidly absorbed into the circulation. This, however, does not apply to seawater drowning where efforts to promote drainage may be helpful.

Because of the atelectatic alveoli, frequent hyperinflation efforts with positive pressure

should be employed once the patient arrives in the hospital. Nebulized alcohol is indicated in patients with obvious pulmonary edema, and steroids and antibiotics for aspiration pneumonia. Each patient will have different clinical requirements because of variations in the composition and volume of aspiration. Arterial oxygen pressure, pH, and carbon dioxide pressure determinations should be made as soon as possible and blood should be drawn for testing the hemoglobin, hematocrit, free plasma hemoglobin, serum sodium, chloride, calcium, and potassium concentration.

In any event, the physician should direct his efforts toward combating acute ventilatory insufficiency as well as arterial hypoxemia and acidosis. This can best be accomplished by effective ventilation, oxygenation, and administration of buffers or bicarbonate.

Whole blood transfusions are indicated only in those patients who have aspirated such *massive* quantities of freshwater as to cause hemolysis and a reduction in the blood's oxygen-carrying capacity.

Warden has documented that there is a marked decrease in lung compliance occurring after near drowning in saltwater. His conclusion is that the respiratory insufficiency is due to a pneumonitis as a result of saltwater aspiration and not from pulmonary edema or reflex airway closure.

Unfortunately, delayed death in dogs after near drowning and subsequent ventricular defibrillation occurs rather often (Redding and co-workers). Delayed death is usually the result of the effects of massive hemolysis, hypervolemia, electrolyte imbalance, and myocardial failure. It is recommended that persons who have nearly drowned in freshwater receive hypertonic sodium chloride slowly. Whole blood should be given, although its use may need to be alternated with repeated phlebotomy. Lower nephron nephrosis may be a delayed complication caused by the marked hemolysis that has occurred, possibly even requiring the use of an artificial kidney.

Prolonged periods of complete anoxia during immersion with subsequent recovery have been recorded. King and Webster report such a case from Prince Henry's Hospital, Melbourne, Australia. The patient, a 21-year-old German seaman, fell over the side of a ship into the tidal reaches of the Yarra River. He was finally recovered by a skin diver at an estimated depth of 32 feet. His immersion was estimated to be 17 to 25 minutes. Cardiac resuscitative efforts were carried out through a thoracotomy and, after an extremely precarious postresuscitative period, the patient was finally discharged on the twenty-sixth postarrest day. Further communications indicate that he has suffered no change in personality. An additional survival after prolonged anoxia from immersion is reported by Kvittengden and Naess of Norway. In this instance the patient, a child, remained immersed for 22 minutes in near-freezing water. External cardiac massage was carried out for 2 hours.

The metabolic abnormalities noted in the first case are of interest. Low serum bicarbonate levels were identified, as was a hypokalemia and a persistently raised serum sodium and chloride concentration. Acidosis was managed successfully by infusion of 1 L. of an M/6 solution of sodium lactate. The low potassium was unexpected in view of the well-documented findings of elevated potassium in most drowning episodes and in severe anoxia. At no stage did gross pulmonary edema occur.

Kylstra suggests that the disastrous complications of water inhalation can be minimized if swimming pools are filled with a balanced saline solution. He mentions that the public swimming pools in Aarhus, Denmark, have been filled with 1% saltwater since 1957.

As an aid in resuscitation of the near-drowning victim, Middleton has designed a practical beach rescue trolley (Fig. 31-3) primarily for use on beaches where lifeguards are available. It is supported by two pneumatic tires that prevent sinking in the sand and provide a comfortable ride over pebbles. When needed for a rescue, the whole trolley is rushed to the scene. The lifesaving reel of the standard type used by the Surf Lifesaving Clubs in Britain and Australia is dismounted by straight lift-off, with the trolley tipped forward on its front leg. The beltman-rescuer swims out to sea in the harness, following the normal surf lifesaving drill. In the meantime, an assistant unloads the equipment, such as airways and oxygen, from the trolley and pushes it out into the sea until the water level reaches the stretcher. The victim is then either floated onto the stretcher or lifted on by the rescue squad. The airway is checked and the victim's head extended over the end of trolley as mouth-to-

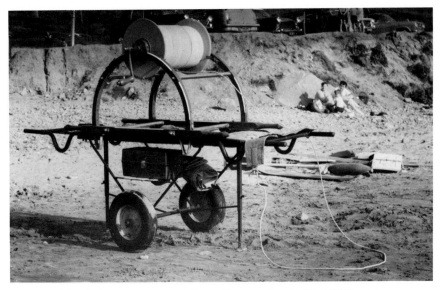

Fig. 31-3. Beach rescue trolley. (Courtesy **Dr. G. W. Middleton.**)

mouth respiration is begun. This is continued as the trolley is wheeled from the sea. The trolley is fixed in a 10% head-down position as soon as it is on dry land. The stretcher gives sufficiently firm support for application of closed-chest cardiac massage.

Some of the obvious advantages of the trolley include providing a rapid means of giving mouth-to-mouth artificial ventilation and avoiding unnecessary handling of the patient. The victim can be maintained in a head-down position and continuous resuscitation can be carried out while the victim is being moved.

One of the dilemmas in the long-term management of the near-drowning victim is the obvious need for a high concentration of oxygen. At necropsy many of the fatalities show evidence of oxygen therapy toxicity such as the presence of pulmonary hyaline membranes.

Gibbs, in England, has suggested a technique immediately applicable for resuscitation of drowned children. The victim is picked up by his thighs, which are put over the rescuer's head, and the rescuer then applies compression of the chest with the patient in the head-down position. This has the advantage of allowing water and aspirate to drain from the lungs and stomach. Any benefit from using this method would be achieved within the first 1 or 2 minutes, the time taken for all unfixed water to be drained from the lung but also allowing head-down artificial respiration for a limited period followed by mouth-to-mouth respiration when the lungs are relatively cleared.

Redding advocates the desirability of cooling the mentally obtunded near-drowning victim to about 30° C. immediately after resuscitation in order to reduce cerebral oxygen consumption and carbon dioxide production. The increased metabolic rate from shivering is prevented by the use of neuromuscular blocking agents or narcotics. The cerebral edema resulting from asphyxia and circulatory arrest may be somewhat reduced by passive hyperventilation or use of a respirator with a resultant respiratory alkalosis and cerebral vasoconstriction. Osmotic diuresis should be attempted. Steroids in large doses are helpful not only in combating cerebral edema but also in minimizing any inflammatory response to the aspiration, whether it be gastric contents or the fluid in which the victim was immersed. An attempt to maintain the arterial oxygen pressure in the range of 60 to 90 mm. Hg should be made, and the percentage of oxygen in the inhaled gas mixture adjusted accordingly. The large areas of nonventilated lung to which pulmonary blood flow is shunted compounds the problem of aeration for at least 48 to 72 hours.

Humidification of the inhaled gas mixture should not be forgotten. For airways maintained by tracheostomy or by an endotracheal tube, one should insist that all suctioning of the trachea be done under most strict aseptic techniques. Many near-drowning victims eventually succumb to a pulmonary infection because damage of respiratory membrane provides excellent opportunity for bacterial growth. Routine, frequent cultures should be obtained.

At the Second International Symposium on Emergency Resuscitation in Oslo, Norway, the question arose concerning the use of hyperbaric oxygenation in drowning. As the pulmonary problem would be more than acute, Modell expressed the opinion that hyperbaric oxygenation would not offer much help since the duration of toleration of lung tissue to 100% oxygen in a hyperbaric chamber is limited.

In a discussion of prognostic factors in patients treated following freshwater immersion, Currin reports no survivors among those who had ventricular fibrillation even though regular sinus rhythm was reestablished. In addition, there were no survivors among fifteen patients who developed delayed pulmonary edema, despite immediate large intravenous doses of methylprednisolone sodium succinate. No patients with hematuria survived. There was, however, a low or normal P_{CO_2} in all survivors. Plasma hemoglobin levels above 65 mg. also suggested a poor outcome.

Steroids theoretically may also be of benefit in the profound disturbance in the microcirculation, much similar to the classic picture of disseminated intravascular coagulation. It is suggested that in freshwater drowning, hemolysis not only increases the potassium concentration in the plasma, but probably releases ADP from erythrocytes, resulting in aggregation. Substances accelerating coagulation may also be derived from hemolyzed blood cells. Jorgensen speculates that these patients might benefit from heparin administration.

Measures necessary in resuscitation of the near-drowning victim

Before considering the immediate measures necessary to resuscitate a submersion or near-drowning victim, the reader should be reminded of several considerations. For one thing, it is no longer considered desirable to spend precious early seconds during the resuscitation period in trying to remove water from the patient's lungs. If the drowning has occurred in freshwater, this hypotonic solution will be rapidly absorbed through the lungs. Although the water is less rapidly absorbed in instances of saltwater near-drowning and drowning in chlorinated water pools, simply establishing an airway and allowing postural drainage will allow any trapped water in the lungs to escape. There is strong evidence in some instances that very little water at all enters the lung because of early occurrence of marked laryngospasm.

To a large extent, resuscitation of the nearly drowned patient is simply an extension of the principles of cardiopulmonary resuscitation with the interjection of several specialized components.

PRIORITIES

What are the immediate priorities that must be met in the resuscitation of the near-drowning victim? Immediate efforts to establish ventilation receive top priority. This may even be instituted before the victim is removed from the water. After removal, the mouth and pharynx should be cleared quickly and mouth-to-mouth ventilation begun. One can use somewhat greater exhalation pressure than ordinarily used because of the beneficial effect of positive pressure breathing on any intrapulmonary shunts and pulmonary edema present. If means are available, the oronasopharynx should be suctioned, an oral airway inserted and ventilation maintained by means of an AMBU bag. Sometimes the victim will already show efforts at breathing. Coughing may be present. In such instances, an improvement of the airway and assisted ventilation are indicated. Postural positioning of the patient will permit draining of what little water there is in the lungs.

Obviously, ventilatory support will be of no benefit unless adequate circulatory efforts are taking place. Using the same criteria for establishing the presence or absence of an adequate cardiac output as mentioned elsewhere in this book, one must quickly make a decision whether or not closed-chest cardiac compression is needed. If there is any doubt, manual compression of the chest as detailed in Chapter 21 is begun, along with the maintenance of artificial ventilation.

For many years it has been customary in most communities to call the fire department whenever a near drowning has occurred with the idea that the fire department was most likely to have a pulmonary resuscitator available. It may be difficult to realize that mouth-to-mouth ventilation along with closed-chest cardiac compression of the immersion victim are measures that have been generally employed around the country for less than a decade. I can recall the drowning of the son of one of our university professors in a pool not far from the Medical Center over 15 years ago. When the young man was discovered on the bottom of the pool, he was quickly pulled out of the water and both the fire department and the local funeral parlor were called because of their oxygen units. In the meantime, ineffective respiratory support was attempted by the old "push-pull" method that was so relatively ineffectual and yet so often employed in the years before the present decade. Today this young man would almost certainly

have survived if present-day immediate care efforts had been employed.

VENTRICULAR FIBRILLATION

During transportation to the hospital, 100% oxygen administration via positive pressure breathing is desirable. Obviously, closed-chest resuscitation should be continued if there is an ineffective or absent cardiac output. If the ambulance is equipped with a portable electrocardiograph and a defibrillator (hopefully, all ambulances should have these), the patient should be defibrillated as soon as possible. Originally it was believed that perhaps half the people who drown in freshwater experience ventricular fibrillation, thought to be a potassium fibrillation. In dogs the increase in potassium was attributed to anoxemia and to hemolysis with subsequent release of intracellular potassium. This increased incidence of ventricular fibrillation in freshwater drowning has not been adequately documented in clinical cases, however. In any event there are undoubtedly many cases of cardiovascular collapse in which a ventricular fibrillatory rhythm may be established during cardiopulmonary resuscitation.

METABOLIC ACIDOSIS

In addition to the prompt establishment of an adequate airway (and if indicated, cardiac resuscitation via closed-chest massage), other immediate efforts are likely to be most valuable. It now appears that there is an almost inevitable metabolic acidosis associated with these patients and the sooner it is corrected by adequate ventilation and administration of sodium bicarbonate, the sooner adequate perfusion will occur. For this reason an adult should get at least one ampule of sodium bicarbonate administered intravenously. Each ampule contains 44.6 mEq. of bicarbonate in 50 ml. of water. If the patient is unconscious or nearly so, two ampules may be given in rapid succession. With small children, intravenously administered sodium bicarbonate may be given in a dosage of 1 mEq. per kilogram of body weight. Often the administration of sodium bicarbonate will result in rather immediate, dramatic clinical improvement of the patient.

Frequent oronasal suctioning should be instituted as soon as a suctioning device is available. In addition, early insertion of a cuffed endotracheal tube is advantageous. Since a large percentage of near-drowning victims vomit during resuscitative procedures, it is desirable to aspirate the gastric contents via a nasogastric tube in order to prevent aspiration of vomitus into the lungs, which are already severely compromised.

EMERGENCY ROOM CARE

Immediately upon the patient's arrival at the emergency room, the effectiveness of ventilatory efforts must be rechecked, electrical activity of the myocardium monitored and closed-chest resuscitation continued as long as necessary following much the same procedural routine as outlined in Chapter 21. Because a marked metabolic acidosis and hypoxemia may not be clinically apparent, blood samples should immediately be drawn for arterial oxygen and carbon dioxide tension along with acid-base studies consisting of blood pH and base excess. Blood pH levels of below 6.96 have been reported in near-drowning victims with subsequent recoveries along with base deficits of minus 26 mEq. per liter. Almost empirically one can administer one ampule of sodium bicarbonate to an adult or a graduated dose to a smaller individual.

It is at this point that a mechanical ventilator will most likely have its first usage. Mechanical ventilators at the scene of the drowning or on the way to the hospital are sometimes ineffective because of the unfamiliarity of the rescuer with the equipment.

CONTINUING OBSERVATION

After the patient has arrived in the emergency room and spontaneous respirations and adequate heart action have resumed, much of the immediate action is over. However, further definitive care is almost always necessary since many near-drowning victims may take a turn for the worse several hours after initially successful resuscitative efforts. Corticosteroids should be administered in large doses if there is any suspicion of prolonged cerebral anoxia and in an effort to reduce subsequent cerebral edema. Steroids may also reduce the inflammatory reaction subsequent to aspiration and the resulting aspiration pneumonitis.

The emergency room physicians should obtain chest films, serial electrocardiographic observations, and repeated blood gas determinations. The blood gases should be monitored carefully in order to determine the need for additional buffer solutions such as sodium bicarbonate.

Antifoaming agents such as 20% to 30% ethyl alcohol as an aerosol may be helpful in treating the patient's pulmonary edema, and there is some rationale for use of isoproterenol to reduce bronchospasm. This may be administered either by aerosol inhalation or intravenously. Antibiotics such as ampicillin are usually given as a prophylactic measure. As mentioned earlier some hemodilution or hemolysis may occur. In most instances in which these factors have been documented, they have been relatively minimal.

An intravenous route is maintained. Ideally, lactated Ringer's solution is given at the rate of 10 ml. per kilogram body weight for the first hour.

SUMMARY

In summary, much can be done for the near-drowning victim. Studies of Dr. J. H. Modell at the University of Florida in Gainesville and Dr. Hasan and associates at Mount Sinai in Miami Beach have placed resuscitation of the near-drowning victim on a more rational plane by their careful clinical observation of large numbers of these patients. It is important to remember that the intensity of the cardiopulmonary resuscitative efforts should be maintained throughout, just as they are when any other etiologic factor is involved. The danger of irreversible brain damage always looms as a potential threat, and its likelihood must certainly not be accentuated by any inadequacies on the part of the rescuer.

For the reader interested in an excellent discussion of the pathophysiology and treatment of drowning and near drowning, attention should be directed to the excellent monograph on the subject by Modell.

Chapter 32

RESUSCITATION AFTER LIGHTNING SHOCK

Injuries caused by lightning

The number of deaths from lightning shock in the United States each year has been estimated at around 300. It is further estimated that approximately three fourths of all individuals struck by lightning will survive. Many of the injuries from lightning result from the fires it causes. Approximately 75% of all reported farm fire losses originate from lightning. Incidentally, more than 80% of all livestock losses from accidents are a result of lightning.

The United States Weather Bureau estimates indicate that lightning strikes the earth about 100 times every second. More deaths are caused by lightning than by hurricanes and tornadoes.

National Safety Council figures indicate that lightning killed 1,792 Americans between 1954 and 1964. At the famous Ascot races in England in 1965, a single bolt of lightning killed fifteen persons and injured forty-five. Although many patients struck by lightning characteristically sustain severe shock and burns scattered over the entire body, an appreciable number die of ventricular fibrillation.

The gigantic electrical discharge involved in a bolt of lightning is well known and can be testified to by all sorts of sequelae. The precise physiologic effect of a bolt of lightning on the heart of a patient is not well known. A remarkable experience is reported by Ravitch and co-workers at the Baltimore City Hospital. Successful resuscitation of a 10-year-old boy struck by lightning was accomplished. Experience encountered in this case would tend to confirm the likelihood that ventricular fibrillation is not necessarily the expected sequel, but that there is a slow relaxation and a gradual resumption of slow but regular cardiac activity, until anoxia (induced by the absence of respiration) results in a secondary arrest of cardiac activity (Pearl). In the case of the 10-year-old boy (who was struck while riding his bicycle), a delay of 22 minutes occurred prior to the resuscitative efforts in the hospital. A pulse had been felt for a brief period after the accident. Marked evidence of neurologic disability was present for the first 2 weeks but gradually subsided. Cardiac massage was carried out by an open thoracotomy approach. The heart action occurred rapidly.

In the postresuscitative period, hypothermia was maintained between 30° and 31° C. Even though convulsions and hemiparesis developed and the patient was comatose for 6 days, he made a subsequent normal recovery except for a minimal speech deformity.

A most interesting and very similar case is reported by Nesmith. A 14-year-old boy was hit by a direct lightning strike while playing golf. While his father performed mouth-to-mouth respiration, his mother ran to a telephone to summon aid. An army corpsman arrived in an ambulance, began external massage, and radioed the hospital for a physician. When the physician arrived the corpsman was performing external cardiac massage, but no artificial respiration was being given. At this point the boy's pupils were dilated and there was evidence of severe burns on various parts of his body. In the emergency room of the hospital, a carotid pulse soon became palpable and a tracheotomy was performed. The patient was treated with steroids, antibiotics, restricted intravenous intake, and hypothermia. During the first 4 days, a comatose state persisted along with decerebrate spasms and a positive Babinski sign on the left side. It was not until 14 days after the injury that the patient first responded to stimuli. Approximately 3 weeks later, he was discharged with very minimal spasticity. Subsequent follow-up has shown no neurologic sequelae.

In both of the above cases the time before the start of artificial respiration and artificial cardiac compression was exceptionally long, but amazingly was followed by complete recoveries. Is there a common denominator peculiar to lightning shocks that contributes to a recovery that would not be expected in the usual case of cardiac arrest? Taussig also has noted this long period of total arrest followed by recovery and speculates that perhaps the cessation of metabolic activity in all cells, including the brain cells, following lightning stroke is so instantaneous that the onset of degenerative processes is delayed. At any rate, ambulance attendants and others likely to participate in resuscitation of these patients have reason to be particularly aggressive and persistent in their efforts.

Often as many as a dozen individuals are knocked to the ground by a bolt of lightning. In such a situation the rescuer should avoid the general axiom that one centers his first aid efforts on the living rather than the apparent dead. If an individual shows signs of life, the chances are good that he will survive. On the other hand many of those individuals who are apparent fatalities can be resuscitated if cardiopulmonary resuscitative efforts are followed.

As Taussig has pointed out in a study on "death" from lightning, metabolic activity, in addition to heart action and respiration, stops almost instantly when a person is struck by lightning. The heart may start again in sinus rhythm. The onset of degenerative changes is apparently delayed by the sudden cessation of metabolic activity to the extent that successful resuscitation may be achieved in the victim who has apparently been "dead" for longer than 4 minutes. Therefore, vigorous efforts at resuscitation following lightning shock are often most rewarding.

An amazing variety of clinical findings may be present immediately following lightning shock even though the patient appears to be only stunned by the lightning. The patient may be unable to move the extremities. Deafness or blindness may be present. Fortunately many of the complications are only transient, but obviously the victim should be transported to the nearest medical center where definitive care can be administered.

Most injuries from lightning do not result from the mainstream of the bolt but are caused by current flowing through the victim from direct contact with the charged ground.

While some individuals may be only momentarily stunned following a lightning shock, others will require cardiopulmonary resuscitation. Artificial respiration, as described elsewhere in this book, should be begun immediately as well as closed-chest cardiac massage. Cardiopulmonary resuscitation may be necessary during transportation to the hospital, and respiratory depression may be such that artificial maintenance of respiration will need to be continued for several days. In addition, cardiac defibrillation may be required in a certain percentage of patients. Originally it was believed that most patients fibrillate following a lightning shock; however, there is now additional evidence that a majority represent simple asystole.

One should assume that multiple skeletal injuries may have occurred from the tremendous repulsive force. The skull and extremities should be checked by the rescuer for the possibility of fractures. Temporary paraplegia may be due either to the effect of lightning on the central nervous system or to a spinal cord injury.

The rescuer should be prepared for the victim to complain of deafness, blindness, and other neurologic deficits. Fortunately most of these are temporary. A postlightning shock psychosis is reported.

A word concerning prevention is always in order. To the golfer in an electrical storm goes the advice to get rid of his clubs, get away from trees or golf carts, and lie down on the ground in the area of greatest depression. A thick woods is a relatively safe spot. During an electrical storm, an automobile (with a metal top) is one of the safest spots. Certainly one should avoid being in a swimming pool, near a single tree, near horses or cattle, or on the top of a hill or mountain. Always avoid being the tallest object or being near the tallest object in a given vicinity. *Never* raise an umbrella over your head in an electrical storm.

Chapter 33

ACCIDENTAL ELECTROCUTION

The specific occupational hazards of telephone and electric lineman include that of accidental electric shock and subsequent cardiac arrest. Obviously, the challenge of adequately resuscitating a victim high on a pole in a maze of wires is considerable. Towne and Dewey, however, have detailed a technique making it possible to begin the cardiopulmonary resuscitation before the 4-minute time limit. In Fig. 33-1 these various steps are enumerated.

Mr. Robert D. Fagg of the Pacific Gas and Electric Company, San Francisco, states that, according to the Edison Electric Institute's annual fatality report for the last decade, there have been over 1,000 deaths due to electric shock or burn accidents. It is for this reason that one of the most extensive programs in lay education of resuscitation techniques has been given to utility company employees. In 1961 the medical task force of the Edison Electric Institute's Accident Prevention Committee unanimously recommended the adoption of external heart massage in conjunction with lung ventilation as a technique that the electric utility industry should teach to its personnel.

There are those who maintain that hospital patients may be in greater danger from electrical shock hazards than are industrial workers. Many of the complex medical instruments used in hospitals represent potentially lethal instruments of accidental electrocution. In 1965 the National Electrical Code and the National Fire Protection Association set standards for electrical wiring in hazardous areas where flammable fluids are stored or used, for example, in x-ray installations and in operating rooms, but no set standards are now available for use in coronary care or intensive care units. There is growing awareness, however, that potentially hazardous circumstances require increasingly safe medical electronic equipment design.

Aronow and associates report a patient thrown into ventricular fibrillation when the control mechanism of his electrically operated bed was accidentally submerged in urine. They stress the hazard of electrocution by hospital apparatus, particularly the increased danger when a wire or catheter leads directly to the heart. In this case, current from a grounded, 120-volt line passed from the bed controller into the urine pool, through the patient's buttocks, back to the ground by way of a precordial monitor electrode pasted to the skin. Continued manufacture or use of beds with such controllers is not justifiable. The fault is easily corrected by a transformer and relay module that places a low voltage across the controller. With external cardiac compression, this patient was restored to consciousness and recovered without evidence of cardiac irritability, but the authors suggest that many such episodes of electrocution have passed unrecognized. No special investigation is usually made into the sudden death of a patient with a documented myocardial infarction and a recent stroke.

There are several reasons for the increased concern with iatrogenic electrocution. Not only are there many more electrical instruments—in the doctor's office, clinic, outpatient treatment area, intensive care unit, operating room, and diagnostic rooms—but two or more instruments are often connected to the patient at one time.

389

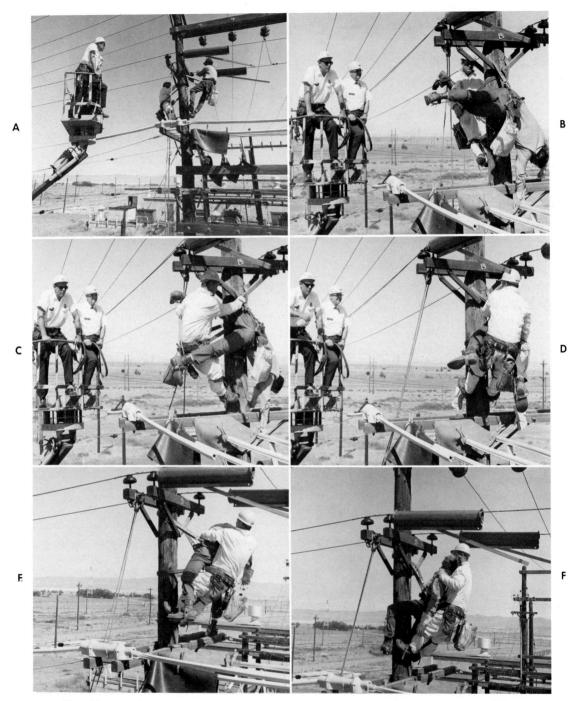

Fig. 33-1. Cardiopulmonary resuscitation for victim high on pole. **B** shows victim, dropped in his safety straps in head-down and sideways position. **C**, Rescuer slides under victim to place one of victim's legs above and one below rescuer's safety strap. Rescuer then pulls victim to a sitting position, **D** and **E**, resting him on his own (rescuer's) safety strap. **F** and **G**, Having removed his gloves, rescuer feels the diaphragm and abdomen-chest area for victim's breathing. He next explores the mouth with bare finger to remove gum or any other loose foreign material.

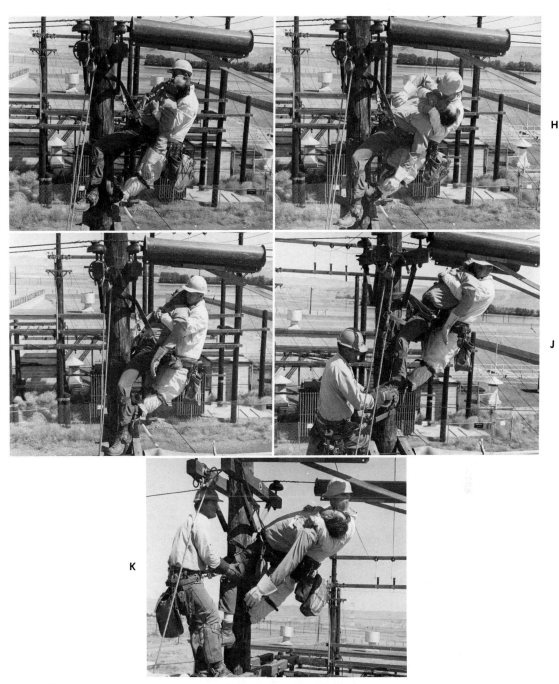

Fig. 33-1, cont'd. H, Mouth-to-mouth ventilation is then begun. If he finds the pupils dilated and there is no pulse, rescuer moves behind victim, **I,** and, with his arms around victim's chest, grasps one of his own wrists with the other hand cocking his wrist so that hand is like a plunger on lower half of victim's sternum. **J,** Rescuer gives fifteen forceful compressions to victim's sternum. After the fifteen cardiac compressions, five pulmonary ventilations, **K,** should be followed by another fifteen cardiac compressions. (From Towne, G. E., and Dewey, L. S.: J. Occup. Med. **13:**398-401, 1971.)

Unsuspected sources of electrical shock are created when "negligible" leakage of current from one instrument occurs by way of a ground path in the second (with the patient as part of the circuit), or when several instruments considered to be "safe" individually accumulate leakage currents to a harmful degree. Also, certain patients are unusually vulnerable to electrical shock even from current levels so low they would go unnoticed if applied to the skin. These patients are being paced with a direct electrical connection to the myocardium.

All equipment connected to a patient should be solidly grounded, and all equipment should be so designed as to minimize leakage of current between those components connected to the A.C. power system and those in contact with the patient.

Animal experiments by Kouwenhoven and Langworthy suggest that ventricular fibrillation from accidental exposure to electrical current may be initiated by considerably smaller voltage between the upper and the lower extremities than when the current flows between the upper extremities. Probably the most common pathway in accidental electrocution in man is from the right hand to the feet.

LaJoie concludes that the postelectrical shock syndrome, consisting primarily of vague discomfort in the chest and arms following electrical shock, results from severe contractions of the pectoral and arm muscles that occur at the time of the shock. He reported a careful follow-up of twenty-nine persons who had received accidental electrical shock. The long-range effect on the myocardium appeared minimal. A direct cardiac reaction to electrical shock could not be shown. There was almost no effect on preexisting myocardial disease.

The intensity of the current, its frequency, its pathway through the body, and the duration of the current—all these factors influence the extent and scope of the patient's injury as well as the development of ventricular fibrillation (Table 33-1). An episode of atrial fibrillation that persisted for several days occurred following the ac-

Table 33-1. Effects of direct and alternating current*

Current range	Direct current (generally produced by voltages from 110 to 800)	Alternating current (generally produced by voltages from 110 to 380, frequency 50 c.p.s.)	Effect
I	<80 milliamperes	<25 milliamperes	Slight contraction of respiratory muscles; no damage to heart
II	80 to 100 milliamperes	25 to 80 milliamperes	Cardiac arrest; increased blood pressure; respiratory spasm; if duration of shock exceeds 25 to 30 sec., cardiac arrest may be followed by ventricular fibrillation
III	300 milliamperes to 3 amperes	80 to 300 milliamperes to 3 amperes	With direct current, ventricular fibrillation occurs only for certain pathways; with alternating current, irreversible ventricular fibrillation generally results except for very short duration of shock from 0.1 to 0.3 sec.
IV		>3 amperes (voltage from 3,000 upward)	Cardiac and circulatory arrest followed by protracted arrhythmia; increased blood pressure; respiratory spasm; if duration > few sec., death occurs as result of serious burns

*From Report of Proceeding, International Labor Organization, Geneva, Switzerland, Oct. 12-23, 1961; Murray, R.: Hazards to health, N. Engl. J. Med. **268:**1127-1128, 1963.

cidental electrocution of a 52-year-old line-man (Wehrmacher). Subsequent recovery seemed complete, and a 2-year follow-up indicated no permanent adverse effect.

Induction of fibrillation in the atrium of the heart is difficult. The fibrillatory threshold of the atrium can be lowered by stimulation of the vagi. It is thought that the vagal stimulatory action shortens the refractory period of the atrium.

Few accurate statistics are available to indicate the true incidence of deaths from accidental electrical contact. However, the toll of accidental death from electrocution annually reaches a tragic figure. Despite increased precautions by manufacturers of electrical appliances, safety warnings, and protective clothing, this catastrophe creates news stories daily.

From a review of the circumstances following electrical shock, it is highly probable that the majority of deaths result from the sudden conversion of normal cardiac activity to ventricular fibrillation. Frequently, the voltage has been minimal, and evidence of electrical burn has been absent. The explanation of this is that the actual flow of current through the body rather than the voltage involved is regarded as the mechanism that causes death from electrocution, although high voltages cause extensive damage to tissue at contact locations. Ohm's law $\left(I = \dfrac{V}{R} \right)$ is applicable in this situation, but it is often hard to correlate voltage and tissue damage because the variations in contact resistance are usually great. This reasoning is that of the majority of biophysicists, engineers, and physiologists concerned with this problem and is the basis for placing the criterion of danger from electrical shock upon the amount of current conducted by the body.

Dalziel, an electrical engineer, has made some interesting observations concerning this problem. He explains that external bodily contacts with electricity, in which the current pathway involves the chest, may produce heart block, respiratory inhibition, ventricular fibrillation, or irreversible damage to the nervous system if the current is in considerable excess of that needed to cause paralysis of the chest muscles and cessation of breathing. Shocks of much greater intensity than those necessary to produce ventricular fibrillation are needed to produce heart block, respiratory failure, and severe damage to the central nervous system.

For short shocks the susceptibility of the heart to fibrillate increases with increasing current until a most dangerous current is reached—then the susceptibility decreases. At relatively high currents the likelihood of producing ventricular fibrillation is almost negligible. The explanation of this phenomenon is that very high currents paralyze the nerve centers in the heart, the heart is contracted and silenced, and fibrillation is prevented. Death is inevitable if the shock is of long duration, but if of short duration and the heart has not been damaged, interruption of the current may be followed by a spontaneous resumption of normal rhythmic contractions. This is offered as explanation for frequent accident cases in which victims apparently withstood relatively high currents. This phenomenon is the basis for countershock, or defibrillation shock treatment to arrest ventricular fibrillation.*

In light of these comments, the feasibility of employing accepted resuscitative measures (massage, artificial respiration, and so on) is readily apparent.

A.C. is more dangerous than D.C. However, A.C. of extremely high frequencies can be used (as in physiotherapy machines) since human nerves and muscles are not sensitive to frequencies as high as 500,000 to 1,000,000 cycles per second. Some physiotherapy machines employ 20,000 to 40,000 volts, from 1 to 2 amperes, and about 1,000,000 cycles per second. Currents of 40 to 150 cycles per second appear to be the most dangerous.

Patients accidentally receiving an elec-

*From Dalziel, C. F.: Effects of electric shock on man, IRE Transactions on Med. Electronics, PGME-5, July, 1956, Institute of Radio Engineers, New York.

trical shock may show ECG evidence of nodal rhythm for several hours to several days after the shock.

In addition to producing ventricular fibrillation, contact with A.C. represents a clinically observed method of producing nodal rhythm.

The following abstracts of newspaper accounts of deaths from electrocution suggest the possibility of ventricular fibrillation or cardiac standstill.

A 22-year-old Irish pop musician was electrocuted in front of a crowd of screaming teenagers in a Dublin ballroom when his electric guitar short-circuited. Efforts at artificial respiration were unsuccessful.

A 29-year-old fireman was standing in an alley fighting a fire at a downtown store when an electric wire fell across a stream being trained on the blaze, electrocuting the fireman.

One young football player was reported dead and at least twelve others were injured after a goal post the high school team was erecting came in contact with a power line. The post touched a high power line running across the edge of the field.

A 14-year-old Dubuque, Iowa, youth died, apparently of electrocution, when he jumped into a swimming pool being drained with the aid of an electric motor.

A 22-year-old Kansas City, Kansas, man was electrocuted when a kite string containing a metallic filament came into contact with a 12,000 volt electric line. The string being used to fly the kite was a nylon crochet yarn containing decorative strands of metal.

The body of a 5-year-old boy was found draped across an electrified fence erected by his father. The potential across the fence was 21 volts.

An 8-year-old boy was killed when he climbed a light pole to examine a bird's nest. He was revived twice on the way to the hospital, remarking once, "I'm going to buy an ice cream cone." Death occurred shortly afterward.

A 10-month-old baby was electrocuted when he stuck his tongue into an extension cord socket. He was pronounced dead after 2 hours of resuscitative efforts by a physician proved of no avail.

A fatal electrical shock was received by a Brooklyn teenager from a hair dryer. She was drying her hair in the shower room at the time of the accident. She was taken to a hospital, but succumbed shortly afterward.

A Long Island man was electrocuted in a swim-

ming pool because of a short circuit in one of the underwater lights. He lived for 20 minutes after being taken from the pool but could not be resuscitated by ambulance crews on the scene.

A bolt of lightning sent a charge of electricity along a water pipe and caused the death of a Charlotte, North Carolina, woman who was drawing a glass of water for one of her children. She was knocked to the floor and, when asked if she was hurt, she replied, "No, but I'm turning blind." She died moments later.

A small boy was electrocuted when he placed his hand in an electric broiler. He was pronounced dead about 45 minutes after receiving the shock. Resuscitative measures at a hospital failed.

A 16-year-old youth developed ventricular fibrillation when he touched an electric lamp while seated on a radiator. He screamed and fell to the floor. He could not be revived.

A 3½-year-old boy was electrocuted while playing near an electrically operated rocking horse in a self-service laundry. It was thought that the boy might have reached under the horse and touched a live wire while standing on the wet floor.

A 39-year-old woman suffered ventricular fibrillation when she was electrocuted while picking up a defective bedside lamp while touching a disconnected radiator pipe with her leg.

A 9-month-old boy in a wet diaper was electrocuted when he grabbed an exposed wire in the living room of his home.

A 19-year-old girl was electrocuted while taking a bath when a lamp was accidentally tipped over and fell into the water.

With increasing dependence on electrical appliances in the home and at work, it is likely that accidental electrocutions will continue to occur and perhaps even increase in frequency. A partial solution may be found in more rigid adherence to high standards of manufacturing, double insulation and rapid-acting differential circuit breakers, and educational aspects of prevention. Nevertheless, ventricular fibrillation from accidental electrocution is likely to continue to take its tragic toll.

The same principles of resuscitation apply in these as in other instances of cardiac arrest. Artificial respiration (mouth-to-mouth) must be started at once along with closed-chest cardiac massage. These measures must be maintained until the fibrillating ventricles are converted to normal rhythm by external defibrillation. The *time factor* will, of course, continue to plague the rescuer. Not all "apparent deaths" after electrical shock will, however, be due to ventricular fibrillation. Some will result from temporary inhibition of the bulbar centers, and some will result from tetanization of the respiratory muscles long enough to produce asphyxia.

Successful defibrillation after accidental electrocution

The remarkable resuscitation of a 4-year-old girl accidentally electrocuted in her home is reported from the Harbor General Hospital (Halpern and Webber). The child received a fibrillating shock when she caused contact between a wet mop and a vacuum cleaner with a known short circuit. Aided by a fortuitous chain of circumstances, the child was in a doctor's office within a matter of 3 to 4 minutes. At this time the thorax was entered and manual compression of the heart against the ster-num was begun after initiation of artificial respiration with the aid of an intratracheal tube. The child was transported across the street to the hospital after manual massage of the heart. When the pericardium was opened, the ventricles were observed to be fibrillating and successful defibrillation was achieved on the third attempt.

Dilated pupils that reacted only slightly to light, pathologic reflexes, and other evidence of CNS depression were present. For these reasons the child was packed in ice, and rectal temperatures of 32.2° to 34.4° C. (90° to 94° F.) were maintained. Chlorpromazine was administered to control shivering. The child made a rapid recovery and was discharged from the hospital on the eighth day postoperative. Tachycardia had disappeared by the third week, and by the fourth week, the ECG was reported as normal. There was no evidence of intellectual deterioration, even though the period without cerebral circulation was estimated to have been from 5 to 7 minutes.

Chapter 34

THE STONE HEART SYNDROME: ISCHEMIC MYOCARDIAL CONTRACTURE

Denton A. Cooley and Don C. Wukasch

Myocardial failure occurring in patients undergoing open-heart procedures with ischemic cardiac arrest may be of two distinct types. The first and most common is a low output failure in which the left ventricle is flaccid, poorly contracting, overdistended and nonresponsive to inotropic drugs (Najafi and co-workers; Robicsek and co-workers). The second and more striking is the "stone heart" syndrome (Cooley and co-workers) in which the heart develops a tetanic contracture or myocardial rigidity and the left ventricular cavity becomes small and the ventricle is literally frozen in systole. The ventricular chamber is decreased, notably in volume because of the contracture, and even vigorous manual compression does not produce an adequate stroke volume. Changes in peripheral resistance, cardiotonic agents, electrolyte solutions, adrenergic blocking and stimulating agents, and assist devices usually have not altered its inevitable course. On palpation the heart is in a contracted state similar to the uterine contraction ring or the tetanic contraction of striated muscle as seen in the experimental laboratory.

Fortunately, the stone heart is rare. Of the 4,732 patients (1,407 for congenital lesions and 3,325 for acquired) who underwent open-heart surgery at the Texas Heart Institute during the 5-year period from July, 1966 to July 1971, only 51 patients (1%) died during operation from acute myocardial insufficiency. Of that group, less than a third (13 patients) experienced severe contracture

of the heart and the criterion we recognize as stone heart.

Recognition

The stone heart syndrome can be easily recognized at the time of cardiopulmonary bypass (see list below). Characteristic of the syndrome is the small fixed-volume left ventricular cavity so that forceful manual compression of the heart produces almost no pressure wave on the arterial monitor. Contracture of the heart may occur almost immediately upon application of the aortic occlusion clamp, during the time of ischemic arrest or shortly after removal of the clamp. We had one patient with severe aortic stenosis and left ventricular pressure over 250 mm. Hg who developed the syndrome while the thoracotomy incision was being made. Another of our cases developed ischemic contracture of the heart in the recovery room (Wukasch and co-workers). At the time of cardiac arrest the patient was resuscitated and returned to the operating room. Severe contracture of the left ventricle was identified, and a left ventricular assist device failed to produce relaxation of the heart. When the heart was opened on the operating table, no outflow tract obstruction could be identified in either valve or from previous lesions. Effective cardiac output could not be obtained when the heart was massaged despite injection of various pharmacologic agents into the aorta or directly into the coronary arteries or myocardium.

*Stone heart: characteristics for recognition**

Firm myocardial muscle mass
Spastic contracted ventricle, frozen in systole
Ventricular volume decreased
No cardiac output on manual massage
Irreversible

Predisposing factors

Two types of patients appear prone toward development of the stone heart during operations using cardiopulmonary bypass: (1) patients with severe aortic valve disease— usually aortic stenosis with extreme left ventricular hypertrophy and (2) patients with end-stage coronary artery disease. A review of the clinical and pathological features of thirteen patients who developed stone heart elucidated a number of features common to patients who developed this complication (Table 34-1).

CLINICAL FEATURES

All patients with manifestations of the stone heart had acquired heart disease. The age range and sex differences were insignificant. Preoperative symptoms were interesting since eleven of the thirteen patients had congestive heart failure, eight had angina pectoris and only three had previously documented myocardial infarction. Ten of the thirteen patients were in Functional Class IV and the remainder in Class III according to the New York Heart Association's classification. These characteristics, however, are seen with equal incidence in patients who develop low output failure and are not unique to those who develop stone heart.

ELECTROCARDIOGRAM

Although electrocardiography before operation was of little importance in anticipating the occurrence of stone heart, the predominant electrocardiographic pattern seen in those patients who developed the syndrome was that of left ventricular strain with left ventricular hypertrophy.

---

*From Wukasch, D. C., et al.: The "stone heart" syndrome, Surgery **72:**1071-1080, 1972.

Table 34-1. Stone heart: primary anatomic diagnosis in 13 patients*

Diagnosis	Number
Calcific aortic stenosis†	8
Periprosthetic mitral valve leak†	1
Noncalcific aortic insufficiency†	1
Syphilitic aortitis and aortic valvulitis†	2
Coronary artery disease	13
Total	13

*From Wukasch, D. C., et al.: The "stone heart" syndrome, Surgery **72:**1071-1080, 1972.
†Eleven of thirteen patients had aortic valve disease requiring aortic valve replacement.

Table 34-2. Stone heart: cardiac catheterization*

	Number in abnormal group	Average value (mm. Hg)	Range (mm. Hg)
Pulmonary artery pressure (>32 mm. Hg)	9/9	59	33-80
Mean pulmonary artery wedge (>14 mm. Hg)	8/9	27	11-50
Left ventricular end-diastolic pressure (>20 mm. Hg)	8/8	34	25-45
Aortic valve gradient (>60 mm. Hg)	4/4†	95	69-30

*From Wukasch, D. C., et al.: The "stone heart" syndrome, Surgery **72:**1071-1080, 1972.
†Aortic valve gradient could not be measured in two of six patients with pure aortic stenosis.

CARDIAC CATHETERIZATION

Cardiac catheterization (Table 34-2) revealed findings indicative of left ventricular failure. No measurement of left ventricular end-diastolic pressure could be obtained in five patients with severe aortic stenosis because of inability to cross the densely calcified aortic valve with the catheter at the time of left heart catheterization. The left ventricular end-diastolic pressure was greater than 20 mm. Hg in the remaining eight patients, and in three of these the pressure was greater than 40 mm. Hg at rest. In patients with aortic stenosis, notable left ventricular hypertension was present with large gradients across the aortic valve in those in whom it could be measured. Since almost all of the patients had pulmonary hypertension, cardiac catheterization data acquired at rest showed significant elevation in peak systolic pulmonary artery, mean pulmonary artery wedge, and left ventricular end-diastolic pressures. Noted also was left ventricular hypertension with large aortic valve gradients.

ASSOCIATED OPERATIVE PROCEDURES

Of the thirteen patients, eleven had significant aortic valve disease and all eleven underwent aortic valve replacement. Among this group, five patients had aortic valve replacement alone, four had aortic valve replacement plus mitral valve replacement, one had aortic valve replacement plus coronary artery bypass, and another had aortic valve replacement plus replacement of the ascending aorta for severe aortitis that extended proximally to occlude the right coronary artery. Two patients had undergone coronary artery bypass procedure for severe coronary artery disease.

PATHOLOGIC FEATURES

Autopsy of these patients demonstrated some common features. In all instances severe myocardial hypertrophy was noted. The average heart weighed 782.2 gm. with a range of 620 to 1,227 gm. (Table 34-3). Two hearts weighed over 1,000 gm. Myocardial hypertrophy was present on microscopic section as well as on gross examination, and concentric hypertrophy resulting in a small ventricular chamber was observed in most specimens (Fig. 34-1). Myocardial fibrosis was present in all hearts but one (Figs. 34-2 and 34-3). Evidence of recent myocardial infarction was observed on microscopic section of three hearts. Severe coronary artery

Table 34-3. Stone heart: pathological findings in 13 patients*

Findings	Patients	
	Number	%
Myocardial hypertrophy†	13	100
Myocardial fibrosis	12	92
Recent myocardial infarction‡	3	23
Severe coronary arteriosclerosis	4	31
Hypoplastic left circumflex artery	1	8
Ostial stenosis right coronary artery	1	8

*From Wukasch, D. C., et al.: The "stone heart" syndrome, Surgery 72:1071-1080, 1972.
†Average heart weight, 782.2 gm. (range 620 to 1,227 gm.).
‡One patient had cardiac arrest postoperatively.

disease was found in only four patients, and mild coronary arteriosclerosis was observed in two. Angina pectoris was present in some patients but did not correlate well with autopsy findings of coronary arteriosclerosis. The common pathological findings thus were myocardial hypertrophy and fibrosis with occasional coronary arteriosclerosis.

Etiology

Elucidation of the exact cause for the contracture has been difficult and explanations are mostly speculative. Factors concerning conduct of the operation including ischemic arrest time, the technique of cardiopulmonary bypass, and medications administered both before and during operations have been similar to other patients undergoing comparable procedures, and none appeared responsible for the production of stone heart. Because of the severe myocardial hypertrophy and interstitial fibrosis, one may assume that a relative coronary insufficiency was present even though gross coronary artery disease was noted in only two patients.

Onset of the ischemic contracture may occur immediately after starting cardiopulmonary bypass, late during the course of the operation, or upon making the first attempts

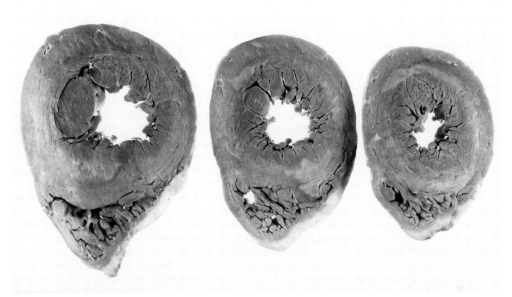

Fig. 34-1. Cross-sectional views of "stone heart" at autopsy showing small cavity size of hypertrophied and contracted left ventricle at different levels from base to apex. Comparison of wall thickness of left and right ventricles is striking in this heart, which weighed 1,227 gm. (From Wukasch, D. C., and others: Surgery 72:1071-1080, 1972.)

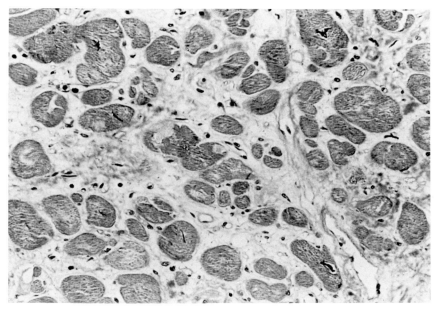

Fig. 34-2. Photomicrograph showing diffuse dense interstitial fibrosis in "stone heart" of 69-year-old man with severe calcific aortic stenosis. Heart weighed 875 gm. (From Wukasch, D. C., and others: Surgery 72:1071-1080, 1972.)

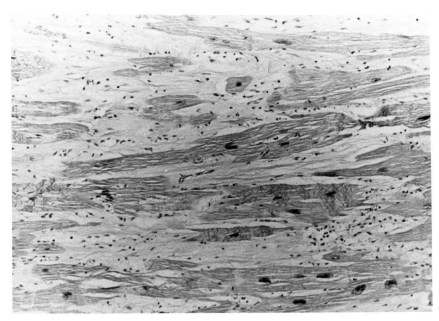

Fig. 34-3. Photomicrograph with section made longitudinal to myocardial fibers showing diffuse cellular fibrosis and overgrowth of collagenous connective tissue in 58-year-old patient with combined mitral and aortic valve stenosis and normal coronary arteries. Heart weighed 950 gm. (From Wukasch, D. C., and others: Surgery 72:1071-1080, 1972.)

at cardiac resuscitation while discontinuing bypass. The contracture appears first in the subendocardial myocardium and progresses peripherally toward the epicardial surface. As the contracture becomes extreme, the vertically directed coronary arteries originating from the epicardial arteries are undoubtedly compressed or squeezed. This mechanical effect plus associated arterial spasm probably accounts for the failure of pharmacologic agents to reverse the condition since the agents never reach the cellular level of the contracted myocardial tissue. Electric countershock and applied heat and cold also have failed.

Lundsgaard-Hansen has suggested that the heart outgrows its blood supply with severe cardiomegaly. Further ischemia at the time of operation may produce early myocardial injury. As demonstrated by Hensen and Morales, one of the early signs of myocardial ischemia following cardiopulmonary bypass is the microscopic presence of contraction bands in myocardial fibers. This state pre-

cedes actual ischemic necrosis. Contraction bands may have a relation to the contractile state in the myocardium since most myofibrils appear contracted when viewed by light and electron microscopy. Moreover, the ischemic period may promote excess catecholamine production, further enhancing the contractile state. Coronary artery perfusion on the cellular level may be reduced irreversibly by closure of the myocardial sinusoids. These facets are presently under study in our laboratories.

The presence of contraction bands in the sarcomeres is interesting. Similar bands may be produced as the first manifestations of myocardial ischemia (Reichenbach). They also have appeared in patients with chronic failing hearts, in animals during hemorrhagic shock preparations, and in patients dying from acute myocardial infarctions, ruptured aortic aneurysm, trauma, and renal disease (Hensen). Contraction bands result when the thick and thin filaments no longer have their usual spatial relation. They represent overlapping of the thin filaments in the sarcomere and usually are thought to occur as "super" contractions ·beyond the usual 50% state to around 80% shortening. Similar contracted states are common to most types of muscle. The tetanic contraction of the fatigued gastrocnemius muscle is analogous. Super-contracted states also may be present in the sea barnacle (Balanus), and extreme shortening of the sarcomere occurs in rigor mortis. These states have shown a relation to a deficiency of adenosine triphosphate (ATP). When human heart weight exceeds 500 gm. 50% of the ATP energy reserve may be lost (Lundsgaard-Hansen). All of the patients with stone hearts had cardiomegaly. Since relaxation cannot be accomplished without ATP, the contracted state may represent a response to ATP depletion.

This possible relationship of the stone heart state to deficiencies of adenosine triphosphate (ATP) has been previously described (Gott and co-workers; Katz and co-workers). Because of massive myocardial hypertrophy, the ATP deficiency state may exist (Fox; Lundsgaard-Hansen; Pool). Tetanic contraction of striated muscle occurs in ATP-deficient states such as fatigue and rigor mortis. The contraction of the myocardial fibrils further compromises the capillary and sinusoidal flow and the contracted state becomes irreversible.

Another interesting facet is the role of calcium ion exchange and the sarcoplasmic reticulum in cycling of the myocardial contractile process. If the calcium ion exchange is disturbed, with the added effect of repeated stimulation of the sarcomere, the calcium may accumulate in the cytoplasm, causing a continued contractile state similar to rigor mortis. According to both Nakamaru and Schwartz, the sarcoplasmic reticulum, calcium ion exchange, and intracellular acid-base balance play an essential role in the contraction-relaxation mechanism of the myocardium. The calcium may become bound to the regulator proteins in the face of intracellular alkalosis. This results in contraction of the heart with failure of relaxation.

Prevention and treatment

Because of recent interest in this complex problem, several methods of prevention and treatment have been considered and some tried clinically. The mechanical obstruction to subendocardial vessels by the contracted myocardial fibers (whatever the underlying cause) must be prevented. The initial ischemia probably begets more ischemia as a result of the myocardial squeeze on the coronary arterioles. After aortic cross-clamping, prompt induction of cardiac arrest to a completely relaxed state of diastole using acetylcholine as the pharmacologic agent could theoretically prevent the contracture and the coronary strangulation. Thus, upon cross-clamping the aorta, acetylcholine injected into the aortic root may be worth a trial (Kirklin). Previous experience in the early years of open-heart surgery, however, revealed that induced cardiac arrest with acetylcholine and potassium or magnesium salts caused delays or failure to restore effective myocardial activity upon restoration of coronary flow— probably because of an extensive depolarization of myocardial fibers. Certainly electrically induced ventricular fibrillation would theoretically be contraindicated in patients with advanced left ventricular hypertrophy because of the increased myocardial metabolism, which increases the oxygen deficit and metabolic waste products in an already undernourished tissue.

If the stone heart state truly represents an ATP-depleted heart, then once the state develops, agents designed to reduce myocardial ATP hydrolysis may reverse the contractile state. Because of the viselike effect of the contracted myocardium and the endogenously induced spasm of the coronary arteries, forced high pressure perfusion through the coronary arteries by direct cannulation may allow entrance of these agents into the myocardium. Therefore, the perfusion of oxygenated blood containing acid solutions, propranolol, or calcium chelators (EDTA) directly into the coronary arteries may be worth a trial. A definite risk of vascular damage exists, however, from forced perfusion (Bloodwell and coworkers).

Another approach has recently been reported by Gerami, who described successful resuscitation of a stone heart by use of sublingual nitroglycerin and intravenous corticosteroids. This regimen was tried in one of our cases without success.

PREVENTION BY HYPOTHERMIA

Gott and associates reported an experiment on the ischemic canine heart in which a "time of rigor" was determined under various conditions. Onset of myocardial rigor occurred most rapidly in the anoxic myocardium at 37° C. and following approximately 50 minutes of ischemia. In Gott's experiments maximum protection of the myocardium was achieved by intermittent perfusion of the heart with a small amount of blood (5 ml. per kilogram of body weight every 10 minutes) or by cooling the heart to 27° C. In both situations, time and onset were more than doubled.

Recently, we have adopted a new plan of operation for patients with severe left ventricular hypertrophy in an effort to prevent this complication. Since October 20, 1971, we have used moderate general hypothermia (30° C.) with topical application of cold saline (12° C.) to the exterior and interior of the heart before and during ischemic arrest. Hypothermia to 30° C. is induced before cross-clamping the ascending aorta and placing the patient on total cardiopulmonary bypass. While the aortic valve is being replaced by a prosthesis, the patient, except for the heart and to some degree the lungs, is being gradually rewarmed to 35° to 36° C. When the clamp is released from the ascending aorta, restoring coronary circulation, the cold heart receives warm blood and cardiac action resumes.

During the ensuing 13-month period, among our total operative cases, 1,173 operations were performed using hypothermia for aortic valve disease and/or coronary artery occlusive disease, often with left ventricular hypertrophy and myocardial decompensation. No deaths from stone heart occurred in these patients. We have concluded that hypothermic cardiac arrest is an important and valuable preventive measure.

Using a variation of the hypothermic method, two patients with aortic valve disease developed stone heart that was reversed by intravenous propranolol (Inderal) 1.0 mg. Cardiac resuscitation was then achieved after a prolonged period using epinephrine cautiously infused during continuous cardiopulmonary bypass. Recently in all patients with severe left ventricular hypertrophy, Inderal 0.4 to 0.8 mg. has been administered prophylactically before bypass. We believe that this medication further protects the myocardium from ischemic contractions.

An experimental model of "stone heart" in the animal laboratory would be useful to elucidate the cause and to define a reliable therapeutic technique. The mechanism of production and various attempts at biochemical reversal could then be attempted with this model. To determine the metabolic effects of hypothermia, studies are now being conducted in our laboratories on intramyocardial temperature, electron microscopy of myocardial biopsies, and on blood pyruvate, lactate, and intracellular enzymes in coronary sinus blood. An experiment using dogs is in progress to ascertain the degree of protection offered by myocardial hypothermia against stone heart. Hopefully these studies may elucidate the pathophysiology and biochemical factors responsible for stone heart.

Summary

Ischemic contracture of the heart, or the "stone heart" syndrome, is an uncommon but extremely serious complication of open heart surgery. Severe aortic stenosis or end-stage coronary artery disease in patients with massive myocardial hypertrophy and fibrosis are the most common predisposing lesions to development of this condition. Usually present are longstanding obstruction to ventricular outflow across the aortic valve with left ventricular hypertension, increased pulmonary artery pressure, increased pulmonary capillary wedge pressure, and large aortic gradients. The electrocardiogram made before operation may not be useful, but left ventricular hypertrophy with strain is present in most cases. Angina pectoris associated with relatively normal coronary arterio-grams, and congestive heart failure resulting from aortic stenosis or severe end-stage coronary artery disease with congestive heart failure, fibrosis, and hypertrophy may set the clinical picture for the production of stone heart. Induced hypothermia of the myocardium by blood cooling and direct application of cold solutions to the epicardial and endocardial surfaces of the heart and the intraoperative administration of propranolol have proved to be effective preventive measures.

Chapter 35

CARDIOGENIC SHOCK

Tony A. Don Michael

Shock is a clinical syndrome characterized by well-recognized signs and symptoms. The clinical picture of shock is familiar to the practicing physician and is recognized by the coolness of the extremities, pallor, cyanosis, diaphoresis, mental obtundation, a rapid, thready pulse, a fall of blood pressure, and reduced urinary output. This profile arises from a combination of decreased tissue perfusion and an associated sympathoadrenal discharge. In accordance with the primary underlying mechanism, shock is categorized as neurogenic, cardiogenic, hypovolemic, anaphylactoid, septic, and so on. Cardiogenic shock arises from and is primarily due to acute dysfunction of the left ventricle. Irrespective of cause, certain abnormalities occur in the shock syndrome. These include lactic acidosis, which correlates fairly well with the severity of the shock. In addition, hypoglycemia, an elevation of endogenous catecholamines and the production of certain biochemical substances such as kinins, has been reported to occur.

Criteria of cardiogenic shock

Since the development of the shock syndrome is related to tissue perfusion, reduced systolic and diastolic blood pressures are conventionally associated with its occurrence. However, the determination of blood pressure, as measured by the indirect Korotkoff method, does not always reflect intra-arterial levels. Thus, Cohn and his colleagues showed that intra-arterial pressures may be within normal levels or even elevated in the presence of reduced or unobtainable indirect blood pressures. Intense peripheral vasoconstriction induced by the production of endogenous catecholamines is responsible for this disparity. Such profound vasoconstriction, however, is not directly related to the severity of the shock syndrome. A fall of blood pressure to normal levels in a hypertensive patient may be consistent with clinical shock.

Mortality

The mortality of cardiogenic shock is of the order of 75% to 90%. In series in which arrhythmias, acidosis, and hypovolemia are reported, the mortality is in the range of 90%, whereas in studies in which these criteria are not specifically included, the reported mortality is somewhat lower (75%). Although widely used and promising in experimental animals, pharmacologic agents have, in general, been unsuccessful in influencing survival in patients with cardiogenic shock. The use of the "balloon" circulatory assists have been reported to reverse the shock state in approximately 75% of patients, but hospital survival is less than 15%. Acute revascularization of the myocardium involved in shock has been reported to be dramatically successful, but the series of patients in whom these procedures have been done is small and precise criteria for the patient selection are, at this time, unclear.

Pathophysiology and pathology

Page and his co-workers have shown that a critical amount of necrotic tissue at variable stages of cell death is present at the time of death. However, there is no evidence in man as to whether or not all the affected myocardium is actually necrotic at the time of onset of cardiogenic shock, nor are data available concerning the temporal sequence of changes in ischemic myocardium in a reversible phase prior to the development of irreversible cell death. Furthermore, while from a pathophysiologic standpoint cardiogenic shock has been considered to be a homogeneous entity, recent studies (Don Michael and co-workers, 1972) have indicated three specific etiologic mechanisms that may underlie the shock syndrome:

1. Sudden occlusion of a major vessel, specifically the left coronary artery or its anterior descending branch
2. Additional infarction of a critical amount of myocardium in a previously diseased heart
3. Rupture of the ventricular septum, of the ventricle, or the development of significant mitral incompetence

In general, peripheral vascular resistance tends to be elevated in states of cardiogenic shock and may be disproportionately raised with respect to the fall in the cardiac output. This may lead to body fluids and blood being trapped beyond severely constricted arteries and veins in areas such as the splanchnic bed. Thus pooling and sludging of blood with intravascular clotting may occur; with production of vasodilator material, resistance may be disproportionately low so that the maintenance of blood pressure is not possible. When diastolic pressure is below a critical level, coronary flow may be grossly reduced, aggravating the state of shock. The cardiac output tends to be low in states of cardiogenic shock and is associated with elevated left ventricular filling pressure (usually above 15 mm. Hg).

Clinical features

The clinical features of shock are well known and have been alluded to previously.

Table 35-1. Criteria for clinical subsets

Factor	Subset		
	I	*II*	*III*
Presenting mode	Shock	Shock with development of lesion	Heart failure and shock
Mechanical lesion	No	Yes	No
Gross cardiomegaly	No	±	Yes
Recurrent failure	No	No	Yes

Table 35-2. Clinical features of subsets

Factor	Subset		
	I	*II*	*III*
Mode of onset	Sudden shock	Signs of lesion	Heart failure
ECG	Anterior myocardial infarction	Nonspecific	Nonspecific
Heart size	Normal to slight enlargement	Variable	Moderate to gross enlargement
Hemodynamics	Nonspecific	Giant V waves in metabolic rate oxygen step-up (ventricular septal defect)	Nonspecific
Coronary angiography	Left atrial duct or left coronary artery occluded	Nonspecific	Nonspecific
Ventriculogram	Apicoanterior akinesis	Mitral regurgitation	Generalized hypokinesis

That clinical subsets may be identified by corresponding pathophysiological changes has recently been demonstrated (Table 35-1). Subset I differs from subset III by the absence of gross cardiomegaly or a history of recurrent heart failure. Subset II differs from subsets I and III by the presence of a mechanical lesion coincidental with that of shock. The clinical features of subset I are illustrated in Table 35-2. Anterior infarction is the rule and isolated inferior infarction was not encountered. Heart size radiographically ranges from normal to slight enlargement and at cardiac catheterization and angiography, apicoanterior akinesis of the left ventricle with left coronary artery obstruction is found. Subset II is characterized by the signs of the underlying lesions and mitral regurgitation, presenting usually with an apical holosystolic murmur and a third heart sound. "Silent" mitral regurgitation, however, has been reported, the diagnosis in this case being made by the presence of giant V waves of 30 to 40 mm. Hg in the pulmonary wedge tracing. A ventricular septal defect may be suspected by the presence of an oxygen step-up between right atrial and pulmonary artery samples obtained via a double lumen catheter. Cardiac rupture is often preceded by intractable pain and the signs of tamponade. Subset III is characterized by gross cardiomegaly, recurrent intractable failure, and a clinical picture akin to an ischemic cardiomyopathy.

Treatment

The treatment of cardiogenic shock may be divided into three main categories: (1) medical treatment, (2) circulatory assists, and (3) surgery. Medical treatment is directed toward the correction of factors that aggravate the shock state. Anoxia and hypercapnia may require the administration of oxygen by mask or following intubation. A volume cycle respirator is preferred to a pressure cycle machine because of mechanical changes in the lung in shock. Metabolic acidosis is corrected by the determination of the absolute base deficit and its replacement

by bicarbonate. The correction of electrolyte imbalance and of arrhythmias by specific therapy as well as of hypovolemia and hypoosmolarity by low molecular weight dextran are other means of therapy.

The use of pharmacologic agents in the treatment of cardiogenic shock is aimed at (1) increasing the performance of the heart without a proportionate increase in myocardial oxygen consumption and (2) altering the peripheral vascular resistance to an optimal level. Inotropic drugs have been used to achieve the former aim. Thus, beta-adrenergic stimulants decrease afterload, increase the inotropic and chronotropic activity of the heart, but have the drawback of inducing tachycardia and arrhythmias as well as of increasing arteriovenous shunting in the lungs. Norepinephrine has a beta-adrenergic effect on the myocardium and a predominant alpha effect on peripheral vessels. Its use, early in cardiogenic shock has been recommended by Corday, Griffith, and others. However, there is no clear-cut evidence that it increases cardiac performance in man and indeed may decrease renal flow and cause arrhythmias. Epinephrine, like norepinephrine, has both alpha and beta effects with a predominant beta effect on the heart and an alpha effect on peripheral vascular resistance. It, too, may induce arrhythmias. Dopamine has a positive inotropic effect on the heart and little effect on the peripheral vascular resistance, and increases renal and mesenteric blood flow. Other inotropic drugs that have been used are digitalis and glucagon. All these drugs, however, have had limited success in the treatment of cardiogenic shock associated with myocardial infarction. The work of Swan and co-workers points out the limitation of using inotropic drugs in patients with myocardial infarction with severe pump failure since the heart is under maximum endogenous catecholamines stimulation. In addition, Braunwald and co-workers have indicated that inotropic drugs may actually extend the area of myocardial infarction by increasing the gap between myocardial oxygen demand and supply.

Drugs that are used to alter the peripheral vascular resistance include the alpha-adrenergic blocking drugs such as phentolamine, phenoxybenzamine, steroids, and smooth muscle relaxants such as nitroprusside. A number of studies have demonstrated that a reduction of peripheral resistance is followed by improved myocardial performance with a fall in left-sided filling pressure. This is especially true in the presence of mitral regurgitation. On the other hand, these drugs may cause a precipitous fall of pressure with a reduction in coronary blood flow, increase in the area of ischemia, and aggravate the shock state. Even though Lillihei and his co-workers have emphasized the dramatic benefits of massive doses of steroids in the treatment of cardiogenic shock following surgery, these results have not been duplicated in the setting of cardiogenic shock following infarction. Drugs that increase peripheral vascular resistance such as norepinephrine, Vasoxyl, mephentermine, and angiotensin have equally proved to be of limited value. In general, it may be stated that drug therapy as a whole has failed to influence the mortality from cardiogenic shock.

Cardiac assists

A number of techniques have been used to mechanically decrease the work of the heart and to increase coronary perfusion. Since coronary flow is maximal in diastole, augmentation of diastole and the reduction of systolic work are the basic mode of action of these devices. This leads to so-called "systolic unloading" of the ventricle and "diastolic augmentation" of the pressure pulse. The balloon counterpulsator has been widely used and is said to reverse shock in 75% of patients. However, long-term survival of these patients has not been correspondingly good because a proportion of patients who recover from shock become balloon dependent. In general, cardiac assists may allow the physician to "buy time" to enable definitive procedures such as cardiac catheterization and surgery to be carried out and may be of additional value in the postoperative man-

agement of patients. They have a limited value as a means of treating shock if used as the sole means of treatment.

Surgery

Surgery has been used in the treatment of cardiogenic shock in a relatively small number of patients. Two difficulties encountered are in (1) the selection of patients and (2) the timing of surgery. The clinical recognition of subsets previously outlined may be useful in the bedside evaluation and selection of patients for definitive measures, that is, cardiac catheterization and surgery. The two specific categories likely to benefit are the patient in whom the left coronary artery occlusion with patent distal vessels has led to cardiogenic shock with a variable degree of ischemia and infarction and the patient who has developed mechanical defects such as mitral regurgitation, rupture of the ventricular septum, or rupture of the myocardium itself. The total experience to date, however, is small. Mundth and his co-workers, by the combined use of balloon assistance and emergency intravenous bypass graft, have had encouraging results in the treatment of patients in cardiogenic shock. The group at Cedars of Sinai Medical Center have reported survival of five to seven patients in whom surgery was performed within 12 hours of onset of shock. All of these patients had proximal lesions of the left coronary artery or of the left anterior descending vessel, and following emergency vein bypass, made complete recoveries from shock. Logistic considerations may, however, limit the role of surgery in the treatment of cardiogenic shock, which predicates the need for and mobilization of an emergency team for cardiac catheterization, circulatory assistance, and emergency surgery.

Summary

In conclusion, the mortality of cardiogenic shock at present lies between 75% and 100%, the condition being responsible for approximately 250,000 deaths each year. Although pharmacologic agents have been used in the animal laboratory with limited success, they have, in general, been unsuccessful in the treatment of clinical cardiogenic shock or in making a significant impact on the mortality of this condition. Current thinking is directed to recognition of the disturbed pathophysiology so that shock may be expeditiously treated by means of the circulatory assist, cardiac cathterization, and angiography, followed by a decision as to the feasibility of surgery. The respective roles of surgery and of the circulatory assist, however, need to be assessed over the next few years. Meanwhile, animal models can provide information concerning the potential reversibility of ischemic tissue and the time intervals that relate to irreversible cell death and damage. Experience with revascularization of patients under emergency conditions may provide additional evidence of the duration of potentially reversible ischemia in man. Logistic problems need to be overcome so that the circulatory assist and surgery may be used early in the treatment of shock. If used with the appropriate selection of patients, these measures may well alter the mortality of this dreaded complication of myocardial infarction.

Chapter 36

RESUSCITATION REQUIRING SPECIFIC SURGICAL APPROACHES

Mechanical circulatory support

Perhaps one of the major advances in the field of resuscitation is in the area of mechanical circulatory support. Its use as a logical extension of cardiopulmonary resuscitation for the cardiac arrest victim has been the concern of many workers. Kennedy has particularly popularized this extended concept and has contributed significantly to its use. While a number of methods of mechanical circulatory assistance have been used clinically (Fig. 36-1), the heart-lung machine has proved most readily applicable in cases of cardiac arrest. As an example, Kennedy cites the case of a 65-year-old woman who suddenly collapsed on the ward in view of a physician, 8 days after an exploratory laparotomy with a jejunojejunostomy for intermittent small bowel obstruction. Closed-chest cardiac compression and mechanical ventilation with a nasotracheal tube were instituted quickly, as was the administration of calcium chloride, sodium bicarbonate, and Ringer's lactate solution. Even though closed-chest cardiopulmonary resuscitative efforts appeared to be effective, the ventricle did not respond. This prompted Kennedy to use a portable lung machine, battery powered and mounted with a disposable bubble-dispersion oxygenator filled with 5% dextrose and water. The right femoral artery and vein were used for cannulation, and within minutes of hookup to the heart-lung machine the patient became responsive and opened her eyes. A markedly reduced serum potassium (1.9 mEq. per liter) was noted, and the patient subsequently received intravenous potassium. After 1 hour of cardiopulmonary bypass the patient was able to be disconnected, had an effective cardiac mechanism, and maintained an adequate arterial pressure. Assisted mechanical ventilation was continued for an additional 12 hours. She awoke without neurologic sequelae, did well, and became partially ambulatory. Fifteen days later she was found dead in bed; a postmortem examination revealed a myocardial infarction with superior mesenteric arterial thrombosis or embolism and an infarction of the small intestine.

Skinner points to significant advantages of a mechanical ventricular assistance device first described by Anstadt, Schiff, and Baue. This cuplike device, applied to the apex of the heart, must obviously be used with open-chest massage but as opposed to this disadvantage, the cup requires no more than 2 minutes to apply, there are no vascular cannulations, no need for heparin administration, and no risk of hemolysis or blood-borne contamination. In laboratory animals, renal function as indicative of the quality of tissue perfusion served to support the effectiveness of this mechanical ventricular assistance device.

Although this book does not attempt to go into detail relative to many related aspects, particularly those involving open-heart surgery, it does appear evident that lessons learned from open-heart surgery may be readily applied to many of our resuscitative techniques. For example, it is a common practice among most cardiac surgeons

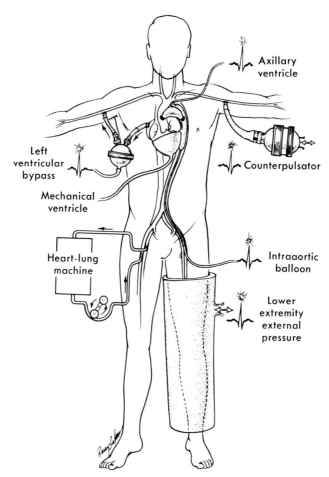

Fig. 36-1. Available means of mechanical circulatory assistance (artist composite summary). (From Kennedy, J. H., and Bricker, D. L.: Am. J. Cardiol. **27:**33-40, 1971.)

to employ a partial venoarterial pump oxygenator support following the completion of definitive cardiac surgery in order to allow the heart to return to a more nearly normal state. Particularly is this true if the coronary circulation has been interrupted by cross-clamping the aorta or if hypothermia has been employed. The postoperative hypotension and myocardial irritability can be, to a large extent, almost eliminated by "weaning" the heart off the pump.

It is almost inevitable that such a technique be applied to cases of cardiac resuscitation unassociated with open-heart surgery. Lefemine and colleagues have extensively investigated the problem of assisted circulation and have included a consideration of pressure work, flow work, and coronary perfusion. It appears that the main advantage of venoarterial bypass is the restoration of normal aortic and coronary artery pressure. Those familiar with cardiopulmonary bypass procedures recognize the disadvantage of venoarterial circulation in that the heart must pump against the machine unless the pump can be synchronized so that the return of the blood to the arterial compartments can be accomplished during diastole.

With the advent of assisted circulation through the use of the left-sided cardiac pump, the scope of cardiac resuscitative possibilities has been widened. Following cardiac resuscitative measures after ventricular defibrillation precipitated by a coronary occlusive episode, the left side of the heart may be assisted to reduce the area of infarction. In addition, the work load of the heart will be considerably reduced, an optimal pressure in the coronary arteries may be maintained, and the likelihood of pulmonary edema developing will be decreased by lowering the pressure in the left atrium.

External cardiac massage

It must be kept in mind that myocardial contractility, although of a rhythmic nature, may be markedly reduced following a period of several minutes of cardiac asystole or ventricular fibrillation, even though resuscitative procedures have been carried out. The effort initiated by resuscitation may, in itself, be of such a depressed nature that ventricular fibrillation or a repeat asystole may occur. It is for this reason that assisted circulation may be helpful. It is our practice to continue with intermittent manual compression of the anterior chest wall, even though a normal sinus rhythm has been restored. This is continued in a much slower fashion for a variable period of time, depending upon the time it takes the heart action to strengthen.

Artificial kidney in treatment of cardiac arrest

Numerous examples of cardiac arrest associated with potassium intoxication have been cited elsewhere in this book. Once arrest of the heart has occurred as a result of hyperkalemia, the usual methods of cardiac resuscitation may be employed; but, unfortunately, they do not effectively alter the existing elevated serum potassium level. Extracorporeal hemodialysis, in such cases, can be effectively employed as a lifesaving adjunct. Lawton and Lardner provide a good example of the benefit derived from dialysis in a patient with a serum potassium level of 9.32 mEq. per liter. After use of the artificial kidney, electrocardiographic evidence of potassium intoxication was all but absent.

Surgical treatment of cardiac arrhythmias
INFARCTECTOMY AND CONTROL OF VENTRICULAR ARRHYTHMIAS

Ligation of the anterior descending coronary artery in dogs regularly produced an infarction, with all animals developing frequent premature ventricular contractions. Sixty-five percent developed ventricular fibrillation. Only 8% of the control group could be defibrillated; but, after infarctectomy, 92% could be defibrillated (Stein and Cordell).

Ectopic activity associated with infarct may be caused by the slowing of conduction in the area of infarction with impulses reentering normal myocardium outside of a refractory period. Surgeons having experience with infarctectomy agree that the removal of a focus of biochemical and electrical instability decreases the incidence of refractory ventricular arrhythmias.

As discussed elsewhere in this book, myocardial infarction with subsequent hypotension continues to remain lethal. Mortality rates for cardiogenic shock range between 70% and 100%. Cardiac augmentation systems have been shown in certain instances to benefit such patients. Closed-chest resuscitation is often of only temporary assistance.

In 1966, a successful infarctectomy was performed on a 56-year-old man with the typical picture of cardiogenic shock. Large infarcts were resected from both left and right ventricles, and a necrotic, perforated ventricular septum was repaired. Heimbecker and co-workers report this case, along with results of experimental infarctectomies in laboratory animals. Only 8% of the calves survived with massage and cardiopulmonary bypass after anterior descending coronary artery ligation. Most of the animals that failed to survive were refractory to defibrillation. Forty-seven percent of the infarctectomized calves survived.

In addition to the mechanical and electrical benefits theoretically possible, Heimbecker speculates that healthy myocardium that is adjacent to areas of infarction may be adversely affected by toxicity arising in the infarcted area. Zones of marginal nutrition may be further depressed by metabolic acidosis. He believes that the ideal patient for emergency infarctectomy is one who shows coronary shock or pulmonary edema, or both, with a first myocardial infarction. Although an anterior infarction is most amenable to resection, a posterior wall resection can be done through a median sternotomy. Since only necrotic material is being resected, one need not be too concerned about interfering with the conduction system of the heart.

A particularly dramatic result of infarctectomy is reported by FitzGibbon and associates and involves the rupture of the free wall of the left ventricle after a myocardial infarction in a 45-year-old man. The patient sustained a rupture of the free left ventricular wall 20 days after an extensive myocardial infarction. A cardiorrhexis occurred in the superficial muscle bundles at the apex of the left ventrical. Although the possibility of infarctectomy was considered for control of arrhythmia on the thirteenth day when the patient underwent selective coronary angiography and left ventriculography, it was not until the twentieth day that external cardiac rupture was detected clinically and confirmed by pericardiocentesis. A venous bypass from the aorta to the right coronary artery to ensure the viability of the remaining ischemic myocardium was necessary to complete the operation. On last report, the patient had done exceptionally well, had learned cross-country skiing and had skied up to 10 miles without cardiac symptoms. FitzGibbon's report contains an excellent discussion and review of the clinical pathologic studies of postinfarction left ventricular rupture.

Emergency infarctectomy seems to accomplish several ends. For one thing, excision of the infarcted muscle removes the focus of electrical irritability. Easier electrical defibrillation and maintenance of sinus rhythm are achieved. In addition, paradoxic systolic expansion of the ventricle is eliminated, thus improving left ventricular function. Effler has repeatedly emphasized that huge sections of the left ventricle can be excised in instances of ventricular aneurysm without a marked impairment of ventricular function. In almost all instances, ventricular function is improved by removal of the paradoxically pulsating segment of the wall.

Excision of the ischemic portion of the left ventricle following ligation of the anterior descending coronary artery proved feasible in an experimental study on dogs by Jude and associates. Immediate and lasting improvement of ventricular function resulted. In spite of a considerable excision of ventricular wall, the remaining ventricular cavity seemed to be of an adequate size. Congestive heart failure was not a problem.

The advantages of excising the ischemic portion of the left ventricle are such that it appears worthy of serious consideration for patients with acute myocardial infarction and cardiogenic shock where the reduction in stroke volume has been markedly decreased because of impaired contractility in the infarcted segment of myocardium. Experimentally, the likelihood of fibrillation is decreased in the operated heart. Ventricular defibrillation is often difficult in the heart with a massive infarct.

A current appraisal of the value of excision of areas of akinesis of the left ventricle in men by Ellis (1971) reviews many of the uncertainties especially with surgical excision of localized areas of chronic left ventricular dysfunction. For example, no safe guidelines have yet been established on the amount of left ventricle that can safely be excised in men. Some remaining area of ventricular asynergy will remain as a result of the suture line. Should revascularization be done concomitantly? How does one adequately identify the area of akinesis? Aids in answering the latter question include preoperative ventriculograms, a technique of exerting a negative pressure within the left ventricular cavity in order to evaginate the thin, scarred, nonfunctioning myocardium, surface electrocardiography, and myocardial biopsies.

So far, results have not been encouraging when patients in cardiogenic shock, unresponsive to medical management, are treated by infarctectomy.

Intractable supraventricular tachycardia

Over 200 cardioversions were attempted without success in a 51-year-old woman severely incapacitated by intractable supraventricular tachycardia and aortic and mitral rheumatic valvular disease. At the time of double-valve replacement, the conduction bundle was divided in the region of the A-V node and a permanent pacemaker was attached to the epicardium. Permanent ventricular pacing at 75 beats per minute followed. It was believed that surgical division of the bundle of His was particularly indicated if there was to be satisfactory functioning of the ball-in-cage valves. Because of the presence of supraventricular tachycardia, it was doubted that there would be adequate opening and closing of the valves. Pulse duplicator data are available to indicate that aortic and mitral valves replaced with the Starr-Edwards prosthesis are competent at rates up to 190 per minute.

Using the heart-lung bypass, a 3-0 vascular silk suture was placed in the atrial wall 2 mm. from the coronary sinus toward the supposed location of the A-V node and at right angles to the course of the bundle of His. The location of the bundle was assumed to be along an imaginary line drawn from the coronary sinus to the ventricular septum at the midpoint of the attachment of the septal leaflet of the tricuspid valve. The suture was tied, and the ECG was observed for A-V disassociation. It did not occur with the first suture, and two additional sutures were placed 2 mm. apart. After placement of the third suture, there was an abrupt change from sinus rhythm to complete A-V

disassociation with a ventricular rate of 54 beats per minute. An incision was made just distal to the sutures and toward the tricuspid valve at a right angle to the course of the conduction system. It was about 8 mm. long and about 3 mm. deep. It was hoped that this would sever the conduction system.

Although it is unusual, periods of total cardiac standstill may interrupt bouts of supraventricular tachycardia. Examples of total cardiac standstill and "pacemaker block" during supraventricular tachycardia are rare (Bradlow).

Surgical treatment of supraventricular tachycardia by electrical stimulation of carotid sinus nerves

Recurrent attacks of supraventricular tachycardia may be promptly and effectively terminated by reflexly increasing vagal activity and withdrawing sympathetic drive to the heart, which is made possible through stimulation of the carotid sinus nerves with a radiofrequency pacemaker (Braunwald and Sobel; Braunwald and co-workers). Patients refractory to the usual medical management and incapacitated by the arrhythmia may benefit from this radiofrequency stimulation, which can be initiated by the patient for brief periods during an episode of supraventricular tachycardia. Vagal stimulation can be produced without traumatizing the carotid artery as theoretically may occur with manual carotid sinus massage. One can thus avoid use of pressor agents such as phenylephrine or metaraminol, which are often effective but carry a risk of cerebrovascular accident from hypertension. Electrocardiographic monitoring during stimulation is not essential.

The technique of carotid sinus nerve stimulation consists of implanting the receiving unit of the radiofrequency carotid sinus nerve stimulator and bilateral electrodes in contact with both carotid sinus nerves. The transmitting unit is powered by a 12.5 volt rechargeable battery that generates a radiofrequency pulse of 0.3 msec. duration and

1.5 to 8.0 volts in amplitude at a frequency of 50 pulses per second (Angistat, Medtronic, Inc., Minneapolis, Minnesota).

Resection of ventricular aneurysm associated with recurrent or intractable arrhythmia following myocardial infarction

The surgical management of ventricular aneurysm can be accompanied by a relatively low rate of morbidity and mortality. Usually the indication for resection is associated with one of the various complications of ventricular aneurysm such as congestive heart failure or peripheral embolism. Both supraventricular and ventricular arrhythmias may also complicate the course of ventricular aneurysm and may be life threatening. Magidson reports three patients for whom the resection of ventricular aneurysm led to termination of a dangerous cardiac arrhythmia. Earlier, Hunt and co-workers successfully removed a ventricular aneurysm in a case of recurrent tachycardia.

Five of six patients operated upon as an emergency with death impending from cardiogenic shock and left ventricular aneurysm are reported by Majafi and associates. Four of the six patients were operated upon during the night. One suffered numerous attacks of ventricular fibrillation and two required external cardiac massage before the operation. In three, an infarctectomy was done in addition to the aneurysmectomy. A cardiac assist utilizing venoarterial bypass during the critical phase of the operation (the period between the induction of anesthesia and the institution of total cardiopulmonary bypass) was used. From the University of Tel Aviv Medical School, Schlesinger and co-workers report a ventricular aneurysmectomy done for severe arrhythmias, including ventricular fibrillation. An undisturbed sinus rhythm followed the surgery without the need for any antiarrhythmic agent.

Surgical treatment of bradycardia

Although this subject is covered in greater detail in other areas of the book, it is appropriate to emphasize here that the surgical management of patients with bradycardia has generally been highly successful. With the development of new types of pacemakers, both atrial and ventricular, the indications for electrically pacing the heart have increased. Predominantly the bradycardiac conditions so managed consist of sinus bradycardia or arrest, second-degree heart block, second-and-third-degree heart block, and third-degree heart block. While the etiologic factor responsible for the conduction disturbance is unknown for many patients, at least $33\frac{1}{3}\%$ of the patients have arteriosclerotic heart disease and perhaps less than 6% of the cases are due to trauma and myocarditis. Generally, bradycardia is a disease of the elderly. Complete atrioventricular disassociation may evolve only over a long period of time. In the St. Louis University series of more than 100 patients, nearly half had third-degree heart block. Adams-Stokes attacks and congestive heart failure were the major indications for treatment.

Cardiac rupture

Among 933 cases of myocardial infarction, the incidence of cardiac rupture during a 10-year period, confirmed at autopsy, is 3.8% (Sahebjami). Cardiac rupture occurs within the first 5 days after the onset of a myocardial infarction in 70% of cases, the majority occurring on the first day. Over half the ruptures are located in the anterior wall of the left ventricle. Cardiac rupture should be suspected when there is a sudden onset of chest pain, progressive dyspnea, or shock in the first few days after a myocardial infarction, especially in an elderly patient with an extensive infarct. The electrocardiogram invariably remains stable. It is almost always true that cardiac rupture complicating myocardial infarction is not a blowout incident; rather, the presence of an initial tear seems necessary. The intraventricular pressure is a critical factor in development of the rupture. Lillehei successfully repaired a ruptured left ventricle following an acute myocardial infarction with a postoperative survival of 38 days. Such surgery usually requires an effective combination of total cardiopulmonary bypass, hypothermia, and total circulatory arrest.

Coronary endarterectomy

The presence of coronary artery obstruction in the cardiac arrest patient represents an added difficulty in successful resuscitation. Electrical defibrillation of the heart may prove difficult, if not impossible. Although several cases of emergency coronary endarterectomy have been performed in this connection, I am not aware of any successful cases to date. Nardi and Shaw report four unsuccessful attempts, although one patient was restored to a normal cardiac rhythm for 52 hours. It is our belief, however, that successful endarterectomy in such cases may proceed hand in hand with other adjuncts in therapy that are becoming available, for example, mechanically assisted circulation.

Coronary artery bypass graft

Hufnagel successfully performed a coronary artery bypass graft on a 51-year-old man suffering an acute myocardial infarction and experiencing five episodes of ventricular fibrillation prior to the bypass graft insertion.

Surgical management of Wolff-Parkinson-White syndrome

A most interesting example of the possibility of surgically relieving dysrhythmia of the heart is seen in the pioneering work of Sealy and his associates at Duke University. By identifying and surgically dividing the bundle of Kent for type B Wolff-Parkinson-White syndrome, they have been able to successfully treat several patients and thus prevent the transmission of atrial dysrhythmias through the anomalous tract to the ventricle. In addition, patients with Wolff-Parkinson-White syndrome may incur a post-tachycardia asystole that may precipitate ventricular fibrillation. The period of asystole results from sinus arrest when the heart changes from tachycardia to sinus rhythm. Unfortunately, in medically treated patients, this period of arrest may be accentuated by the use of beta-adrenergic blocking drugs, digitalis, and cardiac depressant drugs. In the patients managed by Sealy, the episodes of tachycardia were so persistent that congestive heart failure and considerable disability were present. The supraventricular tachycardia seen in patients with Wolff-Parkinson-White syndrome is rather likely a reentry or circus phenomenon, which is dependent upon the presence of a His and a Kent bundle, both of which have different properties of conduction and refractoriness. The tachycardia may be precipitated by a supraventricular premature beat that occurs sufficiently early for the Kent path to be refractory, but for the normal atrial ventricular His system to be receptive. Epicardial mapping, both preoperatively and during the operation, aids in the search for the aberrant conduction tissue. The details of the procedure are described by Sealy in separate publications.

Obviously, many patients with Wolff-Parkinson-White syndrome may not be suitable candidates for a surgical approach. Some are managed successfully with intensive drug treatment with beta-adrenergic blocking agents, digitalis, and various myocardial depressant agents to control the heart rate. A demand pacemaker is effective in protecting the patient from the long periods of sinus arrest that may occur when the heart returns from tachycardia to sinus rhythm.

Chapter 37

ARTIFICIAL HEARTS: TOTAL REPLACEMENT AND CIRCULATORY ASSIST DEVICES

Clifford S. Kwan-Gett and Willem J. Kolff

Within the past two decades, an exciting new family of prosthetic devices called artificial hearts has been introduced. These artificial hearts are much different in character than other prosthetic devices, such as valves or arterial grafts, in that they are active prostheses. Their role is to pump blood or to assist in the pumping of blood in the circulatory system.

The words artificial heart have been loosely applied to a wide range of mechanical devices that act on the circulation of blood. These devices can be classified into two distinct groups:

1. The total artificial heart or orthotopic cardiac prosthesis that totally replaces the natural heart in position and function
2. Mechanical circulatory assist devices that aid or supplement the natural heart in the maintenance of the circulation of blood

These two groups have distinctly different functions; however, many problems that limit more widespread application of artificial hearts are common to both groups.

In one study, it was estimated that each year about 100,000 Americans who would otherwise succumb to heart disease could be returned to active life with the use of an appropriate artificial heart. Despite the compelling need for the use of artificial hearts, the complexity of problems associated with their use has severely limited their clinical application to only a limited but expanding number of hospitals.

The orthotopic cardiac prosthesis or total replacement artificial heart

One of our major goals is to produce a prosthetic heart that can completely and permanently replace the irreparably damaged human heart. Continuous concentrated work toward this achievement has been carried out in only a few laboratories (Cleveland Clinic Foundation, University of Mississippi, and University of Utah). The slow, painstaking, and difficult nature of progress has restricted the number of laboratories able to participate in this research.

Superficially, the requirements of an acceptable research prosthesis appear to be simple. The artificial heart must be able to pump blood to the lungs and to the arterial circulation at a rate of up to say 10 liters per minute, to produce a systemic blood pressure of about 100 mm. Hg mean, while maintaining systemic and pulmonary venous pressures in the range of 0 to 5 mm. Hg. In addition, its physical shape and size must approximate that of the natural heart so that compression of the great veins and lungs does not occur, and the device should induce minimal thrombosis or trauma to the blood it pumps. In practice, these apparently simple specifications have not been met. It is possible that other factors must be introduced as control parameters, such as use of pH, P_{O_2}, P_{CO_2}, acid-base balance, and blood volume to control cardiac flow or pressure wave form.

It is convenient to describe a total artificial heart in terms of its three component subsystems, namely:

1. The heart proper, which contains and pumps blood
2. The control system, which directs the manner in which the heart pumps
3. The power source, which provides energy for the prosthetic heart

In the past, most attention has been directed to the making of the prosthetic ventricles. Almost all artificial ventricles have had an inflow valve that accepts blood from an atrium and an outflow valve that directs blood to the pulmonary artery or aorta. The atria have been simple, passive reservoirs. Some early models (Fig. 37-1) were powered electrically with the electric motor built into the artificial heart. The electrical power activated a solenoid to pump blood or powered a pendulum that alternately squeezed blood from the prosthetic right ventricle, then the prosthetic left ventricle.

The blood-containing chambers have been made of silicone rubber, polyurethane, or natural rubber and other materials. Many varieties of valves have been used, such as ball, leaflet, disc, or tricuspid valve. The control of the pumping of these hearts was inadequate. They often relied on an inadequate response of the heart to fluctuations in pressure and flow. The presence of the electrical motor within the heart also added problems of excessive size, weight, and heat production. These problems were accentuated by the use of a small experimental animal, the dog.

A very significant step was made with the change from an electrically powered device to a pneumatically powered system. The pneumatic system allowed the production of a lightweight heart free of heat generation, which could be connected via light plastic tubes to an external power source of compressed air. The calf and sheep replaced the

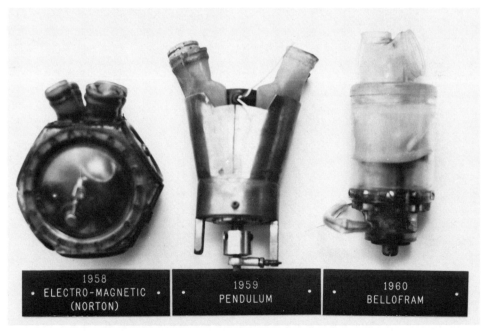

Fig. 37-1. Early model total artificial hearts. Many early hearts were electrically driven with motor contained in same housing as the blood chambers.

dog as experimental animals. These larger animals could be procured in weights approximating that of man. The supply was more dependable, and blood for transfusion of these animals was much more accessible.

Early pneumatically driven hearts for the calf and sheep had sac-type ventricles that were held within rigid housings. During systole, air was introduced under suitable pressure to the space between the housing and sac to compress the sac and expel the blood held within the sac. In diastole, air was evacuated to suck blood into the ventricle.

The cycle was then repeated. The atrium for each ventricle was usually a passive container and the outflow from each ventricle was directed through artificial vessels that were anastomosed to the corresponding pulmonary artery or aorta.

Some of the early control systems were rather sophisticated. One system built for driving pneumatically powered hearts had a wave form synthesizer that allowed the operator to set up various electrical wave forms. The signal from this synthesizer was first directed, either through a manual amplitude

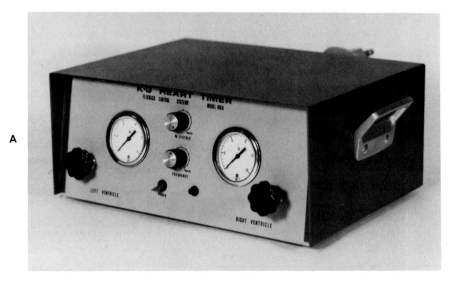

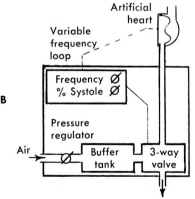

Fig. 37-2. Control system for an artificial heart. **A,** Control panel shows simplicity of controls, which require adjustment. **B,** Control schematic. The inherent automatic response of an increase in output flow with an increase in atrial pressure provides an extremely stable and reliable system.

control or through a small analog computer, then to the servo valves, which translated the electrical wave form into an air pressure wave form to drive each ventricle. Signals from the atrial or arterial pressure transducers could be fed back to the analog computer. The computer could be programmed in a variety of ways. It could be used to allow atrial pressures to control cardiac output. In this mode, an increase in atrial pressure increased the amplitude of the signal to the servo valves, which, in turn, produced a larger amplitude pressure wave form to drive the heart. The system worked well for relatively steady state conditions, but because of the feedback paths within the system, instability often occurred. Excessive suction applied to the ventricles created negative atrial pressures, resulting in air aspiration and early termination of the experiments.

The need for a system that is extremely stable under all conditions led to the redesign of our control systems. Currently, the most successful control system (Fig. 37-2) uses the

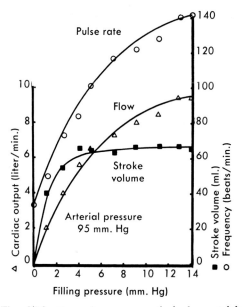

Fig. 37-3. Dynamic response of single ventricle. Left and right sides are similar. Usually the heart is operated at a constant rate. Variable rate operation is possible as shown above.

pressure within each atrium to proportion and determine the amount of blood that enters its corresponding ventricle during diastole. A low filling pressure causes a low volume of blood to enter the ventricle in diastole so that only a low stroke volume is produced in systole. A high filling pressure produces a high stroke volume. Therefore, within a certain range, each ventricle's cardiac output is proportional to the atrial pressure (Fig. 37-3). Since this characteristic applies to each ventricle on a beat-to-beat basis, a very high degree of inherent stability is produced. This characteristic also ensures that the flows from the right and left ventricles are balanced. An increase in flow from the right ventricle increases blood flow through the lungs to the left atrium, thereby raising left atrial pressure. The left ventricle responds to the increase in atrial pressure with an increase in output to match that of the right ventricle. Similarly, a decrease in flow from either ventricle produces a decrease in flow from the other ventricle. A simple diagram of the driving system used at the University of Utah is seen in Fig. 37-2. Although simple in operation, this type of control system has operated artificial hearts that have supported the circulations of calves for days without requiring intermittent manual adjustments.

Diaphragm-type or sac-type artificial ventricles are the most common in use. The sac-type ventricle may damage red cells by crushing them between its opposing walls. A diaphragm-type ventricle is shown in Fig. 37-4. This ventricle has a hemispherically shaped nondistensible housing mounted on a rigid base. Between the rigid base and housing is a flexible but nondistensible diaphragm. Blood occupies the space between diaphragm and housing. During systole, when air is forced into the space between diaphragm and the base, the diaphragm is displaced toward the housing, and it pumps blood out of the ventricle. Even at maximum displacement of the diaphragm, there remains a clearance between the diaphragm and housing. During diastole, the atrial pressure forces the blood into the ventricle and displaces the diaphragm back toward the base. Since the diaphragm is highly compliant, the filling volume during each diastolic period varies directly with the atrial pressure. The inflow and outflow valves are placed in the housing so as to provide convenient connections to the artificial atrium and outflow vessels. Each hemispherical ventricle is con-

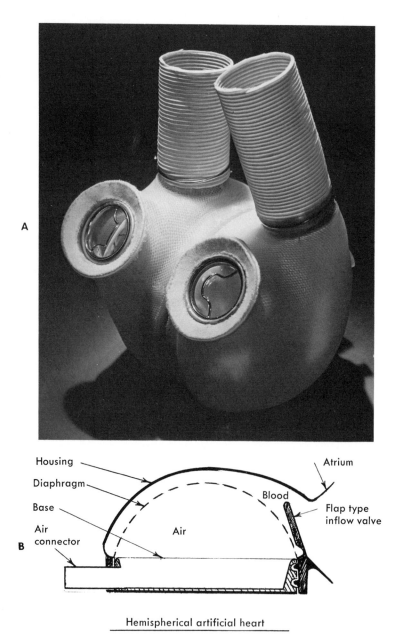

Fig. 37-4. A, Artificial heart showing two hemispherical ventricles. Heart may have any of a variety of prosthetic valves. **B,** Cross section of single ventricle. One diaphragm is highly flexible, but since it is not distensible, the diaphragm cannot touch housing.

nected to the driving system by an air line about 6 feet in length. The characteristics of the ventricle, air line, and driving system are matched so that the combination gives an output flow proportional to atrial pressure. The artificial heart is usually operated in a constant frequency mode. It can also operate in a manner that increases pulse rate with increase in output.

In our early hearts, the diaphragm-type ventricles were made with Silastic surfaces in contact with blood. These hearts created very low levels or negligible levels of hemolysis. Calves implanted with these artificial hearts could stand, walk, eat, and drink. However, there always occurred marked diminution of platelets, occasionally as low as 10,000 per cubic mm.

The longest survival we had with a Silastic surface was over 100 hours. In later work, we coated the Silastic surfaces with Dacron fibrils or Dacron cloth. The changes obtained with the Dacron surfaces were remarkable. The maximum survival time for a calf with a total mechanical heart was extended to 14 days (Fig. 37-5). The changes in blood components were also remarkable. The Dacron surfaces produced marked early hemolysis and clearly visible levels of free

plasma hemoglobin. However, the platelet levels, although diminished, remained at levels much higher than that achieved with Silastic hearts. It was postulated that the Silastic surfaces allowed the continual formation of microthrombi that were shed as emboli distally. Platelets were apparently continually used in the formation of the microemboli. The Dacron surfaces apparently induced the deposition of a fibrin layer that became adherent to its rough surface. The fibrin layer then acted as a boundary layer between the blood and foreign surface, and since no further clot formation was induced, platelet loss was halted. Apparently the rough surface, either because of its much greater surface area or possibly local dynamic effect, produces a high rate of red cell damage that is reflected as a high level of hemolysis. At autopsy, the organs, especially the kidneys, showed many regions of infarction produced by microemboli with Silastic surfaces, but much fewer infarcted areas were seen with Dacron surfaces. Apparently the animals could tolerate the high levels of red cell destruction much better than the lowered platelet levels with multiple microemboli.

With initial normal arterial pressures and blood flows, animals can recover very rapidly

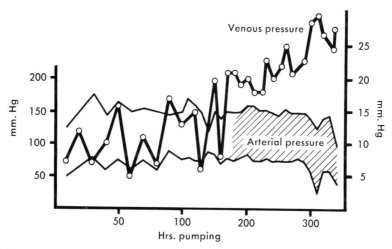

Fig. 37-5. Blood pressure in animal supported for 14 days. Note rise in venous pressure and fairly normal arterial pressures.

from surgery so that they can stand, eat, and drink within a few hours after surgery. Deterioration inevitably begins within a few days. A characteristic finding is a gradual elevation in systemic venous pressure despite apparently adequate blood flow and arterial pressure. At autopsy, the lungs and liver are usually found to be very congested, and marked edema of tissues can be seen. While the exact cause of these changes has not been determined, we postulated that the venous congestion is produced by abnormally high peak pulsatile pressures transmitted to the right atrium and vena cavae. These pulsatile pressures are apparently brought about mainly by the pulsatile nature of a right ventricle that has been operating with a non-pulsatile type of atrium. In very recent work, the prosthetic atria have been made to fluctuate in volume so as to act as a dynamic reservoir to the incoming blood during ventricular systole.

The major problems that slow progress at present appear to be the same ones that have been present since the beginning of research in this field. The most urgent requirement is for suitable materials that may be used for construction of those surfaces that contact blood. All foreign materials seem to promote clot formation or cause blood trauma to a certain degree. A material is required that either has or produces a blood-to-surface interaction similar to that of the natural blood-to-intima interface. Woven and knitted Dacron or Teflon materials have been used for years as replacement for arteries or for coating of prosthetic valves. These prosthetic arteries are relatively immobile and have living material on the side not exposed to blood. The prosthetic heart must have materials that flex and pump blood, and it cannot provide a living tissue interface on the opposite side.

The comparison and evaluation of new surfaces is very difficult. Ideally, materials should be compared under conditions of actual intended use—that is, in a total artificial heart. A material that is tested under different conditions can produce different results with respect to thrombogenesis, hemolysis, or protein denaturation. Even results from two laboratories may differ; for example, we noted with Silastic a marked fall in platelet levels, yet Akutsu did not experience this problem. We have noted low hemolysis rates but great platelet reduction with Silastic surfaces. Dacron cloth or fibril surfaces produce limited platelet diminution but higher degrees of hemolysis. Our preliminary tests with a hydrophilic surface such as Hydron, showed that this surface produced little platelet diminution but generated many peripheral emboli. The emboli may have been produced in part from the geometry of the surfaces. Some of our hearts have had fetal fibroblast tissue one cell layer thick grown on the blood-contacting material prior to introducing it to the bloodstream. We have tried surfaces coated with heparin and others have produced an electronegative surface potential on a surface to inhibit thrombogenesis. The evaluation of these materials is very difficult since the physical configuration of the material may influence the results considerably. Factors such as rough surfaces, junctions, placement with adjacent foreign surfaces, and rate of blood flow may produce variations greater than that produced by the material being tested.

The material must also possess major mechanical characteristics such as high flex life, high compliance, low extensibility, negligible porosity to fluids, electrolytes, and gases, and must have suitable heat conductivity, either to avoid heat loss or possibly to deliberately transfer heat from the power source into the bloodstream.

It is remarkable how difficult it is to construct an artificial heart that can both pump a high output flow and yet fit within the pericardium. The physical size and shape of prosthetic hearts are still cumbersome and inadequate compared with the natural heart. Adequate stroke volume and atrial reservoir capacity are difficult to produce in a heart that does not compress the lungs, the major veins, or arteries.

Adequate controls for a permanent total

artificial heart have not been produced. We have shown that a prosthetic heart having a Starling's law type of response is adequate for survival of a calf for at least 2 weeks. However, in our prosthetic hearts, the function characteristics that compare cardiac outflow with input atrial pressure differ markedly from those of the natural heart. It is not known what effects abnormal aortic, pulmonary, or atrial pressure wave forms will have after long-term pumping. Factors such as control of aortic pressure, P_{O_2}, and P_{CO_2} may become essential parameters for control of heart action.

If reliable percutaneous leads were available, it would be possible to mount the power source exteriorly and, thereby, eliminate major problems of accessibility of internal shape and space limitations. The development of satisfactory percutaneous leads would bring the use of total artificial hearts much closer.

One of the major problems in the development of a totally implantable prosthesis with pump, controls, and power source is the power source. The power expended on the blood to maintain normal flow and blood pressure in man is estimated to be about 4 watts. Assuming an overall efficiency of about 10% for the complete heart, controls, and power source, the power source must expend a power of about 40 watts and operate continuously for about 5 years or more. The power source must be charged with an energy cell with at least a 1,750 kilowatt hour capacity. The power source must be of appropriate shape and size to allow implantation in the body, and provision must be made for the dissipation of heat at the rate of 40 watts. Power sources that are being assessed at present utilize plutonium 238 as the prime source of energy. It is likely that a power source that is worn externally will become available long before a compact completely implantable power pack is manufactured.

In the future, total artificial heart implantations will have two roles in clinical medicine. The earliest application will be as a temporary heart substitute, used to sustain a patient's life until a suitable donor for a heart transplant becomes available. One such application took place in 1969 when a patient's heart was removed and an externally powered orthotopic cardiac prosthesis was implanted. This supported the patient's circulation for 64 hours until a donor heart was located and transplanted.

The most important application will be for permanent replacement of the irreparably damaged human heart. Ultimately, there will become available a completely implantable permanent device complete with atria, ventricles, control system, and power source. The blood-containing chambers will occupy the space of the natural heart while the power source is placed within the chest or in the abdomen. The patient receiving such a cardiac prosthesis should have no symptoms of chronic cardiac failure, and once again, he should be able to lead a normal life.

Circulatory assist devices

Circulatory assist devices are mechanical pumping systems that aid the natural heart in circulating blood around the body. Most of these assist devices are able to support life only in the presence of a heart that is still contracting and pumping blood. Only a few systems are able to sustain the circulation without the assistance of the natural heart.

There is a need for assist devices to provide support both for the heart in acute failure and also for the heart in chronic failure. At present, no functioning assist device has been proved to be suitable for permanent implantation either experimentally or clinically. The clinical use of assist devices has therefore been limited to highly selected patients. These patients were usually considered to be in an acute, severe state of failure with very remote chances of recovery even under the best of conventional medical management. Assist devices have been used most frequently in patients who have developed cardiogenic shock following a myocardial infarction. In addition, use of an assist device is currently limited to those patients who with the aid of the assist device may recover sufficiently within a period of days or weeks to become independent of the device. With continued development of materials and techniques, assist devices will become available for chronic implantation and will be used for those patients in chronic cardiac failure.

The mortality rate for patients in cardiogenic shock following a myocardial infarction has been reported to be as high as 95%. The following simplified situation is considered to be present in many of these patients. An acute coronary artery occlusion blocks blood flow to the myocardium normally supplied by the occluded coronary artery. The contractile ability of this muscle becomes very severely compromised and cardiac output at a low level is sustained by the healthy muscle whose blood supply is not limited by the occlusion. The low cardiac output can sustain only a very low systemic blood pressure. As a result of the lowered blood pressure, blood flow through the remaining patent coronary arteries is reduced. This reduced coronary flow produces further depression of myocardial contractility, with decreased flow into the systemic circulation and further reduction of coronary flow. The depressed myocardial function is also reflected in dilation of the left ventricle, high left ventricular end-diastolic pressure, high left atrial pressure, high pulmonary venous pressure, and high central venous pressure. A portion of the ischemic myocardium becomes infarcted. Some of the ischemic myocardium between this infarcted area and the healthy myocardium is supplied by collateral circulation from the region of the healthy myocardium. In cardiogenic shock, recovery of ischemic myocardium is generally inadequate and continued heart failure occurs.

The goals in the application of temporary assist devices are:

1. To maintain adequate circulation to support other vital organs, especially the brain
2. To prevent further deterioration in the myocardium and pulmonary system and to avoid further failure and pulmonary edema
3. To improve myocardial function

Improved circulation is obtained by increasing total blood flow in the systemic circulation. Further cardiac deterioration is made less likely by relieving overdistension of the left ventricle, by lowering left ventricular end-diastolic pressure. The lowered end-diastolic pressure also results in lowered pulmonary venous pressure with a reduction in stimulus for the production of pulmonary edema. Improved myocardial function is brought about by increasing coronary circulation by raising coronary perfusion pressure. An increased coronary perfusion pressure is intended to produce an increase in blood flow through those coronary arteries that are fully patent and those that are partly occluded. The increase in perfusion pressure in the coronary arteries is also intended to open up or produce collateral blood supply to the myocardium rendered ischemic by the initial coronary occlusion. Improvement in myocardial status is also produced secondary to an improved overall condition of the patient, especially with respect to normalized acid-base balance, normal pulmonary function with high oxygenation of systemic blood, and normal renal function.

It has been difficult to assess improvements in myocardial function, both clinically and experimentally. Some gross measurements have been used experimentally, such as comparison of survivors and nonsurvivors following coronary artery ligation with and without the benefits of an assist device. Other parameters have been used such as myocardial oxygen consumption. It has been shown that myocardial oxygen consumption varies with the work load of muscle fibers and so a reduction in myocardial oxygen consumption is aimed for with the use of an assist device. The tension-time index, which is derived from the area beneath the curve of intraventricular pressure plotted against time, for each contraction has been shown to correlate fairly well with the myocardial oxygen consumption. Other changes that have been regarded as beneficial are: fall in left ventricular end-diastolic pressure, increase in slope of the left ventricular pressure curve during isometric contraction, increased coronary artery blood flow, and increase in cardiac output. Probably more accurate assessments of results would be obtained by comparing the function curves of a ventricle. Curves are plotted at a constant blood pressure to show the relationship of cardiac output versus atrial pressure or left ventricular end-diastolic pressure. Normal hearts have a steep slope and high plateau whereas failing hearts have curves with a low slope and low plateau. These curves are compatible with the clinical concept of improvement in cardiac function. Improvement occurs when a given cardiac output can be obtained with progressively lower atrial pressures.

Comparison of the relative effectiveness of various assist devices is difficult. There are problems involved in producing experimental cardiac failure resembling that met clinically, there are different ways in which a device can be operated, and investigators often use different parameters for the assessment of their assist devices. As a result of these problems, devices that are most likely to be used clinically at present are those that are simple to apply and that do not require extracorporeal circulation of blood.

VENO-ARTERIAL BYPASS

A venous to arterial bypass system takes blood from the venous circulation, passes the blood through an oxygenator, and then pumps the oxygenated blood into the arterial circulation. This type of system has been in use clinically for many years and is the method commonly used for open-heart surgery and other major arterial surgery such as excision and replacement of aneurysm of the ascending aorta. This type of bypass can provide assistance to the right ventricle, the lungs, and the left ventricle. The bubble- and disk-type oxygenators are the ones in common clinical use. However, because of the

blood trauma associated with these devices, the time for which they may be safely and usefully used is limited to about 6 hours. Occasionally following open-heart surgery or surgery to the coronary arteries it is found that the natural heart is initially unable to sustain an adequate circulation. Supporting the circulation for up to several hours with or without the natural heart contracting frequently allows the natural heart to recover sufficiently to maintain adequate output alone without further assistance. When more prolonged support is required, the membrane-type oxygenator must be used. Membrane oxygenators have been used clinically as veno-arterial bypass circulatory assist devices for up to 9 days continuously. The membrane type of veno-arterial bypass is eminently suitable for use when inadequate lung function is present since it can take over the function of the lungs completely. When severe left heart failure is present, this bypass system may in some cases elevate the systemic blood pressure to a level too high for the failing left ventricle. If this occurs, the left ventricular end-diastolic pressure may rise excessively, producing a high left atrial pressure and pulmonary edema. In these circumstances, a left ventricular vent should be provided.

Veno-arterial bypass may be applied by placing cannulas in the patient's femoral artery and vein. The bypass does not usually require opening of the chest, but if there develops a raised left ventricular end-diastolic pressure, thoracotomy and venting of the left ventricle may be essential.

Veno-arterial bypass can provide almost total bypass of blood from the heart, while producing high systemic pressures. It can therefore reduce left ventricular work, reduce tension-time index and increase coronary artery perfusion pressure.

AORTA-TO-AORTA CIRCULATORY ASSIST

This system allows the left ventricle to pump blood at very low pressure into a pumping chamber, which in turn pumps blood into the aorta. The inflow of this assist device is connected to the ascending aorta and its outflow is anastomosed to the arch or descending aorta. The aorta is occluded distal to the anastomosis with the inflow connector. The pumping chamber is activated during diastole to circulate blood in the arterial tree, raising aortic pressure and coronary artery perfusion pressure. It is deactivated at the beginning of systole to provide a very low pressure reservoir into which the left ventricle pumps.

The disadvantage of this system is that a thoracotomy is necessary. It also requires accurate synchronization with left ventricular systole. When the pumping chamber pumps blood, it raises the diastolic pressure, both proximal and distal to itself, and so elevates the pressure perfusing the coronary arteries. Since the left ventricle ejects its stroke volume against a low pressure it produces a

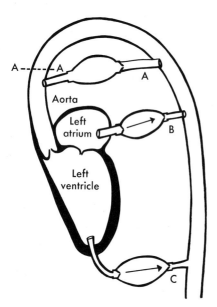

Fig. 37-6. Alternate methods to provide cardiac assistance. *A,* In aorta-to-aorta assist, the prosthetic ventricle assumes role of normal ventricle, which becomes a "second left atrium." The arch of aorta is occluded. *B,* Left atrium to aorta does not compress left ventricle. *C,* Left ventricle to aorta decompresses left ventricle, which becomes a "second left atrium."

higher stroke volume at a low pressure head. Its work load and tension-time index are significantly decreased. With its increased ability to empty, the left ventricle's end-diastolic pressure is lowered. If power to the assist device is removed while the pumping chamber is left in position, blood may flow from the left ventricle directly through the inactivated chamber into the aorta. However, it is then possible for the diastolic pressure for coronary artery perfusion to fall to a very low level since a competent outflow valve in the pump prevents reverse flow from the arterial tree into the coronary circulation (Fig. 37-6).

LEFT ATRIUM TO AORTA BYPASS

A pumping chamber that accepts blood from the left atrium and pumps blood into the aorta has been applied clinically. The left heart bypass pump may take almost all of the total blood flow, leaving the natural ventricle only a small proportion of the total flow. Ideally the bypass pump should be synchronized with the left ventricle's contraction so as to pump during ventricular diastole. If it pumps during systole it will raise the aortic pressure against which the ventricle pumps.

This bypass requires thoracotomy for implantation, and it must be removed when deactivated or the stagnant blood within the pump will clot. Although it may reduce left atrial pressures to very low levels, it does not decompress the left ventricle, and left ventricular pressure overload may occur. Since the bypass may take nearly all of the total flow, it can greatly reduce the work load (pressure × flow) of the left ventricle. It can effectively reduce left atrial pressure to eliminate risk of pulmonary edema and pulmonary congestion (Fig. 37-6).

LEFT VENTRICLE TO AORTA BYPASS PUMP

This pump accepts blood from the apex of the left ventricle and pumps the blood into the descending thoracic aorta. The action of this pump should be synchronized with that of the left ventricle, operating so that it is pumping during left ventricular diastole and relaxing and filling during left ventricular systole. The pumping chamber then becomes a very low pressure reservoir into which the left ventricle pumps its stroke volume. This bypass pump must be removed when inactivated since blood contained in the pump will stagnate and clot.

Total bypass of the left ventricle can be provided by this system so that no blood flows forward through the aortic valve. Since left ventricular systolic pressure can be dramatically reduced with this pump, the total work load and tension-time index of the left ventricle are reduced considerably. It also produces effective decompression of both the left atrium and left ventricle.

INTRA-AORTIC BALLOON PUMP

The intra-aortic balloon pump has a long flexible balloon attached to a long thin pneumatic line that is connected to an external

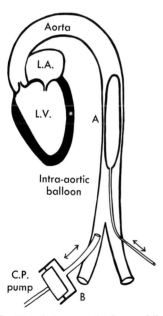

Fig. 37-7. Closed-chest methods providing assistance. *A,* Intra-aortic balloon is inserted via femoral artery. *B,* Femoral counterpulsation pump–effectiveness decreased by long distance from aorta and limited volume exchange per pulse.

driving source. Inflation and deflation of the balloon is effected by alternately passing a gas such as carbon dioxide, air, or helium through the pneumatic tube into the balloon and then aspirating the gas via the same tube. The nonocclusive balloon is inserted via a femoral arteriotomy so as to lie high in the descending aorta. Inflation of the balloon in diastole displaces approximately 30 ml. of blood and therefore raises the pressure in the arterial tree. Deflation of the balloon at the beginning of systole produces a fall in pressure in the arterial tree and so decreases the pressure against which the left ventricle pumps.

As with most other assist devices, a sophisticated triggering system is required to synchronize balloon deflation and inflation with cardiac systole and diastole. The problems involved with ideal triggering of the balloon can become quite complex especially when the balloon must be synchronized with cardiac arrhythmias. There are several potential hazards in the application of this device such as leak or rupture of the balloon with production of air emboli, and trauma to the aortic wall. Heparinization systemically is usually required. The effective volume of the balloon is limited by the dimensions of the aorta and by the problems associated with aspiration and then return of air via a narrow pneumatic tube.

The balloon pump may be rapidly applied to the patient and it does not need to be activated continuously. The balloon may be left in place, inactive while the condition of the patient's unaided heart is reassessed. Blood need not be withdrawn from the circulation and so problems related to hypovolemia and thrombosis or blood trauma are minimized. These favorable factors have made the intra-aortic balloon pump one of the most popular types of cardiac assist devices in use (Fig. 37-7).

FEMORAL-COUNTERPULSATION PUMP

The femoral-counterpulsation pump is operated to produce similar pressure counter-

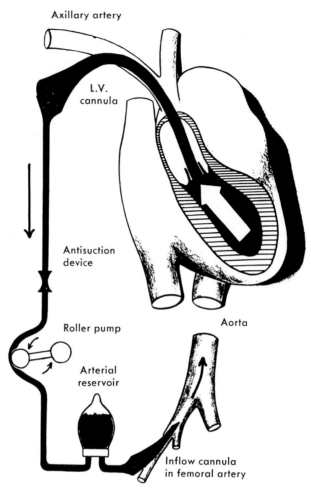

Fig. 37-8. Transarterial left ventricular bypass. This provides decompression of left ventricle and is applied without thoracotomy.

pulsation at the aortic root as is produced by the intra-aortic balloon. A pump is attached to a cannula inserted in the femoral artery. The pump sucks blood from the femoral artery so as to produce a fall in arterial pressure at the aortic root at a time that coincides with the beginning of contraction of the left ventricle. Blood is then returned from the pump to the arterial tree during ventricular diastole. This return of blood helps to propel blood around the circulation and raises the pressure for perfusion of the coronary arteries.

The value of the pump varies with the amount of blood that it can aspirate from a femoral artery of limited size. The blood trauma produced by the pump is probably much greater than that of the intra-aortic balloon pump (Fig. 37-7).

TRANSARTERIAL LEFT VENTRICULAR BYPASS

The transarterial left ventricular bypass provides a left heart bypass from left ventricle to aorta without need for thoracotomy. A thin-walled cannula is passed via an arteriotomy in the axillary artery into the aorta, through the aortic valve into the left ventricle. Blood is sucked from the left ventricle through the cannula and it is then pumped back into the arterial system through a femoral arteriotomy. The return flow may be either continuous or pulsatile.

The volume of blood that this system can pump is limited by the maximum internal diameter of the cannula that can be passed through the axillary artery into the ventricle. It cannot be used when there is an obstruction at the aortic outlet, such as with aortic stenosis or with a prosthetic aortic valve.

This bypass can produce a total left heart bypass by leaving the left ventricle insufficient blood to pump out via the aortic valve. It produces effective decompression of the left ventricle and left atrium and, in the presence of complete bypass, no synchronization with cardiac contraction is necessary. It can produce a great reduction in the work load of the heart and in the tension-time index. It produces low left atrial pressure, and can also support the circulation temporarily in the presence of ventricular fibrillation (Fig. 37-8).

OTHER METHODS

Other methods have also been applied clinically or experimentally. The veno-arterial bypass without pump oxygenator takes blood from the venous system and pumps it directly into the systemic circulation. A closed-chest left heart bypass has been obtained by passing a metal cannula down the jugular vein into the right atrium, across the atrial septum into the left atrium. The blood removed from the left atrium is pumped back into the femoral artery. Counterpulsation similar to the femoral counterpulsation can be more effectively applied by attaching a large diameter connector to the arch of the aorta. The use of the transapical bypass provides a rapid method for instituting left heart bypass, but requires a thoracotomy. A

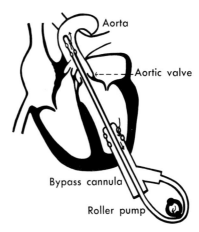

Fig. 37-9. Transapical left ventricular bypass takes blood from left ventricle and pump blood into aorta. This requires thoracotomy but can be applied rapidly.

double lumen cannula is thrust through the apex of the left ventricle so that the inner small-diameter cannula lies across the aortic valve in the aortic root. Blood is now sucked from the left ventricle through the outer cannula into the pump and returned by the inner cannula to the aortic root (Fig. 37-9).

Summary

The use of total artificial hearts and circulatory assist devices is still strictly limited. Further progress in the use of these devices depends partly upon the development of materials and devices that are compatible with blood, that cause minimal blood trauma, and that do not require systemic heparinization. Permanent devices require the development of control systems and compact power sources that can be fully implanted and that may be charged by induction through the skin or that have power packs with stored energy sufficient for several years of continuous use.

Chapter 38

CARDIAC AUGMENTATION BY MEANS OF INTRA-AORTIC PHASE-SHIFT BALLOON PUMPING

Adrian Kantrowitz

For those who manage the patient with acute left ventricular failure, the potential importance of a practical, rapidly applicable circulatory support system is obvious. By reducing or even eliminating demands for external work by the heart while maintaining coronary arterial and systemic perfusion, such a system might restore hemodynamic stabilization, providing time for correction of abnormal myocardial metabolism, effective therapy of rhythm disturbances, or diagnostic efforts to determine the appropriateness of surgical management.

Today there is considerable interest in intra-aortic phase-shift balloon pumping as a method of meeting these requirements. This technique entails only minor surgery and can be applied rapidly to the patient with acute, massive circulatory failure. A growing body of clinical experience, reflecting the efforts of many centers during the last 5 years, indicates that balloon pumping is safe and physiologically effective. Other systems of cardiac augmentation have been

The investigations described in this chapter were supported by Public Health Service research grants HE-06510, HE-11173, and HE-13737 from the National Heart and Lung Institute. *The Cooperative Study: Phase-shift Balloon Pumping in Cardiogenic Shock* was initiated with a planning grant from the David and Minnie Berk Foundation and is supported by the John A. Hartford Foundation, Inc.

devised that require surgical implantation to become operational. Both types of cardiac assist systems can support the failing left ventricle for days, weeks, or longer periods.

The following discussion attempts to summarize the present status of work with representative examples of each of these systems. For more extensive review of the relevant literature, the reader is referred to reports by Kantrowitz, Kantrowitz and others (1971), and Cooper and Dempsey.

Intra-aortic phase-shift balloon pumping

OPERATING PRINCIPLE

Intra-aortic phase-shift balloon pumping is obtained by expanding and deflating a flexible pumping chamber placed within the descending thoracic aorta synchronously and out of phase with the heart. Balloon pumping therefore introduces periodic pressure perturbations into the central aorta at the fundamental frequency of the heart. The action of the assist device may be represented as a change in the afterload on the left ventricle (Jaron and others, 1970). Fig. 38-1 shows a recording of hemodynamic parameters from a canine experiment. Aortic root pressure, its fundamental component (obtained by low pass filtering), aortic root flow, and its fundamental component are shown. When the balloon is inactive, the fundamental components of the pressure and flow wave forms are approximately in phase.

Effect of balloon pump on phase relationship between aortic root pressure and flow

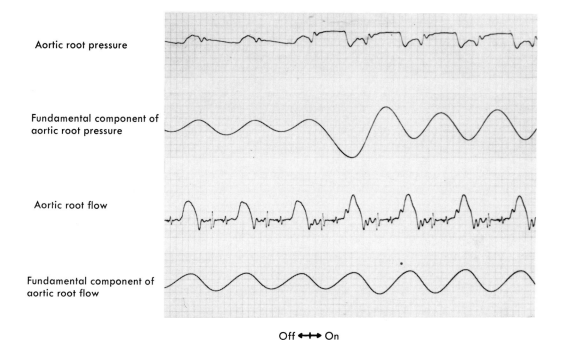

Aortic root pressure

Fundamental component of aortic root pressure

Aortic root flow

Fundamental component of aortic root flow

Off ←→ On

Fig. 38-1. Recording of pressure and flow wave forms and their fundamental components at the aortic root in an experiment on a dog. These variables were recorded before activation of the balloon pump (at left) and during cardiac assistance. Note that flow and pressure wave forms are approximately in phase when the balloon is inactive; slight deviations from perfect phasing reflect essentially instantaneous transmission of flow signal and 30 to 40 msec. delay of pressure signal because of mechanical inertia of fluid in pressure catheter, catheter elasticity and length, and transducer. Activation of the assist device causes the flow and pressure wave forms to be approximately 180 degrees out of phase.

During balloon pumping, the fundamental components of pressure and flow are approximately 180 degrees apart (that is, the maximum of one wave occurs at a time when the other wave is at a minimum). Consequently, the fundamental component of the afterload impedance (pressure/flow) has a phase angle of approximately 180 degrees. Thus, pumping causes a shift in the phase of the aortic root impedance. The precise phase angle obtained depends on the timing of balloon inflation and deflation and has been demonstrated to be a critical determinant of the hemodynamic effectiveness of

in-series assistance (Jaron and others, 1970), as discussed below.

APPARATUS AND METHOD

The principle of balloon pumping was first reported by Moulopoulos and others and by Clauss and colleagues in 1962. At that time a practicable system was not developed. In 1967, our laboratory presented experimental results obtained with a different configuration of the apparatus (Schilt and others). This system (Kantrowitz and others, 1968a and b) utilizes a nonocclusive flexible polyurethane balloon mounted on a

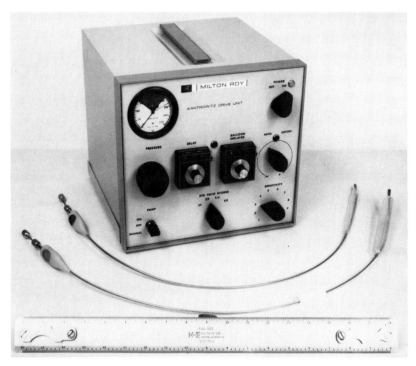

Fig. 38-2. Kantrowitz phase-shift balloon pump and driving unit. For clinical use, balloons of 27 ml. and 33 ml. displacement volume are available, the choice depending on the diameter of the patient's aorta. Control unit operates in both automatic and manual modes, the latter permitting the operator to synchronize balloon operation with resuscitative measures after cardiac arrest. Control unit incorporates defibrillation protection and automatically deflates the balloon when a ventricular premature beat is sensed. This control unit can also be used for circulatory support with the dynamic aortic patch mechanical auxiliary ventricle.

polyurethane catheter (Fig. 38-2). The balloon is threaded through a sleeve of Dacron arterial graft into a femoral arteriotomy and advanced into the descending thoracic aorta until its tip is approximately at the level of the origin of the left subclavian artery. The sleeve is then sutured to the femoral artery incision. This permits release of occlusive snares around the vessel and restoration of circulation to the extremity (Kantrowitz and others, 1968c).

The distal end of the catheter is attached to the pneumatic port of an electronic control unit (Fig. 38-2), also developed in our laboratory. The control unit is triggered by signals derived from the R wave of the electrocardiogram to operate a fast-acting, three-way solenoid valve that admits helium at a pressure of 120 to 150 mm. Hg to the catheter and exhausts it to atmosphere. The solenoid valve is controlled by two adjustable time delays so as to inflate the balloon at the beginning of ventricular diastole and to deflate it at the beginning of systole.

EXPERIMENTAL OBSERVATIONS

In 1953, Kantrowitz and Kantrowitz reported the results of a canine study in which propagation of the arterial pressure pulse was experimentally delayed in order to arrive in the coronary circulation during diastole. The data indicated that coronary flow was markedly increased in this preparation. Following this demonstration, a number of techniques based on this principle have been studied (Clauss and others, 1961;

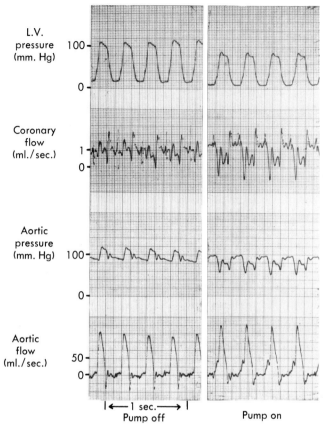

Fig. 38-3. Recording of hemodynamic changes due to balloon pumping in a dog with experimental heart failure. Note reduction in peak and end-diastolic left ventricular pressures, marked accentuation of coronary flow, augmented diastolic pressure in aorta, and substantial increment in cardiac output. Data presented by Jaron and others (1970) indicate that these favorable hemodynamic responses to phase-shift pumping are critically dependent on phasing of balloon and cardiac action.

Goldfarb and others, 1968; Kantrowitz and others, 1966; Kantrowitz and others, 1968; Nachlas and Siedband; Soroff and others).

In animal experiments performed in our laboratory (Jaron and others, 1968, 1970; Schilt and others; Tomecek and others; Yahr and others), a number of hemodynamic responses to phase-shift pumping have been defined (Fig. 38-3). In animals with heart failure induced by successive coronary artery ligation, the following average changes due to balloon pumping were demonstrated: Left ventricular end-diastolic pressure was diminished by 40%, and tension-time index

by 20%. Cardiac output, coronary blood flow, and left ventricular dp/dt were increased by 50%, 100% and 25%, respectively. Reduction in left ventricular peak and end-diastolic pressures and tension-time index reflect a decrease in myocardial wall tension and suggest a reduction in myocardial oxygen demand. In addition, the reduced end-diastolic pressure suggests diminished left ventricular volume, and thus reversal of compensatory cardiac dilatation secondary to failure. The increase in central aortic diastolic pressure enhances coronary artery perfusion pressure. These effects, in concert with decreased systolic ejection time and diminished myocardial wall tension, produce increased coronary flow and myocardial oxygenation.

These observations have been corroborated and extended in a number of other investigations (Brown and others; Powell and others; Talpins and others; Corday and others; Tyberg and others; Urschel and others), which are discussed by Kantrowitz and others (1971).

A number of studies have failed to disclose beneficial effects of intra-aortic balloon pumping (Feola and others; Gallo and others; Tanaka and others). A recent investigation in our laboratory by Jaron and others (1970) may help to account for such findings. The purpose of this investigation was to examine the relationship between the hemodynamic effectiveness of assistance and the adjustment of the times of balloon inflation and deflation. This adjustment has proved to be subjective and difficult to reproduce when based on visual inspection of the central aortic pressure wave form. Balloon pumping was performed at various settings of inflation and deflation before and after induction of experimental acute heart failure. The phase angle of the left ventricular afterload was monitored. The results indicated that most hemodynamic benefits of assistance were strongly dependent on the afterload phase angle, which varies according to the adjustment of balloon inflation and deflation relative to the cardiac cycle (see Fig. 38-1). Improvement in coronary flow, external left ventricular work, work in the aorta, and tension time index was maximal when the afterload-phase angle was approximately 180 degrees. Timing adjustments that resulted in small deviations from 180 degrees were associated with large reductions in hemodynamic benefits. Large deviations from 180 degrees caused changes in some hemodynamic parameters opposite to those desired. Although data for cardiac output followed a parallel trend, the relationship to afterload-phase angle was not as clear-cut as for the other variables.

An additional observation in this study was that an afterload-phase angle of 180 degrees could not be achieved when a balloon with an inflated diameter larger than that of the aorta was used. Hemodynamic effects under this condition were significantly reduced or even lost. The results indicated that a left ventricular afterload-phase angle of approximately 180 degrees is a necessary condition for maximal effectiveness of balloon pumping. Since other in-series devices are based on the same operating principle, this conclusion is expected to hold for them as well. Thus, the findings that balloon pumping has negligible hemodynamic benefits may require reassessment in the light of the above results, as well as other factors enumerated in the report by Jaron and others.

CLINICAL OBSERVATIONS

Our initial clinical work with the balloon pumping method was restricted to patients in medically refractory cardiogenic shock secondary to acute myocardial infarction. Since methods for control of arrhythmias and congestive failure have improved in recent years, the importance of shock as a cause of death in acute myocardial infarction has increased. Mortality in cardiogenic shock has not been determined in a large, prospectively studied population, although the Myocardial Infarction Research Unit investigations now being conducted may be expected eventually to provide this information. In smaller individual series of cases, the incidence of fatal outcome has varied from 85% to 100% (Cronin and others; Scheidt and others; Friedberg, 1966).

Since the pathophysiologic abnormalities in intractable cardiogenic shock have not been completely defined and quantitated, in selecting candidates for our initial studies, we utilized the generally accepted clinical manifestations as a basis for the diagnosis. When transferred to the cardiac assistance group, candidates for balloon pumping had classic symptoms and signs of intractable cardiogenic shock: systolic blood pressure of less than 80 mm. Hg (during interruption of vasopressor therapy), cold, clammy skin reflecting generalized sympathetic hyperactivity, and urine flow of 10 ml. per hour or less, with or without mental obtundation.

Balloon pumping, shown to be effective in initial animal experiments, was attractive for the treatment of cardiogenic shock because of its ability to augment coronary flow while maintaining systemic perfusion, and to reduce left ventricular external work. Because of these effects, the procedure could be expected to diminish myocardial oxygen requirements and consequently favor an improved balance of myocardial oxygen demand and supply. These effects might serve to interrupt the progressive cardiovascular deterioration and loss of homeostatic control mechanisms in shock. At the same time, it appeared that patients in shock unresponsive to vigorous medical management offered an appropriate population in which to test the clinical efficacy of balloon pumping and to identify the possible complications of the method.

In our series of cases treated at Maimonides Hospital (Brooklyn) and Sinai Hospital of Detroit, the results, which have been described in part elsewhere (Butner and others; Kantrowitz and others, 1968a and b, 1969a; Krakauer and others), were as follows: Twenty-five patients had onset of cardiogenic shock soon after myocardial infarction—in most cases, within 12 hours of the acute infarct, and in all, within 30 hours. During pumping, symptoms of shock were reversed in twenty-three, or 92%. Nineteen patients, or 76%, regained hemodynamic stabilization and no longer needed mechanical assistance. The remaining six patients died during pumping.

Of the twenty patients who recovered from cardiogenic shock, eleven were discharged from the hospital upon convalescing from their infarcts and became long-term survivors. The remaining nine patients died 8 hours to 7 days after pumping.

Two case reports will illustrate the course of the assist procedure:

A 48-year-old man was admitted with the diagnoses of acute anterolateral wall myocardial infarction, pulmonary edema, and hypotension. The patient had had an inferior wall infarction 8 weeks previously from which he had recovered uneventfully.

During the first 2 days the patient's condition gradually deteriorated, as manifested by ventricular arrhythmias, decreasing urine output, rising BUN and creatinine, persistently elevated serum enzyme levels and injury patterns on the ECG, and hypotension, which necessitated increasing amounts of vasoactive medications.

Because of the patient's grave condition, phase-shift intra-aortic balloon pumping was requested. Prior to initiation of mechanical assistance, the patient's cardiac output was 2.5 liters per minute during treatment with vasoactive medications. One-half hour after balloon pumping and intermittent administration of chlorpromazine was started, the cardiac output was 4.8 liters per minute. Balloon pumping was discontinued after 5 hours, and the cardiac output did not decline.

Approximately 8 hours later, with the pump inoperative but still in the vascular system, the patient had a cardiac arrest immediately following a tracheotomy. He was resuscitated with closed-chest cardiac massage synchronized with phase-shift pumping; cardiotonic medications were also administered. Pumping was continued for approximately 5 hours longer. After the assist procedure was stopped for the second time, the patient's cardiac output was 4.6 liters per minute, and his blood pressure varied from 120/70 to 100/60 without vasoactive medications.

The patient was then transferred for management of concurrent medical problems. At this time he was thought to have bilateral pneumonia and acute renal failure. Despite large doses of antibiotics and peritoneal dialysis, his condition deteriorated, and he died 1 week later.

A 64-year-old man was admitted with an acute myocardial infarction. His recovery was uneventful until the twentieth day, when cardiac arrest suddenly occurred. After the patient was resuscitated, electrocardiographic evidence of an acute anteroseptal infarction was obtained. The patient was now in cardiogenic shock and had pulmonary edema and anuria. The central venous pressure was 18 cm. H_2O. A constant lidocaine infusion was required to control ventricular tachycardia, and a continuous infusion of levarterenol and Regitine was needed to maintain the blood pressure.

Because of progressive hemodynamic failure, balloon pumping was begun. Vasopressor therapy was immediately discontinued and chlorpromazine, 0.1 to 0.2 mg. per kilogram of body weight, was given periodically. Half an hour after pumping was started, the lidocaine infusion was stopped. Therefore, the arrhythmia did not recur, and the electrocardiogram demonstrated normal sinus rhythm.

After $3\frac{1}{2}$ hours of balloon pumping, the patient had excellent diuresis, the central venous pressure fell to the normal range, and the blood pressure rose to 120/70 mm. Hg; the heart rate was 88 per minute. The patient recovered from his infarction and was discharged from the hospital.

In fifteen patients in this series, signs of shock developed 30 hours or longer after acute myocardial infarction. Shock was clinically reversed during pumping in twelve patients. Six died during the procedure, and thus only nine patients regained hemodynamic stabilization and no longer required mechanical assistance. Death in these cases occurred 12 hours to 6 weeks after termination of balloon pumping.

Complications due to balloon pumping have been relatively minor: two instances of infection at the site of the femoral arteriotomy (Kantrowitz and others, 1969a), and—in the first patient, in whom the Dacron side-arm graft was not used—circulatory insufficiency below the arterial incision (Kantrowitz and others, 1968c). Temporary neuropathic complications with flaccid paralysis and absent deep tendon reflexes at the knee and ankle occurred in a recent long-term survivor; three months after the procedure the patient has completely recovered. On the basis of studies of red cell morphology, serum haptoglobin, plasma hemoglobin, serum bilirubin, serum LDH levels, and platelet and reticulocyte counts, significant hemolysis or other damage to formed elements of the blood has not developed in any patient in this series.

Myocardial rupture was seen in one patient with "early" shock, and in seven of those with "delayed" circulatory collapse. Although the frequency of myocardial rupture was thus higher than that expected in patients with acute myocardial infarction, there was no evidence implicating the assist procedure in its etiology. Since the aortic valve is closed during inflation of the balloon, and since the action of the device is to reduce left ventricular peak systolic pressure, and thereby, myocardial wall tension, it seems unlikely that mechanical assistance causes myocardial rupture. A more reasonable explanation may be that pumping prolongs survival of patients with massive myocardial insults long enough to allow the complete pathophysiologic sequence of events to unfold. This matter, and also the apparent difference in prognosis according to the interval from infarct to onset of shock, needs to be investigated further.

Other groups have also reported clinical studies of balloon pumping in patients with cardiogenic shock after acute myocardial infarction (Summers and others; Mueller and others; Mundth and others; Bregman and others). The most extensive data appear to be those generated by the Cooperative Study: Phase-shift Balloon Pumping in Cardiogenic Shock. The ten institutions participating in this study agreed to manage patients according to a common protocol for diagnosis, treatment, and physiologic and clinical observations, in order to assess the safety and efficacy of the balloon-pumping technique. Patients were admitted to the study only if they met strict diagnostic criteria for refractory cardiogenic shock, as defined in a detailed report prepared by Scheidt and others (1972) (Report to the John A. Hartford Foundation, Inc.). Each group used balloon pumps and driving units developed by our group.*

In an analysis of the cases of eighty-seven patients coming under this protocol, Scheidt and others found that physiologic responses to balloon pumping were favorable in most. Diastolic pressure in the central aorta rose from 53 ± 12 to 83 ± 19 mm. Hg, whereas arterial pressure, or left ventricular afterload, decreased from 76 ± 22 mm. Hg to 57 ± 17 mm. Hg. Cardiac output increased, on the average, 0.4 liter per minute. The heart rate declined from 110 ± 24 beats per minute to 103 ± 21 beats per minute. Of nineteen patients in whom myocardial metabolic studies were performed (Mueller and others, 1970), all but one had decreased production, or increased extraction, of lactate.

Clinically favorable responses to phase-shift intra-aortic balloon pumping were observed in most patients. Thirty-five patients survived balloon pumping, but only fifteen left the hospital, and of these, ten were alive at the time of writing—eight for more than a year.

Scheidt and his associates concluded that balloon pumping is safe and physiologically effective. There was 12% survival in the group of patients totally refractory to conventional medical therapy, a group in which mortality approaches 100%. However, although overall survival of these patients was somewhat improved as compared with patients treated conventionally, mortality nevertheless remained high. The data obtained in the study suggested that earlier initiation of therapy to limit the "massive myocardial damage invariably associated with shock" would be desirable.

*The Milton Roy Company, St. Petersburg, Florida.

As a participant in this investigation, our group concurs in this interpretation of the cumulative results to date. At the same time, it seems clear that a definitive assessment of the role of the technique in patients with established cardiogenic shock cannot be offered until more information is available about the optimal interaction of the assist device with the failing cardiovascular system, and about the most appropriate adjunctive management for these patients. Scheidt and associates stress the requirement for "technical perfection" in the application of balloon pumping. Data in studies discussed above point to the desirability of a quantitative technique for adjusting the timing of the balloon inflation-deflation cycle to the natural heart's cycle, and underscore the inaccuracy and poor reproducibility of currently available qualitative techniques. The variability in clinical outcomes of balloon pumping may reflect (1) lack of quantitative analysis of the effects of in-series assistance, and (2) inability to optimize the device's operation, as well as (3) excessive delay in the application of balloon pumping as a result of which the myocardial damage may progress to the point that restoration of autonomous cardiac function is no longer possible. Investigation of these considerations may lead to an explanation of variability in the clinical outcomes of phase-shift pumping in cardiogenic shock.

A second area that appears to require additional investigation as a prerequisite for definitive assessment of balloon pumping in cardiogenic shock is the adjunctive management, which may vary considerably from investigator to investigator. Although not absolutely established, the effectiveness of certain tentative guidelines is suggested by our observations in these cases (Krakauer and others). Upon initiation of pumping and at regular intervals thereafter, heparin is administered. Efforts are directed toward improving cardiac function and correction of systemic abnormalities due to the shock state and its prior treatment, that is, volume abnormalities, hyponatremia, hemodilution, hypoxemia, and acid-base aberrations, which often are masked by defective myocardial contractility.

1. Vasopressor treatment is withdrawn, if possible, when the assist device has been placed in the vascular system and optimally synchronized with the cardiac cycle (Fig. 38-3). In instances when mean central aortic pressure is below 50 mm. Hg and there is evidence of occlusion of the aorta by the inflated balloon, administration of pressor amines is continued for a brief period. Pressor support is stopped when cardiac assistance alone is capable of producing central aortic pressures sufficient to maintain an aortic diameter larger than that of the inflated balloon.

2. In cases where satisfactory central aortic pressures were obtained but diaphoresis and oliguria tended to persist and capillary filling remained poor, a vasodilating agent, chlorpromazine, was given in a dosage of 0.1 to 0.2 mg. per kilogram (except to patients thought to be in right heart failure). Digitalis was given to all patients who demonstrated evidence of congestive heart failure.

3. When adequate perfusion had been achieved, as indicated by restoration of urine flow, warming of the extremities, and improved sensorium, abnormalities of effective plasma volume, pH, serum osmolarity, and red cell mass were corrected. Functional hypovolemia, hyponatremia, and metabolic acidosis were frequently seen in these patients, but occult right ventricular failure also occurred. In such cases phlebotomy was performed, despite "normal" central venous pressure and hypotension. Hemodilution caused by phlebotomy was corrected by infusion of packed red cells.

4. Severe hypoxemia was observed in all patients and, in most, resisted conventional treatment. When necessary, patients were intubated and ventilation was assisted or controlled with a volume-cycled respirator. Adequate management of this problem has

not been evolved, and further study is needed.

5. Pumping was sustained until shock was clinically reversed and all metabolic aberrations had been corrected. If several hours' additional pumping produced no change in the patient's condition, mechanical assistance was interrupted, and if no immediate deterioration was noted, the procedure was discontinued for half an hour. Pumping was then resumed for 30 minutes. If the patient's condition improved during this period, pumping was continued for several hours more before trial discontinuation was again attempted. On the other hand, if the 30-minute trial of pumping caused no change in the patient's state, pumping was terminated. The balloon was left *in situ* for 24 hours and, if the patient remained stable, was then removed.

6. Just as positive criteria for discontinuing assistance have not been identified, no definite limitations to its duration have been established. Whereas only a few hours were required for restoration of circulatory stabilization in some cases, in others 2 to 3 days and more were needed. At the Barnes Hospital in St. Louis a patient, who ultimately died, was supported with only brief interruptions by balloon pumping over a period of 20 days (G. Wolff, personal communication). Two patients were treated by our group respectively for 34 and 35 days. The first of these patients recovered and was discharged to his home.

COMMENT

Although the ultimate role of intra-aortic balloon pumping as a primary therapeutic measure in medically refractory cardiogenic shock remains to be established, a wealth of evidence is accumulating that demonstrates the safety and physiologic effectiveness of the technique for temporary support of the acutely failing circulation.

Additional considerations supporting the use of balloon pumping as a method of cardiac augmentation include the system's speed of application, mobility, and freedom from complications. Once the decision to undertake mechanical assistance is made, pumping can usually be started within 20 to 25 minutes. All components of the system are completely mobile.

A specific contraindication to phase-shift pumping is incompetence of the aortic valve. Severe sclerosis or aneurysms of the aorta, the iliac arteries, or the femoral arteries may prevent insertion of the pumping chamber.

Except for patients with these conditions, a large number of patients in acute ventricular failure might potentially be candidates for phase-shift pumping. For patients in this category, who presumably account for a significant percentage of those who go into cardiac arrest, ventricular support by means of phase-shift balloon pumping may prove to be a treatment of choice. Indeed, it may be that balloon pumping in these patients helps to prevent cardiac arrest.

For the patient in cardiac arrest, balloon pumping is not an immediate therapeutic procedure, except for the special case of the patient whose cardiac action comes to a halt while the balloon-pumping equipment is in the vascular system. In one instance reported above, arrest occurred while the pumping chamber was *in situ* but inactive. Resuscitation was achieved with closed-chest massage synchronized with balloon pumping. On theoretical grounds, balloon pumping, by increasing coronary flow and maintaining the cerebral circulation during massage, would be an attractive therapeutic adjunct in this situation. More realistically, however, the chief indication for balloon pumping in the treatment of cardiac arrest would be cardiogenic shock as a complication after resuscitation, or its prophylaxis.

Permanent mechanical support of the left ventricle

The possibility of permanent support of the chronically failing left ventricle has been under study for many years (Cooper and Dempsey; Kantrowitz and others, 1966,

1968d, 1971). In principle, a permanently implanted assist device might find application in patients with acute ventricular failure who cannot be weaned from support with a temporary assist technique, as well as in those with medically uncontrollable end-stage atherosclerotic heart disease.

Various experimental configurations of a permanently implantable auxiliary ventricle have been developed in our laboratory during the last 12 years, all based on the principle of introducing external energy into the cardiovascular system synchronously and out of phase with the natural heart, as discussed above. In 1966, a U-shaped mechanical auxiliary ventricle was implanted in two patients. This experience demonstrated the clinical feasibility and the hemodynamic effectiveness of this form of mechanical assistance for patients in chronic left ventricular congestive failure. The demise of the second patient due to a thromboembolism 12 days postoperatively prompted reconsideration of the geometry of the assist device and search for an improved blood prosthesis interface (Kantrowitz and others, 1966, 1968d).

The new configuration, the dynamic aortic patch (Sujansky and others), has an operating principle similar to that of the balloon pump. Since this prosthesis is intended for implantation in the wall of the descending thoracic aorta, it is expected that when inactive, it would interfere minimally with the hydrodynamics of blood flow. Only one artificial material is required for the intravascular interface. For this purpose, we explored the possibility of using a material that would favor tissue ingrowth, leading to a blood interface that would eventually be covered by a pseudo-intima. This would be expected to provide a biological interface having a low potential for thromboembolism.

In its present configuration the dynamic aortic patch (Fig. 38-4) consists of an elliptical silicone rubber pumping chamber, covering materials, and a gas conduit. The covering material used for the intravascular

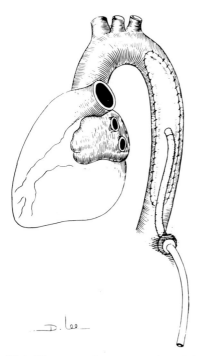

Fig. 38-4. Diagrammatic representation of dynamic aortic patch in situ.

surface consists of Dacron velour backed with a conductive polyurethane (Sharp and others, 1966); plain Dacron cloth is used for the outer surface. The prosthesis is implanted on the lateral surface of the descending thoracic aorta between the origin of the left subclavian artery and the diaphragm. The gas conduit is led to a transcutaneous connector implanted in the left hypogastric area. Electrocardiographic electrodes implanted in the left ventricular myocardium are also brought to the transcutaneous connector. An extracorporeal driving system is attached to the prosthesis through the connector. The driving system consists either of the electropneumatic driver used for balloon pumping or a portable battery-driven compressor built into a vest. Both systems utilize the R wave of the electrocardiogram to trigger the pump.

A report of preliminary studies of this auxiliary ventricle was presented by Sujansky and associates (1969). Results of experiments utilizing the Dacron velour backed with conductive polyurethane for the blood interface showed that in eighty-four dogs in which inactive prostheses had been implanted, an organized layer of pseudo-intima covered most or all of the artificial material. Four to six months were required for complete coverage, but a stable layer of fibrin was deposited within hours after the surgical procedure. In twenty-six experiments in which the prosthesis was activated immediately after implantation and intermittently thereafter, data were obtained suggesting that pumping delayed but did not prevent formation of the pseudo-intimal layer. Hematologic studies disclosed no evidence of hemolysis or gross damage to formed elements of the blood (Kantrowitz and others, 1971).

The hemodynamic effects of the dynamic aortic patch were evaluated in nineteen studies in ten dogs before and during periods of pumping (Kantrowitz and others, 1971). In these studies, each animal served as its own control. The results indicated that left ventricular peak pressure, tension-time index, stroke work, and systemic vascular resistance all decreased significantly when the dynamic aortic patch was activated. Concurrently, there were substantial improvements in cardiac output, left circumflex coronary blood flow, diastolic blood pressure, and mean systolic ejection rate. These effects were comparable to those produced by balloon pumping and previous configurations of the mechanical auxiliary ventricle (Kantrowitz and others, 1966, 1968d).

In view of this evidence of the hemodynamic effectiveness and freedom from thromboembolic potential of the dynamic aortic patch, our group decided that a limited clinical trial of the system was appropriate in patients with severe, intractable chronic heart failure unresponsive to conventional therapy. A patient meeting these criteria was recently referred to us; detailed accounts of this case have been presented elsewhere (Kantrowitz and others, 1971, 1972).

He was a 63-year-old man with chronic congestive heart failure unresponsive to medical treatment. He was bedridden because of weakness, severe dyspnea, and recurrent leg edema. Symptoms had first been noted in early 1967, when the patient developed shortness of breath, two-pillow orthopnea, and leg edema. A conservative medical regimen consisting of digitalis and diuretics provided moderate relief until 1969. Thereafter, his condition deteriorated progressively. Shortly before referral, right and left cardiac catheterization, coronary arteriography, and left ventriculography disclosed severe left and right ventricular failure, severe pulmonary hypertension, enlarged, dilated, poorly contracting left ventricle, 1+ mitral regurgitation, and greater than 70% narrowing of the main right, main left, and anterior descending coronary arteries. Because of the overwhelming evidence of cardiac decompensation and the absence of an anginal syndrome or clear-cut myocardial infarction history, the coronary artery disease was considered inoperable. A permanent transvenous pacemaker was implanted in the right ventricle to control premature ventricular contractions.

To determine whether this patient would be a suitable candidate for implantation of the permanent dynamic aortic patch, we studied his response to intra-aortic balloon pumping. Before cardiac assistance, left ventricular end-diastolic pressure, pulmonary capillary wedge pressure, and pulmonary artery pressure were severely elevated. Lactate and pyruvate studies indicated anaerobic cardiac metabolism. With approximately 2 hours of cardiac assistance, left ventricular pressure, pulmonary capillary wedge pressure, and pulmonary artery pressure returned to near normal. Cardiac output increased by 16%. Lactate extraction indicated aerobic myocardial metabolism. Because of the favorable response to diastolic augmentation, the patient was considered to be a good candidate for the mechanical auxiliary ventricle.

The dynamic aortic patch was implanted without incident on August 10, 1971, during total cardiopulmonary bypass. The patch booster was activated at the end of the operation. It was used without interruption for the first two days and intermittently thereafter.

Postoperatively, the patient's hemodynamic condition stabilized, and he made good progress during the first seven weeks. An atrial arrhythmia during the first postoperative week and a shallow dehiscence of the chest incision, which was repaired under local anesthesia, were the chief problems during this period. The patient's exercise tolerance gradually increased to the point that he could walk several hundred yards without assistance. Repeat catheterization and angiocardiography 5 weeks postoperatively documented objective improvement in hemodynamic parameters; in addition, his cardiac transverse diameter, previously indicative of an enlarged heart, decreased to within the normal range. Hematologic studies, which included the use of scanning and transmission electron microscopy, disclosed no significant deviations from the preoperative state.

The patient was sent home in the sixth postoperative week. Two weeks later, he was readmitted because of low-grade fever, anorexia, and increasing weight loss. Thereafter, his condition progressively deteriorated, despite vigorous efforts to treat an infection that apparently originated in the chest incision, and he died 96 days after the operation. The patch booster had provided effective hemodynamic support virtually until the end.

Autopsy disclosed that the prosthesis was intact. Its intravascular surface was covered by a firm, smooth fibrin layer. Despite meticulous search, no indications of embolization were found anywhere. An extensive infectious process began near the external surface of the prosthesis and extended along a number of planes but did not include the transcutaneous connector. The postmortem examination also confirmed the severity of the patient's underlying heart disease; the heart weighed 558 gm. and contained evidence of three old infarcts involving the left ventricle.

Clearly, much more additional investigation is required before widespread use of a partial artificial heart such as the dynamic aortic patch will become a realistic possibility. The present experience, however, reinforces the conviction that such a goal is attainable within the near future.

Chapter 39

ELECTRIC CARDIAC PACING

John C. Schuder

The early history of experimental attempts to stimulate the heart electrically have been adequately described in *Cardiac Pacemakers* by Siddons and Sowton (1967), in *Principles and Techniques of Cardiac Pacing* by Furman and Escher (1970), and in previous editions of *Cardiac Arrest and Resuscitation* by Stephenson (1958, 1964, 1969).

Two decades of progress

In 1952 Zoll reported upon his experience in two patients in whom electric cardiac pacing was achieved by means of monophasic pulses of about 2 msec. duration delivered via needles placed in the subcutaneous tissue of the chest. This work, which served to initiate the era of clinical pacing, was followed by reports by Zoll and colleagues (1954, 1956) of favorable experience in larger groups of patients. Because of the high value of current, typically 75 to 150 milliamperes, required for pacing with subcutaneous needles or surface electrodes, chest pain, muscle twitch, and skin burns often occurred. Relatively large line-operated units were used for supplying the pacing pulses to the electrodes.

Damage to the conduction system and complete heart block sometimes result from open-heart surgical procedures. In 1958 Weirich and colleagues reported upon favorable results in pacing such patients by means of a myocardial electrode. In their system, a needle was swaged onto a wire and used to attach the wire to the ventricle. The needle was later cut off. The insulated portion of the wire was brought out through the chest and it, together with a lead from an indifferent electrode implanted in the chest wall, were connected to an external stimulator. The voltage and current requirements were much less than for external pacing and low enough that there was no pain associated with the pacing process. After the heart block disappeared, the wire was removed by pulling.

In 1958 Thevenet and co-workers described a technique for the emergency insertion of a myocardial electrode in which a lumbar puncture needle was pushed through the chest wall and 0.5 cm. into the myocardium. A stiff conducting wire was then inserted through the needle and pushed about 1 cm. into the heart. The needle was then removed, leaving the wire in place. For monopolar pacing this wire was connected to one terminal of the stimulator and a wire from a subcutaneously implanted needle was connected to the other terminal.

Furman and Schwedel, in a 1959 report, described the first clinical application of a method of pacing that involved the application of a stimulating pulse directly to the endocardial surface of the right ventricle by means of a wire catheter inserted in a method equivalent to that employed in cardiac catheterization studies. The indifferent electrode was sutured to the right anterior chest wall.

In 1959 Glenn and co-workers reported the clinical application of a system that involved a transistorized radiofrequency pulse generator external to the patient and inductive coupling between a coil on the sur-

443

face of the chest and another coil buried subcutaneously over the lower midsternum. Included with the implanted receiving coil was a tuning capacitor and rectifying diode. Wires within the body were used to connect the receiver to bipolar electrodes attached to the heart.

Chardack and colleagues, in a 1960 paper, described a self-contained pacemaker unit for implantation in the subcutaneous tissue. Wires from the generator, which was powered by a primary battery, led to a bipolar Hunter-Roth (1959) electrode patch attached to the ventricle. Initial clinical experience was detailed. Other early implantable units were described by Zoll and co-workers (1961) and by Kantrowitz (1961).

Abrams and co-workers (1960) described a system that involved close inductive coupling between a coil on the external surface of the chest and another coil buried subcutaneously. This arrangement employed a pulse generator external to the patient. Since a radiofrequency carrier was not utilized, rectification was not required within the chest. Clinical results with this system have been discussed by Norman and colleagues (1964).

In 1962 Cammilli and associates reported clinical experience with a radiofrequency inductive coupled pacing system in which the receiving unit was small enough to be sutured directly to the ventricle. The external coil was excited by a transistorized radiofrequency pulse generator. Schuder and co-workers (1962) have described experimental studies with a similar system, which was later used clinically by Mackenzie and colleagues (1966).

Experience with a completely implanted system in which the ventricular pacing pulse was synchronized (with suitable time delay) with the atrial beat was described by Nathan and colleagues in 1963. Previously, such pacing had been demonstrated on an experimental basis with external units by Folkman and Watkins (1957) and by Stephenson and associates (1959).

In 1963 Lagergren and Johansson described their early favorable clinical results with a transvenous endocardial pacing system in which the pulse generator was completely implanted. Bluestone and colleagues (1965) and Chardack (1965) also made early studies of similar systems.

The concept of paired pacing in which two suitably spaced pulses are used to slow the heart rate was introduced by Lopez and co-workers in 1963. A detailed study of the hemodynamic effect in human patients of slowing the heart rate by paired or coupled pacing of the atria was reported by Lister and colleagues in 1967.

For some patients, it is desirable to stop electrical pacing during periods of normal conduction. In 1966 Parsonnet and co-workers described their clinical experience with a totally implanted "demand" or "standby" pacemaker that took over the pacing function only during periods when the natural rate fell below a predetermined value. This work followed studies by Lemberg and colleagues (1965) in which a demand pacemaker unit was used external to the body. In a related, but somewhat different approach, Neville and colleagues (1966) described a system in which pulses were triggered by the R wave so that they fell into the absolute refractory period. In the event that the interval between R waves exceeded a predetermined value, the pacemaker reverted to a fixed rate.

When normal atrioventricular conduction is present, it is sometimes more appropriate to pace the atria than the ventricles. In a study on postoperative cardiac surgical patients with sinus bradycardia or slow nodal rhythm, Friesen and colleagues (1968) found that in terms of hemodynamic considerations, atrial pacing was considerably more effective than ventricular pacing.

In 1969 Berkovits and colleagues described a bifocal demand pacing system that was controlled by the ventricular depolarization signal. Following the signal and depending upon the needs of the patient, the pacemaker remained quiescent, stimulated the atria only, or stimulated both the atria and the ventricles with a predetermined interval between the pulses.

In 1970 the nuclear-powered pacemaker was first used in humans by a team of French physicians headed by Laurens and Piwnica. The unit was fueled with plutonium 238. The radioactive decay of the fuel released heat that was then converted to electrical energy in a thermopile. It is anticipated that the nuclear-powered pacemaker will have an appreciably longer life than primary battery-powered units. Morrow and colleagues (1970) have reported upon experimental experience with a somewhat similar system that is being developed in the United States.

Schaldach and Kirsch (1970) have reported considerable clinical experience with implanted biogalvanically powered pacemakers. Earlier experimental work with other biologically powered systems has included investigations of electromechanical converters utilizing piezoelectric ceramic transducers (Kennedy and colleagues, 1966) and studies of bioautofuel cells (Wolfson and co-workers, 1968).

Follow-up of patients with pacemakers is necessary in order that units may be replaced before battery exhaustion, component failure, or other problems compromise the ability of the unit to adequately pace the heart. In a 1971 paper, Furman and colleagues described a system in which information concerning the interval between pacemaker pulses could be conveniently and accurately transmitted over an ordinary telephone line to a receiving terminal. Since such information is very useful in predicting the approach of battery exhaustion, the procedure served to complement the type of pacemaker clinic that Furman and colleagues (1969) had previously described.

Current practices

INDICATIONS FOR PACING

The indications for electrical pacing have expanded considerably in recent years. In addition to its early application to the treatment of complete heart block, electrical pacing is now used in the treatment of bradyarrhythmias of a variety of etiologies as well as in the treatment of some tachyarrhythmias. In particular, electrical pacing is widely used in the management of many of the arrhythmias that accompany myocardial infarctions. Although ineffective in the treatment of persistent ventricular fibrillation, electrical pacing is sometimes helpful in establishing an appropriate cardiac rate in the period following defibrillation. A detailed review of the indications for pacing has been presented by Lown and Kosowsky (1970). The ease with which the transvenous approach can be employed and the availability of demand-type generators have contributed appreciably to the wider use of electrical pacing.

PACING SYSTEMS

Of the many approaches to electrical cardiac pacing that have been studied over the past two decades, some have been discarded because of marginal performance, some have passed into disuse because they were awkward or inconvenient for the patient, others are still in the experimental or clinical evaluation stage, and a comparative few are widely employed at the present time. In this section I shall discuss those approaches that are currently (1972) popular in the United States and that can be adequately implemented by commercially available apparatus.

Transthoracic pacing. Because transthoracic pacing can be initiated quickly and conveniently, it is widely used in emergency situations. The basic pulse generator used for transthoracic pacing is often combined with an external defibrillator or cardiac monitoring apparatus, or both. Fig. 39-1 illustrates one such combination. Small metal disks (not shown in the illustration) are used with electrode paste for connection to the chest of the patient. The location of the electrodes is not critical, but one is often placed at the point of maximum cardiac impulse and the other electrode is placed at a symmetrical location on the right chest.

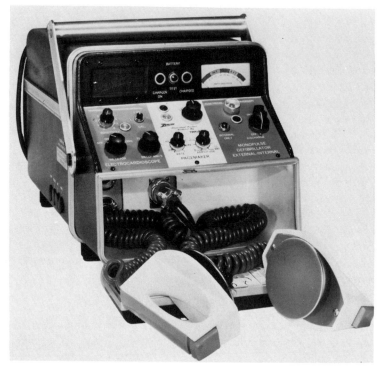

Fig. 39-1. Battery-operated defibrillator, pacemaker, and cardiac monitor. (Courtesy Travenol Laboratories, Inc., Morton Grove, Ill.)

The disks are held in place with a rubber strap. Chest pain and skin burns associated with transthoracic pacing ordinarily dictate that patients who require continued pacing should be switched to percutaneous transvenous pacing as soon as adequate facilities for the insertion of a catheter-type lead are available.

Temporary transvenous pacing. In temporary transvenous pacing, a lead structure with one or two electrodes on its distal end is introduced through a peripheral vein and advanced into the right ventricle or, if atrial pacing is desired, into the right atrium. Unipolar and bipolar leads with a variety of size and stiffness characteristics are available.

As one example, Medtronic supplies a Chardack type 5821 bipolar endocardial silicone rubber covered lead in which two platinum electrodes at the distal end of the lead are 3.2 mm. in diameter and 28 mm. apart. Insulated helical-wound conductors are used to connect the electrodes to the external terminals of the lead set. The stiffness needed for manipulating the tip of the catheter into the right ventricle is supplied by two stainless steel stylets, which are inserted into the lumens of the helical-wound conductors and removed after a satisfactory position has been obtained. A cutdown is required for the insertion of this catheter and the right external jugular vein is often selected. The procedure is best carried out under image intensifier fluoroscopy and the tip electrode is usually wedged into the apex of the ventricular cavity.

As another example, the type 370-210 bipolar lead supplied by the Cordis Corporation is only about 1.6 mm. in diameter and inherently stiff enough to be manipulated. It may be inserted into the vein by either percutaneous or cutdown techniques.

Still other leads are flexible enough that

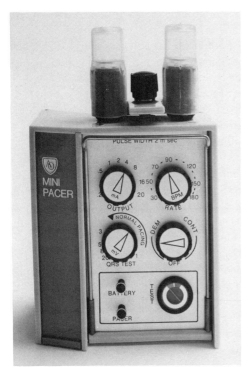

Fig. 39-2. External strap-on demand pacemaker of the type frequently used for short-term pacing. (Courtesy American Optical Corp., Bedford, Mass.)

they may be introduced into an appropriate vein and their distal ends more or less carried into position by the flow of the blood. Suitable positioning can be inferred from the unipolar electrocardiogram.

Small, transistorized, battery-powered pacemaker generators with both demand pacing and asynchronous pacing capabilities are favored for temporary transvenous applications. Such units are available from a number of manufacturers. Shown in Fig. 39-2 is American Optical Corporation's model 2101 Mini Pacer. This particular model has an output rate of 30 to 180 beats per minute, an output current of 0.2 to 20 milliamperes, a pulse width of 1.9 msec., and a refractory period ranging from 190 to 250 msec. In the demand mode, it supplies an impulse only when the heart rate falls below a predetermined value. In the asynchronous mode,

it delivers impulses independent of the cardiac rate. It, and similar apparatus from other manufacturers, can be used with either unipolar or bipolar leads. If a unipolar lead is used, it is necessary to connect the other terminal of the pacemaker to some kind of skin or subcutaneous electrode.

Pacemakers of this type are also widely used to energize atrial or ventricular leads that are brought through the chest wall at the time of cardiac surgery and that are intended for relatively short-term use.

Permanent asynchronous pacing. Although small, primary battery-powered, and completely implantable asynchronous pulse generators no longer dominate the permanent pacing field as they did a few years ago, they are still widely used in patients with established complete heart block. Available in a variety of unipolar and bipolar models, most asynchronous pulse generators can be used with either endocardial or myocardial leads.

In addition to nonadjustable models, asynchronous generators are available in which the rate or the amplitude or the width of the pulse may be manually adjusted before or after implantation.

A Medtronic Chardack model 5858 unipolar pacemaker generator and its myocardial lead are shown in Fig. 39-3. Designed for use in small children, the myocardial electrode is attached to the left ventricle and the generator is implanted in subcutaneous abdominal tissue. A platinum disk implanted in the side of the generator serves as the indifferent electrode. As the child grows, the lead unwinds from its circumferential groove and the generator rotates in its tissue pocket.

A General Electric model A2073AB dual amplitude pulse generator together with a bipolar endocardial lead is shown in Fig. 39-4. By removing an insulating label, this generator may be converted into a unipolar unit.

When endocardial leads are used, the tip of the electrode is ordinarily positioned in the apex of the right ventricle and the pulse generator is placed in a subcutaneous pocket beneath the medial portion of the clavicle. Fig. 39-5 is an x-ray photograph of a typical implantation, performed at the University of Missouri, in an adult of an asynchronous generator and bipolar endocardial lead system.

Permanent demand pacing. Completely implantable demand pacemakers were originally intended for use in patients with intermittent heart block. It was argued that their use would minimize the possibility of pacer-induced ventricular fibrillation resulting from competitive stimulation. Demand pacemakers are now used in the treatment of a variety of arrhythmias. Available from a number of sources and in both unipolar and bipolar models, demand pulse generators may usually be used with either endocardial or myocardial leads.

A Medtronic Chardack model 5942 bipolar demand pulse generator is illustrated in Fig. 39-6. In this particular model, the physician may adjust the rate before and after implantation to any desired value between 50 and 120 pulses per minute. Once the rate is selected, the generator delivers a pulse only when the patient's own heart rate drops below the selected rate. Since interference from external fields is more of a problem in demand pacing than in asynchronous pacing, a titanium housing is used to shield the generator from such fields. Furthermore, the circuit is designed so that

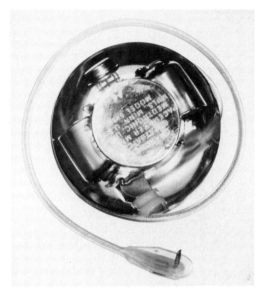

Fig. 39-3. Asynchronous pacemaker with myocardial lead intended for implantation in small children. (Courtesy Medtronic, Inc., Minneapolis, Minn.)

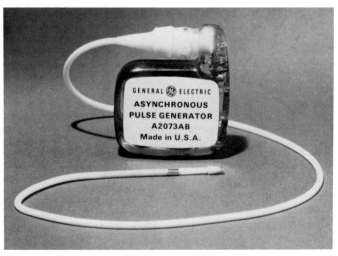

Fig. 39-4. Asynchronous pacemaker with bipolar endocardial lead. (Courtesy General Electric Co., Milwaukee, Wisc.)

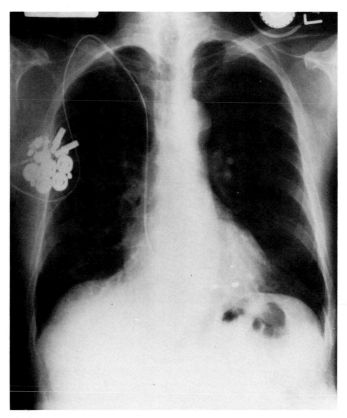

Fig. 39-5. X-ray film showing implanted asynchronous pacemaker with endocardial lead inserted through a vein into the right ventricle.

extremely strong continuous wave fields cause the generator to revert to its fixed rate mode. For the evaluation by the physician, of the viability of the system, a magnet may be held against the skin over the generator. This activates a reed switch and causes the unit to revert to a fixed rate. Upon the removal of the magnet, the generator resumes its normal operation.

Permanent ventricular synchronous pacing. In ventricular synchronous pacing, generator pulses are superimposed upon each detected R wave. In the event that an R wave is absent for a predetermined time following a generator pulse, another generator pulse is delivered anyway. The end result is quite similar to that achieved with demand pacing. If the natural rate is

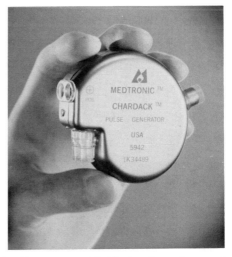

Fig. 39-6. Implantable bipolar demand pacemaker. (Courtesy Medtronic, Inc., Minneapolis, Minn.)

above a preselected value, the output of the pulse generator does not interfere with the rate. Otherwise, fixed rate pacing is realized.

Shown in Fig. 39-7 is a ventricular synchronous unipolar generator that is marketed by the Cordis Corporation under the trade name of Ectocor. Either a myocardial or an endocardial lead may be used. When a myo-cardial lead is employed, a spare lead is often attached to the ventricle and routed along with the active lead to the vicinity of the generator where it is capped for possible future use. A metal ground plate on the generator serves as the anode electrode. This model is ordinarily supplied with a base rate of 70 pulses per minute and with a

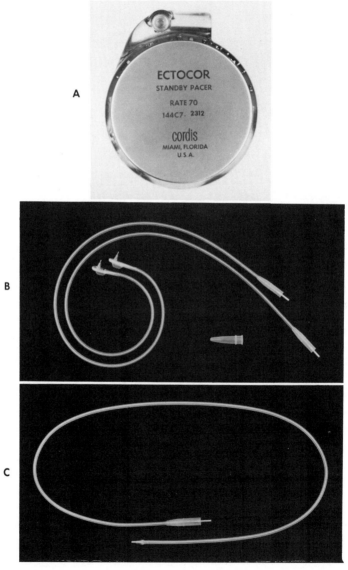

Fig. 39-7. Ventricular synchronous unipolar pacer together with endocardial and myocardial leads that may be used with it.

refractory period of 0.4 seconds so that the generator pulse rate can never exceed 150 pulses per minute.

Permanent atrial synchronous pacing. The unipolar P wave synchronized pulse generator shown in Fig. 39-8 is marketed by the Cordis Corporation under the trade name of Atricor. Of the three leads shown, one is sutured epicardially to the left atrium and the other two are sutured to the left ventricle. One of the ventricular leads is a spare. A metal ground plate on the generator serves as the anode electrode.

In operation, a P wave, which is picked up in the left atrium lead, serves, after a delay of 0.12 seconds, to trigger a generator pulse which is delivered to the left ventricle via the active ventricular lead. Thus, the pacemaker effectively serves to artificially bridge the conduction defect and the ventricular rate ordinarily follows the atrial rate. However, in the event that the atrial rate exceeds 125 per minute, the ventricle is stimulated only once for every two atrial beats. Furthermore, if the atrial rate falls below 60 per minute, the ventricle is stimulated at a fixed rate of 60 impulses per minute.

Patients with complete heart block but having relatively unimpaired atrial and ventricular function are probably the best candidates for atrial synchronous pacing.

Future directions

The completely implantable primary battery-powered pacemakers, which are currently so widely used, require replacement after an average time of about 2 to 3 years.

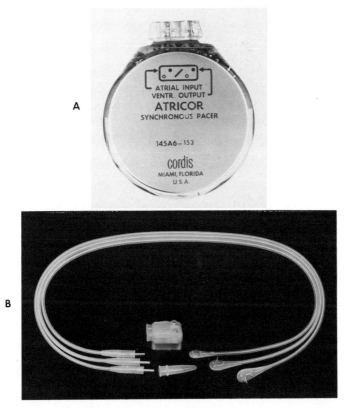

Fig. 39-8. P wave synchronized cardiac pacemaker together with epicardial leads to be used with it.

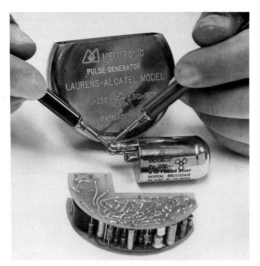

Fig. 39-9. Partially assembled nuclear-powered bipolar demand pacemaker. (Courtesy Medtronic, Inc., Minneapolis, Minn.)

Battery failure is the predominate reason for replacement. The prospects for achieving an appreciable increase in the longevity of implanted energy sources and consequently in the useful life of pacemakers seem excellent.

One promising approach is that exemplified by Medtronic's Laurens-Alcatel nuclear-powered pacemaker, which is currently (1972) undergoing clinical evaluation in the United States and several countries in Europe. Shown partially assembled in Fig. 39-9, this bipolar demand pacemaker that is intended for use with myocardial leads has sufficient plutonium 238 fuel to function for at least 10 years. Whether the actual longevity will, in fact, be limited by the fuel supply or by other factors remains to be seen from the results of the clinical trials.

Primary batteries that are used in pacemaker service fail long before delivering their rated energy. Rather evolutionary development in primary battery design with explicit attention to the specifications inherent in pacemaker service may serve to yield improved units. For example, General Electric is currently evaluating improved mercury-zinc batteries that are projected to give 5 years service.

We should also expect the development of pacemakers with more sophisticated decision-making capabilities. American Optical Corporation's BIFOCAL AV sequential demand pacer represents such a trend. The availability of integrated circuits and the associated technology should serve to facilitate additional developments. It may also prove possible to incorporate ventricular fibrillation detection capabilities and provisions for defibrillation into the pacer package.

Chapter 40

RESUSCITATION OF THE NEWBORN INFANT

Robert Hook and Clarence D. Davis

Introduction

Significant advances in both anesthetic and obstetric care of the parturient have not eliminated the lifesaving value of resuscitation efforts at birth. The factors involved in the production of neonatal depression are many. They may be related to the stress of normal delivery or be the result of normal birth conditions superimposed on a fetus already compromised in utero.

In an attempt to understand the physiologic mechanisms operative in asphyxia neonatorum, respiratory responses to controlled experimental asphyxia have been investigated in newborn monkeys. In the initial phases of asphyxia, the unmedicated experimental animal demonstrates increased frequency and depth of respiratory effort for about 3 minutes. This initial phase of hyperpnea is followed by a period of primary apnea lasting about 1 minute. Following this, a period of regular slow gasping efforts begins. After 4 to 5 minutes the frequency of this gasping decreases, until after approximately 8½ minutes a period of secondary apnea occurs.

In these experimental animals a variety of external stimuli such as cold or slapping can initiate gasping during the period of primary apnea, but such stimuli are not effective during the period of secondary apnea. At this time artificial ventilation and the correction of acidosis are necessary to reinitiate gasping efforts. It is also possible to eliminate the initial period of primary hyperpnea with narcotics and systemic anesthetics administered to the mother. It has been well established in these experimental animals that in the stage of secondary apnea, there is a direct relationship between the duration of the apnea and the degree of difficulty of resuscitative measures necessary to reinitiate gasping. Thus, the longer artificial ventilation is delayed during this stage, the longer the resuscitation will take. Finally, it has been shown that prolongation of asphyxia beyond 4 minutes of the secondary apneic stage results in extensive damage to the animal's brainstem, while monkeys resuscitated before the onset of secondary apnea demonstrated no brain damage.

These experimental animal data serve only as a basic model with which we can attempt to organize data observed under clinical circumstances in humans. Difficulties in resuscitation of the infant occur in about one out of every ten deliveries. The commonly used terms "apnea neonatorum" and "asphyxia neonatorum" can be misleading. It is well recognized that every fetus is subject to a certain degree of "asphyxia" during the course of vaginal delivery and in some cases the asphyxia begins in intrauterine life. It is the degree to which the infants become hypoxic, hypercarbic, and acidotic during an intrauterine catastrophy or a traumatic delivery that determines the severity of the respiratory depression in the newborn infant.

In severe asphyxia, extreme degrees of hypoxia and acidosis may lead to cardiac embarrasment requiring external cardiac massage to support the circulation during the resuscitation. This may lead to the erroneous diagnosis of successful resuscitation of a stillborn infant. The term stillborn in such a situation is a misnomer, since the presence of cardiac electrical activity is impossible to detect without the aid of continuous ECG monitoring of the fetus. Such cases must represent extreme neonatal asphyxia, rather than the true lifeless situation implied by the term "obstetrical stillborn."

Factors involved in the production of newborn asphyxia are multiple and complex. They will be discussed from the point of view of maternal, fetal, and obstetric management considerations.

Maternal factors involved in producing neonatal asphyxia

Age. There seems to be some general correlation between age of the mother and the degree of birth asphyxia. Whether this is only apparent or is real and related to maternal disease factors and/or obstetric management problems is difficult to establish. In any case, as the age of the mother increases it is well to be alert to the possibility of the need for vigorous resuscitation.

Parity. It is not difficult to understand why primiparous mothers deliver more babies that are hard to resuscitate than do multiparous ones. Constant efforts at improvement of obstetric management will eliminate much of this differential. The reason for increased need for infant resuscitation in the grand multipara is more difficult to understand. It may be related to poor placentation, more frequent precipitate labor, a casual attitude on the part of the obstetrician, and/or some yet unknown specific factor.

Maternal condition. A multitude of maternal disease patterns has an effect on fetal welfare before, during, and after the delivery. Preeclampsia, eclampsia, diabetes, hypertension, renal and cardiovascular disease, and many other conditions favor fetal distress. The development of fetal monitoring systems utilizing continuous fetal ECG and intrauterine pressure recordings, together with fetal acid base data obtained through scalp sampling, has contributed much new information. Using such systems, it has been possible to study intrauterine fetal welfare during labor and evaluate the effects of many maternal conditions on the ability of the fetus to tolerate the stresses of labor. Some investigators have been able to predict newborn Apgar scores on the basis of such data with amazing accuracy.

Fetal factors affecting the incidence of neonatal apnea

Prematurity. The premature infant presents a special problem in resuscitation and its magnitude increases in proportion to the prematurity. The premature infant is hypersensitive to the effects of central nervous system depressants used for analgesia and anesthesia. These should be used sparingly, if at all. The premature infant's undeveloped central nervous system and pulmonary immaturity are responsible for various types of respiratory difficulty. The avoidance of undue trauma and large quantities of depressant analgesic drugs is of the utmost importance in the obstetric management of such an infant, and meticulous attention must be given to the details of the resuscitation technique.

Postmaturity. Postmaturity is not a common occurrence. The true postmature baby presents special problems, probably because placental senility has subjected it to chronic intrauterine hypoxia. The babies frequently die suddenly in utero, or when born alive, many tolerate birth asphyxia poorly.

Erythroblastosis fetalis. The problem in this disease is not one of resuscitative difficulties per se, but in severe cases may be one of anemic hypoxia because of destruction of fetal erythrocytes. High output cardiac failure can be a prominent feature of the disease and is often helped by umbilical venous phlebotomy.

Obstetrical management factors contributing to increased neonatal apnea

Conduct of labor. There is a steady increase in neonatal mortality when the duration of labor exceeds 24 hours. So-called conservative obstetrics becomes very radical when the life of the infant is lost because of false pride in a low cesarean section rate. There are fetal as well as maternal indications for abdominal delivery. It may require the wisdom of Solomon to judge correctly whether or when such a procedure should be done strictly on a fetal distress indication. Surely cesarean section should never be delayed until there is already marked fetal embarrassment. One feels very foolish doing a section for a fetal indication and ending up with a nonviable baby. Suffice to say, whenever there has been prolonged and/or traumatic (including precipitate) labor, one should anticipate the need for infant resuscitation. Neonatal apnea should be anticipated in any delivery that is likely to cause undue trauma to the fetal head. In order of decreasing likelihood of asphyxia, the following can be listed: version and extraction, high forceps, difficult midforceps and breech extractions, and assisted breech deliveries.

Cesarean section. Cesarean section offers a special problem in resuscitation because of the indications for the procedure, relative increase in incidence of prematurity, increased likelihood of fetal aspiration, and increase in RDS (respiratory distress syndrome) or hyaline membrane disease. Probably every baby delivered by cesarean section, regardless of whether it seems to be doing well or not, should have both intratracheal and gastric aspiration at birth, plus 12 to 18 hours of 40% oxygen and close observation.

Prolapse of cord. The chances for increased need of resuscitation in this situation seem obvious. One should not violate obstetric rules in the interests of an already severely decompensated fetus.

Placental abnormalities. Neonatal apnea should be anticipated in any instance of placenta praevia, premature separation, tetanic uterine contraction, or other placental anomalies resulting in fetal hypoperfusion.

Anesthesia and analgesia. As obstetric care improves, the contributions of drugs used for analgesia and anesthesia to the development of neonatal apnea are becoming increasingly apparent. The injudicious use of narcotic analgesics in labor causes fetal central nervous system depression and may contribute greatly to an increased incidence of neonatal apnea. General anesthesia with potent inhalation agents significantly reduces the fetal tolerance of hypoxia at delivery by depressing the fetal respiratory center. Babies born after the use of either type of drug (narcotic or general anesthetic) must be observed carefully for moderate to severe degrees of depression at birth.

Fetal distress and its diagnosis. Continuous monitoring of the fetal heart rate during labor has contributed significantly to our ability to anticipate newborn apnea in the clinical situation.

Diagnosis of fetal distress. Whenever the fetal heart rate is below 100 more than 30 seconds after termination of the uterine contraction or thick meconium is being passed, or both (except in instances of breech presentation), some degree of fetal distress should be anticipated. Hon has identified three basic fetal heart rate (FHR) patterns in utero. The cord compression, unless severe, and head compression patterns are generally nonsinister; that is, they are temporary in nature and are not associated with low Apgar scores. The third pattern, uteroplacental insufficiency (UPI), can be lethal, and there is a direct relationship between the total duration of UPI and the predicted Apgar score.

Basic principles of the technique of infant resuscitation

In certain situations where fetal distress in utero is discernible by fetal electrocardiogram, resuscitative procedures can be instituted prior to the delivery. Correction of severe persistent cord compression patterns can frequently be accomplished by positional changes in the mother. Oxygen administration to the mother as well as lateral positioning to correct maternal hypotension can correct fetal bradycardia associated with uteroplacental insufficiency type patterns.

The most commonly used clinical criteria for the assessment of the newborn is the Apgar score (Table 40-1).

After the infant is properly classified according to the Apgar method, his clinical status can be assessed by using the following grouping:

Apgar rating 1 minute after birth	Clinical status
5-8	Mildly-moderately depressed
3-5	Moderately-severely depressed
0-3	Severely depressed

The normal newborn (that is, the neonate who has not been subject to a sufficient degree of hypoxia to produce neonatal apnea) will breathe spontaneously within a few seconds after delivery. When attempts are made at spontaneous respiration the main effort should be directed to clearing the airway and administering oxygen. Suctioning of the oral and nasopharynx with a soft rubber bulb is usually adequate.

Newborn infants should be quickly placed in a semilateral position with a folded towel under the shoulders. The crib should be placed such that the infant's head is lower than the feet. In this position gentle suctioning of the oropharynx and the nose may be carried out. Oxygen should be administered at high flow directly into the infant's face and tactile stimulation in the form of gentle slapping or back rubbing used to stimulate respiration. During all of the preceding maneuvers, care should be taken to keep heat loss from the infant's surface to a minimum by covering the infant with warmed blankets or, better, by using a radiant heating device over the crib.

Passage of a catheter down the nasopharynx is a maneuver of some value to empty the stomach, and prove the patency of the esophagus, however this should not be attempted until the initial hypoxia and hypercarbia have been relieved by a few

Table 40-1. Evaluation of newborn infant (Apgar method of scoring)*

Sign	0	1	2
Heart rate	Absent	Slow (below 100)	Over 100
Respiratory effort	Absent	Slow	Good
Muscle tone	Limp	Irregular	Crying
		Some flexion of extremities	Active motion
Response to catheter in nostril (tested after oropharynx is clear)	No response	Grimace	Cry
Color	Blue	Body pink	Completely pink
	Pale	Extremities blue	

Sixty seconds after the complete birth of the infant (disregarding the cord and placenta) the five objective signs are evaluated and each given a score of 0, 1, or 2. A score of 10 indicates an infant in the best possible condition.

*Quoted with slight changes from Abramson, H.: Resuscitation of the newborn infant, St. Louis, 1960, The C. V. Mosby Co.; based on information from Apgar, V.: Proposal for a new method of evaluation of the newborn infant, Anesth. Analg. **32**:260, 1953, and from Apgar, V., Holaday, D. A., James, L. S., Weisbrot, I. M., and Berrien, C.: Evaluation of the newborn infant—second report, J.A.M.A. **168**:1985, 1958.

minutes of oxygen. When carried out in babies still hypoxic, such a catheter may cause serious ventricular arrhythmias and bradycardia as well as reflex inhibition of respiration (iatrogenic apnea). Endotracheal intubation is seldom necessary in the mildly depressed newborn. When the pharyngeal secretions are stained with meconium or blood and large amounts of either of these are present in the amniotic fluid, gentle endotracheal suction with a plastic catheter to remove stained secretions from the upper airway is indicated.

MODERATELY TO SEVERELY DEPRESSED INFANT (APGAR 3-5 AT 1 MINUTE)

Moderately to severely depressed infants initially may make some spontaneous attempts at respiration or may begin to do so when stimulated mechanically. In many cases the stimulation of airway suctioning and movement may serve to improve the quality and quantity of respiratory efforts to the extent that the methods described may simply have to be continued for a longer period of time before the infant begins to recover. If, at 1 minute after birth, the infant is making no continued efforts at spontaneous respiration and the heart rate falls below 100 per minute, artificial ventilation with oxygen should be immediately instituted. Initially, it is faster and easier to ventilate a newborn with a hand-held positive pressure bag (many such devices are available) and an oropharyngeal airway, if necessary. When using positive pressure ventilation in an infant it is essential that the airways be free of foreign material and that the infant's head be hyperextended to ensure patency of the airway. Secretions in the upper airway can be forced into the periphery of the lung by positive pressure and flexion of the neck obstructs the airway and results in the insufflation of oxygen into the stomach. In order to ventilate the depressed infant, inflation pressures of 25 to 45 cm. H_2O are necessary to expand the newborn lungs. This is a considerable pressure, and, if the airway is not patent because of improper positioning or obstruction by foreign substances, considerable gastric distension may occur. The above maneuvers will, if carried out properly, enable one to easily ventilate the infant. When attempts at artificial ventilation are not successful due to obstruction, or for other reasons, and the infant's condition is deteriorating, an endotracheal tube should be passed to facilitate ventilation. When artificial ventilation has been instituted it should be continued until the infant's muscle tone, heart rate, and color have become normal. At this point, many infants will begin to attempt spontaneous respiration and will eventually return to a normal pattern. Occasionally, however, vigorous artificial ventilation will produce apnea caused by overventilation. This can be corrected by stimulating the infant and allowing short periods (30 to 40 seconds) of apnea to regain the normal respiratory stimulus.

SEVERELY DEPRESSED INFANT (APGAR 0-3 AT 1 MINUTE)

The severely depressed infant (Apgar 0-3 at 1 minute) is usually apneic at birth with no heart rate or one below 100 per minute. The infant is limp and unresponsive and often pale rather than intensely cyanotic.

Such a severely depressed infant should be quickly intubated, after rapid brief suctioning, and ventilated with 100% oxygen. If the heart rate is absent or below 40 per minute, external cardiac massage should be instituted to improve circulation to vital centers. The umbilical artery should be cannulated and an injection of 3 mEq. per kilogram of body weight of sodium bicarbonate mixed with an equal volume of 5% dextrose given over a 2 to 5 minute period. If no cardiovascular improvement occurs with the preceding chemical therapy, 1 to 5 μg. per kilogram of body weight of epinephrine should be injected into the umbilical vein while external cardiac massage is continued. Direct cardiac injection of epinephrine is unnecessary and carries great risk of major trauma in the infant.

After the initial attempts at chemical correction of acidosis described above, further chemical correction should be guided by laboratory determinations of pH, P_{CO_2}, and base deficit. In infants where maternal narcotic administration is a factor in the depression, the use of 0.2 mg. of nalorphine injected into the umbilical vein is indicated. In babies born of mothers who are narcotic addicts, however, narcotic antagonists must be used with great care in the infant, if at all, since they may induce severe withdrawal symptoms.

Summary

Every newborn infant is subject, during labor, to a series of repeated stresses. The normal newborn infant has suffered a mild degree of hypoxia and hypercarbia during birth. The potential for difficulties in the seemingly normal delivery must never be underestimated. The complexity of the difficulties encountered in the complicated situation is great. Any physician working in a delivery room must have a basic knowledge, both theoretical and practical, of the elements of infant resuscitation. The teaching of this and the accompanying skills to interns and residents is a responsibility of major proportions.

Chapter 41

RESUSCITATION AFTER EXSANGUINATING HEMORRHAGE

Successful resuscitation of the patient whose heart has stopped because of exsanguinating hemorrhage requires added information and the employment of additional specific measures beyond those normally employed in most cases of cardiac resuscitation. Although Negovskii and his group in Moscow have been working with the problems of cardiac resuscitation under conditions of exsanguination for years, attention only recently has been directed at this problem in the United States. Many of our current concepts for proper resuscitation of exsanguination have evolved from studies done during the Vietnam war. Complete agreement is still lacking but the material presented to the reader in this chapter is a composite of much of the present-day thought on the subject.

Surprisingly few reports deal specifically with cardiac massage as a lifesaving measure following severe hemorrhage. Connoly details the events in two patients upon whom external cardiac massage was instituted successfully after massive hemorrhage provoked cardiac asystole. I would agree with his conclusion that an attitude of hopelessness has often prevailed when cardiac arrest followed severe hemorrhage. With the advent of external cardiac massage technique, the feebly beating or stopped heart can again be made to propel blood of sufficient oxygenation to postpone irreversible cerebral anoxia until blood volume replacement is accomplished. A dramatic example of this occurred in 1969 at the United States Air Force Academy when a cadet accidentally ran a

javelin through his heart. The victim was running toward the Academy's intramural fields and did not see a fellow cadet ahead of him carrying a javelin. The javelin suddenly became impaled in the ground and the victim ran into the javelin end, which pierced the heart and punctured the vena cava. Bleeding was massive. Mouth-to-mouth resuscitation was started on the field; as no heartbeat was detected, external heart massage was begun. With continued artificial circulation and ventilation, the patient was brought to the hospital for surgical repair of the punctured vena cava and cardiac wound. Blood volume was restored. The cadet was discharged from the hospital 14 days later.

In previous editions of this book I have detailed some of the measures that I have employed in the operating room when exsanguinating hemorrhage was encountered. On several occasions I have used intra-aortic retrograde transfusions. In addition, I have even resorted to intracardiac transfusions. While the above techniques have been used infrequently and perhaps may be most often substituted by intravenous fluids, I have commonly employed aortic compression proximal to the point of bleeding in order to prevent rapid loss of blood and to allow time for blood replacement.

Obviously the achievement of successful resuscitation for patients with cardiac arrest and exsanguinating hemorrhage requires some additional measures other than those usually applicable to most cardiopulmonary resuscitative efforts. A highly esteemed professor of surgery in Montreal told me that every year he would give a lecture to the students on hemorrhagic shock. After great emphasis on the point that the treatment for hemorrhagic shock is *blood,* he would then pull out a unit of blood from the desk and throw it with great gusto at the blackboard, splattering blood over much of the front of the room. Few students in his classes ever forgot that whole blood remains the accepted essential in the treatment of severe hemorrhage.

Nevertheless, in some situations, resuscitation can be initiated with an asanguineous fluid. Such a measure is highly advantageous for several reasons, in addition to the time it allows for adequate crossmatching of blood. As is mentioned above, sludging in the microcirculation and subsequent perfusion diminution occur with pressures under 50 mm. Hg. In addition, fluid replacement helps clear renal tubules by solute diuresis and helps correct functional sodium deficits and possible extracellular volume deficits that may accompany hemorrhage. Even though there will be a degree of hemodilution, the remaining oxygen-carrying red blood cell mass will be allowed to reach the vital organs.

Most commonly, lactated Ringer's solution or physiologic saline solution is the fluid substituted for blood. With the infusion of large quantities of fluid and massive blood transfusions, many considerations and questions arise: Will the lactate in Ringer's solution further accentuate the lactic acidosis present with inadequate perfusion of the tissues? Will hyperchloremia be produced by a large amount of unbuffered saline solution, diluting the buffered base and further worsening the preexisting acidosis? Is it necessary to administer blood that is inadequately warmed? Are there real dangers of hyperkalemia from the high potassium content of stored blood? Do patients receiving large quantities of blood need added calcium during or following blood transfusions? What particular monitoring is essential? How

does one combat the occasional clotting abnormality encountered with massive blood transfusions? These and other questions commonly arise to further complicate the achievement of successful cardiopulmonary resuscitation during and after exsanguinating hemorrhage.

In patients requiring replacement of blood volume under the controlled environment of the operating room, an accurate assessment of the exact status of the circulating blood volume is not always easy. Even more difficult is assessing the needs of patients brought to the emergency room or in situations outside the operating room. While the arterial blood pressure and the ventricular contractile forces are important determinants, the optional amount of fluid or blood required is particularly indicated in the response of the central venous pressure. Although many factors will alter the central venous pressure response, including positive pressure ventilation, cardiac tamponade, and medication, this pressure will be a most helpful guide in indicating adequate restoration of fluid volume.

With a catheter in the bladder, the urinary output should be monitored closely. An output of 30 to 50 ml. per hour, minimally, should be an index of adequate tissue perfusion. When oliguria persists in spite of adequate blood volume, one is prompted to give mannitol intravenously in a dose of 25 gm. per 10 to 20-minute period. Mannitol should not be given in doses exceeding 100 gm. over a 24-hour period. Furosemide (Lasix) (20 to 40 mg.) or ethacrynic acid (Edecrin) (50 to 100 mg.) may be given intravenously if an adequate response to mannitol does not occur.

As one proceeds, the goals are improvement in color of the patient, return of normal level of consciousness with a strong pulse volume, urinary output of 30 to 50 ml. per hour, systolic pressure of 100 mm. Hg and central venous pressure of at least 2 to 10 cm. of water.

With the patient exsanguinating, with no

blood pressure or pulse, and showing absent or agonal respirations, closed-chest cardiac massage should be given at once and an adequate airway with artificial ventilation should be instituted. Intravenous routes should be made available with at least two to four large-bore catheters, one being used to mark central venous pressure. Blood should be immediately drawn for typing and crossmatching, for venous and arterial blood sampling, and an indwelling catheter should be placed in the bladder. Ringer's lactate or physiologic saline solution should be begun as soon as an intravenous route is available. The primary goal at this point is that of reestablishment of cerebral perfusion as well as a near-normal tissue perfusion to the rest of the body. Irreversible metabolic derangements occur if perfusion is too long delayed.

Lowery and associates considered the effects of electrolyte solutions in resuscitation in human hemorrhagic shock and conclude that the infusion of exogenous lactate does not seem harmful nor does it obviate the usefulness of blood lactate determinations. Acid base disturbances or electrolyte imbalances are not a serious consideration in the use of Ringer's lactate.

Kirimli and associates in their excellent studies on resuscitation of cardiac arrest due to exsanguination reviewed the matter of respiratory and metabolic acidosis seen after the resumption of spontaneous circulation and believe that the acidosis is the result of washout of lactacidemia after struggling, agony, and clinical death. They believe that their data strongly indicate the need for hyperventilation and prolonged administration of bicarbonate, titrated by frequent arterial pH determinations during the postresuscitation period.

When a coagulation laboratory is not immediately available, such tests as Lee-White clotting time, platelet count, and observation of clot lysis can be performed. If the platelet count is below 30,000, platelet concentrates or fresh blood less than 4 hours old can be given. If the platelet count is satisfactory, however, low levels of factor V, factor VII, or fibrinogen may be responsible and can usually be restored with fresh frozen plasma or fresh blood. Excessive fibrinolysis as shown by clotting in a test tube may be treated with ε-aminocaproic acid (Amicar).

Thus it would seem that the warming of transfused blood to body temperature is of particular importance, omission of calcium salts is important, as well as the administration of sodium bicarbonate (44.6 mEq. for every 5 units of bank blood). Finally, Wilson recommends the use of steroids (up to 50 mg. per kilogram hydrocortisone intravenously) in severe, persistent, unresponsive shock when blood volume, acid-base balance, and calcium needs appear to have been rectified.

Recent work by Drucker and associates at Toronto indicates that pancreatic blood flow and insulin output are considerably altered in severe hemorrhage. At first, despite a markedly impaired blood flow, the pancreas is capable of releasing insulin in response to minimal hyperglycemia during the early phase of shock. With continued hypovolemia, a fall in insulin output indicates possibly impaired insulinogenesis.

A ruptured abdominal aortic aneurysm is not a rare clinical entity. Cases of retroperitoneal rupture with a subsequent tamponade by the peritoneal structures often are seen in the hospital in time for successful control. An anterior rupture directly into the abdominal cavity represents such a massive blood loss that only optimal circumstances will allow for salvage. I saw such a case on ward rounds one day when a patient with a preoperative abdominal aneurysm suddenly was found pulseless and with agonal respiratory movements. The pupils were dilated. He was immediately rushed to the operating room where the chest was opened within 2 minutes of the original discovery. The left fourth interspace was entered and the aorta was squeezed between the fingers at a point just above the diaphragm. The heart was then in asystole. Since 8 units of blood were available in the blood bank in preparation for the patient's surgery the next day, it was rapidly administered following Ringer's lactate. After brief external compression efforts, the heart resumed its regular rhythm. In the meantime, the rest of the operating team were opening the abdomen and removing the sequestered blood to identify the proper level for placing the aortic clamp above the aneurysm, which was subsequently resected. A bifurcation graft was inserted and the patient was discharged in a satisfactory condition on the ninth postoperative day.

Such a direct approach to the aorta has several advantages. By opening the chest one can easily obtain control of the aorta either by fingertip compression or by placing a clamp across the aorta above the diaphragm. In addition, the actual status of the heart can be ascertained and direct cardiac compression can be instituted. Such an approach obviates the blind application of an aortic clamp within the abdomen in the presence of several thousand milliliters of blood but allows the clamp to be placed after the blood has been suctioned and a direct visualization of the aorta allows for avoidance of injury to structures in the upper abdomen such as the pancreas or renal vessels.

What is the sequence of events during exsanguination? Do respirations stop first? Does the heart stop in fibrillation or asystole? Changes observed during exsanguinating hemorrhage are not as well documented as one might suspect, but Kirimli, Kampschulte, and Safar have contributed significantly to an understanding of the pattern of experimental death from exsanguinating hemorrhage. All the experimental dogs were in asystole except approximately 6%, which spontaneously developed ventricular fibrillation after 4 to 5 minutes of pulselessness. Invariably pulselessness preceded respiratory arrest.

Pupillary and corneal reflexes remained active until after the pupils started to dilate, which is in contrast to that noted under conditions of asphyxia or increasing depth of anesthesia where cessation of lid and corneal reflexes usually precedes pupillary dilatation. Maximal pupillary dilatation coincided with the last gasp. No changes in the retinal arteries were noted until mean arterial pressure declined to 50 mm. Hg; at that time sludging began, and it became increasingly greater as the pressure fell. Retinal capillary blood flow ceased altogether when aortic pressure fell to 25 to 30 mm. Hg, and blood columns in arteries and veins of the retina began to fragment when the aortic pressure was approximately 15 mm. Hg.

The animals, surprisingly enough, reached death in a state of alkalemia with normal arterial P_{O_2} and low arterial P_{CO_2}. The lactacidemia from progressively inadequate tissue perfusion was compensated by hyperventilation as far as the blood pH was concerned. Significantly, sludging of blood in the renal arteries began when the arterial pressure was near 40 mm. Hg and capillary blood flow ceased at an aortic pressure of 15 mg. Hg. Gasping respirations started with cessation of arterial pulsations and continued for 2 minutes during pulselessness (agonal state); this was followed by apnea and cessation of circulation (clinical death).

The prognosis in patients receiving 20 or more units of stored blood is poor. Boyan and co-workers have reduced their mortality in such patients from an earlier 30% mortality to 11% and suggest the following general guidelines:

1. Rapid blood transfusion with stored, cold bank blood requires warming of the blood to body temperature.
2. Sodium bicarbonate should be administered to buffer the acid bank blood when given to a patient in hemorrhagic shock or to one receiving rapidly more than 2500 ml. of citrated blood.

In this connection Collins and associates, from the U.S. Army Surgical Research Team, report on their experience in Vietnam with resuscitation using stored blood and the related acid-base status of seriously wounded combat casualties. In thirty-five combat casualties acid-base changes were studied and it was concluded that patients who responded well to transfusion easily handled the infused acid load of the stored blood with reversed preexisting metabolic acidosis, when present. Increasing acidemia during transfusion was associated with uncontrolled hemorrhage and was more likely due to shock than to transfusion. Routine empiric administration of alkalizing solutions during rapid or sustained transfusion is not always necessary in previously healthy, vigorous individuals.

3. Hypercapnia can be prevented by hyperventilation in patients receiving large amounts of bank blood.

4. Patients with normal calcium metabolism do not need the addition of calcium salts. This rule does not apply to infants.

There is still some disagreement as to the need for added calcium during or following blood transfusions. Generally speaking, most patients not in shock do not need calcium, regardless of the amount of blood they are given, but patients in shock may be unable to mobilize sufficient amounts of calcium to maintain levels necessary to optimal cardiovascular functions. Wilson and co-workers in discussing this matter, state that they have had several patients in shock refractory to all forms of therapy until adequate quantities of calcium chloride were given intravenously for every 2 to 4 units of blood. Citrate reduction of the level of ionized calcium is especially likely to occur when the perfusion of the bone is reduced by hypovolemia (Eustace and others). Eustace ascribes much of the success in very successful resuscitation after cardiac arrests due to hemorrhage to the repeated administration of ionized calcium along with the stored blood that was being given.

5. If the patient is normothermic and good tissue perfusion is reestablished, the citrate in bank blood is not a problem.

6. No significant increase of potassium occurs with massive transfusion.

Although blood stored for as long as 21 days may have as much as a fivefold increase in serum potassium level, large volumes of bank blood preserved in A.C.D. (sodium citrate, citric acid, and dextrose) solution apparently do not play a significant role in the development of increased levels of serum potassium concentration during operation. Actually the level of serum potassium concentration may be more a product of the acid-base balance of the blood and the degree of tissue trauma that has taken place (Vogel).

In addition, there is reduced potassium excretion associated with oliguria. In Wilson and co-workers' analysis of their experience with massive blood transfusions over an 8-year period, they were able to report that most patients were normokalemic. In fact, almost as many of their patients were hypokalemic (10.1%) as were hyperkalemic (12.1%). In any event, it seems wise to obtain frequent potassium determinations, particularly if the patient is receiving digitalis.

7. When the blood transfusion approaches 8 to 10 units, 500 ml. of fresh frozen plasma, containing all plasma clotting factors but platelets, should be given. Again, Wilson and associates emphasize that blood stored for more than 24 hours has no effective platelets and has grossly reduced amounts of factor V and factor VIII. They, in fact, urge that a unit of fresh blood, not more than 24 hours old, should be given after every 3 units of stored blood as a prophylactic measure to prevent any clotting abnormalities associated with massive transfusion.

8. Water and electrolyte balance should not be overlooked.

9. Surgery and manipulations of abdominal or thoracic viscera create a "third space" to which plasma or interstitial fluid are translocated. A trans-

fusion of 5% solution of human plasma protein (Plasmanate) or dextran 75 will replenish the plasma loss.

10. A thromboelastogram provides a quick and readily available test for clotting deficiencies encountered during massive blood transfusions.

Although cardiac asystole most commonly occurs first with exsanguinating hemorrhage, ventricular fibrillation may soon develop during resuscitation efforts. We know that fibrillatory thresholds are considerably reduced with hypothermia and metabolic acidosis and their correction may aid considerably in the ease with which the heart may be defibrillated.

Following the recommendations of Negovskii from his work with arterial reinfusion of warm, heparinized shed arterial blood plus epinephrine without cardiac compression, Safar and his group add epinephrine, 1 mg. or more, intravenously to rapid venous infusion combined with cardiac massage.

Circumferential pneumatic pressure

The use of external counterpressure through the use of circumferential pneumatic pressure applied about the lower extremities and abdomen has attracted attention since Crile originally described his pneumatic suit in 1903. Initially used to combat postural hypotension in patients being operated upon in a semirecumbent or a sitting position, it was later used (1909) to treat a patient in hemorrhagic shock.

G SUITS*

The principle of circumferential pneumatic compression is, of course, exemplified in the modern aviation antigravity suit and was used during World War II by fighter pilots to combat retinal ischemia from centrifugal forces.

---

*An excellent article on the control of abdominal hemorrhage by external counterpressure using the G suit is found in the July, 1972, issue of *Resuscitation* (Lewis, D. G., Mackenzie, A., and McNeill, I. F.: Resuscitation 1:117, 1972).

Gardner employed an aviation antigravity suit to prevent postural hypotension during certain neurosurgical operations carried out with the patient in the sitting position. Gardner describes the use of the antigravity suit in a case of a postpartum intra-abdominal hemorrhage requiring fifty-eight transfusions. In another case the G suit was used in a postpartum hemorrhage that required twenty transfusions. In each instance only one additional unit of blood was required after application of the G suit.

The employment of the G suit has been shown to control bleeding from a longitudinal wound of the abdominal aorta without interrupting circulation. The effect of circumferential pneumatic compression with the G suit to 10, 20, 30, and 40 mm. Hg has disclosed identical increases in intraperitoneal pressure. This type of pressure is transmitted equally in all directions to structures below the diaphragm (Figs. 41-1 and 41-2). There is reduced abdominal aortic flow and increased venous return to structures above the diaphragm (Gardner and Storer). It would seem that a major contribution of the G suit would be in its ability to buy time in an emergency; for example, one would be able to transport a patient to obtain appropriate care. Certainly it would seem that the G suit should be investigated as a worthwhile adjunct to the equipment available in ambulances and emergency rooms.

Gray and associates studied the effects of G suit inflation on the cardiovascular dynamics of twelve normal volunteers. They conclude that the usefulness of the G suit in preventing syncope may be related to occlusion of the peripheral vasculature and to possible redistribution of cardiac output. Changes following sudden G suit release suggest that peripheral vasodilatation occurs, creating a situation that could cause syncope in the erect or semirecumbent individual.

The antigravity suit should not be used when there is respiratory embarrassment or

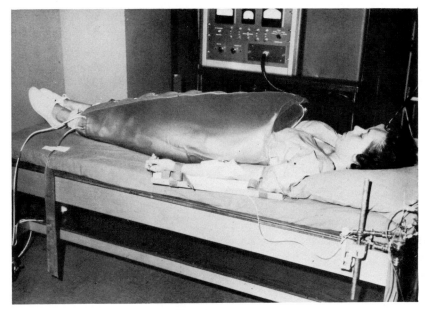

Fig. 41-1. G suit.

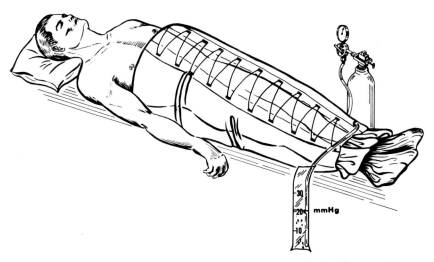

Fig. 41-2. Clinical modification of G suit consists of wraparound vinyl bag applied up to the epigastrium. Air introduced through inlet tube escapes when the pressure equals the height of the column of water in escape valve, the U tube shown hanging from the side of the table. In the healthy person, a pressure of 26 to 39 cm. of water—20 to 30 mm. Hg—causes little reduction of vital capacity.

chest injury. When bleeding is occurring above the diaphragm it is not effective.

In addition, the detrimental effects of the G suit in hemorrhagic shock as studied by Wangensteen and co-workers ·showed significantly lower venous pH measurements in blood samples obtained from several sites during G suit inflation—indicating significantly lower values from the lower extremity when compared with values from other sites. It was concluded that the G suit probably impairs perfusion to the lower extremities. It is for this reason that the G suit may have its greatest value in helping to slow or arrest active hemorrhage by causing a reduction in transmural blood pressure and laceration size. G suit application for a period of several hours may accelerate the development of severe metabolic acidosis and subsequently a decreased chance of survival.

The use of a G suit and its lifesaving value in emergency situations have been documented, however, a number of times. Pelligra and associates present the successful use of an anti-G garment cutaway in a 25-year-old woman who had received 46 pints of whole blood and 64 units of plasma during a 5-week period for internal venous ooze. It was not until the G suit was applied and the patient was exposed to an average of 30 mm. Hg circumferential pressure for a total of 10 hours that the hematocrit promptly stabilized and the size of the pelvic hematoma diminished. A subsequent recovery is reported.

The effect of external counterpressure on venous bleeding and also on aortic bleeding is a subject of two reports by Ludewig and Wangensteen. In vena caval hemorrhage, the arterial blood pressure of dogs with counterpressure remained substantially higher and significantly less blood was lost than in control dogs. It is believed that the beneficial effect results from a reduction in effective laceration size, reduced venous transmural pressure, and decreased venous blood flow. In a group of dogs subjected to longitudinal laceration of the abdominal aorta, a significant prolongation of life occurred with external counterpressure of between 30 and 40 mm. Hg.

In summary, it would seem that use of external circumferential pneumatic pressure does have lifesaving potentialities in certain selected cases of uncontrollable exsanguinating hemorrhage. It is my practice to have such a G suit available in the emergency room as well as in the mobile emergency units.

The use of balloon catheter to arrest hemorrhage

An often forgotten, frequently revived, and somewhat ingenious method of preventing cardiac arrest from exsanguinating hemorrhage is the use of the balloon catheter. Described at least two decades ago by both Burch and Hughes, the principle of the technique involves a balloon catheter inserted within the lumen of a vessel for temporary control of the bleeding distal to the point of a balloon distension. A balloon catheter can be inserted in the abdominal aorta proximal to its rupture at the time of the exploration of the abdomen. Under other conditions it can be placed percutaneously. The balloon catheter can be used to prevent blood from escaping from a laceration in the atrium or even placed in the splenic artery to control bleeding from a ruptured spleen. Wholey describes a double-lumen balloon catheter with an external diameter of approximately 2.6 mm. When expanded with contrast media, the balloon has a maximum diameter of 1.5 cm. It is possible to inject contrast medium into the vessel beyond the balloon to monitor angiographically the changes in the occluded vessel.

Intra-arterial blood transfusions

With a demonstration that blood can be given intravenously almost as effectively as intra-arterially, the use of the latter route has become relatively rare in this country.

The intra-arterial blood transfusion has not enjoyed great popularity during the last decade and has, indeed, fallen into a certain degree of disrepute. It would seem, however, that some of this attitude may be partially due to lack of knowledge of the indications and the limitations for the use of this technique.

Intra-arterial transfusion may be justified in cases of massive arterial bleeding in which the arterial tree can be refilled faster with less blood than by the intravenous route. This is particularly true in patients with certain cardiac lesions such as mitral stenosis, where an intravenous transfusion is likely to provoke pulmonary edema, and situations in which venous transfusion does not return blood pressure to normal (Saba).

In patients requiring rapid resuscitation, the preoxygenation of blood by the addition of hydrogen peroxide (1 ml. of hydrogen peroxide per 1,000 ml.) has been proposed. This allows oxygenation in 15 to 30 seconds. Negovskii gives 1 ml. of 3% hydrogen peroxide for each 200 ml. of blood and also bubbles oxygen through the blood before it is pumped into the artery. He believes that the intra-arterial route is indicated for the rapid compensation of blood loss and the restoration of cardiac activity after rapid and massive hemorrhage.

Intra-arterial transfusions have been well discussed by Negovskii in his book *Resuscitation and Artificial Hypothermia.* During a visit to Negovskii's laboratories in the summer of 1962, I was pleased to observe his work in this regard. Exsanguination arrest was observed, with subsequent total resuscitation by means of intra-arterial transfusion and artificial respiration.

The other tissues of the body are able to extract oxygen as thoroughly as does the myocardium from the coronary circulation. It follows that the most effective way to increase the oxygen supply to the myocardium is to increase coronary artery flow. Intra-arterial blood transfusions with oxygenated blood have achieved dramatic effects. However, it now appears that the work that is being done with the venoarterial-bypass-assisted circulation has most of the advantages of simple intra-arterial transfusion without some of the disadvantages. One of the main disadvantages of intra-arterial transfusion is that it produces volume overloading. Although at this time venoarterial bypass is typically more complicated than a simple intra-arterial transfusion, it does appear that the technique will have an increasingly important role in future resuscitative advances, particularly if the venoarterial bypass can be synchronized for arterial return to occur during asystole so that increased work will not result (Lefemine, Lunzer, and Harken).

Callaghan and Watkins applied their technique of orthophase postsystolic myocardial augmentation for severe shock in animals with an 80% survival rate compared with a 14% survival rate in the control animals.

INTRA-AORTIC TRANSFUSION

The following case illustrates the use of the intra-aortic transfusion route:

A 36-year-old man was admitted to Bellevue Hospital on August 6, 1952, with massive hematemesis and melena of several hours' duration. There was a history of proved duodenal ulcer, demonstrated by x-ray, for which he had been under conservative therapy.

Despite repeated transfusions and passage of a Sengstaken tube, bleeding continued, and a subtotal gastrectomy was deemed advisable. At operation, 36 hours after admission, exploration of the abdomen revealed a large penetrating posterior ulcer of the duodenum as well as an anterior ulcer of the first portion of the duodenum. A subtotal gastrectomy, removing 70% of the stomach, was begun. Because of the position of the common duct in relation to the adhesions about the ulcer, a common duct exploration was performed. An anterior Polya short loop anastomosis was carried out. During the anastomosis the patient's blood pressure rapidly dropped to zero and the pulse was not palpable by the anesthetist. The operator could palpate a pulsation in the abdominal aorta. Intravenous needles in both arms had become dislodged. Cutdown procedures were carried out on each arm at once but were technically unsatisfactory, as was an attempt to enter an ankle vein. After a period of 35 minutes without blood pressure or peripheral pulse, the aortic pulsation became perceptibly faster and weaker.

Because of the danger of prolonged hypoxia from shock as well as the imminent possibility of death, it was felt that no further time could be consumed waiting for administration of blood via the extremities. At this point the operator introduced a 15-gauge needle into the abdominal aorta just above its bifurcation at the pelvic brim and 720 ml. of whole blood was rapidly introduced under pressure toward the heart with pressure on the distal aorta (Fig. 41-3). Within 3 minutes the blood pressure had risen to 170/120. The needle was removed and two fine cotton sutures were used to close the needle hole in the aorta from which blood was rapidly escaping. A piece of gelatin sponge was placed over the bleeding site as suggested by Jenkins and associates. The operation was completed uneventfully. Postoperatively the urine output was satisfactory, and the patient showed no signs of prolonged cerebral anoxia.

Seeley, in mentioning the intra-aortic route as an acceptable method in instances of severe shock, describes a case in which an intra-aortic transfusion was given for a massive hemorrhage from a duodenal ulcer.

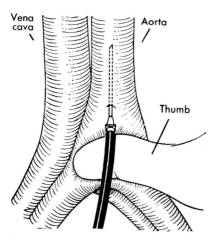

Fig. 41-3. When introducing blood into aorta for an intra-aortic transfusion, finger should be placed distal to needle in order to assure maximal flow toward heart. (From Stephenson, H. E., Jr., and Hinton, J. W.: J.A.M.A. **152:**500, 1953.)

Altogether, over 6,000 ml. of whole blood was given via the arterial route before an adequate blood pressure could be maintained. The patient later died from a lower nephron syndrome. White and Stubbs described their technique of intra-arterial transfusion using the radial artery but believed that the femoral artery or aorta (abdomen open) would be equally effective.

Petrovsky used the common carotid for blood transfusion in four cases of cardiac arrest. Constantini and associates used an intracarotid transfusion in one case, but directed the stream of blood toward the brain. Cardiac pulsations and respirations resumed but the patient died 25 hours later without regaining consciousness.

In a discussion of resuscitation of the neonate, Miller advocates the use of intra-arterial transfusion. He points out that in deep asphyxia, when cardiac efficiency is impaired, the intravenous route is ineffective since the blood accumulates in the liver and portal and caval systems. When the blood reaches the heart it tends to embarrass coronary circulation by distending the heart and thereby compressing cardiac veins against the pericardium. An intra-arterial transfusion passes directly to the coronary arteries and up into the respiratory centers of the medulla via the carotid, vertebral, and basilar vessels. Because of the preferential perfusion of the heart and brain he suggests that intra-arterial transfusions should be used more frequently in resuscitation of the neonate.

Advantages. There would seem to be several advantages of the intra-aortic route for transfusion:

1. During abdominal or chest surgery, the aorta is the most accessible vessel in the body.
2. There need be no delay in starting the transfusion, as in the case of transfusion through the radial or other peripheral route, which requires a cutdown and a short period of dissection.

3. By keeping a hand on the aorta the surgeon can tell at once when an adequate response is being achieved and thus there is less danger of a too rapid infusion of blood.
4. Before and during the transfusion, the surgeon can compress the aorta distal to the point of needle insertion and thus increase blood flow to the cerebral, coronary, hepatic, and renal vessels.
5. No extra equipment is needed.
6. No additional personnel is needed other than an assistant to pump the blood.
7. The vessel need not be ligated as is often done after the use of the radial artery.
8. The danger of ischemic necrosis of the member distal to the site of the arterial puncture is avoided.
9. No extra skin incision need be closed.
10. An extremely prompt response can be anticipated.

In addition to the advantages of the intra-aortic route, the following advantages of the intra-arterial transfusion route in general may be listed. These are suggested by Yee, Westdahl, and Wilson, based on the work by Kohlstaedt and Page:

1. Blood pressure is more rapidly elevated and with a lesser quantity of blood than by intravenous transfusion.
2. When blood pressure is raised, the coronaries are perfused more adequately. With the relief of myocardial ischemia the heart function improves and blood pressure is further supported.
3. When the patient is apneic before the infusion, he will take a deep breath due to the stimulus of filling intracranial arteries.
4. Arterial transfusion is accompanied by a minimum elevation of venous pressure.
5. Latent bleeding which causes blood pressure to fall off rapidly is detectable within minutes rather than hours.*

Disadvantages. Disadvantages include the following:

1. A retroperitoneal hemorrhage may result from improper placement of the needle.
2. The needle puncture (if of sufficient caliber for rapid transfusion) may require a suture for closure.
3. A difficult tear in the aortic wall may occur under conceivable circumstances. A severely arteriosclerotic aorta may tear beyond the point of puncture, either from the needle or from the closing suture.
4. Strict precautions against air embolism are necessary.

The elevation of arterial pressure in the aorta contributes beneficially to the prevention of irreversible cerebral damage from anoxia. Blood pumped under pressure up the aorta toward the heart will fill the coronary arteries in a most satisfactory manner. In 1903 Velich described a method of intra-arterial infusion suggested by Professor A. Spina of Prague. Spina injected warmed physiologic salt solution into the external iliac artery. According to Velich, "Professor Spina . . . injected 200 cc., directing the stream toward the heart. It forces the blood along before it, and when the semilunar valves are reached, the stream closes them. This closes the entrance into the left ventricle and drives the blood into the coronary arteries." Langendorff and later Kuliabko apparently utilized similar methods in their experiments on resuscitation of the isolated heart.

It remained for Kohlstaedt and Page to compare experimentally the intra-arterial and intravenous routes. They show that blood pressure can be restored by arterial route with little more than half the amount of blood given by vein. Page demonstrated conclusively with use of Kiodan injected into the femoral artery in dogs that the renal, coronary, hepatic, and cerebral vessels fill rapidly.

INTRACARDIAC TRANSFUSION

Both the indications and the opportunities are relatively few for either intracardiac transfusion of blood or infusion of a suitable fluid. McLennan cites such an example, however. He found it necessary to resuscitate a 13-year-old boy admitted to

*Yee, J., Westdahl, P. R., and Wilson, J. L.: Gangrene of the forearm and hand following use of radial artery for intra-arterial transfusion, Ann. Surg. 136:1019-1023, 1952.

the emergency room with a stab wound of the heart. While a cutdown was being started, the patient's heart stopped. No additional trained personnel were available to continue cutdown while the chest was opened in an attempt to restart the heart. The left ventricular laceration was quickly repaired, but it was obvious that resuscitation would be impossible without body fluid replacement. This was accomplished by inserting a No. 14 catheter just above the sutured area of the left ventricular apex. The catheter was passed through the valve into the aorta. After 10% dextran in saline and seven group O blood units were pumped in, the blood pressure returned to 100 mm. Hg and the pulse was 110 beats per minute. The catheter in the left ventricle was maintained with the right hand. The danger of producing air embolism was recognized but was fortunately avoided. The patient subsequently died; at autopsy, undigested food particles were found in the left mainstem bronchus and at the carina.

In two cases of cardiac arrest we have resorted to rapid administration of blood into the heart itself. In both instances the blood was administered into the left ventricle.

On August 28, 1950, a 36-year-old woman was being anesthetized prior to a proposed thoracolumbar sympathectomy for hypertension when asystole of the heart occurred. Thoracotomy was performed, and the heart was found to be arrested. The usual resuscitative measures were carried out, including rapid manual massage of the heart, 100% oxygen administration through an endotracheal tube, 0.5 ml. of 1:1,000 epinephrine and 6 ml. of 1% procaine into the left ventricle, and positioning of the patient in the Trendelenburg position. A nodal rhythm was resumed, but was weak and failed to continue. Cardiac refill seemed markedly inadequate. Two hundred fifty milliliters of whole blood was pumped into the left ventricle via a 19-gauge needle. Massage was resumed and a temporary improvement in the tone of the myocardium was noted. Further attempts at resuscitation were unsuccessful.

A Brock procedure for tetralogy of Fallot was being performed upon a 3-month-old infant. Arrest occurred following excessive hemorrhage. A total of 400 ml. of whole blood was given rapidly into the left ventricle. Myocardial tone increased and weak contractions began. Ventricular fibrillation, however, ensued after 2 ml. of barium chloride was given intracardially. Attempts at defibrillation were unsuccessful.

An intracardiac transfusion appears to have been the key to successful resuscitation in a case of cardiac arrest following administration of neostigmine (Lawson). Following the unsuccessful use of subdiaphragmatic massage, a long wide-bore needle was inserted into the heart in the fourth intercostal space. Within 3 minutes, 500 ml. of whole blood was given rapidly into the left side of the heart. Within a matter of seconds, the heart was beating vigorously.

SUMMARY

My own experience, although limited, with the intra-arterial route, and particularly the intra-aortic route, for rapid transfusion has given me some encouragement for its use. It must be realized that only in carefully selected cases should it take the place of the intravenous route. In those cases of cardiac arrest in which asystole occurs following rapid exsanguination or when inadequate refill of the heart is present, it would seem indicated. The intra-aortic route is especially effective when the surgeon is operating in the abdomen and when rapid blood transfusion is needed. The clinical results with the intracardiac transfusion route have not been encouraging.

As mentioned elsewhere, the prevention of air emboli is important in any type of intra-arterial transfusion, particularly the intra-aortic transfusion route. Wilkinson described a simple device to prevent air emboli in such cases. One must be certain that all air is out of the distal tubing and that an air trap is present between the blood container and the patient. It should be obvious that all pumping must be discontinued before the blood transfusion has been completed.

Rapid massive transfusions of cold stored blood have been given to dogs, and the effect of the intravenous route as compared with the intra-arterial route has been noted. Cold stored blood given by an artery shows a higher rate of survival than if given by vein. One explanation is that the cold blood is circulated through the body, warmed, buffered, and the citrate removed before it returns to the heart.

In cases of cardiac arrest with direct massage of the heart through the opened thorax, occasions will present themselves that call for rapid transfusion. In my experience, the intracardiac route has not proved of sufficient value either in the human being or in the dog to warrant our advocating its further use at this time. In cases of cardiac arrest, it requires that massage be interrupted since massage about the needle is inadequate and obviously traumatic and the trauma from the needle is located at a fixed point in the myocardium. Injury to a coronary artery is possible if the needle is not inserted properly.

Iokhveds, however, found at postmortem examination that a needle that was present in the contracting heart for about 15 minutes left only a minute puncture.

In cases of severe shock or cardiac arrest, the effectiveness of restoring the intra-coronary pressure by intravenous infusion was compared with the effectiveness of restoring the pressure by intra-arterial infusion. The response to intra-arterial infusions was more rapid and less blood was given than if administered intravenously. I agree with Veal's statement that "In the extreme stages of shock, when the heart was dilated and the peripheral coronary arterial pressures were near the zero level, the intravenous infusions were usually ineffective. It often overloaded the venous circulation and caused complete right heart failure and pulmonary edema." Seeley called attention to the work of Moyer and the latter's conclusions that effective perfusion of the aorta serves to "suck" the lungs dry and aids in overcoming pulmonary edema.

PART FIVE

PHARMACOLOGY
OF RESUSCITATION

Chapter 42

PHARMACOLOGY OF RESUSCITATION: VASOPRESSORS

Both the pharmacologic goals of and the supportive action needed in cardiopulmonary resuscitation have expanded. Unquestionably, the proper use of drugs (including their timing during the resuscitative procedure, proper dosage, and intended pharmacologic action) has provided the necessary measure for success in many instances. The varied pharmacologic goals in resuscitation include those aimed at an improvement in cardiac conduction time, an improved degree of myocardial contractility, a reduction of myocardial irritability, elevation of perfusion pressure, lowering of defibrillation threshold, reduction of vagal tone, and enhancement of ventricular excitability. In addition, it is usually necessary to combat metabolic acidosis with pharmacologic agents, and pharmacologic support of the arterial pressure is generally thought beneficial.

A discussion of the pharmacology of resuscitation inevitably turns our attention to the four basic properties inherent in a normal beating heart: excitability, contractility, rhythmicity, and conductivity.

A sizable group of vasoactive or pressor drugs are now available to the clinician. All of the pressor drugs are derivatives of epinephrine, but they differ from it in their potency and predominant mode of action. In addition, their stability varies in the presence of amine acidosis. Because of their differences in molecular structure, some act primarily as vasoconstrictors, and some act principally upon the heart and may cause vasodilatation. Of the two kinds of receptors at sympathetic nerve endings, the alpha receptors are concerned with excitatory effects such as pupillary dilatation, peripheral vasoconstriction, and mobilization of glucose from liver glycogen. The beta receptors at the nerve endings are chiefly concerned with inhibitory effects and thereby produce vasodilatation of blood vessels that supply skeletal muscles, reduction of tone of the smooth muscle supplying the bronchial tree, and an increase in the rate of the heartbeat and cardiac output. Because epinephrine stimulates some nerve endings while inhibiting others, it is regarded as both an alpha and a beta receptor. Levarterenol (norepinephrine) or norisoprenaline (a synthetic derivative of levarterenol) produces its effect chiefly by action on the alpha receptors. It increases the rate of contraction of the heart in the presence of heart block (see Table 42-1). In addition to causing vasoconstriction, pupillary dilatation, and a rise in blood glucose level by liberation of glycogen from the liver, levarterenol also increases coronary flow and may produce slowing of the heart through reflex vagal inhibition as the blood pressure rises. Marked constriction of the vessels of the gut and reduction of bowel motility may occur with levarterenol infusion. Alpha-adrenergic blocking agents, such as phenoxybenzylene and phentolamine, are able to block the alpha receptors but are not effective in blocking the beta receptors, while propranolol blocks beta but not alpha receptors.

Among the pressor amines, other drugs

Table 42-1. The mode of action of some of the commonly used sympathomimetic amines*

Class of drug	Generic name	Trade name in U.S.A.	Mode of action	Comments
Alpha receptor agonists: direct action	Methoxamine	Vasoxyl	Direct action on smooth muscle receptors producing vasoconstriction	Constricts veins and arteries; increases work load of myocardium; no direct inotropic or chronotropic effects
	Phenylephrine	Neo-Synephrine	Similar to methoxamine	Some inotropic and chronotropic effects in very large doses
	Levarterenol	Levophed	Marked constriction of arteries and veins; direct stimulant effect on cardiac receptors	May be used in cardiogenic shock since it increases myocardial contractility; reflex bradycardia may limit cardiac output
Alpha receptor agonist: indirect action	Metaraminol	Aramine	Releases epinephrine and norepinephrine from tissue; constricts smooth muscle of arteries and veins; positive inotropic effect	Ineffective in patients treated with reserpine and guanethidine; tachyphylaxis may occur
Alpha receptor antagonists	Phentolamine	Regitine	Depresses sympathomimetic responses at alpha receptor sites	No effect on beta receptors; releases epinephrine and norepinephrine from tissue stores; rapid onset and short duration of action
	Phenoxybenzamine	Dibenzyline	Relaxes smooth muscle of arteries and veins; marked increase in vascular volume	No effect on beta receptors; slow onset and long duration of action; does not block metabolic effects of epinephrine in dogs
Beta receptor agonists	Epinephrine	Adrenalin	Both alpha and beta receptor effects; in doses used in man the beta effects are dominant	Usually reserved for anaphylactic shock; stimulates anaerobic metabolism and causes metabolic acidosis
	Isoproterenol	Isuprel	Decreases systemic and pulmonary vascular resistance; marked direct inotropic and chronotropic effects; short duration of action	Useful in Adams-Stokes attacks; elicits myocardial stimulation without vasoconstriction; effective in cardiac resuscitation
	Nylidrin	Arlidin	Causes smooth muscle relaxation in all blood vessels; direct positive inotropic and chronotropic effects	Longer duration of action than isoproterenol; increased cardiac output for more than one hour following single intravenous injection
Beta receptor antagonists	Pronethalol	Nethalide	Causes cardiac slowing and systemic vasodilatation	Carcinogenic effect in rodents; some complicating sympathomimetic effect in dogs; not available for clinical use
	Propranolol	Inderal	Similiar to pronethalol	Of value in treating tachyarrhythmias induced by digitalis and anesthetics

*From Marshall, R. J., and Darby, T. D.: Shock, pharmacological principles in treatment, Springfield, Illinois, 1966, Charles C Thomas, Publisher.

Table 42-1. The mode of action of some of the commonly used sympathomimetic amines—cont'd

Class of drug	Generic name	Trade name in U.S.A.	Mode of action	Comments
Ganglion block-ing agents	Mecamyla-mine	Inversine	Decreases transmission at autonomic ganglia	Does not block humoral stimulation of adrenal output of epinephrine
	Pentolinium	Ansolysen	Same as mecamylamine	Unpredictable dissociation of the salt when given intravenously
	Trimethaphan campho-sulfonate	Arfonad	Same as above	Continuous infusion allows vasorelaxation for short intervals
Other vaso-constrictor	Angiotensin II	Hypertensin	Stimulates smooth muscles of arteries; does not con-strict veins	Does not stimulate heart; probably should not be used in cardiogenic shock

are phenylephrine, methoxamine, and metaraminol. By acting mainly on the alpha receptors, this group of drugs raises the systemic arterial blood pressure during vasoconstriction of peripheral vessels. Except with metaraminol the force of contraction of the heart is not appreciably altered, but coronary blood flow and cerebral blood flow are increased when hypotension is present (Fig. 42-1).

A category of mixed alpha and beta receptors could also be added to Table 42-1. This would include metaraminol, epinephrine, levarterenol, and mephentermine (Wyamine).

Other pressor amines, in addition to epinephrine, that act mainly upon the heart and in the production of vasodilatation are ephedrine, methamphetamine, and mephentermine.

In administering vasopressors during cardiac resuscitation and in the immediate postresuscitative period, care should be taken to avoid local tissue necrosis by using large catheters in large veins and by using dilute solutions. Obviously, one should use the smallest dose that will provide the desired effect. The action of pressor amines is less effective in the presence of uncorrected metabolic acidosis. Use of intravenous

hydrocortisone may also potentiate their action.

Pearson and Redding stress that vasoconstrictors increase diastolic pressure during cardiac resuscitation and materially improve the chances for return of spontaneous circulation. The vasopressors, which act mainly on the alpha receptors, do raise diastolic pressure; their value seems to lie primarily in the improvement of the peripheral vascular tone.

One of the important outgrowths of the interest in resuscitation of the acutely arrested heart has been advancement of the knowledge of drug action on the heart. Even so, much confusion still exists in the application of our knowledge of the pharmacology of cardiac resuscitation.

It has been my observation that, too frequently, drugs are used in cardiac resuscitation without knowledge of their precise indications, their correct dosage, and the pharmacologic response likely to occur.

Intercardiac or intratracheal injections

Under competent hands and in controlled situations, the intracardiac injection of drugs during cardiac arrest emergencies may prove most effective. For the individual inexperienced in such techniques, however, more harm may be done than good. For one thing, the delay in seeking the appropriate spot to insert the needle and the time required for repeated blind stabs through the chest wall may be excessive. While not common, a tension pneumothorax may be provoked as may a laceration of a coronary artery. Pericardial tamponade has been experienced. One thing is obvious: marginal cerebral circulation should not be compromised even further by an interruption of closed chest massage.

As stressed elsewhere in the book, drugs may be injected intravenously through such routes as the central venous catheter, if available. One should not forget that the intratracheal administration of cardiotonic drugs diluted in water or saline provides an effective and relatively rapid rate of absorption, provided there is adequate circulation. If an intravenous route is not immediately available, epinephrine (1 to 2 mg./ml. sterile water) can be effective if instilled into the tracheobronchial tree, usually through an endotracheal tube. Likewise, lidocaine can be instilled as a dose of 50 to 100 mg./10 ml. sterile water. Ventilation should be delayed briefly to prevent the drug's being swept back up.

Intracardiac injections of any drug during cardiac resuscitative techniques carry with them the risk of damaging a coronary artery or vein. An intravenous infusion of large amounts of saline solution with epinephrine,

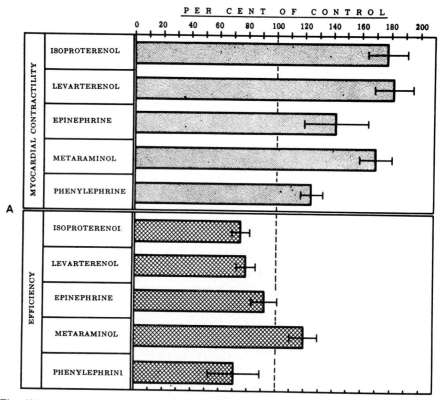

Fig. 42-1. Comparison of the action of catecholamines on the heart. **A,** Changes in myocardial contractility and cardiac efficiency. **B,** Changes in coronary blood flow and heart rate. **C,** Changes in total peripheral resistance and coronary vascular resistance. (From Waldhausen, J. A., and others: Arch. Surg. **91:**85, 1965.)

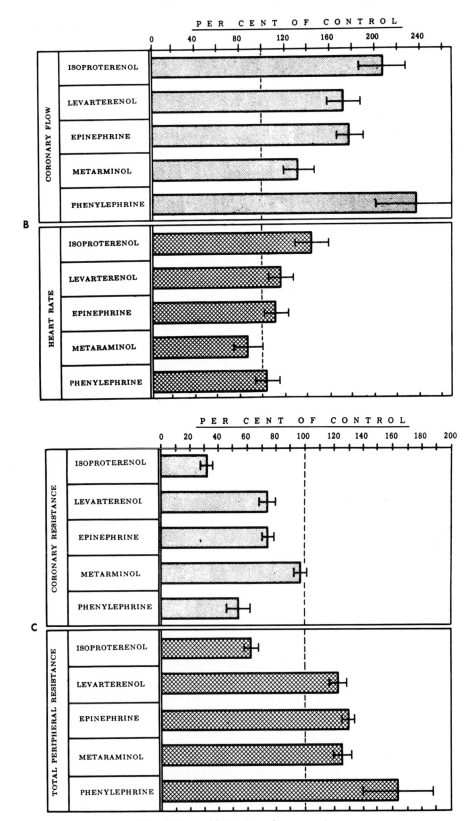

Fig. 42-1, cont'd. For legend see opposite page.

given in combination with circulatory assist techniques, may often accomplish the same result as an intracardiac injection. In patients with large, thick ventricles, it is not always easy to inject the drug into the lumen of the ventricle. Necrosis of conduction tissue may result if the interventricular septum is injected. On the other hand, an intravenous injection may not always be available; in these instances, the intracardiac route will be the only practical one.

Epinephrine (Adrenalin, Supranol, Vasodrine)

There is much to recommend the immediate and empirical administration of 0.5 mg. of epinephrine through an indwelling intravenous catheter at the time of cardiac standstill or even fibrillation.

It is estimated that 30 ml. of oxygenated blood per 100 gm. of brain tissue per minute are required to prevent irreversible brain damage but that the brain may tolerate a cerebral blood flow of as little as 15 to 18 ml. per 100 gm. per minute (Jude). Approximately 15% to 22% of the normal spontaneous cardiac output constitutes cerebral blood flow. In a patient with cardiac arrest where the average cardiac compression is usually 20% to 30% of normal (0.84 to 2.8 liters in young adult males), a minimum cerebral flow of 420 ml. per minute or about 30% of the average cardiac output is needed. It is for this reason that Jude recommends improved perfusion of the central nervous system by increasing arterial pressure through intravenous or intracardiac Adrenalin injections. His studies show that epinephrine, when compared with metaraminol, phenylephrine, levarterenol, and isoproterenol, has the greatest consistent pressure elevation at both minimal and maximal dosage levels, but had the least persistent duration of effect. Jude suggests that epinephrine, when indicated, be given repeatedly at 4 to 5 minute intervals. The other drugs just mentioned, also have effective cardiotonic actions with the exception of phenylephrine.

Although quantitative values for improved cerebral or coronary blood flow are difficult to obtain, signs of improved circulation in the central nervous system and heart support the belief that such improvement must be taking place. For example, the myocardial tone definitely improves and can be palpable under the compressing hand after the use of cardiotonic drugs. In addition, pupillary constriction almost regularly occurs. As noted elsewhere, easier defibrillation and return of spontaneous functional cardiac activity is facilitated.

Not only does epinephrine improve coronary perfusion by coronary vasodilatation and increased peripheral resistance but it also improves myocardial conduction, as is evidenced by the fact that stimulation of the origin of impulses in the right atrium is encouraged. I agree with Swan that epinephrine does not appear to predispose to subsequent ventricular fibrillation when it is used to set the stage for successful defibrillation.

Epinephrine exerts a direct effect on the myocardium and on the conduction tissue, producing more forceful contractions of the myocardium. It increases myocardial irritability and markedly affects the metabolic rate and oxygen consumption of the heart muscle. It increases the speed of atrioventricular conduction.

Following the administration of epinephrine, a reduction in cardiac size is noted, with an impressive shortening of systole. Stroke volume, in spite of the brief duration of systole, increases because of the marked acceleration of ejection. Cardiac peak power, defined as maximum work per unit of time, is considerably increased by epinephrine. Epinephrine particularly shortens the atrial-His interval. The His-Purkinje-intramyocardial conduction time is less actively affected.

Although the effectiveness of epinephrine has been known for a long time, its dangers have been also recognized. The occurrence of ventricular fibrillation after intracardiac injection of epinephrine has been frequently observed and is well known.

Even so, for years we have not hesitated to use epinephrine in cases of ventricular fibrillation. Following work in the animal laboratory, we repeatedly observed that the chances of successful electrical defibrillation were enhanced if the myocardial tone was improved by injection of epinephrine into the left ventricle, followed by massage to disseminate the drug through the coronary arteries. A clinical experience bore this out rather dramatically. During an exploratory celiotomy on an elderly woman, the heart suddenly went into cardiac arrest at the very instant the endotracheal tube was inserted. A thoracotomy was performed and, after several minutes of cardiac massage, the heart went into ventricular fibrillation. Electrodes were applied and the heart was shocked by serial defibrillation, the method recommended by Wiggers. After ten or twelve separate shocks, the heart failed to show any signs of defibrillation and the myocardial tone failed to improve in spite of continual compression of the myocardium. Following the injection of 0.5 ml. of 1:1,000 epinephrine, it required but a single electrical shock to adequately defibrillate the heart; resuscitation of the heart was subsequently achieved without difficulty. The chest was closed and the operation was completed. A similar experience has occurred in additional cases personally encountered.

With adequate means for electrical defibrillation available, I give little consideration to the possibility that ventricular fibrillation will result from the use of epinephrine. I do not use procaine as a prophylactic measure against the fibrillary action of epinephrine. The heart in ventricular fibrillation presents a problem as simple as that of asystole; in fact, the prognosis is generally better.

Epinephrine should not be used routinely in all cases of cardiac arrest but should be reserved for periods following adequate cardiac compression in which the heart has failed to show any evidence of a return to normal rhythm and in instances when the cardiac musculature continues to remain flaccid as revealed by direct observation, if possible.

By combining epinephrine with sodium bicarbonate, Kirimli, Harris, and Safar note greater success than when bicarbonate or epinephrine is used alone. All experiments were carried out in dogs. Successful defibrillation had lower average energy requirements in the bicarbonate-epinephrine group than in the epinephrine-alone group. Ventricular fibrillation did not recur in any of the bicarbonate-epinephrine groups. Thirty minutes after defibrillation, mean carotid blood flows were approximately 100% of normal in the bicarbonate-epinephrine group, as compared with a control group of 55% and an epinephrine group of 65%.

Epinephrine increases the force of myocardial contraction, which is accompanied by a decrease in cardiac glycogen and an increase in oxygen consumption. The increased excitability of the ventricular myocardium is mediated by induced shifts in potassium. The drug produces a positive flux of potassium ions into the myocardium. A marked rise in serum potassium is a result of the release of potassium by the liver in response to epinephrine. Thus epinephrine alters the ventricular myocardium so that it is more susceptible to fibrillation in response to a variety of stimuli.

It has been my practice since 1951 to recommend the use of epinephrine via an intracardiac injection, or occasionally intravenously, in patients with ventricular fibrillation resistant to defibrillation attempts.

It has become a rather common practice for cardiac surgeons to use vasopressor agents in resistant cases of ventricular defibrillation. A study on dogs at the University of Mississippi by Crowell and associates, however, takes an opposite approach. They conclude that large amounts of epinephrine and norepinephrine are liberated from sympathetic discharges produced by the severe anoxia of cardiac arrest. After about 30 seconds of cardiac massage, the released pressor substance is allowed to circulate and produce a "vasopressor response," as evidenced by an increased blood pressure during cardiac massages as well as a more firm ventricular mass. Elevated levels of epinephrine and norepinephrine in the blood are found during this period; but within 3 to 4 minutes, these levels have subsided along with the vasopressor response. It is at this time that electrical ventricular defibrillation can be accomplished with much greater ease than during the period of the vasopressor response. Crowell and his co-workers state that it is far better "to massage the heart for three to four minutes, allow the vasopressor response to run its course, dissipate the vasopressor catecholamines and improve the oxygenation of the blood."

Although it is not surprising, Bailey in England 35 years ago reported intracardiac injection of epinephrine in forty cases without a single incident of success. The difficulty, of course, resulted from the lack of any associated effort to move the drug into the myocardium by means of either closed- or open-chest cardiac compression.

Swan and his co-workers, in studies on resuscitation in dogs, report much the same conclusion. They injected epinephrine into the right ventricle of dogs in which circulatory failure had occurred, and their experience was that epinephrine proved to be completely ineffectual in restoring the circulation. Swan emphasizes that the reason for this is obvious, since, if the circulation has failed, the cardiac contractility cannot possibly be restored by intracardiac epinephrine injections because the drug cannot get to the place where it would be of value. During systemic circulatory failure, there is no blood flowing from the ventricles to the myocardial tissues; therefore, epinephrine injected into the lumen of the heart could never be circulated to the myocardium unless the heart is massaged.

Laboratory and clinical observations confirm the generally accepted belief that epinephrine is a valuable adjunct in cardiac resuscitation using the indirect, or closed-chest, approach. In discussing his method of closed-chest compression, Dr. George W. Crile, over 60 years ago, advocated the combined technique of intra-arterial epinephrine injection, closed-chest compression, and artificial respiration. Crile's suggested approach was by the use of a cutdown on the axillary artery. Epinephrine was then injected directly into a stream of normal saline solution. In his book *Anemia and Resuscitation,* Crile states that arterial rather than venous injections should be employed because the blood pressure is dependent on the resistance offered by the muscles of the arteries. If injected into the vein, the epinephrine must pass through the right auricle, the right ventricle, the pulmonary circulation, and then to the left auricle and the left ventricle before it enters the aorta and subsequently the coronary circulation. Not only is this a circuitous route, entailing loss of time, but also the epinephrine itself must be somewhat dissipated. It wholly lacks the directness of effect secured by injecting it toward the heart through an artery. Saline-epinephrine arterial infusion toward the heart, combined with rhythmic pressure upon the thorax, proved most efficient in animals.

I have often injected epinephrine directly into the lumen of the left ventricle, with the heart exposed by a thoracotomy incision. Not only can the site for injection be well chosen with direct visualization but, with a drug injected into the left ventricle (Fig. 42-2), it also requires only several compressive actions on the heart to force the blood out into the aorta and into the coronary arteries. If the aorta is compressed beyond the coronary ostia for several seconds, a larger percentage of the drug will reach the myocardium.

Gerbode and associates, believing that the drugs will reach the coronary arteries more steadily after passing through the

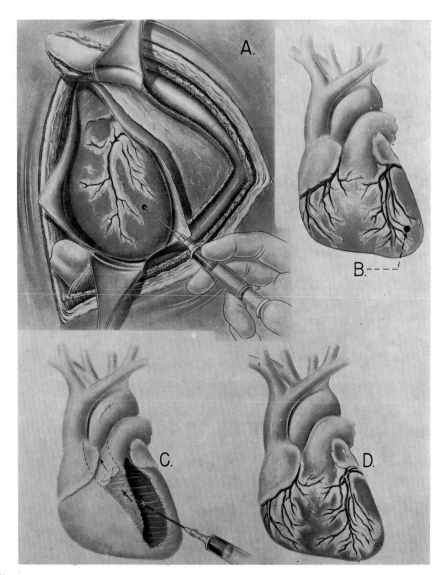

Fig. 42-2. A, Administration of drugs intracardially can be done best in this fashion and into the most readily available site of the heart. **B,** Site for needle injection, being cautious to avoid coronary vessels. **C,** Drugs such as epinephrine can be injected into left side of heart without ill effects and with a more rapid course into the coronary vessels. **D,** The sooner drug reaches myocardium via coronary arteries, the quicker will be its expected action. Drugs injected through closed chest may not always enter intended area. Usual landmark used is one just to left of sternum in fourth or fifth interspace. (From Stephenson, H. E., Jr., Reid, L. C., and Hinton, J. W.: Arch. Surg. **69:**37, 1954.)

lungs, advocate the right ventricle or pulmonary artery for drug injections.

Because of the intraluminal pressure in the heart, it is advantageous to inject the needle through the heart muscle at a slant rather than at right angles to the surface of the heart. By so doing, bleeding is less likely to occur when removal of the needle takes place because the intraluminal pressure will tend to close off the hole caused by the needle.

Another objection to the left ventricular route is that it is more likely to produce ventricular fibrillation. With a large group of patients, however, fortunately we have seldom seen this occur. Kay states that he injected drugs into the left ventricle over 150 times in dogs without a single case of ventricular fibrillation being produced. With closed-chest resuscitation, an injection in the fifth left interspace next to the sternum will usually be satisfactory—especially if the needle is pointed in a cranial direction.

Beck believed that the atria do not bleed as easily as the ventricles. In addition, he believed that the right ventricle is preferable to the left since it has fewer coronary vessels on the surface. Then too, the right ventricle wall is much thinner than the left and does not have the large papillary muscles.

DOSAGE

In the average adult patient receiving epinephrine for indicated circumstances in cardiac arrest, a dose of 0.5 ml. of a 1:1,000 solution diluted to 10 ml. with sterile normal saline, or 5 ml. of a 1:10,000 solution, should be effective. The dose may need to be repeated every 5 minutes.

EPINEPHRINE DOSAGE IN INFANTS

Rahter and Herron report an attempt at cardiac resuscitation, using the thoracotomy approach, that failed to produce a response to manual massage until after the second injection of 0.5 ml. of 1:1,000 epinephrine into the myocardium. The infant was successfully resuscitated, and 7 months later appeared to be a normal, healthy child. Such large doses are seldom required. Usually an intracardiac dose of 0.3 to 2.0 ml. diluted to 1:10,000 (0.1 ml. per kilogram) will suffice.

Phenylephrine hydrochloride

Use of phenylephrine hydrochloride (Neo-Synephrine) in cardiac resuscitation is of minimal value since its effectiveness is not as great as that of epinephrine. There would seem to be little indication for its use in the usual clinical case.

Isoproterenol hydrochloride (Aludrine Hydrochloride, Asdrin, Isopro, Isuprel, Norisodrine Aerotrol, Proterenol)

The effectiveness of isoproterenol is related to its ability to increase the contractility and excitability of the heart while reducing peripheral vascular resistance. It is considered to be the drug of choice in cardiogenic shock resulting from acute myocardial infarction. More and more centers use isoproterenol as the first drug in cardiogenic shock due to myocardial infarction. Gunnar and co-workers, however, point to the ineffectiveness of isoproterenol as compared, for example, with levarterenol. They theorize that isoproterenol may decrease effective coronary artery flow while, at the same time, it increases myocardial oxygen requirements. Although the drug elevates the systolic pressure and the cardiac output by its inotropic actions, isoproterenol also lowers the diastolic and mean pressure by peripheral vasodilatation.

Gunnar and associates consider patients with myocardial infarction to be in shock if there is a reduction in mean arterial blood pressure to less than 70 mm. Hg (or less than 80 mm. Hg in previously hypertensive patients). In addition, the clinical picture is associated with evidence of shock, including oliguria, mental confusion, diminished pulse, diaphoresis, and cyanosis.

Isoproterenol is an effective drug for

improving cardiac dynamics, even during severe acidosis (Silberschmid and others). This drug, because of its known inotropic and chronotropic effect, is useful in instances of a low perfusion state.

Cardiogenic shock caused by myocardial infarction is distinguished from other types of cardiogenic shock by its pressure-dependent coronary flow. It would seem, therefore, that it is imperative to elevate the arterial pressure to at least the lowest level compatible with adequate cerebral, coronary, and renal blood flow in patients with myocardial infarction and cardiogenic shock.

Isoproterenol is a most satisfactory therapeutic agent for treating the patient with an acute episode of Adams-Stokes syndrome. Commonly, it is used prior to placement of the temporary cardiac pacemaker. A dosage of 1 to 10 ml. of a solution of 1 mg. in 500 ml. of 5% dextrose and water is initiated intravenously. The rate of infusion is determined by the amount necessary to restore a ventricular rate of forty to fifty beats per minute. Ventricular extrasystoles or tachycardia may occur; therefore careful observation is necessary.

Epinephrine stimulates higher and lower ventricular foci, whereas isoproterenol stimulates more particularly the higher foci. This fact makes isoproterenol extremely useful in profound bradycardia as a result of atrioventricular heart block, Adams-Stokes syndrome, and certain ventricular arrhythmias. Because isoproterenol stimulates only the higher ventricular foci, it may allow the normal cardiac pacemaker to take over and the heart to return to normal rhythm. At this point, it should be emphasized that no drug is a substitute for transvenous pacing in the Adams-Stokes syndrome. The drug is only a temporary emergency measure; pacing should be initiated as soon as possible.

Isoproterenol may be administered sublingually or by subcutaneous, intravenous, intramuscular, or intracardiac injection. It should not be given in conjunction with epinephrine, but the two drugs may be used alternately.

Metaraminol (Aramine)

The search continues for the ideal drug as a useful agent in cardiogenic shock. Most agree that such an agent should improve coronary artery flow and myocardial contractility as well as raise the blood pressure and increase the cardiac output. At the same time, myocardial oxygen consumption in relation to work load (efficiency) should not be increased. Tests on a variety of catecholamines with inotropic effects are discussed by Waldhausen and his co-workers. In summarizing their excellent study, it can be noted that metaraminol (Aramine) most closely fits the qualification for an ideal drug because it does indeed increase myocardial contractility without a fall in efficiency and with very little increase in heart rate, as well as with only moderate increase in total peripheral resistance. Isoproterenol (Isuprel), on the other hand, decreases the work load by peripheral resistance, but this advantage is overshadowed by the marked fall in cardiac efficiency due particularly to an increase in heart rate. Phenylephrine shows the least efficient inotropic response and is predominately effective as a vasopressor. It would seem to have little value in the management of cardiogenic shock according to these studies.

Methoxamine hydrochloride (Vasoxyl)

Methoxamine, an alpha-adrenergic agent, is useful in ventricular fibrillation because of its negative chronotropic effect on the heart as well as its useful antiarrhythmic effect coupled with a potent vasoconstrictive action.

Chapter 43

PHARMACOLOGY OF RESUSCITATION: ANTIARRHYTHMIC AGENTS

In this section we will briefly consider various drugs available for the management of cardiac arrhythmias. At the onset, it is obvious that the search for the ideal agent must still go on. Some antiarrhythmic agents require more than once-daily doses, others need to be administered intravenously. A marked difference in blood level may be seen with some agents (quinidine). Procainamide can cause lupus erythematosus, fever, leukopenia, or bone marrow depression.

Lidocaine (Xylocaine)

Hitchcock and Keown, working at the University of Missouri in the late 1950s, predicted the increasingly important role of lidocaine as an antiarrhythmic drug after witnessing its beneficial effect on ventricular extrasystoles and on ventricular tachycardias in patients in the operating room, particularly those undergoing open-heart surgery.

Lidocaine is an unusually effective drug in the treatment of arrhythmias after myocardial infarction, particularly so for ventricular tachycardia or multiple premature ventricular beats. It will raise the fibrillation threshold. Gianelli and associates recommend an intravenous bolus of 1 to 2 mg. per kilogram of body weight initially (approximately 50 to 100 mg.). If there are recurrent premature beats, a constant intravenous infusion at the rate of 1 to 3 mg. per minute is given. Gianelli's group was able to terminate twenty episodes of ventricular tachycardia in twenty-nine coronary patients after a 25 to 100 mg. bolus was injected.

Although lidocaine is effective because of its antiarrhythmic properties, it has an advantage since it has no vasopressor action and can thus be used with such drugs as epinephrine. Lidocaine is particularly effective in depressing myocardial irritability in instances when successful myocardial defibrillation repeatedly reverts into a fibrillatory state. Lidocaine is useful in suppressing and terminating ventricular arrhythmias, whether digitalis induced or not. Its use is of limited value in atrial arrhythmias.

Not only is lidocaine effective in treating ventricular arrhythmias but it also appears to be effective and relatively safe as a means of reducing the frequency of—or preventing—ventricular arrhythmias after myocardial infarction when given intravenously as constant infusion.

Although the routine use of lidocaine for the prevention of ventricular arrhythmias in acute myocardial infarction has been advocated, its use is not innocuous, as is apparent from the occasional case of sinus arrest following the infusion of lidocaine under certain conditions (Jeresaty and others). These authors caution against its use in elderly patients, particularly if they have sustained an inferior wall myocardial infarction which is often associated in itself with sinus bradycardia. Depression of diastolic depolarization of the sinoatrial node (in suppression of impulse formation) may be enhanced by interaction with other antiarrhythmic drugs such as quinidine and diphenylhydantoin.

When injected intramuscularly, lidocaine reaches an effective plasma level for the prevention of ventricular arrhythmias within 10 minutes (1 to 1.5 mg. per ml.). It is rapidly metabolized by the liver.

Contraindicated in the "sick sinus syndrome." If one is overly enthusiastic about abolishing certain arrhythmias, occasionally one may abolish the function of the sinus node when that node is already injured. Lippestad and Forfang emphasize this danger in reporting the detrimental effect of lidocaine on the sinus node in such a patient with a "sick sinus syndrome." This syndrome is often characterized as having a defect in elaboration or conduction of sinus impulses manifested by chaotic atrial activity, changing P wave contour, and bradycardia interspersed with multiple and recurrent ectopic beats, with runs of atrial and nodal tachycardia. In their patient, with no signs of previous myocardial infarction or other myocardial disease, sinus rhythm alternated with ectopic atrial rhythm. Almost immediately after an intravenous dose of lidocaine, sinus node activity ceased completely with an exit block in the nodal pacemaker. Sinus activity was reestablished after 0.6 mg. of atropine was given intravenously. These Norwegian physicians speculate that lidocaine and sick sinus node may depress the depolarization of the impulse-creating fibers, so that they never reach the potential necessary to release the pacemaker impulse. In addition, atrial nonresponsiveness due to subthreshold sinus impulse may occur.

Procaine and procainamide

Several years ago it was generally assumed that procaine hydrochloride was the drug of choice for ventricular fibrillation, used to reduce the irritability of the myocardium and to allow for electrical defibrillation. After frequent experiments with procaine hydrochloride and procainamide (Pronestyl) in the animal laboratory over a period of several years, we have been unable to find evidence that either one of these drugs has a great deal to offer in the treatment of ventricular fibrillation. We

have been particularly unimpressed with procainamide. In almost all instances we have found it considerably more difficult to defibrillate a dog's heart after procaine hydrochloride had been used than if no procaine were used at all. Not only does it appear more difficult to defibrillate but also, once fibrillation has ceased, the problem of restoring effective and spontaneous cardiac rhythm is made more difficult. Clinically, our experience has been much the same, and the result is that the use of procaine during cardiac resuscitation has fallen into disrepute as far as we are concerned. This also appears to be the consensus of other physicians.

That there is still disagreement is noted by quoting Gerbode, who states:

> I would use procaine amide in any difficult case of ventricular fibrillation if I could not promptly restore sinus rhythm with electrical shocks to the heart. It has been shown experimentally that procaine amide is of aid in defibrillating the heart. The dosage is somewhat in question, but I think 100 to 250 mg. is a good dose in this situation.

Harken states that he has had unusually good results with procaine hydrochloride in successfully defibrillating sixteen patients. His procedure was to inject 10 ml. of a 1% solution into the left atrium; success was noted after a brief period of massage. All were during cardiac operations.

Hinchey and Straehley wrote that they include procainamide in their emergency resuscitation kits and that they have used the drug with what they consider to be good results. Doses varying from 150 to 300 mg. were given intravenously.

Three cases have been described by Meyer and associates, however; they emphasize the apparent aid provided by procainamide in electrical defibrillation. In each instance, defibrillation could not be accomplished after prolonged massage, and in one instance defibrillation followed the use of epinephrine. A total of 500 mg. of procainamide was given to the first patient intravenously before defibrillation was accomplished. In the second patient, 200 mg. was required, and in the third patient only 100 mg. of procainamide, intravenously administered, was necessary. The last two patients had also received epinephrine. In each of these three cases, it was the opinion of the surgeon that successful defibrillation could not have been accomplished without the use of procainamide.

Much of the cardiac action of procainamide is similar to that of quinidine, in that the excitability of all areas of the heart is reduced and conduction in the bundle of His and throughout the myocardium is slowed. It is said, however, that procainamide does not depress contractility of the heart (Meyer and others). Those who employ procainamide for assistance in electrical defibrillation believe that it is superior to procaine hydrochloride in that there is a lower toxicity and a more favorable ratio between cardiac and CNS effect. In addition, there is a longer duration of action following such administration by the intravenous route.

Procainamide appeared to be particularly beneficial in the treatment of a 52-year-old woman with repeated episodes of ventricular fibrillation in the absence of heart disease. She received high doses of procainamide without untoward effects. Initially, she was given 500 mg. of procainamide intravenously. During the first 72 hours of treatment, the patient received 7.5 gm. intravenously and 6.5 gm. orally. She later had an uneventful recovery.

It is argued that the antiarrhythmic action of procainamide resides principally in its ability to depress the excitability of the heart rather than in its ability to prolong refractoriness. The hypotensive action of procainamide should be noted. In addition to depressing the myocardium (more so than lidocaine), it decreases peripheral resistance.

Milstein and Brock (1954) state they were able to abolish nine episodes of ventricular fibrillation using procaine hydrochloride in doses of 50 to 200 mg. It is their impression that there is a place for the use of procaine hydrochloride in cases of ventricular fibrillation, and they discount the possibility that it weakens the heart beat after defibrillation. In addition, they encountered no difficulty in starting the heart after defibrillation when procaine hydrochloride had been used. Stephenson and Main studied various antifibrillary drugs and concluded that low doses of quinidine give the most highly significant protective action—considerably more than atriocaval block with lidocaine.

In summary, it can be stated that the use of procaine in preventing and treating ventricular fibrillation is still in question. As far as I am concerned, the use of procaine, particularly procainamide (Pronestyl), in the treatment of ventricular fibrillation should be discontinued.

Propranolol hydrochloride (Inderal)

Propranolol has been used in this country only a few years, although British physicians have been working with the drug rather extensively. In 1962 Black and Stephenson suggested the possibility of beta-adrenergic receptor blocking agents in the use of certain cardiac arrhythmias. Considerable experience has now been reported to indicate that propranolol hydrochloride may have a role in the prevention and management of certain cases of cardiac arrest. Propranolol has a number of beneficial actions that include decreasing cardiac output and heart rate, a reduction of the total body and myocardial oxygen consumption during exercise, increasing arteriovenous oxygen extraction, and reducing of the detrimental effect of catecholamines on the myocardium. Propranolol is believed to decrease pacemaker activity by arresting membrane potential, maximum depolarization rate, and conduction velocity while increasing the diastolic threshold and refractory period of the myocardium. The drug has been of particular value in suppressing or preventing ventricular fibrillation that recurs persistently in patients with acute myocardial infarction and in whom lidocaine or procainamide hydrochloride has been unsuccessful in suppressing the arrhythmia (Rothfield and others). It has been demonstrated that ouabain-induced ventricular fibrillation can be prevented by the use of propranolol. Propranolol has also proved its usefulness in preventing ventricular fibrillation associated with both the toxic effects of digitalis and isoproterenol overdosage.

For suppressing persistently recurring ventricular fibrillation, 5 mg. of propranolol hydrochloride may be given by an intravenous drip. The effect of the drug should be monitored closely, since severe hypotension, cardiac failure, and profound bradycardia may be observed. Dreifus and co-workers have combined the use of propranolol and quinidine in the management of ventricular fibrillation. In one case, they used propranolol hydrochloride in a dose of 40 mg. every 6 hours (orally), coupled with quinidine sulfate, 200 mg. four times daily.

It is emphasized that propranolol hydrochloride plays a significant role in the prevention of ventricular fibrillation occurring as a primary electrical event in acute myocardial infarction.

The use of propranolol for treating the "stone heart" is discussed in Chapter 34.

Bretylium tosylate

Experimentally, Bacaner indicates the significant protection of the heart against electrically induced fibrillation with the use of bretylium tosylate. Apparently, the drug lengthens the period of tolerance to fibrillatory stimulation between three and several hundred times. The arrhythmia is often limited solely to the region of the electrode and, when the electrode is removed, sinus rhythm returns in timings varying between a fraction of a second

and 20 seconds. In the untreated heart defibrillation requires several counter shocks but, after the use of bretylium, Bacaner notes that only one shock is necessary. Bacaner considers bretylium to be the only antiarrhythmic agent known to augment rather than depress the strength of cardiac contraction. It produces a positive inotropic effect and elevates the fibrillation threshold. It does not block myocardial response to catecholamines.

Bretylium tosylate may be effective when refractory ventricular arrhythmias follow myocardial infarctions. Aravinbakshan, in a clinical study, found that the intramuscular route is preferable to intravenous administration since the latter almost always produces hypotension and vomiting. That the drug be reserved for only serious refractory ventricular arrhythmias is suggested by Mansour because of its likelihood of transiently increasing ectopic beats and reducing arterial pressure.

Diphenylhydantoin sodium (Dilantin, Denyl Sodium, Diphentoin, Diphenylan Sodium)

Diphenylhydantoin has proved to be useful in patients with cardiac arrhythmias such as supraventricular and ventricular arrhythmias arising from digitalis excess. It seems to be particularly effective in patients with multifocal, premature contractions and in those with bigeminal rhythms. It should not be used in patients with bradycardia or a high degree of atrioventricular block, and it is apparently of very little value in patients with atrial flutter and fibrillation.

Although diphenylhydantoin sodium (Dilantin) is effective in treating ventricular tachycardia and is thought to be a potentially valuable antifibrillatory drug, it was given a thorough trial in the experimental laboratory as a prophylactic agent against ventricular fibrillation during intermediate and deep body cooling induced by immersion in ice water (Swan and Sawyer). It was concluded that the drug exerts no significant changes that would be useful in the management of hypothermia.

Effect of quinidine in defibrillation

Levine, Van Dongen, and other investigators have reported the use of quinidine as an effective agent in raising the "fibrillation threshold" following electrical stimulation of the living ventricle or after other procedures, such as injection of epinephrine. Laadt and Allen, working in the Department of Physiology at Northwestern University Medical School, report on their work to determine the effect of quinidine on the incidence of ventricular fibrillation induced in dogs by ligation of the left coronary artery at the origin of the circumflex branch. Their results, after experiments on fifty dogs, indicate that quinidine does not exert a favorable effect upon ventricular fibrillation, at least, not when it is produced by coronary artery occlusion. The results even indicate, on the contrary, that quinidine increases the mortality. Two dogs died from cardiac asystole after having received rather large doses, and were thought to have suffered from quinidine poisoning since Gordon and co-workers have shown that toxic doses of quinidine may produce all forms of heart block and even cardiac arrest. On the other hand, one physician reported a case of ventricular defibrillation that he attributed to the beneficial effects following the use of quinidine sulfate.

Scott and associates report on the protective action of quinidine in raising the fibrillation threshold following electrical stimulation in animals. Wegria and Nickerson, in 1942, also report that quinidine reduces the susceptibility of the heart to ventricular fibrillation if the dose is not too large or given too rapidly.

Bernreiter cautions against the use of quinidine when there is extreme prolongation of a Q-T interval in connection with premature ventricular contractions. In Q-T prolongation, the premature ventricular con-

tractions fall of necessity in the vulnerable zone regardless of the cause of the Q-T extension. Quinidine may produce excessive Q-T duration. In the case Bernreiter describes, the patient showed severe prolongation of a Q-T interval with premature ventricular contractions occurring in the vulnerable period of the cardiac systole as a subsequent onset of a ventricular fibrillation that did not respond to therapy.

Effect of neostigmine in defibrillation

Interesting observations have been made at the University of Colorado in Swan's laboratory by Holmes and Montgomery on the effect of neostigmine on ventricular fibrillation. They also studied the effect of acetylcholine. For control studies they used twenty-three animals; they produced ventricular fibrillation in all of the animals by making a ventricular incision under hypothermia. Montgomery and others, working with dogs, found that when given 1 ml. of 1:4,000 neostigmine intravenously at about 30° C. during the cooling process, ventricular fibrillation occurred in only seven of fifteen animals. When neostigmine was given to the animals by coronary perfusion (injection directly into the coronary system at the time of occlusion of the circulation) none of the sixteen operated upon fibrillated. Reasoning that, as an anticholinesterase, neostigmine might be affected by its potentiating action on acetylcholine, the effect of simply giving acetylcholine was noted. None of the animals given acetylcholine developed ventricular fibrillation as produced in the control group.

Effect of potassium in defibrillation

d'Halluin, in 1904, conducted experiments in the treatment of ventricular fibrillation by giving intravenous injections of a 5% solution of potassium chloride solution in doses of 0.2 gm. per kilogram body weight. Defibrillation would promptly develop, and then he would inject Locke's solution through the artery toward the heart. With persistent massage, he often was able to restore a normal beat to the heart. Frequently, it was necessary for him to inject a 5% calcium chloride solution intravenously to increase the tone of the myocardium.

In 1930 Wiggers injected 40 to 110 mg. of potassium chloride solution (5%) per kilogram body weight into twenty-one experimental animals. The drug was injected into the ventricular cavities and, within 1 to 6 minutes, ventricular fibrillation was abolished without the use of countershock or massage. Forty milligrams or less per kilogram of body weight similarly introduced in an additional group of experimental animals did not abolish fibrillation; and Wiggers concluded that in these animals 50 mg. of potassium chloride per kilogram represented the minimal effective dose that could be relied upon to abolish ventricular fibrillation. Wiggin and colleagues state that potassium relaxes the myocardium and may produce cardiac inhibition that stops the ventricular fibrillation.

At a meeting of the International College of Physiology at Boston in 1929, Wiggers showed a motion picture demonstrating that ventricular fibrillation could be abolished by intracardiac injection of 5% potassium chloride, and that normal rhythm and blood pressures could be restored by the intraventricular injection of a 5% solution of calcium chloride to which a small amount of heparin had been added.

Practically speaking, the use of potassium to abolish fibrillation did not satisfactorily fulfill the requirements listed by Wiggers. Not only did it rapidly depress conductivity of the heart but it also depressed contraction and rhythmicity. When calcium was given, it frequently reawakened too many pacemakers and the heart reverted to fibrillation.

Winkler and associates, in 1938, after studying the effects of potassium on the mammalian heart, believed that its main action is to promote relaxation of the myocardium, and, when present in excess, causes arrest in diastole. In addition, potassium was found to produce widespread, progressive, intracardiac block noticeable first in the atrium, then at the atrioventricular node, and finally in the ventricle. In man as well as in other animals, maintenance of the blood pressure begins to fall only after the intraventricular block becomes pronounced. Correlation of the electrocardiographic changes with the level of potassium in the serum is perhaps the first such observation made.

It is interesting to note that Adams and Hand used procaine to accomplish the first successful defibrillation in man in 1942.

Drugs provide a major and worthwhile adjunct to successful ventricular defibrillation. The list of drugs potentially valuable in resuscitation is long. Their precise relationship to cardiac resuscitation as well as an accurate determination of the optimal dosages still remains a generically empirical consideration. Redding and Pearson have contributed significantly to a better definition of the proper place of drugs in resuscitation. Using various drugs and various combinations of drugs on groups of dogs experimentally fibrillated, they were able to make several conclusions. The combination of epinephrine and sodium bicarbonate is as effective in restoring circulation as any other drug or combination of drugs and, in addition, there is a higher rate of permanent survival. Methoxamine hydrochloride (Vasoxyl) is almost equally as effective except for the long-range survival rate. Epinephrine alone or in combination with lidocaine is not as effective. Sodium bicarbonate used alone is less successful than if no drugs are used. (This fact is not to be confused with the overall effect of sodium bicarbonate in combating metabolic acidosis.) The addition of procainamide hydrochloride does not alter results in the treatment of ventricular fibrillation.

Effect of epinephrine in defibrillation

In spite of warnings to the effect that epinephrine hydrochloride may throw a heart that is in cardiac asytole, or even one that is beating normally, into ventricular fibrillation, and in spite of warnings that epinephrine hydrochloride is contraindicated when ventricular fibrillation is present, we have found (both experimentally and clinically) that epinephrine hydrochloride is of distinct value in successful defibrillation procedures. On one occasion over thirteen trials of electrical countershock were attempted unsuccessfully on a fibrillating heart in a middle-aged woman. In spite of manual compression of the heart and repeated attempts at countershock, the tone of the myocardium remained feeble. However, after the injection of 0.5 ml. of a solution of 1:1,000 epinephrine hydrochloride, it was possible to defibrillate the heart with the very next electrical countershock. This matter is discussed in more detail elsewhere in this book.

Chapter 44

PHARMACOLOGY OF RESUSCITATION: MANAGEMENT OF THE ACIDOSIS OF CARDIAC ARREST

There is complete absence of body perfusion during either cardiac asystole or ventricular fibrillation. This state is often followed by the marginal perfusional status of cardiopulmonary resuscitative efforts, and both situations add up to a severe metabolic acidosis. The acidosis contributes to atony of the myocardium, to decreased peripheral vascular tone, and to interference with catecholamine (endogenous epinephrine and norepinephrine) production and action. When severe metabolic acidosis is present in association with attempts to resuscitate the fibrillating heart, success is unlikely since the arrhythmia rapidly recurs even after defibrillation.

Nearly all studies concerned with pH determination made during resuscitative attempts concur in finding rather marked metabolic acidosis as a result of oxygen deficit and accumulation of carbon dioxide and fixed acids. Under such conditions, catecholamines are interfered with. Once the pH is elevated to normal, however, endogenous epinephrine and norepinephrine again act on the vascular tree. Although not likely to be available under emergency situations outside the hospital, antacids, once available, should be given probably at least every 10 minutes during resuscitation.

The beneficial effects of maintaining near-normal blood pH and blood gases are multiple. For instance the ventricular fibrillation threshold is considerably higher in an alkalotic heart than in an acidotic heart. The incidence of spontaneous defibrillation is also considerably higher in an alkalotic heart (Dong, Stinson, and Shumway).

It is not altogether clear whether or not it is a hydrogen ion concentration per se that determines the ventricular fibrillation threshold or whether it is other effects such as potassium or calcium changes. Certainly, the change in carbon dioxide concentration has a definite effect on the ventricular fibrillation threshold.

The marked vagotonia of severe acidosis probably results from inhibition of cholinesterase activity as well as from reduced responsiveness to endogenous catecholamines at low pH.

A more accurate definition of the acidosis of cardiac arrest is urged by Chazan, Stenson, and Kurland. To date, the acidosis that accompanies cardiac arrest has not always been well defined. Use of sodium bicarbonate has been urged on an empirical basis, regardless of the type of acidosis. Metabolic acidosis is present at least to some degree in most patients with cardiac arrest because of the admittedly ineffective perfusion during closed-chest massage, accompanied by hypoxia, anaerobic metabolism, and the production of lactic acid. There is a group of patients, however, in whom the predominant derangement is due to a respiratory acidosis from inadequate ventilation, causing a rise in carbon dioxide tension and the development of hypercapnia.

Regardless of the etiology of the acidosis,

myocardial contractility is decreased, as is the responsiveness of the myocardium and the peripheral vasculature to catecholamines. Chazan carefully studied twenty-two patients during cardiac arrest. Atrial blood was drawn and analyzed at frequent intervals during resuscitative efforts. Whole blood pH and total carbon dioxide were measured, and the partial pressure of carbon dioxide was calculated as well as the plasma bicarbonate concentration. An element of metabolic acidosis, as reflected by a reduction in plasma bicarbonate concentration, was observed in all patients. However, in almost half of the patients studied, respiratory acidosis seemed to be the predominant problem, as indicated by a significant elevation of carbon dioxide tension (hypercapnia) with only a slightly depressed plasma bicarbonate concentration and metabolic acidosis. Thus Chazan notes that respiratory acidosis occurs perhaps more frequently than might be suspected. Respiratory acidosis with hypercapnia is usually more difficult to treat. While metabolic acidosis responds rather promptly to sodium bicarbonate therapy, the hypercapnic patient can compensate for the fall in pH only by lowering carbon dioxide tensions, since significant elevations in bicarbonate concentration cannot occur for many hours. Also, many of these patients have problems of the cardiovascular system that will not tolerate the amount of exogenous bicarbonate required to raise the pH. Therefore, for the treatment of acidosis due to respiratory hypercapnia, one should concentrate on requiring an adequate airway, frequent tracheal aspiration, and, occasionally, tracheotomy. Alkali therapy may prove to be of some small benefit.

Ventilation must be adequate not only to prevent respiratory acidosis but also to correct metabolic acidosis (by the administration of sodium bicarbonate). Sodium bicarbonate decreases the acidosis by combining with the lactic acid to form carbonic acid. This acid then dissociates into carbon dioxide and water. The reaction can be completed only if carbon dioxide is eliminated from the lung.

Arterial blood samples

In order to guide therapy and evaluate resuscitative efforts early in the course of resuscitation, arterial blood samples should be obtained for pH, oxygen pressure (P_{O_2}), and arterial carbon dioxide pressure (P_{CO_2}). Significant acidosis will be present in most patients although inadvertent overventilation leading to significant hypocapnia and alkalosis is occasionally seen.

After considerable clinical experience in cardiac surgery and with problems relating to cardiac arrest, Wilson suggests a rule of thumb in the administration of sodium bicarbonate to protect against the devastating actions of metabolic acidosis upon the rhythmicity of the heart. He suggests administering 44 mEq. of sodium bicarbonate at the first opportunity following cardiac arrest and then an additional 44 mEq. every 5 to 10 minutes until adequate circulation is reestablished. In addition, he suggests 1 ml. of 1:1,000 epinephrine diluted to 10 ml., injected directly into the ventricular chamber to increase excitability or contractility and to increase peripheral resistance with selective flow to vital organs.

Use of base-buffer solutions

The preponderance of studies indicate that open-chest resuscitation is hemodynamically more effective in supporting circulation than is closed-chest resuscitation. For example, cardiac and stroke indices are greater. Circulation time is shorter. Regardless of the method used, however, metabolic acidosis occurs rapidly because of the relatively poor perfusion rate.

Numerous clinicians have observed the rather dramatic and beneficial effect of pharmacologic agents acting to reduce the metabolic acidosis present in certain cases of cardiac resuscitation, particularly in cases refractory to the usual resuscitative measures. The acidosis may have been present before the arrest and may have been a contributing factor to the arrest. Metabolic acidosis may, on the other hand, have resulted from prolonged and ineffective tissue perfusion by means of artificially maintained circulation by cardiac massage. Most evidence seems to point to some depression of the ventricular contractile force as well as vasomotor tone under such conditions.

Sodium bicarbonate

As mentioned, cardiac arrest represents a *zero* perfusion state. During resuscitative efforts, this situation may improve only to the point that a *low* perfusion state exists. In any event, metabolic acidosis enters the picture along with its own inherent adverse features such as decreased arterial pressure, reduction in cardiac output, and a gradual rise in both central venous pressure and peripheral resistance. Cardiac slowing, sinus arrhythmias, sinus pauses, and sinus arrest (all suggestive of increased vagal activity) may be seen. Certainly the threshold for ventricular fibrillation is lowered.

How may metabolic acidosis associated with cardiac resuscitation best be managed? Both the severe hypoxia and the anaerobic glycolysis (which produce metabolic acidosis in the cardiac arrest patient) further potentiate ineffective myocardial function.

The routine administration of sodium bicarbonate to the patient with cardiac arrest was early advocated by Brooks and Feldman of Westminster Hospital, London. Many observations have now been recorded to indicate considerable support for this practice, particularly in patients with cardiac arrest who have been subjected to prolonged resuscitative efforts. Ventricular defibrillation has often been considerably facilitated. In the postresuscitative period, the elevation of a depressed blood pressure, the correction of an arrhythmia, the improvement in the patient's color, and an apparently improved cardiac output may

all be beneficially influenced by alkaline infusion.

Brooks and Feldman's early report considered the case of a 59-year-old man whose heart stopped on the way to the hospital after a myocardial infarction. Closed-chest resuscitation was employed until he arrived at the hospital at which time a direct approach to the heart was employed. Despite cardiac massage, the patient's pupils were dilated and the extremities showed inadequate perfusion. Regardless of efforts to defibrillate the heart, 50 minutes elapsed before it was decided to give an infusion of sodium bicarbonate. After 400 ml. of a 2.74% solution had been given, a marked lessening in the peripheral cyanosis occurred, and electrical ventricular defibrillation was successful. The blood pressure rose to a normotensive level, and not only did a sinus rhythm return but the patient also showed signs of returning consciousness. An attempt to perform an endarterectomy of the anterior descending coronary artery under profound hypothermia was subsequently made, but the patient died 14 hours after admission.

Numerous observers have noted extreme metabolic acidosis resulting from the suboxygenation occurring during cardiac resuscitative efforts. If cardiac asystole or ventricular fibrillation persists for some time, metabolic acidosis will usually have occurred. In a child, 1 ml. (0.9 mEq.) per kilogram of sodium bicarbonate diluted 1:1 with sterile water is a satisfactory dose.

Fifty milliliters of sodium bicarbonate solution will increase the pH of the blood approximately 0.1 of a pH unit. Therefore, if the pH of the blood is 7.0, four doses of sodium bicarbonate are usually necessary to correct the metabolic acidosis. This dosage can be given rather rapidly over a period of 5 or 10 minutes. With the elevation of the pH, catecholamines become relatively more effective, and the ventricular fibrillation threshold rises.

Roe cautions against overtreatment of acidosis with sodium bicarbonate. Acute alkalosis, with resulting ventricular fibrillation, may result from hypokalemia. Silberschmid and co-workers produced low perfusion acidosis by severe hemorrhagic hypotension in laboratory animals under controlled respiration. They were amazed at the speed with which acidosis develops and also with the rapidity with which the acidosis disappears simply by restoring blood volume and, hence, tissue perfusion.

A warning against too much reliance on sodium bicarbonate is voiced by Redding and Pearson. They observed from their animal studies that sodium bicarbonate alone did not promote return of circulation. Correction of the acidosis was not feasible until circulation was restored. In spite of the contention that sodium bicarbonate potentiates the action of endogenous catecholamines, they failed to notice a potentiation resulting from the effects of a suboptimal dose of epinephrine. As a matter of fact, in their experience, epinephrine given intravenously was definitely effective in restoring circulation when the pH was as low as 7.0 to 7.2. Their plea is for a greater reliance on epinephrine supplemented by, or in combination with, sodium bicarbonate.

Sodium bicarbonate may not be necessary if ventricular defibrillation attempts are carried out immediately following the onset of the arrhythmia. Parkinson and Dickson failed to note any derangement in blood pH in 204 separate successful defibrillation efforts.

When heart failure limits the use of sodium bicarbonate it may be wise to deliberately hyperventilate the patient who has carbon dioxide retention and metabolic acidosis.

Tris-(hydroxymethyl)-aminomethane (THAM)

Measures to correct the hypoxic acidosis include several possibilities. One promising base-buffer agent is Tris-(hydroxymethyl)-aminomethane (THAM). Lee and co-workers had an opportunity to study fifteen patients who were considered refractory to usual methods of resuscitation. After 15 minutes of failure to respond to the usual treatments, base-buffer solutions were injected into the left ventricle. A rather dramatic improvement was noted in the coarsening and strengthening of refractory ventricular fibrillation. This allowed prompt electrical defibrillation. Blood acid-base values in twelve of the fifteen patients were studied 5 minutes after the arrest and revealed a marked lowering of the arterial pH, the average being 7.23. The total carbon dioxide content was also considerably depressed with the average being 13mM./L. as compared with the normal 23 to 28 mM./L. The ability of the whole blood to combine with carbon dioxide was likewise lowered. Blood lactic acid values averaged 5.2 ml. (normal is equal to 0.55 to 1.1). The usual dosage by this group of investigators was in 20 ml. increments of a 0.3M solution. The largest dose required to restore cardiac rhythm was 60 ml. of a 0.3M solution. An additional effect resulting from a correction in the acidosis is an improvement in the response to sympathomimetic amine therapy.

THAM is an organic amine buffer. When administered intravenously, it acts as an amine proton acceptor that corrects acidosis. The drug readily attracts hydrogen ions, and their associated acid anions. THAM also acts as a diuretic, increasing urinary pH and excretion of electrolytes, fixed acids, and carbon dioxide.

Dosage is 1 mEq. (120 mg.) per kilogram of body weight of a 0.3M isotonic solution.

A critical appraisal of the usefulness of THAM has been provided by Bleith and Schwartz. From their appraisal, they conclude that theoretical, experimental, and clinical evidence fail to support THAM as a significant therapeutic agent. They see no reason for it to supplant the use of sodium bicarbonate. In fact, they contend that

THAM compares unfavorably with sodium bicarbonate in the treatment of metabolic acidosis from the standpoint of both efficacy and safety.

Bleith and Schwartz deny that a rapid alkalinization of intracellular spaces is desirable. In fact, they are of the opinion that rapid correction of intracellular acidosis may not be as desirable as correction of extracellular acidosis. THAM, when administered to a patient for the treatment of respiratory acidosis, depresses ventilation and thus increases the severity of hypoxemia. The depression of ventilation leads to a further retention of carbon dioxide. These authors state that THAM is of questionable value in the treatment of metabolic acidosis in patients with sodium-retaining conditions. (The reader is referred to the article for more detailed information.)

THAM is intensely alkaline and is likely to produce severe spasm, phlebitis, or thrombosis of muscles into which it is injected. Subcutaneous extravasation of THAM may produce necrosis of tissues and sloughing of overlying skin.

Other drugs, in addition to THAM, that are useful in the treatment of hypoxic or metabolic acidosis are sodium bicarbonate, $\frac{1}{6}$M sodium lactate, and 3% sodium chloride. The advantage of THAM over the other agents mentioned is that extra sodium is not added. An additional advantage of THAM over sodium buffers is that they modify intracellular as well as extracellular pH. Also, THAM is not dependent for its effect on the presence of normal alveolar exchange. The buffering action of agents such as sodium bicarbonate and sodium lactate occurs particularly in the extracellular space, where diffusion time is prolonged. In addition, equilibrium with the intracellular fluid may be minimal (Moore and Bernhard). By avoiding the additional sodium volume, there is no risk of expanding the extracellular fluid volume with its subsequent effect upon heart action. Jordan and co-workers conclude from experiments that sodium lactate beneficially affects resuscitation by direct effect on cardiac action rather than by increased pH or by presence of the sodium ion.

Sodium lactate

One-sixth molar sodium lactate, commonly used in the treatment of acidosis, has been employed in the management of cardiac arrest in the past few years. A report by Bellet and associates showed that 1M and 0.5M solutions of sodium lactate were helpful in treating patients in instances of cardiac arrest, ventricular standstill occurring during repeated Adams-Stokes seizures, and complete atrioventricular heart block.

The beneficial effect of increased ventricular rate in complete atrioventricular heart block and the return of the heartbeat in cardiac arrest are often transitory, lasting only as long as the sodium lactate is being given. As soon as metabolism of the drug occurs, the previous abnormal cardiac activity usually returns. Continuous intravenous or, in some instances, oral administration of sodium lactate has tended to prolong the improvement in cardiac activity, according to these workers.

Bellet and co-workers believe that sodium lactate causes rapid pH changes, which occur earliest in the vicinity of the heart. Any local cardiac acidosis is balanced by the sodium lactate, and a shift toward alkalosis is the result. Campbell disputes the value of sodium lactate and believes sodium bicarbonate is much preferred. Sodium lactate seems to be contraindicated because of its slowness of action (Harden and colleagues).

Chapter 45

VAGOLYTIC, CARDIOTONIC, "ANTI-SLUDGING," AND GLUCOSE-LOADING AGENTS

Atropine sulfate

Upon restoration of rhythmic contraction of the heart, the beat may be considerably slowed. In such instances, atropine sulfate intravenously administered (0.4 mg.) may reduce vagal tone, if present, and initiate a more normal rate of contraction.

The ability to reverse the cardioinhibitory effects of acidosis with atropine is an important clinical application in the treatment of shock and low perfusion syndromes, which are frequently associated with bradycardia and eventual cardiac arrest. Atropine, in this setting, should improve myocardial function pending correction of the underlying disease state (Walker, Silberschmid, and Smith).

In infants, a high degree of protection from cholinergic stimuli for 60 minutes can be provided by the use of atropine in doses of 0.05 mg. per kilogram body weight (0.014 mg. per pound) by intramuscular injection (Gaviotaki and Smith).

Should atropine be used routinely by ambulance and paramedical personnel on the basis that it will suppress ectopic activity? Lown believes that the patient with infarction is in a hypercatecholic state and undue rate acceleration produced by vagolytic agents may produce serious complications. Atropine should be reserved for situations when bradycardia is present and especially when accompanied by ventricular premature beats or by evidence of hemodynamic compromise.

Methantheline (Banthine)

Methantheline is sometimes used in place of atropine. Although it is a good drying agent, it is not the potent vagolytic agent in preventing cardiac arrhythmia and asystole as found in atropine and its action is more prolonged.

Cardiotonic agents

CALCIUM CHLORIDE

Since the revival of interest in the use of calcium chloride for cardiac resuscitation by Kay and Blalock several years ago, this drug has been enjoying increasing prominence as an adjunct in cardiac resuscitation. d'Halluin was probably the first to report encouraging results with calcium chloride in patients with cardiac arrest.

Kay and Blalock report on their work with calcium chloride in dogs. They believe the drug is a better cardiac stimulant than barium chloride, chiefly because the effect is more rapid. In no case were they able to find satisfactory action achievable when calcium had failed. In discussing the effect of calcium, Kay and Blalock state:

The calcium cation increases the contractility of the heart and prolongs the systolic phase of the heart. Winkler's experimental evidence suggests that as the serum concentration of the calcium ion rises progressively, there is an initial bradycardia followed by higher concentrations by a direct action of calcium on the ventricular muscle, increasing its excitability and producing foci of idiopathic ventricular rhythm and ventricular extrasystoles of large and unusual form. This effect resembles both the accelerator stimulation of epinephrine hydrochloride and the muscular stimulation of digitalis.*

*Kay, J. H., and Blalock, A.: The use of calcium chloride in the treatment of cardiac arrest in patients, Surg. Gynecol. Obstet. **93**:97-102, 1951.

Although calcium chloride has much to offer in resuscitation, it must be remembered that, in certain doses, it will inhibit normal sinus formation. Several cases of sudden death following intravenous injection of calcium chloride are reported by Sherf.

Calcium chloride may be given in a dose ranging from 0.3 to 1.0 gm. Particularly is calcium chloride indicated in resuscitation of patients who have lost a considerable amount of blood and received citrated blood for replacement. Sealy recommends 0.5 gm. of calcium chloride per 500 ml. of blood administered.

The usual dose of calcium chloride is 5 ml. of a 10% solution given either intravenously or by the intracardiac route. If calcium chloride is not available, calcium gluconate (10%) may be administered. Ten to fifteen milliliters of calcium gluconate is equivalent to 5 ml. of 10% calcium chloride.

Calcium chloride may be used repeatedly in instances of ventricular asystole, along with one of the cardiotonic-vasopressor drugs, as an agent to combat the metabolic acidosis that results from a low perfusion state.

Wolff, in 1950, advised the use of calcium chloride in the treatment of cardiac standstill when the heart is dilated or flaccid. He suggested the use of calcium chloride when epinephrine fails. Beck also suggests that, following electrical defibrillation of the heart, calcium chloride should be injected into the right ventricle if the fibrillation had been converted into a ventricular standstill without restoration of any signs of contractility. Beck and his colleagues recommend that the calcium be given into the right ventricular cavity. They suggest repeated doses, if necessary. Mautz found that calcium chloride is of aid in the heart where extreme dilatation is present following a toxic dose of procaine.

Kay and Blalock suggest that calcium chloride may be more effective than is epinephrine for treating cardiac arrest in patients with congenital heart disease. The usual dosage recommended for the adult heart is 2 to 5 ml. of a 10% solution of calcium chloride.

Calcium chloride is an aid in improving the tone of defibrillating hearts and is particularly indicated when ventricular fibrillation has occurred after a massive blood transfusion.

BARIUM CHLORIDE

As early as 1908, Pike and co-workers employed barium chloride in several experiments in resuscitation. They abandoned the drug, believing that it was too uncertain and too dangerous in its action.

Caution should be exercised in employing even small doses of barium. Ventricular fibrillation is often the complication of on overdose. The pharmacologic effect of barium on the heart consists first of a vagal bradycardia, followed by ventricular arrhythmias and ventricular fibrillation.

Cooley, in reporting on cardiac resuscitation during pulmonic stenosis, writes that barium chloride in a 0.5% solution had been employed in a few patients and produced an apparent increase in the force of amplitude of the systolic contractions. Fauteux was also an advocate of barium chloride.

The action of barium chloride is to strengthen the contractions of most forms of muscles—probably by direct action on the contractile tissue. It is likely, also, that it increases the irritability of the cardiac ventricles. Cohn and Levine, in 1925, suggested its use in the Adams-Stokes syndrome or atrioventricular block. Since the soluble salts of barium are all active poisons for both striated and unstriated muscles, their dosage must be well controlled. The action of the blood vessels is one of contraction; consequently, the blood pressure is elevated. It is also likely that barium chloride acts as a coronary vasoconstrictor. Two milliliters of a 0.5% solution of barium chloride is probably a satisfactory dose in the usual case when barium is indicated.

I have used barium chloride a great deal on cardiac arrest experiments in the animal laboratory. Although my experience has been at variance with most on this point, I have been rather impressed with barium chloride as an effective agent in cardiac resuscitation. One particularly effective clinical illustration occurred in a 45-year-old man on whom attempts at cardiac resuscitation were carried out by intermittent manual compression of the heart for over 2 hours. In spite of repeated doses of epinephrine, the successful electrical defibrillation of an episode of ventricular fibrillation, and long periods of massage, no apparent benefit was noted. It was decided to employ barium chloride. After waiting for the pharmacy to prepare the solution, it was finally given into the left ventricle and within just a few seconds after injection and subsequent cardiac compression, normal rhythm of the heart abruptly resumed. The blood pressure returned to 120 systolic and respirations became regular. The chest was closed and the patient lived for a period of about 14 hours, at which time he suddenly went into collapse. At autopsy, it was found that the underlying pathology had been a massively bleeding gastric ulcer. (An emergency gastrectomy had been scheduled for that morning.)

"Anti-sludging" agents and the microcirculation

LOW MOLECULAR WEIGHT DEXTRAN

Not only is plasma expansion produced by the volume of low molecular weight dextran itself but also by the osmotic attraction of interstitial fluids into the vascular channels. With a reduction of blood viscosity, peripheral flow is improved and sequestered blood cells are released. Cardiac output increases subsequent to an increase in venous return to the heart.

MANNITOL

A 20% solution of mannitol reduces elevated cerebrospinal fluid pressure, intraocular pressure, and cerebral edema by establishing intravascular hyperosmolarity. The total dose (1.5 to 2.0 gm. per kilogram of body weight) is to be given in a period of 30 to 60 minutes. Mannitol is contraindicated in patients with severe impairment of renal function unless the kidneys respond to a test dose of 0.2 gm. per kilogram of body weight administered within 3 to 5 minutes. An adequate response measured by urinary output, is at least 40 ml. per hour, measured over a 2- to 3-hour period. The useful range for adult dosage within a 24-hour period is 50 to 200 gm.

If the urinary output, as collected by an indwelling catheter in the bladder, is less than 15 ml. per 30 minutes, a test dose of mannitol (1 ampule contains 12.5 gm.) can be given. If this increases the output, then an additional 50 to 200 gm. per 24 hours can be given. If no diuretic response occurs to the test dose, mannitol should not be used.

Experimentally, mannitol does not appear to have the protective influence against cerebral edema that is shown by prolonged hypothermia.

HEPARIN

Several studies have demonstrated consistent changes in blood coagulation time after cardiac arrest in dogs. In the University of San Carlos School of Medicine in Guatemala City, cardiac arrest was experimentally produced in thirty-seven dogs. Anatomic studies revealed thrombosis in vessels of the brain, lungs, and kidneys to the extent that anticoagulant therapy was urged in the postresuscitative treatment phase in patients (Arroyave and others).

Ripstein stresses the value of heparin in patients with cardiac arrest as a means of preventing thrombosis and maintaining the fluidity of the blood. I have seldom used heparin, but from a theoretical standpoint it may have merit. Heparin is always available as part of the mobile cardiac resuscitation unit.

Although heparin has been used in the postresuscitative period and although advocates of its use have been convinced of effectiveness in prevention of secondary thrombosis following stasis of circulatory arrest, a clear-cut case for the use of heparin has not yet been established.

Glucose-loading agents

SODI-PALLARES REGIMEN

The Sodi-Pallares regimen is designed to encourage the return of potassium into the myocardial cell, as, for example, in postinfarction heart block cases. The regimen consists of the infusion of 1,000 ml. of 5% dextrose containing 40 mEq. potassium and 20 units of soluble insulin.

Burke and co-workers demonstrated that, during ischemia of the myocardium, an increased arterial concentration of glucose reduces myocardial potassium loss and the incidence of serious ventricular arrhythmias.

Glucose and insulin are given in addition to potassium because of experimental evidence that glucose and insulin favor potassium entry into damaged and hypopolarized cardiac cells, and that they may help restore the cells to a normal state of polarization. Mittra studied 170 patients with acute myocardial infarction. Eighty-five were used as controls and eighty-five were treated with the Sodi-Pallares routine. After 14 days, the mortality in the control group was 28.2%, as compared with 11.7% in the treated group.

The value of a polarizing solution in treatment of myocardial infarction has been a subject of considerable controversy among cardiologists and, in spite of comments to the contrary, considerable interest in its potential value exists. Bisteni of the National Heart Institute of Mexico in Mexico City reports a death rate of 6% in 250 patients treated with the solution of a mixture of glucose, potassium, and insulin. Apparently the death rate is 12% to 15% among patients in coronary centers elsewhere in Mex-

ico (patients who are receiving forms of treatment other than the polarizing solution). Experimentally produced heart attacks in dogs treated with the polarizing solution indicated to Maroko that there is some reduction of heart damage or even prevention of damage. This University of California medical group at San Diego furthermore states that when propranolol is used, heart damage can be forestalled even when treated with the polarizing solution as long as 3 hours after the attack. They indicate that further studies are warranted to clarify the potential usefulness of the solution. Bisteni's regimen consists of the administration of 2 quarts of the solution within a 24-hour period following admission to the hospital. It is theorized that sodium, which is normally outside the cell, rushes in when the potassium leaks out of the injured cell. The infusion is combined with a low-sodium diet. The glucose helps additionally to supply energy to the damaged cell while the insulin serves to guide potassium return to the cells.

GLUCOSE

Theoretically, by reducing initial myocardial edema and by forcing potassium back into the cell when aberrations are caused by myocardial hypoxia, hypertonic glucose solutions may be effective in increasing conductivity and contractility.

Danilov, in 1936, advocated the addition of glucose for its effect on cardiac musculature. Negovskii adopted his routine after Kirsch showed that respiration of the cardiac muscle is raised 27% by the addition of 1% glucose in Ringer's solution. Other Russian physicians have also thought that the addition of glucose gave excellent results and have even continued its use in the postresuscitative period. Hall and associates conclude that hypertonic glucose, even with added insulin, is an adjunct in cardiac resuscitation by the action of providing the myocardium with a readily available energy source.

Hydrogen peroxide as an adjunct in cardiac resuscitation

An infusion of 0.12% hydrogen peroxide may be a useful adjunct in cardiopulmonary resuscitation. Urschel has reported on this subject after several laboratory investigations and some clinical experience. In the pig heart, hydrogen peroxide infused through the coronary artery or applied directly to the epicardium decreases the incidence of ventricular fibrillation. Hydrogen peroxide supersaturates the plasma and tissue fluid with oxygen, much as occurs under hyperbaric oxygenation.

The effect of hydrogen peroxide on the cardiovascular system has been the subject of an extensive investigation by Urschel and associates. It was their original intent to find a method for oxygenating tissues in the way that hyperbaric oxygenation does. Using dilute solutions, they note that hydrogen peroxide undergoes decomposition to oxygen and water by catalase and peroxidase and that more oxygen is recovered from the tissues than one would expect from 100% saturation with oxygen at 1 atmosphere.

Hydrogen peroxide is capable of releasing dissolved oxygen equivalent to that which one would find in solutions under oxygen at 3 to 8 atmospheres of pressure. Obviously, hydrogen peroxide administration does not require lung transport and can be given continuously over long periods of time without use of expensive equipment.

Hydrogen peroxide was used to treat a 60-year-old woman on whom attempts at cardiac resuscitation were being made without success. A cardiac catheter was passed through the right brachial artery to the root of the aorta. ECG and blood pressure were monitored. Within 1 minute after the infusion of 0.12% hydrogen peroxide, the ECG reverted from a nodal to a regular sinus rhythm and the mean arterial pressure rose to 70 mm. Hg.

A communication from Urschel states his belief that hydrogen peroxide used intrapericardially in low concentrations will be of great benefit as an adjunct to cardiac resuscitation, particularly when the arrest is secondary to coronary artery obstruction.

Chapter 46

PHARMACOLOGY OF RESUSCITATION: A SUMMARY

Table 46-1 lists a group of over forty drugs that may have a therapeutic role in cardiopulmonary resuscitation. A summary of the rationale for their use is included, along with suggested dosage schedules for specific situations. The reader is cautioned that any drug should be used only with the *full* knowledge of its characteristic activity and varied responses.

Caffeine, picrotoxin, cocaine, nikethamide (Coramine), and pentylenetetrazol (Metrazol) have no place in resuscitation of the heart.

Text continued on p. 509.

Table 46-1. Summary of drugs related to cardiac arrest and resuscitation*

Drugs	Usual adult dose	Route of administration	Rationale
Acetylcholine chloride	50 to 150 mg. 20 mg.	Hypodermic Intravenous	Raises fibrillary threshold of the ventricle; mainly of experimental value
Atropine sulfate	0.5 mg. 0.3 to 0.5 mg. previous to anesthesia	Intravenous Intramuscular	For reduction of vagal tone, to enhance A-V induction, and to accelerate heart rate in cases of bradycardia
	0.4 to 0.6 mg. 1 mg. few minutes before ECT in patients with cardiovascular disease	Oral Intravenous	
	2 mg. 30 min. before ECT in patients with normal hearts	Intramuscular	Increased dosage for patients with jaundice
	0.4 to 0.65 mg., repeat in 15 min. if necessary	Intravenous	Helps reverse cardioinhibitory effect of acidosis
	Infants: 0.1 to 0.2 mg.	Intramuscular	May provide protection from cholinergic stimuli for 60 min.
Barium chloride (extremely toxic and seldom used)	2 ml. of 0.5% solution	Injection into ventricular *lumen* or intravenously	Increases ventricular irritability and rate Strengthens muscular contractions (asystole) Adams-Stokes syndrome

*The drugs listed above are those commonly used in connection with clinical problems of cardiac arrest and resuscitation. Unfortunately, some drug dosages in resuscitation are still somewhat empirical. Dosages listed are for adults unless otherwise specified. Also see Appendix for drug dosage in cardiopulmonary resuscitation.

Continued.

Table 46-1. Summary of drugs related to cardiac arrest and resuscitation—cont'd

Drugs	Usual adult dose	Route of administration	Rationale
Bretylium tosylate (still experimental; not released for general use)	5 mg. per kg. 5% ml. of 5% dextrose in water (slowly over 5 min.)	Intramuscular Intravenous	Postganglionic sympathetic blocking agent; effective in suppressing ectopic foci such as premature beats, bigeminal and trigeminal rhythm, and second-degree heart block; increases myocardial sensitivity to catecholamines; enhances effect of countershock in ventricular fibrillation; elevates fibrillation threshold; promotes hypotension
Calcium chloride	5 ml. of 10% solution (9.1 mEq. Ca^{++}) 0.5 gm./500 ml. of transfused blood 50 to 100 mg. (5 to 10 ml. of 1% solution), can repeat every 3 to 4 min. *Infants:* 1 ml. per 5 kg. diluted 1:1 with saline	Intravenous

Intracardiac | Stimulant (when compression plus epinephrine ineffective, in asystole) Increases amplitude of contractions in feebly beating heart (may cause ventricular fibrillation); prolongs systole; increases ventricular excitability; synergistic with epinephrine; antagonist of acidosis-induced hyperkalemia

Use caution in digitalized children **Do not use in digitalis intoxication** |
Calcium gluconate, 10% solution (calcium chloride preferred to calcium gluconate; latter poorly ionized)	10 ml. of 10% solution (4.8 mEq. Ca^{++})	Intravenous or intracardiac	Often given after blood transfusion to maintain calcium-potassium ratio Increases amplitude of contractions in feebly beating heart
Chlorpromazine (Thorazine)	25 mg. every 6 hr.	Intramuscular or oral	Facilitates hypothermia during postresuscitative period Provides autonomic and general sedation
Corticosteroids (prednisone)	60 mg./day 100 mg., repeat if needed	Oral Intravenous (prednisolone)	Antishock properties For complete heart block with Adams-Stokes attacks Beneficial effect on A-V conduction in absence of organic heart disease Antiinflammatory effect of drug may be helpful May maintain idioventricular pacemaker
Dexamethasone phosphate (Decadron)	8 mg. initial dose; 4 to 8 mg. every 6 hr. for 4 to 5 days	Intramuscular	For prevention or attenuation of cerebral edema; postoperative pneumonitis or "shock lung"
Dextran 40 (low molecular weight) (Rheomacrodex, LMD, Gentran 40)	500 ml. @ 20 to 40 ml./min. (may repeat at intervals)	Intravenous	Prevents sludging during circulatory impairment; increases capillary blood flow

Table 46-1. Summary of drugs related to cardiac arrest and resuscitation—cont'd

Drugs	Usual adult dose	Route of administration	Rationale
Digitalis (lanatoside C)	0.8 mg., repeat in 2 hr.	Intravenous	For certain postresuscitation arrhythmias (supraventricular tachycardia) Myocardial support To decrease heart rate (when tachycardia is caused by heart failure or atrial fibrillation or flutter *only*)
Diphenylhydantoin sodium (Dilantin) (250 mg., 5 ml. vial)	100 mg. as bolus given over 3 to 4 min. period (2 to 4 mg. per kg. of body weight)	Intravenous	Useful in supraventricular and ventricular arrhythmias arising from digitalis excess For multifocal ventricular ectopic beats in postresuscitative period Contraindicated in bradycardia Of little value in atrial flutter or fibrillation For postresuscitative convulsions
Ephedrine sulfate	25 mg. every 4 hr.	Oral	As a sympathomimetic amine, it improves atrioventricular conduction and speeds up heart For Adams-Stokes syndrome
Epinephrine (Adrenalin), 1:1,000 (1 mg./ ml., 1 ml. ampule) 1:10,000	0.5 ml. of 1:1,000 solution Occasional larger doses	Intravenous every 5 min.	Ventricular standstill May be used in ventricular fibrillation when heart dilated and flabby, making defibrillation difficult (lowers defibrillation threshold) Increases myocardial tone, conduction, and heart rate, elevates perfusion pressure Peripheral vasoconstriction Mobilizes potassium when glucose released from liver—may induce fibrillation
	Usually best to increase volume by diluting to 10 ml. in normal saline solution (5 ml. of 1:10,000 solution)		
	Newborn infant: 0.1 to 0.2 mg.	Intracardiac	
	0.1 mg. in 10 ml. dextrose	Intracardiac	Effectiveness improved by combining with sodium bicarbonate
	0.3 to 0.5 mg. aliquot (effective for about 5 min.) *Children:* 1 ml. per 5 kg.		
Ethacrynic acid (Edecrin)	50 to 100 mg.		Potent diuretic agent
Ethamivan (vanillic acid diethylamide)	100 mg. initially (1 to 2 mg. per kg. of body weight in infant); may repeat dose	Intravenous over 20 to 30 sec.	Used as a respiratory stimulant; increases tidal volume with subsequent improved alveolar ventilation
Furosemide (Lasix)	20 to 40 mg.	Slowly if intravenous	Potent diuretic agent

Continued.

Table 46-1. Summary of drugs related to cardiac arrest and resuscitation—cont'd

Drugs	Usual adult dose	Route of administration	Rationale
Heparin	100 units/lb. body weight	Intravenous	Counteract increased blood coagulability after resuscitation May be too risky after direct method of resuscitation
Hydrochlorothiazide (Hydrodiuril)	50 mg. twice a day	Oral	For heart block with Adams-Stokes syndrome Kaluretic effect Hypokalemic effect (hypokalemia tends to improve A-V conduction)
Hydrogen peroxide (still experimental)	0.12%	Intravenous	Supersaturate plasma and tissue fluid with oxygen
	0.12%	Intrapericardial	Adjunct in resuscitation, especially when arrest is secondary to coronary artery obstruction
Isoproterenol hydrochloride (isopropylnorepinephrine, Isuprel), 1:5,000 (0.2 mg./ml.) (1:15,000, 0.2 mg., 1 ml. ampule)	10 to 15 mg. t.i.d. 10 to 30 ml. of 1:50,000 (by adding 9 ml. normal saline solution to 1 ml. of 1 to 5 mg. per 100 ml. 1:5,000)	Sublingually (for prevention of Adams-Stokes attacks) Intravenous injection Intravenous drip	Stimulant (S-A node) Adams-Stokes syndrome Ventricular standstill (less likely to cause ventricular fibrillation than is epinephrine) **Should not be given with epinephrine**
	2 mg./500 ml. of 5% glucose solution	Intravenous, prior to placement of cardiac pacemaker	Probably to be avoided in cardiogenic shock
	0.1 to 0.2 mg.	Intravenous, every 3 to 5 min.	In association with ventricular asystole and myocardial infarction
Levarterenol bitartrate (Levophed) (1 ml. = 2 mg., 1 ml. ampule)	16 mg. in 500 ml. of 5% glucose in water 0.1 to 0.2 mg. *Children:* 2 mg. per 500 ml. of 5% dextrose in water	Intravenous	For pressor effect during resuscitation effort (may cause tissue slough)
Lidocaine (Xylocaine)	50 to 100 mg. as slow intravenous bolus Repeat if necessary or follow with continuous infusion of 1 to 3 mg. per min. (not over 4 mg. per min.) 500 mg. in 500 ml. of 5% dextrose in water gives solution of 1.0 mg. per 1 ml. for infusion	Intravenous	For ventricular irritability after myocardial infarction—ventricular tachycardia or premature ventricular beats Raises fibrillation threshold Effective for digitalis-induced ventricular arrhythmias Limited value in atrial arrhythmias once ectopic beats cease

Table 46-1. Summary of drugs related to cardiac arrest and resuscitation—cont'd

Drugs	Usual adult dose	Route of administration	Rationale
	Infants: 0.5 mg. per kg. (not over 100 mg. per hour)		
Mannitol, 20% solution (1 ampule contains 12.5 gm.)	1.5 to 2 gm./kg. body weight in 30 to 60 min. 50 to 200 gm. within 24-hour period	Intravenous	Reduces elevated cerebral spinal fluid pressure and cerebral edema Produces intravascular hyperosmolarity Contraindicated with severe renal impairment (give test dose) Diuretic for postresuscitative oliguria
Meperidine (Demerol)	50 to 100 mg.	Intravenous	To help prevent shivering under hypothermia Given with promethazine hydrochloride (Phenergan)
Mephentermine sulfate (Wyamine)	2 to 5 mg. every 10 to 15 min.	Intravenous	Cardiotonic action Liberates noradrenalin
Metaraminol bitartrate (Aramine) (10 mg./1 ml., 10 ml. ampule)	15 to 100 mg. (1.5 to 10 ml.) in 500 ml. sodium chloride or 5% dextrose injection Can be given 2 to 5 mg. every 5 to 10 min. *Children:* 25 mg. per 100 ml. of 5% dextrose in water	Intravenous titration (slowly)	For postresuscitative hypotension Vasoconstrictor-positive inotropic effect
Methacholine (Mecholyl)	20 mg. doses (repeat in 30 minutes if needed)	Subcutaneous	For postresuscitative supraventricular tachycardia if digitalis, quinidine, or procainamide fail
Methoxamine hydrochloride (Vasoxyl)	3 to 5 mg. every 10 to 15 min. 5 to 15 mg.	Intravenous titration (slowly) Intramuscular	Vasopressor effect Depresses myocardial excitability Negative chronotropic effect on the heart
Methylprednisolone sodium succinate (Solu-Medrol)	125 mg. initially, 40 mg. every 6 hrs. (5 mg. per kg.)	Intramuscular	For use in postresuscitation cerebral edema, cardiogenic shock, or "shock lung"
Neostigmine	2 ml. of 1:4,000 solution	Intravenous	Raises fibrillary threshold of ventricle To counteract "neomycin arrest"
Papaverine hydrochloride	30 to 60 mg.	Slow intravenous administration (too much induces coarse fibrillation)	Of unproved value in raising fibrillary threshold of the ventricle Possible increased cerebral blood flow
Phenylephrine hydrochloride (Neo-Synephrine)	3 to 5 mg. (40 to 50 mg. in 500 ml. dextrose in water)	Intravenous Intravenous titration	Alpha-adrenergic To support arterial pressure (little action on heart)

Continued.

Table 46-1. Summary of drugs related to cardiac arrest and resuscitation—cont'd

Drugs	Usual adult dose	Route of administration	Rationale
Procainamide hydrochloride (Pronestyl) (100 mg./ml., 10 ml. vial)	100 to 200 mg. increments (may give up to 500 mg. initially; start with 50 mg.)	Intravenous or intracardiac (slowly)	Indications: Myocardial irritability Adams-Stokes syndrome Occasional case of ventricular fibrillation Longer duration and less toxic than procaine, also less effect on CNS **Do not use with epinephrine**
	250 to 500 mg. every 4 hours	Intramuscular or oral once ectopic beats cease	Diminishes excitability of both atria and ventricles and slows conduction Elevates fibrillation threshold
Procaine hydrochloride, 1% solution (Novocain)	2 to 5 ml. of 1% solution	Intracardiac	Defibrillary action (when countershock fails, not as a substitute therefor) May depress cardiac output
Promethazine hydrochloride (Phenergan)	50 mg. in 500 ml., slowly	Intravenous	Sedation to prevent shivering under hypothermia (while treating cerebral anoxic sequelae)
Propranolol hydrochloride (Inderal)	1 mg. (may be repeated to 3 mg.)	Intravenous (not to exceed 1 mg. per min.)	As beta-adrenergic blocking agent may suppress persistently recurring ventricular fibrillation (May cause bradycardia, hypotension, and cardiac failure); negative chronotropic and inotropic action Resort to lidocaine or procainamide first Good in treatment of arrhythmias resulting from digitalis intoxication Useful for tetanic heart contraction (stone heart)
Quinidine gluconate (80 mg./ml., 10 ml. vial)	In increments of 240 mg.	Slow intravenous administration (too much induces coarse fibrillation; monitor with ECG)	Raises fibrillary threshold of the ventricle Inhibits vagal influence Permits sinus node acceleration Postresuscitative extrasystoles
Sodi-Pallares regimen	1,000 ml. of 5% dextrose containing 40 mEq. potassium and 20 units soluble insulin	Intravenous	To encourage return of potassium into myocardial cell—postinfarction heart block
Sodium bicarbonate, 4.75 gm. (44.6 mEq) (50 ml. ampule)	1 mEq. per kg. 50 ml. (one ampule) injected as bolus or over 10-min. period Repeat every 10 min. if arrest persists Give half initial dose at 10-min. intervals if no blood gas and	Intravenous (avoid intracardiac route)	To combat metabolic acidosis

Table 46-1. Summary of drugs related to cardiac arrest and resuscitation—cont'd

Drugs	Usual adult dose	Route of administration	Rationale
	pH determinations available		
	Children: half dose		Counteracts myocardial atony from metabolic acidosis
Sodium lactate, 1M solution	Up to 250 ml. of 2.5M solution Increments of 10 ml. of 1M solution/kg. body weight	Intravenous	Indication: metabolic acidosis resulting from prolonged circulatory arrest or inadequate cardiac output (sodium bicarbonate preferred) Reduces interventricular block Is slow to become effective
Sucrose, 50%	300 to 500 ml. in divided dose	Intravenous	Possible effect: decreasing cerebral edema (probably transient)
Tris-(hydroxymethyl)-amino-methene (THAM)	20 ml. increments of 0.3M solution; after heart activity restored, 0.3M until arterial pH 7.35 to 7.5	Intravenous	Strengthens and coarsens ventricular fibrillation, leading to successful electrical defibrillation Corrects metabolic acidosis May not be as effective as sodium bicarbonate
Urea, 30% solution (Urevert)	1 gm./kg. body weight (40 gm. in 250 ml. of 5% dextrose) b.i.d.	Intravenous, 60 drops/min.	Following resuscitation in cases associated with prolonged cerebral anoxia Lowers cerebrospinal fluid pressure Induces osmotic diuresis (contraindicated in renal shut down)

Drugs in heart block

Drug therapy in the treatment of heart block is directed at improving both the rate and stroke output of the heart. Since the rate is dependent upon the fibers of the specialized conducting system of the heart and since the stroke output reflects the functional status of the contractility property of the myocardium, drug action is designed to be twofold.

Increasing cardiac output by accelerating pulse rate and building up stroke volume can be aided by beta-adrenergic drugs such as isoproterenol. A relative hypokalemia produced by thiazide diuretics and dietary restrictions on potassium may enhance the conductivity and contractility of the ventricle. Anticholinergic drugs that block vagal stimulation may provide a relative increase in sympathetic nerve stimulation. The antiinflammatory property of cortisone-like drugs may help shrink the edema that surrounds the conducting tracts and may thus remove a block to conduction as in acute myocardial infarction and in cases of sarcoid heart disease. Cortisone-like drugs also stimulate potassium loss. Quinidine and other myocardial depressants are usually contraindicated in complete heart block. Digitalis should be used with extreme caution.

However, at present no drug is an effective alternative to placement of a transvenous pacemaker either prophylactically or in an emergency. Drugs in this situation are largely of historic interest.

PART SIX

ORGANIZATION AND APPLICATION OF EFFECTIVE RESUSCITATION

Chapter 47

THE LOGISTICS OF RESUSCITATION WITHIN THE HOSPITAL

Glenn O. Turner with the assistance of Dick Ames

Introduction

The next significant reduction in the number of sudden and unexpected deaths occurring inside and outside of hospitals is not likely to occur until we have succeeded in breaking the logistics barrier that now often intervenes between the patient who needs resuscitation and the resuscitation he needs.

Probably no one doubts that the resuscitation techniques developed during the 1950s and 1960s could save many more lives than they now do if they were employed more quickly on more patients. The logistics barrier that prevents this has two major elements: first, patients do not seek help quickly enough, if at all; and second, hospitals are often not prepared to provide these life-saving procedures efficiently, swiftly, and economically (Fig. 47-1). The result is waste—waste of hospital plant and waste of human lives.

In Springfield, Missouri, we have developed during the past 12 years two promising techniques for avoiding this waste. One, at St. John's Hospital, is concerned with amplifying and organizing hospital facilities in a way that will assure more effective resuscitation when the patient arrives. The other, by the Greene County Heart Association, is concerned with mobilizing more patients to act faster when they need help. In combination, these techniques have enabled us to reduce in our region the number of sudden and unexpected deaths caused by a wide range of cardiovascular and surgical emergencies.

We use two acronyms to designate our techniques: CVCU and EWS. CVCU stands for a comprehensive cardiovascular care unit and refers to our expanded version of the traditional CCU, or coronary care unit, which we have redesigned to treat not only heart attack patients but all others who have any type of acutely life-threatening cardiovascular condition, both in the acute phase of the illness and in the intermediate and convalescent phases as well. EWS stands for early warning signs of heart attack and refers to a community-wide, multimedia educational program through which we have attempted to increase public awareness of premonitory symptoms of this major cause of death in the United States. With the EWS program we have speeded the response of patients and increased the number who call for aid; with the CVCU we have significantly increased the numbers of successful resuscitations among patients who reach the hospital.

Because of the spectacular results achieved by modern methods of resuscitation, we tend to forget that our present resuscitation programs rest upon only a few relatively simple procedures: techniques to keep the airway open, such as suctioning and either mechanical or mouth-to-mouth ventilation; and techniques to maintain circulation, such as

513

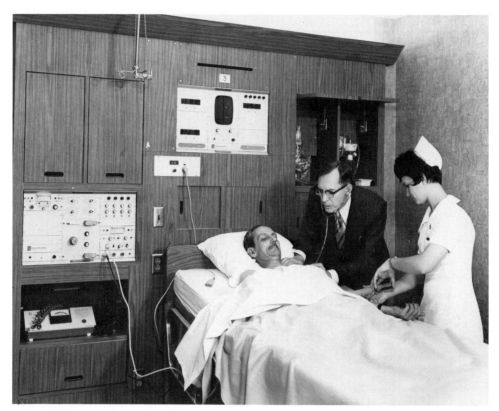

Fig. 47-1. In an optimum setting for resuscitation, backed by the Springfield Wall and its array of the latest equipment for monitoring and treatment, this heart patient receives far better than the "fighting chance" he would have had just a few years ago. All necessary resuscitative equipment is housed in the wall, including defibrillator at left, monitor scope above patient's head, and oxygen and suction on both sides of the bed, in the open cabinets at right and in the closed cabinets at left. All required medications and supplies are in drawers at the bedside.

closed- or open-heart massage, electronic monitoring of heart rhythms, and drug or replacement therapy.

The very simplicity of these procedures has helped account for their effectiveness and widespread use. Increasingly, resuscitative tasks are being performed by nurses and aides, rather than by doctors, with no appreciable decline in success rates. The two procedures discussed in this article have a similar simplicity. They can be applied by any hospital, from the largest to the smallest, without requiring an unfeasible increment in equipment or staff.

"Grouping" is the key word in explaining why these procedures succeed in breaking the logistics barrier. The EWS program creates a larger group of patients applying for treatment, and the expanded CCU groups the necessary number of beds, adequately equipped, staffed, and interrelated, to handle this increased population of critical patients. Instead of being scattered on different general and specialty halls ill-designed and ill-equipped to manage them, these patients are grouped in one section, where the hospital's full lifesaving potential can be brought to bear on them. Because these lifesaving machines and personnel are worked to full capacity, or near it, they soon are honed to perform their tasks with maximum success and minimum cost.

This chapter discusses the evolution of the CVCU concept at St. John's, and describes the operation of the present unit. It concludes with a description of the EWS program, together with guidelines as to how such a program can be carried out elsewhere. The CVCU section begins with a brief description of the first three generations of traditional CCUs, with emphasis on the specific characteristics of each; describes how the first "fourth generation" CCU was built at St. John's by simple remodeling of existing bed space; and concludes by explaining how the increased demand for intensive care facilities, stimulated by the success of this first 42-bed progressive care unit, led to construction of the new 90-bed unit.

Both the remodeled and the newly constructed units differ radically in function and design from the earliest CCUs. It is the new unit, the CVCU, that we in Springfield regard as the wave of the future in resuscitative care, not only for cardiac patients but for all patients who face acutely life-threatening cardiovascular emergencies.

At first blush it may seem that description of the EWS program is extraneous to a discussion of current resuscitation facilities in hospitals. But it is not. In the future, I am convinced, hospitals and individual physicians will be called upon to engage increasingly in efforts to acquaint the public at large with the early signs of life-threatening emergencies and to motivate them to seek appropriate medical aid. Traditionalists may look askance at these educational efforts, regarding them as unethical attempts to "drum up trade." I submit that this attitude is both untimely and unproductive and that it serves the interests neither of the public nor of the medical profession.

"Consumerism," the right of the consumer of goods to have a voice in determining what he shall receive, and when, and under what conditions, and at what cost, is today the dominant trend in medicine as in many fields. We ignore this trend at our peril. In

years to come the public is going to become ever more aware of the health dangers it faces and the means of avoiding them. Hospitals that are equipped to provide less than the best level of care—commensurate with their natural limitations in size, equipment and staff—may find themselves bypassed. In collaboration with public and private agencies, the hospital of the future will play a vigorous role in recruiting patients by educating the public, and it must therefore prepare itself to handle an increased load of medically sophisticated patients. It can do this well only by providing an adequate number of beds suitably equipped and staffed to accommodate every type of life-threatening emergency at a price the public can afford.

This, at least, is the "bet" of the Springfield group, whose collective experience is summarized here. What follows is an attempt to explain why we think as we do and to explain how our ideas can be realized by hospitals of any size, from the smallest to the largest.

The concept of a CVCU

"Many coronary care units now being built will be obsolete before construction is complete." These words were spoken in 1970 by Dr. Irving S. Wright, Chairman of the Inter-Society Commission for Heart Disease Resources. The challenge he then voiced to CCU planners was to create units "which would still be up-to-date in 1980."

That challenge remains valid today. But what exactly does it mean? Dr. Wright implies that the CCU concept is undergoing some process of evolution, in terms of which some CCUs now being constructed can be considered anachronisms. But what is that process of evolution? Toward what ideal is it tending? What guidelines can planners of future CCUs rely on to ensure that they will be in the vanguard of resuscitative medicine?

I am convinced that the CCU as originally conceived and as presently operating in many hospitals is virtually obsolete, both in design and function. So I am proposing that some radical changes be made in the traditional CCU concept. This has always been a glamorous concept. Wondrous machinery producing wondrous results—this was and still is a fascinating event for any physician accustomed to feeling that nothing can be done for certain types of patients. But perhaps we have been so mesmerized by the machinery and its early successes in treating "hopeless" coronaries that we have arbitrarily limited our concept of a CCU. Most of us probably still think of such a facility only as an electronically equipped ward of 3 to 6 beds designed for detecting and reversing cardiac arrhythmias, particularly those associated with myocardial infarction. Because CCUs do that job so well, we may have failed to ask ourselves, "Can they do more?" The fact is that they are already doing more in a few hospitals throughout the United States. The CCU concept is experiencing an evolution. One purpose of this chapter is to describe that evolution and, if possible, assist it on its way.

We already have on hand the necessary information and expertise to improve CCUs; what is lacking primarily is liaison between the various groups responsible for hospital development. We need a full sharing, in an ecumenical spirit, of the best that has been thought and done about CCUs in the past decade. Few specialists and even fewer laymen have had the time or means to make a tour of the nation's top CCUs; therefore, many may still be unaware of the advances being made in providing more effective intensive care.

I was first made aware of the stirrings of change when, beginning in 1967, as a member of a multidisciplinary team financed by the Missouri Regional Medical Program, I was privileged to visit sixteen outstanding CCUs throughout the United States and later to make personal visits to over thirty more. The purpose of these visits was to enable the team to accumulate data they

would need to plan and design a contemplated 75- to 100-bed total-care CVCU for St. John's Hospital, a 700-bed facility serving 1,000,000 people in Springfield and the surrounding predominantly rural area of the Missouri-Arkansas Ozarks. As part of an undertaking known as the Comprehensive Cardiovascular Care Unit Project, the team had been charged to draw on the experience of the best CCUs in the country in order to design a type of unit that was to have broader functions than the traditional CCU.

As a result of experiences accumulated since 1960 with a special type of multidisease progressive care unit at St. John's, we had formed the notion that a CCU might well be expanded in function and size to deal with all types of cardiovascular emergencies, without neglecting its original commitment to coronary artery disease. We wanted to broaden the goals of our new CCU to provide for management not only of heart attack but also of congestive heart failure, miscellaneous arrhythmias, acute stroke, pulmonary embolism, thrombophlebitis, acute and chronic pulmonary insufficiency, noncardiac medical illness in patients with heart disease and in certain instances pre- and postoperative care for patients with cardiovascular disease admitted for surgical procedures. Furthermore, we wanted a "progressive" system, able to provide all services required not only in the acute phases of these diseases, but in the intermediate and convalescent phases as well. In short, we wanted a facility that would provide portal-to-portal care, from admission to discharge, for a far wider spectrum of patients than had formerly been considered proper candidates for a CCU. In fact, we didnt want a CCU at all. What we wanted was a CVCU —a comprehensive cardiovascular care unit.

But we appreciated that a CVCU would necessarily differ in design from the traditional CCU. At the very least it would require more beds, more monitoring and resuscitative equipment, and a larger staff.

Some of these needs we knew how to meet. Other solutions we could intuit. But nothing like a CVCU had been established before and the cost was to be 3 to 4 million dollars, so we felt that we should take the careful long road home and see first what others were doing.

What we found was that the type of unit we were contemplating was actually a fourth generation CCU. The first generation was represented by Day's unit at Bethany Hospital in Kansas City, Kansas (Fig. 47-2, *A* to *E*), established in 1962 and soon followed by similar units at Presbyterian Hospital in Philadelphia, under Dr. Lawrence Meltzer and Rose Pinneo, RN (Fig. 47-2, *B* and *G*), and at Peter Bent Brigham Hospital in Boston, under Dr. Bernard Lown. These were the realizations of a brilliant idea in modest settings, geared to provide a level of acute heart care that had never before been possible. The essential feature was the grouping in one hall of all equipment and specially trained staff required to detect, prevent, or treat life-threatening arrhythmias. But little or no attempt was made to modify the environment beyond installation of the monitoring and resuscitative equipment.

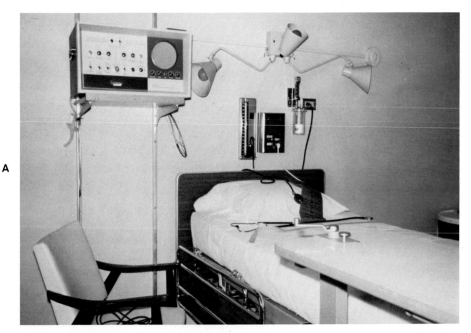

A

Continued.

Fig. 47-2. A, A revolution in resuscitation techniques took place in this room, one of four in the first CCU, established by Dr. Hughes Day in 1962 at Bethany Hospital, Kansas City, Kansas. Private rooms were used for routine, less complicated patients. **B,** The 8-bed intensive care unit was set aside for more complicated coronary cases. Day's pioneer effort reduced in-hospital coronary death rates by about one third, a potential saving of 50,000 lives a year. **C,** Dr. Hughes Day in his office. **D** and **E,** Though the physical setting of Day's unit was not elaborate, the equipment was highly sophisticated. With these instruments, including the 24-hour ECG tape recorders shown in **D,** Day contributed to the discovery that ventricular fibrillation is preceded by a series of premature ventricular beats. **F** and **G,** at Presbyterian Hospital in Philadelphia, Dr. Lawrence Meltzer was making his contribution to first generation CCUs in surroundings as modest as those of Day's unit. In addition to contributing to the discovery of premature ventricular beats as a precursor of ventricular fibrillation, Dr. Meltzer has written a textbook on modern coronary care nursing education systems.

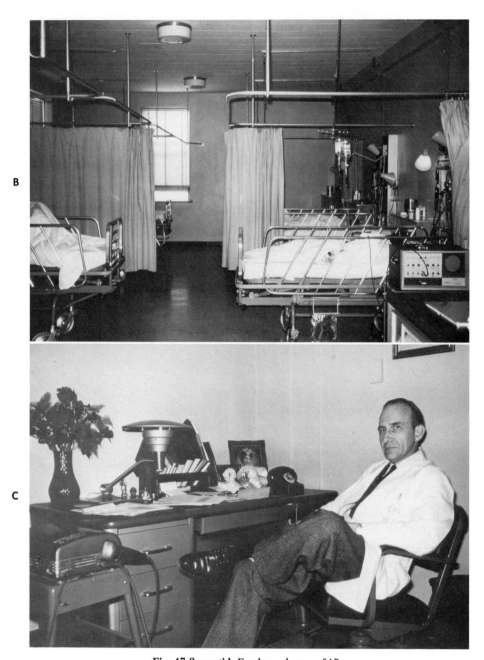

Fig. 47-2, cont'd. For legend see p. 517.

The second generation of CCUs was introduced when a unit specifically designed to provide acute heart care was created by Dr. Paul Unger and Adeline Jenkins, RN, at the Miami Heart Institute, Florida (Fig. 47-3, *A* and *B*). This unit provided a central nursing station with direct vision to all beds and was constructed with full concern for the patient's psychological needs—it was attractively decorated in restful colors, and

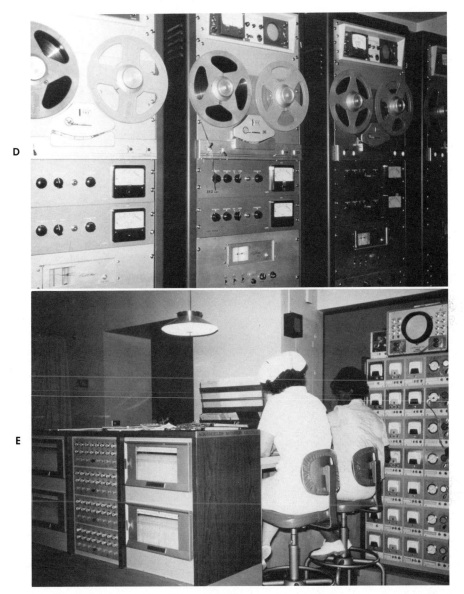

Fig. 47-2, cont'd. For legend see p. 517. *Continued.*

sound and light were carefully controlled.

The third generation CCU was characterized by an attempt to link the CCU with other sections and services in the hospital and to provide contiguous bed space for "step-down" care once the acute phase of illness had passed. The originators of this type of unit were Dr. G. S. Grier, III, and Phyllis Wertz, RN, at Riverside Hospital, Newport News, Virginia (Fig. 47-4, *A* to *C*); and Dr. Lewis Young and Sister Mary Rosa at Sisters of Charity Hospital, Buffalo, New York (Fig. 47-5, *A* to *D*). The Riverside CCU was one of the first "round units," designed to provide full visibility and minimum walking distance from the central nursing station to each bed. Sisters of Charity Hospital was one of the first to provide

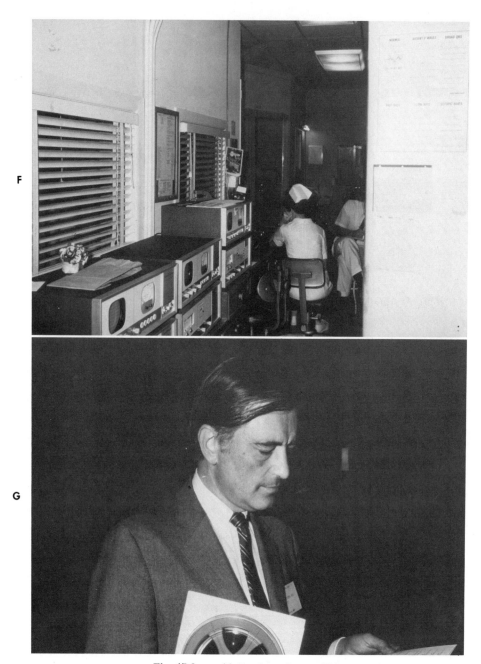

Fig. 47-2, cont'd. For legend see p. 517.

radiotelemetry between the central nursing station and the intermediate phase-two area and to provide an ECG monitoring hookup between the CCU and the emergency room, operating room, surgical recovery room, and general intensive care section. This hookup placed the skills of the CCU nurses at the disposal of patients in all sections of the hospital where life-threatening cardiovascular incidents were likely to happen. This

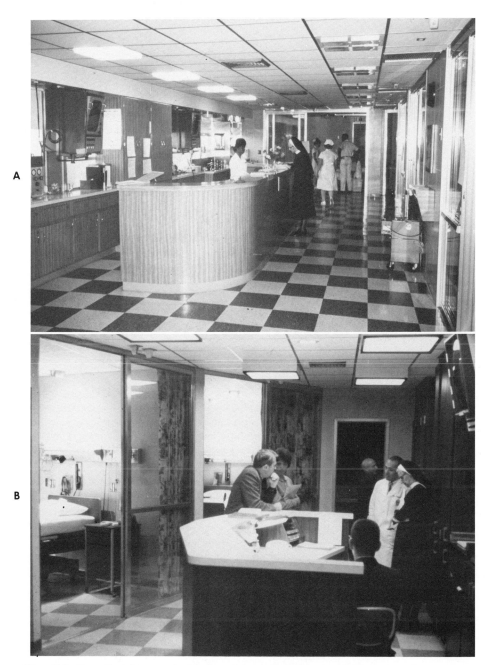

Fig. 47-3. Overall architectural planning characterized the second generation of coronary care units, illustrated here by the Miami Heart Institute, developed by Dr. Paul Unger. The original unit, **A**, contained eight glass-enclosed rooms with light and sound control and full visibility of the patients from the nursing station. After two additional 4-bed units, **B**, were opened for less complex admissions, the original unit was restricted to the most complicated cases requiring medical and surgical cardiovascular care.

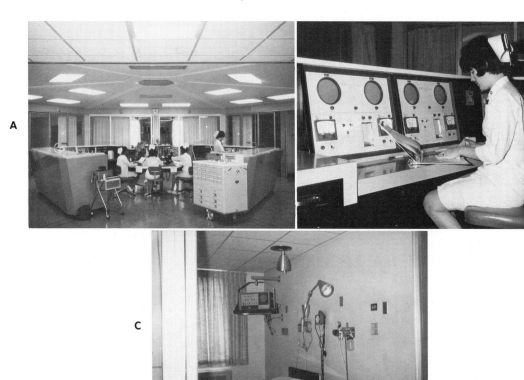

Fig. 47-4. A, The third generation unit at Riverside Hospital, Newport News, Virginia. Good lighting, spaciousness, and superb decor in a "round" design. Opened by Dr. G. S. Grier III, this unit provided a less stressful environment. **B,** Central monitor scopes were placed under the counter top at the nursing stations so that the nurse could watch the rhythm patterns closely while she did her charting. **C,** Each room has an outside window to preserve visual contact with the outside world, and a bathroom between each two rooms.

hospital also was among the first to provide videotaped instruction programs for nurses and physicians.

In 1960, at the very time that Dr. Day was evolving the first generation unit, a fourth generation unit was slowly taking shape at St. John's Hospital in Springfield, Missouri. It was conceived from the outset as a three-phased progressive care system in which all patients with acutely life-threatening cardiovascular diseases could be grouped for better care by nurses and physicians. Success of this original unit led to the planning and construction of the present 90-bed comprehensive cardiovascular care unit, which

opened in 1972 and is the first completed example of a fourth generation CCU.

The traditional CCU is well known even to most laymen. Day's idea was to assemble in one hall or ward all severely ill heart patients who required intensive care and who formerly had been housed in many different parts of the hospital. In this location he assembled all the special staff and equipment required to deal with cardiac emergencies— essentially a team of cardiac nurses and a battery of electronic equipment for monitoring heart rhythms, for resuscitating patients whose rhythms had become dangerously erratic, or for predicting and preventing

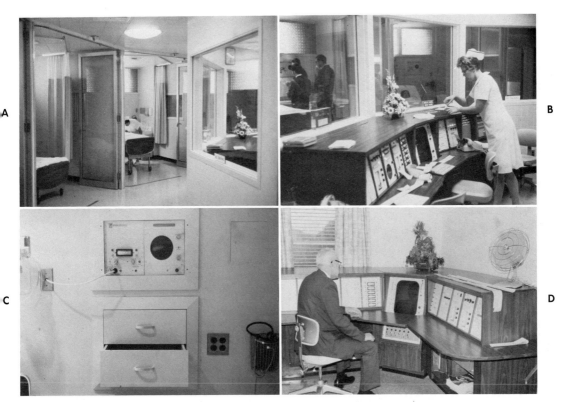

Fig. 47-5. Another third generation unit at Sisters of Charity Hospital in Buffalo, New York, under the direction of Dr. Lewis Young. **A,** The 6-bed phase-one area featured glass-enclosed nursing station and patient rooms to ensure sound control. **B,** A factory-constructed nursing station-monitor console, placed low so that the nurse can see her patients even when sitting at her desk. **C,** Bedside monitor and drawers containing emergency supplies are fully recessed. Observation of this feature led to the conception and development of the Springfield Wall in which *all* gear is recessed. **D,** A second customized monitor console receives telemetered heart rhythm patterns from ambulatory patients in the 20-bed step-down or phase-two unit.

these rhythm disturbances. With this one idea, Day reduced in-hospital heart deaths from 30% of all such patients to 20% and demonstrated the feasibility of a system capable of saving 50,000 lives or more each year.

Not as well known is the intermediate coronary care unit, or ICCU. This is essentially a part of the hospital contiguous with the CCU that functions as a CCU but less so, having a less highly trained staff and less sophisticated monitoring and resuscitative equipment. This section is reserved for patients who have passed the acute phase of heart attack and so can "step down" from the CCU, or for patients whose condition on admittance is less critical.

Even less well known and less prevalent is the facility for third-phase care, the convalescent unit. This section is located next to the acute and intermediate units, in case the patient should regress and require additional intensive care, but its function is to prepare the patient for resuming a full life. Here he receives appropriate physical therapy, including graded exercise, and instructions on medication, diet and other matters affecting his life style after he leaves the hospital.

And finally, almost unheard of as yet, is

Table 47-1. Analysis by disease categories of 886 consecutive patients treated in St. John's Hospital cardiovascular care unit, September 1, 1972 to March 1, 1973

Disease category	No. of patients	No. of deaths	Mortality (%)
Heart attack	229	50	21.8*
Acute myocardial ischemia	170	1	0.6
Chest pain: heart attack suspects (noncardiac disease diagnosed in 48; no organic disease diagnosed in 47)	95	0	0.0
Congestive heart failure	106	6	5.6
Arrhythmias	64	1	1.6
Pulmonary embolism	24	1	4.2
Pulmonary insufficiency	34	4	12.0
Acute stroke	35	4	12.0
Special procedures (pacemaker, cardioversion, angiogram, etc.)	30	0	0.0
Medical illness with coexisting cardiac disease	21	1	4.8
Syncope	19	0	0.0
Surgical disease with coexisting cardiac disease	10	3	30.0
Pericardial disease	9	0	0.0
Peripheral vascular disease	6	0	0.0
Miscellaneous (bacterial shock, ASHD, hypertension, GI bleeding, overdose, cardiovascular surgery, rheumatic heart disease, digitalis intoxication, renal failure, pancreatitis, etc.)	34	9	26.5
Total	886	80	9.0

*This 6-month sample shows our peak (winter) heart attack mortality. Other 3-month samples during 1972 show death rates as low as 10%, illustrating seasonal and other variations. Only annual figures will be meaningful in determining overall mortality for myocardial infarction. The primary point illustrated by this table is that a CVCU of adequate size can accommodate the full range of life-threatening cardiovascular and pulmonary cases liable to appear at the hospital at any one time, and can manage them with excellent results. Mortality for the 886 cases in all categories is 9%; if myocardial infarctions are excluded, the rate drops to 4.6% for the remainder.

the system that embodies all three of these phases—acute, intermediate, and convalescent. Such a system is able to provide comprehensive care for all phases of a life-threatening emergency, from the time the patient enters the hospital until he leaves and—if he follows instructions—even beyond.

The Springfield idea is to place in such a comprehensive unit all high-risk, or acutely life-threatening cardiovascular cases, many of whom, although known to be subject to sudden, unexpected or unexplained death, are now scattered throughout the hospitals on general or specialty halls, ill equipped and inadequately staffed to deal with them. (At St. John's, the same "grouping" concept has been applied to high-risk surgical patients through the establishment of a progressive care postoperative division, bringing together the recovery room, surgical intensive care, and a step-down unit for intermediate and convalescent care.) Such a unit—a comprehensive cardiovascular care unit—is, I am convinced, the unit of the future. It behooves all those concerned with financing, constructing, equipping, and staffing cardiac care facilities to face up to their responsibility to make some crucial decisions if their system of care, so costly to put together, is not to become obsolete at a very early date, perhaps even before construction or remodeling is complete.

Few of the fifty-odd hospitals I visited

from 1967 to 1972 had allocated enough beds to meet the progressive care requirements for heart attack alone, to say nothing of the rest of the spectrum of life-threatening cardiovascular diseases. To further compound the problem, the costs were so high in some units that even this less-than-ideal number of beds was not adequately utilized, thus further escalating the cost per patient.

The essence of the progressive care system is "phasing of care" in such a way as to provide high-intensity service at one end of the system; and at the other end, as the patient's needs diminish, a minimum of service. The object is to place patients in this system wherever their individual needs can be met most efficiently and economically.

Notwithstanding the widespread recognition of the progressive care principle, it has not yet been adequately applied to coronary or cardiovascular care in very many hospitals. The result, I believe, is that nursing care costs are higher than they should be, thus discouraging use of intensive care facilities and initiating the spiral of nonuse and even higher cost that leads to abandonment or neglect of our greatest single weapon against sudden and unexpected death in the hospital.

I want to suggest, as emphatically as possible, that comprehensive systems of care, modified appropriately to fit particular circumstances, are feasible for any large or intermediate size hospital and many that are smaller; and further, that even the smallest hospitals and individual physicians can secure the benefits of the system for their patients by tying into the larger institutions through a network of remote monitoring, consultation, and referral.

I am not unaware of the possible theoretical objections to a CVCU. To restrict 10% to 20% of a hospital's beds to cardiovascular care—and this is the ideal—may shock conservative administrators and raise the eyebrows of physicians whose normal concern is not with emergency situations. The necessary costs, and the need for an expanded staff of highly trained nurses and aides, may seem insurmountable obstacles to anyone familiar with the nation's present apparent dearth of health dollars and health personnel. To such skeptics I can only say that I was of your party until I became convinced that what I am proposing is not a luxury or mere medical adornment but the minimum expression of our professional concern for the nation's well being and of respect for our own skill.

In order to illustrate the concept of a fourth generation CCU—that is, of a CVCU—I have drawn heavily on our experiences at St. John's. My purpose is not to draw unbecoming attention to my own hospital (though I have no hesitancy in expressing my admiration for it), but to demonstrate in all relevant detail how a CVCU can be brought into being, what steps in planning and execution are essential, and how the unit can supply superior care at modest cost to the entire spectrum of cardiovascular patients.

Our first progessive care unit was assembled by remodeling existing structures and so may provide tips for hospitals planning their first steps in expanded intensive care facilities. Our present system, the full CVCU, was an entirely new construction, offering possibilities for innovation and for adaption of the best ideas we were able to accumulate from others. It is our present ideal.

Remodeling: our first progressive care unit

Like most happy stories, the story of the development of St. John's cardiovascular care unit begins with a clutch of unsolvable problems and the merest glimmerings of a solution. It's a story worth telling just as it happened, because much of the experience gained there can be applied by others now engaged in enlarging or improving their hospital's cardiovascular care capability.

The problem at St. John's in the 1950s was the same as that faced by all other hospitals at the time—we had no really effective means to meet the threat of sudden and un-expected death that could spring at any moment from any section of the hospital, usually signalled by extreme ventilatory or circulatory distress. The result was that only 5% of these patients survived.

But the first elements of a solution appeared in the mid 1950s with the appearance of the defibrillator, a device that enabled us to regulate abnormal heart rhythm by delivering an electric shock to the heart; and with the development of simple but effective techniques of cardiopulmonary resuscitation.

But techniques are useless without men who know how to use them, and St. John's was fortunate in having two such men on its staff. One was Dr. Oral B. Crawford, an anesthesiologist, who established the first resuscitation team effort at St. John's and sustained it for years. As a result of the efforts of Dr. Crawford and an increasing number of his colleagues, the hospital-wide resuscitation rate climbed from 5%, then the national average, to 25%.

Dr. Crawford's experiences of the 1950s resulted from his being often exposed in the operating room to patients with overdoses of anesthetic agents and the obligation to resuscitate them at that site. And, he states, he had the wherewithal in the operating room to do it—tubes, machines, drugs, and the constant feasibility of open-chest cardiac massage. After spectacular early successes, impetus was gained by the introduction in 1960 of closed-chest massage.

Dr. Crawford capsulizes the reason for the success of the early program as "simplicity and awareness." Be aware, he says, that before anything else can be done, one must get the patient breathing and must start the heart through massage. With only 350 cc. of oxygen in the lungs at one time, enough oxygen must be continuously introduced to bring about oxygen saturation of the blood and this can be done only through adequate ventilation. Through cardiac massage, circulation can be restored and sustained. With

these simple steps promptly undertaken, there is then time to attempt to correct the underlying problem.

The successes of Dr. Crawford and of his anesthesiologist colleagues and nursing supervisor Sister Mary Avilla became known throughout the hospital and this team began to be called to other areas to revive all manners of cases. With simplicity still the first consideration, they simply packed the essentials for their mission in a picnic basket for easy portability. This included an AMBU bag, endotracheal tubes, necessary drugs, intravenous catheters, and a variety of other essentials. Once circulation and ventilation were restored, the remainder of the resuscitation effort could be carried out with ample time for assembling needed personnel and equipment.

In contrast to many resuscitation efforts, which had been termed elsewhere the "galloping exercise that results in failure," the record of Dr. Crawford and his associates became the "galloping exercise that results in success," primarily through their ability to get to patients within two minutes of the catastrophe and frequently within one minute, regardless of the area of the hospital in which the disaster occurred.

Dr. Cecil Auner contributed to this story as the first chairman of St. John's Cardiac Instrumentation Committee, established in the mid 1950s. Dr. Auner had been a naval electronics technician during World War II and had entered medical school after the war, bringing to Springfield the unique combination of electronics and cardiologist's skills. It was he who provided the instrumentation backup to anesthesiologist Crawford's sustaining and holding action.

Notwithstanding the successes of this team effort, the logistics barrier came clearly into view. Many patients failed to survive because of the time factor and because of the difficulty in assembling not only the new machines but people experienced in their use.

For one thing, the defibrillator went unused most of the time because there never seemed to be someone at hand who knew how to operate it. Even when a doctor was available, more often than not he had never used the equipment on human subjects and so shied away from it. Defibrillation by nurses was unheard of then and, in this hospital of 450 beds without a house staff, it was highly unlikely that a doctor would be at the patient's bedside precisely when cardiac resuscitation was required.

A series of shattering experiences in the late 1950s made us painfully aware of our problems. The most heartbreaking was the case of a man in his 50s, the father of a young attorney. He sustained a heart attack at his home some 3 miles south of the hospital while I was at my office 2 miles to the north. A prompt call to me permitted immediate assembling of equipment, and within about 1 minute of each other we all arrived at the hospital's best-staffed hall—the patient, the EKG machine, nurses, oxygen equipment, and myself. But not the defibrillator! This was safely stored in a closet one floor below and halfway down the building. As you may have guessed, this patient died within the first minute, presumably of ventricular fibrillation, before the ECG could be taken. Even if the defibrillator had been at hand, I could not have used it because I did not know how! In my attempt to console the attorney and to try to show him that efforts were being made to remedy this sad type of occurrence, I told him that we had in that very hospital the means of saving his father's life were it not for the logistic problem of getting equipment and a trained operator to the bedside. In his characteristic courtroom cross-examination style, he almost snarled at me, "Doc, you had better do something about that!" That is probably the most vividly recalled statement ever made to me by a patient or a family member. It is ironic that this attorney, also a patient with rheumatic heart disease, died suddenly at home one night not many months later, presumably of an arrhythmia.

At about that time, a highly respected and revered dentist from a nearby community with known coronary artery disease underwent a very necessary hemorrhoidectomy and on his first postoperative night was diligently treated on a surgical hall from midnight until daylight with colon tube, enemas, and various medications for "gas," only to suddenly expire of a heart attack before my morning rounds. Obviously, his real problem had not been "gas"; but at that time we were not sufficiently alert to the warning signs of heart attack to appreciate his danger or equipped to combat it quickly. So a very valuable and beloved man was needlessly lost.

A pharmacist from the same community suddenly and unexpectedly expired on a general hall while undergoing treatment for a rather prolonged episode of paroxysmal atrial tachycardia as a complication of rheumatic heart disease. I remember sadly that I had given his family strong assurances that he would almost certainly be relieved of his arrhythmia by drug therapy.

About that same time, Springfield's most highly respected automobile-rattle-removal expert, who was soon to have ministered to my aging Oldsmobile, suddenly died on the orthopedic hall, of pulmonary embolism, as he was nearing dismissal following treatment involving prolonged bed rest in a body cast for a compression spine fracture. Resuscitation of many such patients is now a matter of routine in intensive care units. But at that time, no such unit existed.

Also indelibly impressed on my mind is the memory of the night on the gynecology hall when the entire nursing staff was usurped for a period of hours by a middle-aged woman who had developed severe pulmonary embolism after a vaginal hysterectomy complicated by hypotension. She was having breathing problems and required both prolonged ventilatory support and a continuous intravenous norepinephrine drip that had to be closely monitored. Because the gynecology hall was not set up to handle such emergencies, the whole nursing staff was tied down by this one case, and other patients were virtually abandoned. This sort of experience occurs frequently in any hospital that does not have special intensive care facilities.

I could multiply such unnecessarily tragic instances almost endlessly, but these few should suffice to illustrate the general problem. Note particularly that many of these cases were not heart attacks but circulatory complications arising from noncardiac conditions. Our problem, as we conceived it, was to provide definitive care for the entire range of such cases.

Because I was then the junior associate of one of the city's busiest cardiologists, it was my duty to receive all after-bedtime calls. On many occasions I was informed that such and such a patient had been found dead in bed by the nurse on her hourly rounds. It was I who had to contact the family and try to explain why this had to be. In those days, as a result, I established a routine practice of setting a 24-hour-a-day watch, by family and friends, over all high-risk patients. Often I recruited volunteers from churches to fill the roster. Most Ozarkians could not afford a full shift of private duty nurses and there had to be someone on hand to alert the nurses. But the sudden deaths still occurred, even with watchful companions at the bedside.

This was the setting and atmosphere in which we received a startling proposal from Sister Mary Chrysostom, St. John's administrator, and her assistant administrator, Mr. Leo Bargielski. They proposed that St. John's should establish an intensive care unit and progressive care division. For me, it was a most exhilarating experience to take a call from Dr. William I. Park, the president of St. John's medical staff, requesting that I head a multidisciplinary Intensive Care Committee to establish this unit in a recently vacated 42-bed hall.

The matter of sudden, unexpected death was presented to the committee at its first meeting, and members were told that the proposed unit would provide a setting into which could be channeled all categories of patients, both medical and surgical, but particularly cardiovascular, who carried a high risk of sudden death and who could be resuscitated by existing teams. What was lacking was adequate instrumentation with which to monitor the initial intensive unit, which was to contain 7 beds. This would cost thousands and no such funds could be spared from the hospital budget for such an untested idea. But St. John's Ladies Auxiliary, when informed of our need, donated $12,000 for equipment, thus establishing a tradition of special gifts to cover fixed equipment costs that has enabled us to improve care at St. John's without greatly increasing patients' costs.

Dr. Auner was charged with the responsibility of assembling this gear and all doctors attending national meetings were asked to survey the market of electronics equipment. But there were no central monitoring systems available for purchase in 1960. The top engineer of one company heard this story, however, and at enormous expense fabricated a central system with display at the nursing station. This was installed during 1961, but it didn't work. Dr. Auner, spending hundreds of hours away from his practice did make the valuable contribution of determining what was unsatisfactory, and . ultimately, in 1963, obtained for us a workable system of bedside units. But meanwhile very few if any lives had been saved as a result of this expensive new idea that I, as chairman of the Intensive Care Committee, had touted so highly.

The unit was noisy because it accommodated all types of patients requiring intensive care, including many head injuries, most of whom were patients of an avid devotee of intensive care, neurosurgeon John L. K. Tsang. Had it not been for Dr. Tsang and a few other physicians, the unit would soon have failed financially. Meantime, I was still faced with the daily unpleasantness of having to confront one after another of the members of the Ladies Auxiliary, reporting "no progress" on electronic monitoring. With this personal embarrassment stalking me, I felt required to admit acute cardiacs of all types to the unit, notwithstanding the noise and clutter, so as to keep it from failing.

So perhaps it was the need to keep our first intensive unit financially solvent that led us to the conception of the present comprehensive cardiovascular care unit. If we wanted to keep a promising idea alive, we had to admit all types of high-risk patients, tumbling them together with no clear conviction—and certainly no objective evidence—that this procedure would help reduce the number of sudden and unexpected deaths in the hospital.

But with a census of fifteen to twenty cardiac patients in those days, I soon acquired enough experience to become impressed with the value of the unit. Despite the noise and clutter, and despite the lack of electronic monitoring, my patients and those of Dr. Tsang were doing better than they would have done on general halls. They appeared to be less apprehensive in spite of the notorious psychological disadvantage of a small, open-ward curtained unit. Fewer catastrophies arose, and routine procedures, such as medication, graded activity regimens, and diet, went off more smoothly.

Within a very few months we identified the two reasons for this improved state of affairs. One was the grouping of high-risk patients; the other was the presence at all times of an excellent, specially trained staff of nurses.

Grouping all patients with life-threatening conditions had seemed at first to be risky. Would a patient become more anxious and depressed if placed in a section of a hospital known to be reserved for emergency situations and filled with the sounds and signs of the acutely morbid? We weren't really sure. Our original idea had been to bring the patients close to the monitoring equipment and we were willing to take the risks involved in order to give them this improved facet of care. But with no monitoring equipment, we were really skating on thin professional ice, and we knew it. That's why the improvement we saw in our patients was enough to bring great pleasure to us.

For the patients were good for one another. They provided each other a kind of therapy, and its effects were striking. In time, we came to understand that seriously ill persons are not a source of distress to one another but in many ways a comfort. Perhaps the answer lies in the adage, "Misery loves company," but I doubt that that is the whole answer. Surely they are also consoled by seeing that others with problems as severe as their own are "making it," and can conclude that they can, too. And if they see those who are beyond help, and beyond the reach of consolation, surely they must conclude that their own is a better, happier state and a cause for self-congratulation. They are drawn gratefully to those who are near their own level of health. I have seen many friendships that have lasted long after discharge from the hospital develop in this reputedly grim environment.

But it was the nurses who really saved the day. For 10 years, from 1950 to 1961, I had been in charge of teaching cardiovascular nursing in the 3-year diploma nursing school at St. John's. By the time our intensive unit opened, we had an ample supply of these specially trained persons. I cannot repeat too often that without such nurses neither our unit nor any other can hope to succeed. An intensive unit is not just a collection of bricks, mortar, and electronic gear; it is a setting in which persons with a need for special care can find other persons who have the skill, compassion, and dedication to offset that need. On the floor of the unit, it is the nurse far more than the doctor who plays that ministering role.

Because our nurses had been trained to deal with cardiovascular emergencies, and because they were exposed daily only to patients who might experience such emergencies, they rapidly became even more expert than most doctors in observing, interpreting, and treating dangerous symptoms. We found ourselves giving nurses increasing authority to make treatment decisions and this greatly expedited handling of hour-to-hour emergencies when we were not in the hospital.

In addition to their specific medical duties, the nurses began to assume a crucial role in the less tangible process of educating patients and families to the nature of cardiovascular disease and the value and necessity of various treatment programs in and out of the hospital. In daily informal conversations, the nurses learned how to convey, in a non-frightening manner, kinds of information that were often fear provoking when they came from physicians. Now at St. John's we are preparing a formalized program of education for patients and families; much of the content of these films, tapes, and slides has been derived from the practical experience of our nurses. We know it works. Channeling this experience into patient- and family-useful audiovisual material is a current activity of cardiologist J. William Cheek, who arrived in 1966 with a zeal for nurse, physician, and patient education equaling his leadership in resuscitation. (As Drs. Crawford and Auner's ideas took hold and many more cardiac candidates for resuscitation became logistically available, Dr. Cheek became the new Resuscitation Committee chairman.)

The nurses also indirectly benefited patients by expediting our rounds. When high-risk patients were scattered throughout the hospital, we often had to make rounds alone, and even when a nurse was available she was usually not specially trained to understand or care for this type of patient. Now, with a cardiac nurse at our shoulder, we could make chart entries and issue instructions quickly and confidently, knowing that they would be comprehended and carried out. The result was that we had more time to deal with the psychological dimensions of our patients' problems and to form unhur-

ried, daily impressions of their response to treatment. Surprisingly, even though we were less rushed on rounds than we had been, we found that we were saving from half to a whole hour each day.

Two other indirect benefits flowed from the grouping of high-risk patients and high-capacity nurses. One was that we could dispense with the 24-hour watch by families and friends and thus save them this additional stress. They could share our confidence that the patient's welfare would be better served when left to professionals highly skilled in the gruelling work of watching and waiting.

The second benefit was that these professionals were never rattled by the emergencies that were bound to arise. They expected them. They dealt with them quickly and accurately, one or two nurses at a time, never herding themselves fearfully or abandoning their other patients. They were able to demonstrate time and again that the battle of life and death is not won by huffing and puffing, but by precision and poise.

But, surprisingly, most physicians were disinclined to admit any acute cardiac patients, especially heart attack patients, to a less-than-quiet, always lighted open ward. And our unit was still less than quiet since we were admitting all categories of critically ill patients, especially patients with head injuries, neurosurgical procedures, general surgery problems, gastrointestinal hemorrhage and the like. A unit that had opened with the high hope that it would serve as a setting for resuscitation of all cardiopulmonary patients seemed to have overextended its function in such a way as to exclude these very cases.

Even when I reported my extremely favorable and enlightening experiences to sessions of the medical staff, I almost always got either a neutral or adverse response. For instance, when I told the staff that it was totally feasible to identify high-risk cases of all categories, particularly cardiovascular conditions, and to treat them in one location, one influential member discounted the idea and told the group bluntly, "It can't be done!" But very unexpectedly, another prominent member stood up in support of the concept and suggested that the staff give it a try. That person was Dr. Walter W. Tillman, Jr., an anesthesiologist, who was a member of the Advisory Council of the Missouri Regional Medical Program, which later allocated funds for planning the present large comprehensive cardiovascular care unit.

From the day of Dr. Tillman's endorsement of the idea, things went forward, though there were still hurdles to leap.

First, of course, we had to get the monitoring equipment going. Then we had to lick the noise problem. We also had to find a way to convince skeptical staff members that there was a real need for the large unit we had in mind. And, finally, we had to find a way to deliver on our promise of progressive, step-down care, from the acute phase of illness to the convalescent phase.

Even when the unit was patronized by only a few doctors, we soon had to face the problem of providing beds for patients when they left the 7-bed intensive unit. Such trans-

fers had to be placed wherever there happened to be a bed, and often this was in an undesirable location since most good spots would already have been filled by patients who came in with a reservation. Complicating this problem was the reluctance of my patients to move from the intensive unit, particularly to some remote area of the hospital. They and their families had come to feel protected in the unit and protested being "tossed out into the cold." Fortunately, this problem was settled by Sister Mary Rene Higgins, the new St. John's administrator. She gave us special dispensation to use the entire contiguous area as an intermediate and convalescent unit, where we could transfer patients without removing them dangerously from the intensive unit's facilities. With the addition of this new 35-bed area, once reserved for a miscellany of medical and surgical cases, our unit now totalled 42 beds, which in those days, as in many hospitals even today, was an unheard-of allocation of beds for intensive and step-down cardiovascular care (Fig. 47-6). The new dispensation allowed us to move noncardiac patients out of the contiguous area whenever we needed beds for cardiovascular pa-

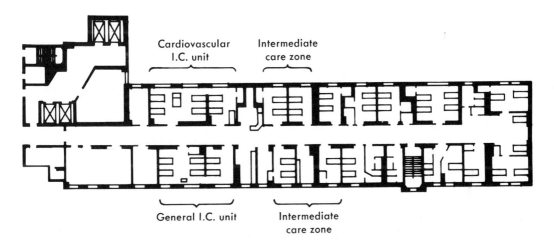

Fig. 47-6. Floor plan of the original cardiovascular care unit at St. John's Hospital, showing sections reserved for cardiovascular intensive care, general intensive care, intermediate care, and convalescent care. Once functioning, this 42-bed unit soon proved too small to accommodate the number of eligible patients in what was then a 450-bed hospital.

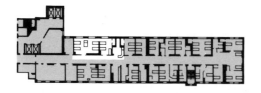

Cardiovascular I.C. unit (7 beds)

A

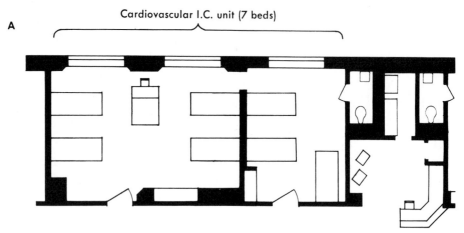

Fig. 47-7. A, This 7-bed cardiovascular intensive care unit was created by cutting large windows and a door between existing 4- and 3-bed rooms. From the nursing station in the center of the 4-bed section, all patients were directly visible. The nursing station at lower right served the intermediate and convalescent sections, but it was close enough to the intensive care section that nurses at both locations could exchange information and support each other in emergencies. B, This was the 1965 version of St. John's CVCU. Families wait outside doors to the 7-bed intensive care section at left. Beyond them nurses gather at the nursing station serving the intermediate and convalescent care sections. The man at right has his back to the 6-bed unit for intensive care of "noisy" patients. C, The 7-bed intensive care section; the central nursing station—desk at right—provided full visibility of all patients, as well as space for charting. One portable defibrillator-ECG machine served all patients in this unit. (B, Photograph by Joe Baker, Medical World News.)

tients who were ready to leave the intensive unit but were still in need of special treatment.

Finally, in 1963, Dr. Auner got the electronic equipment working, and we were able to provide the bedside monitors that had prompted us to construct the intensive unit in the first place (Fig. 47-7).

The noise problem was solved for us by Dr. Hughes Day. On a visit to his unit in Kansas City, we learned that we should form two intensive units, next to but soundproofed from each other, one to contain the "quiet" cardiovascular cases, the other to contain "noisy" cases of any type. He also gave us

fervent support for the concept of progressive care for all high-risk patients, and, armed with this information and prestigious approval, we returned to Springfield elated.

Our first step was to set up a second 6-bed unit for noisy cases (Fig. 47-8), leaving the 7-bed unit exclusively for "quiet" cardiovascular care. Our second was to undertake a survey of the entire hospital to determine whether there were enough high-risk cardiovascular cases in the house to occupy the entire 42-bed floor. Much to my amazement, using the criteria that had been employed in designating that hall as the proper place for my own patients, we found a total of seventy-

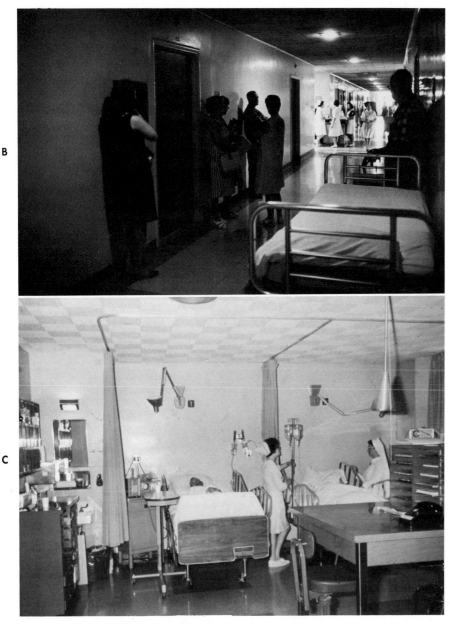

Fig. 47-7, cont'd. For legend see opposite page.

five such cases scattered throughout the several halls. Clearly, if all patients were to be dealt with according to our concept, we would need even more beds than we had already been allowed! We would be over-subscribed.

And that's exactly what happened. Within

30 days after we got the machines working, established objective evidence of the need, licked the noise problem, and set up facilities for both intermediate and convalescent care, we had more requests for admission to the unit than we had beds. We actually had to open up another floor for convalescent pa-

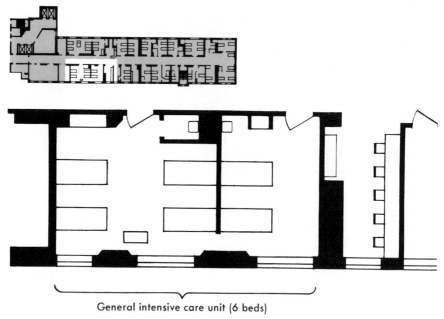

General intensive care unit (6 beds)

Fig. 47-8. Floor plan of the 6-bed intensive care unit for "noisy" cardiovascular and general cases. Separating these cases from "quiet" coronaries was essential to securing the patronage of cardiologists reluctant to put their patients in a stressful setting. At right is physician's dictating area.

tients adjudged able to move away from the monitoring equipment altogether. This space problem was later to be solved by construction of the present 90-bed CCU, but at that time we had to make do with what we had and rest content with the reflection that we were at least doing miraculously better than we had before.

Not that there was much time to rest. Our new system quickly broke down. The night supervisors and admitting office personnel seemed always to run out of beds for accident cases and for acute surgical problems during the night. Much to our dismay, they would then fill up all available beds on the new cardiovascular division, depriving us of the space needed to guarantee admission of cardiacs. However, as in so many other crises, a nurse finally came to the rescue. Upon arriving each day at 7:00 A.M., charge nurse Clara Leteux would demand that these noncardiac patients be moved off the hall immediately so that there would be space to

receive cardiacs. Top-level approval was often necessary to get the patient moved, but very soon the futility of bucking Miss Leteux became apparent to everyone.

Word about this unit quickly spread, and an unexpected public demand for care in that part of the hospital followed, with a sharp increase in total cardiovascular admissions. All other Springfield hospitals then promptly mobilized to develop their own three-phased cardiac treatment units.

But we still had problems. Occasionally conflicts arose as to whose patient would have to be moved out of the acute or intermediate area (Fig. 47-9) in order to accommodate admissions, and eventually these conflicts led to appointment of a referee, Dr. John J. McKinsey, Chairman of the Cardiovascular Care Committee. It was Dr. McKinsey who correlated the activities of internists, surgeons, anesthesiologists, and others, and it was he who established a mechanism by which they all shared in at-

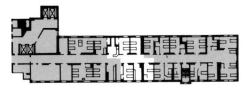

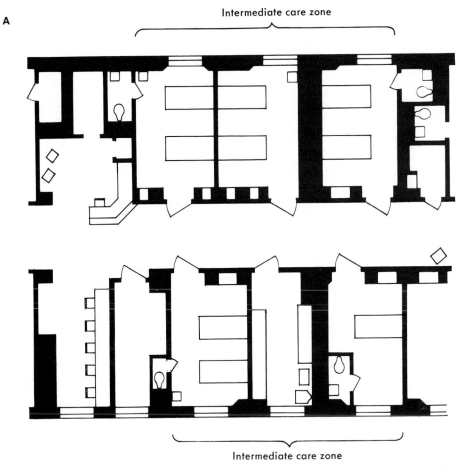

Intermediate care zone

A

Intermediate care zone

Continued.

Fig. 47-9. A, The intermediate care section; the four beds nearest the nursing station—two on each side of the hall—were monitored by direct wire into two multichannel ceiling-mounted scopes, shown by the obliquely positioned boxes in the nursing station at top left. These scopes also received rhythm tracings from six units of radio telemetry used anywhere in the division. **B,** These scopes in the intermediate and convalescent section nursing station monitored four patients by direct wire and six by radiotelemetry. Nurses at this station were only steps away from the intensive care section and could provide speedy backup. **C,** At right center, a mirror reflects nurse and patient on the same side of the hall as nurse (blurred outline at right) who is sitting at the nursing station in the intermediate care section and has direct vision into the 2-bed room seen through the doorway. Such mirrors enhance visibility in remodelled units, where the cost of removing walls might be prohibitive. **D,** As the patient moved from left to right down this hallway, he could feel that he was graduating into health. Even in the convalescent section, at right, he was not far from the intermediate and intensive care sections, and could be "stepped-up" quickly if his condition required reversing the normal step-down procedure. (**C,** Photograph by Joe Baker, Medical World News.)

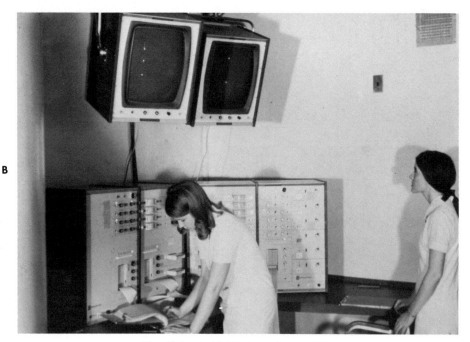

Fig. 47-9, cont'd. For legend see p. 535.

For legend see p. 535.

tending to all the duties incumbent upon doctors, thereby enabling us to get by without a full-time salaried director of the unit. Actually, it seemed to us that this system of rotating duties among staff members was a far more suitable approach than hiring a director. Since all staff physicians could admit patients to the unit and participate in its activities, there was always an abundance of manpower on hand. We strongly disagree with many published recommendations to the effect that a unit cannot earn a top functional rating without a salaried director. Our way of doing things is no different from the method used in the operation of such sophisticated services as surgery. All qualified people traditionally have operating room privileges, and it would be considered preposterous in any hospital to restrict to one or even a few chiefs the privilege of operating on patients. Also, rotation of services serves as a mechanism whereby cardiovascular-care skills can be acquired by the less experienced internists and by the generalists, who learn not only from daily contact with

their medical colleagues but also, and perhaps more importantly, from the highly skilled nurses who have been trained by cardiologists.

To sum it up, we finally demonstrated at St. John's that there are always in the hospital a very large number of cardiovascular patients of several categories who are in danger of sudden death and who can effectively be grouped in a single division, *provided that* two decisions are first made by the medical staff and the administration: first, to allocate the necessary number of beds to care for those cases in a specially staffed and equipped division and, second, to prohibit admission of any other types of cases in order to guarantee space for new cardiovascular patients.

This story has been presented in some detail to show that such progressive cardiovascular-care systems can be installed in hospitals through remodeling and without a huge outlay for bricks and mortar. This kind of unit can serve as a stopgap until a more satisfactory system can be constructed. The

C

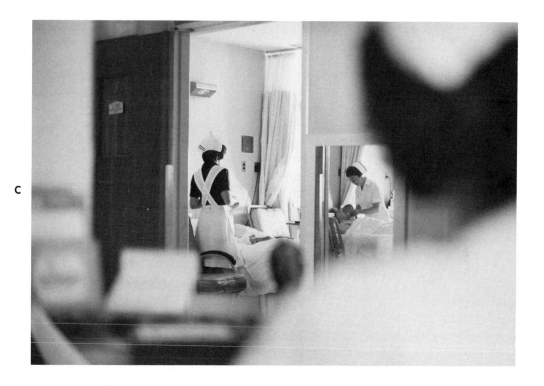

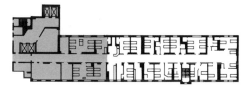

Intermediate care zone

D

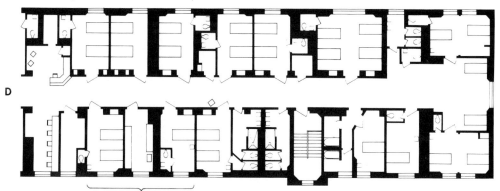

Intermediate care zone

Fig. 47-9, cont'd. For legend see p. 535.

Table 47-2. Cardiovascular disease census, St. John's Hospital, by division, February 5, 1965*

Conditions	Divisions											Total
	4N	Int	5W	4W	3W	2W	GW	4E	3E	2E	Pius	
Acute myocardial infarction and/or ischemia	6	1	2	1		3	4		1	2	1	21
Chronic coronary disease	3						1				2	6
Congestive failure	2		1	1		1	1		3	1	1	11
Stroke	3		3	1			1					8
Seizures, miscellaneous			1	2				1				4
Chronic cor pulmonale	1						1	1				3
Pulmonary embolism												
Complicating leg fracture				3								
Complicating abdominal surgery	1											
Complicating phlebitis, without surgery									2			
Total pulmonary emboli												6
Arrhythmias, acute				1						1		2
Arrhythmias, chronic				1								1
Hypertension				1								1
Congenital heart disease								1				1
Acute rheumatic fever								3				3
Pericarditis	1											1
Bleeding esophageal varices	1											1
Ruptured CNS aneurysm		1										1
Chronic coronary disease, in for surgery			1				1			1	2	5
Total	18	2	8	11	0	4	9	6	6	5	6	75

*This simple tally sheet can be used by any hospital to determine quickly the total cardiovascular patient load present at any one time. The tally shown here, indicating a population of seventy-five patients, provided an objective basis for recommending that the original 42-bed unit could be expanded. Later tallies invariably showed a population of 90 to 115 likely candidates for grouped cardiovascular care, and confirmed the decision to more than double the size of the unit. (From Turner, Glenn O.: The community approach to reduction of cardiovascular deaths, Mo. Med. 65:746-749, 753, 1968.)

floor plans of the pilot division have been presented to illustrate its simplicity. All that a hospital requires is a set of rooms that can accommodate intensive care equipment, a central nursing station close by, and contiguous bed space to provide for progressive, step-down care.

The next step in this chapter should be description of our present CVCU, but before providing this I want to make a digression. I have mentioned that a CVCU is designed to accommodate all types of high-risk cardiovascular patients, not just heart attacks. This policy is controversial and requires some explanation, which I shall attempt in the next section.

Our view is that all high-risk cardiovascular patients can benefit from the same type of monitoring and resuscitative service that has been demonstrated to be so effective with actual, threatened, or possible heart attacks (Table 47-2). This is our key recommendation and the policy regarding function of the CVCU that accounts for its size and design. We are convinced that this policy is also the key to reducing sudden and unexpected in-hospital deaths.

Sudden deaths are not altogether sudden; death accumulates at a slow rate in most patients and can often be detected in its manageable infancy.

Too often, the "unexpected death of a patient" is actually the "unnecessary death of a neglected patient."

The range of patient categories

What finally made the intensive care unit so popular with doctors and nurses alike was that it provided some larger measure of hope for such a broad range of life-threatening cases. No one doubted that monitoring-cum-nursing capability would reduce heart attack deaths. Day and others had already demonstrated this, and no one then or now would question our decision to admit all cases of possible, suspected, impending or actual heart attack; rhythm disturbances, acute and chronic; or congestive heart failure. Where

we fell afoul of some doctors and administrators was in admitting patients with chest discomfort of undetermined etiology, and patients with known heart disease hospitalized for diagnosis and treatment of other medical illness. I can only say that undiagnosed chest pain is such a frequent forerunner of heart attack that any doubt about its cause should be resolved as soon as possible, by angiography if necessary, and that many noncardiac illnesses can trigger acute cardiac episodes.

When a known heart patient is admitted for other disease, don't be content with conventional treatment methods. We had one 78-year-old woman with long-standing but well-controlled rheumatic heart disease who was admitted with severe pneumonia and a fever of 104° F. She was placed in the intensive unit and kept under continuous visual surveillance. After she recovered from the pneumonia she developed ventricular fibrillation and had to be defibrillated by the nurse *thirty-five times* (Fig. 47-10). Hers was the kind of problem that today could have been anticipated by determination of blood-gas and acid-base relationships, but in those days this invaluable predictive tool had not been adequately utilized. While she was in the hospital, by the way, we first heard about the value of intravenous lidocaine for suppressing impending arrhythmias. We put her on this medication immediately and soon had her home. Without doubt, she would have died on a general hall.

We have also seen known heart patients with gastrointestinal bleeding, and a frequent dispute has been whether we should consider this bleeding "cardiovascular" in origin and admit the patient to the CVCU. I'm for that. Even if the bleeding is due to other causes, I know it can be controlled best in a unit accustomed to dealing with diseases involving the blood vessels and circulation, whether the circulatory system be involved primarily or secondarily. Why take chances? I sometimes feel that the only resistance to the idea of admitting such patients to inten-

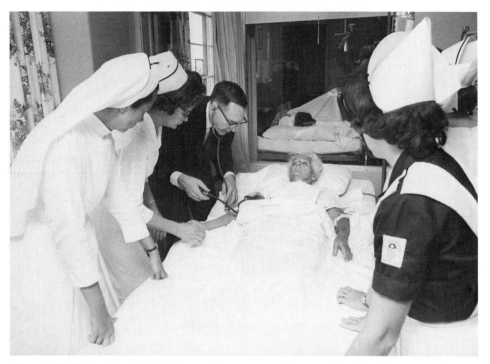

Fig. 47-10. Thirty-five defibrillations and constant nursing care brought this woman through pneumonia complicated by preexisting heart disease. (Photograph by Joe Baker, Medical World News.)

sive care comes from doctors and administrators who don't have the beds to accommodate the need. But the need remains. And its answer is "Get more beds." Don't make a physical lack the occasion for a scantly defensible medical judgment.

That same reasoning holds for many other conditions where the presenting symptoms are not arrhythmias or other signs of acute or impending heart attack. I refer in part to a number of peripheral vascular diseases, including thrombophlebitis, pulmonary embolism, arterial occlusion, cerebrovascular insufficiency and stroke, and syncope and seizures possibly attributable to circulatory abnormalities. But I would go farther and include cases of pulmonary insufficiency; surgical cases involving known cardiacs, whether the surgery is on the heart or elsewhere; and any diagnostic cases in cardiacs requiring the often stressful techniques of endoscopy or other penetration of the body

with potentially damaging instruments. The same applies to many angiography procedures, especially coronary cineangiography.

In regard to peripheral vascular disease, one of the most gratifying early experiences at St. John's was the recognition by Clara Leteux of a femoral artery embolism in a 90-year-old man. The first thing she noticed after the patient complained of severe leg pain was an abrupt disappearance of the femoral pulse at the groin—she could feel it just above but not below. The result was that she provided the doctor with a diagnosis before he had seen the patient himself. Within slightly more than 1 hour after her first observations, the embolus was removed successfully.

Probably no one would challenge the statement that patients with pulmonary embolism, or embolism in the lung, need to be managed in an intensive setting, with monitoring and other surveillance comparable to that provided for heart attack. However, we doctors seem somehow able to forget that many cases of pulmonary embolism begin with clot formation in other parts of the body, usually the legs, from which the clot migrates to the lung where it can do its deadly worst. Four cases of pulmonary embolism found in our original survey of the hospital's total cardiovascular case load were discovered on the orthopedic division. Clots had developed in the legs as a result of prolonged immobilization for fractures. Since the orthopedic nurses were not trained to recognize pulmonary embolism, the cases either had gone unrecognized or had been inadequately treated. We now adamantly contend that patients with any variety of thrombophlebitis that creates the potential for pulmonary embolism should be managed in a CVCU where full treatment for this complication can be mobilized immediately if needed. We have had quite enough well-documented sudden deaths from such a cause. It is perhaps time that all hospitals provide orientation on this subject to their entire staff of nurses and doctors, particularly orthopedists, surgeons, and obstetrician-gynecologists. At least it's a challenge worth thinking about.

Another treatment challenge is acute stroke or cerebrovascular insufficiency. Pilot "stroke units" have yielded generally good results, if we can judge from the present variable data. Yet stroke patients, like heart patients, are often admitted to whatever bed is available, or, as they say at St. John's "down the hall and around the corner," far removed from nurses trained for intensive care. And this occurs even though failure to treat stroke may be even more disastrous than failure to treat heart attack.

Another aspect of the problem of treating strokes is that the cause of the stroke is frequently obscure. Cerebral ischemia may be a "pure stroke" but it may also be the consequence of impaired cardiac output due to acute myocardial ischemia. Until the chain of events leading to a stroke has been identi-fied, the patient is entitled to the same type of care he would receive if he had had a heart attack.

There is a third consideration. Patients with primary cerebrovascular disease who enter with strokes frequently have associated heart disease not yet manifested by myocardial infarction and deserve management in a cardiac unit. With this in mind, some time ago we in Springfield appointed a Committee on Cerebrovascular Disease to consider how to handle stroke patients in relation to the CVCU. We had space elsewhere in the hospital that could have been used to set up a separate stroke intensive care unit, but we ultimately agreed it would be better to manage acute strokes in the CVCU, since otherwise we would have to duplicate staff and equipment and this would escalate costs for the patients without providing them any additional benefit. So we made provision in the CVCU for controlling the noise associated with stroke, and we agreed that patients in the convalescent phase of stroke, those hospitalized primarily for physical therapy or other rehabilitation, should not be admitted to the CVCU unless we had on hand nurses and therapists specially trained in stroke rehabilitation. Nevertheless, as I shall explain elsewhere, there is merit in structuring a CVCU to provide better physical therapy than is now feasible, so perhaps some means should be devised for offering this phase of treatment if our CVCU is to be truly "comprehensive."

An equally "iffy" problem is presented by syncope and seizures secondary to circulatory abnormalities. The symptoms of these diseases are often mild and unspecific, a fainting spell or "nervousness" that may remain undiagnosed for a long time. But if these patients are put into an intensive care unit under constant ECG monitoring, one can often detect transient and otherwise unrecognizable rhythm disturbances that account for the faintness, dizziness, or actual syncope. That, at least, has been our gratifying experience at St. John's. I have to acknowledge guilt for having misdiagnosed some of these patients in the days before we had the intensive unit. I remember hospitalizing one patient, for instance, because of what I called "anxiety," thinking that his condition was probably psychogenic. In other more fortunate cases, when assisted by our present bevy of nurses and machines, I have been able to locate the actual cause of the syncope, whether it was cerebral ischemia, a labyrinth disturbance, or some variety of epileptic seizure. Fortunately, at St. John's we have an abundance of neurologists, neurosurgeons, and neurologically oriented internists closely involved with the CVCU, so that misdiagnoses are now rare.

Primary bronchopulmonary disease should also be treated in an intensive care unit, but in many hospitals it is not. We found from the first that such patients could be treated in the intensive unit without greatly disturbing patients with heart attacks or pure cardiovascular problems. I say "pure" because often pulmonary disease has a secondary cardiac component and can rightly be regarded as a cardiovascular disease. Perhaps very large hospitals can consider having a separate pulmonary intensive care unit, but for most hospitals this is not feasible. Also, since many of these patients are old and have developed concurrent primary heart disease, and since impaired ventilation has a more serious effect on a heart that is already damaged, we believe that pulmonary patients are entitled to the same type of care given to the acute and chronic cardiacs. Keep in mind, too, that these patients require a great amount of laboratory work, particularly blood-gas studies: doesn't it seem practical, then, to house them in that section of the hosptial, the intensive care unit, where a blood-gas laboratory and facilities for inhalation therapy are right next door? And if these facilities are not adjacent to the intensive unit, shouldn't a hospital administrator take thought in the matter and see that they are?

Another class of patients that, in selected instances, might well be handled in the CVCU are cardiacs in for surgery. Preoperative evaluation and postoperative care in an intensive care unit should be welcomed by surgeons, internists, and generalists alike (Fig. 47-11). It offers them a means to reduce operative risk. In the preoperative stage, patients should receive continuous ECG monitoring and roentgenograms should be taken to detect and evaluate any degree of rhythm disturbance or heart enlargement. Even if fairly early surgery is indicated, we feel that these patients should pass through the CVCU for evaluation, provided that the nurses are competent in surgical care. If such a condition as congestive heart failure is detected, operative and anesthetic risk can be rapidly decreased by prompt and vigorous attention to the problem. Furthermore, our experience in Springfield has been that it is feasible to transfer operated patients directly to the CVCU from the recovery room. At any rate, we strongly recommend that there be adequate monitoring capability in both the recovery room and the surgical intensive care unit.

Many hospitals have found, however, that it is usually not possible to staff recovery rooms and general or surgical intensive care units with nurses as skilled and as actively and totally involved in cardiac surveillance as those in a CVCU. Some of my most gratifying experiences have been with surgical patients who, just a few years ago, would have been considered inoperable had not excellent cardiac surveillance and management been available through the CVCU's nurses and machines. In general, surgeons aware of the near-prohibitive risks presented by such patients are pleased to have the CVCU made available to their patients. For example, recently a 70-year-old professor who had had a slight ischemic ECG abnormality for about 5 years was admitted to the emergency room at 7:00 A.M. with obvious acute cholecystitis requiring surgery. Immediately he was transferred to the CVCU and was found to have a stable and normal heart rhythm with no angina or evidence of con-

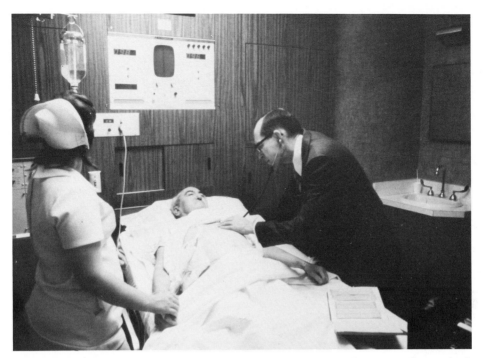

Fig. 47-11. This 64-year-old diabetic patient had a 20-year history of coronary disease. Angiography 2 years earlier revealed inoperable triple vessel disease, followed by severe nocturnal angina and congestive failure. The "problem" at the time of this admission was a hypernephroma of the right kidney. The stress of an infusion IV pyelogram produced severe ischemic pain on the x-ray table, requiring nearly 1 grain of IV morphine for relief, followed by mild enzyme rise. The question was whether to let him die of his carcinoma or to operate and risk death from heart complications. We decided to operate, primarily because we knew he would receive excellent cardiovascular nursing care in an unstressful environment. Surgery and the postoperative course were smooth.

gestive heart failure. Thirty hours later, after surgery, he was moved from the recovery room to the acute care section of the CVCU. There, during the first night, he developed paroxysmal intermittent atrial flutter, which was promptly managed and which subsided completely within the next 12 hours. The next event, a few days later, was acute widespread myocardial ischemia, detected and managed with ease in the CVCU. Needless to say, the surgeon was extremely pleased.

A second patient, a 65-year-old man with obvious acute myocardial ischemia but without infarct, was shown on roentgenogram to have a lung carcinoma. The difficult problem was to decide whether to release him for sev-

eral weeks, clean up the heart situation, and then operate, perhaps too late to remove the lung cancer, or whether to operate at once notwithstanding the risk of triggering a heart attack. We decided to operate. Two weeks after admission he was operated on and then brought to the CVCU for postoperative surveillance. Unfortunately, his carcinoma had proved to be inoperable and he later died of it, but our monitors showed that he had sustained no cardiac complication as a result of surgery.

I have given these examples of surgeons' use of the CVCU to counter the opinion I have heard in some hospitals that surgeons would never entrust their patients to such a facility. The truth is that surgeons, if properly oriented, will strongly support this mechanism for reducing the risk of death or disability in their patients.

As to the last class of patients whom I recommend be treated in the CVCU—those in for endoscopy or angiography of many sorts—no one, I think, would argue against providing intensive care for patients requiring angiography, since this procedure, even in the best hands, is tricky and carries its own calculable death rate. But the pertinence of the CVCU for patients undergoing other types of endoscopy might be open to question.

I would add to the "must" list, however, any patient with known serious heart disease, no matter which endoscopic procedure had been prescribed.

New construction: the CVCU

In 1965 and early 1966, the new progressive care unit was so enthusiastically supported by physicians, nurses, patients, and administrators that we began to think we should develop a much larger unit, a complete cardiovascular care system, that would require 75 to 100 beds. But this ambition was thwarted because of lack of funds for

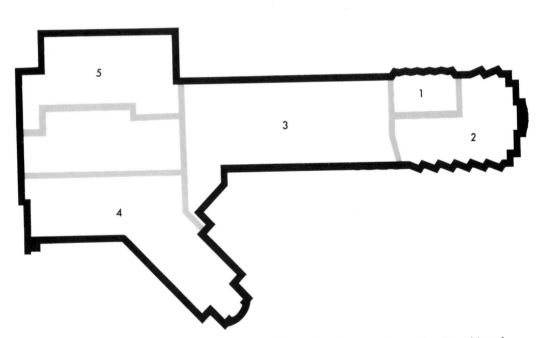

Fig. 47-12. An adequate number of beds suitably equipped to provide varying intensities of care is the key to improved delivery of in-hospital cardiovascular care. At St. John's, the saw-tooth area at right is reserved for acute care and is divided into two sections: Section A (1), containing 6 beds, for the most complex cases and Section B (2), with 14 beds, for less complicated heart and vascular cases; it has a slightly lower nurse-patient ratio. In both sections, the Springfield Wall contains full monitoring and resuscitation equipment. All patients are visible by nurses from their station. In the 32-bed intermediate section (3), patients are placed in private or semiprivate rooms serviced from one nursing station with two teams. Rhythm monitoring by radiotelemetry, available for as many as ten patients, is recorded on scopes at the central station. Less intensive nursing service is provided in the 38-bed convalescent section (4). Patients can be admitted to any section, or moved from one section to another, as their needs require. All necessary ancillary services are located a few steps away in the special section (5).

planning, building, and instrumenting such an expanded layout. Grant money might never have been obtained had we not secured the aid of three members of the staff of the Missouri Regional Medical Program (MoRMP): Dr. Vernon E. Wilson, Coordinator; Dr. George E. Wakerlin, former Medical Director of the American Heart Association, Director of Planning for MoRMP; and cardiovascular surgeon Earl M. Simmons, Jr., MoRMP Director for Heart. They assisted in the preparation of a successful proposal for planning a new total-care, admission-to-discharge CVCU. We received a $67,000 first-year planning grant on April 1, 1967, and began, among other activities, the tour of leading CCU's that I have already mentioned.

What evolved was a three-phase system of progressive care capable of handling all the types of cardiovascular conditions just described (Fig. 47-12).

THE ACUTE CARE SECTION

The acute care section is the first port-of-call for all categories of cardiovascular and pulmonary patients requiring the highest intensity of service (Fig. 47-13). On the basis of our experience with the first unit, we divided the acute section into two areas, embracing two levels of intensive care, which could be called maximum and median. Although all patients entering the section were either severely or critically ill, the majority of these, including actual, threatened, and possible heart attack, congestive failure, certain rhythm disturbances, acute stroke, pulmonary embolism, and certain surgical and noncardiac cases with severe cardiovascular disease, could generally be expected to stabilize rather promptly and to do well. For this group of patients we provided a 14-bed private room area occupying about three fourths of the roughly oval 20-bed section (Fig. 47-14, *A*).

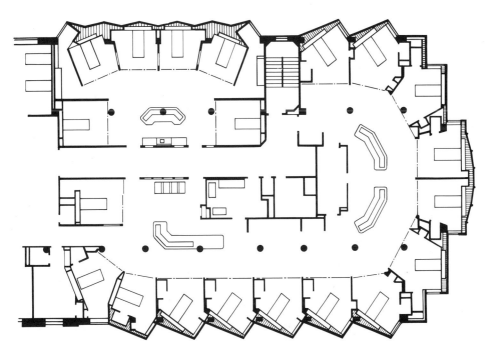

Fig. 47-13. In Sections A and B of the acute care section, a nurse is never more than a few feet away from the patient, whom she can see directly at all times. Closely placed nursing stations enhance staff backup.

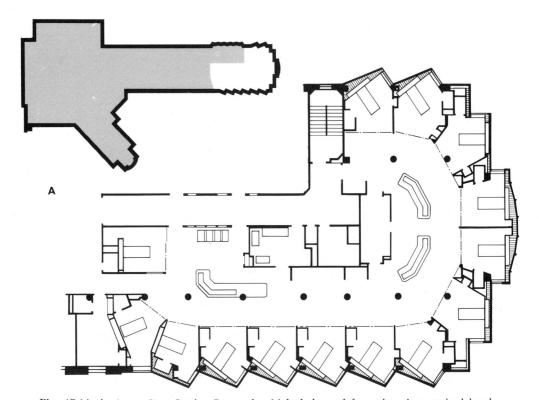

Fig. 47-14. **A,** Acute Care Section B contains 14 beds in oval formation characterized by the sawtooth design. The section is served by three nursing stations, two next to each other at the right and one at the left. **B** and **C,** Each of the nursing stations in Section B serves five patients, arranged in a semicircle that allows direct vision into each room. A third nursing station for the remaining four patients is located around the corner to the right. **D,** The privacy of a motel room and the reassurance of a hospital are enjoyed by patients in the CVCU. Clocks, TV, and the sights and sounds of visitors and nurses all help keep the patient oriented in space, time, and person. Yet with a flip of his finger he can separate himself from any disturbance by closing his drape. He remains in partial control of his environment and thus avoids the "infantilism" of being a purely passive recipient of services in an unvarying setting. **E,** All rooms in Section B have a wide opening for easy access and full visibility from the nursing station, with sliding glass doors and power-operated drapes to ensure privacy when desired; a window made possible by the sawtooth design; a closet for personal effects, so that the patient need not be deprived of them; the Springfield Wall; a lavatory and medicine cabinet; and an enclosed bathroom. The design combines privacy and quiet with exposure to the outside world and to the nursing station. The rooms are large enough to accommodate portable x-ray, ventilation, and other equipment that might be needed from time to time. **F,** At one of the nursing stations, nurses and aides go about their business quietly, even though this houses severely ill patients and in many hospitals is a tense and stressful environment. **G,** This unposed picture reflects the easygoing but alert spirit of the nurses in all sections of the CVCU. **H,** Sunlight streams into the hallways from windows in Section B, and space, light, and quiet surround the nursing station (1). Double-monitoring, by direct vision and by scope, is illustrated in **I** and **K.**

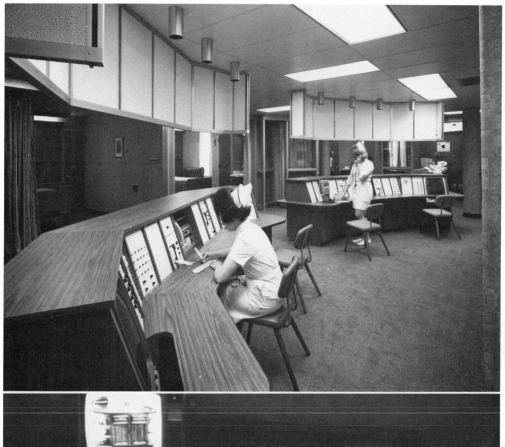

B

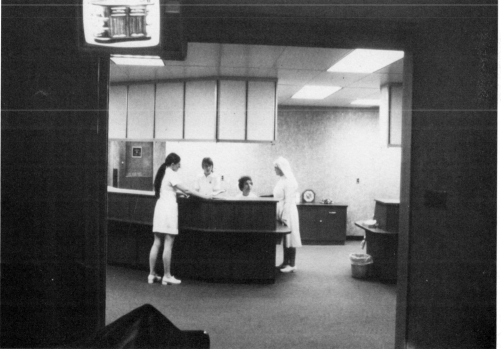

C

Continued.

Fig. 47-14, cont'd. For legend see opposite page.

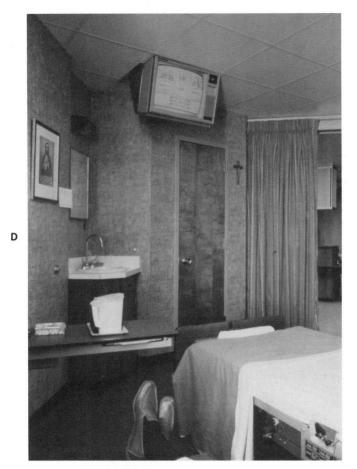

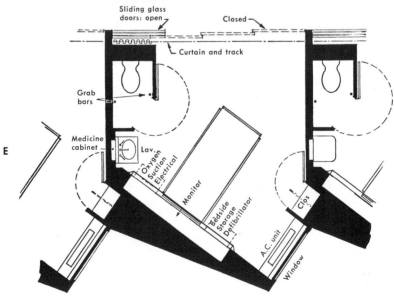

Fig. 47-14, cont'd. For legend see p. 546.

For the more dangerously ill patients, we set up the 6-bed maximum-care area (Fig. 47-15).

Many new patients are not admitted to the acute section. If their condition requires a lesser intensity of care, they are admitted directly to the intermediate, or even to the convalescent section, with advantages that I will detail later.

It is a frequent practice for a patient to

Text continued on p. 554.

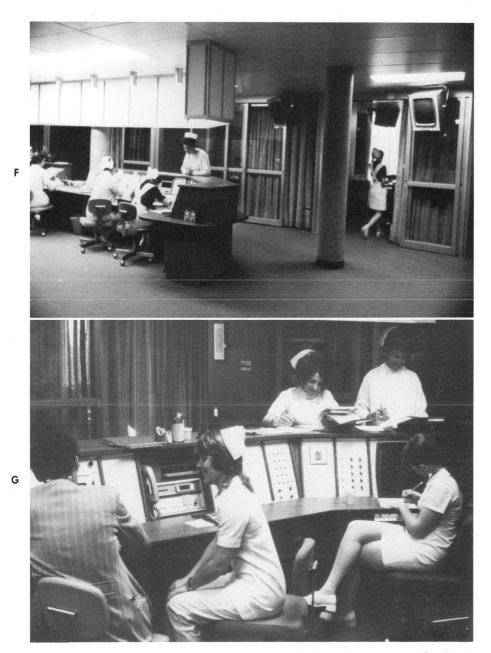

Continued.

Fig. 47-14, cont'd. For legend see p. 546.

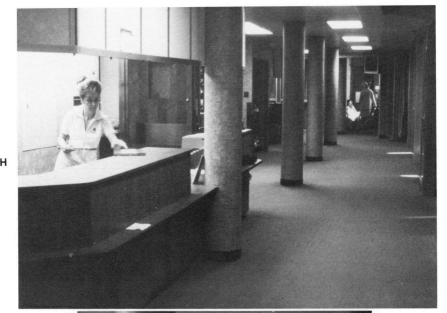

H

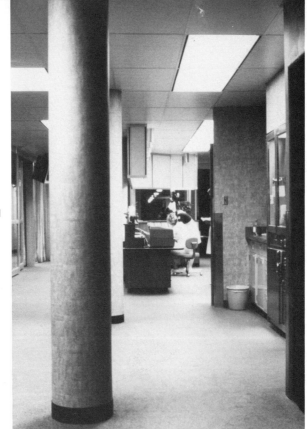

I

Fig. 47-14, cont'd. For legend see p. 546.

Fig. 47-14, cont'd. For legend see p. 546.

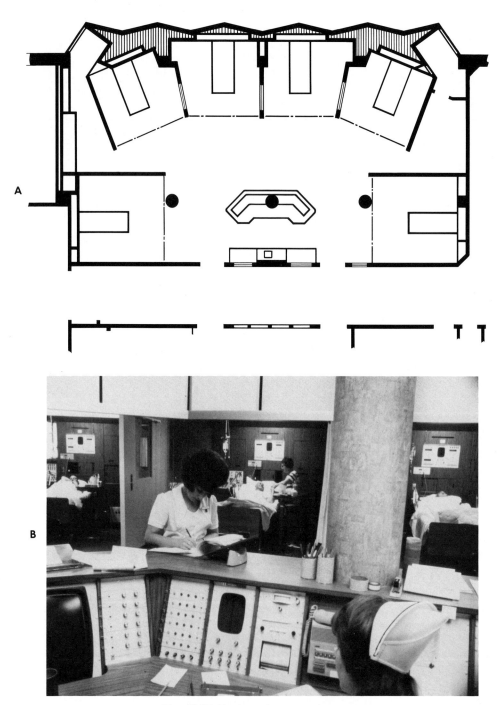

Fig. 47-15. For legend see opposite page.

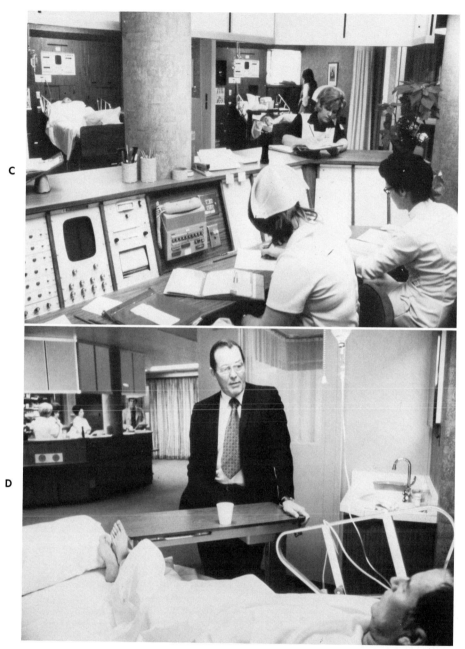

Fig. 47-15. A, Acute care Section A, reserved for the most complicated cases, combines compactness and full visibility to ensure continuous surveillance and instant response to emergency. Compartments at extreme right and left are glass enclosed to provide isolation for noisy or infected patients. **B** and **C** show the calm, spacious, reassuring atmosphere generated by the design of Section A. Normally such a section, reserved for the most seriously ill, is a jungle of wires, tubes, scopes, and lights; here all equipment is recessed in handsome but inexpensive cabinetry. Patients are separated from each other by a wall, but have a full view of the nursing station unless their drapes are drawn. Carpets, drapes, and an acoustic-board baffle at the top of the nursing station mute noise. **D,** A patient's view of the nursing station and the ever present nurses. Just left of the visitor's shoulder, drapes are drawn on one of the rooms reserved for noisy or infected patients.

be moved from the 6-bed unit to the 14-bed private room area as soon as his condition improves, and thence to intermediate; but transfer may be direct from the 6-bed unit to intermediate. Or, if a patient in the private room area worsens substantially, he may be moved to the more critical area.

While the 6-bed unit was designed for the more critically ill and the 14-bed for the less ill, either unit can actually accommodate either type of patient, thus giving flexibility to the system in terms of patient placement.

The total number of beds in the acute section was determined by a number of factors, one being our experience with the previous progressive care unit. We had found a need in that unit for at least 9 acute beds at all times; now that the hospital was increasing total beds from 450 to 700, a 55% increase, we assumed that intensive bed requirements would also increase proportionately, from 9 to 14.

We also made allowance for the significant but not exactly determined number of patients who could not be admitted to the progressive care unit because it was usually full.

Still another increment of beds was considered necessary to provide reserve space during peak patient loads, such as in winter and during the hot summer months.

We also took into account the anticipated increase in patient admissions that would result from the Early Warning Signs of Heart Attack Public and Professional Education Program. Statistical analysis of the EWS program up to the time of this publication indicate an approximate 20% increase in total, hospital-wide, heart attack and acute myocardial ischemia admissions, with a somewhat smaller increase in heart attack suspects who proved not to have ischemic heart disease. An additional interesting point about the early warning signs program, derived from the original 42-bed division, is that there was an over 50% increase in number of patients admitted to the acute section. It would appear that the EWS program, by

focusing sufficient attention on acute cardiac care, caused a greater proportion of heart suspects to be processed through the CVCU. These additional patients were accommodated through shortening the stay of patients cared for in the acute intensive units. Although this information did not become available until after plans for the new unit were finalized and construction was actually complete, it proved to be very fortuitous that the probable impact of the EWS program had been taken into account in determining the number of beds in the acute section of the new division.

Still another factor considered in determining size of the unit was the probability that prestige of the hospital, through establishment of the more modern facility, would attract more patients. Somewhat offsetting this factor, however, was the prediction that other hospitals in the region, both large and small, would make comparable improvements which would ultimately offset some of the initial increase in patronage of St. John's. Furthermore, it was felt that the EWS program, in itself, could well stimulate more patients to seek care closer to home since the emphasis of the program was on the securing of immediate attention to possible heart attack symptoms.

Still another ingredient in the process of determining the size, not only of the acute section but of the intermediate and convalescent sections as well, was a series of patient counts throughout the hospital for the purpose of determining how many patients were in the house at given times who might most appropriately be cared for in a CVCU for high-risk cases. The first such count, in early 1965, with a total patient census of 450, indicated that there were then in the hospital seventy-five patients who would benefit from group, specialized care for actual or possible high-risk cardiovascular disease. Subsequent counts, by other individuals, showed this number to increase to 100 or above. Although it had early been learned that well under a third of the total hospital stay of heart attack patients, comprising the largest single category, was spent in the acute section, it was felt that one should plan for up to 5 days' average stay in the acute section. Dividing 100 patients by five gave a figure of 20 beds needed. Diminishing this number somewhat was the knowledge that certain categories of patients, such as congestive heart failure, might require a lesser period of time in the acute unit. Still another minus factor to be applied to this 20-bed total was the anticipation that not all physicians would utilize the CVCU as extensively as others.

It is to be noted from the foregoing multi-faceted discussion concerning determination of bed needs that no fixed formula system, such as has been advocated by some for determining the number of CCU beds, has been applied; on the contrary, day-to-day experience in the previous unit, plus an assessment of factors to probably come into play later, led to determination of unit size. It should further be stressed that this same type of reasoning is applicable to all hospitals and that this broad approach should replace, or at least augment, the formula proposed by the Inter-Society Commission for Heart Disease Resources, which suggests that the number of CCU beds be based on 5 days' occupancy for each heart attack admitted during the year, plus a factor of 50%.

Although smaller hospitals will not find it feasible to establish two levels of intensive care in the acute care section, larger hospitals should give some consideration to determining the ratio between the two differing levels of intensity of care in respect to bed needs. At St. John's, this ratio was based chiefly upon estimates by a number of physicians and nurses, doubtless primarily influenced by the ratio of cases handled in the original two units of the pilot 42-bed division, the lesser number being in the more critically ill category.

While the new division has been in operation only 7 months at the time of this writing, it would appear that the size of the acute section at St. John's was correctly estimated,

both in respect to total beds and to the 6- to 14-bed subdivisions within the unit. On this date, prior to the predicted acute cardiovascular patient load peak of January, February, and March, there are 4 of 6 beds occupied in the area for more critical patients and there are eleven patients in the 14-bed private room area.

While this type of discussion may appear tedious, it is my strong conviction that the acute care sections in most of our hospitals are undersized and therefore do not meet total needs. For example, the PAS* systematic sample of acute myocardial infarction patients, derived from a great number of hospitals, showed that during January to June, 1970, only 64.5% of patients with heart attack were managed in CCUs. This sample makes no reference to those patients with acute myocardial ischemia or to patients with other life-threatening cardiovascular diseases. Figures at St. John's prior to opening the new CVCU showed that while the average acute heart attack mortality in the old CVCU was 16%, that for patients managed outside the CVCU was 28%. This may be a reflection of the tendency of some not to admit more or less hopeless cases to the CVCU, but I feel that this high death rate outside the unit is more likely the consequence of less adequate care being rendered on general halls than in the CVCU. Therefore, it seems inappropriate not to create adequate bed space for these patients and to accompany this with an intensive educational program designed to induce all staff physicians to routinely admit actual, threatened, or possible heart attack patients to the CVCU, as well as to include other high-risk cardiovascular patients.

A final point concerning bed needs in the acute care section is one that cannot yet be stated as a fact but that should be given serious consideration: at St. John's, where

---

*Professional Activities Study, companion service to Medical Audit Program (MAP), both sponsored by Commission on Professional and Hospital Activities, Ann Arbor, Michigan.

there is great ease of patient transfer from acute to intermediate and to convalescent, preserving the opportunity for similar ease of transfer back into a higher level of care, it is beginning to appear that there is a significantly shorter stay in the acute section than is customary at many hospitals. I feel that this is due to the availability of radio telemetry in the intermediate section, which permits patients doing well after the first day or two to be transferred out of the more expensive acute section. I believe that there may be some bias of judgment in determining length of stay in the acute section as a consequence of the almost ever present shortage of beds there, more or less forcing doctors to move patients along more rapidly than might actually be desirable. While a number of surveys are showing in-hospital mortality to be less than previously expected with shortening of hospital stay, it is very difficult to gather good data on what the later course of such patients is. Based on my own personal estimate of a very large volume of patients managed with the previous traditional 3-week average stay for heart attack, and the opportunity for a reasonably close observation of patients of a number of other doctors who use a shorter stay, I feel that the tendency to advance and discharge patients more rapidly is not sound. Recognizing that numerous competent cardiologists might well challenge this statement, I simply make these comments to stimulate thought and to suggest that doctors reconsider what their decision as to length of patient stay might be if there were no bed shortage.

Certain features are common to the entirety of the acute care section. Like the unit as a whole, the acute care section is fully carpeted. This is viewed at St. John's as one of the most important decisions made. Soilage in the rooms and compartments has not been a problem; spills of staining liquids, particularly coffee, have been much more common in the corridors. Lighting is chiefly fluorescent, incandescent lighting being used only to focus on nursing station desk areas and for

ceiling-recessed, airplane-type reading lights above each patient's bed. Fluorescent lighting above each bed, switchable to two intensities (two or four tubes) has proved very adequate for all procedures requiring high illumination and at much less cost than the traditional quartz lights. Fluorescent cove lights at the top of each headwall provide adequate general illumination, also switched to provide a choice of intensities. Code Blue call buttons are located in each headwall and transmit a signal to the main telephone switchboard so that a page is enunciated by the operator as to precise location of the patient without voice communication between nurse and operator being necessary.

Each room and compartment in the acute section is to be supplied with a battery-powered clock that has a calendar mechanism. An attractive walnut-framed prototype was built in Springfield. Cost of each unit will be about $40. Dr. Hughes Day and his staff feel that a clock and a calendar do much to preserve time orientation in confused patients.

An intercom system connects all nursing stations in the acute, intermediate, and convalescent sections as well as laboratory, department of electrocardiography, and all other areas. Not only is this quicker than dialing a telephone but response can be given at the receiving end from a distance of several feet from the receiver-transmitter, making it unnecessary for the recipient of the call to leave her duties to go pick up the telephone. This appears to be a great time-saver throughout the unit.

All nursing station cabinetry is factory built, accommodating monitoring equipment, ECG paper printout equipment, chart holders, intercom, patient-nurse call, and an abundance of drawers for storage. This system of nursing station design is considered in Springfield to be one of the most important advances by electronics firms, pioneered by the supplier of the equipment used in St. John's.

Even though each room and compartment

has a bedside defibrillator, there is also provided a conventional crash cart with plug-in defibrillator. In addition, there is a battery-powered portable (hand-carried) defibrillator with built-in oscilloscope, a "must" item of equipment. This has been vividly demonstrated at St. John's already. Notwithstanding elaborate planning of an emergency alternate power source, this has been found not to work on two occasions and this unit has already saved two lives. One should also be placed in the emergency room.

Continuously stored in the acute care section, in the corridor, is a portable x-ray machine with capacitator discharge, permitting chest x-ray films to be made at one sixtieth of a second. Quality of films made by this unit is usually indistinguishable from films made in the x-ray department. Since 20% of deaths in CCU's occur as a result of congestive heart failure, I strongly feel that early detection of failure by appropriately spaced chest x-ray films is possible and should alter survival figures. This machine and the increasingly favorable reputation it has achieved have resulted in much accelerated utilization of portable chest radiography at St. John's in the acute care section.

The 20-bed section basically consists of a multiple of four patient care units, one of 6 beds in acute section A, and, in the 14-bed acute section B, two of 5 beds each and one of 4. This is consistent with the usually accepted ideal of having four to six, and not more than eight, patients served by one team. Accordingly, there is one nursing station in the 6-bed unit and three nursing stations in the 14-bed area. While each team has full responsibility for patients in its own service area, all stations are so close to one another that excellent backup and interchange are afforded during times of work overload and staff absence caused by holiday, vacation, or illness. This opportunity for backup and interchange also applies to the entire system, acute, intermediate, and convalescent, and is valuable from the standpoint of staff satisfaction and economy of operation, with the probable

added benefit of improved staff tenure. This is believed to be one of the very most important features of the CVCU. Smaller hospitals should determine the number of patient care units needed on the basis of numbers of patients to be served.

Staffing of each team includes graduate nurses, licensed practical nurses, and aides, with secretaries serving one or two teams each.

Certain design features, in addition to differing staffing levels, distinguish the 14-bed private room area from the 6-bed portion of the section for the more severely ill. The former has three-section sliding glass doors, most rooms providing a recess for the stacking of these sections when the doors are opened. It should be noted, however, that the noise level is so low that these doors are rarely closed. Each room has moderate weight, single-thickness drapes that are power operated by switches at three points: in the patient's nurse call handset, on the wall at the entry to the room, and at the nursing station. Cost for each unit, less wiring and switching, is about $70.00.

Each room has an outside window, preserving contact of the patient with the outside world. There is a bathroom for each patient. Monitor cables are long enough to extend into the bathroom, making it unnecessary to have a separate monitor plug in the bathroom. There is a ceiling-mounted radio/television in each room. The Springfield group feels that providing television for all routine acute heart attack admissions is very worthwhile. The sets at St. John's carry all local radio broadcasts, as well as closed circuit television for patient and family education. Each room has a closet for the storage of clothing and personal effects. The patient and the headwall in each room are visible from the nursing station serving that patient. There is a triple monitor display: above the head of each patient, at the nursing station, and in the corridor. The last is actually a dual display, one multichannel screen facing in either direction so as to increase staff surveillance. All rooms are provided with the

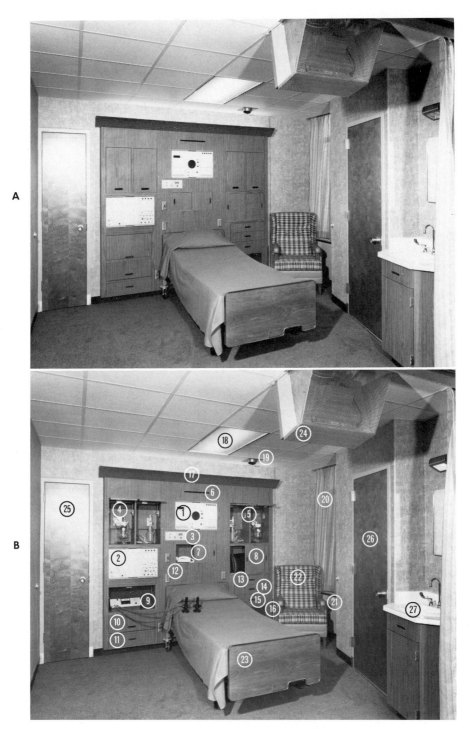

Fig. 47-16. For legend see opposite page.

"Springfield chair," a specially researched and built chair selling for about $100, less ottoman, designed for patient comfort, durability, and ease of cleaning. There is a washbasin in each room, built into a Formica-covered cabinet that also accommodates various basins and supplies.

Room sizes and shapes vary somewhat but contain a minimum of 132 square feet, within the 130 to 150 square foot recommendation of the National Conference on Coronary Care Units. Shown in Fig. 47-14, *E*, is the design of a typical room of smaller size. A model of this room was built in 1968 and was thoroughly tested over a period of 4 years, proving to be adequate in all respects for all services to be performed, including resuscitation, assisted ventilation, and portable chest radiography.

The 6-bed unit, while compartmented, actually has somewhat more space per patient than do the smaller private rooms. For the sake of compactness, bathrooms and outside windows are not provided. Nor is there a television. I personally regret this decision and plan to utilize a specially built support for a small TV set, the lower extremity of

which will be inserted into the intravenous pole socket at the midportion of either side of the bed. The Springfield Wall in this area is more heavily instrumented than in the private rooms. Closure is by standard curtains, without a power mechanism except for two of the six compartments that have sliding glass doors, in addition to drapes, for better sound control when noisy patients are in the unit. Each compartment has the same washbasin-cabinet unit that is seen in the private room area, a great convenience to the nurse. Chairs are not provided as a standard item but are frequently moved to the bedside. It has been found that even some of the more critically ill patients need to be up in the chair at times. There is an overhead intravenous support trolley, not included in the private room area for esthetic reasons. Between patient compartments and the nursing station there is excellent proximity of patient and nurse. The nursing station of this unit is just across another corridor from one of the three nursing stations in the private room area, affording good contact between the two nursing teams.

The Springfield group feels that one of its

Fig. 47-16. A, Springfield Wall with equipment recessed. **B,** Springfield Wall with equipment in action. *1,* Recessed, two-channel monitor display panel (the six compartments and rooms in the area for more critically ill have four-channel displays). *2,* Control panel for monitor at a level easily accessible to nurse. *3,* Patient's control panel contains a plug-in point for hand-control piece, which allows patient to call nurse, operate television, and open and close drapes. Panel also contains emergency call button connected directly to hospital switchboard. *4,* Oxygen and suction recessed in cabinets. *5,* Duplicate oxygen and suction for opposite side of bed. Compressed air can easily be added to either side without crowding. *6,* Slot for warm air exhaust. *7,* Recess for plug-in telephone. Compartment also contains space for water pitcher, dentures, reading matter, etc., all within easy reach of patient. *8,* Added storage space for personal effects or bottles of intravenous fluids. *9,* Fixed-position, slant-mounted defibrillator with paddle storage, right, atop airtight automatic-opening electrode jelly container. *10,* Storage compartment below defibrillator. Door opens to horizontal position as additional work shelf. *11,* Storage space. *12,* Electrical outlets, 120 volt (220-volt current was considered unnecessary but could be provided). *13,* Drawer for emergency medication and supplies. Drawer has shelf that slides to either side to expose items underneath. *14,* Drawer for aneroid blood pressure instrument, stethoscope, etc. *15,* Storage space. *16,* Panel for connections to ground-bus electrical safety system. *17,* Indirect cove light, which can be switched for choice of light intensity. *18,* Four-tube fluorescent ceiling light, which can be switched for two intensities. Bright light is adequate for patient care, cut-downs, and most minor surgical procedures. *19,* Inexpensive airplane-type reading light. Switch is at left, near telephone. *20,* Outside window. *21,* Air handling unit of heating and cooling system. *22,* Springfield chair. *23,* Electric bed. *24,* Overhead TV. *25,* Clothes closet. *26,* Door to bathroom. *27,* Washstand.

most effective and best appreciated achievements was the development of the Springfield Wall, a headwall that completely recesses all gear (Fig. 47-16). The idea of recessing was first seen at Sisters of Charity Hospital, Buffalo, New York, where the monitor was completely recessed. Building on that observation, we began in 1968 to develop a wall that would house all the electronic gear and equipment and would provide space for telephone, personal effects, emergency supplies, and examination instruments, including stethoscope and sphygmomanometer.

This undertaking attracted top engineers from a number of firms manufacturing equipment and represents the bringing together of some of the nation's finest talent. The purpose was to create a motel-room appearance, doing away with the traditional gruesome mechanical jungle of monitors, oxygen and suction apparatus, lights on derricklike supports, cables, and tubes. One by one, it became possible to incorporate all these features in the wall at modest cost and with great efficiency of function.

Separate oxygen and suction cabinets are on either side of the bed. Compressed air is not included, for cost reasons. This omission appears justified, since portable compressors are less expensive to acquire and operate than a pipeline system.

The first bedside defibrillator was seen in the unit of Dr. Henry Cooper at Broward General Hospital, Fort Lauderdale, Florida. Dr. Day terms the bedside defibrillator one of the most important developments in coronary care unit design and function in recent years. Each of the twenty private rooms and compartments in the acute care section has a defibrillator in the wall to the right of each patient. It is in a fixed mount, in a slanted position, with space for the paddles at the side of the unit, one of which sits atop an automatically opening electrode jelly container, developed in Miami, Florida, by an electronics firm designer.

An earlier version of the wall had an "eyeball" reading light recessed in it beside the monitor screen but there was glare, which competed with the visualization of the monitor. Consequently, this light was moved into the ceiling and now is an extremely worthwhile feature. There is a ground-bus electrical safety system, with plug-ins just above the floor to the left of the patient. Cove lighting at the top of the wall provides a choice of level of illumination for day or night.

Thickness of the wall is $14\frac{1}{2}$ inches, with a $1\frac{1}{2}$ inch ventilation space behind for cooling of the monitor. A very quiet fan provides for adequate air movement, intake being at the bottom of the wall and exhaust through a slot at the top of the wall. Although the wall as installed at St. John's sets into a plastered recess, it would be very simple to attach such a unit to a flush wall in new or remodeled construction, simply facing over the space on either side for closets and/or storage. Access to much of the pipes and wires leading to items in the wall is through a large removable panel behind the head of each bed.

Particularly in remodeling, this manner of instrumenting a cardiovascular patient room should simplify and hasten the job. The wall, built in Springfield, is in modular form, in three sections, and is easily shippable. Current cost, less equipment, is about $1,250.

When the move was made at St. John's from the old unit to the new, the nursing staff was almost ecstatic over the convenience afforded by this one feature. Several made special effort to express individual personal appreciation. Just recently, I observed, once again, the harrowing delays in the process in attempting to defibrillate a patient on a general hall with a good crash cart—the first problem was getting the unit plugged in, the second was getting the cables and paddles out of the drawer, and the third problem was that there was no electrode jelly in the drawer.

In the new unit, patients can be defibrillated within several seconds and the nurse may even have to wait until the patient becomes drowsy, which is said to take about ten seconds, before applying countershock. I feel that the bedside defibrillator, always ready to go with the touch of a button and without the necessity of assembling paddles and jelly, will rank in importance with the grouping concept as a whole in increasing success of resuscitation efforts.

The telephone, which can be plugged in to the personal effects compartment above the head of the bed, with easy access to the patient, has a dial in the handset and is a much appreciated feature. I strongly feel that more acute cardiac patients, including those with heart attack, should be allowed access by telephone to their family and business associates. Touch tone dialing would add to the convenience of this instrument.

The oscilloscope in the fourteen private rooms can handle two channels of information. Those in the 6-bed unit are larger and can display four channels. The instrumentation layout in the 6-bed unit includes a variety of other added features, including intravenous drip regulators.

The question most frequently asked by visitors is, "How much does all this cost and how can you possibly afford it?" The fact of the matter is that daily room rates in the 14-bed private room area are $90.00 and those in the 6-bed area, $95.00. It is true that there have been grants and gifts that covered a portion of the cost, but it is felt that exposition of such a program can generate substantial gifts in other communities as well and that the entirety of the system, as described, can be put together at a cost not inconsistent with a much lower daily patient charge than is customary for intensive cardiac care in most hospitals. This lower rate is due to a number of factors, one of which is greatly increased utilization. The greatest benefit of the lower rate is, in actuality, the greater utilization that results from it, bringing more benefits to more people in need and, in addition to other patient advantages, enabling more people to be resuscitated and, more importantly still, making it possible to attend to more problems before resuscitation is necessary.

One has to actually spend some time in such an acute care section to fully appreciate

the less harried appearance of the nurses, the quieter tempo, the more efficient performance of duties, and the more relaxed state of the patient, in contrast with the conventional intensive care unit. I feel that among the dominant reasons for improved staff satisfaction and performance are the adequacy of beds for any occasion, the low noise level and improved decor.

INTERMEDIATE CARE SECTION

The simplicity of the intermediate section is the reason for its success and also for its feasibility in practically any hospital (Fig. 47-17, *A*). It must be contiguous with both the acute care section and the convalescent section unless, as is very practical in many hospitals, especially small institutions, intermediate and convalescent care are combined. While reference has been made by others to the importance of monitoring, usually by radiotelemetry, it must be emphasized that the presence of a nursing staff skilled in cardiovascular disease is a close second if not actually even more important. It is the nursing staff that is the mechanism for the impressive benefits that accrue to patients over and above mortality reduction through detection, correction, and prevention of arrhythmias.

The first prerequisite of the system is an adequacy of beds. The Springfield teams observed a number of "step-down" or intermediate care units during their travels, but these, like most of the acute care sections, were too small to meet total hospital needs even if the progressive care system was intended only for coronary heart disease. At St. John's, calculation of intermediate bed needs was determined along the lines already discussed in detail under the acute care section. The larger size resulted from the experience in the earlier unit; doctors and nurses preferred to keep patients in the intermediate area longer than in the intensive acute section. Actually clinching the decision for a unit of 32 beds were two factors: the first was an architectural limitation, since the floor was built on top of a previous expansion, with all dimensions being predetermined; the second was the fact that plumbing and other facilities for the two original floors underneath were positioned in a manner that dictated that approximately half the rooms be private and the other half be semi-private. Whereas there is an apparent trend toward having all patient rooms in new hospitals be private, with a uniform daily rate, there seemed to be no alternative to a dual rate structure at St. John's with a higher rate for a single room than for a double. This price differential is believed to be one major reason why there is less demand for private rooms in the intermediate section. Another possible reason is an apparent tendency in this region for patients to want to have a roommate. Some doctors have expressed the opinion that the "buddy system" gives some psychological protection to each of the two occupants of a room. Regardless

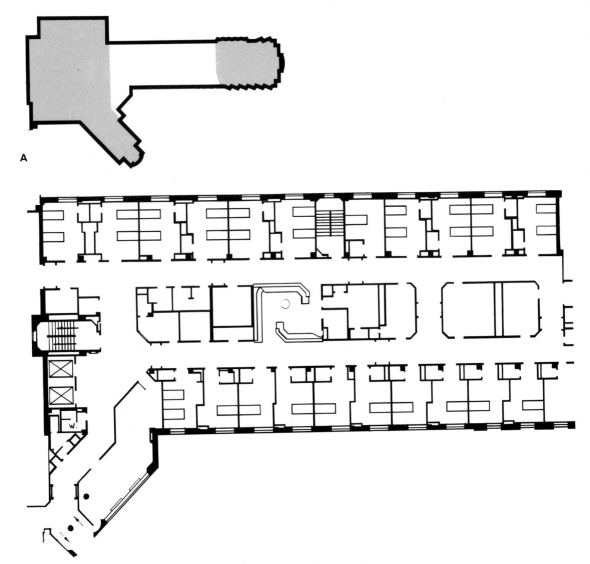

Fig. 47-17. For legend see opposite page.

of the reasons, a number of the single rooms at St. John's in the intermediate section have to be assigned to patients requesting semi-private accommodations and at the lower semiprivate rate, as "only available" accommodations. This led to a decision in the con-

valescent section to have only 8 private rooms for a total of the 38 patients, although this ratio can be adjusted more flexibly than in the intermediate section.

Actual design features of patient rooms are no different from those of conventional

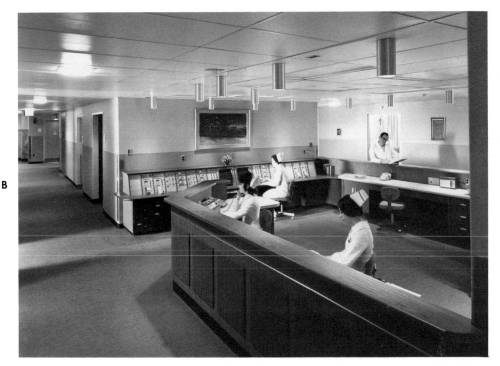

B

Continued.

Fig. 47-17. A, The 32-bed intermediate care section provides private rooms, bottom, and semi-private rooms, top, and is served by a central nursing station that faces both corridors. Many less complicated cases are admitted directly to this section. The proximity to the acute care section is a boon to nurses who must switch patients from one section to the other, and a source of reassurance to the patients, who know they are never far from maximum care if they need it. B, The console at the end of the nursing station picks up radiotelemetered rhythm patterns from ten patients. Despite a double team of nurses and the almost constant presence of doctors and visitors near this station, noise levels are low and traffic flows smoothly. C, Within 20 feet of the nursing station, and yet in an environment of her own, this patient enjoys maximum security and privacy. In her left hand is a radio that broadcasts her heart rhythm to the central nursing console; on the bed to her right is the switching device that enables her to control her TV and summon the nurse. Through the window she can see the world to which she will soon return. In an actual admission of a patient, I check heart sounds in the emergency room, D, assist in rushing the patient through the hallway, E, then out the elevator into the CVCU, F, and into a bed in the intermediate care section, where a nurse and an orderly transfer the patient to his new bed, G. Finally, with two nurses caring for his immediate needs, the patient and his wife can begin to relax (H). This man was admitted directly to the intermediate care section since his condition did not warrant intensive care at the time of admission. He was discharged in stable condition 12 days later.

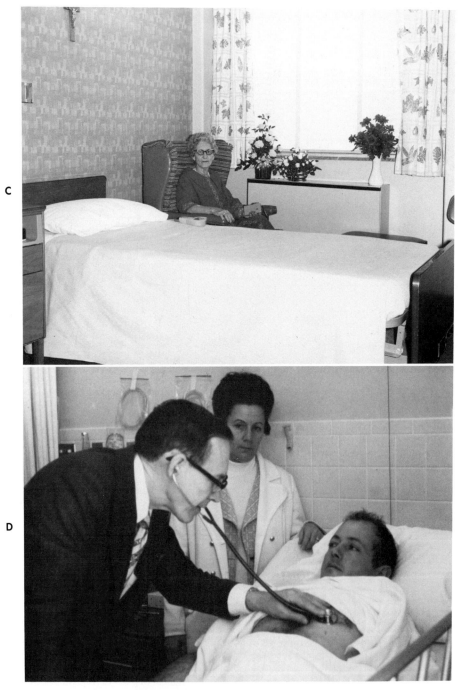

Fig. 47-17, cont'd. For legend see p. 563.

hospital construction (Fig. 47-17, C). There is a television in a recess in cabinetry which, like the units in the acute care section, carriers radio as well as closed circuit television. Each room has a closet, bathroom, an outside window, and a Springfield chair with ottoman. Space does not permit having two of these chairs in the 2-bed rooms and there is competition between roommates for this comfortable chair.

As should be the case in all hospital design, every possible effort was made to reduce

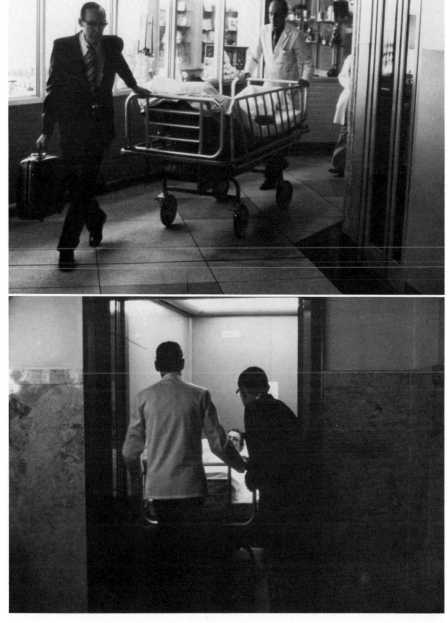

E

F

Continued.

Fig. 47-17, cont'd. For legend see p. 563.

nurse-to-patient travel distance. While there are some round designs that might reduce the time-consuming walking by nurses to see patients in distant rooms, such a design would require new construction from the ground up and was not feasible at St. John's. As has been emphasized by architects, the rectangular design with the greater dimension not being overly long, appears to be the best solution for many hospitals.

Although direct wire monitoring could be provided at lesser cost if conduitry could be installed at the time of initial construction or remodeling, this has the distinct disad-

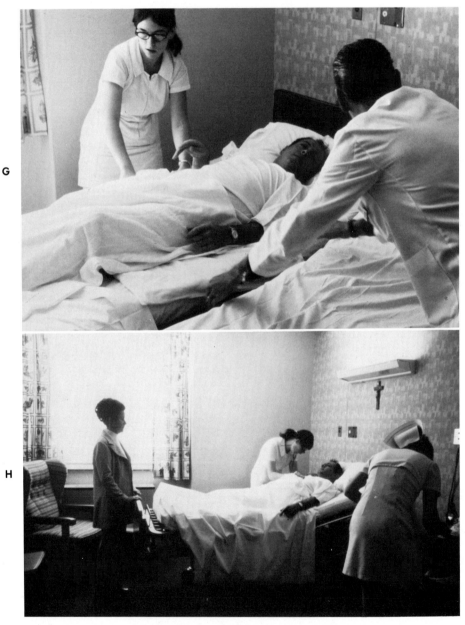

G

H

Fig. 47-17, cont'd. For legend see p. 563.

vantage of preventing mobility of the patient. For this one reason, telemetry appears to be much more preferable and has been very satisfactory at St. John's, with continued use of the brand of equipment selected in 1968, 4 years prior to the move into the new division. Actually, the same patient transmission units are still in use and serviceable. Initial cost and maintenance are somewhat higher, and "down time" is greater, but the benefits of the system far outweigh these disadvantages and it is planned at St. John's to steadily expand the number of monitor units from the present ten. It is felt that ultimately the entire patient population in the intermediate section will be monitored.

Distinguishing design characteristics of the intermediate section involve the nursing station (Fig. 47-17, B) and certain supporting services. A large bank of instrumentation and controls is placed against the wall in a location that provides maximal surveillance by the several members of the staff, from graduate nurses to secretaries. The monitor display cabinet has a work space that makes it convenient to do chart work there so as to increase monitor observation. My observation of the nursing staff has been that there has been almost continuous presence at this area of one or more members of the staff, making it impractical to have a separate ECG monitoring technician. In addition to this surveillance, there are ceiling-mounted monitors in the corridors, although there are not as many displays as in the acute section (two multichannel scopes are used, one in each of the double corridors).

The second point of emphasis in nursing station design is that all nurse work areas are situated so that they are always facing the patient rooms, in contrast to an arrangement seen in some hospitals where the nurses have their backs to patients and corridor traffic, presumably to increase the efficiency of their desk work.

Supporting services include an office for the division director (a graduate nurse) and for the unit manager. A final decision has not been made as to whether there will be such a manager but I feel that this will prove to be wise. There are two staff lounges, one at the point of juncture with the acute care section, for the staff of that unit, and the second for the intermediate section staff. These are roomy, pleasant, and well furnished. At the point of entry into the intermediate section is a spacious relatives' lounge and, across the corridor, a conference room for discussion with individual families. The intercom system will summon relatives from the lounge to either the intermediate nursing station or to the acute care section, a great time-saver.

Patients cared for in the intermediate section include all those in the categories previously enumerated as eligible for treatment in the acute section. In addition, less ill patients in a number of these categories are frequently admitted direct to intermediate or transferred there from general halls once their condition has been recognized (Fig. 47-17, E to H). Specific examples of this latter group are worsened angina without clearly impending infarction; rhythm problems, especially those for elective cardioversion or drug treatment; congestive heart failure; thrombophlebitis; acute stroke; and, importantly, patients for coronary angiography. In addition to these direct admissions, there are transfers from the acute section and, occasionally, from the convalescent section. The feasibility of immediate transfer back to acute, together with the provision of radiotelemetry, are the dominant features that expedite the passage of patients through the acute section. If a patient transferred out of acute early because he is doing well should unexpectedly worsen, he can be promptly moved back. This "step-up" feature, as emphasized by Dr. Fred Ownby of Nashville, is just as important to a progressive care division as is the more often publicized "step-down" capability.

In actual practice, the intermediate care section has been abundantly shown to be the "backbone" of the entire progressive care system. For this reason, it is well staffed with nurses specially trained but at a lesser level than those in the acute section. Patient morale is excellent because transfer into this section is regarded as an important promotion. Nurses from the acute section, who meant so much to the patient during his initial stay in the hospital, visit the patient after transfer and, conversely, patients in this area, as part of their exercise program when this is feasible, take advantage of the proximity to the units to visit their nurse friends back in the acute section. And, staff backup between the two sections, as well as with convalescent, is an impressive feature.

Cost considerations are of great appeal to hospital administrators, medical staff, and patients alike. At St. John's, room rates in this section are only modestly above those on general halls, with the exception that there is an additional daily monitor charge of $7.50. This gives incentive for moving patients out of the acute area and also gives reason for direct admissions to this section when the case does not require the intensity of service available in the acute section, which does increase the cost. And, it is this reasonable daily rate that makes it feasible to admit the full spectrum of cardiovascular cases to this area. Whereas it has been said by some authorities that a hospital cannot afford to provide specialized cardiovascular nursing care to the entirety of the cardiovascular patient population, it has been clearly shown at St. John's that this is feasible and with clear patient benefits.

These benefits include better recognition of and attention to problems peculiar to cardiac patients. One major benefit is the proximity to lifesaving measures, whether that be full resuscitation or simply the better prevention of those developments requiring resuscitation. During their stay in this section, patients acquire from the nursing staff, and from other patients as well, a better understanding of their disease process and what is necessary to be done in the future in respect to better care and better prevention of recurrence of the acute episode. This patient education will be greatly accelerated when the closed circuit television programming is initiated in the near future. And there is a benefit for the doctor—through this grouping and through having a skilled cardiovascular nurse with him on daily rounds, his instructions are better understood by the nurse and better carried out with less time spent by the doctor. Not only can the doctor do a better job, with not so much stress on himself, but he can do this in less time than on a general hall. Still another benefit to all, and this was repeatedly shown in the pilot St. John's unit, is the fact that should the acute care section be full, it is very feasible for an uncomplicated heart attack patient to be admitted to the intermediate section provided a monitor unit is available. This opportunity for acute care in this fashion is the same as is routinely employed for acute care in some institutions where there is no direct vision acute section. It should be stated, however, that the Springfield group feels that direct visual observation is so important that direct vision units should be provided for initial care in heart attack as well as in any other serious acute cardiovascular situation.

THE CONVALESCENT SECTION

With all the foregoing discussion, the nature of the third phase, or convalescent section, should by now be apparent. At St. John's this is an unmonitored area into which patients are transferred after it has been clearly demonstrated that they are doing well and there is no reasonable likelihood of their requiring resuscitation or other emergency care although these possibilities do always exist in all cardiacs regardless of whether they are in the hospital or out (Fig. 47-18, *A*). The dominant features of this unit are the provision of intensification of patient and *family* education and initiation of rehabilitation, including physical reconditioning through exercise and, as needed, formal physical therapy. Although the matter

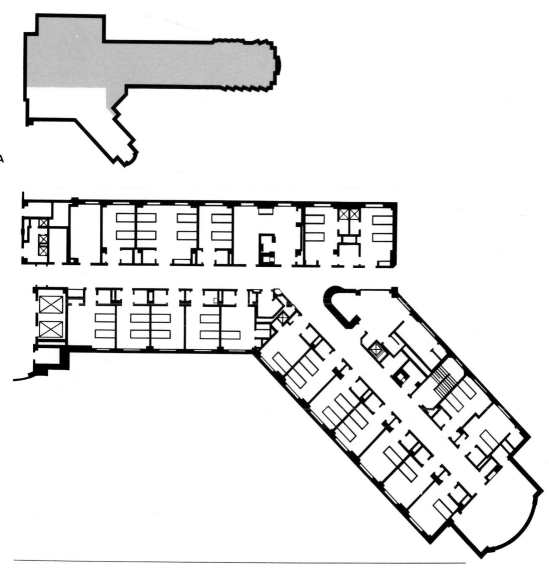

Continued.

Fig. 47-18. A, The 32-bed convalescent care section branches out compactly from a central nursing station. At lower left is large room that serves as recreational lounge and as classroom for patient and family education. **B, C,** and **D,** In the convalescent care section the patient finds the same restful decor that he had become accustomed to in the intermediate or acute care sections. He is not shunted off into a strange section of the hospital, and he is never far from intensive care facilities. Some patients are admitted directly to the convalescent section if their primary need is for observation or, in some cases, terminal care.

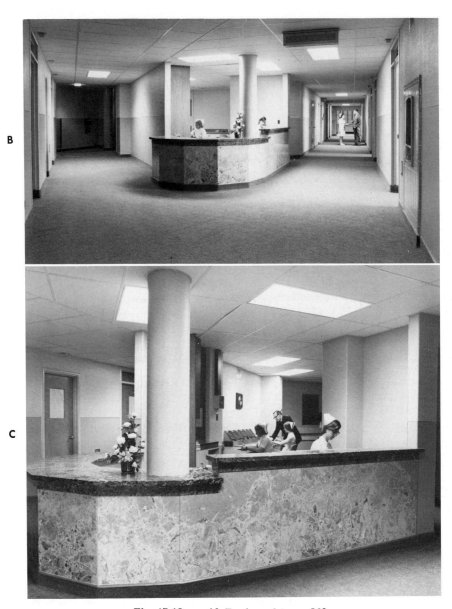

Fig. 47-18, cont'd. For legend see p. 569.

of what to do with chronic stroke patients during rehabilitation has not been settled at St. John's, it appears probable that certain of these patients can be accommodated in this section.

Lounge areas are provided, visitors' hours are much more liberal than in the intermediate and acute sections, and emphasis by the nursing staff is on the patient being up and about all that he is able. In the original St. John's unit, the saying among patients was that "the nearer you get to the statue at the end of the hall, the better you are," and this applies equally to the promotion into the new convalescent section. The atmosphere in this area is one of increased cheerfulness and anticipation and must be seen to be appreciated (Fig. 47-18, *B* to *D*). This is in contrast to the situation that exists when a patient must be "bumped" out of

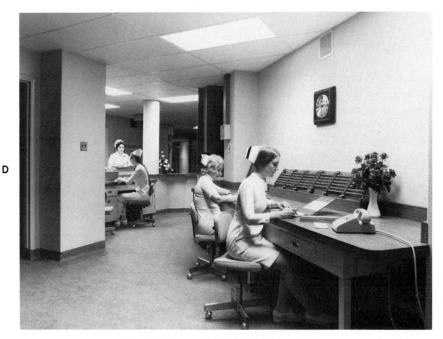

Fig. 47-18, cont'd. For legend see p. 569.

the acute or intermediate section into a totally foreign section of the hospital, where he must entirely reacquaint himself with staff and surroundings. These are some of the intangibles that we feel are very significant in the future psychological, and perhaps physical, recovery of the patient.

Physical design, as regards room sizes, construction features, and nursing station design, is exactly the same as in the remainder of the hospital, including the intermediate section. However, important to the feeling of continuity of progression is the complete refurbishment of the convalescent section. The addition of the new, "dropped" ceiling, vinyl wall covering identical to that in the acute and intermediate sections, and extension of the same carpeting throughout the division makes this remodeled area practically indistinguishable from the new construction. This continuity of tasteful decor seems to "validate" the promotion theme as patients are moved into this area. Before the convalescent section was opened, there was great resistance on the part of the patient

and the physician to move into distant areas of the hospital, which were less attractive and often much noisier. One vivid example of the undesirability of moving patients into a strange, noisy, and somewhat less pleasant area was that of a woman who was admitted with markedly increased frequency of angina, and reinfarction appeared to be impending. The patient did extremely well in the acute and intermediate sections but, prior to completion of remodeling of the convalescent section, it was necessary that she be moved out of intermediate to accommodate a transfer from acute. She was transferred into an uncarpeted, noisy hall. She slept very little that first night and promptly again began to have frequent angina, necessitating transfer back to the intermediate section. She again improved and was held for the remainder of her time in the hospital in the intermediate section and has done extremely well since discharge.

It is into the convalescent area that cardiovascular patients with minimum nursing care needs can very appropriately be admitted.

We have been asked about what we do with our hypertensive patients in for study and for initiation of treatment (this category of patient was selected for discussion because these patients do not represent acutely life-threatening cardiovascular conditions). If there is space, such patients should be accommodated in a cardiovascular division because there, orders and procedures are more accurately and efficiently carried out and there is the opportunity for exposure to educational materials that would not be available on other halls.

Although emphasis in this division is on cardiovascular care, should there be excess of bed space, it would be less wasteful of cardiovascular nursing skills for non-cardiac patients to be admitted to the convalescent area than to the intermediate section. Conversely, should there be an excess of patients so that it is necessary to transfer a cardiac patient off the floor, such a transfer is less objectionable if from the convalescent section than from the acute care section or intermediate.

There is not as great a cost differential between intermediate and convalescent as there was between acute and intermediate; however, rates are a few dollars a day lower in the convalescent section. We feel that the reasonable rates in this area will encourage doctors to keep their patients in the hospital for as long a period of time as is actually beneficial, thus hopefully offsetting what I feel to be premature dismissal because of cost and lack of space considerations. There is an ongoing statistical analysis that will ultimately throw more light on these points.

THE PROGRESSIVE CARE POSTOPERATIVE SURGICAL DIVISION

From the outset of the comprehensive cardiovascular care unit planning program at St. John's, involvement by and interest from surgeons was brisk. This unexpected interest from general, thoracic, and cardiovascular surgeons emphasized the point that the modern treatment of cardiovascular disease is no longer the private domain of the internist and that especially in locations remote from university medical centers, it is time that surgeons be more broadly involved in acute and chronic heart care than has previously been customary.

A further tying together of the interests of the medical and surgical camps was a vigorous involvement of anesthesiologists, particularly in the persons of Dr. Gordon Wise and his senior associate, Dr. Oral B. Crawford. While anesthesiologists serve surgeons in the operating room and in immediate postoperative care, they also, as already shown, are crucial to the resuscitation effort in nonsurgical cases. These participants in the original program seemed to help bring medical men and surgeons into a more warmly cooperative relationship.

Benefit of this relationship was mutual. Not only did the medical men get very provocative ideas from the surgeons but the surgical participants in the program picked up the progressive care idea and applied it to creating a postoperative division, one floor beneath the CVCU.

Briefly stated, the final design situated the recovery room contiguous with the cardiovascular surgery suite, which abutted the surgical intensive care unit next to a "step-down" area for the continued care of more severely ill postoperative surgical cases (Fig. 47-19).

As might be expected, a high percentage of patients entering the new surgical division are patients who have had cardiovascular surgery (Fig. 47-20). The intensive care unit is staffed by nurses who have had the same course of instruction as received by nurses staffing the cardiovascular division. However, these are nurses who are primarily attuned to surgical problems and the type of care rendered in the surgical intensive unit should not be confused with that in the predominantly medical division.

While no valid statistical information as to frequency and success of resuscitation or, for that matter, success of surgical care in

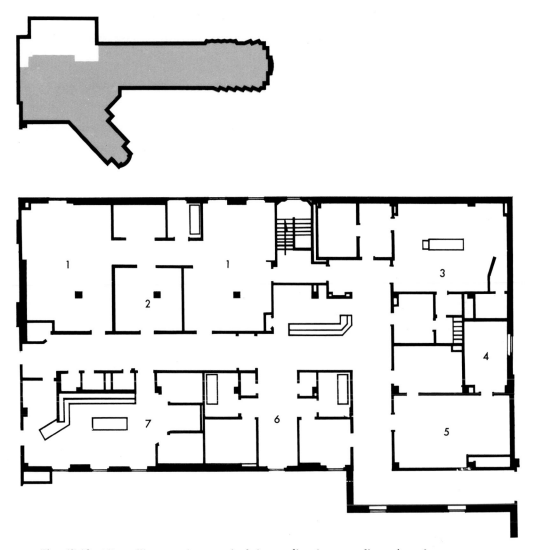

Fig. 47-19. All ancillary services required for cardiopulmonary diagnosis and treatment are provided in a laboratory only a few steps from the CVCU and on the floor immediately above the surgical intensive care section and recovery room. The numbers indicate areas reserved for *(1)* pulmonary function testing, *(2)* blood-gas determinations, *(3)* coronary and large vessel angiography, *(5)* ECG laboratory, *(6)* doctors' offices and patients' waiting rooms, and *(7)* inhalation therapy.

general, has become available, material from doctors, nurses and patients concerning the success of the new division is extremely favorable and parallels the kind of gratifying personal experiences that have been gained in the cardiovascular division. Therefore, even with no more to support this recom-

mendation than the logic of these theoretical considerations, hospitals with any opportunity to modernize or revamp the surgical areas in such manner as to provide grouping of high-risk pre- and postoperative surgical cases are urged to do so. (Figs. 47-21, *A* and *B,* and 47-22, *A* and *B*).

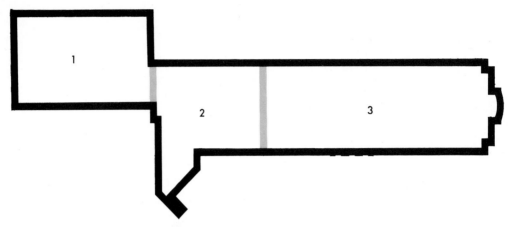

Fig. 47-20. Built on the same general principles as the CVCU, the surgical intensive care division is on the floor immediately below and is divided into three sections: operating rooms and recovery room *(1)*, intensive care section *(2)*, and beds for intermediate and convalescent care *(3)*. Operating rooms are directly below the laboratory housing all ancillary services, including facilities for angiography, ventilation therapy, and blood-gas determinations.

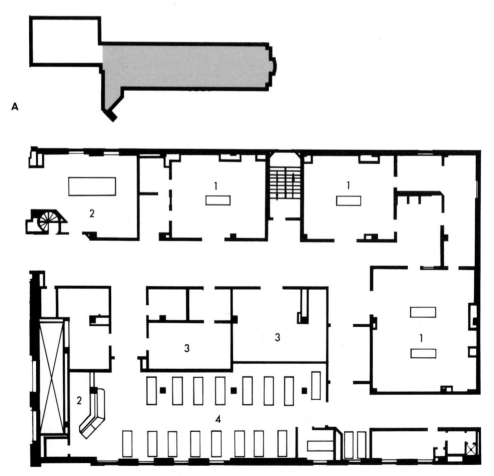

Fig. 47-21. For legend see opposite page.

It should be noted that there are certain exceptions to my recommendation that high-risk postoperative, or for that matter pre-operative, surgical patients be managed in the surgical division. These are those patients whose predominant problem is a nonsurgical cardiovascular difficulty, one in which the highest degree of skill is desirable for the survival and full recovery of the patient. Therefore, in such cases, and where the surgical nursing requirements are not major, I urge that such patients be handled pre- and postoperatively in the cardiovascular division. One recent example of such a situation, with a highly successful outcome, was a patient with a long history of ECG abnormality and episodes of acute ischemia who required cholecystectomy for severe acute cholecystitis. He was managed up to the hour of surgery in the cardiovascular acute care area. Upon transfer out of the recovery room, he was brought back to the

acute care section. There, he promptly developed paroxysms of atrial flutter and not long after, developed severe, acute myocardial ischemia. While he probably could have been managed in the surgical division, the ease with which he was handled in the cardiovascular division by full-time cardiac nurses was impressive. Surgeons who have had an opportunity to understand that their operative mortality can be reduced by this special type of handling of those patients with severe cardiovascular disease warmly welcome this approach.

THE CARDIOPULMONARY SPECIAL DIAGNOSTIC PROCEDURES UNIT

Fortuitous was the opportunity to construct this unique layout accommodating special diagnostic, as well as therapeutic, facilities in a location contiguous with the cardiovascular division. Such a section was not originally planned but several observa-

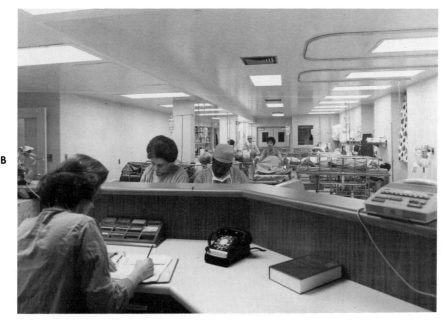

Fig. 47-21. A, Floor plan of the surgical suite shows compact arrangement of operating rooms *(1)*, nursing stations *(2)*, anesthesia section *(3)*, and recovery room *(4)*. **B,** Staff of the recovery room easily accommodate a heavy load of patients. Light, cleanliness, spaciousness, and easy availability of all required equipment—these are the dominant features of the surgical unit.

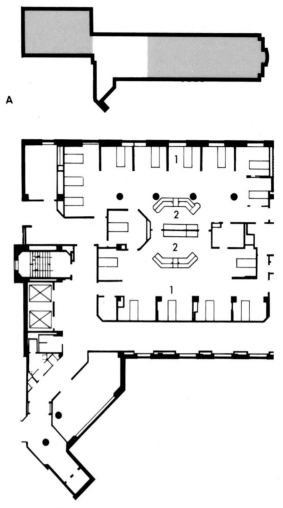

Fig. 47-22. A, Sixteen beds *(1)* and two nursing stations, situated back to back *(2),* are provided in the intensive care section of the surgical division. **B** shows central monitoring console at one of the nursing stations and the direct vision from the station to each of the patients in the section.

tions in visits to other units led to the conclusion that an ancillary services area was obligatory (Fig. 47-23).

One of the earliest stimulants to this thinking was a conference with Dr. Mason Sones, at the Cleveland Clinic, in which he expressed great interest in our proposed comprehensive cardiovascular care unit, adding his own recommendation that there be included provision whereby acute heart attack patients could be readily angiogrammed

and then, if necessary, operated on at that point. He stressed that to accomplish this would require the very closest proximity of the patient treatment area, coronary angiography unit, and the cardiovascular surgery suite. This recommendation was made even before we had decided to do coronary angiography.

Next was a conference with Dr. Tom Noto at Mercy Hospital, Miami, who stressed the necessity of the close proximity of the inhala-

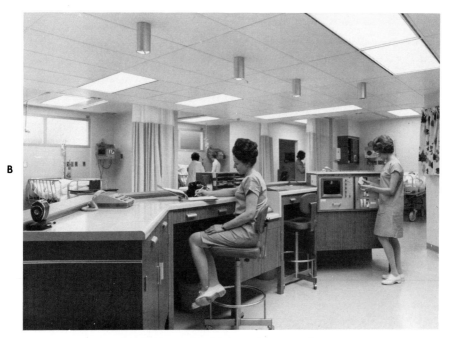

Fig. 47-22, cont'd. For legend see opposite page.

tion therapy department to the cardiovascular care unit. He added to this recommendation another to the effect that pulmonary function testing should be also adjacent. He emphasized that the greatest volume of services of these two departments was in caring for cardiac patients, who often have a ventilatory impairment component. He also recommended that the department of electrocardiography be in close proximity.

Next was the observation at Methodist Hospital, Rochester, Minnesota, that the blood-gas laboratory had been moved next door to the acute cardiac care area, being placed in what previously was a cloakroom since not much space was required.

The outcome of all this was that a block of space that had earlier been slated for a new maternity division was preempted for the newly conceived ancillary services area.

As shown on the diagram (Fig. 47-19), this area includes coronary angiography, the department of electrocardiography (with adequacy of space for central recording and computerization if deemed desirable), blood-gas laboratory, pulmonary function, inhalation therapy, stress testing, and a classroom for the teaching of inhalation therapy for Springfield and Ozarks region hospitals. The latter is very essential to the resuscitation program because conferences with smaller hospitals have consistently shown that the biggest deficiency in resuscitation programs is the lack of skilled personnel to properly ventilate the patient.

A review of revenues from the new supporting unit shows that the venture has been adequately successful financially to justify a strong recommendation to other hospitals that this kind of arrangement be duplicated, either through new construction or by remodeling. Essential to this decision is an agreement with the director of the clinical laboratories that a substation be established in proximity to the cardiovascular division for blood-gas determinations. To expedite this agreement, it can be pointed out that the greater volume of services, and therefore

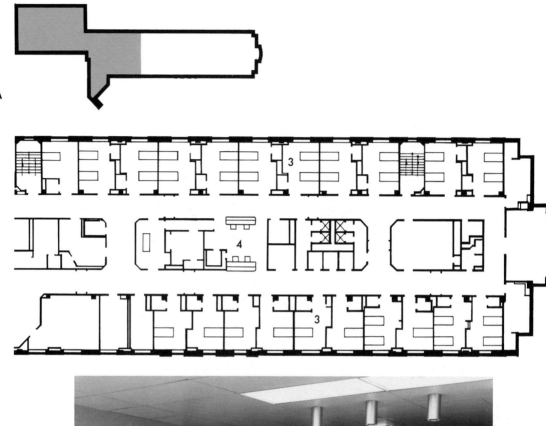

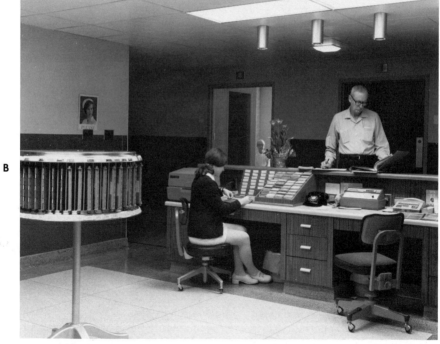

Fig. 47-23. A, The 34-bed intermediate and convalescent section of the surgical unit *(3)* is serviced from a centrally located nursing station *(4)* shown in **B** and **C. D,** Private and semi-private rooms are decorated in the same tasteful style employed in the CVCU.

the greater revenue, makes it financially feasible to appropriately staff such a unit and provide equipment.

To date, there have been about 2,000 coronary angiograms done at St. John's since the angiography unit was opened in temporary quarters in early 1970. It is felt that this valuable means of clarification of the status of patients will do much for the better defining of patient care needs as a con-

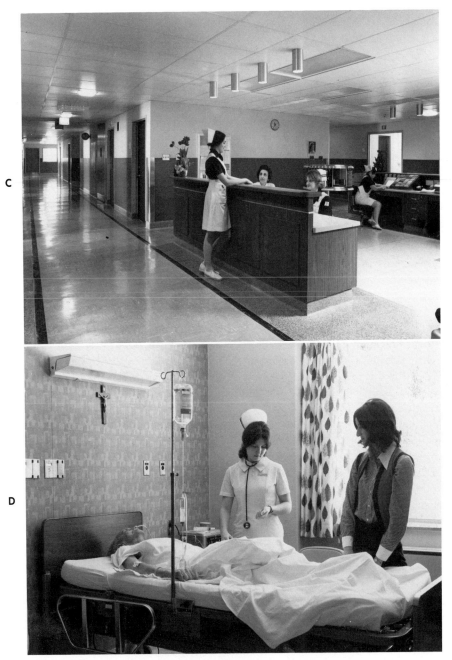

Fig. 47-23, cont'd. For legend see opposite page.

sequence of more accurate diagnosis. This improved accuracy of diagnosis in potentially life-threatening acute or chronic cardiovascular disease should, in the long run, enable us to more efficiently and more effectively channel crucial special care services to more of those in need. It is much better to enhance a resuscitation program through prevention of the need of resuscitation than to actually have to carry out resuscitation for a condition that was preventable.

It is nothing short of astounding how promptly a full resuscitation team can be assembled anywhere in the cardiovascular division with the proximity of these special services. From time to time in this presentation, the comment has been made that one has to see a feature or observe a service or circumstance in order to be fully appreciative of it, but this applies most strikingly in the case of patient resuscitation at St. John's, so enhanced through the grouping concept, not only of patients but also of all needed physical and staff resources.

The early warning signs of heart attack: public and professional education program

A vigorous educational program dealing with the early warning signs of heart attack has been conducted in southwestern Missouri since July, 1971, and is now being adopted enthusiastically in many other regions of the country. The program utilizes newspapers, radio, and television to beam serialized educational messages about the kinds of chest discomfort that presage heart attack. So far it has produced results in excess of expectations (Fig. 47-24). When these messages are repeated continuously in the mass media, both the lay public and professionals are alerted to the problem to a degree that has not previously been possible, or at least observed. Early statistics accumulated at St. John's show that the program has speeded both patient and physician responsiveness, increased the number of hospital admissions for actual or suspected heart attack, and very probably decreased cardiovascular deaths

among the more than 1,000,000 population centered in Springfield.

If instituted nationwide and continued indefinitely, there is little reason to doubt that such a program could be expected in time to produce results as exciting as those that flowed from Day's original development of the CCU. Treatment facilities must be provided, of course, but these are less than maximally effective if patients fail to get there on time. The logistics barrier now responsible for tens of thousands of deaths in the United States each year has two major components: human delay and hospital inadequacy. The CVCU can equip hospitals to provide adequate care; the EWS program can mobilize patients and physicians to act before it is too late. One can hardly doubt that if all heart attack victims were to get to a hospital within one hour after onset of symptoms, and if all hospitals were able to give them optimal treatment, the present alarming out-of-hospital death rate could be reduced by 50% or more.

But the point that must be stressed is that neither the CVCU nor EWS program will get up and walk by itself. Each must be carefully conceived, unselfishly financed, and diligently administered, not just for a few weeks or months, but indefinitely. Complacent acceptance of present heart attack mortality is no longer defensible. The fault is not in our stars but in ourselves—and can be largely corrected by ourselves.

This at least was the thinking of a group of Springfield health leaders who banded together in 1966 to take advantage of the then newly available Missouri Regional Medical Program funds. The group wanted to devise methods for reducing cardiovascular deaths throughout the Ozarks Region and agreed on a three-pronged program: first, to develop an expanded cardiovascular division that would demonstrate more fully the ideas that had proved so successful in St. John's first cardiovascular care unit; second, to enable all Springfield's hospitals to upgrade their cardiovascular service and to act as consultants and a motivating force for the remaining thirty-five hospitals in the region; and third, to institute a public and professional education program on the early warning signs of heart attack that would bring about earlier arrival of patients at the hospital.

Although the importance of the EWS program was not questioned, the group could not immediately devise a workable mechanism for carrying out such an untried and untested venture and hence did not at first ask Regional Medical Program for EWS funds. The program actually began quite fortuitously when an enterprising local reporter wrote an article synopsizing a public address in which one of the group had outlined the early warning signs. Public and professional response to this and a follow-up article on the same subject was so satisfactory that the group began to draft a series of such articles, coupled with radio and TV spot announcements, and submitted a proposal to Missouri Regional Medical Program for a 3-year saturation program. This was approved at the state level but rejected at the national level on the grounds that it might cause an adverse "panic" reaction and might overload doctors and hospitals in the region. But continued successful efforts to secure support for the idea from national health figures and from the American Heart Association led to eventual funding by the Missouri Heart Association, Missouri Regional Medical Program, and other sources.

Two weeks in advance of our proposed launch date for the program, we alerted all hospitals and physicians in the region so that they might be more responsive to what might well be an unprecedented increase in chest pain patients. Shortly before launch date, we held a dinner meeting with media representatives, doctors, nurses, hospital administrators, and the local Heart Association board and gave them a preview of all media materials we planned to use.

The program was launched on July 18, 1971, with release of eight television spot announcements, eight radio spot announcements, eight newspaper stories, wallet-purse cards bearing the EWS message, appearances on talk shows, and several interviews on radio and TV. Television and radio stations declared the EWS spots to be the most important public-service material they had ever received, and they used it heavily. These spots included four 60-second announcements emphasizing, respectively, all early warning symptoms, harmless chest-wall pain often felt by tense individuals, abdominal pain, and sweating; and four 30-second announcements dealing with arm pain, back pain, neck and jaw pain, and left chest-wall pain.

The newspaper stories, written by Springfield newspaper writer Hank Billings, ran daily and were clipped for reference by some readers. These stories, suitable for use in any area with slight modifications and chapterized for serial presentation, were accompanied by artwork, reproducible in color or in black and white, showing the locations of pain and discomfort. Similar illustrations were employed in animated form and in full color on the television spots.

These materials were prepared with due consideration for the (untested) presupposition that any public message about heart attack would have an adverse public effect. We included not only specific details of the nature and location of heart attack pain but also reassuring information about the harmless chest-wall discomfort of tense individuals. This latter information, not included in any other education program that we knew about, proved invaluable in helping reassure many patients who had erroneously feared that they were having a heart attack.

Results of the program have so far exceeded expectation. A 6-month preprogram statistical analysis of heart attack suspects admitted to the 7-bed cardiovascular intensive care unit at St. John's showed that the *average* patient-physician reaction time (time from onset of persistent symptoms until starting to the hospital) for proved heart attack

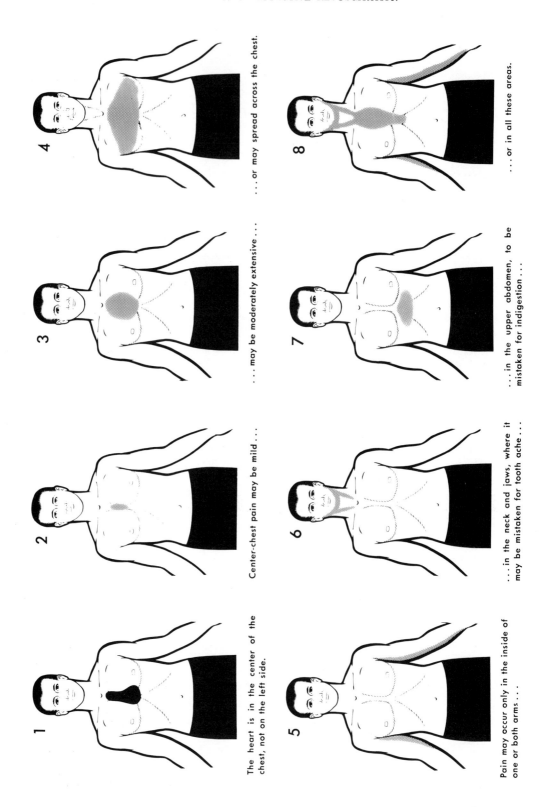

Fig. 47-24. The heart of the EWS program: diagrams of pain patterns arranged in "lessons."

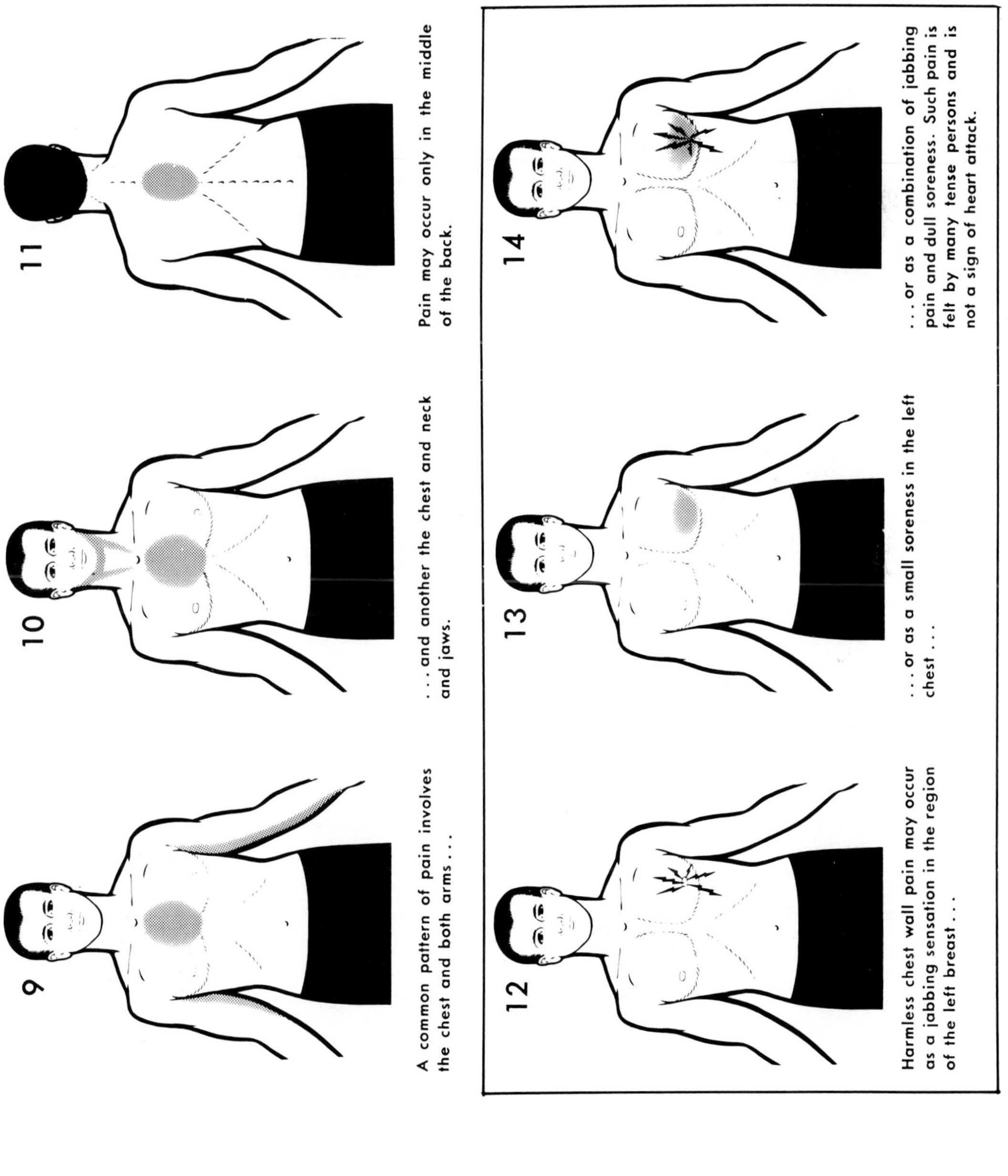

9
A common pattern of pain involves the chest and both arms . . .

10
. . . and another the chest and neck and jaws.

11
Pain may occur only in the middle of the back.

12
Harmless chest wall pain may occur as a jabbing sensation in the region of the left breast . . . .

13
. . . or as a small soreness in the left chest . . .

14
. . . or as a combination of jabbing pain and dull soreness. Such pain is felt by many tense persons and is not a sign of heart attack.

and ischemia cases was 13¾ hours, with travel time averaging 36 minutes for an average travel distance of 30 miles (*median* reaction time was 4⅗ hours). Although it was not feasible at that time to accurately determine *physician* promptness of availability and his reaction time, it was shown that those patients who contacted their physician first took over twice as long to get to the hospital as those whose initial contact was with the hospital emergency room.

A series of samplings of patient-physician reaction times following inauguration of the multimedia program yielded a good 5-month period of apparently very valid data to compare with the preprogram 6-month survey. At the time of this writing the data are still undergoing study but certain information has been derived.

Most significant is a shortening of the patient-physician reaction time from 13¾ hours average to 7⅗ hours (shortening of median time was from 4⅗ to 2¾ hours).

Total hospital admissions of heart attack and acute ischemia cases increased by approximately 20%, as determined from PAS figures. Such cases admitted to the 7-bed acute care, cardiovascular intensive unit increased by over 50%, as determined from data gathered within the unit, separate from PAS. We interpret this as an indication that the intensive focus on acute heart attack care has resulted in a greater proportion of heart attack suspects being channeled through the cardiovascular division. Of further significance is the fact that data gathered from within the unit and independently from PAS show an approximate doubling of the number of cases admitted with acute myocardial ischemia, without evidence of infarction. This is being interpreted as an indication that earlier hospital arrival is yielding more patients for treatment before actual infarction occurs.

Of great interest is the finding that, after the program was initiated, those patients who contacted their doctor first arrived after almost exactly the same time lag as in the case of those who came directly to the hospital, without physician contact. This suggests that the process of physician contact and response has been markedly shortened, the number of cases involved being large enough to be statistically significant. Probable factors in this shortening of response time in the physician-first contacts are diminished reluctance of the patient to call his doctor, the improved accessibility of the physician to the patient as a result of physicians being heavily exposed to the saturation news media program, and accelerated physician decision time. Physician-first contacts before the program were 71% of the total and, after the program, 64%. Developers of the program had felt that the news media approach would probably have a very favorable influence on physician responsiveness and it appears that this has been the case. Also, in view of the marked shortening of the reaction time in the physician-first contacts, the validity of the decision to heavily stress that patients attempt to reach their doctor first, going to the emergency room only if he is not immediately available, appears to be confirmed.

This last point is emphasized because there has been an insistence in some quarters elsewhere that the American Heart Association should delete from early warning signs messages the recommendation that the patient attempt to contact his physician first and, instead, only recommend that the patient with possible heart attack symptoms go to the hospital emergency room. To further amplify on the reasoning behind the Springfield decision to urge that the doctor be contacted first, if possible, we felt that this contact would introduce the physician's judgment in screening out obviously noncardiac chest discomfort cases, thereby helping to avoid emergency room overload and also easing the burden on doctors. It is easier for them to receive a telephone call from patients with noncardiac symptoms than it would be to leave their offices or homes and tend to the patient at the hospital. Also, this early involvement enables the doctor to give specific instructions direct to the patient or family concerning immediate care, including selection of mode of transport. Additionally, an interesting theory has evolved in Springfield, to the effect that the "Call your doctor first" instruction in the television, radio, newspaper, and other announcements may be paying off because there is less patient resistance to calling the doctor than to the possibly more stressful decision to go to the hospital. If all patients with acute, possible cardiac symptoms go to the hospital, we in Springfield feel that they could well overload the emergency room and the physician as well.

Although hospital admissions of patients with noncardiac chest discomfort did substantially increase, the number increase was less than that of proved cardiac symptom cases, but the noncardiac cases were not sufficient in number to overload the hospital.

Before the program, 55% of patients came to the hospital by car and 45% by ambulance. After the program, 58% came by car and 42% by ambulance. It should be noted that this program was and is being conducted in a predominantly rural area, with patients being derived from a 100-mile radius of Springfield. Many of the patients coming to Springfield come from farms and small communities where ambulance service is not promptly available, leading us to feel that it should be urged that emphasis be on selection of the most prompt method of transport, time being the critical element. This contention is further supported by the fact that travel time is a very small percentage of total elapsed time from onset of symptoms to arrival at the hospital. This does not, however, negate the pressing need for improved ambulance transport and the broader availability of it in rural regions as well as cities.

Responses prompted by the news media were up to 25% after the program, the highest figure being in those under age 50; there were no news media–prompted responses before the program. It is felt that "subliminal" influence resulting from news-media exposure would raise the total after the program to a considerably higher figure.

Area physician reaction, based on a poll of the over 300 doctors in the area, with good questionnaire response, was far better than anticipated, 94% indicating no overload. There was a similar good reaction from area hospital administrators, 97% indicating no overload. Public reaction was enthusiastic and widespread.

Of interest to all those who have a stake in increased heart research and programming through the Heart Fund is the fact that the 1972 Ozarks Region Heart Fund increased by 45.4% whereas the other five rural Heart Association regions in Missouri increased only 9%.

We in Springfield predict that early warning signs programs will do more to catalyze the emergence of truly adequate emergency heart care than anything that has yet happened—simply because once you create a vigorous public demand for service, something has to give. Until now, the barrier to such programs has been the presupposition that doctors and hospitals would be flooded with heart cases and unable to respond. Our follow-up study of 117 consecutive heart attack suspects demonstrates objectively for the first time that there *has* been an increase in both real and "false" heart cases, but that doctors and hospitals have been able to handle the load. We feel that an EWS program does not create "nervousness" in laymen as some have feared but simply brings in people who are already "nervous" and should have come in for diagnosis anyway. If the person does not have heart disease, we do him an incalculable service by delabeling him and correcting his erroneous "self-diagnosis." The process of delabeling can be so complex that we may have to resort to angiography; this should not be considered a wasted procedure if the result is negative, since obviously a little discomfort and some expense is preferable to a lifetime of anxiety, and that is what such patients face.

And, extremely important to those who

have devoted so much to the cause of cardiac resuscitation and emergency heart care, getting possible heart attack patients into the hospital earlier should render treatment efforts more successful, at a point in the patient's illness when resuscitation, on the one hand, is less likely to be necessary and, on the other hand, more likely to be successful if it is needed.

We urge the nationwide, intensive, and prompt utilization of community-based early warning signs programs.

Chapter 48

A HOSPITAL PLAN OF ACTION
FOR CARDIAC ARREST

There has been more than a decade of experience with external cardiac massage, artificial ventilation, closed-chest defibrillation, and the pharmacologic adjuncts available in resuscitation. It seems obvious now that the stakes are sufficiently high and the amount of available knowledge is sufficiently large for proper medical care, but this also requires a commitment by the hospital and its staff before the full potential of cardiopulmonary resuscitation can be realized and extended to all patients. Such a commitment demands an actively functioning and effective cardiac resuscitation committee supervising a day-and-night resuscitation team, a continuing in-hospital training program, and proper maintenance of all resuscitation equipment, along with a meaningful record system.

It is easy to imagine potential medical-legal problems that may result from a hospital's inability to provide an effective resuscitation program. It would seem logical that the Accreditation Committee of the Joint Committee on Hospital Accreditation would view with alarm any hospital that would fail to utilize a cardiac resuscitation program.

As a requirement for complete accreditation, most hospitals are developing their own plan of action in event of a cardiac arrest within the hospital. These plans will naturally vary considerably with the size of the hospital, the type of patient being treated, the personnel available, and the *leadership exerted*.

Each hospital interested in establishing a workable overall plan in preparation for cardiopulmonary resuscitation will have its own specific problems to consider. Obviously,

large university medical centers and hospitals with a sizable number of residents for round-the-clock staffing will have a plan somewhat different from that of a small community hospital in which there are considerable periods of time during which no physicians may be present. The equipment and physical layout of hospitals will vary considerably, as will their organizational patterns. Nevertheless, all hospitals do, of course, share common problems and common responsibilities. Each hospital, regardless of its size, staffing, physical plan, and other variations, must have at the core of its plan of action a determination and an ability to mobilize its resources in a matter of seconds. It must be able to do this on a 24-hour basis.

Cardiac arrest can no longer be regarded as an emergency confined to the operating room and its immediate environs. Sudden cardiac standstill or ventricular fibrillation will occur in other parts of the hospital. These cases may occur in such areas as the x-ray department, the admitting and receiving rooms, the emergency treatment room, the eye, ear, nose, and throat examining room, on the medical wards, in the patient's room, in the obstetric units, and especially in the recovery room, intensive care units, and coronary care units.

If cardiac resuscitation is to be successful, some of the responsibility must rest with the hospital in addition to that shouldered by the individual physician. Definite steps of a positive nature can be taken. They are as follows:

1. The hospital should assume the responsibility of seeing that all members of

its staff have been properly oriented as to the correct method of cardiac resuscitation regardless of the particular specialty with which the physician is concerned.

2. Staff conferences relating to cardiac resuscitation should be held at regular intervals. Attendance should be required.

3. If at all possible, practice sessions in the procedures of cardiac compression, electrical defibrillation of the heart, artificial respiration, and other emergencies should be available to all members of the staff. This could be carried out in the animal laboratory.

4. Proper resuscitative equipment should be readily available in various parts of the hospital. All members of the staff should be well acquainted with the use of any specialized equipment.

Hospital residents should be taken to the postmortem room and, at the autopsy table, should be given an opportunity to approach the heart in a manner suitable for use in cardiac resuscitation. Practice sessions on electrical defibrillation of the dog heart are essential. There is no better way to acquaint the house staff with the technique of cardiac resuscitation than by actual experience in the animal laboratory.

The chief of the surgical service, the anesthesia service, the hospital administrator, or other members of the hospital staff might well take the initiative in inaugurating formal periods of instruction on cardiac arrest and resuscitation for the members of the medical and surgical staff of the hospital (Fig. 48-1). In September, 1950, such a program was initiated at the New York University Post-Graduate Medical School under the direction of Dr. J. William Hinton. For those desiring a more detailed knowledge, a course in cardiac arrest and resuscitation was presented at frequent intervals during the subsequent years. A course in cardiac resuscitation was inaugurated in November, 1950, by the Cleveland Area Heart Society, which reports

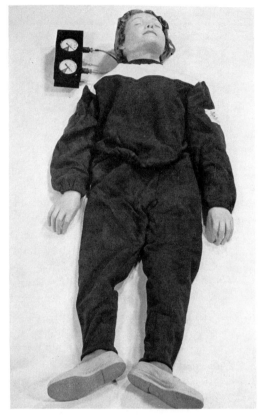

Fig. 48-1. Example of manikin useful in demonstrating mouth-to-mouth respiration and closed-chest massage technique. Lungs will not expand unless proper position of head and neck is achieved. (Courtesy Smith, Kline & French Laboratories, Philadelphia, Pa.)

gratifying experiences of the subsequent success in the management of this problem by the large number who have attended the course.

In summary, the chief measures that the hospital should take to be prepared for cardiac arrest revolve around those of creating an atmosphere of preparedness through encouraging proper instruction of all branches of the hospital, providing adequate well-kept equipment, and correcting environmental situations that would be conducive to poor resuscitative attempts. It is logical that necessary measures be carried out to protect the patient from procedures likely to produce cardiac arrest.

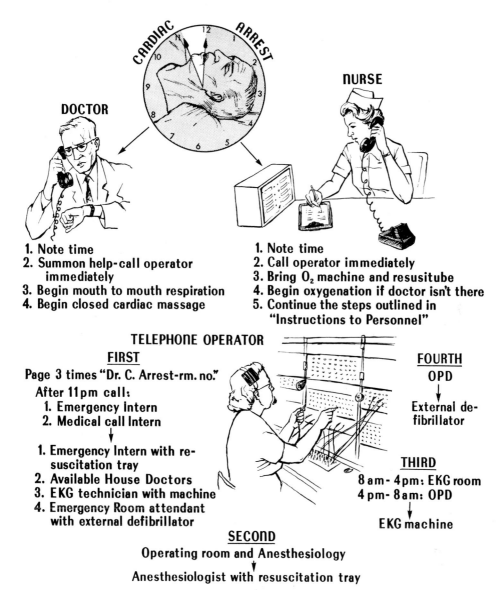

DOCTOR
1. Note time
2. Summon help-call operator immediately
3. Begin mouth to mouth respiration
4. Begin closed cardiac massage

NURSE
1. Note time
2. Call operator immediately
3. Bring O₂ machine and resusitube
4. Begin oxygenation if doctor isn't there
5. Continue the steps outlined in "Instructions to Personnel"

TELEPHONE OPERATOR

FIRST
Page 3 times "Dr. C. Arrest-rm. no."

After 11pm call:
1. Emergency Intern
2. Medical call Intern

1. Emergency Intern with re-suscitation tray
2. Available House Doctors
3. EKG technician with machine
4. Emergency Room attendant with external defibrillator

FOURTH
OPD
External de-fibrillator

THIRD
8 am - 4pm: EKG room
4 pm - 8am: OPD
EKG machine

SECOND
Operating room and Anesthesiology
Anesthesiologist with resuscitation tray

Fig. 48-2. Plan of operation in cardiac arrest. (Based on procedure used in Latter Day Saints Hospital, Salt Lake City, Utah; courtesy J. Johnson; from Ritchie, M. N.: A nurse's responsibility in cardiac arrest, New York, 1962, American Nurses' Association, Inc.)

A plea to the subprofessional corpsmen and technicians of the armed forces has been made by Allen, relative to their duties in the event of cardiac arrest. Much of what he says has equal application to all operating room technicians in addition to the surgeon, anesthetist, or nurse. He stresses that all of the operating personnel should, of course,

make sure they know where the cardiac arrest equipment is being kept and that they should make efforts to have it immediately available. Allen appropriately urges that all concerned become familiar with the problems of resuscitation so that they may contribute to the team effort.

Fig. 48-2 illustrates a workable plan of

operation for hospitals to use in care of patients with cardiac arrest. Many varied plans are in use in hospitals. The previously mentioned plan has many desirable features.

As an example of a concerted effort to prepare for cardiopulmonary resuscitation, the 217-bed Community Hospital at Glen Cove, New York, has made it mandatory for all the attending and courtesy staff to take part in the cardiopulmonary program. Each member is required by a medical board ruling to demonstrate closed-chest massage on manikins under the direction of a special cardiopulmonary resuscitation committee.

In the treatment plan for every case of cardiopulmonary resuscitation within the hospital, it would seem wise to include a surgeon experienced in open-chest massage, should efforts at closed-chest compression be unsuccessful.

The magnitude of an effective hospital training program for resuscitation is reflected in the experience of the Toronto General Hospital where over 1,300 persons are trained annually. These include hospital assistants, nursing assistants, ward helpers, physical and occupational therapists, x-ray and laboratory technicians, and dieticians.

The day-to-day review of resuscitation efforts within the hospital will inevitably upgrade the technical aspects of resuscitation, will spot areas of weakness in communication and equipment needs, and areas that need further emphasis in the training program.

The dividends from an active cardiac resuscitation program in a teaching or community hospital will soon be apparent. Such is the case at DeKalb General Hospital in Georgia where an 18% discharged-alive rate in 104 cardiac arrest cases is reported. A key aspect in their repeated 6- to 9-month resuscitation courses involved the training of coronary care nurses.

New Zealand has had a Standing Committee on Resuscitation since 1952. It is now called the Advisory Committee on Resuscitation and coordinates the teaching of resuscitation techniques in New Zealand. Its members are nominated from the Departments of Health, Defense, Education, and Electricity, the Society of Anesthetists, the New Zealand Surf Life Saving Association, the New Zealand Branch of the Royal Life Saving Society, and the New Zealand Red Cross Society.

Cardiac resuscitation committee

The resuscitation committee should be set up as a permanent hospital committee. It should meet regularly and with a degree of frequency sufficient to consider all resuscitation attempts, analyze deficiencies, and make suggestions for their correction. It should actively supervise the resuscitation team. The resuscitation team composition will vary with the type of hospital being served. Most often, the medical resident or fellow on cardiology, a surgical resident, an inhalation therapist, and an anesthesiologist will be immediately available. It is the responsibility of the cardiac resuscitation committee to see that a continuing program of resuscitation instruction is being provided to hospital personnel. The rapid turnover of personnel as well as the well-documented need for frequent retraining makes it essential that the cardiac resuscitation committee assume this responsibility.

The composition of the cardiac resuscitation committee will vary depending upon the special interests of individual participants. Generally speaking, however, it should consist of senior members of the departments of medicine, cardiology, surgery, anesthesiology, inhalation therapy, and nursing.

Regardless of the location of the arrest and the personnel involved, adequate data should be made available to the committee in each instance. An effective cardiac resuscitation committee will have the cooperation of all nursing units and physicians and a brief report on each resuscitation effort will be an automatic function of the resuscitation team or of the specialized unit. Cross-checks with records kept by the telephone operator and with data available in morbidity and mortality conferences may locate an occasional stray case. As the efforts of the committee become more sophisticated, records may be maintained on a computerized data-retrieval system to facilitate periodic evaluations.

It is particularly desirable that an office be specifically designated and devoted to the effort of the cardiac resuscitation committee. In some hospitals this will justify the employment of a full-time secretary to maintain the records of all resuscitation events and to collect data for the committee. The secretary will obtain information relating to the eventual discharge of the patient and long-term follow-up of the patient and will work closely with the medical record department. Additional time by the secretary should be spent in maintaining an effective medical library on resuscitation references, specifically catalogued to allow for their most effective use by anyone desiring specific information. Books and monographs on cardiac arrest and related subjects should be available.

Within this office should be kept all cardiac resuscitation teaching slides, training films, manikins, and other teaching devices. It is the responsibility of the secretary to see that they are maintained in proper working order and that they are returned promptly when checked out to various groups. As an employee of the cardiac resuscitation committee, she should maintain records of instruction given to hospital personnel and it will be her responsibility to schedule retraining sessions at periodic intervals.

Cardiac arrest team

We hear a great deal these days about the "delivery of health care." Prompt and effective cardiopulmonary resuscitation is certainly an appropriate place for a hospital to begin this delivery.

Since adequate personnel and sophisticated equipment are almost always present, the need to summon a resuscitation team is seldom encountered in the operating room, coronary care unit, intensive care units, or cardiac catheterization laboratory. Nor should it be necessary in a fully staffed and equipped emergency room.

How many cardiac arrests will the average 300- to 400-bed hospital encounter each year? Obviously the patient-mix will determine, to some extent, this figure. A preponderance of older individuals subject to myocardial infarction will influence the number of emergency resuscitation efforts. It does seem likely, however, that the average 300-bed hospital is either not attempting resuscitation in a significant number of instances or is not locating and reporting such cases if there are fewer than 75 to 100 cardiopulmonary resuscitation efforts each year. These should include cases occurring in the operating room, coronary care units, emergency room, cardiac laboratory, and in the general medical and surgical wards.

In our own hospital we maintain a monthly schedule showing the daily assignments of each member of the resuscitation team. It is the responsibility of each team member to remain in the hospital at all times when he is on call, and he should not be tied up in an operating room or otherwise unavailable for emergency duty. Periodically, drills are conducted to determine the efficiency and promptness of the team's ability to respond to a resuscitation call.

Since it is often the most junior member of the house staff who gets night duty, it is particularly essential that the cardiac resuscitation team feel confident that each member of the house staff or attending staff, regardless of how junior, be well versed in all aspects of resuscitation.

Most importantly, the cardiac resuscitation team must have the full support of the administrative structure of the institution or hospital with enough delegated responsibility to carry out the task. The team's budgetary needs should receive high priority.

In addition to those listed as members of the cardiac resuscitation team there should also be included the head nurse of the floor where the cardiac arrest occurs and, in many instances, the electrocardiogram technician.

If prompt artificial ventilation and closed chest massage have not already been instituted by the time the resuscitation team arrives then there is obvious deficiency in the system.

Evaluation

The sooner a critique session is held after a cardiac arrest the more significance it will probably have. Technical errors will more likely be spotted, suggestions will be more pertinent, and the overall benefit to the house staff, nursing staff, and attending staff will be increased.

Examination for cardiopulmonary resuscitation proficiency

Standardized examination for determining the competency of an individual performing cardiopulmonary resuscitation is difficult since so much of the proficiency is dependent upon one's technical ability. Nevertheless, hospital personnel who are involved with high-risk patients and those who have been instructed in cardiopulmonary resuscitation should be given both a written and an oral examination. This should cover basic anatomy and physiology, pulmonary resuscitation, including various measures of expired air ventilation and maintenance of an open airway, all aspects of cardiac massage, and, in addition, the pharmacology of resuscitation. One should demonstrate an ability to diagnose the various significant arrhythmias as well as a knowledge of the purpose and function of specialized equipment.

Communications

The matter of *communication* deserves particular attention and emphasis. Doctors and hospital personnel may be notified by a variety of means, including the telephone, public address paging system, pocket page system, or visual paging system. In areas of the hospital covered by a single nurse, this nurse is diverted from her role of initial resuscitative efforts while she notifies the switchboard. A single telephone operator frequently must notify individual house staff members in numerous on-call rooms; during this period, the switchboard is diverted from other functions. Nobel notes a human error of about 8% in the reporting of the proper room location of the stricken patient.

In describing an ideal emergency alert system, Nobel urges that the emergency dialing code for resuscitation alerts should consist of multiples of the digits 1 or 2. This results in a rapid dialing sequence and a low number of dialing errors.

In the telephone equipment room, the dial-switching equipment immediately connects the initiating telephone to an announcement machine and activates a distinct tone at the telephone switchboard. The alert initiator, after hearing a tic tape tone, gives the standard message and the patient location— "code blue" and the appropriate room number—replaces the telephone hand set and then immediately returns to support the patient. This has been timed to require only 4 to 6 seconds instead of perhaps a minute.

Various code calls have been used in hospitals to announce a cardiac arrest. Included among the code calls are: "Calling Dr. C. Arrest," "Dr. Haste," "Dr. Blue," "code 10," "code blue," "CRT" (cardiac resuscitation team), and "code 99." In the usual instance, the location of the appropriate nursing station or of the patient's room is announced.

After the initial emergency alert is given, automatic mobilization of personnel is accomplished when the dial-switching equipment activates a paging alert override circuit that stops normal public address paging. The recorded alerting code and room number are then repeatedly broadcast over the paging system.

Certain vital hospital telephones, which have been previously designated, are automatically and simultaneously activated by the dial-switching equipment and intermittently ring for 15 to 30 seconds with a distinctive pattern. When the hand set is lifted, the recorded alert message is heard. If that particular telephone is in use, the dial-switching equipment transmits a tone to indicate that a high priority call is waiting. Nobel suggests the inclusion of such high priority telephones in the anesthesia department, the anesthesia on-call room, the emergency room, the physicians' on-call room, the heart station, the intensive care unit, the interns' quarters, and certain other on-call rooms or physicians' offices. In addition, it would seem wise to include, in some hospitals, the inhalation therapy offices, certain conference rooms where physicians are likely to be, and certain outpatient facilities. This, of course, will vary from hospital to hospital. In hospitals where pocket radio page systems are in use, the dial-switching equipment automatically activates the transmitter.

In another method to permit more efficient utilization of personnel responding to "stat" paging from the telepage system, a special announcement is used over the loud speaker system to signify the specific emergency condition of cardiac arrest. Since time and speed are of the utmost importance, the operator announces the code for cardiac arrest and the number of the room where the arrest has occurred over the telepage system; for example, "code blue—West 516." Such a paging system alerts such various members of the medical staff as inhalation therapists, nursing personnel, and ECG technicians. Obviously, in hospitals that have a visual paging system, a number signifying cardiac arrest is flashed and held until the operator has been notified that adequate aid has arrived.

The hospital administration must be responsible for a workable system of emergency alert. With increasing sophistication of telephone equipment, a variety of possibilities is provided. Since time continues to be the key factor in all successful resuscitations, any hospital-prepared plan of action is doomed at the onset unless an almost instantaneous alert system is provided.

In many hospitals a major roadblock in successfully mobilizing personnel and equipment for resuscitation is the inability of the elevator system to function in an effective fashion. Depending on the type and number of elevators, several methods of solving this problem are available. Nobel, in his excellent discussion of the hospital emergency command system, explains automatic control of elevators. The dial-switching equipment si-

multaneously activates a locking-relay that interrupts an electrical current normally continuously transmitted via two circuits to both the automatic elevator controller and the emergency cart storage location. This signal to the elevator automatically overrides the standard controller and sends the elevator to the floor where the emergency equipment cart is located. The elevator controller automatically chooses the most appropriate elevator, depending on the location of the other elevators.

The Emergency Care Research Institute of Philadelphia has developed what is termed the "hospital emergency command system." Its goal is to quickly and simultaneously mobilize personnel, equipment, and elevators during clinical emergencies by utilizing existing telephone equipment, paging systems, and elevators. The system allows anyone to initiate an emergency call by dialing the proper code on any telephone in the hospital. This automatically activates a recorder, which simultaneously is connected to telephones in key areas of the hospital. The hospital public address and radio pocket page systems also automatically broadcast the recorded message. The system allows for automatic control of the elevators: one car automatically travels to the floor where the emergency equipment is stored and a second car transports personnel by responding to a special set of coded call buttons that are functional only for the 3 minutes following initiation of the alert.

A variety of methods can be used for notifying the telephone operator in the event of an arrest. We have found that the most dependable system utilizes a transistorized radio contact with each member of the team.

Care of equipment

In order to avoid the problem of nonfunctioning resuscitation equipment, outdated drugs, and inadequacy of vital pieces of equipment, the central service department may provide the necessary coordination. An active role has been assumed by central ser-

Time	Blood pressure mm/Hg	Heart rate per min	Levarterenol bitartrate	Metaraminol bitartrate	Epinephrine 1:10,000	Isoproterenol hydrochloride	Calcium chloride 10 cc of 10% solution/vial	Sodium bicarbonate 44.6 mEq/ampule	Procainamide hydrochloride	Lidocaine hydrochloride	Lanatoside C	Electrical cardioversion	Others	Comments
9 30	0	0												Airway inserted. Bag breathed, external cardiac massage. Pupils dilated.
31	0	0	4 cc in 500 cc 5% D/W		5 cc									Asystole. Venous catheter inserted, right arm.
32	0	0										100 watt-sec		Ventricular fibrillation.
33	70/50	120	2 cc/min							50 mg				NSR with numerous VPCs. Spontaneous respirations. Pupils constricted.
36	90/60	100												Awakening. Color good. NSR with occasional VPC.
38	0	0						1 amp						Respirations stopped. Cyanotic. 20-second seizure. Pupils dilating. Resuscitation started.
39	0	0							1,000 mg in 500 cc 5% D/W			100-watt sec		Ventricular fibrillation.
40	80/50	100	1 cc/min											NSR, spontaneous respirations. Pupils constricted.
44	100/70	100							2 cc/min					Strong radial pulses. Color good. Rare VPC.
50	108/75	100	stop											Awake. Moving well. Sweating. NSR.

Simple flow chart for recording pertinent observations and drug therapy during cardiac arrest (an illustrative case situation). D/W = dextrose in water, NSR = normal sinus rhythm, and VPC = ventricular premature contraction.

Fig. 48-3. Example of flow chart, which provides simple, readily accessible, and accurate commentary of medical management and patient response in cardiac arrest. This type of chart is of particular value for postresuscitation studies. (From Duke, M.: J.A.M.A. 202:143, 1967.)

vice in the 1,350-bed Jackson Memorial Hospital in Miami. It is responsible for the complete and standardized resuscitation set-ups rotated on seventy-five separate units of the hospital. Kelley and Mason estimate that this equipment is utilized approximately 600 times per year. Central service also assumes the responsibility for cleaning, replacing, and checking the equipment. Used equipment is returned to central service with a tray voucher after each emergency and a clean, sterile setup is immediately issued to replace the used equipment. Defibrillator paddles and patient electrodes are conscientiously cleaned. The monitor-defibrillator units are checked twice a week by a specially trained central service technician who goes to each area in which a unit is located. Each machine is plugged into a standard electrical outlet, turned on, and the patient leads connected to a heart simulator to test its effectiveness.

Record keeping

So far there has not been a generally accepted cardiac arrest report form. Part of the reason for this stems from the wide variations in the many aspects of each case. Obviously, each record form should have basic identifying data, information of the events leading to the arrest, and underlying pathology of a possible contributory nature. How was the arrest diagnosed and under what conditions? What were the initial resuscitation efforts and how soon after the arrest were they employed? What type of ventilation and cardiac massage was given? Particularly difficult is an accurate progress report on drugs given, at what time, and in what dosage.

For the arrest form to be meaningful, it should supply concise and complete data. It must be reasonably easy to fill out.

It is imperative that each hospital maintain a cardiac arrest data sheet in order to record systematically all events taking place prior to, during, and after resuscitation.

Any physician who has concerned himself with the collection and study of clinical cardiac arrest and resuscitation data is aware of the difficulties in evaluating data from the charts of these patients. A comprehensive picture of the sequence of events is seldom available. Subsequently, many of such studies can only approximate any satisfactory degree of accuracy.

Duke has suggested a simple flow chart (Fig. 48-3) that provides a continuous record of events as they occur and that allows simplicity of recording and ease of review. Each patient chart in a coronary care unit is provided with such a chart.

Data sheets on cardiac arrest should be reviewed each month by the cardiopulmonary resuscitation committee of the hospital. At this time, any obvious shortcomings or deficiencies in the program should be noted, and steps should be taken toward their correction.

Chapter 49

RESUSCITATION BY THE NURSE

Nowhere has the emerging pattern of increased responsibility in nursing practice been more dramatic than that now occurring in the coronary care unit. The expanding scope of nursing practice witnessed within the last several years is a strong testimony to the desirability that the nurse serve not only as a skilled observer but also as one prepared to make key judgments, decisions, and take action of a lifesaving nature. The highly trained and confident nurse practitioner of a coronary care and intensive care unit is due much of the credit for one of the major breakthroughs in emergency-care medicine. This degree of increased precision in nursing observation has its effect throughout the hospital. Lessons learned from the highly skilled and technically knowledgeable coronary care unit diffuse throughout other nursing units to further enhance the skills with which all patients can be observed.

The nurse today is a more vital member of the medical team than at any point in history. Developments in intensive care, in coronary care, and other areas of patient care have moved the nurses to a crucial position where, more than at any time in the past, their efforts may be of a lifesaving nature. This is particularly exemplified in the immediate handling of certain "malignant" arrhythmias, the immediate defibrillation of the patient, or the artificial maintenance of the cardiorespiratory system until the physician arrives.

It is estimated that the majority of all cardiac arrests are first suspected and diagnosed by the nurse. It is becoming increasingly evident that the nurse's initial efforts are extremely meaningful in determining the eventual successful resuscitation of the patient.

The degree to which nurses have become involved in resuscitative techniques and procedures varies considerably from hospital to hospital. How vocal have the state Nurses' Associations and state Medical Associations been in defining the role and responsibility of the nurse in cardiopulmonary crises? How much training have the registered nurses been given and how much supervised practice is provided? Is there a written statement of policy regarding the conditions under which lifesaving measures may be performed by registered nurses? How well defined is the preparation and training necessary for registered nurses who perform lifesaving measures?

Three hundred eighty-five nurses from 152 hospitals were involved in a survey in England on the nurses' responsibility in resuscitation. Resuscitation had been needed by 1,001 patients in 302 different wards. Most interestingly, twelve visitors to wards had required resuscitation as well as had one member of the staff. Twenty patients in a male medical ward required resuscitation within a year. In a majority of instances, resuscitation was initiated by the nurse, although in some instances it was a student nurse. Others who were involved in the initial effort, other than doctors, included cardiology technicians, nursing auxiliaries, ward orderlies, dental assistants, and ambulance drivers. The survey also brought to light the fact that the presence of a cardiac resuscitation team is not necessarily known to all members of a hospital nursing staff.

A significant opinion was frequently voiced that hospital policies regarding resuscitation have not been well defined. Many nurses are hopeful that better guidance can be given as to what patients should *not* be resuscitated. Some hospitals are stated to have an upper age limit above which patients are not to be resuscitated (varying between 60 and 70 years of age). It should be pointed out, however, that age has not been a major determining factor in the success of resuscitation.

The survey generally reported an agreement on a satisfactory level of instruction that had been provided. Others in the hospital who had been offered cardiopulmonary instruction included physiotherapists, radiotherapists, ward orderlies, x-ray technicians, EEG technicians, medical students, clerks, and various nursing auxiliaries.

In the second edition of this book (1964) it is stated: "With expanding application of cardiac resuscitative techniques including the closed-chest resuscitative approach, it is inevitable that other members of the health team, particularly nurses, will be concerned with the general problems of resuscitation of patients with cardiac arrest."

Events have moved rapidly in this direction during the last 10 years. Of particular significance was the action taken by the American Medical Association at its annual clinical session in Houston, Texas, on November 26 to 29, 1967. First introduced by the Nevada delegation, the House of Delegates of the American Medical Association approved a resolution *recognizing the importance of utilizing properly trained, competent, registered nurses to institute lifesaving measures in the hospital setting when a physician is not immediately available during coronary emergencies.*

The American Medical Association's House of Delegates realized the importance of minimizing resultant legal risks for the hospital, the medical staff, and the nurses by drafting procedures or guidelines of assistance to the hospital medical staff. Their resolution is as follows:

Resolved, That with the intent of promoting good patient care, the American Medical Association recognizes the propriety of registered nurses using monitoring, defibrillation, and resuscitative equipment, and instituting immediate lifesaving corrective measures, if a licensed physician is not immediately available to do so, providing that:

1. The techniques to be used by a registered nurse in a hospital setting shall have been specified for the hospital by the medical staff on the basis of counsel by a committee representing authoritative medical and nursing opinion; and that
2. The registered nurse has been competently instructed in the techniques to be used; and that
3. The registered nurse performs the authorized procedures upon: (a) the direct order of a doctor of medicine, or (b) pursuant to standing procedures established by the medical staff, these procedures to include for immediate summoning of a physician and such other personnel as may be needed.

Mrs. Mignon N. Ritchie summarized this problem at an annual meeting of the American Nurses' Association.

The nurse's early recognition of the arrest and her immediate action in summoning help and making the emergency equipment readily available may make the difference between life and death for the patient. The development of the technique for cardiac arrest resuscitation requires the nurse to be an effective assistant to the physician who is employing artificial ventilation and circulation.*

Formerly, in May, 1962, three organizations—the California Medical Association, the California Hospital Association, and the California Nurses' Association—issued a joint statement for qualification of their position with regard to closed-chest cardiac resuscitation and the nurse.

A nurse making the judgmental decisions when a physician was available to make them would be running the risk of violating the medical practice act, even if she was thoroughly familiar with the physical aspects of the technique. Such decisions are a part of "diagnosis and prescribed treatment" the essence of medical practice. Her choosing closed-chest cardiac massage in such circumstances might well be termed unreasonable.

If a physician was not available and would not be available before significant brain damage occurred, the emergency exception in medical practice acts would protect the nurse who had been

---

*American Nurses' Association, Detroit, 1962.

taught closed-chest cardiac massage. However, until the technique has gained broad recognition as a standard procedure in cases of cardiac arrest of the type confronting the nurse, the potential for liability for negligence in choosing to use the technique would exist. Surmounting the medical problem does not do away with the negligence problem.

Consider the situation of the nurse who has only a vague familiarity with closed-chest cardiac massage. Would it be reasonable for such a nurse, under almost any circumstances, to attempt it? The medical practice issue is clearly present if a physician is available to make the decision about closed-chest massage and either perform it himself or closely direct its performance. Aside from this, there is a great danger of liability for negligence arising out of performing a technique with which one is not familiar.*

By October, 1968, six state nurses' associations had adopted a policy concerning the role of the nurse in performing cardiac defibrillation. The Massachusetts Nurses' Association's policy statement states:

Defibrillation should always be performed within the framework of designated preparation and practice of the nurse established for the hospital or agency by a committee composed of representatives for the medical staff, department of nursing and the administration. This framework of preparation and practice is to be reproduced in writing and made available to every member of the medical and nursing staffs.

One thing seems clear: the medical and nursing staff must work together in each hospital to develop a practical plan of operation in case cardiac resuscitation is needed. It should be a well-defined plan of action with responsibility specifically designated, it should be a well-rehearsed plan of action, and it should be a realistic and practical plan to fit the needs of that particular institution.

The placement and maintenance of resuscitation equipment is often a responsibility assumed by the nursing service. This implies that the equipment is checked regularly, that all components of the equipment are intact, and that it is in functioning condition. The

suggested equipment for resuscitation units is described elsewhere in this book.

A well-developed "plan of operation" for cardiac resuscitation has been developed by the Latter Day Saints Hospital in Salt Lake City, Utah. The nurses have been instructed as follows:

The success or failure of attempts at resuscitation on your division will depend largely on you, how well you understand the problem, how well you have organized your equipment and your employees to meet the emergency. Since time is of the utmost importance, it will be your responsibility frequently to diagnose cardiac arrest and call the operator. Unless you know that the patient's prognosis does not warrant resuscitative attempts, resuscitation should be attempted on any patient who dies unexpectedly. Within five minutes, a doctor familiar with the patient's care will either be present or can be located to decide whether resuscitation should be continued.*

At several hospitals, it is the practice to signify by means of a red star or some other identfying mark on the chart and on the bedside if the patient's personal physician does not believe that the patient's underlying pathology warrants a resuscitative effort, should cardiac arrest occur. Since a physician other than the patient's personal physician will often be the only doctor available at the time the arrest occurs, it is helpful to be forewarned about factors that may influence resuscitative techniques.

Responsibilities of the nurse in charge of a patient at the time of cardiac arrest include careful observation and subsequent recording of the time of onset of the arrest and either calling the telephone operator or seeing that the operator is immediately notified so that the plan of operation of the hospital may be immediately put into action. Pulmonary resuscitative equipment, including the resuscitube, should be brought to the patient's bedside. If the doctor has not yet arrived, mouth-to-mouth respiration should

---

*Calif. Med. Assoc. Bull., May 23, 1962.

*Joyce Johnson, M.D., Director, Outpatient Department, Latter Day Saints Hospital, Salt Lake City, Utah (personal communication).

be instituted immediately after clearance of the airway has been established, the head hyperextended, and the patient's nose closed. Numerous things can be done to assist the physician employing resuscitation, such as a frequent check of the peripheral pulses. The pupils should be observed to note their relative dilation.

Since the crux of all resuscitative efforts in cardiac arrest centers around the *time factor,* it is obvious that the responsibility and the role of the nurse in cardiac resuscitation can be a major one. The immediate judgment of the nurse may be crucial to the outcome of resuscitative efforts. It is unlikely that the percent of successful resuscitation accomplished outside the operating room will be high unless the nursing service is knowledgeable and effective. Nurses must be particularly oriented to the concept that cardiac resuscitation is essentially a 3- to 4-minute emergency and that there will be few successful resuscitative efforts if this time limit is exceeded.

Although inadequately applied closed-chest resuscitation has resulted in many adverse effects and complications (liver lacerations, ruptured large vessels, multiple rib fractures, and traumatized lungs), few, if any, untoward effects will result from artificial ventilation of an apneic patient. Mouth-to-mouth respiration, in such an instance, should be started immediately. In an occasional case, this alone may serve to resuscitate the patient. Already, however, nurses are initiating closed-chest resuscitation in coronary care units throughout the country.

Both mouth-to-nose and mouth-to-mouth respiration should be taught to nurses, since some will find it easier to apply mouth-to-nose respiration. The details of artificial respiration have been outlined elsewhere in this book. Mention should be made that pressure over the epigastrium may be indicated when overdistension of the stomach has occurred from hyperventilation. An additional effort, which can be extended by the nurse in the first phase of resuscitation outside the operat-

ing room, is placement of the patient upon a firm surface so that some resistance may be afforded when downward compression of the anterior chest wall and sternum is applied to the myocardium.

From many standpoints it is inappropriate to suggest a special area of knowledge requirement for the nurse as contained in a single chapter. A large number of nurses have gone far beyond in developing a new degree of competency and confidence in understanding and applying their contribution to the prevention and treatment of cardiac arrest. Their ability to start intravenous fluids, initiate respirations, secure and interpret electrocardiographic information and apply other emergency equipment may in some instances outstrip the physician's. Such nurses will find much of this book relevant to their interests.

The recent practice of placing the coronary care unit nurse in a position of responsibility to initiate electric countershock as well as to use a variety of antiarrhythmic drugs is most significant. In some institutions, approximately half of the defibrillations are carried out by the nursing staff.

Because of the nurse's responsible role and increasingly accurate monitoring and interpretation of responses of the patient, many coronary care units include the nurse's observations and recording of significant events as an integral part of the medical progress notes. The nurse's observations from oscultation of the heart and lungs, observations of signs of venous distension, and calculations of urinary output changes and patterns of fluid balance and psychologic response are extremely relevant to the patient's clinical course.

At the time of the publication of the last edition of this book, only a limited number of states gave the nursing profession encouragement to initiate electrical ventricular defibrillation. Today, just a short while later, sophisticated training experiences for nurses in arrhythmia recognition, pacing, defibrillation techniques, and preventive drug therapy have been instituted to create an amazingly effective first echelon of assault against one of the great killers of the day. Many of these training courses are cooperative efforts by groups or institutions or by other resources in the area such as Regional Medical Programs. The American Heart Association is one of the many groups that sponsors programs. Certainly the nursing profession can be extremely proud of the manner in which it has accepted the challenge and responsibility.

Inhalation therapists

In some hospitals, resuscitation procedures are delegated to well-trained inhalation therapists, since physicians are often unavailable within the time demanded. The inhalation therapists represent a logical group, as they are already competent in dealing with emergency ventilatory assistance. In some hospitals, a continuous educational program in resuscitation is conducted under the department of inhalation therapy.

Chapter 50

MOBILE CARDIAC RESUSCITATION CART

The need for a mobile cardiac resuscitation unit has been dramatically demonstrated many times. On one occasion, even though cardiac arrest occurred in one of the main operating rooms of a large teaching hospital, resuscitation was hindered greatly by complete absence of any prepared plan on the part of the physicians present and an almost total lack of necessary equipment. On another occasion, cardiac arrest occurred in the anesthesia induction room, and a cardiac consultant was called before it was considered necessary to open the chest. The stethoscope was passed around among a number of the physicians present. Subsequently, it was decided that a mobile unit should be constructed containing all of the conceivably necessary equipment and that it should be available at a minute's notice. In addition, its presence in the operating room or on the wards would serve as a constant reminder to the physician of the possible danger of sudden cardiac arrest and of the necessity to have an effective, readily applicable plan of action.

Our first mobile cardiac resuscitation unit was built by A. S. Aloe Company and was given to Barnes Hospital, St. Louis (1949); several months later, a more complete model was constructed (Fig. 50-1). The mobile cardiac resuscitation unit employed in Bellevue Hospital has been used many times on the wards, in the operating room, in the admitting and emergency rooms, during angiocardiographic studies, in the x-ray department, and elsewhere. It is complete with all necessary cardiopulmonary resuscitative tools. There is a positive-negative pressure pulmonary resuscitator that can be adjusted for alveolar pressures suitable in both infants

and adults. The rate of respiratory exchange is easily adjusted, and, following return of spontaneous respirations, the unit may be placed on "assisting respirations." Two oxygen tanks are attached, one serving as an auxiliary unit. The concentration of oxygen can be adjusted, but 100% oxygen is almost universally used. A tracheal suction apparatus, which can allow low pressure both in and out of the bottle, is also present. If an obstruction occurs in the patient's airway, a clicking sound will be heard, indicating that an obstruction exists. The airway can be attached to either a face mask or an endotracheal tube.

All necessary instruments, consisting principally of two scalpels, two pairs of scissors, several clamps, and some hemostats, are kept in a sterile instrument tray on the top of the machine. Interval time clocks are attached to the panel; as soon as cardiac arrest is diagnosed, the knob under each clock is turned to its maximal distance. One clock rings at the end of 3 minutes, whereas the others ring after 2 minutes have elapsed. Each signals a warning that so much time has passed and that the period of irreversibility is near at hand unless artificial maintenance of the circulation has been established. On one end of the machine, an electrical defibrillation unit is installed. The current and voltage can be regulated by hand and can be checked easily on the voltmeter and ammeter. Both a foot switch and a hand switch are available for control of the duration of current flow. The electrodes are plugged into the machine, and the faces of the electrodes are then ready to be applied to the myocardium. Three sets of electrodes are included for adaptability to size and

601

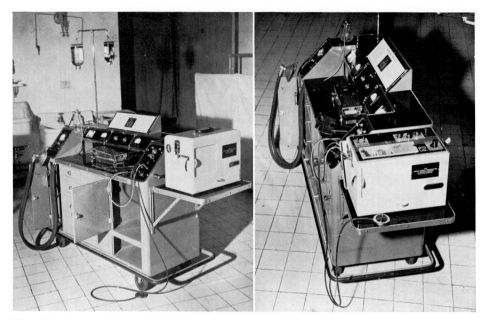

Fig. 50-1. First mobile cardiac resuscitation unit. Such a unit is supplied with all of the necessary equipment for resuscitation, including positive-negative equipment for artificial respiration, an electrical defibrillation unit, various drugs, instruments, tracheal suction unit, electrocardiographic, and interval timers.

shape of the heart. When the current is on a green light shines; when defibrillation is being attempted a red light shines. In addition, all of the necessary drugs that might be of use are kept in the drawer of the machine. These drugs include epinephrine hydrochloride, procaine hydrochloride, heparin, calcium chloride, barium chloride, procainamide, and quinidine sulfate. Endotracheal tubes, mouth gags, and face masks are in the drawers. A direct-writing ECG, if also on hand, can be placed on the folding table that is attached to the machine. An electrophrenic stimulator is included. A special drawer for pediatric resuscitative equipment is also included, and there is space provided for an intra-arterial transfusion unit. Space for transfusion bottles, intravenous glucose bottles, and other articles has been provided. A standard is attached to each end of the machine. A long extension cord is available so that outlets some distance from the machine may be utilized. Directions for

the use of the machine are prominently placed.

Undoubtedly, the average case of cardiac arrest does not require such a large outlay of equipment, but almost invariably most of the equipment will be used within a space of several months. Resuscitative equipment has been compared with other first-aid measures: "Like life preservers on a ship and fire extinguishers in a theater, this equipment may stand idle for long periods, but when needed, its value is certainly beyond the price." The mobile cardiac resuscitation unit has proved to be a teaching aid during the courses presented on cardiac arrest and resuscitation. Because of the emergency elevator bell system, it can be readily transported between the floors of Bellevue Hospital.

At the Grace–New Haven Hospital, according to Turk and Glenn, cardiac resuscitation kits are wrapped in bright red drapes to identify them easily as "cardiac-arrest kits." These kits are kept at critical points

Text continued on p. 610.

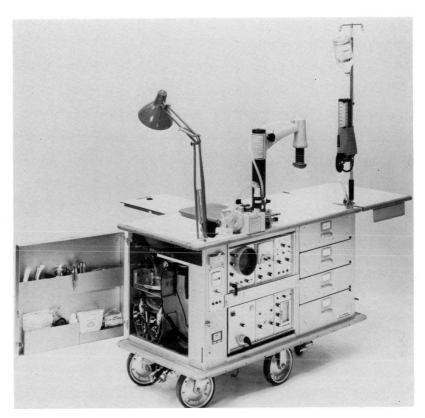

Fig. 50-2. MAX Emergency Life Support and Resuscitation System is, in effect, an assembly jig for rapid and effective emergency care. Its pneumatic external cardiac compressor with synchronized ventilator, aspirator, extensive electronic equipment, storage system, and accessories are all prepositioned efficiently in relation to the patient and operating personnel. (Courtesy Corbin-Farnsworth, Inc., Palo Alto, Calif.)

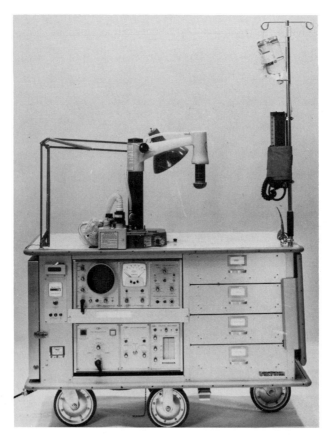

Fig. 50-3. When stored at its base station, the **MAX** Emergency Life Support and Resuscitation System is two thirds the size of a conventional litter. Its self-contained power supply is automatically energized when the battery-charging umbilicus detaches as the cart is moved to an emergency site. (Courtesy Corbin-Farnsworth, Inc., Palo Alto, Calif.)

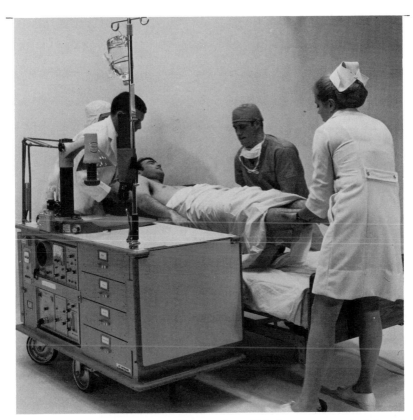

Fig. 50-4. Patient is placed on MAX's litter surface. This is tantamount to being placed in an assembly jig for emergency care because of the highly efficient operating relationships between equipment, patient, and team members. (Time: zero.) (Courtesy Corbin-Farnsworth, Inc., Palo Alto, Calif.)

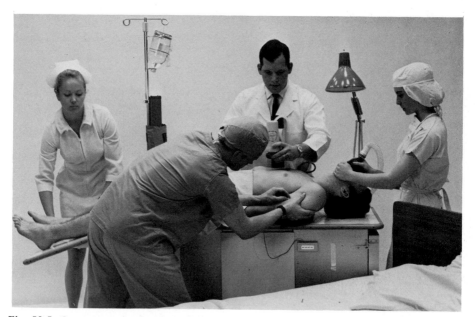

Fig. 50-5. Oxygen-supplemented respirator synchronized with pneumatic external cardiac compressor and ECG needle electrodes are rapidly applied. Folding leg board is elevated to form a full-length litter. (Time: plus 8 to 9 seconds.) (Courtesy Corbin-Farnsworth, Inc., Palo Alto, Calif.)

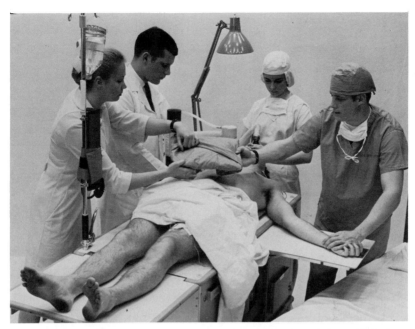

Fig. 50-6. Patient is ventilated with respirator and mask, the last of three ECG electrodes is attached, and a venous cutdown tray is passed to the surgical resident. The mode of arrest is visible on the oscilloscope. (Time: plus 15 to 17 seconds.) (Courtesy Corbin-Farnsworth, Inc., Palo Alto, Calif.)

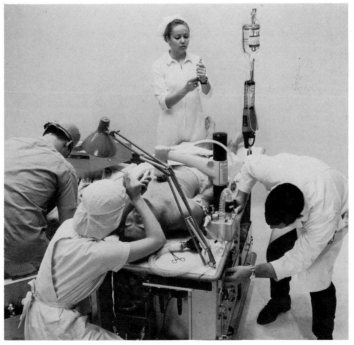

Fig. 50-7. Patient is intubated, drugs are prepared, and the cutdown is under way. (Time plus 35 to 40 seconds.) (Courtesy Corbin-Farnsworth, Inc., Palo Alto, Calif.)

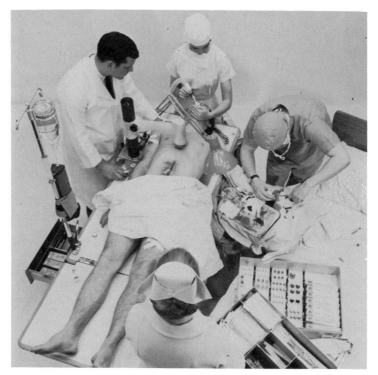

Fig. 50-8. Overhead view of patient's ventilation via endotracheal tube, operation of external cardiac compressor, cutdown procedure, and preparation of drugs. (Time: plus 65 to 70 seconds.) View demonstrates absence of mutual interference by team members engaged in various tasks and obvious accessibility to the patient by all personnel. (Courtesy Corbin-Farnsworth, Inc., Palo Alto, Calif.)

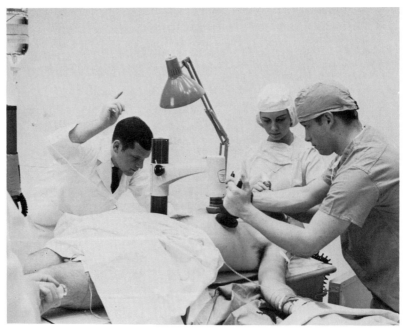

Fig. 50-9. Defibrillation is carried out during continuous perfusion by the cardiac compression unit. (Courtesy Corbin-Farnsworth, Inc., Palo Alto, Calif.)

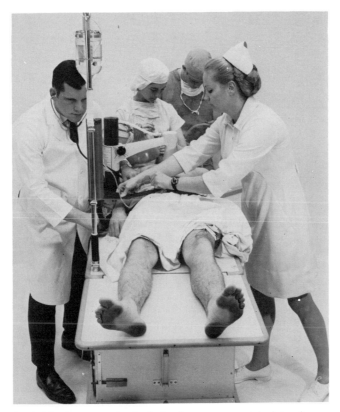

Fig. 50-10. Patient's blood pressure is checked prior to transport to intensive care unit. (Courtesy Corbin-Farnsworth, Inc., Palo Alto, Calif.)

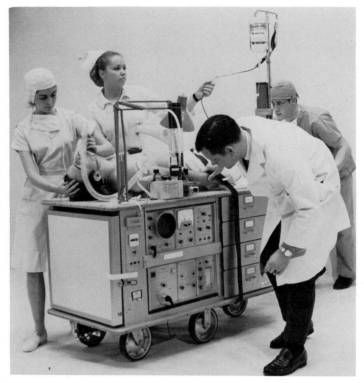

Fig. 50-11. Self-contained oxygen and electrical power permit transport of patient with concurrent operation of respirator, aspirator, external cardiac compressor, cardioscope, pacemaker, defibrillator, and intravenous drip. Patient may then be moved to an intensive care unit for postresuscitation care or to an operating room for emergency surgery with all essential functions sustained in transit. (Courtesy Corbin-Farnsworth, Inc., Palo Alto, Calif.)

in the hospital and contain sterile gloves, sterile knives, a pharyngeal airway, and other instruments. A sterile kit has been of value in closing the chest incision under sterile conditions after the resumption of heart action.

Today most hospitals have developed special resuscitation units of their own, and many elaborate and worthwhile units are available commercially. Newer units employ elaborate electronic monitoring devices, as well as pacing and defibrillating instruments. The MAX Emergency Life Support and Resuscitation System and its use are shown in Figs. 50-2 to 50-11.

Pediatric resuscitation unit

A portable resuscitation apparatus for babies, consisting of an oxygen cylinder with contents gauge, pressure regulator, mucus aspirator, and unit to give continuous or positive pressure oxygen, is described by MacRae. The positive pressure unit can supply continuous oxygen at the rate of $1\frac{1}{2}$ to 2 liters a minute and allows expired air, or excess oxygen, to escape through air vents. The entire unit weighs 5 pounds.

Chapter 51

AMBULANCE AND MOBILE RESUSCITATION CARE

Frank L. Mitchell

The prehospital medical care of acute illnesses and injuries represents the greatest medical care deficiency in our country today. Acute myocardial infarction is the leading cause of all prehospital fatalities. In 1966 Drs. J. F. Pantridge and J. S. Geddes of Belfast, Ireland, first demonstrated the feasibility of *mobile coronary care units* in reducing prehospital cardiac deaths. Previously, the lack of immediately available equipment, with the resultant delay in time, accounted for the usual failure in cardiac resuscitation outside the operating room. The success of closed-chest cardiac massage and mouth-to-mouth ventilation, as initial resuscitative measures on hospital wards, stimulated interest in expanding resuscitation capabilities to community life outside the hospital.

The great majority of myocardial infarctions with their associated arrhythmias and arrests do not occur in the hospital. Typically, the myocardial infarction patient comes under intensive medical care after the greatest risk has passed. Even though most deaths from myocardial infarction occur within 12 hours of the onset of symptoms, the average cardiac patient is admitted to the hospital more than 12 hours after the onset of symptoms. McNeally found that the majority of deaths attributable to coronary thrombosis occur within 3 hours after the onset of symptoms (Pantridge). Yater estimates that more than 50% of the individuals with coronary thrombosis die before reaching a hospital and that 60% die within the first hour after infarction.

Pemberton and McNeally surveyed the deaths from myocardial infarction in Belfast, Ireland, over a 1-year period (1965 to 1966). Of 901 individuals who had fatal coronary insufficiency, less than 50% reached the hospital and 25% of these were dead on arrival (Pantridge).

If emergency resuscitative measures could be made immediately available to such individuals, the potential survival and salvage would be very rewarding. As many as 95% of the patients who survive their first acute myocardial infarction are alive 2 years later. A 60% 10-year survival can be expected if the patient is less than 50 years of age at the time of infarction (Shailand; Pell).

In most communities the individual who develops ventricular fibrillation outside the hospital is a fatality. However, Pantridge (1967) reviewed fifty patients who survived ventricular fibrillation complicating ischemic heart disease. Seventy-eight percent were still living almost 1 year later, and a 2-year survival was projected to be 55%. These patients had been resuscitated in their homes, in ambulances, in emergency rooms, in medical wards, and in intensive care units. The residual disability among survivors of ventricular fibrillation approximates that of patients whose myocardial infarction is not so complicated (Geddes).

Lethal arrhythmias frequently precede the onset of ventricular fibrillation. Tachyarrhythmias predominate in hospital coronary care units. However, bradyarrhythmias frequently precede the onset of ventricular fibrillation in the prehospital or early infarction patient. The control of these arrhythmias is much easier and more effective than the treatment of the subsequent ventricular fibrillation.

A study of a rural community ambulance service demonstrated that patients with cardiovascular disease who were carried by ambulance more than 10 miles had a higher mortality rate than those carried less than 10 miles. Only 20% of the patients transported had cardiovascular disease, but 50% of the patients who died in the ambulance had cardiovascular disease (Waller).

The desirability of providing immediate medical care for the cardiac victim is obvious. The need for continuous cardiac stabilization and support during transportation should be equally obvious. The best way to save the lives of patients in traumatic emergencies is to begin resuscitation at the scene of injury, stabilize the patient before movement, and continue support during transportation to the hospital. The same methods should apply to myocardial ischemic problems. The ambulance must essentially be a hospital emergency ward on wheels and must be staffed with medical personnel able to perform the necessary cardiac stabilization and resuscitation.

At the present time there are not enough physicians available to carry out this type of ambitious service, and few ambulances are designed or equipped for modern cardiac care. The problem is generally being attacked through three major approaches:

1. Modification of ambulances to provide an extension of the hospital environment
2. Training of ambulance paramedical personnel in advanced methods of emergency medical care, especially airway control and cardiac resuscitation
3. Development of advanced communications between ambulance and hospital

Mobile intensive care unit (MICU)

Most ambulances, in the past, have been designed and equipped primarily for simple transportation of patients. The commonly used hearse-type ambulance is satisfactory for transporting the human body in the prone position. However, it is generally inadequate for the procedures and treatments demanded by the newer concepts in total emergency care. In order to provide an intensive care unit on wheels, modifications in ambulance design and equipment are essential. Safar and Brose have most adequately described the desirable modifications:

1. Access to the patient from his vertex for respiratory resuscitation
2. Access to the patient's side for external cardiac massage
3. Hand-operated self-inflating bag-valve-mask units for use with oxygen—to replace automatically cycling resuscitators, which have proved cumbersome and less effective
4. Powerful suction—powered from the ambulance engine, electric motor, or battery
5. Large reservoir of oxygen
6. Transparent bag-mask unit for oxygen inhalation
7. Oropharyngeal tubes
8. Portable equipment for ventilation, oxygen inhalation and suction*

Additional resuscitation equipment is desirable when well-trained paramedical emergency medical technicians or physicians are available:

1. Direct-writing ECG
2. Defibrillator
3. Mechanical heart-lung resuscitator
4. Intravenous fluids
5. Cardiac drugs

The van-type and camper-body type vehicles are gaining widespread support as emergency medical care mobile units. The major advantages are (1) increased space for needed patient care, (2) increased residual space for convenient equipment storage, (3) 30% to 50% less purchase price, and (4) less complicated and expensive upkeep.

In order to apply effective cardiac resuscitation, some minimum interior dimensions must be considered. Ideally, the interior

---

*Safar, P., and Brose, R. A.: Ambulance design and equipment for resuscitation, Arch. Surg. **90:** 343-348, 1965.

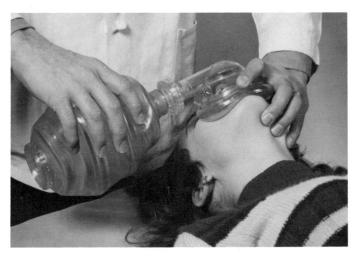

Fig. 51-1. Laerdal bag is self-inflating with one-way valves. Mask is clear, which allows visualization of any regurgitation.

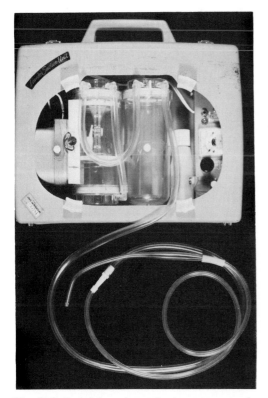

Fig. 51-2. Laerdal suction unit. Apparatus may be powered by self-contained battery or attachment to 12-volt ambulance circuit. Unit contains 16-ounce collection bottle.

height should allows the attendant to stand, since closed-chest compression can be more effectively carried out from the standing position. At the minimum, the attendant should be able to sit upright and be erect when on his knees. This generally would require a floor-to-ceiling height of over 50 inches. In order to effectively deliver artificial ventilation, the patient compartment must be no less than 110 inches in length. This allows the attendant access to the patient's head from the vertex. From the vertex position, the attendant can most effectively use the bag-mask-valve ventilator, maintain the proper patient head tilt for open airway, and accomplish oropharyngeal suctioning. In order to perform cardiac massage, the width of the compartment must allow the attendant sufficient space at the side of the stretcher. The minimum comfortable compartment width would be 50 inches.

In May, 1971, a committee of experts in the emergency health field reported to the National Highway Traffic Safety Administration a comprehensive recommendation on ambulance design criteria. The measurements of the patient compartment requirements were:

1. Length—25-inch clear space at head and 15 inches at foot of a 76-inch litter

2. Width—25-inch clear area to side of patient
3. Floor to ceiling—minimum 54 inches, preferably 60 inches

AIRWAY MAINTENANCE EQUIPMENT

Bag-mask-valve units. Immediate and adequate ventilation can be produced using the simpler methods of artificial ventilation such as mouth-to-mouth and bag-mask-valve equipment. An example of a satisfactory bag-mask-valve unit that is not dependent upon a supply of oxygen and can very effectively use room air is shown in Fig. 51-1.

Safar nicely demonstrates that the widely used automatic cycling, pressure-set oxygen resuscitators are not the best choice for emergency artificial ventilation. Common problems encountered with this type of equipment are (1) pressure-set resuscitators do not compensate for changing airway resistance, lung-chest compliance, and mask leak; (2) start of resuscitation is delayed by setting up the equipment; (3) airway obstruction, leakage, and improper setting of the mechanical switches may go unnoticed; (4) oxygen resuscitators are heavy and are not easily portable; and (5) oxygen resuscitators stop when the oxygen supply is exhausted.

Suction equipment. The suction unit should supply approximately 300 mm. Hg suction with a flow of 30 liters per minute (Safar, 1965). This suction can be obtained by attaching the unit to the ambulance engine manifold. Good suction can also be obtained from a standard hospital machine

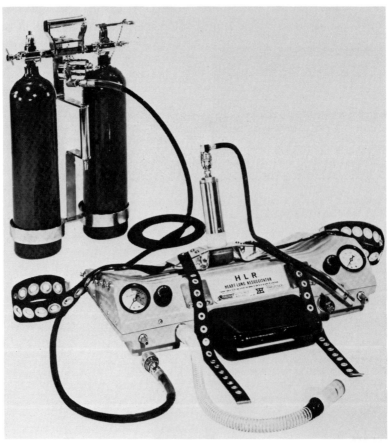

Fig. 51-3. Heart-lung resuscitator with oxygen pack power source. Oxygen continues through system for patient administration. Note straps to prevent lateral or distal displacement of plunger. (Courtesy Travenol Laboratories, Inc., Morton Grove, Ill.)

driven by an inverter in the ambulance. A portable suction unit that can be driven by either a self-contained battery or the ambulance's electrical power is ideal and has recently become commercially available (Fig. 51-2). These battery-powered units allow good suction capabilities both in the ambulance and away from the vehicle. Suction of 550 mm. Hg can be developed with a flow rate of 6 liters per minute.

Miscellaneous supportive airway equipment
1. Oropharyngeal airways—various sizes
2. S tubes for mouth-to-mouth ventilation
3. Laryngoscope with endotracheal tubes
4. Tracheotomy set with various tube sizes
5. Oxygen cylinders—portable and fixed
6. Clear semiopen oronasal face mask with deep-breathing bag

CARDIAC RESUSCITATION EQUIPMENT

1. Cardioscope and direct-writing ECG
2. Portable defibrillator
3. Pacer
4. Heart-lung resuscitator

External cardiac compression machines, or heart-lung resuscitators, do not replace manual external massage (Fig. 51-3). However, they should approximate the performance of manual cardiac massage (Fig. 51-4). They are primarily indicated when prolonged resuscitation or transportation is required. Successful resuscitation has been reported after machine massage of 2½ hours. The design of the machine should provide for quick application and positioning of the plunger as well as facilitating backward head tilt for airway maintenance. Some type of stabilization between the patient and the machine must be present to prevent accidental displacement of the plunger during transportation. If the positive pressure breathing apparatus is used, it should be volume regulated and programmed to inflate the lungs after each fifth cardiac compression.

Training of emergency medical technicians

A minimum of two highly trained persons is necessary to handle a mobile resuscitation unit. The most effective units include a physician, but the luxury of a physician attendant is not universally possible or practical.

It is possible to train paramedical emer-

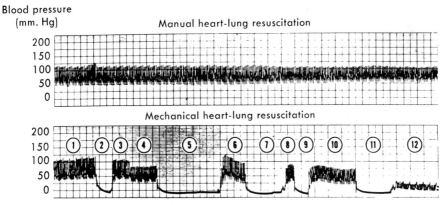

Fig. 51-4. Comparison of uninterrupted blood pressure achieved during movement of patient with a mechanical heart-lung resuscitator *(top)* versus interrupted and inadequate blood pressure resulting from manual CPR under the same circumstances *(bottom)*:

1. On floor	5. Moving down 10 steps	9. Through outside doors
2. Move to stretcher	6. Stop on landing	10. Across yard
3. On stretcher	7. Moving down 10 steps	11. Into ambulance
4. Moving down 50-foot hall	8. Moving through downstairs hall	12. In ambulance

(From Gordon, A. S., editor: Cardiopulmonary resuscitation conference proceedings, 1967.)

gency medical technicians to provide effective cardiopulmonary resuscitation. The Baltimore city fire department units have demonstrated the success possible without physicians in direct attendance (Wilder). The Baltimore study of cardiopulmonary resuscitation by trained ambulance personnel revealed not a single fatal injury produced by the resuscitation measures.

One study demonstrated the unsuspected reluctance of police and fire fighters to use mouth-to-mouth breathing because of fear of exposure to contagious disease, apprehension over possibility of legal liabilities, and esthetic distaste for the procedure. The use of S tubes and bag-mask resuscitators should overcome these obstacles (Weingarten).

The advanced Red Cross first aid course must be a minimum requirement for every ambulance attendant. In addition, all ambulance attendants should be certified in cardiopulmonary resuscitation. Manikin practice and periodic refresher courses can be continued under paramedical instructors.

Advanced programs for intensive training of paramedical emergency medical technicians are developing throughout the United States. These programs generally require 75 to 81 hours of instruction time after the advanced Red Cross certification. The curriculum varies considerably in emphasis, but the topics are reasonably obvious and consistent. The Department of Transportation Basic Training Program for Emergency Medical Technician-Ambulance is the most widely accepted initial EMT curriculum. The total course consists of 71 hours of classroom instruction, practice, and examination plus 10 hours of in-hospital observation and training. Fifteen hours are devoted to cardiopulmonary resuscitation and shock.

Such a training program has been initiated at the University of Missouri School of Medicine. Approximately half of the instruction is given in the local communities. The remainder of instruction is given during a 4-day course at the University Hospital. Twenty percent of the instruction time is devoted to airway maintenance, cardiac resuscitation,

and shock. The ability of paramedical personnel to develop technical ability and judgment has been encouraging.

The Oregon Coronary Ambulance Project (Rose) admirably demonstrated the practical and successful training of emergency medical technicians to recognize ECG arrhythmias and proceed with defibrillation. The EMTs worked without radio telemetry in their ambulances. Seven of fourteen patients with ventricular fibrillation were resuscitated and subsequently discharged from the hospital. This capability conserves medical manpower, reduces MCCU expense, and allows much more effective prehospital medical care.

During the training period, technicians should be encouraged to rotate shifts in the emergency room, operating room, heart station, recovery room, intensive care units, psychiatric wards, and delivery suite. This allows additional experience to be gained on a practical basis. Some hospital-based ambulance services use emergency technicians to provide help to the nursing services through-

---

Oregon curriculum for training ambulance attendants in emergency cardiac resuscitation*

Didactic: 16 hours
  Anatomy and physiology
  Cardiac emergencies, recognition, and treatment
  Electrocardiography
  Monitoring and defibrillating equipment
  Review of principles and practice of resuscitation
Observation and tutoring in coronary care unit: 40 hours
Animal laboratory: 8 hours
  Effects of life-threatening arrhythmias
  Defibrillation, cardiopulmonary resuscitation
Instruction by anesthesiologist: 4 hours
Weekly 2-hour drill sessions, quizzes, and examinations: 16 hours

*From Rose, L. B., and Press, E.: Cardiac defibrillation by ambulance attendants, J.A.M.A. **219**:63-68, 1972.

Oregon Coronary Ambulance Project: Standing orders for patients with suspected coronary occlusion*

1. Attach monitor; observe cardiac rhythm
2. Take blood pressure, apical rate, respiration rate, listen for rales; start oxygen
3. Give analgesic authorized, or if blood pressure more than 90 mm. Hg, and the patient under 70 years of age, give 75 mg. of meperidine hydrochloride; over 70 years of age, give 50 mg. of meperidine hydrochloride
4. If sinus rhythm or controlled atrial fibrillation is present and patient more comfortable move to ambulance, with monitor on during movement and in transport
5. If marked sinus bradycardia, give 0.4 to 0.8 mg. atropine sulfate intravenously or intramuscularly
6. If heart block is present, start isoproterenol hydrochloride intravenously, 0.5 mg. in 250 ml. of 5% dextrose in water, and keep rate above 40 beats per minute
7. If premature ventricular contractions are frequent and heart rate above 70 beats per minute, give 50 mg. of lidocaine hydrochloride intravenously every 30 minutes as needed; if multifocal premature ventricular contractions or ventricular tachycardia, start lidocaine hydrochloride infusion 1 gm. in 250 ml. of 5% dextrose in water at 15 to 30 microdrops per minute; do not give lidocaine if heart block, hypotension below 80 mm. Hg, or severe bundle branch block.
8. In case of cardiac standstill
   a. Percuss chest
   b. Turn on external pacer previously attached
   c. Cardiopulmonary resuscitation
   d. Start isoproterenol
9. In case of ventricular fibrillation
   a. Defibrillate
   b. If unsuccessful, cardiopulmonary resuscitation, debrillate again
10. In case of pulmonary edema
    a. Elevate head
    b. Start rotating tourniquets if blood pressure more than 100 mm. Hg

*From Rose, L. B., and Press, E.: Cardiac defibrillation by ambulance attendants, J.A.M.A. **219**:63-68, 1972.

out the hospital. This provides continuing education for the technician and much needed support to the nursing personnel. In addition, emergency technicians rotate blood drawing and intravenous fluid duties to maintain technical competency.

As radio telemetry between the ambulance and the hospital-based physician develops, the ambulance attendant will be performing more advanced lifesaving measures. Therefore, advanced training of ambulance attendants or emergency medical technicians will be essential if we are to succeed in the new concepts of emergency medical care and the mobile intensive care unit.

Emergency medical communications

Constant radio contact between the mobile emergency unit and the hospital is essential for an efficient and effective operation. The emergency room should always be alerted to the impending arrival of a seriously ill patient. Delays in availability of personnel and equipment are averted and continuity of medical care is preserved.

Radio contact with the hospital-based physician should permit more definite therapy by the ambulance attendants. Two-way radio telemetry of vital signs, ECG, and EEG is already being used in pilot projects. The use of television surveillance and other communications systems in connecting ambulance attendants to hospital-based physicians is being explored. With the development of radio telemetry, hospital-based physicians have been able to direct paramedical personnel to perform defibrillation, drug administration, intravenous infusion, tracheal intubation, and other advanced lifesaving measures.

In Miami, Florida, the fire department rescue service has been extensively trained in cardiac resuscitation. ECGs are radioed to Jackson Memorial Hospital. Physicians at the hospital use a radiotelephone to communicate instructions back to the rescue team.

The University of Missouri Emergency Medical Service is working with direct radio telemetry of ECGs, pulse rates, and respiratory rates. Doppler measurement of blood pressure for radio transmission is under study.

The future of communications as a vital adjunct to cardiac problems is just beginning to be studied. As an example, small portable cardiac monitors have been devised that sound a radio alert when arrhythmias develop. These could be worn by high-risk cardiac patients and more quickly summon emergency medical care.

ACTIVE MOBILE INTENSIVE CARE UNITS

Since 1966 when Pantridge described his mobile coronary care unit (MCCU) in Belfast, over 60 MCCU's have been established in larger metropolitan areas of the United States. Concurrently, many general ambulance services have been established that incorporate skilled cardiac resuscitation as well as the other parameters of advanced emergency medical care. The duplication of vehicles and manpower necessary to have a specialized MCCU and a general ambulance service has raised some questions of the desirability of MCCU as such. This is especially so, since about 50% of emergency calls to MCCU are for noncardiac problems. Conversely, many "noncardiac" conditions become complicated by cardiac problems. There is a gradual realization that mobile intensive care units are effective with cardiac problems and have the additional capabilities of emergency medical care for *all* acute illnesses and injuries.

It is not possible to discuss every MCCU or advanced EMS presently operating. However, we should mention several that have made unusual contributions to the advancement of concepts.

Belfast, Ireland. One of the most significant advances in the management of acute myocardial infarction took place in Belfast, Ireland, in 1966. A mobile coronary care unit was developed to serve a population of approximately a half-million people. The mobile unit is an ambulance containing monitoring and resuscitation equipment, including a D.C. defibrillator and bipolar pacing catheters. The staff is from the cardiac department of the Royal Victoria Hospital. Monitoring and therapy in the patient's home is often necessary to establish a stable rhythm before it is considered safe to transfer the patient to the ambulance. During transport to the hospital, monitoring and treatment are continued. Pantridge and Geddes state that the response of the unit has been so increased that 78% of patients are reached within 15 minutes of telephone notification. Of 101 patients seen within 4 hours after symptoms of myocardial infarction, twelve developed ventricular fibrillation before or during transport. Seven of these patients were successfully resuscitated. It is suspected that more would have developed ventricular fibrillation during transport if preliminary rhythm stabilization had not been obtained. *No patient died during transit to the hospital.*

New York. St. Vincent's Hospital and Medical Center of New York used the first MCCU in the United States. The MCCU consists of a standard hospital ambulance with battery-powered defibrillator monitor, battery-powered electrocardiograph, and cardiac medications. Personnel include physician, nurse, ECG technician, and two drivers. There is a 4½-minute team response to calls and an average 8½-minute response to site. In the first 161 calls, forty-one patients had acute myocardial infarction. Three patients had ventricular fibrillation and there was successful resuscitation of one. Fifty-two patients had arrhythmias: eleven bradyarrhythmias, twenty-two tachyarrhythmias, and twenty premature beats. It is difficult to objectively evaluate the lifesaving potential of early control of arrhythmias, but the benefit should be obvious.

Rancho Santa Fe. Dr. Quentin Wood from Rancho Santa Fe, California, modified a large step-in van to act as an elaborate mobile hospital (Fig. 51-5). Rancho Santa Fe is a medically isolated community of predominantly older retired people. The nearest hospital is 20 miles away. The emergency unit is maintained in the local area. Myocardial infarction patients are taken immediately to

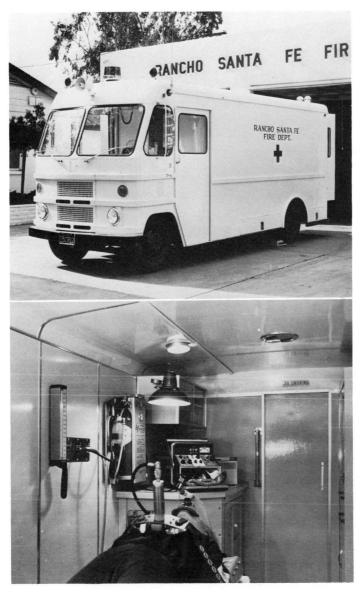

Fig. 51-5. Mobile intensive care unit, Rancho Santa Fe, Calif.

the vehicle, where they are stabilized and then transported in the vehicle to the hospital. Intensive training of the paramedical staff is provided in all aspects of emergency care. The equipment is as sophisticated as in a major hospital; the unit carries a heart-lung resuscitator, a defibrillator, an electrocardioscope, a pacemaker, a synchronizer, a recording electrocardiograph, an adjustable examining table, suction, oxygen, a refrigerator, drugs, airways, a tracheotomy set, and intravenous solutions.

Mainz, Germany. In Germany, Ahenfeld has developed the Clinomobile (Fig. 51-6), which is a hospital emergency ward on wheels. The unit is staffed by an anesthesiologist and cardiologist. The equipment within the vehicle is capable of providing extensive

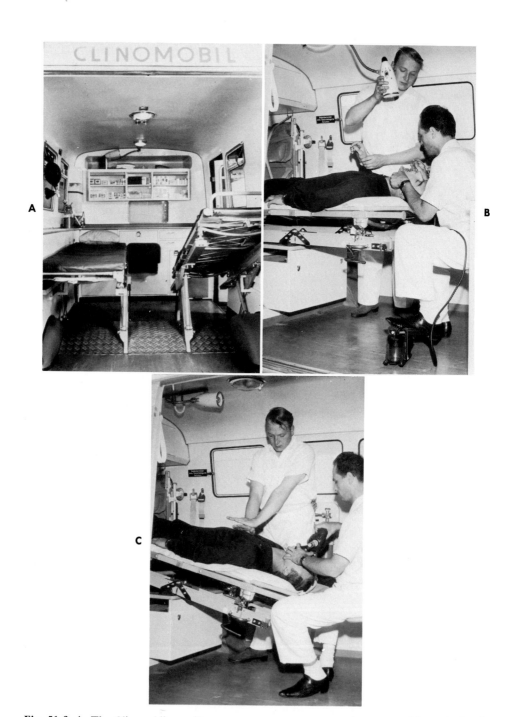

Fig. 51-6. A, The Clinomobil can, if necessary, carry two prone patients, accessible at the head and from one side. The heads of both stretchers can be lowered. B, Suction equipment in action. C, Cardiopulmonary resuscitation on the stretcher of this vehicle. Note the adequate head room.

Clinomobile modules		
	Paramedical module	*Physician module*
Respiration		
Free airway	Suction equipment	Emergency intubation set
Reestablishment of respiration	Self-inflating bag-mask-valve unit	Emergency tracheotomy set
	Two 3-liter oxygen cylinders	
	One portable oxygen inhaler	
	Guedel airways	
	S tubes	
Hemorrhage and shock treatment	Bandage material for compresses	Two Kocher forceps
	Four triangle bandages	Plasma expanders (4)
	Tourniquet	Injection set
		Syringes
		Compartment for circulator stimulants and analgesics
Cardiac resuscitation	Hard, flat surface for thoracic portion of stretcher	Compartment for cardiac stimulants
		Cardiac puncture cannulae
		D.C. defibrillator
		Venous cutdown

emergency medical care. The equipment is listed in two modules. One module contains everything that trained paramedical personnel would need for treatment. A second module is restricted to use by physicians.

University of Missouri. The University of Missouri School of Medicine at Columbia is in a rural area. A van-type ambulance (Fig. 51-7) has been developed that has all the capabilities of the emergency room to maintain life and prevent complications. The EMTs have received over 200 hours of training, including "Medication course for the LPN." When not on an ambulance call, the emergency medical technicians work in the University Hospital—emergency room, recovery room, intensive care units, and delivery suite. The EMTs are not only equipped to perform the manual aspects of cardiopulmonary resuscitation, but start intravenous fluids, administer medications, and defibrillate upon radio instructions from the emergency room physician. ECGs are radio transmitted directly to the emergency room to allow the emergency room to monitor the incoming patient's condition and permit the hospital-based physician to more intelligently advise the EMT of any immediate indicated treatment. The equipment carried that relates to cardiac care includes:

Stethoscope	Syringes and needles
Blood pressure cuff (aneroid)	Cardiac drugs
Recording ECG and transmitter	Bag-mask-valve ventilator
Electrocardioscope	Oxygen
Pacemaker	Oropharyngeal airways
Heart-lung resuscitator	S tubes
Intravenous fluids	Laryngoscope
Defibrillator	Tracheotomy set

Drugs

Meperidine (Demerol)	Digoxin
Atropine	Lanatoside C
Lidocaine	Furosemide (Lasix)
Quinidine	Epinephrine
Metaraminol (Aramine)	Isoproterenol (Isuprel)
Diphenylhydantoin (Dilantin)	Dextrose 50%

Intravenous fluids

(Always started with blood-filter tubing)

5% dextrose in water

5% Ringer's lactate

Dextran

Seattle, Washington—Harborview Medical Center and Seattle Fire Department. By a cooperative effort, the Medical Center and fire department have developed a unique system of response to emergency calls that reduces travel time to the patient. When the central dispatcher determines an emergency call to be a life-threatening situation, he simultaneously dispatches a fire department

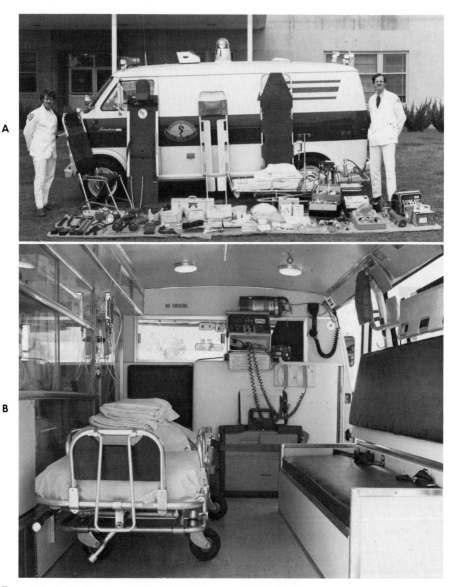

Fig. 51-7. **A,** University of Missouri Emergency Medical Services van-type vehicle. All of the equipment seen is carried in the vehicle. Cost of this type vehicle is much less than other types of emergency vehicles. **B,** The equipment stores nicely within the patient care area. Airway and cardiac resuscitation equipment is placed at vertex position.

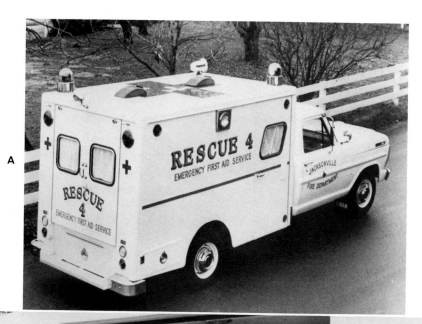

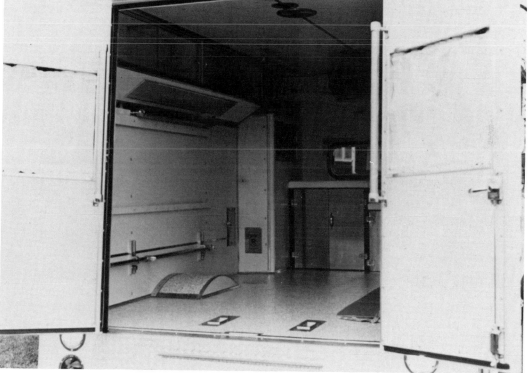

Fig. 51-8. A, Jacksonville, Florida, ambulance. Patient compartment may be transferred to a new truck chassis. **B,** Interior dimensions are 116 inches long, 72 inches wide, 56 inches high. (Courtesy Swab Wagon Co., Elizabethville, Pa.)

aid car from a neighborhood fire station and a more distant centrally located MCCU. The aid cars are within 2 to 5 minutes of any point in the city and perform triage and early life-sustaining measures using basic cardio-pulmonary techniques. The MCCU will arrive in several more minutes and proceed with definitive resuscitation. The patient is then transported to a hospital coronary care unit, but only after radio confirmation of space available at the specific hospital. This system seems to be very practical and reduces time delays in initial care as well as hospital administrative delays. The results are also encouraging. Three-hundred-twenty-four patients had ventricular fibrillations *at the time of arrival of the MCCU.* Thirty-six percent were resuscitated and returned to a hospital. Thirteen percent left the hospital as long-term survivors.

Jacksonville, Florida. One of the most comprehensive emergency medical systems in the world. Mobile intensive care units are housed in the fire stations. Patient entry into the system is by a single telephone number or public emergency phones, which have replaced the usual fire pull alarms. Central dispatch sends a two-man unit from the closest fire house. If the patient has arrested, a second supporting unit is dispatched. Duplex ECG telemetry is constantly available from all units to Memorial Hospital. Defibrillation, administering of medications, and intravenous fluid therapy are all performed by the emergency medical technicians. The vehicle used is a truck chassis with a detachable patient compartment (Fig. 51-8). Patient compartment space is excellent. The good maneuverability and handling make these vehicles suitable for urban and rural use. These vehicles cost more initially but considerable savings eventually ensue when the chassis needs replacement and the patient compartment can be transferred to a new chassis.

Chapter 52

STADIUM RESUSCITATION
(A LIFE-SUPPORT UNIT)

Stephen W. Carveth with the assistance of H. E. Reese and R. J. Buchman

Introduction

In 1966 a combined mobile and fixed life-support unit was organized at the University of Nebraska Memorial Football Stadium in Lincoln, Nebraska. The purpose of this unit was to rapidly recognize and treat football spectators who develop a cardiopulmonary emergency. In the fall of 1965, the year before its inception, at least three football fans suddenly collapsed and died and neither emergency nor definitive resuscitative attempts were carried out in the stadium. In the fall of 1971 the stadium life-support unit was integrated into Lincoln's stratified system of treatment for patients with a suspect acute myocardial infarction.*

The fixed stadium resuscitation unit was built in 1966 in conjunction with a stadium expansion and was specifically located near an entrance and exit drive of the stadium (Fig. 52-1). An externor sign indicated that it was a first aid and life-support unit. The unit was built of concrete blocks and the interior was well ventilated with heat and air-conditioning units.

This unit is strategically located with proper identification and with specific capabilities to render life support to persons with cardiopulmonary emergencies. As such, the unit follows the guidelines of minimal standards of a fixed and mobile life-support unit as indicated by the American Heart Associa-

*Lincoln Area Mobile Coronary Care Unit

tion standards for emergency cardiac care. This life-support station is really a combination of a fixed and a mobile unit. It is a fixed unit in the sense that the spectator is transported from the stadium seat to the fixed installation during which time emergency cardiopulmonary resuscitation is carried out. Once the spectator is brought to the unit, definitive measures of monitoring, establishment of intravenous lifelines, drug therapy, and defibrillation are administered. After the condition of the patient stabilizes, the unit becomes mobile and the patient, personnel, and appropriate equipment are transferred to one of the three coronary care units in Lincoln.

Method of development

By 1966 it was known that prompt immediate artificial ventilation and external cardiac massage could often resuscitate a stricken person provided the equipment and personnel arrived at the site of the emergency within 3 to 5 minutes. It is now suspected that at least half of the people who die of a myocardial infarction do so before reaching a hospital. Therefore it was theorized that if the appropriate personnel and equipment from a coronary care unit were taken to the scene of the emergency, many of these out-of-hospital deaths from myocardial infarction might be saved.

Certain advantageous resources were present in Lincoln, Nebraska, at that time and in

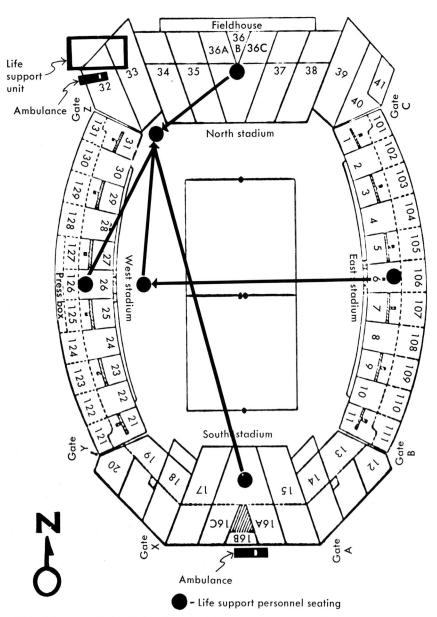

Fig. 52-1. Diagram of the University of Nebraska Memorial Stadium. Life-support unit is located on ground level under the north stands. Black dots indicate approximate location of Red Cross and Boy Scout volunteers during game. Black arrows indicate line of communication via walkie-talkie radio between personnel of Red Cross, emergency medical technicians, and life-support unit. This plan is provided for rapid identification of location of spectator who needs help.

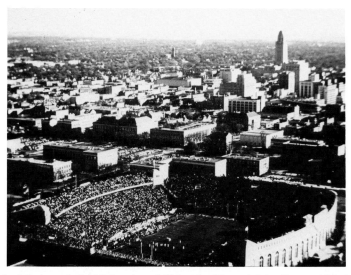

Fig. 52-2. Aerial view of the University of Nebraska Memorial Stadium, which has a seating capacity of 76,000.

particular at the football stadium on Saturday afternoon. These resources consisted of a well-organized Red Cross team who managed medical emergencies in the best fashion they were capable of at the time. In addition, approximately 100 policemen were on duty in the stadium to assist in the management of a frequently overenthusiastic crowd (Fig. 52-2).

With the realization that the need was present to improve emergency cardiac care and the resources were present to accomplish this, a plan was formulated to coordinate a variety of community volunteer efforts that eventually culminated in an effective and successful plan of management of a football spectator who collapsed on a Saturday afternoon. Initially in 1966 the plan of action was presented and wholeheartedly agreed upon by Mr. Tippy Dye, Athletic Director of the University of Nebraska. More recently the unit has the complete support of Mr. Robert Devaney of football coaching fame. The unit has operated under the auspices of the Student Health Center, which is under the direction of Dr. Samuel Fuenning. He has assisted in many ways and in particular by the coordination of the personnel of the

campus and Lincoln police departments, Red Cross, Boy Scouts, and the Lincoln Mobile Heart Unit. In addition members of the Executive Committee of the Lancaster County Medical Society enthusiastically supported the idea and provided much appreciated endorsement in the early, formative years.

From 1966 through 1970 the unit was staffed by volunteers from the Cardiopulmonary Laboratory of Bryan Memorial Hospital. In the following 2 years the unit was staffed by members of the Lincoln Area Mobile Heart Team. It is necessary to have two teams of personnel and equipment present Saturday afternoon to manage efficiently. Both units are at the stadium. One covers the stadium while the other covers the Lincoln area and acts as backup in case two emergencies occur at the same time in the stadium. The latter happened in 1966. The personnel of the Mobile Heart Team consisted of a skilled coronary care nurse and two cardiopulmonary technicians. The stadium unit had adequate physician backup at all times from cardiovascular surgeons who acted as medical directors and advisors. The equipment was loaned each fall by the Car-

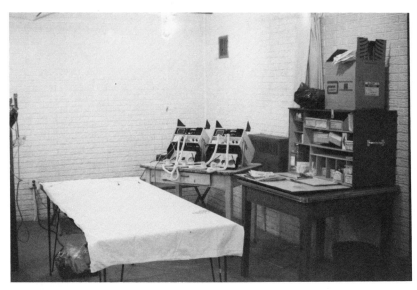

Fig. 52-3. View of stationary equipment in life-support unit at stadium.

diopulmonary Laboratory Section of Bryan Memorial Hospital and included cardiac monitor, portable D.C. defibrillator-monitor, intravenous solutions, emergency ventilation equipment, and drugs. Except for the portable ventilator, suction, monitor, and defibrillator, all pieces of equipment and supplies were brought to the life-support unit at the beginning of each season and remained at the unit in a compartmentalized plywood box (Fig. 52-3). Equipment is listed on p. 629.

In addition to the life-support team, approximately thirty Red Cross volunteers are scattered throughout the stadium in strategic areas of high density of adult population. Six of these Red Cross volunteers act as supervisors and carry walkie-talkies, which allows instant communication with the personnel who staff the unit that includes the emergency medical technicians. Over fifty Boy Scout ushers assist the Red Cross people when needed. In addition, the Lincoln police force supplies 100 or more men with their own communications system. Either interns or physicians are stationed in sections of the stadium where a high density of adult population exists. Their location is known by the

Red Cross volunteers and these physicians are called upon when needed.

Emergency medical technicians, portable stretcher, and oxygen remain at each end of the stadium and can be summoned for assistance when needed at the site of a collapsed spectator. The training of all personnel who manage the collapsed spectator is stratified and follows closely that outlined by the American Heart Association for emergency and definitive cardiopulmonary resuscitation. The skilled coronary care nurse has had from 2 to as many as 7 years' experience in coronary care nursing. The cardiopulmonary technicans are trained according to the American Heart Association guidelines in the emergency management of cardiopulmonary resuscitation. Some of the firemen and policemen have had training in emergency cardiopulmonary resuscitation as outlined by the American Heart Association. The ambulance personnel and emergency medical technicians vary between Level 1 and Level 2 of training as outlined by the National Research Council. The Red Cross and Boy Scout personnel have had training in rescue breathing according to American Heart Association standards.

Equipment and medication for stadium life-support unit

Equipment
- 2   ECG monitors
- 2   Patient cables—2 each needle and paste electrodes (8 sets)
- 2   Defibrillators and saline sponges
- 1   Temporary pacemaker unit with electrode for transthoracic pacing
- 1   Portable suction machine

Respiratory therapy supplies
- 1   AMBU bag with adult- and child-size face mask
- 1   Large oxygen cylinder
- 1   Oxygen regulator
-    Plastic airways of various sizes for adult, child, and infant
-    Tongue blades, padded and plain
- 1   Laryngoscope handle
-    Laryngoscope blades, curved and straight; long, medium, and small
-    Endotracheal tubes with cuff, No. 12 through No. 40
- 1   Hemostat
- 2   6 ml. syringes
-    Extra set of batteries
-    Extra bulbs for laryngoscope
- 2   Each, oxygen masks, cannula, and connecting tubes
-    Xylocaine lubricant
-    Stylet

Prepackaged syringes
- 10   Sodium bicarbonate
- 3   Epinephrine 1:10,000/10 ml.
- 3   Lidocaine 100 mg./5 ml.
- 3   Lidocaine 1,000 mg./25 ml.
- 3   Isuprel 1:50,000/10 ml.
- 3   Atropine 1 mg./10 ml.
- 3   Demerol 75 mg.
- 3   Morphine 10 mg.
- 2   Calcium chloride 10%/10 ml.
- 2   Calcium gluconate 10%/10 ml.
- 1   Dextrose 50 ml./25 ml.
- 1   Aminophyllin 500 mg./10 ml.
- 2   Valium 10 mg./2 ml.
- 2   Benadryl 50 mg./5 ml.

I.V. and medication supplies
- 1   I.V. stand
- 1   Sterile gloves
-    Variety syringes (disposable) 50 ml., 12 ml., 6 ml., 3 ml.
-    Variety of needles: 25 gauge × ⅝", 21 gauge × 1½", 18 gauge × 1½"

Suction supplies
- 2   No. 16 suction catheters
- 2   No. 18 suction catheters
- 2   No. 18 Levin tubes
- 2   Connecting tubing

Medications and intravenous fluids
- 5   250 ml. 5% G/H_2O
- 2   500 ml. 5% G/H_2O
- 1   500 ml. 10% G/H_2O
- 1   500 ml. 5% Sodium bicarbonate solution

Other parenteral medications
- Lasix
- Lanoxin
- Cedilanid
- Solu-Cortef
- Solu-Medrol
- Aramine
- Compazine
- Reserpine
- Pronestyl
- Glucagon
- Dilantin
- Inderal
- Sterile H_2O (30 ml. vials)
- Sterile saline (30 ml. vials)
- Xylocaine 2%, 50 ml.

Miscellaneous
- Blood pressure cuff
- Stethoscope
- Emesis basin
- Linens (treatment towels and sheets)
- Unsterile hemostat
- Alcohol sponges, 1 box

Continued.

Equipment and medication for stadium life-support unit—cont'd

I.V. and medication supplies—cont'd
- 2   Tubexes
- 3   Intracardiac needles, 20 gauge × 6″
- 2   Subclavian needles
- 2   Scalpvein needles
- 2   C. R. Bard 14 gauge intracatheter
      Plastic needles 18 gauge, 20 gauge
      (6 each)
- 6   Microdrip I.V. tubing sets
- 4   Tourniquets
      Sterile hemostat
      I.V. arm board

Miscellaneous—cont'd
    Variety sizes, paper and adhesive tape
    Bandage scissors
    4 × 4's unsterile
    Mobile unit patient forms
    Extension cord

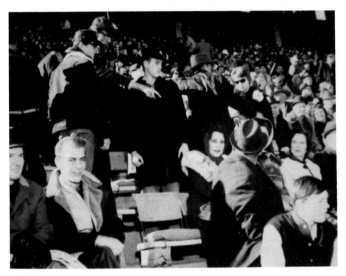

Fig. 52-4. Red Cross volunteer and Boy Scout relay exact location of spectator before administration of artificial ventilation.

Mode of operation

The plan of action for the management of a spectator who either develops a cardiac arrest or who complains of chest pain was practiced by the volunteers on several occasions prior to commencement of the program. The following is a description of the usual sequence of events during one of these emergency situations. The collapsed spectator was usually noted by a nearby fan who summoned either Red Cross personnel, physician, or Boy Scout. These first-line action personnel were trained in the recognition of cardiopulmonary collapse and immediately initiated the emergency measures of cardiopulmonary resuscitation (Fig. 52-4). Using walkie-talkies, the Red Cross personnel immediately notified the Red Cross supervisor on ground level who in turn notified the emergency medical technicians of the exact location of the emergency (Fig. 52-5). These skilled emergency medical technicians rushed to the collapsed spectator with a stretcher, oxygen, and ventilator. The patient was transferred to

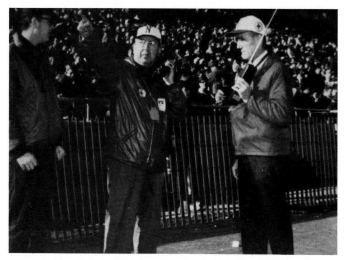

Fig. 52-5. Red Cross supervisor notifies emergency medical technicians of location of collapsed spectator.

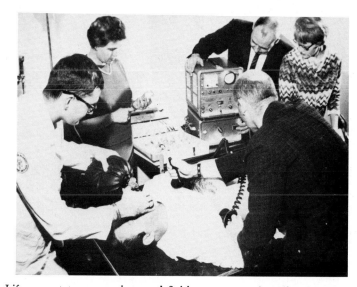

Fig. 52-6. Life-support team carrying on definitive measures of cardiopulmonary resuscitation.

the stretcher and emergency measures were continued while the spectator was transported to the fixed installation. The patient was usually transported down the ramp and, at intervals, more efficient mouth-to-mouth ventilation and external massage were carried out until the crew reached ground level. At this point the stretcher wheels were lowered and the stretcher was rolled to the fixed unit.

Once the patient was brought to the unit he was transferred from the stretcher to the table and cardiac monitoring was immediately instituted. At this point definitive measures of cardiopulmonary resuscitation were carried out, according to the specific situation. Intravenous fluids were instituted, tracheal intubation was carried out on the unconscious victim, and drug therapy and defibrillation were done when necessary to convert the patient to as near a stable sinus rhythm as possible (Fig. 52-6). When his condition stabilized, he was transported to one of the three functioning coronary care units in Lincoln. During his transportation he was accompanied by monitor-defibrillator, durgs, cardiopulmonary technician, and a coronary care nurse. While one spectator was transferred, the second life-support crew was available to manage a second stadium emergency should it arise.

Results

By the end of the 1973 football season the stadium life support unit had completed its eighth year of operation. This unit serviced forty-six home games. The personnel in the unit saw a total of eighteen spectators who developed either a cardiac or a pulmonary emergency while attending the game. Four of the eighteen people had only moderate to severe chest pain without cardiovascular collapse. One of the spectators had an acute myocardial infarction and developed ventricular tachycardia after transfer to a coronary care unit. He was cardioverted successfully and made a good recovery. One person had severe angina, but signed himself out of the hospital shortly after admission and returned to see the ballgame. The other two people did not prove to have an acute myocardial infarction. Four patients developed cardiopulmonary emergency, were successfully resuscitated but died in 1 to 7 days with a primary diagnosis of stroke. One patient had a definite transient cerebral ischemic episode and was told to see her physician. The remaining nine spectators developed cardiac arrest at the game secondary to acute myocardial infarction. Eight

Table 52-1

Year	Spectator	Date	Cardiac arrest	Success-ful CPR	% Success-ful CPR	Chest pain without arrest — MI	Chest pain without arrest — No MI	Follow-up
1965	3		3					No CPR available
1966	W. P.	9/24/66	1	1	100			Expired next day, CVA
	C. S.	10/15/66	1	1	100			Expired 10/68, DOA, E.R.
	W. S.	10/15/66				×		L & W, attends games
	M. W.	10/29/66	1	1	100			L & W, attends games
1967	E. D.	11/4/67	1	1	100			Expired 8/72, Heart ?
	W. S.	11/11/67	1	1	100			Expired 7/68, Heart ?
1968	None							
1969	A. P.	9/21/69	1	1	100			L & W, attends games
	D. T.	10/20/69						
1970	J. C.	10/10/70	1	1	100			L & W, attends games
	E. S.	10/10/70	1	1	100			L & W, attends games
	J. S.	10/10/70					×	
1971	None							
1972	H. H.	10/14/72	1	1	100			Recovery slowed by aspiration
	H. K.	10/28/72	1					Failed to respond to CPR
	J. B.	10/28/72					×	
1973	G. R.	9/22/73					×	Expired 9/73, CVA
	D. A.	9/22/73				×		Signed himself out of hospital
	R. S.	9/22/73						L & W
	J. F.	9/29/73	1	1	100			L & W
Total			13	12	92%			

were successfully resuscitated on a long-term basis. Three of these eight survivors subsequently died 6 months to 2 years later. More detailed information about the results can be seen in Table 52-1.

Comment

In eight years following the initiation of the unit, all but one patient who collapsed at the Memorial Football Stadium were resuscitated. The two major concerns at this time appear to be the ability to maintain (1) continued and effective method of communication between the Red Cross volunteer who initially locates the collapsed spectator and the emergency medical technician who brings the spectator to the fixed unit and (2) effective emergency cardiopulmonary resuscitation of the patient from the time of collapse in the stands to and during transfer to a fixed life-support unit. The solution to these problems was the repeated practice by all volunteers. This improved rapid communication from the Red Cross worker to the emergency medical technician crew. Daily practice by the emergency medical technicians, who are professionals, allowed effective and efficient emergency cardiopulmonary resuscitation of the collapsed spectator while en route to the fixed unit. Because of the success of the current mode of operation we have not seriously contemplated the transportation of a portable ventilation and external massage unit to the spectator in the stands. It would appear that during the commotion and uproar of an exciting football game, the ability to connect one of these units to the patient in the stands would be a formidable task. However, if this were possible, a more efficient form of emergency cardiopulmonary resuscitation might well be executed. At the present time with only one mortality in a very serious cardiac patient and nine successful resuscitations on the other spectators, the management of these people appears adequate. However, it is important to constantly stress the necessity of immediate and continued emergency cardiopulmonary resuscitation and the expeditious transportation of the spectator to a fixed life-support unit within the stadium where definitive cardiopulmonary resuscitation can be administered.

The incidence of development of a serious cardiopulmonary emergency in football spectators was fourteen patients in forty games. The National Collegiate Sports Services indicate that more than 25 million sports fans attend intercollegiate football games per year. Our incidence of serious cardiopulmonary emergency is one out of every 180,000 fans, which would mean that close to 140 spectators develop a cardiopulmonary emergency throughout all collegiate stadiums each fall season. These figures of course do not include high school and professional football stadium spectators. The latter particularly has a high incidence of cardiac emergencies as indicated from the Atlanta report. Judging from our report as well as that of others it would seem appropriate that all major stadiums have a life-support station within the stadium. Certainly all those communities that have a mobile life support unit should manage to incorporate their coverage to include any sports arena, civic auditorium, or racetrack in their area.

Since its inception this project was supported by the Red Cross, Boy Scouts, Lincoln Mobile Heart Team, Bryan Memorial Hospital, University of Nebraska, Nebraska Heart Association, and Lancaster County Medical Society. Some of these institutions have provided funds and others have provided assistance in the education of personnel. Neither federal, state, nor local funds or grants were utilized because this unit was part of a stratified system of management of the acute myocardial suspect within the Lincoln community. Funding must be from and at the community level. Since the people are the recipients of the improved medical care, they should, through tax dollars, provide the bulk of the monetary fundings of such a system in any community.

Chapter 53

ADJUNCTIVE TECHNIQUES AND EQUIPMENT FOR CARDIOPULMONARY RESUSCITATION

Archer S. Gordon

Cardiopulmonary resuscitation (CPR) is a combination of emergency lifesaving measures, which can be divided into *basic life support* and *advanced life support*. These consist of the following A-B-C-D steps:

Cardiopulmonary resuscitation (CPR)

A	Airway	
B	Breathing	Basic life support
C	Circulation	
D	Definitive ℞	
	D Diagnosis	
	D Drugs	Advanced life support
	D Defibrillation	
	D Disposition	

The basic life-support measures (A-B-C) provide artificial ventilation and artificial circulation that can be applied immediately without the need for any adjunctive equipment in cases of cardiac arrest. In the emergency situation, this consists of direct mouth-to-mouth resuscitation and manual external cardiac compression.

Numerous adjunctive techniques and devices have been recommended for use in conjunction with or as replacements for these basic life-support measures. Some of them are useful and some are not. Most of them do *not* increase the effectiveness of CPR. They are *not* required, and emergency arti-ficial ventilation and artificial circulation should not be delayed in order to provide them. They should be used when they become available, if their effectiveness has been demonstrated, and only by individuals who have been specifically trained in their application.

Various adjunctive techniques and devices will be discussed in this chapter. This will include only those that relate to the A-B-C measures. It will not include equipment involved in providing advanced life support (that is, oscilloscopes, electrocardiographs, defibrillators, drugs, telemetry, and so forth). Since the use of adjuncts must be related to the emergency A-B-C measures, it is important to review the basic principles of CPR before discussing these devices.

Principles of cardiopulmonary resuscitation

The primary factors affecting a successful outcome following the application of cardiopulmonary resuscitation are (1) the underlying pathophysiology of the cardiac arrest, (2) the speed of application of CPR, and (3) the effectiveness with which the method is applied. The first factor cannot be altered in the emergency situation; but speed in starting and optimum technique of performance can make the difference between life and death.

The optimum technique for two rescuers is illustrated in Fig. 53-1. The rescuer performing artificial ventilation lifts the patient's

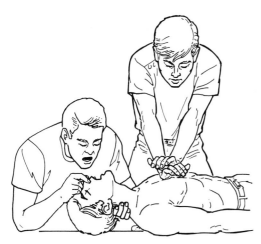

Fig. 53-1. Cardiopulmonary resuscitation (CPR) performed by two rescuers.

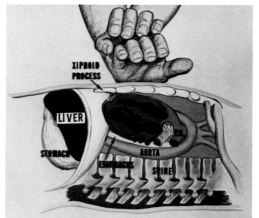

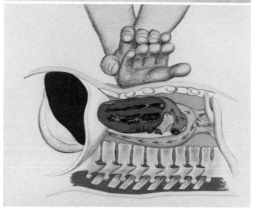

Fig. 53-2. A, Correct hand position for external cardiac compression; **B,** 1½ to 2 inches compression of lower half of sternum.

neck with one hand and tilts the head back into maximum extension with his other hand on the forehead. He seals the nose with his thumb and index finger, takes a deep breath, opens his mouth widely, makes a tight seal with his lips around the patient's mouth, and inflates the lungs until he sees the chest rise. He then removes his mouth and allows the patient to exhale passively while he hears and feels the air escape and watches the chest deflate.

The rescuer performing external cardiac compression positions himself at the patient's side, places the heel of one hand over the lower half of the sternum but not over the xiphoid process, places the other hand on top of the first one, rocks forward so that his shoulders are directly over the chest and, keeping his elbows straight, exerts pressure vertically downward to move the lower sternum 1½ to 2 inches at a rate of once a second. The rescuer performing artificial ventilation "interposes" a breath after each five chest compressions without any pause in compressions.

The hand position and position of the rescuer performing external cardiac compression are of critical importance. His shoulders must be directly over the patient and he must press straight downward to achieve optimum

sternal movement. His fingers must be kept off the chest in order to reduce the incidence of rib fracture. Fig. 53-2, *A,* illustrates the correct hand position and Fig. 53-2, *B,* reveals the importance of not placing the hand on the xiphoid process of the sternum. Pressure here can drive the xiphoid into the liver and result in lethal lacerations.

The circulatory effects of external cardiac compression have been studied extensively on experimental animals in induced ventricular fibrillation. Determinations of blood pressure, blood flow, and cardiac output have indicated that the most effective artificial circulation is achieved with external cardiac compression rates between 60 and

Table 53-1. Results with various techniques for CPR by over 1,000 trainees performing on Resusci-Anne manikins

Two-person CPR				
Compression-ventilation ratio	Compression rate	Ventilations	Achieved	
			Compressions	Ventilations
5:1	60	Interposed	60	12
	60	One-beat pause	45	9
	80	Interposed	80	16
	80	One-beat pause	68	13
15:2	60	Four-beat pause	48	6 (2 × 3)
	80	Four-beat pause	60	8 (2 × 4)

One-person CPR			
Compression-ventilation ratio	Compression rate	Achieved	
		Compressions	Ventilations
10:2	60	40	8
	80	48	10
15:2	60	45	6
	80	54	8
	90	60	8

80 per minute, using a regular, smooth rhythm, with no interruptions for interposing artificial ventilation between each series of 5 compressions.

Comparable studies have been performed on myocardial infarction patients in end-stage cardiogenic shock with ventricular standstill that did not respond to transvenous pacing or in electromechanical dissociation. These patients have been kept alive with prolonged resuscitation and have had arterial and venous lines in place prior to the arrest state. Measurements of stroke volume and cardiac output in duplicate with cardiac green dye during external cardiac compression using manual compression, a manually activated compressor (Rentsch), and a mechanical compressor have revealed comparable values of 30 ml. per stroke with compression rates of both 60 and 80 per minute with all three methods of compression.

The above observations that the stroke volumes are equal with compression rates of 60 and 80 per minute and that optimum flow results from compressions that are uninter-rupted has instigated a comparative study of variations of the standard two-person CPR technique (5:1 compression-ventilation ratio and rate of 60 per minute) and the one-person CPR technique (15:2 compression-ventilation ratio and rate of 60 per minute) using over 1,000 trainees performing on Resusci-Anne manikins. Table 53-1 summarizes the results of that study.

From these findings the following recommendations can be made regarding two-person CPR and one-person CPR:

TWO-PERSON CPR

Optimum compression and ventilation are achieved at a rate of 60 with a 5:1 ratio and breaths interposed without a pause. Theoretically superior results are obtained using a rate of 80 with breaths either interposed or given during one-beat pauses. However, it is very difficult to interpose breaths when a rate of 80 is used so this variation is impractical. The 80 rate with one-breath pauses is more tiring than the 60 rate and promotes interruptions that tend to become extended

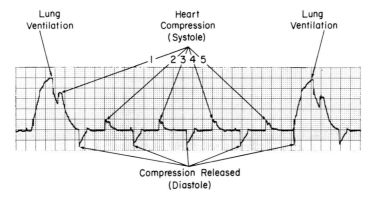

Lung Ventilation   Heart Compression (Systole)   Lung Ventilation

Compression Released (Diastole)

Compression Rate = 60 x /Min
Ventilation Rate = 12 x /Min
Systole : Diastole Ratio = 50 : 50

Fig. 53-3. Airway pressure tracing during CPR performed at a rate of 60 per minute using a 5/1 ratio of compression to ventilation with breaths interposed between each five compressions.

resulting in interruptions in blood flow and lowering the minute rate back toward 60. The 15:2 ratio at a rate of 80 only provides four pairs of two breaths each. Thus, there is less ventilation and the pauses required for these impair circulation.

It has been found that almost all trainees can be taught to interpose breaths using a rate of 60 compressions per minute. This, therefore, is the optimum technique. Fig. 53-3 shows airway pressure tracings taken during two-person CPR at a compression rate of 60 with breaths interposed without a pause after each 5 compressions.*

ONE-PERSON CPR

The use of a 15:2 ratio at a compression rate of 60 per minute is completely inadequate. A 15:2 ratio at a rate of 90 is much more effective but is quickly exhausting. Therefore, the preferred technique for one person should be 15 compressions at a rate of 80 per minute followed by two quick inflations after each 15 compressions.

---

*This is the standard technique recommended by the 1973 National Conference on Standards for Cardiopulmonary Resuscitation (CPR) and Emergency Cardiac Care (ECC).

Special aspects of cardiopulmonary resuscitation

EFFECT OF POSITION ON ARTIFICIAL CIRCULATION

Various techniques have been evolved for performing cardiopulmonary resuscitation in the vertical position under special circumstances, such as cardiac arrest cases with a lineman on a telephone pole, a victim trapped in a vehicle, in a dental chair, or sitting in an inaccessible stadium seat. However, experimental animal studies have indicated that there is no manual technique that is capable of providing any effective blood flow or blood pressure in the carotid arteries when the patient is in the vertical position during cardiac arrest.

Fig. 53-4 illustrates the results with one of eight experimental animals in which comparative studies were performed in the horizontal and the vertical positions during cardiac arrest. Although blood pressure and blood flow in the carotid arteries is little affected by change in position under normal circumstances, when the animals were in induced ventricular fibrillation external cardiac compression provided the usual amounts of flow and pressure in the horizontal posi-

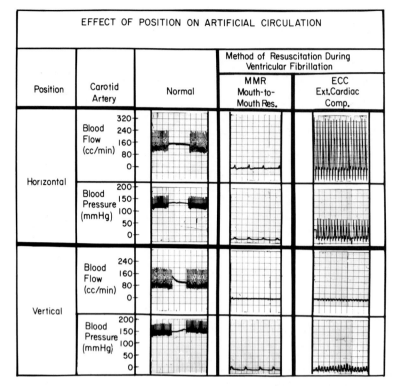

Fig. 53-4. Effect of CPR on blood pressure and blood flow in horizontal and vertical position.

tion, but essentially *no flow or pressure* in the vertical position. Mouth-to-tube resuscitation provided effective ventilation in both positions, but was ineffective in moving blood or providing perfusion pressure in either the horizontal or the vertical position.

This makes it obvious that it is pointless to develop techniques for performing CPR on patients who are in the vertical position. In order to provide blood pressure and flow to the brain, the patient must be placed horizontal under all circumstances before CPR is started.

CPR DURING MOVEMENT OF PATIENT

Ideal management of the cardiac arrest case includes advanced life support at the scene with defibrillation, drug therapy, intravenous fluids, and stabilization prior to movement. However, this is possible only with properly trained and equipped mobile life-support teams. In other instances, it may be necessary to continue cardiopulmonary resuscitation during movement of the patient. This can be best achieved with completely mechanical units for providing artificial ventilation and artificial circulation. These are discussed in detail later in this chapter. When they are not available, it is necessary to continue effective manual CPR during movement to a properly equipped hospital or advanced life-support unit. There are a number of special considerations when this is done (Fig. 53-5).

1. CPR should always be started immediately wherever the patient is located. Two-person CPR using a ratio of 5:1 and a rate of 60 is preferred.

2. A spine board should be used beneath the patient on the wheeled litter. This provides a firm support during CPR. (It can also be used for extrication, movement of patients with possible neck and back injuries, and so on.)

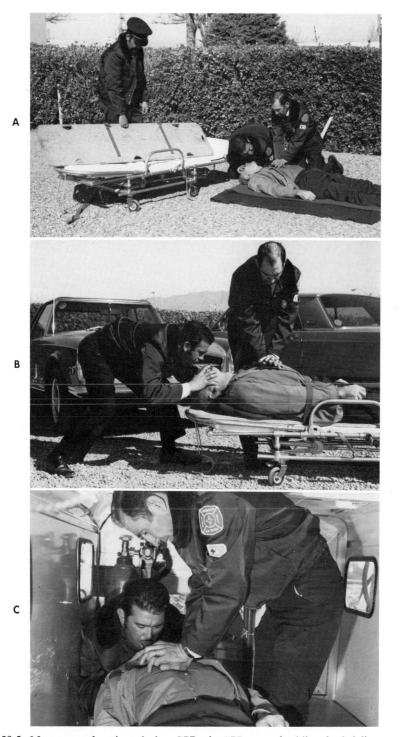

Fig. 53-5. Movement of patient during CPR. **A,** CPR started while wheeled litter and spine board are prepared; **B,** CPR during movement of patient with litter in low position; **C,** CPR in rescue vehicle with rescuer pressing straight downward on patient's sternum.

3. When ready, the patient should be transferred quickly to the wheeled litter, and CPR resumed immediately.

4. The litter should be kept in the low position during movement. This allows proper and adequate external chest compression, provides stability on rough terrain,

and facilitates movement either up or down staircases.

5. The litter should be moved slowly enough to allow effective CPR. Pause briefly at the top or bottom of stairways while continuing effective CPR. Then, at a given signal, CPR should be discontinued while

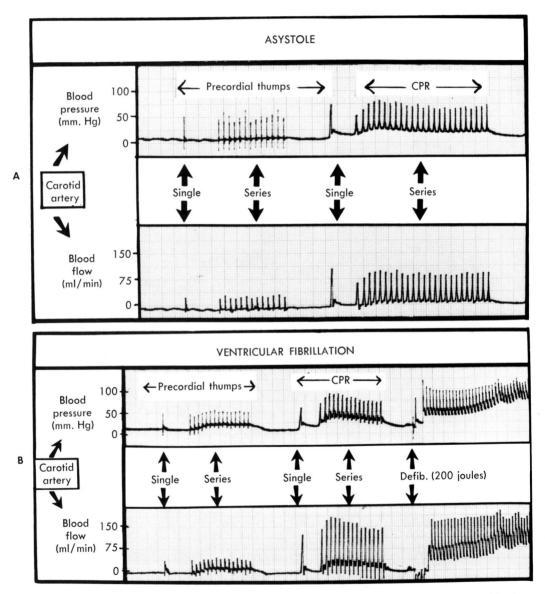

Fig. 53-6. Comparison of effects of single and multiple precordial thumps versus CPR on blood flow and blood pressure. **A,** During asystole; **B,** during ventricular fibrillation.

the patient is moved quickly up or down the stairs. Effective CPR should be resumed immediately at the next level.

6. In the ambulance or rescue vehicle, CPR should be continued by two rescuers whenever possible. If necessary, one-person CPR can be performed. The rescuer performing external cardiac compression must position himself so that he is properly braced to resist movement of the vehicle and has his shoulders directly over the patient so that he can direct his chest pressure vertically downward on the sternum.

MANUAL PRECORDIAL THUMP

An initial thump on the patient's chest with the rescuer's fist is an effective first maneuver in some cases, but its use should be restricted to specific circumstances. Such a blow generates a small electrical stimulus in a heart that is reactive. This may be effective in restoring a beat in cases of heart block or in reversing ventricular tachycardia. However, it is seldom useful for asystole, which is essentially an anoxic phenomenon, and it cannot be depended upon to interrupt or reverse an established ventricular fibrillation.

Human and animal studies have established that a precordial thump also generates a mechanical stimulus, but that this is not as effective as external cardiac compression in producing blood pressure and blood flow in the major arteries (Fig. 53-6, A and B). The important consideration here is not the thump, which can be given quickly, but rather the action taken after the thump. Too often, the patient does not respond immediately and valuable time is lost with repeated thumps, pulse checks, pupil size determination, and a wide assortment of procrastinations. For these reasons, it is recommended that an initial thump on the chest be restricted only to situations where patients are being monitored or where a rescuer actually witnesses a sudden cardiac arrest and appropriate action can be started immediately. When this occurs, the rescuer should perform the following steps in the order indicated and within the first few seconds.

1. Deliver a single, quick, effective precordial thump. To accomplish this, place the fleshy part of the fist over the precordium or lower sternum, flex the elbow, raise the fist 8 to 12 inches off the chest, and rapidly extend the elbow, giving a thud with the fist (Fig. 53-7).

2. If there is no immediate response, tilt the head into maximum extension and give four quick, full lung inflations in rapid succession without allowing time for full deflation between breaths.

3. Quickly palpate the carotid pulse.

4. If carotid pulse is absent, begin external cardiac compression.

5. Continue CPR by one or two rescuers.

In situations other than with monitored patients or witnessed cardiac arrests, CPR should be started as the initial step. It will be equally effective, assures minimal delay, and provides continuing support.

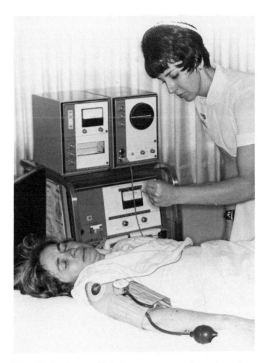

Fig. 53-7. Precordial thump on monitored patient in coronary care unit.

BED BOARD

A firm support should be provided beneath the patient's back when CPR is performed on a bed. This is to prevent loss of the compressive force into an underlying soft mattress. Simple serving trays or supports of comparable size have been recommended, but these are *not* adequate and they must not be relied upon for this purpose. Newer hospital beds have headboards that are removable and can be placed beneath the patient during CPR. To provide adequate support, a bed board should extend from the shoulders to the waist and across the full width of the bed.

Arrangements should be made to have sufficient numbers of properly designed shoulder lifts, headboards, or bed boards at each bed or at strategic locations in the hospital, life-support unit, or rescue vehicle. They should be used as soon as available, but when they are not available, CPR should be started immediately without any delay to seek this adjunct.

Simple airway adjuncts

OROPHARYNGEAL AIRWAY

Oropharyngeal airways are simple devices that should be used on all unconscious patients. They should also be inserted whenever a mask is used in any form on an unconscious patient (mouth-to-mask, bag-valve-mask, mechanical ventilation, anesthesia equipment, and so forth). It keeps the tongue away from the posterior pharyngeal wall and assists in maintaining a patent airway, particularly when fluids collect in this area.

The airway should only be used on unconscious patients. If introduced into a conscious patient, it may promote vomiting. Care and training is required in the placement of the airway because incorrect insertion can displace the tongue into the pharynx and produce airway obstruction. It should be introduced with the tip directed toward the cheek or the hard palate until it enters the pharynx after which it should be rotated 180 degrees.

Various types of oropharyngeal airways are available, but the Berman design, which is shaped like an I beam, is preferred for routine use. All doctors, nurses, and paramedical rescue personnel should be trained in its insertion, and it should be available in infant, child, and adult sizes.

S TUBE

The S tube is a double oropharyngeal airway designed specifically for resuscitation purposes (Fig. 53-8). It can usually be used effectively with only minimal training. It does not provide more effective artificial ventilation, but it does overcome the unaesthetic and possible contagious aspects of direct oral or nasal contact. Its major draw-

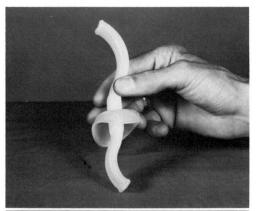

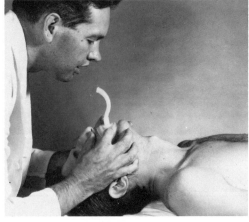

Fig. 53-8. A, S tube; B, S tube in patient's airway for artificial ventilation.

back is difficulty in providing a leakproof seal on some patients, since it is essential to maintain head tilt, jaw elevation, nose seal, and flange seal around lips during mouth-to-tube resuscitation.

MASKS

Well-fitting face masks have proved to be the most effective simple airway adjuncts available for artificial ventilation. The optimal mask may be either a standard anesthesia design or a folding pocket mask (Figs. 53-9, *A,* and 53-10, *A*) and should have the following characteristics: (1) transparent, to allow observation of the color of the lips, the presence of vomitus, and the condensation of exhaled air; (2) easily inflatable

cuff; and (3) available in one average size for adults and additional sizes for infants and children.

Data collected during ventilatory studies on unconscious patients during performance by doctors, nurses, and professional paramedical personnel have revealed that mouth-to-mask ventilation provided greater ventilatory volumes for these nonanesthesiological personnel than did direct mouth-to-mouth or mouth-to-nose resuscitation, or the use of the S tube or bag-valve-mask devices (refer to Table 53-2). The reasons for this are apparent in Figs. 53-9, *B,* and 53-10, *B.* When the rescuer is properly positioned above the patient's head, as shown, he has two hands available to tilt the head back-

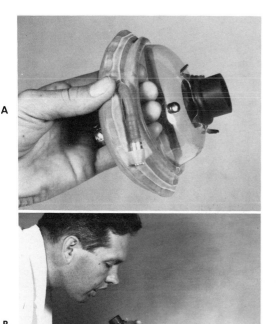

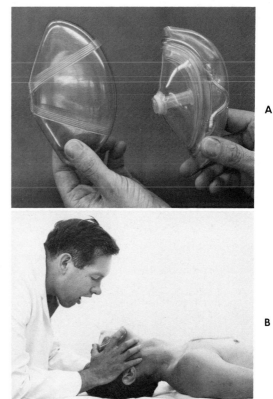

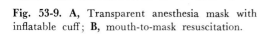

Fig. 53-9. A, Transparent anesthesia mask with inflatable cuff; **B,** mouth-to-mask resuscitation.

Fig. 53-10. A, Transparent folding pocket mask; **B,** mouth-to-mask resuscitation.

Table 53-2. Pulmonary ventilation with artificial respiration*

Ventilatory gas	Ventilatory technique	Ventilatory volumes† (ml./breath) rate: 12/minute
Room air (21% O_2)	Normal resting tidal volume	475
Exhaled air (16% O_2)	Mouth-to-mouth	1125
	Mouth-to-nose	1050
	Mouth-to-S tube	1075
	Mouth-to-mask‡	1200
Room air (21% O_2)	Bag-valve-mask	400
Automatic devices (100% O_2)	Manually-triggered ventilator (Elder)	1350
	Mechanical compression-ventilation unit (HLR) (set at 1200 ml. per breath)	1125

*Mean values for thirty (nonanesthesiologist) professional rescuers (ten M.D.s, ten R.N.s, ten parameds) performing on fifteen anesthetized patients.
†Ventilatory volumes measured on Sanborn Recorder with calibrated pneumograph.
‡Esophageal airway tested on some patients. Ventilatory volumes were slightly greater in all cases where used.

ward, maintain elevation of the mandible and encircle the mask with thumbs and index fingers to provide a leakproof seal. An alternative and equally effective technique is to place all four fingers of both hands beneath the mandible and use the heel of the hands and the thumbs to seat the mask on the face. Use of an oropharyngeal airway beneath the mask enhances ventilation by allowing simultaneous inflation through the patient's mouth and nose.

Mouth-to-mask ventilation can be practiced on most approved resuscitation manikins and should be required for all personnel who will use a mask for mouth-to-mask ventilations.

Gastric distension

All forms of positive pressure lung inflation can produce gastric distension. This applies particularly to those methods that result in high airway pressures and/or high flow rates and includes mouth-to-mouth, mouth-to-nose, and mouth-to-mask ventilation, various mechanical ventilators, and automatic compression-ventilation devices. An awareness of the problem does not necessarily help in preventing its occurrence.

The techniques that produce gastric distension cannot be discarded because they are all useful for providing effective lung ventilation. The gastric distension is a secondary consideration, but it is important because the stomach may become massively distended and produce a number of deleterious effects: (1) the distended stomach elevates both hemidiaphragms, which compresses both lower lungs and reduces the effectiveness of artificial ventilation; (2) the elevated hemidiaphragms may also distort the position of the heart and great vessels and impair venous return; (3) the enlarged stomach compresses intra-abdominal viscera and reduces venous return and ultimately cardiac output; (4) the distended stomach may promote vagal reflexes that are deleterious to the circulation; and (5) the distended stomach is prone to sudden regurgitation, which carries liquid gastric contents into the pharynx followed frequently by aspiration into the tracheobronchial tree. For these reasons, it is desirable to prevent or remedy the gastric distension as quickly as possible. This can be accomplished by: manual decompression, passage of a nasogastric tube, endotracheal intubation, or passage of an esophageal obturator airway.

MANUAL DECOMPRESSION

In the unconscious patient with gastric distension, the stomach can be decompressed manually by the rescuer exerting moderate pressure over the patient's epigastrium with his fingers between the costal margin and the umbilicus. CPR should be interrupted briefly and the patient turned on his side prior to this maneuver so that liquid gastric contents that are expelled with the gas that has been forced into the stomach will not be aspirated into the lungs. This maneuver is very simple in infants and children, and it can also be accomplished in adults. Reaccumulation of gas will occur unless some pressure is maintained in this area or other therapeutic measures are taken.

NASOGASTRIC TUBE

Passage of a nasogastric tube provides a more definitive and lasting effect. This can be accomplished simply by trained medical, nursing, or paramedical personnel, and passage from the nostril to the stomach can be achieved without any interruption in artificial ventilation or artificial circulation. When the nasogastric tube is in place, all air is expelled and further air should not accumulate. A bulb syringe can be used to aspirate the fluid gastric contents.

One criticism of the use of nasogastric tubes for such cases is that the tube may tend to keep the esophagogastric sphincter patent and allow fluids to run up into the pharynx since the patient is in the supine position. However, early passage and rapid decompression of the stomach should eliminate this possibility.

ENDOTRACHEAL INTUBATION

Ventilation of the lungs by direct oral or nasal artificial respiration with or without adjuncts should always be accomplished as quickly as possible and should precede attempts at endotracheal intubation. However, optimal ventilation and prevention of gastric distension are best achieved by endotracheal intubation, and this should be accomplished by trained personnel as soon as practical.

Endotracheal intubation requires a detailed knowledge of the upper airway and extensive training in the nontraumatic and rapid passage of the tubes. Corpses cannot be used for this purpose and even well-designed manikins only provide an introduction and orientation to the trainee. Training can best be accomplished on anesthetized patients prior to surgery or on patients who arrive at the emergency department dead on arrival (D.O.A.) or succumb following cardiopulmonary resuscitation. The training of personnel in intubation for cardiopulmonary resuscitation emergencies is further complicated by the following considerations: (1) It is not sufficient just to train personnel in this technique. The trainee must either have continued and repeated experiences in passing an endotracheal tube or he must be retrained periodically. (2) Well-oxygenated patients prior to surgery can tolerate some delay in intubation, but intubation must be done very quickly on the anoxic cardiopulmonary resuscitation patient.

The effectiveness of bag-valve-mask devices and other adjuncts is enhanced significantly by endotracheal intubation. Oxygen-enriched atmospheres can be delivered via the endotracheal tube and aspiration of liquid gastric contents can be prevented by use of a cuffed tube. However, all of these advantages are thwarted by the problem of adequate training and retraining for significant numbers of the medical, nursing, and paramedical professions.

A simpler technique would be useful and the esophageal obturator airway appears to provide this.

ESOPHAGEAL OBTURATOR AIRWAY

The esophageal obturator airway is a new resuscitation concept. It provides a simple airway adjunct that can be passed with ease following minimal training, provides excellent lung ventilation, and prevents aspiration of gastric contents. The characteristics of the device are shown in Fig. 53-11.

The device is essentially a modified endotracheal tube designed for insertion into the esophagus instead of the trachea. The tube

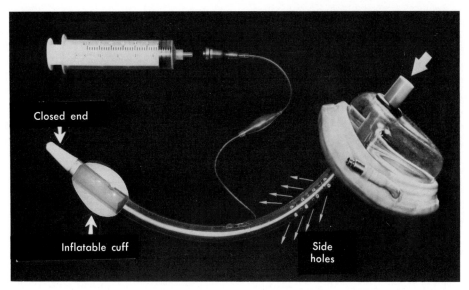

Closed end

Inflatable cuff

Side holes

Fig. 53-11. Esophageal obturator airway. (Brunswick Manufacturing Co., North Quincy, Mass.)

is mounted on a transparent mask that has an inflatable cuff. There is also an inflatable cuff just proximal to a soft rubber obturator, which blocks the distal end of the tube. This cuff is Silastic and distends in a symmetrical fashion when 30 ml. of air is injected from a 30 ml. plastic syringe via a one-way check valve. The syringe can be removed and the air does not escape. A series of sixteen openings are located in the upper third of the tube. The sum of the diameters of these exceeds the diameter of the tube itself.

The esophageal obturator airway is designed for insertion into the esophagus. In contrast to endotracheal intubation, no visualization of the anatomic structures is required. The rescuer merely grasps the mandible between the thumb and index finger of one hand and lifts, as illustrated in Fig. 53-12, *A,* and with the other hand he inserts the tube into the mouth and pharynx and advances it into the esophagus (Fig. 53-12, *B*). The mask is then seated on the face and the rescuer performs mouth-to-airway resuscitation. Since the distal end of the esophageal airway is blocked by the obturator, the air escapes from the openings in the upper portion of the tube and inflates the lungs. Since

the cross-sectional area of the sixteen openings exceeds the cross-sectional area of the tube itself, there is no restriction to inflation. The openings are located in the posterior portion of the mouth and the upper portion of the pharynx, so that even moderate amounts of fluid do not interfere with ventilation.

The tubes are reusable and have the advantages of providing as much ventilation (or slightly more, since air does not pass into the stomach) as mouth-to-mask ventilation (Table 53-2) and of being much easier to introduce than the standard endotracheal tube. Medical, nursing, and paramedical personnel who plan to use the esophageal airway should first train on an anatomically correct adult intubation manikin such as the one shown in Fig. 53-12. It is recommended that they also have additional training on D.O.A. patients, patients who have been anesthetized for surgery, or during actual CPR emergencies. The airway should never be introduced into a conscious patient.

Fig. 53-13 illustrates the anatomical relationships of the esophageal airway after it has been introduced. The mask provides a leakproof seal on the face, the side holes are

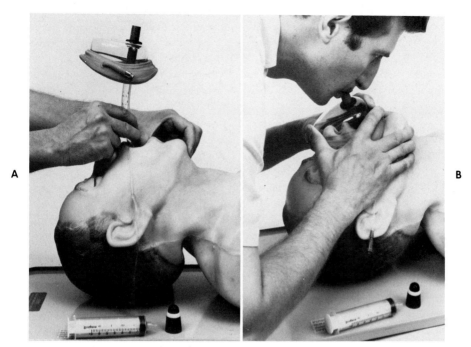

Fig. 53-12. A, Insertion of esophageal obturator airway into adult intubation manikin; **B,** ventilation of manikin via esophageal obturator airway.

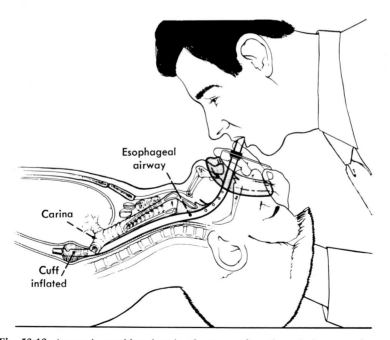

Fig. 53-13. Anatomic considerations in placement of esophageal obturator airway.

located in the mouth and upper pharynx, and the inflated cuff lies distal to the carina of the trachea. This latter observation is of critical importance since inflation of the cuff above the carina could compress the posterior membranous portion of the trachea and produce some obstruction of the airway. The tube is designed so that even with tall individuals, the cuff will always lie below the carina.

It might be anticipated that blind intubation of the esophagus would result in inadvertent intubation of the trachea in some cases, such as occurs with relative frequency during nasogastric intubation. However, this did not occur during preliminary studies of the device by doctors on anesthetized patients, and it has not been reported during over a thousand insertions on actual CPR cases by highly trained paramedical personnel. Apparently, the rescuer senses the position of the larynx and easily directs the curved tube posteriorly into the esophagus. However, it is anticipated that inadvertent tracheal introduction may occur occasionally. As soon as the rescuer introduces the esophageal obturator airway, he immediately seats the mask on the face and inflates the lungs. If the chest rises, the tube is in the esophagus; if the chest does not rise, the tube is in the trachea. In the latter case, it is immediately removed and some other form of artificial ventilation used until it can be replaced properly.

The cuff on the esophageal tube does not need to be inflated prior to starting mouth-to-airway ventilation. The diameter of the tube is such that minimal air passes into the stomach, even before the cuff is inflated. It should be inflated quickly with 30 ml. of air as soon as convenient so that further gastric distension and/or regurgitation of stomach contents do not occur. If regurgitation and aspiration have occurred prior to introducing the esophageal obturator airway, lung ventilation may not be possible due to blockage of the tracheobronchial tree with aspirated material. This situation has occurred clinically on a number of occasions.

The airway is provided with standard fittings so that standard anesthesia equipment, bag-valve-mask devices, and automatic breathing devices can be used for ventilation, if desired. It is important to remember that the mask must be firmly seated on the face when any form of artificial ventilation is being applied. When the patient resumes spontaneous respiration, the mask may be removed, but the tube should be left in place until the patient is reacting or is conscious enough to permit extubation. Supplemental oxygen can be administered into the tube either with or without the mask in place.

The effectiveness of the esophageal obturator airway in preventing regurgitation is demonstrated by the fact that most patients vomit as soon as it is removed. Therefore, it should not be removed until appropriate plans have been made. The patient should be conscious or reactive; he should have been turned on his side; emesis basins should be available; and adequate suction should be present to clear the airway if necessary. The cuff on the esophageal airway should always be deflated prior to its removal.

Some individuals desire to decompress the stomach prior to removal of the esophageal airway. This can be accomplished in one of two ways:

(1) A nasogastric tube can be passed to the area of the cuff in the esophagus. The cuff can then be temporarily deflated while the nasogastric tube is passed into the stomach, and then reinflated while the stomach is being decompressed.

(2) In the unconscious patient, an endotracheal tube can be introduced while the esophageal obturator airway remains in place. After the cuff on the endotracheal tube has been inflated, the esophageal airway can be removed without any hazard of aspiration of stomach contents.

The esophageal obturator airway is available in one adult size only. Experience to date has not indicated any need for several sizes. As mentioned previously, the tube size does not overdistend any normal adult, flaccid esophagus. The inflatable cuff always lies central to the carina of the trachea even in tall individuals. In small or short patients, it lies deeper in the esophagus, but not in the stomach. The cuff should be inflated with only 30 ml. of air. This does not overdistend the esophagus.

Damage to the esophagus has not been reported in over a thousand clinical uses of the esophageal airway by well-trained medical, nursing, and paramedical personnel on cardiopulmonary resuscitation cases. However, the mucosa and wall of the esophagus are delicate and it is only reasonable to assume that rapid and careless introduction in an emergency situation by less than well-trained personnel may result in damage to this structure in some cases. This should not occur with proper training and care and it should not be a deterrent to use of the airway. It is estimated that 40% to 60% of patients vomit at some time during their resuscitative emergencies. Many potentially successful rescues are lost because of this, and it is reasonable to assume that numerous lives can be saved by the early and proper application of this device.

Foreign body obstruction of the airway

Foreign body obstruction of the airway is common in both children and adults. Mucus, blood, pus, or small particulate matter can be quickly removed from the upper airway by gauze-covered fingers or effective suction devices. However, solitary foreign bodies such as food, candy, gum, dental work, marbles, or beads pose much graver problems.

Upper airway obstruction usually results from a foreign body being lodged either at the base of the tongue just above the epiglottis, or just below the epiglottis at the entrance to the larynx above the vocal cords. (Refer to Fig. 53-19.) The response varies in accordance with the size of the foreign body. When these are small, the patient usually chokes, gags, or coughs in an effort to expel them. This is a normal physiological mechanism and he should be neither assisted nor restrained during these efforts at expulsion. When the foreign body is a large piece of food, it completely blocks the upper air passage, and is unable to be either swallowed or coughed up. The patient's efforts may be further impaired by the depressant effects of alcoholic intake prior to eating.

Foreign body obstructions are not usually present in most resuscitative emergencies and the rescuer should not take time to seek them initially. He should start artificial ventilation and his first efforts will indicate whether or not airway obstruction is present. If present, he can then attempt to remove the obstruction. However, when it is known or strongly suspected that foreign body obstruction exists, the initial emergency measure should be to remove it.

The victim's mouth should be opened widely and one or two fingers swept back towards the base of the tongue and the epiglottis. This action should be deeply into the throat and from one side to the other in an attempt to dislodge and withdraw any large foreign bodies. It is estimated that there are several thousand deaths in the United States each year from this cause, and that many of them result from pieces of food large enough to be grasped and removed in this manner.

Smaller foreign bodies usually cannot be removed with this action of the fingers. Their presence in the throat promotes reflex spasm of the vocal cords and muscles of the upper airway. When this occurs in children, the child should be picked up and inverted over one arm of the rescuer while he delivers firm blows over the spine between the shoulder blades with the heel of the other hand. After a brief series of blows the child should be placed supine and attempts at mouth-to-mouth ventilation repeated. In some cases, the airway is only partially obstructed and slow, forceful inflations may be effective in providing enough ventilation to partially inflate the lungs and sustain the patient until he recovers or more definitive action can be taken. If unable to be adequately ventilated, the child should again be inverted and firm blows delivered over the spine. In many of these situations, the key to success is persistence. This is because, when the patient becomes more anoxic, the muscles of the throat relax and it may then be possible to dislodge a foreign body that was previously impacted by muscular spasm.

This same maneuver can be used for adults. They should be rolled toward the rescuer onto their side so that firm blows can be delivered with the heel of the rescuer's hand over the spine between the shoulder blades. Repeated attempts at forceful ventilation followed by additional firm blows on the back are useful.

Various types of adjunctive equipment have been developed and recommended to cope with foreign body obstruction situations. Some of them are ineffectual or dangerous, and most of them are usually not available when and where needed. However, some of these adjuncts may be useful in the emergency room and/or in advanced life-support units. Fig. 53-14 shows several simple devices that are recommended for extrication of foreign bodies from the supralaryngeal area.

The instrument at the top of Fig. 53-14 is a plastic Choke Saver and has been promoted widely. However, the plastic construction is flimsy, the tongs are curved excessively, and at their tips there are several sharp barbs. It has been demonstrated that this device is easily broken and it is felt that its use would be hazardous, particularly by nonmedical and paramedical personnel.

The long, slightly curved hemostat and the broad-tipped Russian forceps shown at the middle and bottom of Fig. 53-14 are more practical instruments for such emergencies. If a patient with a foreign body obstruction is placed in the supine position with his head elevated and tilted backwards, a rescuer positioned at the top of his head can use a tongue blade to depress the base of the tongue forcefully in order to visualize the area of the epiglottis and remove a foreign body under direct vision with the curved hemostat or the broad-tipped forceps.

When total or near-total obstruction of the upper airway persists as a result of foreign body obstruction, macroglossia, edema of the larynx or chords, acute laryngotracheobronchitis, and so forth, it may be necessary to

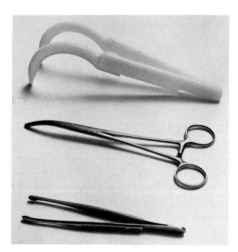

Fig. 53-14. Instruments for removing foreign body obstruction from upper airway. Top, Choke Saver. Middle, long curved hemostat. Bottom, broad-tipped forceps.

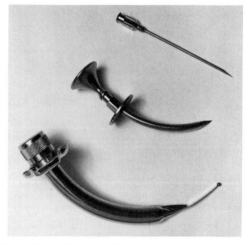

Fig. 53-15. Top, needle for needle tracheotomy. Middle, cricothyrotome. Bottom, tracheotome.

establish a direct passage into the trachea below the vocal cords. The use of needles or special knives or tubes has been recommended for this by some. Fig. 53-15 shows a large bore needle, a cricothyrotome, and a tracheotome, which are available for this purpose.

NEEDLE TRACHEOTOMY

For some time, many physicians and nurses have carried a large caliber hollow-bore needle (No. 12) for use in establishing a needle tracheotomy when required in cases of airway obstruction. Their thesis was that this could be quickly thrust into the trachea and would allow the patient to breathe spontaneously until further action could be taken (Fig. 53-16). In an attempt to substantiate this, arterial blood gas studies were performed on a series of 40 to 50 pound experimental animals with endotracheal tubes that were totally obstructed. When a No. 12 needle was inserted into the trachea, the arterial P_{O_2} fell to 66 mm. Hg in 3 minutes and continued down to a P_{O_2} of 50 at the end of 5 minutes, and thereafter. The P_{CO_2} rose to 55 and the pH to 7.58 at 5 minutes

and thereafter. A comparable study performed with a No. 8 needle showed that the P_{O_2}, P_{CO_2} and pH remained at essentially normal levels when animals of this size were used. However, three No. 12 needles were required to maintain normal blood gas levels in this size animal, and it is reasonable to assume that three No. 8 needles would be required to achieve the same for an average size adult. This makes the technique impractical, especially when one considers the potentiality for damage to adjacent structures when introducing this number of large-gauge needles in an emergency situation. This danger is further amplified in the following section.

TRACHEOTOMES AND CRICOTHYROTOMES

Realization of the ineffectiveness of needle tracheotomy led to the development of cricothyrotomes and tracheotomes that could be quickly forced into the trachea and would provide a more adequate opening. These are pictured in Fig. 53-15 and the application of a tracheotome is demonstrated in Fig. 53-17. The tracheotome consists of a metal cannula in which is housed a trocar

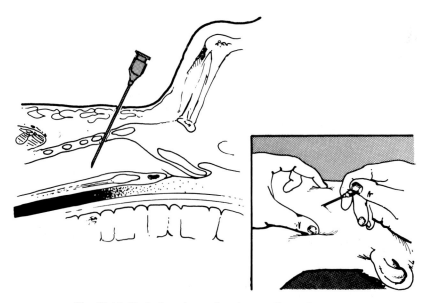

Fig. 53-16. Technique for performing needle tracheotomy.

that carries a short, sharp blade terminating in a small metal ball. For introduction of the tracheotome, a large-caliber, slotted needle is first thrust into the trachea (Fig. 53-17, *A*). The ball on the trocar is introduced into the slot on the needle and, as the tracheotome is advanced, the ball slides down the slot. As the blade follows the ball it incises the skin, the underlying structures, and finally the trachea itself (Fig. 53-17, *B*). The trocar with blade and ball is then removed leaving the cannula in place in the trachea (Fig. 53-17, *C*).

The theory and the design of this equipment are excellent, but there is a serious flaw with use of the device. The trocar is smaller and fits inside the cannula. Therefore, there is a bulge or enlargement where the trocar emerges from the cannula. During insertion, the incision made by the blade is large enough to admit the trocar—but not the cannula. In order to pass the cannula through the incision in the skin, which is smaller than the diameter of the cannula, an extra force or thrust must be exerted. When the skin gives way, the entire instrument is driven posteriorly. Sometimes it is driven into the esophagus, and tracheoesophageal fistulae result. Sometimes it is driven into the carotid artery, and exsanguinating hemorrhage results. And, sometimes it is driven into the apices of the lungs

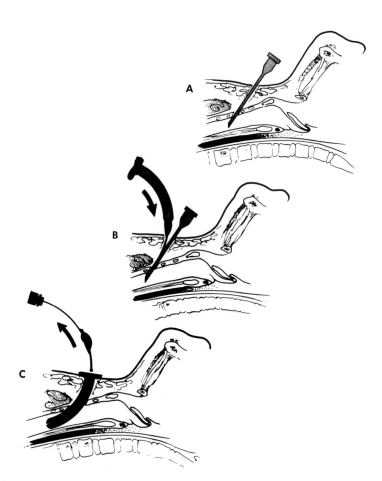

Fig. 53-17. Technique for use of tracheotome. **A,** Insertion of slotted needle; **B,** insertion of tracheotome obturator; **C,** removal of tracheotome obturator.

resulting in pneumothoraces. We have seen patients with all of these complications from use of tracheotomes, and occasionally multiple complications of this type have been observed in the same patient.

Accordingly, it is recommended that this type of device *not* be used. The same flaw and objection exists as regards cricothyrotomes with the same design features.

EMERGENCY TRACHEOTOMY

If these relatively simple instruments are hazardous and should not be used, is it reasonable to recommend emergency tracheotomy for the type of upper airway obstruction described above?

The steps in a routine emergency tracheotomy are illustrated in Fig. 53-18. This procedure can be truly lifesaving when an individual is in acute respiratory distress and it is imperative to establish an improved airway. However, in the emergency CPR situation in which the patient is severely anoxic and probably unconscious from total upper airway obstruction and in whom time has already been spent attempting artificial ventilation, sweeping the fingers through the throat, pounding on the back, making further attempts at ventilation, and so forth, there is not sufficient time to perform an emergency tracheotomy. Those who have had experience realize the problems of adequate instrumentation, light, suction, retraction, bleeding, and so on that can beset this procedure. To attempt it at "the end of the line" of a CPR emergency is less than prudent. A simpler and easier procedure under these circumstances is emergency cricothyrotomy.

CRICOTHYROTOMY

The basic anatomy of the upper airway is illustrated in Fig. 53-19. It can be readily

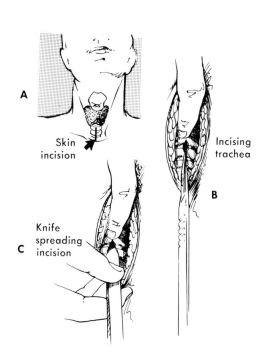

Fig. 53-18. Steps in emergency tracheotomy.

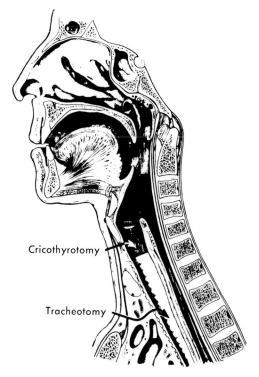

Fig. 53-19. Anatomic considerations in cricothyrotomy and tracheotomy.

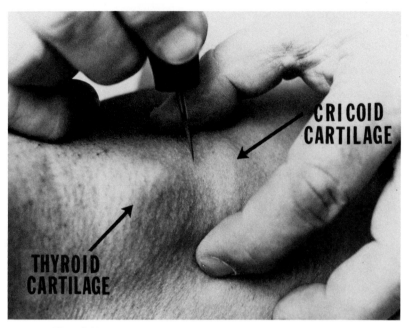

Fig. 53-20. Technique for performing emergency cricothyrotomy.

appreciated that the airway lies closer to the surface in the laryngeal area than anywhere else in the system. The closest access to this area from the outside is between the thyroid cartilage (Adam's apple) and the cricoid cartilage just beneath it. In this area, only skin, subcutaneous tissue, and the cricothyroid membrane separate the airway from the surface. An opening in this area avoids the vascular structures, thyroid gland, muscles, and subcutaneous tissues that separate the skin from the trachea in the area of classic tracheotomy.

A logical question may be why this area is not used routinely instead of performing emergency or elective tracheotomies lower in the air passage. The answer is that the cricothyroid membrane tends to stenose following removal of a cannula that is left in place over 8 to 12 hours. Accordingly, cricothyrotomy should only be used in a desperate situation, and it should be converted to a standard tracheotomy as soon thereafter as possible.

For performing an emergency cricothy-

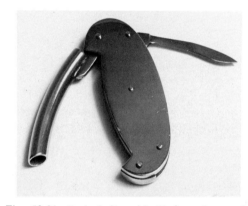

Fig. 53-21. Pocketknife with blade and cannula for emergency cricothyrotomy.

rotomy, a support should be placed beneath the patient's shoulders so that his neck is extended. As illustrated in Fig. 53-20, the skin between the thyroid and cricoid cartilages should be stretched and secured, after which a sharp scalpel blade or knife should be inserted about 1 to 1½ inches. A cannula measuring $\frac{3}{16}$ to $\frac{1}{4}$ inch should then be inserted.

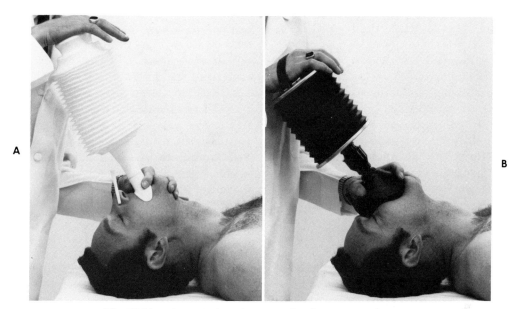

Fig. 53-22. Bellows devices. **A,** Res-Q-aire; **B,** Kreiselman bellows.

Fig. 53-21 shows a pocketknife with cricothyrotomy cannula that can be carried by rescue-conscious personnel.

Mechanical adjuncts for artificial ventilation and CPR

Acceptance and widespread application of CPR has resulted in the development of a number of mechanical devices for emergency artificial ventilation and cardiopulmonary resuscitation. These include: bellows, bag-valve-mask units, automatic breathing devices, and automatic devices for cardiopulmonary resuscitation.

BELLOWS

During the past several years, plastic bellows devices have made their appearance and have been promoted widely to the public through over-the-counter sales in drug stores and department stores. They apparently have a great appeal to the public, but they are almost useless in actual practice. The unit shown in Fig. 53-22, *A,* has an adequate capacity, but the noseclip is ineffective in blocking escape of air; the flange around

the lips does not provide a leakproof seal; the bite-block that is inserted into the mouth results in trauma to the lips, teeth, tongue, and gums; there is no valving system so it is necessary to remove the device from the mouth after each breath to allow for exhalation; and inflation of the lungs requires the hand to cover an open port at the upper end of the bellows during each inflation. Aside from these completely unacceptable design features, the basic ventilatory concept is wrong. One hand is pulling up the lower jaw, while the other hand is pushing down on the bellows. This antagonism results in inadequate ventilation. Furthermore, it is a virtual impossibility for the one hand of the rescuer to provide simultaneous head tilt, elevation of the mandible, and a leakproof seal of the flange around the lips.

The design is poor and the basic concept is incorrect. Bellows devices of this type should not be used. This unit and similar ones have been removed from the market by action of the U.S. Food and Drug Administration on several occasions during the past few years.

A well-designed unit with rubber bellows and mask is illustrated in Fig. 53-22, *B*. This was widely stockpiled by the military services during World War II, but it never received widespread use. Although it has an adequate volume and is provided with a well-fitting face mask with an inflatable cuff and a valving system for escape of exhaled air, it is also a relatively useless device. Again, the basic concept is wrong, and it is difficult for everyone except experienced professional anesthesiologists to provide a good mask seal with one hand tilting the head, elevating the mandible, and holding the mask on the face. It is also completely impractical to be pushing the bellows down with one hand and trying to hold the mandible up and the head back with the other hand. Comparative studies of the actual ventilatory volumes achieved with these units when used on unconscious, anesthetized patients by trained (nonanesthesiologist) doctors, nurses, and professional paramedical personnel revealed values of less than the normal resting tidal volumes and rates, which averaged between four and six per minute.

This well-designed unit only further enhances the observation that bellows devices are inadequate and should never be used.

BAG-VALVE-MASK VENTILATORS

Bag-valve-mask ventilators are manually operated, self-inflating units for providing artificial ventilation. There are at least six to eight well-entrenched units on the market, and these provide wide variations of the optimum features.

Bag-valve-mask units can be recommended if: (1) they are properly designed to provide high concentrations of inhaled oxygen, (2) if they are actually used with supplemental oxygen, and (3) if their use is restricted to highly trained professional personnel. Bag-valve-mask devices do *not* provide any more ventilation than direct mouth-to-mouth (or nose), mouth-to-adjunct, or various mechanical ventilatory devices. A review of the data in Table 53-2 clearly reveals that medical, nursing, and professional paramedical personnel who are not anesthesiologists achieve ventilatory volumes with the bag-valve-mask that are less than the normal resting tidal volumes of the test subjects and only about one third as much as is achieved with exhaled air methods and with automatic breathing devices.

The low values achieved with the bag-valve-mask units are related to several factors. One of these is the skill required to maintain the head in extension, to keep the mandible elevated, and to secure an optimum mask fit, all with one hand while the other hand is squeezing the bag. This can only be achieved by highly trained physicians, nurses, and such professional paramedical personnel as inhalation therapists, EMTs, and so forth, who receive extensive training on manikins and actual patients, and who maintain their capability by continuous practice or periodic retraining. Other factors are the volume of the bag and the size of the hand squeezing it. Some commerical bag-valve-mask units only have a volume of 1,000 ml. and even this volume cannot be provided since it is impossible to completely empty the bag with each squeeze. Even where the bag is larger, operators with small hands are restricted in the amount of ventilation that they can deliver. More effective ventilation with a bag-valve-mask can be achieved by using two rescuers, one to hold the bag, and one to squeeze it. Other than using two rescuers, the problem of achieving effective ventilation with a bag-valve-mask device can only be solved by endotracheal intubation. The problems associated with this have been discussed previously.

Since these units do not provide optimum ventilatory volumes, their purpose should be to provide oxygen enrichment and to have them available for use when endotracheal intubation has been accomplished. Inhaled oxygen concentrations of 50% or over should be delivered. These can only be attained by attaching to the intake valve a reservoir tube with a capacity equal to the tidal volume and an oxygen inflow rate greater than the delivered minute ventilation.

A complete discussion of the features of various bag-valve-mask units is beyond the scope of this chapter. However, most of the ideal features are illustrated by the unit in Fig. 53-23. An ideal bag-valve-mask should have the following characteristics:

1. Transparent mask, to allow visualization of the lips, observe for presence of vomitus, and see condensate on inside of mask during patient's exhalation
2. Inflatable cuff on mask to assure leakproof seal
3. Truly nonrebreathing valve
4. No pop-off valve, except in pediatric models
5. Flex tube between mask and bag to provide greater mobility and enhance emptying of the bag
6. Self-inflating bag that is transparent or semitransparent
7. Available in adult and pediatric sizes
8. No sponge rubber inside of self-inflating bag because of difficulty in cleaning, disinfecting, and eliminating ethylene oxide
9. Delivers high concentrations of oxygen with the oxygen inlet at the back of the bag or via an oxygen reservoir
10. Oxygen reservoir that assures high inhaled concentrations of oxygen
11. Provided with an oropharyngeal airway
12. Provided with standard 15 mm. fittings
13. Can be used with or without head straps
14. Statisfactory for practice on manikins

OXYGEN-POWERED AUTOMATIC BREATHING DEVICES

Automatic breathing devices that are activated by oxygen can be classified on the basis of their cycling mechanism into pressure-cycled ventilators, time-cycled ventilators, and volume-cycled ventilators.

Automatic pressure-cycled ventilators (resuscitators) can be programmed to deliver either intermittent positive pressure breathing (IPPB) or positive-negative pressure breathing (PNPB) (see Fig. 53-24, *A*). They are available as emergency models for rescue work and as hospital models for inhalation therapy. These devices are effective for providing artificial respiration or assisted breathing. However, they should *never* be used in conjunction with external cardiac compression because effective cardiac compression elevates the airway pressure to the cycling level and triggers termination of the inflation cycle of the device prematurely, producing shallow and insufficient ventilation. The instantaneous flow rates of these units are usually inadequate and attempts to ventilate between series of external cardiac compressions results in long and unwarranted interruptions in CPR.

Oxygen-powered manually triggered (time-

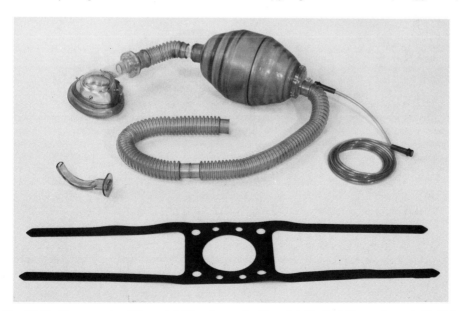

Fig. 53-23. Components of Resusci-folding bag unit. (Laerdal Medical Corp., Armonk, N. Y.)

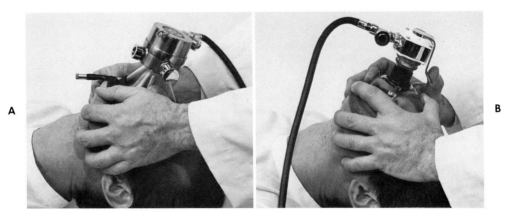

Fig. 53-24. A, Pressure-cycled resuscitator; **B,** manually triggered (time-cycled) resuscitator.

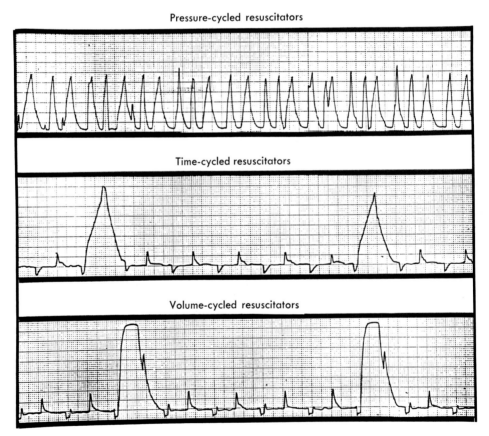

Fig. 53-25. Automatic breathing devices with external cardiac compression (airway pressure tracings).

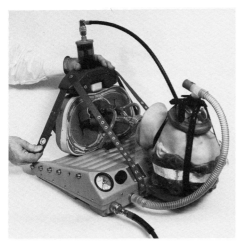

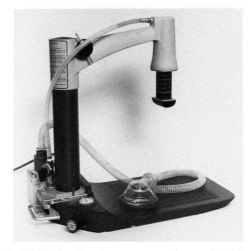

Fig. 53-26. Heart-lung resuscitator. (Courtesy Brunswick Manufacturing Co., North Quincy, Mass.)

Fig. 53-27. Cardiopulmonator resuscitator. (Michigan Instruments, Grand Rapids, Mich.)

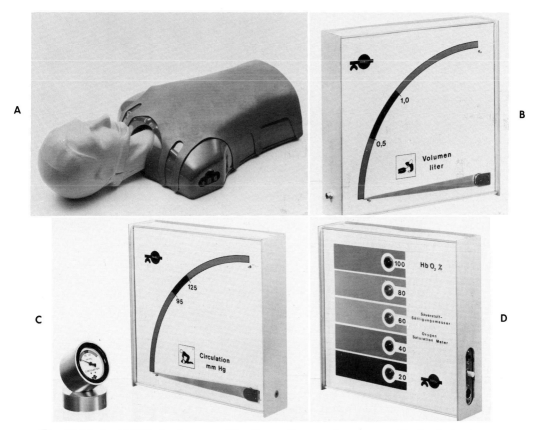

Fig. 53-28. A, AMBU simulator manikin; B, ventilatory volume meter; C, circulation meter; D, Hb O₂ meter.

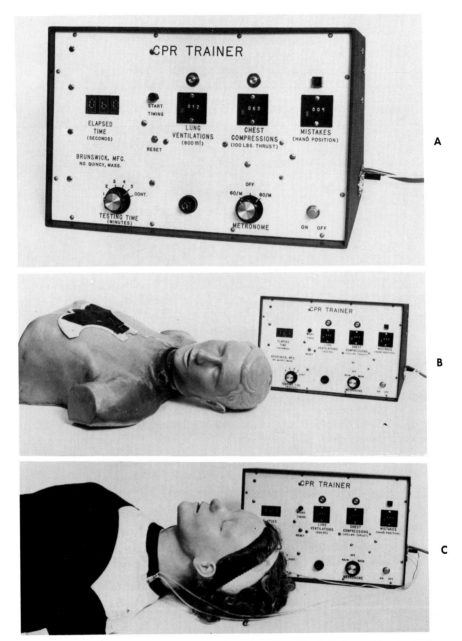

Fig. 53-29. A, CPR Trainer (Brunswick Manufacturing Co., North Quincy, Mass.) which can be adapted to a CPR-Mani manikin, **B,** or a standard Resusci-Anne manikin, **C.** It provides auditory time signal as well as signal lights and digital counter indicating correct chest compression, correct lung ventilation, and mistakes in hand position. Trainee can be timed for various periods and receives grades at end of performance. Can be adapted for self-instruction purposes.

cycled) automatic ventilators are acceptable for artificial respiration alone or in conjunction with external cardiac compression if they are capable of providing instantaneous flow rates of 100 liters per minute, or more, for adults (Fig. 53-24, *B*). A safety valve release pressure of 50 cm. of water should be provided. Ideally, these ventilators should permit the use of high concentrations of oxygen and support of the airway and mask with both hands. For use on infants and small children, specialized mechanical breathing devices producing lower flow rates are required.

Volume-cycled resuscitators include mouth-to-mouth and bag-valve-mask techniques in which cycling depends upon the volume delivered being adequate to cause the chest to rise. Most mechanical volume-cycled ventilators are used for paralyzed, apneic, or critical respiratory care patients who are sustained in controlled respiration. The only unit for CPR that is volume-cycled is the HLR (heart-lung resuscitator), which provides adjustable volume and cycled ventilation interposed between each five chest compressions of a mechanical compression-ventilation unit. It is discussed in a subsequent section of this chapter.

The actual airway pressure tracings obtained with these three types of resuscitators are illustrated in Fig. 53-25. This illustrates the ineffectiveness of ventilation achieved with pressure-cycled resuscitators when used in conjunction with external cardiac compression.

Mechanical devices for external cardiac compression

MANUALLY ACTIVATED CHEST COMPRESSORS

Simple, hinged, manually-operated mechanical chest compressors can be used for effective external cardiac compression. They should provide an adjustable stroke of 1½ to 2 inches and be capable of application with only 5-second interruptions in manual CPR. Such devices are relatively inexpensive and make it easier for one individual to provide prolonged effective external cardiac compression, but they have the disadvantage that a second rescuer is required to provide simultaneous interposed artificial ventilation.

AUTOMATIC DEVICES FOR CARDIOPULMONARY RESUSCITATION

As indicated previously, optimum life support should provide stabilization and definitive therapy for the patient prior to movement. However, until adequately trained and

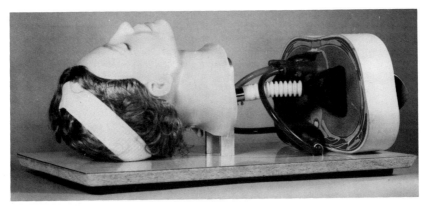

Fig. 53-30. Anatomic Resusci-Anne has features that allow observation of blood flow in circulatory system during external cardiac compression and interposed ventilations of lungs between chest compression. (Laerdal Medical Corp., Armonk, N. Y.)

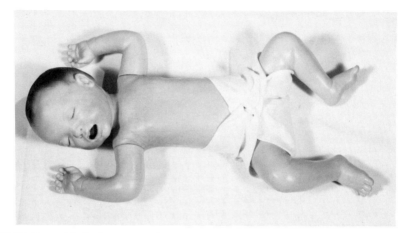

Fig. 53-31. Resusci-Baby has normal infant proportions that allow mouth-to-mouth and mouth-to-nose resuscitation, external cardiac compression, and cardiopulmonary resuscitation to be performed. Air can be blown into stomach and cause distension. (Laerdal Medical Corp., Armonk, N. Y.)

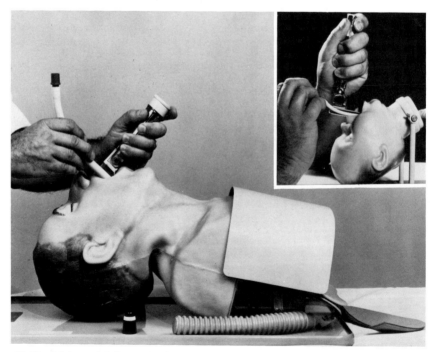

Fig. 53-32. Adult and infant intubation manikins. Anatomic upper airway structures permit complete visualization during endotracheal intubation. On adult model, larynx can be replaced, lungs can be inflated, stomach is also provided. This manikin is also useful for practicing intubation of the esophagus with the esophageal airway. (Laerdal Medical Corp., Armonk, N. Y.)

equipped advanced life-support units are available, it will continue to be necessary at times to use mechanical compression/ventilation devices to sustain patients until advanced life support is available (See Figs. 53-26 and 53-27.)

These machines perform both artificial ventilation and artificial circulation mechanically. They are no more effective than the manual methods, and they should only be used when they become available after the manual technique has been started. However, where prolonged CPR or continued CPR during movement of the patient is required, they provide the facilities required for this. The units should, wherever possible, provide as many of the A-B-C features as possible, and according to the standards detailed for the manual methods. They should be portable, self-contained, oxygen-activated, operate on both tanked or wall oxygen sources, provide independently adjustable ventilation

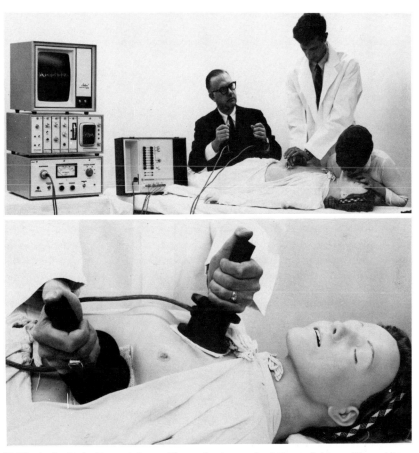

Fig. 53-33. Arrhythmia Resusci-Anne. Uses a basic standard Resusci-Anne. Chest skin overlay used for practice of DC defibrillation or elective cardioversion. Electronic heart can be used with any standard DC defibrillator, oscilloscope, and monitoring equipment. Allows selection of normal sinus rhythm, first degree block, second degree block, third degree block, auricular fibrillation, auricular flutter, ventricular tachycardia, ventricular fibrillation, ventricular asystole, PACs and PVCs at the option of operator. Trainees can perform artificial ventilation, artificial circulation, defibrillation, and an infusion arm is available for drug injection practice, if desired. (Laerdal Medical Corp., Armonk, N. Y.)

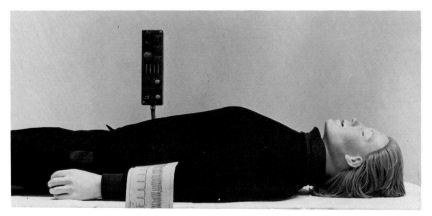

Fig. 53-34. Recording Resusci-Anne. Involves a completely different internal mechanism for artificial ventilation and artificial circulation. Lights on box denote correct ventilation, correct compression, and mistakes in hand position. Internal strip chart simultaneously records ventilation, compression, and mistakes, and provides permanent written record.

and compression, allow defibrillation of the heart without interruption in mechanical CPR, be capable of application with only 5-second interruptions in manual CPR, and be adequately secured to the patient to prevent malposition of the compressor plunger during movement of the patient.

When an automatic mechanical CPR device is used, one rescuer must always remain at the patient's head to monitor plunger action and ventilation continuously, as well as to check the pulse and pupils, to support head tilt and mask fit manually, and to assure adequate ventilatory exchange via mask or endotracheal tube. External cardiac compression must always be started with the manual method first. Medical and paramedical personnel who will be using the automatic equipment must have careful and extensive training and manikin practice in the manual method, the mechanical method, and the proper technique for changing from the former to the latter.

Training devices for cardiopulmonary resuscitation

Optimum performance of CPR can only follow adequate training. Since CPR is a team activity, it should be taught to teams of trainees at all levels, whenever possible. CPR should be taught in the schools and to as many members of the general public as possible. Professional paramedical trainees must ultimately be instructed in advanced life support as well as basic life support. At the hospital level, it is recommended that every hospital be required to have a CPR committee, consisting of a surgeon, anesthesiologist, cardiologist, nurse, and administrator, charged with the responsibility of providing CPR teams in the hospital on a 24-hour-a-day basis.

There are many essentials of adequate training programs in CPR. The most important are well-designed manikins that allow proper training and practice in all of the basic principles. Manikins that are acceptable for training in cardiopulmonary resuscitation must have the following minimum characteristics:

1. Obstruction of the airway when the neck is flexed and patency of the airway when the neck is extended
2. Proper rise and fall of the chest associated with inflation through the mouth or nose (mouth and nose for infant or child)
3. One and one-half to 2 inches movement of the lower sternum and thorax when 80 to 100 pounds of pressure are applied

4. A carotid pulse synchronous with external cardiac compression, an advantageous but not essential feature

These features, plus a number of additional ones, are provided by various manikins and training aids that are currently available and acceptable. They are illustrated in Figs. 53-28 to 53-34 in order for the instructor and trainee to be aware of what is available.

PART SEVEN

POSTRESUSCITATIVE CARE

Chapter 54

POSTRESUSCITATIVE CARE: GENERAL CONSIDERATIONS

Attention is now directed to the period following resuscitation of the heart. In many instances, the diagnosis will have been promptly made and correct resuscitative measures will have been sufficiently carried out. If such is the case, the patient should require little further care and no discernible change will be noted except for the thoracotomy incision if the heart was directly massaged. On the other hand, the postresuscitative period may often demand considerable judgment and ability. This chapter will emphasize certain important points in the postresuscitative care of the patient.

Postresuscitation shock

Postresuscitation shock presents one of the greatest challenges in cardiopulmonary resuscitation. Of the many patients successfully resuscitated, a large percentage succumb in the postresuscitative shock period. It is also in this area that a great deal of investigation is being conducted. The numerous reports by Del Guercio merit careful reading.

Cohn and associates discuss cardiovascular dynamics in high cardiac output shock associated with hypotension and inadequate tissue perfusion in a group of thirty-eight patients. Five of these represent postcardiac resuscitation cases. The syndrome of high cardiac output shock was characterized by an elevated cardiac index, rapid mean circulation time, low total peripheral resistance, high mean systolic ejection rate, and diminished effective oxygen transport. The syndrome resulted in death in every instance.

It is not an uncommon experience to have resuscitated an acutely arrested heart and subsequently be faced with the problem of maintaining an adequate peripheral blood pressure even though cardiac action appears adequate. We have frequently resorted to the use of norepinephrine (Levophed) or other vasopressors following the resuscitation of the acutely arrested heart when hypotension remains. The effectiveness of norepinephrine results from its almost immediate action, its low toxicity, its elevation of both the systolic and diastolic pressures without significant change in the cardiac output, its absence of coronary artery constriction, and its action arising from and mediated by normal physiologic mechanisms—all in marked contradistinction to the effect of epinephrine. There is some evidence that norepinephrine may cause a striking rise in the oxygen tension in areas of myocardial ischemia in those patients with coronary artery obstruction. The incidence of ectopic beats is rare with norepinephrine. It should be administered in 5% dextrose in distilled water or 5% dextrose in saline solution. It is usually recommended that it not be given with whole blood or plasma. The blood pressure should be checked every 2 minutes from the time the drug is started until the desired blood pressure is obtained, and then about every 5 minutes after administration of the drug has begun. The patient should never be left unattended while receiving norepinephrine.

Epinephrine, on the other hand, acts as an overall vasodilator and causes hypertension only by an increase of cardiac output. There is less CNS effect with norepinephrine than with epinephrine. Its hyperglycemic action is much less than epinephrine. Its safety ratio is estimated to be four times that of epinephrine.

Serial ECG and EEG tracings

When abnormalities are seen on the routine postresuscitative ECG reading, they should be followed serially for evidence of any signs of improvement or deterioration. Barclay from New Zealand reports the case of a 65-year-old woman on whom cardiac massage had been performed on the ward some hours after an exploratory laparotomy. A successful resuscitation resulted. ECGs suggestive of bundle branch block (lead III) were seen on the first day. There was a tachycardia. Two days later, typical left bundle branch block was still present, but 16 days later the tachycardia had disappeared as well as a slurring of the S-T segment and evidence of bundle branch block.

Frequent EEG recordings may provide some prognostic help; however, there is no specific EEG pattern that indicates certain irreversible brain damage.

Serum transaminase levels

Considerable serum enzyme elevation was noted after D.C. countershock by Conttinen and associates in Finland. It is their opinion that skeletal muscle appears to be the origin of the enzyme elevations after electroconversion of the heart.

A unique opportunity for observing the effective serum transaminases of closed-chest cardiac massage in cardiac arrest was presented to Adrouny and associates. Five con-

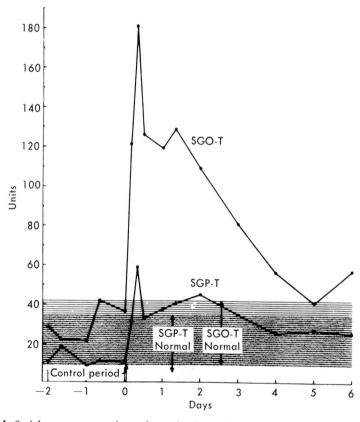

Fig. 54-1. Serial serum transaminase determinations before and after cardiac arrest encountered during left ventricular catheterization. Arrows indicate start of procedure. (From Adrouny, Z. A., and others: Circulation **27**:571, 1963.)

trol blood samples were obtained from a 39-year-old man during retrograde left ventricular catheterization. Cardiac arrest occurred and closed-chest resuscitation was successfully instituted. Fig. 54-1 shows the transaminase values before and after cardiac arrest. Although closed-chest resuscitation was carried out for only 3 or 4 minutes, a marked rise of serum glutamic oxaloacetic transaminase (SGOT) and a modest elevation of serum glutamic pyruvic transaminase (SGPT) appeared immediately after resuscitation. The highest levels occurred 8 hours after the procedure. Adrouny and his coworkers considered all of the possible factors likely to cause elevated SGPT and SGOT levels and conclude that the most likely possibility is a result of trauma to the chest wall. They rule out such factors as contusion of the heart muscle, trauma to the liver, hypotension, myocardial infarction, and effects of catheterization of the heart as being significant in this patient.

SGOT levels have been determined after D.C. electroshock in a series of eighteen patients (Levin and Cohen). Their data indicate that, regardless of the number of shocks administered or the maximum watt-seconds applied, there is no significant elevation of SGOT during either the immediate or the more remote (18 to 24 hours) postconversion phase, despite the fact that patients requiring cardioversion almost invariably have underlying cardiovascular disease. Patients requiring emergency cardioversion because of arrhythmias associated with acute myocardial infarction were excluded from the study.

Although we have had little experience with transaminase levels in patients following episodes of cardiac arrest and resuscitation, it is recommended that the serum transaminase level be determined whenever possible. Although SGOT levels do not seem to be appreciably influenced by elective cardioplegia during operations requiring cardiopulmonary bypass, the comparison between the two types of arrest may not be valid. Fraser and associates record a significant in-crease above preoperative values in the mean SGOT of all patients undergoing cardiac surgery with cardiopulmonary bypass. Quinn's data indicate that the magnitude of the elevation of SGOT is proportional to the duration of the arrest. In Flynn's series of seventeen patients, the changes in the serum glutamic oxalopyruvic transaminase, serum lactic acid dehydrogenase, and aldolase are slight to moderate.

Fluid intake and output

A careful intake and output record should be maintained on all cardiac arrest patients for several days following resuscitation, particularly if the patient has a period of unconsciousness and evidence of considerable neurologic sequelae. It is possible for a patient to become dehydrated easily in such instances. A retention catheter should, in most instances, be placed in the bladder, and urinary output thus kept under careful surveillance. The urinary catheter should be changed at intervals of every 48 hours or so.

Postresuscitative convulsions

Postresuscitative convulsions may arise from cerebral anoxic complications. Seizure may be controlled by intravenous administration of 300 mg. sodium amobarbital (Amytal) during the acute phase. A daily maintenance dose of 500 mg. diphenylhydantoin (Dilantin) can then be given. Valium may be useful in prolonged convulsions.

Use of mannitol in postresuscitation oliguria or anuria

Mannitol may be administered as a 20% solution given at 4 ml. per minute until 100 ml. has been administered or until urine volume of 1 ml. per minute is established. A diuretic response to mannitol will often occur within 1 to 1½ hours.

The mechanism of action of mannitol as a diuretic is open to some debate. Lilien and Mueller find the effect to be that of a fluid shift away from the red blood cells and extravascular compartments, with a fall in hematocrit. Subsequently, decreased blood viscosity and renal vascular resistance occur. They believe that the resulting increased renal blood flow reduces medullary osmolarity and increases urine flow.

Blood chemistry determinations

If there is suspicious evidence of lower nephron nephrosis or other signs of renal damage, the patient should be followed with repeat nonprotein nitrogen determinations. Following resuscitative procedures, a routine hemoglobin determination should be obtained. In some instances, chloride and potassium levels should also be investigated.

Postresuscitative chemotherapy

Even though the chest, if entered, appears dry, underwater chest-tube drainage procedures should be initiated and streptomycin and penicillin placed within the chest cavity. It is usually necessary to place the patient on rather large doses of wide-range antibiotics for at least 1 week or longer. As mentioned before, postoperative infections have been infrequent, in spite of repeated instances of septic technique being used.

Respiratory depression

The use of respiratory stimulants for patients who experience respiratory arrest secondary to cardiac arrest has seldom been employed in the past. Kratzl and Kvasnicka synthesized a corticomedullary-stimulating agent in 1950. It has subsequently received considerable clinical trial and has been named ethamivan (Fig. 54-2). Ethamivan, or vanillic acid diethylamide, is now thought to be

effective as a respiratory stimulant. Following its administration, orally or by a parenteral route, the depth of respiration is increased and, to a lesser degree, the rate of respiration is increased. No known direct cardiovascular effects from the drug have been recorded. The effectiveness of the drug response partially results from the increase in the tidal volume with a subsequent improvement in the alveolar ventilation. This results from the increase in the depth of respiration.

Miller, working in the cardiopulmonary laboratory of the University of Texas Southwestern Medical School, reports considerable clinical experience with the drug. He suggests that the initial intravenous dose be 100 mg. in the average adult (1 to 2 mg. per kilogram body weight in an infant) and that the drug be injected over an interval of 20 to 30 seconds. Since the effect of the drug is not long lasting, repeat doses may be necessary. A continuous intravenous drip may be the most effective means of administration.

Prolonged mechanical artificial ventilation controls hyperventilation in the postresuscitative period. It is also used to further reduce brain size or at least to prevent cerebral congestion and edema during the recovery phase. Artificial ventilation combats the metabolic acidosis which follows cardiac arrest, and it helps to abolish the work of breathing (Safar).

Postresuscitative nutrition

Although many patients will have little interruption in their regular routes of nutrition after cardiac resuscitation, some patients will present feeding problems and will require a period of intravenous nutrition for several days and/or the passage of a tube into the stomach for gastric feeding by means of a constant drip.

Postresuscitation following accidental electrical shock

In addition to the possibility that the patient may have received soft tissue burns, cardiac arrhythmias and ECG abnormalities

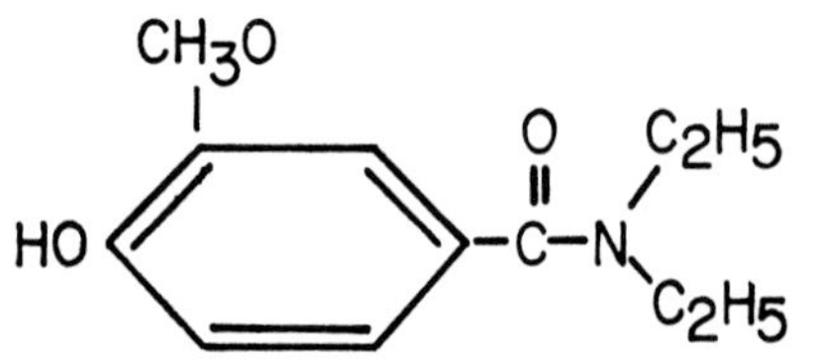

Fig. 54-2. Chemical structure of ethamivan (Emivan), a respiratory stimulant.

may be noted for some time following electrical shock. Traumatic myositis has been described as a frequent complication resulting from the severe contractions of the muscles of the shoulders, arms, chest, and shoulder girdle.

Tracheal suction

In the immediate postresuscitative stage, the patient may need almost constant tracheal suctioning to prevent the complications resulting from aspirated or retained secretion. If necessary, a tracheotomy may be performed to facilitate the tracheal suctioning.

Tracheotomy complications

For those physicians not often involved with patients requiring prolonged endotracheal intubation, it is appropriate to sound an alert regarding numerous potential complications. Cuffed tubes as the cause of tracheal stenosis is well recognized. A cuff is used on an indwelling endotracheal tube or tracheostomy tube in order to ensure the adequate function of the respirator. Several factors play a part in the etiology of tracheal stenosis including infection, incorrect placement and excessive movement of the tube, and excessive cuff pressure. Pressure necrosis may develop from overinflation of cuffed tubes. Patients with hypotension may be particularly prone to develop such complications. Probably the principal causes of tracheal stenosis are ischemia resulting from the actual pressure exerted on the tracheal wall by the cuff and the duration of the pressure (Shelly and co-workers). Strides are being made in the development of improved tracheostomy tubes that allow for sealing the trachea with much less lateral pressure and with minimal occluding volume. An intermittently inflated tracheal cuff produces less tracheal damage than does a cuff that is constantly inflated.

When a tracheotomy is employed, it is important for the physician to be aware of the many complications that may result. For example, a fatal case of hemorrhage from erosion of the innominate artery by pressure of the tracheostomy tube is reported. We have had success with one such case.

A high frequency of posttracheotomy stricture of the trachea has been emphasized by Pearson at the University of Toronto. Many of these strictures subsequently require surgical correction. Many complications from the use of the tracheostomy tube may be avoided if the tube is of the proper size to avoid pressure upon any portion of the tracheal wall. With the use of an inflated cuff, one must be careful to avoid continued pressure. This is accomplished by releasing the cuff at intervals of 1 to 2 hours. Minimal inflation should be employed.

Prolonged nasotracheal intubation

Although tracheotomy is an effective means of maintaining an open airway over a prolonged period of time, nasotracheal tubes can also serve as an effective airway, provided precautions are taken to avoid improper positioning. Positive pressure ventilation and humidification are easily compatible with the nasotracheal tube, but a tracheostomy tube connected to a respirator usually makes it easier to obtain a tight system. The hazards of hemorrhage, pneumothorax, and subcutaneous or mediastinal emphysema are less likely with a nasotracheal than with a tracheostomy tube. The decreased resistance in the nasotracheal tube as compared with the tracheostomy tube is an added advantage, also. Airway management in the immediate postresuscitative period often lends itself advantageously to the use of a nasotracheal tube.

Oxygen under increased pressure

Although few reports have appeared concerning the effect of exposure to increased oxygen tensions following cardiac arrest, oxygen pressure chambers are now available in a number of research centers where physiologic observations are being recorded on a variety of conditions. It is now known that oxygen breathed at twice the normal atmospheric pressure will raise the partial pressure more than tenfold. (The partial pressure of oxygen in mixed arterial blood is approximately 87 mm. Hg when air is breathed at normal atmospheric pressures.) Tissues that have been deprived of oxygen or that may continue to be receiving inadequate oxygen supply may benefit from exposure to increased partial pressures between the plasma and the anoxic tissue. The markedly increased rate of diffusion in such instances may, for example, serve to reduce the cell death and myocardial damage following cardiac arrest and resuscitation. Illingworth and others demonstrated the protection afforded the dog by breathing oxygen at 2 atmospheres pressure. They reduced the mortality from ligation of the left circumflex coronary artery from 56% to 10% in a small series of dogs by the use of increased oxygen pressures. They speculate that oxygen administered under such conditions may tide the heart over until such time as a collateral circulation may be established.

It has not been established what will be the effect of breathing oxygen under increased pressure in patients who show cerebral edema from a period of anoxia. It is interesting to speculate on its possible effect.

Pifarré and associates find no evidence, either experimental or clinical, however, to the effect that the mortality from acute myocardial infarction among patients in shock or in heart failure can be significantly reduced by the use of hyperbaric oxygenation. In their experiments (1970) they conclude that exposure to toxic levels of oxygen (3 atmospheres of pressure) in the presence of acute myocardial infarction results in an acute exudative response, followed by a proliferative phase, and a subsequent death rate of 70% in dogs. They concede that treatment with hyperbaric oxygenation may have reduced the incidence of early mortality by preventing ventricular fibrillation.

Oxygen intoxication

It is well to remember that oxygen-enriched gas mixtures delivered by mechanical ventilation with volume-cycle respirators introduce oxygen intoxication as an iatrogenic complication. Soloway presents several patients with pulmonary hyaline membrane disease thought to result from oxygen intoxication. Once alveolar-capillary block is initiated, the process is self-perpetuating. It requires increased concentration and volumes of oxygen to maintain the Pa_{O_2}. Pathologic findings in the cases included pulmonary hemorrhage, interstitial edema and fibrosis, swollen alveolar A cells, and characteristic hyaline membrane.

Psychologic testing in the postresuscitative period

Determinations of the patient's intelligence quotient should be made at intervals in every instance of suspected neuropsychiatric trauma following resuscitation from cardiac arrest. Evidence of improvement in repeated examinations occurs. Freeman and associates mention one case in which an intelligence quotient rose over a period of 2 years from a reading of 52 to 73 in an individual having received severe cerebral damage following a period of prolonged anoxia.

Use of left heart pump for postresuscitative assist

Following prolonged efforts at cardiac resuscitation, myocardial function may be severely depressed. This is particularly likely if repeated efforts at ventricular defibrillation have been made. It is probable that the left heart bypass pump will come into greater use in this connection to assist the weak or failing heart in the postresuscitative period.

The advantages of the left heart pump include effecting a reduction of the work load on the heart, maintenance of the pressure in the coronary arteries, maintenance of adequate oxygenation of tissue, and reduction in the pressure of the left atrium. This results in a decrease in the likelihood of pulmonary edema and gives general support to the body circulation.

Chapter 55

EFFECT OF CARDIAC ARREST ON RENAL FUNCTION

Alex L. Finkle

General remarks

When cardiac arrest occurs, either during a surgical procedure or with myocardial infarction, it is axiomatic that the shorter the period of ischemia, the less likely the possibility of irreversible damage to vital tissues. Resuscitation from cardiac arrest does not necessarily restore normalcy; a residuum of physiologic problems may present serious challenges in aftercare of the patient. The physician must be fully cognizant of the potential systemic problems and, especially, of the renal sequelae of decreased blood supply to the kidneys during cardiovascular collapse.

Most of the patients successfully and permanently resuscitated from cardiac arrest exhibit few or no ill effects, immediate or delayed. Most instances of acute urinary suppression are reversible if the patient can be supported long enough. In essence, the renal problems encountered after cardiac arrest are the same as those following any shock-producing cardiovascular collapse (Uldall and Kerr; Yeboah and co-workers). The older the patient, the greater the danger from sudden cardiovascular failure and its renal sequelae. The higher the preoperative blood urea nitrogen, the greater the probability of renal failure after open-heart surgery, although no direct cause-and-effect relationship is involved (Yeboah and co-workers).

Likelihood of cardiac arrest

Because of the unexpectedness of cardiac arrest during surgical operations, few clinical studies of renal functional status under such circumstances have been made (Miturzynska-Stryjecka and Widmoskaba-Czekajska). However, in patients with myocardial disease and with uremia (Jude and associates) for whom a possibility of cardiac arrest exists, provision can be made for a thorough study of disturbed renal function—as has been done in conjunction with open-heart surgery (Yeboah and others) and in resuscitation following myocardial infarction (Fillmore and co-workers). Should protracted hypoxia develop during an operation, pulmonary and cardiovascular-renal functional studies should be instituted, whether or not the fear of cardiac arrest is realized (Chazan and co-workers; Clark and Caedo; Hamby; Petty and Neff). Impairment of renal function during acute, severe hypoxia with associated metabolic acidosis (Petty and Neff) and hyperkalemia (Chazan and associates) represents a serious threat to life. The acidosis aggravates the hyperkalemia, imposing additional burden upon already overtaxed and precarious renal function. Thus, judicious therapy and careful management of fluid and ionic balance are mandatory (Clark and Caedo). The fact that potassium can shift from cells to blood very rapidly (Finkle) poses severe danger to myocardial function—and thus dictates vigorous therapeutic action.

Definitions

Acute renal failure is defined as abrupt and nearly complete loss of renal function because of profound renal ischemia. This is usually characterized by oliguria, namely, production of less than 400 ml. of urine daily—despite sometimes deceptively "normal" urine volume for a day or two. Linear increase in blood urea nitrogen and serum creatinine ensues for several days, reflecting accelerated production and impaired excretion of nitrogenous metabolites.

Prerenal failure (prerenal azotemia) involves the pathophysiologic mechanisms just described, that is, sharply curtailed urinary output secondary to inadequate renal circulation. However, the cause is readily reversible.

It should be emphasized that renal ischemia cannot be assessed solely by recording peripheral circulation. The physiologic responses that protect systemic blood pressure during clinical shock involve shunting blood away from the kidneys.

Pathophysiology of renal damage

The mechanisms by which temporary renal ischemia produces acute renal failure are still under debate. They include prolonged vasoconstriction, intrarenal shunting, edematous occlusion of nephrons secondary to increased intrarenal pressure, tubular obstructions by casts and/or amorphous debris, leakage of tubular fluid into the renal interstitium, and disseminated intravascular coagulation (Uldall and Kerr).

Whether a single mechanism or a combination of mechanisms is involved, it is known that even after 1 hour of warm renal ischemia in the kidney of a human donor, that kidney is salvageable and transplantable (Belzer and Kountz). Hemodynamic and angiographic studies by Hollenberg and his associates disclosed that patients with nephrotoxin-induced acute renal failure show patterns identical to those induced by shock or hemolysis. This suggests a final common pathogenetic pathway involving undefined mediators that lead to severe sustained preglomerular vasoconstriction. Thus, diffuse and homogeneous reduction in renal cortical perfusion ensues. The histopathologic picture is described as acute tubular necrosis.

Clinical steps and observations in the diagnosis and treatment of renal ischemia

Immediate efforts are instituted to restore cardiac function by various techniques generally involving closed-chest methods designated as "mechanical ventricular assistance" (Skinner and co-workers).

A urethral catheter is inserted at once and left indwelling to measure urinary volume, electrolytes, creatinine clearance, and osmolarity.

Immediate and frequent analyses of serum and of urinary sodium, potassium chloride, and carbon dioxide are procured. By means of flame photometry, results can be obtained within 5 to 15 minutes. Blood gases, pH, and blood sugar are measured repeatedly. Hyperglycemia could spuriously affect sodium in the form of lower than true value.

Immediate and continuous monitoring of the ECG is arranged, if not already routinely instituted at the start of most surgical operations.

Introduction of a small plastic catheter into any available jugular, carotid, subclavian, or brachial vein for continuous monitoring of central venous pressure is performed as soon as feasible.

Of all these tests, the most important evaluations seek to delineate any development of *hyperkalemia* and *metabolic* (lactic) *acidosis.* (Hypokalemia can be caused inadvertently by overventilation during use of a respirator.)

Endotracheal intubation is invaluable for maintaining an open airway (Fillmore) and for providing oxygen or carbon dioxide, as indicated by serial blood gas measurements.

Experimental and human data pertaining to preservation of renal function

In the past decade, increasing experience with renal transplantation in animals (Persky; Skinner and co-workers) and in man (Belzer and associates) has provided significant data regarding function of ischemic and anoxic kidneys. Renal tissue possesses great resuscitative capacity after sudden ischemia such as follows cardiac arrest

(Skinner and others) or ischemia of longer duration, such as follows delay in instituting resuscitative measures. Hypothermia, mannitol with heparin infusion, and beta-adrenergic blocking agents have been evaluated experimentally in preserving function of canine kidneys in situ (Persky). Ethacrynic acid and furosemide have improved glomerular filtration rate in patients postoperatively (Stahl and Stone), in contrast to the known 30% decrease in glomerular filtration rate found in patients undergoing routine abdominal exploration. By giving ethacrynic acid and furosemide during operation, Stahl and Stone could accomplish *increase* in glomerular filtration rate after abdominal exploratory operations. Indeed, none of their patients thus treated developed any postoperative renal failure.

Agonal vasospasm in pigs' kidneys, following experimentally induced anoxia and hypercapnia was believed to be humorally mediated (Keaveny and co-workers). This spasm was preventable by phenoxybenzamine. Finally, the combination of this drug and of procaine administered intra-arterially (Belzer and Kountz) could prevent renal vascular spasm in dying donor-patients before excision of their kidneys. Mechanical pulsatile perfusion of excised cadaver kidneys with cryo-precipitated plasma will allow storage of these kidneys for as long as 50 hours before successful transplantation in human recipients. These techniques have now become recognized measures to broaden availability of cadaver kidneys (Belzer and associates).

Experimental study of renal functional parameters in dogs by Finkle and Smith led to the suggestion that free water clearance (C_{H_2O})* be evaluated in patients as a critical index of renal revivification. Usefulness of C_{H_2O} for this purpose was verified by Jones and Weil who studied thirty-six patients in shock. C_{H_2O} was found to be a valuable indicator of renal injury and of response to therapeutic measures.

$$*C_{H_2O} = \frac{V_u - mOsm_u \times V_u}{mOsm_p}.$$

Treatment

In general, therapeutic action should proceed from simple maintenance of urine flow by reestablishing circulating blood volume (replacing blood loss) to encouraging urine flow (40 to 120 mg. furosemide, intravenously*), combating acidosis (intravenous sodium bicarbonate infusions†) and preservation of acid-base balance by maintaining pulmonary patency and by frequent analyses of urinary acidity. If prolonged support of the patient becomes necessary and maintenance of renal function becomes more difficult, conservative therapeutic measures should be abandoned in favor of more vigorous treatment, such as peritoneal dialysis or hemodialysis. In essence, progressively more intensive treatment must be promptly applied, as outlined in the review by Schreiner and Teehan on dialysis for the detoxification of patients who have been poisoned or who have been involved in overdosages of drugs.

Although peritoneal dialysis is now rather widely used (Kuruvila and Beven) and even hemodialysis is becoming commonplace since introduction of arteriovenous shunts

*After giving 40 to 120 mg. furosemide intravenously the urine flow within 10 minutes should reach 10 ml. or more per minute—accomplishing the desired result. If less urinary output is noted, the furosemide dosage may be repeated twice, at 10-minute intervals. Thus, if 120 mg. additional furosemide fails to stimulate active urinary flow within 30 minutes, consideration of peritoneal dialysis is in order.

†The rationale by which 50 ml. ampules of 7.5% aqueous sodium bicarbonate solution is administered intravenously is as follows: Each mole (180 gm.) of glucose is catabolized to two moles of lactic acid. Since an average patient burns 20 gm. carbohydrate hourly, about 220 mEq. of lactic acid would be formed hourly in a "noncirculatory" state of cardiac arrest or with feeble cardiac output during efforts at resuscitation. In other words, about 1 ampule of sodium bicarbonate would compensate for approximately 10 minutes of complete anaerobic acidosis. The concentration of serum bicarbonate should be raised back to approximately 20 mEq. per liter, with caution to observe for sodium and water retention, as well as overshoot alkalosis (Bennett and co-workers; Britton and co-workers; Reidenberg).

(Thompson) and home-care arrangements (Siemsen and co-workers; Tenckhoff and Curtis), it is reasonable and practical to recommend that patients whose renal dysfunction requires such measures be transported by ground- or air-ambulance to a center specializing in these techniques (Schreiner and Teehan) rather than to undertake dialysis at smaller hospitals. The value of vigorous dialysis in what was previously considered irreversible renal failure is emphasized by the recent report on acute renal failure in malignant hypertension by Mattern, Sommers, and Kassirer.

Evaluation of resuscitation: immediate and long-term results

In mid-1972, Lemire and Johnson asked and answered the question, "Is cardiac resuscitation worthwhile?" Citing a decade of experience, they found that of 1,204 patients resuscitated at Montreal's Royal Victoria Hospital, 19% survived to be dismissed from the hospital. Among this group 74% lived for 1 year and 51% were still alive 3 years later. A random study of 15% of the survivors showed unchanged functional capacities after resuscitation. Thus, these authors concluded that a definite prolongation of life in a productive age group had been accomplished. Their success was commended by Kravitz and Killip who urged other physicians and institutions to acquire the necessary skills to emulate these authors' results.

Similar success in a group of 161 patients was reported by Dupont and others, most of whose patients left the hospital; about half survived for 1 year. Minuck and Perkins studied twenty-six of twenty-seven resuscitated patients through questionnaires sent to them and to their physicians. Their answers led to the conclusion that cardiac resuscitation was justified on the basis of recovery of physical and mental health—and, in many instances, return to gainful employment. Of fourteen cardiac arrests experienced during anesthesia in 17,000 operations reported by Jude and his associates, eight were resuscitable to prearrest status (57%) and six were discharged from the hospital (43%).

Summary

Rapid accretion of data in the past several years, particularly in connection with human renal transplantations, underscores the need for prompt diagnosis and thoroughgoing treatment of early renal failure following cardiac arrest. Comprehensive monitoring of key blood and urinary factors is emphasized. Control of hyperkalemia is of paramount importance. Prevention of acute tubular necrosis is the goal of therapy. If conservative measures prove ineffective, prompt application of dialysis is warranted in treatment centers properly staffed and equipped.

ADDENDUM

Of 507 open-heart operations performed at the Massachusetts General Hospital in 1972, a mortality rate of 30% was encountered postoperatively when BUN or serum creatinine rose to over 50 mg. or 2 mg. per 100 ml. respectively. This compared with a mortality rate of only 1.6% in the same series wherein renal function remained "normal" according to BUN and creatinine values. Possible causes, methods of evaluation, and treatment of renal dysfunction were cited (Abel and others).

Grateful thanks are extended to Drs. Alan J. Coleman and Frank A. Gotch, of San Francisco, for their review of this chapter. The invaluable assistance of Mrs. Kathryn L. Kammerer, Medical Librarian at Mount Zion Hospital, San Francisco, in seeking out current references is acknowledged with great appreciation.

PART EIGHT

PITFALLS, PRECAUTIONS, AND COMPLICATIONS IN CARDIAC RESUSCITATION

At the 1962 meeting of the American College of Surgeons, a case was presented that encompassed a large number of the complications that have been reported following closed-chest resuscitation. This particular patient experienced a ruptured liver, a ruptured spleen, a hemopneumothorax, and a flail chest from multiple fractured ribs. Multiple areas of atelectasis were also present. Tracheotomy had been performed. The arrest had originally occurred during anesthesia for a hemorrhoidectomy.

There is also the case of the man who entered a hospital in Buenos Aires to have a bunion removed and ended up with a broken leg and collar bone, a heart attack, and a ruptured stomach. Fearing the pain during the bunion treatment, the patient asked for a general anesthetic; this led to a heart attack, the newspaper *El Mundo* reports. Doctors revived him by opening his chest and massaging his heart. He was then put in an oxygen tent, where he suffered a stomach contraction followed by a rupture of the stomach and peritonitis.

After more treatment, the patient fell off a stretcher, broke a leg and a collar bone, and suffered further damage to his heart, which made a tracheotomy necessary. At this point, he had a breathing tube in his throat, a drainage tube in his stomach, a leg in plaster, an arm in a sling—and the bunion still unremoved!

Attempts at cardiac resuscitation, by either direct or indirect approach to the heart, require a close review of certain pitfalls, precautions, and complications that are frequently associated with these attempts. In this section, specific note will be taken of those complications that are particularly inherent in either the closed-chest or the open-chest approach. Unless one is familiar with these hazards, the golden opportunity to restore the normal heartbeat may be lost, and the consequent death of the patient becomes the result of a sincere but nevertheless tragically futile attempt to maintain life.

Chapter 56

CEREBRAL ANOXIA AND NEUROLOGIC SEQUELAE AFTER CARDIAC ARREST

Introduction*

Cardiac arrest, by depriving the brain of circulation, has a rapid and severe effect on the central nervous system. The time the brain will withstand complete ischemia without any permanent damage has never been established with certainty, and even if such a time could be deduced, it would be dependent upon many factors—age, state of the brain at the time, and temperature.

At birth and for about 30 days afterward, the brain is extremely resistant to anoxia of any form, but around the age of puberty, it is very sensitive. During adult life the resistance returns, but a sensitivity develops with old age. This variation in sensitivity is partly in keeping with the rate of general body metabolism, except that with old age, the brain becomes more sensitive because, with the approach of senility, it is beginning to disintegrate.

Brains that have already been poisoned by anesthesia or that are suffering from any other form of anoxia will tolerate ischemia less well than a conscious brain, as will brains that have been injured immediately prior to the cerebral ischemia.

At normal body temperature, the accepted standard time for cerebral ischemia (with subsequent recovery) is 4 minutes, although this figure was arrived at on a purely.arbitrary basis. If a safe time for all ages has to be stated, it is probably nearer 3 minutes in the anesthetized subject at normal temperature. With reduction in temperature, the

safe ischemic time can be increased, but it is impossible to give a standard time. At 32° C., the total body metabolism is known to be reduced by half; therefore the ischemic time may be doubled. However, in clinical hypothermia for cardiac surgery it has been found that 6 minutes is an underestimate of the safe ischemic time, and on occasions the circulation has been arrested for as long as 11 minutes at 30° C. without ill effects. Since a patient is cooled rapidly under such circumstances, complete equilibrium is not necessarily reached by the time the circulation is arrested; subsequently, such temperatures can be taken only as a guide. With lower temperature, the ischemic time can be further increased, and with the technique of profound hypothermia, the circulation can be stopped for as long as 1 hour at 15° C. without ill effects.

What exactly happens in the brain following cerebral anoxia is difficult to determine. The effects can be listed under two headings—those associated with the area of the brain most likely to be injured by the anoxic insult and the type of damage to the nerve itself.

The part of the brain most sensitive to anoxia from any cause is the hippocampus, followed by the thalamus, cerebellum, and cerebrum. From knowledge of oxygen consumption as related to phylogenetic evolution of the brain, it would be expected that the cerebellum and cerebrum would be affected most. That they are not so affected is due to the type of blood supply in the basal ganglia and hippocampus. This blood supply

*By B. G. B. Lucas, M.D., F.F.A., R.C.S.

is unable to increase under anoxic conditions, being an end artery system rather than an aggregation of vessels such as that on the surface of the cerebellum and cerebrum. Since the most sensitive part of the cerebrum is the occipital cortex, transient blindness sometimes occurs following cardiac arrest, but this is rarely the end result in an otherwise normal victim.

The cellular change in the brain is related to the time intervening between the anoxic insult and the histologic study. A large number of cellular alterations have been ascribed to cerebral anoxia, but they have been shown to be variants of the same change. During the first 24 hours, it is difficult to identify any alterations in cell structure, but after 48 hours, the nerve cell is apparently swollen with a somewhat ragged nucleus. This swelling increases in the third day and then gradually diminishes until about the fifth day, when the cell has a typical homogenized appearance. This swelling was originally thought to be in the nerve cell itself, but it is now considered to be an accumulation of fluid in the oligodendroglia that envelopes each nerve cell. After the fifth day, the oligodendroglial swelling disappears and the nerve cell either recovers or disintegrates, so that after 2 weeks, the histologic findings are predominantly cell loss with otherwise fairly normal neurons.

The immediate effect of cerebral anoxia is to produce unconsciousness. The length of time this persists and the depth of the unconsciousness depend upon the severity of the anoxic insult. Cerebral ischemia of less than 1 minute will only produce unconsciousness of a few minutes' duration, whereas 3 minutes or more of ischemia may result in a coma lasting several days.

With deep unconsciousness, the body is flaccid with no reflexes, respirations are quiet, and pupils are dilated and do not react to light. Sometimes respiration may be absent or may be jerky in character. The EEG may show predominantly slow activity or may be silent. Apart from the nervous system, the only organ likely to show alteration is the heart, which may show electrocardiographic evidence of anoxic damage to the myocardium as evinced by a raised S-T segment or inverted T waves.

Because of the changes that occur in the neuron during cerebral anoxia, the clinical pattern is usually a neurologic alteration both increasing and decreasing in severity up to a period of 4 to 5 days, followed by partial or complete recovery. Temporary blindness, already mentioned, may last for a week or two, but spasticity or tremor may remain indefinitely. With such neurologic aftereffects, there is nearly always some disturbance of intelligence similar to that of senility. When there are no neurologic disturbances, there may be an alteration in personality, but whether this is permanent or not is difficult to prove. There are well-documented cases of personality changes that have continued over long periods, but most psychiatric evidence suggests that the change is of a temporary nature.

Prognosis is dependent upon the length of time of cerebral ischemia, but it is impossible to be dogmatic during the first few hours following the insult. Recovery is unlikely if, 12 hours after the insult, spontaneous respirations have not returned and there is hyperthermia. Another bad prognostic sign is a constant level of coma, particularly if it persists for more than 5 days. If there is no recovery of consciousness after 2 weeks, it is unlikely that such will ever occur, and these patients usually continue for some months or years as decerebrate "vegetables." Death, if it occurs, is usually associated with hyperthermia.

Apart from general nursing care with special attention to the care and feeding of the unconscious patient, specific treatment should be directed toward the maintenance of adequate ventilation, if need be, by means of a tracheotomy and intermittent positive pressure respiration, maintenance of electrolyte balance, and close attention to kidney function, which may be disturbed during the first few days. Whether there is any specific treatment for the damaged brain is not yet proved. If it is assumed that the reason for the disintegration of the nerve cell is that it has been squeezed by the surrounding edema so that it is unable to metabolize effectively after the insult, then it would be reasonable to cool the patient for some days postoperatively so that the brain's oxygen demand is reduced and so that some attempt may be made to remove the edema by dehydration therapy as quickly as possible. Hypothermia of 32° to 30° C. has been practiced in many instances and an impression has been gained that this is valuable, but for obvious reasons, a controlled clinical trial is not feasible. Nor has it been possible to make such observations experimentally. Clinically, the results of dehydration therapy either by the use of triple-strength human plasma, 50% sucrose, or urea (all given intravenously) have been equivocal. There is no experimental evidence that dehydration is of any value in altering the histologic picture of edema. All that can be said about treatment by hypothermia and dehydration is that during the past few years, when such treatment has been routine, more recoveries from cardiac arrest have occurred than formerly, but this may be due to the fact that the cardiac arrest itself is now treated more speedily and not because of specific treatment of the later condition.

Illustrative case histories

A boy, 8 years of age, suffered cardiac arrest during bronchography under general anesthesia, and cardiac massage was not started for at least 6 or 7 minutes. Ultimately, the heart and respiration restarted, but 24 hours later, the child was deeply unconscious and completely flaccid. During the next few days, he showed all the signs of decerebration, with slowly increasing spasticity. Gradually his spasticity lessened, and after 1 year he was a typical "decerebrate vegetable." He would cry in response to painful stimuli and would eat if food were placed in his mouth, but he was incapable of making any coordinated movements. Twelve years later, he had grown to normal height and weight for his age, but was un-

changed neurologically. The only sensation he appeared to have was that of hearing, inasmuch as he would start at a loud noise. He had the typical appearance of a person whose brain has been destroyed (Fig. 56-1).

A woman, 45 years of age, had cardiac arrest for an estimated 7 minutes during partial gastrectomy for duodenal ulcer. She was unconscious for 7 days, then slowly recovered and was discharged from the hospital 3 months later with the clinical appearance of pseudobulbar palsy. She had typical spastic speech, slow, clumsy movements of all limbs, and mild spastic tetraplegia with brisk jerks and flexor plantar responses. There was marked intellectual impairment. During the next 6 months there was some neurologic improvement, but 1 year later, she was mentally senile and showed many of the ordinary physical signs of old age. Eight years after the cardiac arrest, she looked and acted like a woman of 90 and was completely incapable of doing anything for herself.

A woman, 53 years of age, about to have a stitch abscess incised following subtotal thyroidectomy 3

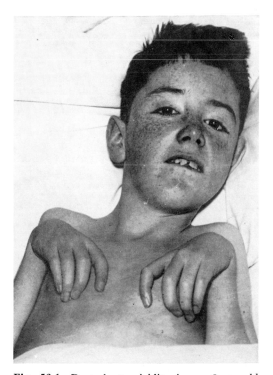

Fig. 56-1. Decerebrate rigidity in an 8-year-old boy following cardiac resuscitation. (From Lucas, B. G. B.: Anoxic states and their treatment. In Evans, F. T., and Grey, T. C.: Modern trends in anaesthesia, London, 1958, Butterworth & Co.)

weeks previously, was induced with 400 mg. of thiopentone. Almost immediately her heart stopped. The abdomen was opened within 4 minutes; her heart was palpated and found to be dilated and inactive. Massage was started and, at the same time, an intracardiac injection of epinephrine was given. Immediately following the injection, the heart started beating and within a few seconds produced an adequate carotid pulse. Respiration did not return for a further 20 minutes. By the time the abdomen was closed, the patient was breathing quietly and had normal pulse and blood pressure, but she was unconscious and had no reflexes. She did not recover consciousness for 2 days, during which time she passed through stages of being acutely spastic and apparently decerebrate. When consciousness returned, she was neurologically normal but was completely deluded and irrational. During the next 2 months she improved slowly. She first passed through a phase of being completely childlike, remembering only her maiden name and incidents of her early life; later, she remembered being a young married woman. She continued to improve, and 3 months after the original cardiac arrest, she was discharged from the hospital as normal, apart from having a somewhat facile personality. One year later, there was no psychiatric, neurologic, or other evidence that she was in any way different from prior to the cardiac arrest.

A woman, 20 years of age, suffered cardiac arrest for an estimated 8 minutes during manual removal of the placenta. She was unconscious for 3 days and then very confused for a further 5 days. She appeared facile and childlike in temperament, and 1 month later a psychologist reported that there was definite brain damage resulting in deterioration of intellectual function. Three months later, however, she had improved and was apparently normal.

Time factor

On March 18, 1948, a 15-year-old girl was nearing the end of a rather minor orthopedic procedure on her arm when suddenly previously normal blood pressure and pulse disappeared. After some delay, the chest was opened and manual compression of the arrested heart was begun. Cardiac resuscitation was successful.

During the spring of 1956, this girl was 23 years of age, beginning the ninth year since sudden cardiac asystole. She still occupied the same bed of previous years; she was almost totally blind; feeding was by syringe; her appearance remained that of a young girl; no cerebration was evident, and she was completely paralyzed. Endocrine imbalances were evidenced by complete atrophy of the previously normal mammary tissue.

There has not been a high reported incidence of severe neurologic damage from resuscitative attempts outside the operating rooms and with closed-chest techniques. External cardiac massage was of sufficient effectiveness to allow recovery with normal neurologic status in twenty-six of fifty-three patients following resuscitation after myocardial infarction (Robinson). Two of the patients remained unconscious for almost 24 hours, with spastic extremities, only to subsequently recover without any evidence of neurologic deficit.

The incidence of major neurologic sequelae following cardiac resuscitation is not accurately known. One report describes a 20-year-old girl who had cardiac arrest during a tonsillectomy. Seven and one-half years later, she died without having regained consciousness. The sociologic and economic ramifications of such cases are rather overwhelming.

Perhaps the reader has been called as consultant to see a patient suffering the ill effects of cerebral anoxia caused by sudden cessation of the cerebral circulation. Perhaps he has wondered about prognostic signs and therapeutic measures.

In 1950 the Cardiac Arrest Registry was begun.* This study was made possible through the cooperation of many physicians in all parts of this country, England, Canada, Australia, New Zealand, France, and several other countries. Many different avenues of investigation have subsequently been followed. Of particular importance is that, for the first time, an opportunity was afforded to study the effect on the human brain produced by total and complete anoxia resulting from sudden absence of cardiac output and subsequent cessation of cerebral circulation. From over 1,700 patients who have experienced sudden cardiac standstill, an attempt was made to correlate neurologic sequelae

*This study was aided by funds from the Institute of Neurological Diseases and Blindness of the National Institutes of Health of the United States Public Health Service and the John and Mary R. Markle Foundation.

experienced by these patients after known periods of exposure to complete oxygen lack.

How long can the brain withstand complete oxygen deprivation without signs of irreversible damage? Surprisingly enough, as late as 1915, it was frequently regarded that the human brain could survive complete anoxia for a period of 15 minutes without permanent injury to the brain. Some of these erroneous conclusions result from transference to human beings of information received by experimental observations on laboratory animals. Many of these conclusions were inaccurate because they were produced by a ligation of the vessels, which failed to consider an abundant collateral circulation. Some were concerned with carbon monoxide poisoning, asphyxia, drowning, or other noxious agents.

Therefore it is of particular importance to consider the role of the time factor in the survival of patients experiencing cardiac arrest. It has been noted that 94% of those who were successfully resuscitated (and left the hospital) were those on whom artificial augmentation of the circulation was begun within 4 minutes of the time of the arrest. It is from the 6% revived after a delay of more than 4 minutes that many of the neurologic difficulties arose. I think it is safe to state that there is sufficient evidence to indicate that somewhere between 3 and 4 minutes lies the threshold of time necessary for the reversibility of the effects of cerebral anoxia and the return of central nervous system function.

Although it is true that few patients will survive a period of complete cerebral anoxia under normothermic conditions for longer than $3\frac{1}{2}$ to 4 minutes, the inference that the cells of the cerebral cortex are irreversibly damaged is not necessarily valid.

Work done at the Bogomolets Physiological Institute of the Ukranian Academy of Sciences has been reported by Yankovskii on the experimental use of Bryukhoneko's auto-injector for resuscitating dogs killed by exsanguination. It is concluded that irreversible lesions are not found in the cells of the cerebral cortex of the dog after clinical death of more than 5 to 6 minutes. In fact, after complete exsanguination at normal temperatures for as long as 10 to 15 minutes' duration and resuscitation by the auto-injector, complete restoration of the central nervous system occurs. The Russian workers have used the conditioned reflex method to evaluate central nervous system activity. Yankovskii believes that as the body dies, the cells of the central nervous system perish not from anoxia caused by stoppage of the heart but mainly by the accumulation in the brain of cellular metabolites during the period of agony and clinical death, metabolites resulting from the consumption of the oxygen present in the blood cells by the brain cells, and from biochemical processes that endure in the brain tissues after circulation stops.

Torskaya, working at the same institute of physiology in Russia, attempted to study histologic data on the nature and extent of the lesions seen in cells of the central nervous system that had been subjected to different periods of anoxia and different methods of resuscitation. As has been the experience of others, it proved difficult to reproduce the same picture in laboratory animals subjected to the identical period of insult. It follows, of course, that if the cells are studied immediately after the anoxic period, many of the histologic changes will not yet be evident. When cerebral anoxia was produced by exsanguination and the animal was subsequently resuscitated, the following findings were reported: the nerve elements of the cerebellum (Purkinje's cells) are the main sufferers, and, following them, the cells covering the minor and medial pyramids in the cortex of the cerebral hemisphere. Pyknosis, marginal vacuolation, marginal lysis, and shadow cells were noted.

Brierley presents an exhaustive examination of the neuropathology in fourteen patients who survived circulatory arrests but who died from severe brain damage. He indicates that there is a generalized loss of neurons, or at least severe neuron damage, in the cerebral cortex. The brunt of the damage centers upon the occipital and parietal lobes rather than upon the temporal and funnel areas. In addition, he notes that necrosis in the hippocampi is always present, as is destruction of Purkinje's cells of the cerebellum. Damage in the adult brainstem is rare. On the other hand, he reports considerable evidence of brainstem injury in infants and young children, while cerebral cortical damage is slight in these patients.

The value of external cardiac massage, even of a prolonged nature, is well documented by many survivors of periods of lengthy cardiac compression. Cleveland continued closed-chest cardiac compression for more than 3 hours on a 14-year-old boy whose heart stopped shortly after a venous thrombectomy. Despite the fact that the boy's pupils remained widely dilated and fixed during the entire resuscitation episode (he had had atropine previously), he showed no neurologic sequelae the following day. Now, several years later, he is leading a normal life, playing school football, and in every way appears to be quite healthy.

Patients with hyperthyroid states who are hypothermic are more likely to have neurologic sequelae after cardiac arrest than a patient who is myxedematous or hypothermic at the time of the arrest. It is estimated that the newborn maintain a resistance to hypoxia for approximately 30 days after birth. As pointed out elsewhere, patients with tetralogy of Fallot who have adapted to chronic hypoxia tend to withstand cardiac arrest somewhat longer.

At the Second International Symposium on Cardiopulmonary Resuscitation, Rosomoff suggested a simple clinical test to indicate brainstem function. It involves instilling ice-cold water into the ear. The eyes deviate to the opposite side if the brainstem is intact— a response referred to as the oculo-encephalic reaction.

There seems to be general agreement that children suffering anoxia for varying periods of time, with subsequent coma, very often make rather dramatic recoveries even after a number of months. I have seen several such cases. One was a young boy who was areflexic, markedly hyperthermic, deaf, and blind for a period of several weeks and yet who made an eventual recovery with minimal neurologic deficit. Progress notes by the resident staff referred almost daily to the "near terminal" state of the patient.

Neurologic sequelae

A remarkable exception to the usual 4-minute period before cerebral irreversibility has been reported by Professor Benson Roe of the University of California in San Francisco. His communication on this patient follows:

The patient was a 23-year-old girl who sustained anterior blunt chest injury in an automobile accident, became shocky and was given several units of blood at the County Hospital. Pericardial tamponade was verified by needle aspiration, and she was transferred here. Although she had a high venous pressure and a narrow pulse pressure, she was in remarkably good shape without significant circulatory deficit or neurological abnormality except for retrograde amnesia. Her circulation deteriorated somewhat during induction and sternal splitting incision.

When the pericardium was opened she began to exsanguinate until I felt a huge, uncontrollable rent in the postero-superior aspect of her right atrial appendage. Electrical ventricular fibrillation was instituted in desperation, but her large venous pool continued to pour through the vena cavae. Slings were rapidly passed around the cavae, and we went to work to sew up the four centimeter hole. During this time she was being rapidly infused with (refrigerated) bank blood and got one or two ventricular squeezes from my hand, but certainly had no effective circulation. When the slings were removed, she defibrillated spontaneously and restored effective cardiac action within less than ten minutes of massage. The time interval between exsanguination and fibrillation to effective massage is fairly well documented to be twenty minutes which is supported by the anesthesia record, the neurosurgeon and two other uninvolved members of the house staff. There is some uncertainty about whether the heart defibrillated spontaneously and might have provided a little circulation while we were fighting to get the slings on, but certainly the period of circulatory arrest was no less than twelve minutes. The factor of unplanned cooling from the refrigerated blood doubtless played a role, but her total body temperature did not get below 35° C.

Needless to say, we were very surprised that she woke up within three to four hours and was completely lucid the next morning—her retrograde amnesia persisting but later resolving.

The whole experience is so untenable with established experience that I have hesitated to report it knowing full well that it would be thoroughly disbelieved. It is of interest, however, that her free communication between the pericardial space and the right atrium resulted in an equilibrium which maintained effective right ventricular filling over a twelve hour period from injury to operation.*

The experiments of Neely and Youmans have stimulated considerable interest in the detrimental effect of anoxic blood flow to the brain, as compared with the considerably less damaging effect of anoxia in a brain deprived of blood. By elevating intracranial pressure in dogs, they "squeezed" the blood out of the brain and simultaneously prevented entry of arterial blood. Thus they theoretically prevented clotting in the presence of acidotic blood. In addition, since no blood glucose is present, no anaerobic glycolytic conversion into lactic acid occurs. Some dogs in this series were able to withstand up to 25 minutes of cerebral circulatory halt without subsequent neuorologic sequelae.

Suspension of CNS activity is not well understood. The relationship to pH changes is well known, as is alteration of glucose metabolism of the brain during hypothermia. The block in glucose mechanism appears to be the crux. In the absence of oxygen, anerobic metabolism produces lactic and carbonic acids. The lowered pH is thought by some to cause coagulation of the blood in the small vascular channels.

From the present study, I think that it can also be stated that the period of time may itself be compromised by various factors. Of first importance is the effectiveness of the physician in his ability to compress the heart

*Roe, B. B.: Personal communication, 1968.

manually. Practice in the animal laboratory should be made available to all physicians. During cardiac massage, one should be able to maintain a systolic blood pressure of at least 85 mm. Hg, produce an easily palpable pulse in the peripheral vessels, maintain normal color of the patient, and keep the pupils constricted. If such is not the case, the likelihood of neurologic damage is increased, regardless of the original time factor. (These remarks are repeated in this book to emphasize their extreme importance.)

Other factors influencing the significance of the time factor would include the position of the patient. There is sufficient evidence to indicate that a 15 degree Trendelenburg position will add seconds to the period of reversibility. Premedication, if of sufficient depth, may add a beneficial effect by reducing somewhat the metabolic demands for oxygen by the cortical cells. Conversely, CNS stimulants may reduce the period of reversibility. Although it would seem so, I cannot find evidence in our study that the condition of the cerebral vessels necessarily plays a major role. The temperature of the patient at the time of the arrest is still another factor, as is the blood pressure. Hypothermic patients withstand longer periods of anoxia than do patients whose body temperature is normal. The converse also appears true. Although I have no explanation, an unexpectedly high number of patients with pulmonary tuberculosis have seemed to show unusual resistance to long periods of anoxia (discussion to follow). Therefore the crux of the entire problem lies in a realization of the importance of the time factor.

The overall survival rate in the first 1,710 cases studied proved to be 536—almost 30%. These cases did not all occur in the operating room. This emergency is likely to be encountered nearly any place in the hospital. Seventy-two of these originally resuscitated patients have been located and have contributed to the study's long-term information. What is the eventual outcome of the patient subjected to cardiac asystole? Of the seventy-two patients, 88.5% were living at the time of this follow-up study. Sixty-five percent of all the patients have been followed over 4 years, 11% have been followed over 8 years. One was followed for 15 years. Of the total, 66⅔% were as well physically and mentally as they ever were thought to be.

The cause of death in the nine fatal cases showed one patient a suicide; two died from cardiac pathology; and one each from cancer, peritonitis, and urinary tract infection. Two died in a decerebrate state. The cause of one death was unknown.

Sex incidence was not remarkable: thirty-one were female; forty-one were male. The incidence of cardiac arrest has continued to maintain this ratio.

As previously stated, if one excludes coronary artery disease, the incidence of cardiac arrest is greatest in the first decade of life, the sixth decade being next in frequency. The neurologic sequelae proved to be a different thing. In the statistical study presented in the first edition, 50% of the patients in the first decade of life showed definite and often severe neurologic sequelae. On the other hand, 100% survival without neurologic sequelae was noted in the patients in the sixth decade of life.

There is still some question in my mind as to whether the prognosis following prolonged periods of cerebral anoxia with resultant cerebral edema is appreciably better in a child or young adult than in an older person. Certainly, this difference has not been well documented, although many physicians consider that children have a better prognosis in terms of residual neurologic deficits than do adult patients.

A breakdown of the 16% with neurologic sequelae shows three patients to be in an almost decerebrate state, eight suffer marked mental retardation, one needs psychiatric care, one (a young boy) has had unusual nightmares regularly since the arrest.

Of interest are two patients hospitalized in psychiatric institutions before experiencing the cardiac arrest. Both improved soon after the arrest sufficiently to be discharged. Two others were considered "neurotics" formerly; now they seem more stable!

A favorable prognosis can usually be made if effective cardiac massage is known to have been started within 2 to 3 minutes of the onset of arrest. If massage is adequate, survival may be expected regardless of the length of the massage period. In the group were patients experiencing massage for 82 and 45 minutes. The rapid return of spontaneous respirations is encouraging. Two patients awoke during cardiac massage.

Immediate postresuscitative hyperthermia is a bad prognostic sign, although there are several exceptions, some patients reaching temperatures as high as 105° F.

Of those who die, 92% will succumb in the first 24 hours. Only 2% die after 6 days. In the sixty-four cases with which I have personally been involved, there were two who were decerebrate for 27 and 36 days before death.

Among patients with immediate CNS sequelae, a long-term follow-up frequently points to many encouraging examples of progressive and definite improvement 6 months to 1 year later. In the group of 66% now judged to be normal, there were such early findings as unconsciousness for 10 days, amnesia, loss of libido for 6 months, convulsions, spasticity, asphasia, complete blindness, and muscular rigidity. IQ tests failed to indicate regression. Seven patients had serial EEG studies. Progressive returns to normal were noted after an elapse of even several months.

In none of our cases have we exactly duplicated the experience reported by Kral from Montreal. His case represented a 6-year follow-up on a young boy. Three different phases were described. The first consisted of gradual recovery from an almost decorticate state. An extrapyramidal syndrome, cerebellar dysfunction, and neurologic findings referable to a lesion of cervical segments of the spinal cord were mentioned. The improvement lasted 7 months. It was followed by a 1-year maintenance period and then by a period of gradual deterioration for at least 4 years. One woman considered to have accomplished an excellent job of rehabilitation later required permanent hospitalization.

Incidentally, cardiac complications have been minimal. Two English patients are now 85 and 86 years of age after exposure to cardiac arrest in their seventies; both had had previous coronary artery insufficiency. Angina was alleviated in one case. Two patients had multiple arrests; one died following the third episode, whereas the other seems quite well after a second arrest several years subsequent to the first. Several women have had children since the arrest. A patient with severe hypertension was improved. One patient experienced cardiac arrest in 1939, fought through all of World War II, and is living and well today.

The American College of Surgeons made public a request by William H. Sweet, Boston, chairman of the Committee on Management of the Unconscious Patient. The committee was eager to know the longest periods of coma followed by useful survival as it has been encountered clinically. It is its belief that the ability of physicians to maintain life for very long periods in the unconscious patient raises the question as to how long such skills should be employed. It is relevant to know the longest periods of coma that have been followed by useful survival. The committee of the Massachusetts General Hospital is seeking to determine pertinent features in all patients who, despite coma for over 5 weeks, have made a useful recovery. Any well-documented patient in this category should be brought to its attention.

Generally speaking, the incidence of severe permanent cerebral damage following resuscitation continues to be low. There was only one such case in the large series reported from the Royal Victoria Hospital in Belfast in which 173 patients were successfully defibrillated following a myocardial infarction and survived to leave the hospital.

In a group of 237 patients only four patients with irreversible cerebral damage survived for more than 1 week (Jeresaty). Ninety percent who failed to respond to cardiopulmonary resuscitation died with 24 hours.

Varying degrees of neurologic damage, many of a transient nature, were estimated to occur to 50% of 305 cardiac arrests evaluated during a 6-year period at the Hospital of the Good Samaritan Medical Center in Los Angeles (Stiles and co-workers). Significantly, however, the frequency of brain damage in surviving patients decreased considerably during the 6-year evaluation of the active resuscitation program. By a combination of monitoring devices and adequately trained personnel capable of recognizing the premonitory symptoms, the time factor was reduced.

During a 4-year period at the University Clinic in Copenhagen, 164 cases of cardiac arrest were encountered (Sandoe and co-workers). Significant residual brain damage was detected in only one of forty-one patients followed for a period of 1 to 4 years. One patient required resuscitation for $3\frac{1}{2}$ hours and yet survived without detectable brain damage. There were no patients with severe neurologic damage among the survivors after cardiopulmonary resuscitation in a group of 368 cases studied at the University of Virginia during a 3-year period. One of twenty patients surviving in 100 consecutive cardiac arrests treated by external cardiac massage was discharged to a nursing home because of permanent brain damage (Jung and co-workers). It would appear that there is little reason for concern whether widespread applications of cardiopulmonary resuscitation techniques outside of the controlled environment of the operating room will lead to a high incidence of permanent neurologic damage.

Low versus absent perfusion rates

The difference between very low perfusion rates and completely absent perfusion rates of the brain can be quite significant as far as recovery is concerned. Belsey, for example, in a report of over 300 open-heart operations, was able to maintain hypothermic cardioplegia up to 2 hours by maintaining a low perfusion throughout the procedure.

Brain ATP levels

Since the functional capacity of the intact brain is reflected by the absolute concentration of the high energy phosphate, adenosine triphosphate (ATP), Sealy and his group at Duke may have made a most significant contribution in defining the extent and duration of ATP disappearance under varying conditions such as ischemia, anoxia, hyperoxia, and profound hypothermia. It is highly possible that they have found the threshold of irreversible damage as measured in the ATP content of the biopsied brain specimen. Nonrecovery of brain ATP can be predicted when there is a reduction of ATP stores to approximately 20% of control levels. With profound hypothermia this occurred after 90 minutes of hypothermic arrests. At the 90% level the electroencephalographic pattern flattens.

Adenosine triphosphate, as a primary source of chemical energy in brain tissue serves as a reliable indicator of the extent of metabolic activity. As a precise measurement of cerebral metabolic activity it surpasses oxygen and glucose utilization and lactate and carbon dioxide production studies. It more nearly reflects the functional state of the brain and its determination may afford, under certain situations, a rational basis for predicting the probability of cerebral recovery following prolonged periods of circulatory arrest. The interdisciplinary effort at the Duke University Medical Center (Kramer, Sanders, Lesage, Woodhall, and Sealy) is a most significant one in that they were able to develop an improved method of sequential cerebral biopsies permitting the accurate determination of ATP during various periods of circulatory insufficiency to the brain. Within 3.8 minutes of complete cerebral circulatory arrest, there is a 50% decrease of cerebral ATP as reflected in brain biopsies. The protection afforded by hypothermia is attested to by their findings that it took 13.3 minutes for a 50% reduction in cerebral ATP under conditions of hypothermia (5° to 11° C.). Recovery of ATP after 30 and 60 minutes of hypothermia and subsequent rewarming occurred but not after 90 minutes. Since, as they point out, ATP is required for the maintenance of electrical activity, membrane integrity, the "sodium pump," protein, nucleic acid, and lipid synthesis, and glucose utilization, it is highly important to quantitate the effect on ATP production during periods of varying degrees of circulatory arrest, particularly when investigating adjunctive techniques that may be of value in forestalling the onset of the "irreversible phase" of ischemic brain damage.

Effect of transient cardiac arrest upon the spinal cord

Although it is generally assumed that the cerebrum and cerebellum are usually damaged before the brainstem and spinal cord during episodes of anoxia associated with cardiac arrest, spinal cord injury may occasionally occur by itself. An excellent study on the vulnerability of the spinal cord in cardiac arrest is provided by Gilles and Nag from the Department of Pathology and Neurology at Harvard Medical School. Studies of infants coming to autopsy after varying periods of survival following cardiac arrest allow several generalizations to be made: When inadequate perfusion is present in the spinal cord, susceptibility to anoxic change increases caudally and is more marked in the anterior horns than in the posterior ones. The damage is more prominent deep within individual subnuclei.

Even though it is well established that the cerebral hemispheres are the most vulnerable to anoxia in cases of cardiac arrest, several cases of paraplegia have occurred without evidence of permanent cerebral damage. Jennings and Newton report on a 63-year-old man who was admitted to the hospital after a myocardial infarction. At least a dozen episodes of ventricular fibrillation and several ventricular asystoles occurred while the patient was in the hospital. Subsequent cerebration was gradually improved although a permanent paraplegia did result. The main lesion was in the lower cord where there was evidence of anterior horn damage at L3 and L4; and sensory levels were established at D8 on the left and D10 on the right. A similar case has been reported by Henson and Parsons. In both cases it is suggested that the cord infarction was precipitated by temporary circulatory impairment and the presence of local vascular disease.

As might be expected, the detrimental effects of ischemia on the spinal cord may be somewhat comparable to those seen in cerebral tissue. Feldman and associates at Ohio State University measured lactate production in the spinal cord of Rhesus monkeys following varying periods of complete anoxia. Anoxic spinal tissue lactate was markedly elevated above controls at periods of 5 to 10 minutes after circulatory arrest.

Prognostic value of the electroencephalogram

Since the last edition of this book, accumulating interest in the electroencephalographic studies following cardiac resuscitation has been sufficiently productive to indicate that the EEG is now a most valuable tool for predicting the eventual outcome of cardiorespiratory resuscitation. In fact, Binnie and co-workers state that when the outcome of known cardiac arrest is established as well as might be, death or survival could be reliably predicted on the basis of a single EEG with a confidence level better than 99.8%. Within a week of cardiac resuscitation, ninety-three electroencephalograms were recorded from forty-one patients. The subsequent outcome was known to be either recovery of cerebral function or death, with associated pathological evidence of gross anoxic brain damage. A statistical analysis of the observations of these EEGs yielded a discriminant function for predicting death or survival. A method of visual assessment and coding was developed that included forty-nine variables. These include the presence, prominence, and distribution of a wide range of EEG phenomena. In addition to isoelectric tracings, the regular recurrence of any particular EEG phenomenon was regarded as a particularly adverse sign. The slower the repetition rate, the worse the prognosis. Other unfavorable signs included paroxysmal activity (spikes, either single or multiple, sharp waves, or complexes of these together with slow components). In addition, consistently low amplitude was regarded as an adverse sign. Episodic reduction in amplitude, however slight in degree, signified a poor prognosis. Although less consistent, signs of asymmetries, lack of theta or alpha activity, and the absence of EEG response to painful or auditory stimulation are noted. It is also noted that resuscitation following barbiturate intoxication often gave a confused EEG pattern that was difficult to evaluate. These workers at St. Bartholomew's Hospital in London have now established a routine service for predicting outcome following resuscitation.

Other criteria for predicting survival after EEG inspection following cardiac resuscitation have been devised by Hockaday and co-workers and Pampiglione and Harden.

Complete cerebral ischemia in dogs was produced by occluding the superior vena cava above the azygous vein, the inferior vena cava, and the aorta. Zimmerman and Nielson varied the duration of complete cerebral ischemia in an effort to determine brain damage as tested by maze and psychomotor performance in dogs. They demonstrate that electroencephalography is not a precise method of determining the effect of cerebral ischemia, since there is no difference in the recovery pattern of the EEG following 6 and 8 minutes of blood flow occlusion. By contrast, however, severe impairment of learning, but without effect upon retention or psychomotor performance, is experienced by dogs after 8 minutes of complete cerebral ischemia. No changes in learning, retention, or psychomotor performance are noted after a 6-minute period of ischemia. Spoerel has presented an excellent review of the EEG after cardiac arrest.

Paroxysmal depolarization of the cortex in cerebral ischemia was studied by Grossman and Lynch, who found that a 10 to 30 mv. potential develops between the cortex and the white matter 4 to 6 minutes after cerebral ischemia, which may indicate that this voltage is a better acute indicator of irreversible brain damage than is the preceding electroencephalographic silence.

Neurologic sequelae from electroencephalogram monitoring

Following a cardiac arrest with resuscitation of the victim, electroencephalographic tracings may offer valuable prognostic information. The importance of "suppression-burst activity" has been reviewed by Delamonica. Its presence strongly suggests the likelihood of severe diffuse cerebral damage. One may define suppression-burst activity as an electroencephalographic pattern characterized by recurrent periods of marked voltage depression, or isoelectric activity, associated or not with bursts of moderate to high voltage, sometimes intermixed with spike discharges. The duration is usually short, from 1 to 3 seconds. While suppression-burst activity has been observed transiently in conditions of temporary hypoxia, the pattern is most usually found with profound alterations in the central nervous system. The presence of suppression-burst activity does not necessarily predicate a vegetative status of the patient but warns strongly of its possibility. Fig. 56-2 illustrates EEG suppression-burst activity.

Adverse prognostic signs as recorded by the electroencephalogram in the postresuscitation period include (1) regular recurrence of any particular EEG phenomenon—the slower the repetition rate the worse the prognosis, (2) paroxysmal activity, (3) con-

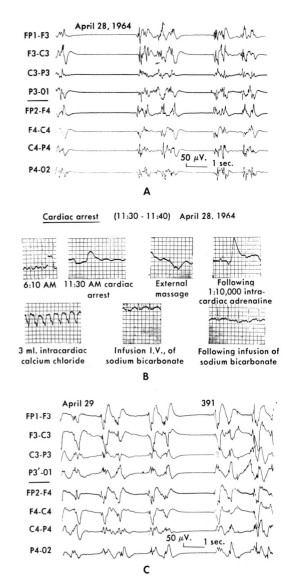

Fig. 56-2. A, EEG showing suppression-burst activity the first day after the patient's first cardiac arrest; B, patient's second cardiac arrest; C, suppression-burst activity following second cardiac arrest. (From Delamonica, E. A.: Suppression-burst activity in a case of cardiac arrest, Dis. Nerv. Syst. 30:618-621, 1969.)

sistently low amplitude, (4) episodic reductions in amplitude, (5) a lack of theta and alpha activity, (6) absence of an EEG response to painful or auditory stimulation (Binnie and co-workers).

The effect of increased cerebral spinal fluid pressure

The devastating effects of high intracranial pressure on the cerebral circulation are apparent when one realizes that vessels supplying the central nervous system must cross a fluid space to get to the brain. The brain, being a semifluid organ, can transmit pressure in all directions. The blood vessels entering the cranial vault and the entire central nervous system are collapsed by high intracranial pressure. Neely and Youmans have shown that cerebral spinal fluid pressures of 400 mm. Hg in dogs can completely shut off cerebral blood flow.

Cerebral venous pressure

One should carefully avoid measures that might lead to an increase of cerebral venous pressure. For example, when a patient is comatose, the pressure of assisted ventilation should be limited to the minimum required to maintain adequate ventilation in order that increasing cerebral venous pressure may be avoided (Wilson). This cardiac surgeon also makes the very excellent suggestion that elevation of the head of the bed 20 or 30 degrees will not only improve ventilation but will also reduce cerebral venous pressure.

Factors affecting oxygen consumption

Oxygen extraction from blood, percentagewise, is increased with a delayed passage, such as in cerebral blood flow. Krainer states that the oxygen consumption of the brain may be reduced to as much as 20% of its normal consumption, with cerebral function returning to normal after an unlimited revival time.

Chlorpromazine or promethazine (Phenergan) as neuroplegic drugs facilitate hypothermic induction and greatly reduce the increased oxygen demand provoked by shivering. Chlorpromazine probably also decreases cerebral metabolic activity and is said to favor the entrance of potassium into the cells. High serum potassium levels occurring with considerable tissue injury may, at times, be significant.

Treatment of cerebral anoxia

Much of the therapeutic effort to overcome the manifestations of cerebral anoxia is directed toward reduction of cerebral edema, which is generally considered responsible for much of the depression that follows a cerebral anoxic episode such as that which follows cardiac arrest.

Brierley emphasizes that a majority of patients who suffer irreversible brain damage from acute circulatory collapse and subsequent resuscitation die within a few days. In only a minority of these patients is there unequivocal evidence of increased intracranial pressure.

In general, treatment to date is difficult to evaluate, especially when the pathology is not altogether clear. From well over 100 autopsies on such patients, the findings are of an extremely variable nature as are the neurologic sequelae. In a death on the thirty-sixth postresuscitative day, no significant gross or histologic findings could be found by the pathologist. Warburg's studies indicate that cortical cells survive well beyond their ability to function. Therapeutic measures such as glutamic acid, nicotinic acid, thiamine, intravenous procaine, carbogen, stellate ganglion blocks, hypertonic glucose, serum albumin, and histamine have all had their advocates.

Crowell and co-workers present an extremely interesting piece of work that challenges the supposition that CNS damage and destruction are directly due only to periods of anoxia. They found that periods of marked hypercoagulability occur in the dog following cardiac arrest.

It appears, therefore, that it is not necessarily the central nervous system that imposes the limiting factor in the duration of arrest tolerated by these experimental animals, but, instead, it is the development of small blood clots in the vascular system. As demonstrated in the figures at the beginning, these small blood clots form in the vascular system during periods of circulatory arrest or during periods of extreme anoxia. However, it is approximately thirty minutes later that the majority of them are washed out to block the flow of blood through the pulmonary sytesm. At this time the arterial pressure begins to fall; thus, there results a time of "irreversible" shock.

It also appears that some of the central nervous system destruction formerly attributed to the primary effects of anoxia may be due to the formation of these small blood clots in the central nervous system. . . .*

These workers were able to present evidence that heparinization of the animals during the period of circulatory arrest greatly decreases the mortality rate and that the duration of arrest can be practically double that in the unheparinized animal. These men present this provocative statement:

If the degree of cerebral destruction were determined by the phylogenetic structure of the brain, then it would be logical to assume that a period of circulatory arrest would allow degeneration of certain portions of the brain, but in all cases the animal would live until such time as the arrest were of sufficient duration to affect the vital centers. This phylogenetic theory of cerebral destruction has not been conclusively confirmed, and, indeed, some pathologic evidence is to the contrary.*

Streptokinase-streptodornase (Varidase) has shown promise of protecting the dog from cerebral damage during cardiac arrest. Crowell notes this preparation to be even more effective than heparin and attributes this to the fact that coagulation may continue in the presence of heparin. Human plasma was added to the streptokinase-streptodornase for activation.

UREA

In addition to generalized hypothermia, limitation of fluids to 600 to 800 ml. per square meter of body surface area per day should be carried out. Osmotic diuretics can be administered by intravenous infusion of urea (20 to 40 gm. of a 40% solution). A

*From Crowell, J. W., Sharpe, G. P., Lambright, R. L., and Read, W. L.: Mechanism of death after resuscitation following acute circulatory failure, Surgery 38:696-702, 1955.

case is reported by Parkhouse from Oxford, England, that illustrates the advantageous effect of urea in reducing intracranial tension. The patient was a 24-year-old woman whose heart stopped during a tympanoplasty procedure. In spite of successful restoration of the heart action, the patient remained apneic, but spontaneous respirations returned almost immediately after administration of 300 ml. of 30% Urevert (a solution of 30% urea lyophilized in 10% invert sugar in water).

Young and Javid, of the University of Wisconsin Medical School, studied the effects of intravenous urea on cerebrospinal fluid pressure and brain volume following simulated cardiac arrest in dogs. Cardiac arrest was produced by inducing ventricular fibrillation via external electrodes. The simulated arrest was carried out for periods varying between 6 and $10\frac{1}{2}$ minutes. Half of the dogs received intravenous 10% invert sugar, and the other half received intravenous 30% urea (a dose of $1\frac{1}{2}$ gm. per kilogram of body weight in 10% invert sugar). Elevation of the cerebrospinal fluid pressure in the control group of dogs remained for as long as 18 hours. Urea routinely reduced cerebrospinal fluid pressure and brain volume. Dogs survived up to 7 minutes of occlusion with or without urea. Occlusion of more than $8\frac{1}{2}$ minutes produced such severe damage that all died. Within the period of occlusion, depending upon the rectal temperature, there was a definite suggestion that the administration of urea favored survival. A marked shrinkage in the brain volume could be noted grossly in dogs treated with urea.

Safar cautions against the use of urea following an anoxic insult. Although the volume of brain tissue is decreased by urea at the expense of an increase in intracranial blood volume, rebound brain swelling may occur.

GLYCEROL FOR CEREBRAL EDEMA

Considerable neurologic inprovement and reduction in cerebrospinal fluid pressure is noted in a group of thirty-six patients with cerebral infarction and cerebral edema and in seventeen other patients with edema of the central nervous system when glycerol was given, either via the oral or intravenous route (Meyer and co-workers).

GLUCOSTEROIDS FOR CEREBRAL EDEMA

Some prefer the use of dexamethasone to intravenous urea in the treatment of cerebral edema resulting from excessive anoxia and hypoxia at the time of cardiac arrest. While dexamethasone takes somewhat longer (about 5 hours) to be effective, there apparently is not the rebound effect so often experienced with urea administration.

Dexamethasone (Decadron) is a glucosteroid. French recommends that the drug be injected initially as an 8 mg. dose intramuscularly, followed by a 4 mg. dose every 6 hours. The dosage may be gradually decreased after 3 or 4 days. The agent probably produces its effect more slowly than does urea or mannitol, but its effect seems to be more prolonged. In addition, it can be given over a longer period of time.

Long, Hartmann, and French conclude that dexamethasone definitely reduces the amount of brain swelling, particularly in terms of astrocyte cytoplasm and the extracellular accumulation of fluid in the white matter. The edematous brains are returned toward a normal configuration by the administration of dexamethasone. The reader is referred to their work for an excellent discussion of the hypothesis for a mechanism of action of the steroids in the treatment of cerebral edema.

Galicich and French presented the first account of the specific use of steroids for the treatment of cerebral edema in 1961.

Hammargren and associates report experimental studies in which cerebral damage was produced with the intracarotid injection of sodium diatrizoate (Hypaque). Premedication with low molecular weight dextran or with dexamethasone resulted in a significant reduction in cerebrovascular permeability to dyes concomitant with less cerebral edema and a lower mortality rate. Premedication with both drugs simultaneously produced almost complete protection against cerebral damage from the intercarotid injection of sodium diatrizoate.

The pathophysiologic understanding of cerebral edema is the subject of great debate and voluminous literature. Vascular stasis and various other mechanical factors are often used to explain the appearance of edema. More recently, Long, Hartmann, and French considered cerebral edema to be the result of a deranged water and electrolyte transport mechanism within the brain. They believe that the disruption probably occurs at the capillary-glial interface but may also be present elsewhere at levels as yet unknown. Abnormal accumulation of fluid, electrolytes, and possibly other substances occurs primarily within the astroglia and in the white matter extracellular space. The continued accumulation of this fluid may result in tissue disruption, compression, and ischemia and may well account for certain of the latter features present in severe brain swelling. They believe that the administration of large quantities of glucosteroids is capable of reversing these abnormalities and of reducing the amount of structural change present in the edematous brain.

Lysosomal membrane integrity is important in the prevention of irreversible brain damage. Free lysosome enzymes and subsequent protein degradation occur under conditions of cerebral anoxia. Steroids are thought to have a role in protection of the lysosomal membranes. In addition to the theoretical benefit of steroids in cerebral edema other immediate beneficial effects would warrant their use. These include its inotropic effect on myocardium and its vasodilating effect as an augmentation of the circulation and increase of vital organ perfusion.

Monitoring of cerebral fluid pressure

Cushman and colleagues have developed an intravenous technique for measuring cerebral blood flow in patients with depressed consciousness. Their patients include controls and those with brain tumor, cerebral vascular concussion, and head injury. (Apparently no patients were followed in a postcardiac resuscitation period.) They indicate that superimposed small vessel occlusion, presence or absence of adequate collateral flow, and increased intracranial pressure are among several factors of critical importance in a return of consciousness. Gosch and Kindt have used a simplified method of monitoring intracranial pressure in experimental animals as well as in patients. The method is similar to that used in measuring central venous pressure and involves making a twist drill hole 4.22 mm. in diameter through the cranial vault, opening the dura, and inserting the standard plastic intravenous tubing, which is attached to a standard spinal fluid monometer in a position level with the ventricular system. The height of the column of saline that stabilizes with the intracranial fluid indicates the intracranial pressure and provides an excellent means of monitoring the effects of intracranial pressure of hyperventilation, intravenous 50% glucose, mannitol, and other efforts being made to lower intracranial pressure.

Increased cerebral blood flow with papaverine hydrochloride

Inhalation of a mixture of 5% carbon dioxide in oxygen is known to be temporarily effective in increasing cerebral oxygenation. Meyer and associates demonstrate that intravenous administration of papaverine hydrochloride increases cerebral blood flow and oxygenation for prolonged periods in patients with cerebral thromboembolism. The amount of oxygen made available to the brain is increased in cases of cerebrovascular disease, anoxic encephalopathy, and carbon dioxide narcosis. Papaverine increases cerebral blood flow even in the presence of carbon dioxide narcosis, which indicates that its vasodilator effect is independent of any vasodilator action of carbon dioxide. The documentation

of increased oxygen was made by continuous measurement of cerebral arteriovenous differences for oxygen pressure and saturation. Both oxygen pressure and saturation showed significant increases. Cerebral venous carbon dioxide pressures decreased, and the central venous pH increased significantly.

The cerebral arterioles are most responsive to partial pressure carbon dioxide and to some extent to the changes in partial pressure of oxygen. With hyperoxia and hypocapnia, vasoconstriction occurs in patients with cerebral vascular disease associated with mild to moderate neurologic deficit, and inhalation of 100% oxygen decreases cerebral blood flow by about 10%. Carbon dioxide is the most effective cerebral vasodilator. Intermittent inhalation of 5% carbon dioxide and 95% oxygen (15 minutes each hour) will cause a marked increase in cerebral blood flow and in the amount of oxygen available to the brain. Papaverine has been found of some value in the treatment of acute stroke caused by cerebral infarction and may theoretically have some benefit after cardiac arrest. It may be administered at the rate of 1 gram every 24 hours by constant intravenous drip for 4 to 5 days.

Controlled hyperventilation

There is considerable controversy as to the value of controlled hyperventilation in patients suffering episodes of cerebral ischemia. Working at the Karolinska Hospital in Stockholm, Gordan noted that there is a significantly greater recovery in patients with traumatic brain injury who are treated with controlled hyperventilation following the injury. In support of controlled hyperventilation, Gordan points to its ability to compensate for low intracerebral pH, its ability to relieve patients from energy-consuming and exhausting respiratory overwork, and its effect in lowering intracranial pressure. Controlled hyperventilation facilitates a more favorable distribution of the cerebral blood flow by the so-called inverse steal effect and permits an effective increase of the oxygen tension and saturation in the arterial blood and thereby the maintenance of higher oxygen supply to the brain. However, it would seem that further study will be needed.

Hypothermia for alleviation of neurologic sequelae

Generalized hypothermia for patients with cardiac arrest was introduced shortly before the first edition of this book (1958). After more than 15 years of clinical trial, it seems evident that the survival rate has been appreciably improved. Deep hypothermia, on the other hand, has been associated with evidence of increased brain damage, as encountered after extracorporeal cooling.

Zimmerman and Spencer report that the survival rate of dogs subjected to 10 minutes of circulatory arrest is raised from 25% to 50% by the use of hypothermia. Wolfe was able to show marked protection in only 33% of dogs cooled at 31° C. after 5 minutes of ventricular fibrillation.

The clinical use of generalized hypothermia in patients with evidence of neurologic injury following cardiac arrest was reported from Johns Hopkins in 1958 by Williams and Spencer. Generalized hypothermia is achieved with a temperature no lower than 31° to 32° C. Patients are cooled with a refrigeration blanket or with chipped ice. Temperatures below 31° to 32° C. have apparently not added any additional benefit to the patient, and it is well known that cardiac arrhythmias are more frequent below temperatures of this level. Hypothermia does not need to be maintained beyond 2 to 4 days, as beneficial effects beyond this time are rarely observed. Chlorpromazine or promethazine is often indicated to prevent shivering. Shivering may increase cerebral metabolism over 100%, even at lowered temperatures.

With hypothermia, a decreased pressure in cerebrospinal fluid occurs, accompanied by decreased cerebral blood flow, diminished cerebral metabolic activity, decreased brain volume (increase of 30% intracranial space), and depression of electrical activity of the brain.

In a group of dogs under hypothermia, cerebral circulation was arrested for 8 minutes to determine the subsequent neurologic sequelae and to compare the therapeutic benefits of postischemic, prolonged hypothermia with those of mannitol infusion. Brient and colleagues failed to note any reduction of neurologic sequelae in the dogs treated by mannitol infusion. In the dogs managed by prolonged hypothermia there was a marked decrease in significant neurologic findings. It is suggested that hypothermia protects against the mortality of experimental brain injury by means other than a reduction in cerebral spinal fluid pressure and cerebral edema. Both mannitol and hypothermia reduce cerebral edema.

A remarkable case of profound neurologic depression after cardiac arrest with subsequent recovery is reported by Nargiello and associates. The patient, a 26-year-old woman, experienced a cardiac arrest on the operating room table. The heart was restored to a normal rhythm after manual massage for 90 seconds. The exact duration of cardiac arrest was unknown since the chest had been closed prior to the arrest. The patient was in a period of profound coma for 28 days. Hypothermia was maintained between 91° and 95° F. for the first 96 hours. On the thirty-second day following the arrest, the patient became conscious, and, after 123 days of observation, she was discharged at her own request. The patient appeared to be normal except for a mild ataxia and a slight speech defect.

Brient compares postischemic, prolonged hypothermia with continuous mannitol infusion in a group of twenty-three dogs observed for neurologic sequelae following 8 minutes of cardiac arrest and total cerebral ischemia. The dogs treated with hypothermia showed considerably fewer neurologic sequelae than did either the control group or the mannitol-infusion group. Brient speculates that hypothermia exerts its protective effect through some mechanism other than the reduction of cerebral edema. Cerebrospinal fluid measurements fail to show a correlation between mortality and the degree of cerebral edema.

Fay (1943) treated patients with severe cerebral injury with generalized hypothermia (32° C.) for 24 to 48 hours.

A 12-day-old infant was operated upon for bilateral harelip associated with cleft alveolus and cleft palate. Following the operation, cardiac arrest occurred. A thoracotomy with direct cardiac massage was instituted and cardiac action was resumed almost immediately after massage was started; however, spontaneous respiration did not return. The child was placed in ice, and the temperature was rapidly lowered. Cheyne-Stokes respiration began 15 minutes later; subsequently, normal respirations returned. The child has been followed, and there is no evidence of permanent damage.

The temperature of the patient may be monitored continuously by a rectal thermometer. Because of the severe vasoconstriction present with hypothermia of 30° to 32° C., blood pressure determinations may be difficult to obtain. The patient's condition may be indicated by the hourly urine volume. If the urine output is below 10 to 15 ml. per hour, renal malfunction may be presumed.

In discussing the management of the patient following cardiac arrest, Safar states that, in his opinion, the oxygen tension should be raised immediately following an anoxic insult and the carbon dioxide tension should be lowered slightly by controlled hyperventilation. The venous pressure should be decreased by keeping the mean airway pressure low and by elevating the head. Early cooling may minimize cerebral edema.

Not only is hypothermia a theoretical aid in minimizing cerebral edema but is also of value in preventing hyperthermia that often follows periods of cerebral anoxia.

What effect has hypothermia in the prevention of neurologic sequelae after infant resuscitation? Because of the effect of hypothermia in decreasing metabolic demands and possible brain damage during asphyxia, Westin presents a strong case for the use of hypothermia in newborn infants who are given ventilatory support in cardiac massage for resuscitation. Zywicka-Twarowska has shown that late neurologic sequelae may be present if apnea is prolonged for more than 4 minutes during the neonatal period. In Westin's group, sixty infants treated with cooling did not deviate from the normal with regard to growth and motor and speech development. The first nine of these have been examined at the age of 10 years and all had completely normal audiograms in spite of being apneic for a mean time of 17 minutes. None exhibited any signs of late neurologic damage.

Low molecular weight dextran

For some years we have suggested that low molecular weight dextran may provide an effective adjunct in the correction of the altered hemodynamics following cardiac resuscitation. Its unique anticoagulation and antisludging properties, as manifested by its apparent coating of blood vessel walls, red blood cells, and platelets, make it an effective means of treating or preventing disseminated intravascular coagulation.

Cerebral blood flow is aided by the administration of low molecular weight dextran since it decreases cerebral edema and cuts down on platelet adhesiveness within the smaller vessels of the brain. Additional evidence indicates that low molecular weight dextran has a definite beneficial effect on reducing the size of the infarction after experimental occlusion of the middle cerebral artery in dogs (Cyrus and co-workers). Here again, the beneficial effect of low molecular weight dextran is ascribed to the drug's action in preventing sludging and keeping the vascular bed fluid. Collateral circulation may in this manner also be favorably influenced. Ten percent low molecular weight dextran in normal saline solution is used.

Low molecular weight dextran may prove to have a place in the postresuscitation regimen.

Hyperbaric oxygen following cardiac arrest

For some time it has seemed logical to expect that cerebral edema may be effectively treated by exposing the patient to oxygen under increased atmospheric pressure.

Sukoff attributes the beneficial effect of hyperbaric oxygenation in cerebral anoxia to a reduction of edema by the cerebral vasoconstricting elements of hyperbaric oxygenation as well as to the actual increase in available oxygen. He was able to decrease the mortality in animals with experimentally produced cerebral edema and compression. After a treatment session, previously semicomatose animals were able to walk away unaided from the hyperbaric chamber.

Smith and associates, Glasgow, Scotland, reason that hyperbaric oxygenation may be of benefit in clinical conditions associated with cellular anoxia and edema of the brain if anoxic damage is minimized by breathing oxygen at increased pressure, thereby fully saturating hemoglobin, increasing the plasma-dissolved oxygen, and increasing the diffusion gradient of this gas between capillary bed and anoxic cell. Smith and his group occluded both common carotid arteries and both vertebral arteries at the root of the neck until loss of EEG activity occurred in dogs breathing air at normal atmospheric pressure. When, however, the same procedure was carried out on dogs breathing oxygen at 2 atmospheres of pressure, no alteration of cerebral cortical activity was identified by EEG patterns. They conclude that collateral channels rapidly open up and prove adequate to carry on cerebral activity if the dogs are protected by superoxygenation during the period of experimental vascular shutdown. Enough oxygen is dissolved in the plasma to tide the brain over the initial postocclusion period and until the rapid opening up of collateral channels between the subclavian and brachiocephalic arteries and the vertebral vessels, chiefly through the agency of the costocervical and omocervical trunks.

A note of caution regarding the clinical use of hyperbaric oxygenation is raised by Fuson and co-workers at the Duke University hyperbaric unit. It is their experience that most patients tolerate the usual hyperbaric oxygenation exposure satisfactorily; however, serious lung oxygen toxicity may occasionally occur, usually under conditions of prolonged hyperbaric oxygenation. The development of profound pulmonary oxygen toxicity is difficult to distinguish from mild atelectasis or pulmonary embolism. They urge extreme care in the application of hyperbaric oxygenation and believe that exposures to hyperbaric oxygenation should be brief.

The use of hyperbaric oxygenation in the management of cerebral air embolism is discussed in the section on management of air embolism. Although the cerebral gas embolisms associated with diving accidents have been treated for more than 35 years by increased pressure in a decompression chamber by the U. S. Navy, recent workers suggest the use of hyperbaric treatment in air embolisms arising from a variety of etiologic factors, such as those associated with cardiac surgery. Takipa reports the use of hyperbaric oxygenation in the treatment of a cerebral gas embolism complicating open-heart surgery. Their patient developed an extensive involvement of the right cerebral hemisphere after air had entered the ascending aorta, passed through the innominate and right carotid arteries, and blocked the branches of the right middle and anterior cerebral arteries. When the patient was placed in the hyperbaric chamber, the pressure was first raised to 2.8 atmospheres absolute; but it was not until after the pressure was raised to 6 atmospheres absolute that the patient seemed to show improvement.

A case of cardiac arrest with severe cerebral damage was treated with hyperbaric oxygen by Koch and Vermuelen-Cranch.

The case of cardiac arrest occurred on September 8, 1961, in Amsterdam, Holland. The patient was being operated upon for bleeding duodenal ulcer, and cardiac arrest occurred at the conclusion of the skin suture placement. The heart was immediately visualized by a thoracotomy and was found to be in marked diastole. It was thought that the cardiac arrest had occurred due to ballooning of the cuff of an endotracheal tube with an occlusion of the left bronchus. Cyanosis of the patient had not been apparent due to the low hemoglobin content of the patient's blood.

About 3 hours after cardiac resuscitation, it was thought that moderately severe brain damage was present and hyperbaric oxygen was considered. Because of some disagreement among consultants, it was agreed to wait for a while and instead to use intravenous urea (equal portions of 60% urea and 20% invert sugar). Even though some improvement was noted following the use of urea, it was decided to place the patient in the high-pressure tank. This was carried out for approximately 4 hours. Reflexes were almost normal and the patient was able to pronounce simple words following removal from the high-pressure tank. It was concluded that administration of oxygen in the hyperbaric oxygen chamber was of definite benefit to the patient, even though he had received urea prior to the hyperbaric oxygen.

It remains to be seen if tissues deficient in oxygenation, such as may occur after cardiac arrest, will be influenced favorably by hyperbaric oxygen drenching of the cerebral tissues. Such saturation of cerebral tissues occurs when the patient breathes oxygen at a pressure of 3 atmospheres absolute. The oxygen, in such instances, is in solution and is sufficient for tissue requirements.

A therapeutic adjunct in the utilization of increased oxygen tension shows promise of considerable reward in such instances. Although clinical experience with this modality is limited, there is evidence that increased oxygen diffusion to the hypoxic cerebral cells may occur if the patient is allowed to breathe oxygen at a high pressure. Surgeons working at the Western Infirmary in Glasgow, Scotland, speculate that oxygen breathed at increased tension produces an increased oxygen-diffusion gradient to the extent that the hypoxic cerebral tissues are no longer prevented from getting oxygen by the edema barrier that has been produced. Not only have the cerebral cells been injured by anoxia but also the blood vessels supplying the tissues have been subjected to hypoxic

damage. The intercellular space becomes filled with fluids that have escaped from the vessels as a result of increased permeability of the vessel walls. With the diffusion barrier established, the vicious circle continues by creating an increased pressure gradient; however, more oxygen can be transferred to the damaged tissue before irreversible damage occurs.

A hyperbaric bed system (see Fig. 56-3), produced by Vickers Ltd. of England, has recently become available through the Bethlehem Corporation. It is designed to treat patients in the sitting position with 100% oxygen at pressures up to 2 atmospheres absolute. The dome consists of a double shell of Perspex. The lower half of the bed is made of steel, and the upper half is made of a double skin of aluminum filled with foamed plastic. Portholes at the foot and at the top of the bed permit viewing of the patient's extremities. Communication with the patient is maintained by an open microphone and speaker mounted on the chamber wall in front of the patient's face. Connections are provided for monitoring ECG, EEG, blood pressure, and temperature. One important advantage of the chamber is that it eliminates the exposure of hospital personnel to any hazards of increased pressure. Although experience with the hyperbaric bed has not been great as yet, there are indications that it may be of benefit in reducing the incidence of myocardial arrythmias in association with myocardial infarction. The hyperbaric bed system may prove to have a valuable place in the immediate care of the postresuscitation patient. At the Westminster Hospital in London, forty patients with acute myocardial infarction were treated one to three times daily with hyperbaric oxygen at 2 atmospheres absolute for periods lasting up to 2 hours. It was noted that dyspnea caused by acute left ventricular failure was uniformly relieved and that no drugs or digitalis needed to be used. Cardiac arrest did not once occur during the periods when the hyperbaric oxygen was being used. Cardiac

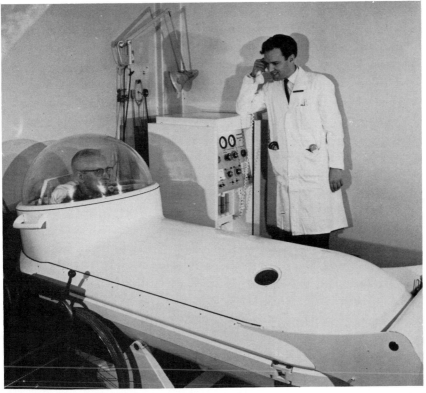

Fig. 56-3. Hyperbaric bed. (Courtesy Vickers Ltd., Medical Group, London, and the Bethlehem Corp., Bethlehem, Pa.)

arrest did occur in one patient outside the hyperbaric bed.

Factors affecting cerebral blood flow

Normal cerebral blood flow in the average male adult is estimated to be 54 ml. per 100 gm. per minute. Cerebral circulation may not be as dependent upon the head of pressure provided by the systolic blood pressure as are the other tissues of the body. A tremendous increase in cerebral blood flow can result from alterations in blood tensions of oxygen and carbon dioxide. For example, a 75% increase in cerebral blood flow may occur in a patient breathing a mixture of 5% to 7% carbon dioxide in air. Breathing a 10% oxygen mixture may cause a rise in cerebral blood flow of approximately 40% (Graham). Since carbon dioxide is the most potent vasodilator of the cerebral circulation,

it may actually be more logical, in some situations, to place the patient in a carbon dioxide–enriched environment rather than in an oxygen tent. Lowering the carbon dioxide tension will produce vasoconstriction and a reduced cerebral blood flow.

It should, of course, be remembered that the cardiac output and the level of blood pressure are major extrinsic factors in regulating blood flow to the brain.

Although of questionable statistical significance, I would like to call attention to the observation that a suprisingly high percentage of the patients surviving periods of complete cerebral anoxia for over 4 minutes consisted of individuals who had pulmonary tuberculosis. Several of these patients made rather spectacular recoveries following cardiac resuscitation even though the duration of arrest had been most prolonged. Kountz made the observation (from a group of 127 patients whose hearts he studied by the perfusion technique) that those who had died of tuberculosis were revived more easily than were those of any other group whose death was due to a single cause. Apparently, this was not limited to individuals with pulmonary tuberculosis alone but was applicable to generalized tuberculosis.

Another case, in which ventricular fibrillation lasted 5 to 10 minutes before cardiac massage was begun, was reported by Southworth and co-workers. Cardiac catheterization precipitated the fibrillation. Continuous ECG tracings were made; therefore a relatively accurate appraisal of the time period was available. This prolonged period of absent cardiac output is, of course, notoriously inconsistent with permanent survival. The patient was a 25-year-old white woman whose diagnosis was that of a patent ductus arteriosus and a congenital anomaly of the vessels arising from the aortic arch. Resuscitation was accomplished after 40 minutes of massage. Surprisingly enough, the patient had almost no mental deficiency and was rational within a period of several minutes following the return to normal cardiac activity. There were no postoperative complications. This patient had had pulmonary tuberculosis diagnosed during her youth, which had required 4 years' treatment before it was arrested. At the time of the cardiac arrest, there was no clinical indication of activity of previous tuberculosis.

Severe cerebral anoxia with subsequent recovery

A successful case of cardiac arrest in association with a ruptured uterus and subsequent recovery is reported by Harris and associates. A rather advanced picture of CNS derangement followed in the postresuscitative period. Twelve months later, changes were noted in the patient's temperament, along with perhaps some persistent cerebellar dysfunction.

Zoll mentions three patients with cardiac arrest who survived without permanent brain damage even though arrest lasted for more than 6 minutes. The time durations were recorded on running ECG paper. All were fibrillary arrests.

It is important to recall that permanent and irreversible brain damage may occur even though cardiac resuscitation is started within seconds after cardiac arrest occurs. In these instances, the CNS is irretrievably damaged by asphyxia before the heart stops.

Wolff's unusual case is worth mentioning at this point.

The patient was a 45-year-old black man with moderately advanced chronic pulmonary tuberculosis. He was prepared for a right-sided thoracoplasty and on June 16, 1949, was taken to the operating room after premedication with morphine sulfate (0.015 gm.) and scopolamine hydrobromide (0.004 gm.). Cardiac arrest occurred during regional block procedures. Following unsuccessful intrathoracic injection of 1 ml. of epinephrine without any benefit being noted, an upper midline abdominal incision was made and subdiaphragmatic massage was carried out. Although it was thought that an interval of 7 to 8 minutes had elapsed between arrest and resumption of oxygenation to the cerebral cortex, the figure of 6 minutes was decided upon in order to be on the conservative side. The respiratory center did not resume spontaneous respiration until 1 hour and 15 minutes later. The immediate postrecovery period was characterized by incontinence of urine and lethargy. On the following day, the patient was fully conscious and well oriented, although neurologic examinations showed generalized hyperreflexia, active cremasterics, an intact position sense, and no gross sensory disturbances. No asteriognosis was demonstrable. Memory was intact, and there were no ECG abnormalities. On the second day, the patient's sensorium was entirely clear. From then on, the patient made an uneventful recovery except for a postoperative complication of a hemopericardium that required aspiration. The pericardial sac had been closed tightly because of the pulmonary tuberculosis. The patient's subsequent course was satisfactory. Psychometric studies showed no abnormalities. Three months later a three-stage right posterolateral thoracoplasty was carried out with the patient under general ether anesthesia. The patient did well and was discharged from the hospital about 1 year later.

The remarkable variability in the sequence of events following different periods of cerebral anoxia is of considerable interest. An example is provided by the following case (Elton):

The heart was restarted following asystole during ligation of a patent ductus arteriosus. Following resuscitation, the ECG was flat. Convulsions were almost continuous, but could be controlled with phenobarbitone. No motion of the patient's limbs was noted during the first 2 weeks. The head was hyperextended. At the end of 1 month, little change was noted, except that the patient would turn her head toward noise. It appeared that the patient was blind. Two years later, however, the child appears to be a bright, intelligent girl. A neurologist states that the patient is in the normal range of intelligence.

The interesting case of Dr. Lev Landau, Russian winner of a Nobel prize in physics, has received attention in the lay press. Landau experienced four episodes of cardiac arrest on the fourth, seventh, ninth, and eleventh day after an automobile accident. Despite the multiple periods of cerebral anoxia, in addition to the neurologic damage from the accident, he is reported to have made a remarkable recovery.

Neurologic sequelae of cardiac resuscitation

Considerable clinical experience and the observation of much variability of the neurologic picture following almost identical episodes of cerebral anoxia leads us to believe that factors are involved other than simply time. There are well-recorded cases of decerebrate rigidity following cardiac arrest that lasted less than 3 minutes. Some of these cases have provoked medicolegal controversies since it was assumed that, if this degree of neurologic damage resulted, the physician was negligent in starting prompt resuscitative efforts. Many of these cases have occurred in the operating room under direct monitoring where the time element was carefully recorded.

Although arteriosclerotic vascular changes and vascular anomalies may play a part in the physiologic and anatomic mechanisms attempting to maintain adequate circulation in the face of hypertension, a more likely explanation seems related to the microcirculation of the brain and its tendency toward progressive aggregation and sludging during periods of transient cardiac arrest. Experimental support is provided by continuous photography of the microcirculation of the brain with an intravital microscope following 7 minutes of cardiac arrest in dogs. Matsumoto, Wolferth, and Hayes monitored the dogs with ECG, EEG, P_{O_2}, P_{CO_2}, pH, coagulation time, and phospholipids. The dogs were allowed to fibrillate 7 minutes, at the end of which some were given medication into the carotid artery. One group received no medication, the second group received phenoxybenzamine, a third received 5% glucose (30 ml. in 6 seconds), and a fourth group reecived phenoxybenzamine following 5% glucose (30 ml. in 6 seconds). Progressive aggregation and sludging of the cellular elements in venules with increased A-V shunting was seen after 5 minutes in the control group. In the fourth group, two of five dogs survived for more than 72 hours without residual pathology; complete recovery of the microcirculation within 1 minute after medication was noted. The second and third groups had a considerably better microcirculation than did the control group.

The ultrastructure and the metabolism of the cerebral cortex are affected both during the anoxic period and in the postresuscitation period. During anoxia, increased glycolysis produces local lactic acidosis while augmenting the damaging effect of anoxia (Cohen and co-workers). Acidosis increases the ultrastructural damage as judged by mitochondrial changes and preferential shrinkage of cell processes. Oxygen consumption of the cerebrocortical cell as well as glucose consumption is decreased with severe acidosis.

The predictability of recovery following neurologic injury continues to be quite haphazard and with few reliable guideposts. A case reported by Parkhouse is illustrative.

The patient was a 24-year-old woman who remained comatose for 3 weeks following a cardiac arrest episode that occurred while she was under general anesthesia in the operating room. Intense, generalized muscular spasm was present, and it was thought that the prognosis was hopeless. After 3 weeks, however, sudden improvement was noted and subsequent progress was rapid. Six months later her general return to normal was nearly complete, except for a somewhat spastic gait and clumsy movement of the small muscles of the hands.

The anoxic susceptibility of the visual centers of the cerebral occipital lobes has been noted repeatedly. Although cortical blindness is a most distressing neurologic sequel of cardiac arrest, return of vision may occur even after as long as 3 months. Weinberger and colleagues describe three such cases, all in children under 3 years of age. A detailed discussion of this complication is provided by Hoyt and Walsh.*

McNeill and associates document a 9-year follow-up on a woman who had a cardiac arrest during a radical mastectomy in 1947 at the age of 49 years. Even though her heart was resuscitated in the immediate postoperative period, she was confused and had periods of fluctuating consciousness. Her memory appeared to be impaired after a month, but her personality seemed to be well preserved and her ability for conceptual thinking was intact, as was her insight into her memory loss. After discharge from the hospital and return to her job, she was unable to cope with her situation, and, during the ensuing years, her condition gradually deteriorated. Her deterioration was marked by decreased drive and concentration and by marked emotional lability. Subsequently, in 1963 she developed bouts of disturbed behavior associated with hallucinations and required hospitalization. EEGs taken 3 years after the cardiac arrest were normal. Seven years after the arrest, however, they were markedly abnormal. It was agreed that some form of cortical degeneration was occurring.

It is heartening to see evidence of increas-

---

*See Hoyt, W. F., and Walsh, F. B.: Cortical blindness with partial recovery following acute cerebral anoxia from cardiac arrest, Arch. Ophthalmol. **60:**1061-1069, 1958.

ing investigative studies of the cerebral circulation and of the changes of the microvasculature of the brain. There has been some crossover of information from studies of the pathophysiology of cerebral ischemia and infarction as related to "strokes." As has been pointed out by Waltz from the Cerebral Vascular Clinical Research Center at the Mayo Clinic, cerebral ischemia does a great deal more than affect just the neurons and glia of cerebral tissue. Ischemia produces significant changes in the cerebral microvasculature. These changes are related to decreases of perfusion pressure and cerebral blood flow as well as slowing of the flow on both the arterial and venous side. This diminished blood flow in the microvasculature of the brain under gross examination shows pallor of the cortex, sludging or aggregation of the platelets and formed elements of the blood, darkening of the venous blood, and venous stasis. Platelet thrombi may be seen in the veins or platelet emboli in the arterial vessels. Unfortunately, perivenous hemorrhage may occur if systemic blood pressure changes occur in the face of venous obstruction from stasis or platelet thrombosis. Subsequent edema develops and venous drainage from ischemic portions of the brain may appear to be quite oxygenated.

A highly significant observation is reported by Neely and Youmans at the University of Mississippi Medical Center that lends considerable support to the idea that the brain can withstand longer periods of complete anoxia than 3 to 4 minutes, yet still recover. By markedly increasing the cerebrospinal pressure in dogs, they were able to completely occlude the cerebral circulation of the brain. Most significantly, however, in doing so they were emptying the brain of blood through the sequential squeezing out of blood in the veins, venules, capillaries, arterioles, and arteries. These dogs, which were subjected to total anoxia for up to 25 minutes, were able to see, stand, and hear the next day and survived for at least 48 hours. The difference between these dogs and others reported in studies of cerebral anoxia is that the latter group have included hypoxic blood in the brain. Neely and Youmans postulate that brain failure in such situations of cardiac arrest is not specifically caused by the period of anoxia but instead by the presence of anoxic blood with its high propensity for clotting and minute thrombi formation with a fall in blood pH. In addition they were able to prevent the production of anaerobic metabolism of lactic acid, which will not accumulate in a bloodless brain because there is no glucose present to be converted to lactate by anaerobic glycolysis.

Hartveit and Halleraker, from the Department of Pathology at the University of Bergen in Norway, have given support to this view with their study of 500 successive autopsy records at the Gade Institute. A small but significant number of patients was finally collected. Patients of comparable age and sex with a similar length and treatment of terminal illness and a similar period of time between death and necropsy were selected. The patients were divided into two groups with the only known systemic difference being that in one group external cardiac massage had been administered at the time of the sudden death, and in the second group sudden death had occurred without external cardiac massage. A clear-cut difference in the histologic findings between the two groups is reported. Changes strongly indicative of intravascular coagulation were present in the blood in the pulmonary and renal glomeruli of the patients who died from acute cardiac infarction and who had received external cardiac massage. These changes were not found in a similar group of patients in whom cardiac massage was not instituted.

Histologic findings indicated changes in composition and physical properties of the blood in the smaller vessels of those patients given external cardiac massage; the changes were most marked in the kidneys. For example, the glomerular capillaries were often overfilled with amorphous eosinophilic material without reactive changes in the surrounding tissues. The afferent arterioles were often plugged with fibrin. The lungs also presented a somewhat similar picture in that the capillaries also were filled with amorphous eosinophilic material that, upon hematoxylin-eosin staining, appeared amorphous and in places hyalin. Consistently small round balls, like beads, filled the capillaries. Some conformed to the size of the capillary and others dilated the lumen of the capillaries. These are illustrated in Fig. 56-4. What triggers this intravascular coagulation? Hartveit and Halleraker suggest several possibilities including the fact that the particulate matter from bone marrow emboli might trigger the coagulation mechanism. Sedimentation and aggregation of formed elements of the blood with subsequent stasis provide another possibility. Endothelial damage from anoxia might favor the formation of platelet thrombi.

The significance of these observations is obvious. Do these phenomena also occur in the brain? Is the cerebral anoxia caused not only by pump failure but by the intravascular coagulation preventing delivery of oxygenated blood during cardiac resuscitation? Should intense anticoagulation therapy be initiated once cardiac arrest has occurred? Certainly the concept has great appeal and needs to be confirmed by additional controlled studies.

The red venous blood sometimes seen under a period of ischemia in the brain is not thought to be caused by arteriovenous shunts since there are no major arteriovenous shunts in the brain. It is probably explained by a decreased uptake of oxygen by brain tissue since there is an impairment of the usual aerobic metabolic processes from ischemia, caused by damage to the enzyme systems and to the mitochondria.

Further support for the contention that greater attention must be directed to the microvasculature during and following periods of ischemia is given by a look at the

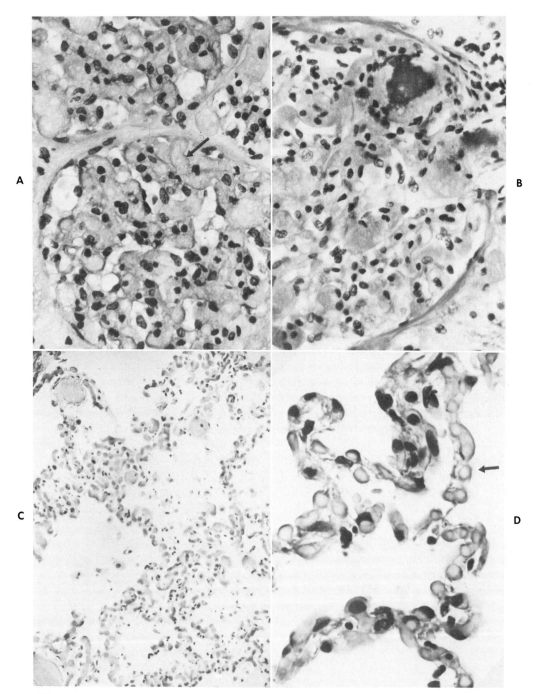

Fig. 56-4. **A,** Glomerular capillaries filled with amorphous material *(arrow)* in kidney from patient treated by external cardiac massage. **B,** Note fibrin plug in glomerular arteriole in another patient treated by external cardiac massage. **C,** Lung from patient treated by external cardiac massage. Note "beads" of amorphous material in pulmonary capillaries. **D,** Magnification of "beads" *(arrow)*.

cerebral microvasculature during ischemia. Waltz points out that under such conditions there is a marked decrease of perfusion pressure and cerebral blood flow caused by slowing of blood flow in arterial and venous vessels and manifested by pallor of the cortex, darkening of venous blood, and sludging or aggregation of the formed elements of the blood with platelet thrombi developing in veins or platelet emboli passing through arterial vessels. Thus a vicious circle is continued once ischemia occurs.

On the basis of present knowledge it would seem logical that major efforts should be directed toward an interruption of this cycle through whatever means are available. Presently, steroids, low molecular weight dextran, and heparin seem likely candidates for the job.

When cardiac arrest occurs, and during the subsequent period of resuscitation when less than desirable brain perfusion may occur, ischemic changes will obviously take place that may considerably influence the overall return of the central nervous system function and overall recovery of the patient. As Waltz points out in an excellent study on cerebral circulation, not only does ischemia produce changes within the lumen of cerebral blood vessels such as the aggregation of formed blood elements previously mentioned, but it also markedly interferes with the regulatory reactivity and responsiveness of the arterioles in the brain. This sophisticated autoregulation system is probably not well understood except by those working intimately in the field.

Ordinarily the regulatory system in the cerebral blood vessels maintains a constant blood flow despite changes of mean systemic arterial blood pressure in the range of 60 to 100 mm. Hg or changes of venous or intracranial pressure that produced similar changes of cerebral perfusion pressure. The significant forces allowing for this autoregulation of cerebral blood flow are probably more of theoretical knowledge than actual. Waltz attributes the response either to a direct effect of transmural pressure on the smooth muscle cells of the vessel wall or to transient changes of cerebral blood flow in response to changes of tissue pH caused by local concentration of acidic metabolites or by changes of arterial carbon dioxide tension. Both of these mechanisms appear to be severely impaired or abolished by ischemia— at least for a period of hours or days. This probably explains why the administration of carbon dioxide, ordinarily an effective cerebral vasodilator, may be of little benefit in the initial period after acute cerebral ischemia. It also would lend little support for the use of vasodilators such as papaverine in the treatment of the cerebral ischemia.

Chapter 57

CARDIAC COMPLICATIONS

ECG changes and myocardial damage following cardiac resuscitation

ECG patterns following cardiac resuscitative efforts have been reported by some authors as suggestive of myocardial infarction. Bloomfield and Mannick are of the opinion that these ECG changes reflect manipulative trauma from the cardiac massage rather than an actual myocardial infarction.

That these ECG changes need not result from cardiac massage has been documented by Nickel and Gale from the records of six living patients who had previously experienced cardiac arrest. All preoperative ECGs were normal. Even after cardiac massage, repeat ECGs showed no deviation from the norm.

A number of pathologists have commented on having seen rather severely traumatized hearts following intermittent manual cardiac compression. As pointed out elsewhere, rupture of the myocardium can easily occur, especially in elderly patients, in patients with coronary artery disease, in those individuals having previous myocardial infarcts, or in persons upon whom prolonged cardiac massage has been performed in an unsatisfactory manner, that is, by persistent and incorrect pressure with the tips of the fingers. On the other hand a number of postmortem studies that I have observed failed to show any evidence of appreciable damage to the myocardium after varying periods of massage. One heart was massaged almost 2 hours without showing signs of epicardial hematomas or other gross trauma. There seems to be considerable difference in the findings noted if the pericardium was not opened. In these cases, the degree of trauma is appreciably less.

Guevara and colleagues, in an effort to assess the traumatic damage to the heart from direct cardiac massage, studied twenty-eight consecutive deaths after cardiac arrest. With one exception, all represented cases in which direct cardiac massage had been applied when death followed anesthesia. Twelve of the patients were children; of this group, nine (or 75%) showed conspicuous evidence of heart trauma at autopsy. Six of these patients had undergone intrathoracic operations. The evidence of trauma included a diffusely ecchymotic extracardial surface, epicardial hemorrhage (particularly over the posterior aspect of the left ventricle and the anterior surface of the right ventricle), and gross hemorrhage scattered through the muscles of the ventricular walls. Microscopic examination revealed interstitial hemorrhages extending through the myocardium, with fragmentation and disruption of muscle fibers. In half of the cases, interstitial hemorrhage involved the interventricular septum (Fig. 57-1).

The remaining sixteen cases were adults. Of this group, 33% showed gross evidence of myocardial damage after direct cardiac massage. Evidence of trauma was less conspicuous than in the pediatric group. Although difficult to determine from the findings described previously, it is possible that myocardial damage may have contributed to some of the deaths.

Bernier describes cardiac arrest in a 63-year-old man on whom closed-chest massage was maintained for 35 minutes. The SGOT rose to 360 units on the day following resuscitation, and gradually returned to normal within the next week.

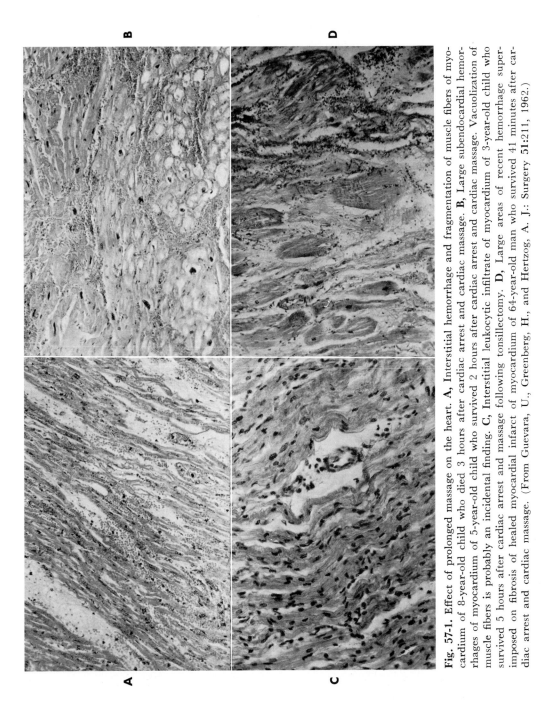

Fig. 57-1. Effect of prolonged massage on the heart. **A,** Interstitial hemorrhage and fragmentation of muscle fibers of myocardium of 8-year-old child who died 3 hours after cardiac arrest and cardiac massage. **B,** Large subendocardial hemorrhages of myocardium of 5-year-old child who survived 2 hours after cardiac arrest and cardiac massage. Vacuolization of muscle fibers is probably an incidental finding. **C,** Interstitial leukocytic infiltrate of myocardium of 3-year-old child who survived 5 hours after cardiac arrest and massage following tonsillectomy. **D,** Large areas of recent hemorrhage superimposed on fibrosis of healed myocardial infarct of myocardium of 64-year-old man who survived 41 minutes after cardiac arrest and cardiac massage. (From Guevara, U., Greenberg, H., and Hertzog, A. J.: Surgery 51:211, 1962.)

Postmortem findings in infants after arrest (Greenberg) show evidence of rather marked trauma in six of eight cases.

Rupture of the anterior wall of the right atrium

Wolf and co-workers report the case of a 69-year-old woman upon whom cardiopulmonary resuscitative efforts were unsuccessful. At autopsy, the patient not only had fractures of six ribs with hemorrhage into the pectoral muscles bilaterally, bilateral hemothorax, and ascites, but she also had a hemopericardium from a 4.5 cm. supravalvular laceration on the anterior wall of the right atrium extending through the endocardium, myocardium, and epicardium to the epicardial fat.

Rupture of the ventricle

Through-and-through rupture of the heart, with hemopericardium and cardiac tamponade was present in nine cases of ninety autopsied hearts following acute myocardial infarction. Six of the nine cases were in the group of forty-one patients who died of an acute myocardial infarct and who had been subjected to external cardiac massage. This incidence of 14.6% is considerably higher than that generally reported in the literature. Postmortem studies indicate that complete through-and-through ruptures occur in the area of necrosis in the infarcted ventricle. The compression pressure from closed-chest cardiac massage may be great enough to tear the already weakened infarcted area of the ventricular wall (Yamada and Fukunaga). Thirty-eight per cent of eighty-six autopsies performed on patients who had undergone external cardiac massage following an acute myocardial infarction were found to have pulmonary bone marrow embolism consisting of adipose tissue and blood-cell-forming elements. There is a positive correlation between the severity of the embolism and the duration of the resuscitation attempts. When the emboli are small and diffusely scattered, only localized tissue reaction, hemorrhage, and edema occurred; but if the embolism is extensive, pulmonary congestion and respiratory failure may be significant mortality factors.

As discussed elsewhere, a number of damaging effects can occur if closed-chest massage is carried out on patients with heart valve prostheses and the valve ring is compressed between the sternum and the vertebral bodies. These complications have included myocardial hematomas, disruption of the ventricle, rupture of coronary arteries, and intractable conduction disturbances. Prevention would seem to lie most feasibly in immediate defibrillation without massage or with open-chest direct cardiac compression if prolonged closed-chest compression seems likely.

Rupture of the ventricle is not necessarily a fatal complication. Gutenkauf, Hosler, Haight, and Sloan have all reported survival following rupture of the ventricle during cardiac massage. Many of these cases occurred in patients with a previously infarcted heart. In one patient, the right ventricle was described as being "paper thin." Another patient, a 59-year-old man who previously had a myocardial infarction, was hospitalized for removal of a cystic mass on the left side of the neck. Ventricular fibrillation occurred during induction of anesthesia. After the pericardium was opened and the heart massaged, the right ventricle was perforated, with blood pouring out of an opening approximately 3 to 4 cm. in length. Closure was accomplished by placing Gelfoam over the closure site and reinforcing it with fat. The patient lived approximately 7 weeks following the cardiac arrest and died suddenly in his bed at home. The actual instance of rupture of the myocardium following direct cardiac massage is difficult to estimate. In the first 1,700 cases of cardiac arrest that I studied, only eleven such cases were present. Cole and Corday reported two cases from a series of 132 patients (both of the patients died). Six cases of ruptured myocardium were reported from a series of sixty patients studied by Adelson.

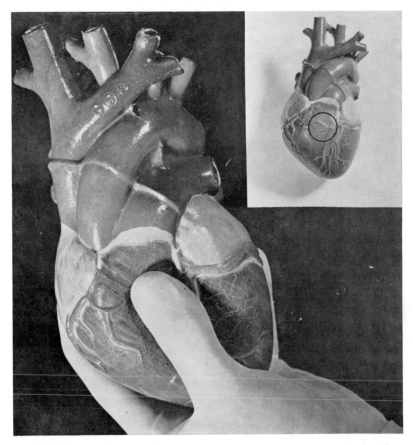

Fig. 57-2. Rupture of upper and anterior portion of right ventricle may occasionally occur in elderly and arteriosclerotic patients following prolonged and excessive pressure with left thumb in the area indicated in the inset. (From Stephenson, H. E., Jr., Reid, L. C., and Hinton, J. W.: Arch. Surg. **69**:37, 1954.)

Fig. 57-2 (inset) illustrates the site most likely to weaken and rupture during compression of the heart by direct massage. Rupture is most commonly caused by prolonged, localized, and excessive thumb pressure on the myocardium. The most likely site is the upper portion of the right ventricle, as pictured in the inset. The anterior wall of the right ventricle may already be weakened by preexisting cardiac pathology, especially in the elderly patient. This may be from excessive myocardial fibrosis, previous myocardial infarct, or coronary arteriosclerosis. In all but one of the cases, the pericardium had been opened.

To prevent such a complication, several precautions might well be noted:

1. Remember that intermittent cardiac compression does not entail pressure with the tips of the fingers, particularly the thumb.

2. Compression of the heart should be done, if possible, through an intact pericardium in order to take advantage of the lubricating effect of the fluid in the pericardial sac.

3. In addition to the lubricating effect of the pericardial sac, one should consciously endeavor to prevent prolonged pressure on one area of the heart. Movement from one spot to another is desirable.

Even if rupture of the myocardium occurs during resuscitation, it is conceivable that all is not lost. In a case of cardiac resuscitation personally encountered on a ward at Bellevue Hospital, a rupture occurred but was small enough that a fatal result was not immediately incurred. The patient's heart was resuscitated; however, cortical damage was too severe, and death resulted in 12 hours.

Medford reports that, in two instances, ventricular rupture occurred, the rupture being in areas of infarction.

Laceration of the heart

If laceration of the myocardium occurs, management can be carried out in a somewhat similar fashion as with an elective incision of the myocardium. In most instances, however, the myocardium may be quite friable adjacent to the actual laceration. In these instances, wide through-and-through sutures may be placed and tied over a piece of Dacron or Teflon sponge.

Although it is an extremely rare complication, I know of at least one case in which the heart was severely lacerated at the time of a particularly energetic skin incision. Resuscitation was quite impossible, and the patient did not survive. Fortunately, this was in an individual suffering from far-advanced, inoperable malignancy.

Xanthine oxidase inhibition in cardiac arrest

Cardiac arrest experimentally produced in dogs results in an increased uric acid level in plasma, dependent to a large extent on the length of the cardiac arrest (Parker and Smith). High blood uric acid levels are also seen after hemorrhagic shock and may be related to the irreversibility that occurs during prolonged hemorrhage. Parker and Smith believe that the uric acid level increase represents a rapid depletion of the high-energy nucleotide pool and an increased formation of uric acid caused by the catabolism of these high-energy nucleotides. Adenosine triphosphate is being dephosphorylated at a faster rate than it can be replenished by approximization of adenosine diphosphate

(ADP) in the hypoxic state. Eventually, deaminization produces hypoxanthine. Xanthine oxidase catalyzes oxidation of hypoxanthine first to xanthine and then to uric acid. Parker and Smith gave allopurinol, a xanthine oxidase inhibitor, to depress the irreversible steps in purine catabolism to uric acid so that more purine base would remain for nucleotide formation. Pretreatment with allopurinol improved survival rates, presumably through the maintenance of intracellular high-energy nucleotides.

Hematoma of ventricle

Jung reports two patients with hematomas of the anterior walls of the left ventricle. One of the two patients also had a hemopericardium that was thought to result from laceration of coronary vessels during intracardiac injection. In Saphir's group of 123 consecutive patients with circulatory arrest treated by external cardiac massage, nine patients had a hemopericardium as a complication of the external massage. Both authors suggest a judicious use of intracardiac needling in patients who have been anticoagulated.

Cardiac tamponade

Pericardial temponade has been present following resuscitation in several patients and has been noted by others in cases when needle injection of the heart through the unopened chest was performed. Its presence may be detected by a pulsus paradoxus, a reduction in cardiac output during inspiration, and an increased venous pressure. The liver may be enlarged. Williams and Soutter mention that the best way to test for a pulsus paradoxus is by noting the top systolic blood pressure during normal breathing. The patient is then requested to breathe deeply, and systolic pressure slowly falls. Ordinarily, one should note a decrease in pressure of only about 5 mm. Hg. In patients with tamponade, the drop may be so great that the pressure cannot be measured.

In addition, venous pulsations may be

noted. In the patients I have studied, there has usually been subjective evidence of substernal pain. Electrocardiographic as well as roentgenographic findings may be of some help.

Treatment, as a rule, may be accomplished simply by pericardial needle aspiration, repeated aspirations having been necessary on occasion. It is possible that the reaccumulation of fluid may be so rapid that a pleuropericardial window is necessitated. Cardiac arrest in a hemophilic child has been described (McKay), along with the added problems involved.

Gradual or sudden elevation of the venous pressure, decrease in the pulse pressure and in cardiac output with signs of shock, and, finally, syncope may be noted when there is an accumulation of fluid or air in the intact pericardial sac. As mentioned previously, this complication follows cardiac massage in which the pericardial sac has been opened and, following successful restoration of the normal heart rhythm, has been tightly closed. Serosanguineous fluid may accumulate within the pericardium following its closure. It is for this reason that it is desirable to have the opening in the sac communicate freely with one of the pleural cavities so that the fluid may pass into the pleural space where it can be readily aspirated, if necessary. The possibility of cardiac tamponade should be suspected.

An interesting case of a hemopericardium that complicated cardiac resuscitation has been recorded by Wolff.

Following the usual resuscitative procedure on a 45-year-old man with chronic pulmonary tuberculosis, an excellent response resulted even though it was estimated by the physician that the period of arrest was between 6 and 8 minutes. The pericardium had been opened. Spontaneous respirations did not return for 1 hour and 15 minutes after the arrest. Because of the presence of bilateral pulmonary tuberculosis, the pericardium was closed by means of a continuous catgut suture.

The patient had neurologic findings compatible with a period of cerebral anoxia. These included generalized hyperreflexia, absent cremasterics, and loss of memory for recent events. Because of the periodic recurrences of substernal pain that did not respond to nitroglycerin, and because of a prolonged circulation time, pericardial aspiration was attempted. Thirty-five milliliters of blood-tinged fluid was aspirated on the eleventh postoperative day. On the fourteenth postoperative day, 60 ml. of a somewhat similar appearing fluid was obtained by pericardial aspirations. This was followed by striking symptomatic relief, and the subsequent course of the patient was one of progressive improvement.*

Herniation of the heart

A potential, but fortunately uncommon, complication following direct cardiac resuscitation is herniation of a portion of the heart through an opening in the pericardial sac. This complication usually arises when an aperture in the pericardial sac has been left that is of sufficient size to permit the rotatory movements of the heart to cause protrusion of its apex. Such a case was reported by Dr. William W. Shingleton of Duke University School of Medicine. The patient was a 4-year-old boy, and a craniotomy was being performed. Following a biopsy of an intracranial lesion, the heart suddenly ceased beating. The patient had been under open-drop ether anesthesia for 1 hour and 15 minutes prior to the arrest. Following the recognition of the arrest by the anesthesiologist, the scalp wound was rapidly compressed and the child was turned over on his back. A thoracotomy was performed and intermittent compression of the heart was employed. The heart appeared dilated on inspection, and after opening the pericardial sac, further massage was carried out. Subsequent to this, the heart responded with a resumption of normal nodal rhythm. The chest was then closed and the remaining portion of the craniotomy was completed. The patient was returned to his room in a satisfactory condition and made a subsequent postoperative recovery, having had no

*From Wolff, W. I.: Cardiac resuscitation, complete recovery after over six minutes of true circulatory arrest, J.A.M.A. 144:738, 1950.

sequelae from the cardiac arrest. (Over a year later, the child died from an intracranial neoplasm.)

Chest x-ray films were taken during both the preoperative and postoperative periods and are shown in Fig. 57-3. A postoperative roentgenogram shows a marked convexity of the left border of the heart, which was interpreted as a herniation of the heart through the pericardial sac. Fortunately, the effect of the herniation did not prove to be of clinical embarrassment to cardiac function.

An additional case of cardiac arrest caused by ventricular herniation (Munchow and associates) involved a 26-year-old woman who was first treated for hemopericardium and cardiac tamponade following an ice-pick stab wound in the left anterior chest. Cardiac arrest was caused by the tamponade, but the heart was successfully resuscitated after the chest had been opened and the heart and the pericardial sac had been decompressed. Sixty-two hours later, a second arrest occurred after a brief period of gradual deterioration. A thoracotomy was again performed, and the left ventricle was found to have herniated through the drainage opening from the previous resuscitative efforts. Following the successful restoration of heart action, the pericardium was left completely open. The patient made a subsequent recovery and was well 10 months later, without neurologic or cardiovascular sequelae.

ECG artifacts during cardiac massage

Electrocardiograms taken during closed-chest resuscitation have been a source of confusion, and their interpretation has been difficult. Saphir and Falsetti have clarified the nature of these electrical complexes and conclude that there is a primary mechanical etiology responsible—the ECG artifacts are directly related to the method, duration, and force of sternal compression employed.

Myocardial burns from direct defibrillation

If the electrodes are well moistened with saline solution or distilled water before their

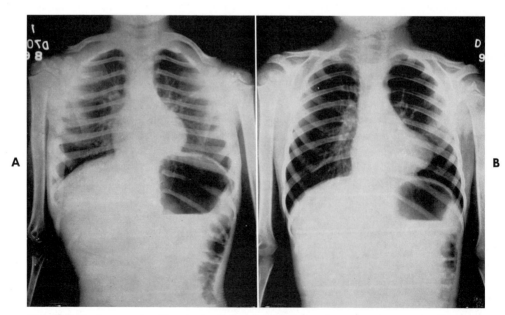

Fig. 57-3. A, Preoperative film obtained on 4-year-old boy prior to craniotomy. Cardiac arrest occurred during the procedure. **B,** Postoperative film showing what was interpreted as a herniation of the heart through the pericardial sac. Clinically, herniation did not seriously affect the function of the heart.

application, if they are sufficiently large, and if they conform to the contour of the heart, the likelihood of a burn is lessened, especially when the current is applied for but a fraction of a second. In many instances, a very small electrode plate has been used. Sometimes the heart can be defibrillated through the unopened pericardium; in such instances, the likelihood of a myocardial burn is reduced.

The electrodes should be applied snugly to the surface of the heart, MacLean's studies show that the risk of burns can be considerably decreased if the electrodes are large and also if the duration of shock is approximately 0.15 second. Temperature elevations over 149° F. are achieved with shocks of over 170 volts. This study concerns A.C. applied directly to the heart. The frequency of myocardial burns may be decreased with D.C. application.

Rivkin did a control study on myocardial temperature elevations with defibrillation and myocardial burns from the accompanying electrical shock. His study encompassed intraventricular and intramural temperatures following the application of 480 shocks to twenty dog hearts. Intraventricular temperature varied directly with the total energy of the shock applied in watt-seconds. Temperatures were related to the contact of the electrode. With the A.C. defibrillator and good contact of sponge-covered electrodes, the maximum temperature rise was only 2° C. Temperatures rose to 44° C. when bare electrodes and good contact were employed. If contact was poor and bare electrodes were employed, temperatures rose to 51° C. No significant intramural temperature elevations were encountered at voltages less than 200 or with any sponge-covered electrodes. With the D.C. defibrillator and good contact with sponge-covered electrodes, no significant temperature elevations were noted. Rivkin concludes that cardiac burns are an expected consequence of internal cardiac defibrillation, particularly if electrode contact is poor and if the energy of the defibrillating current is high. He recommends that the defibrillator electrodes be enclosed in a saline-saturated envelope of polyvinyl sponge, which is conductive and which will conform to the cardiac surface. Padded electrodes accompanying A.C. defibrillators and shocks of 0.1 second's duration or less yield a very insignificant incidence of burns. Similarly, D.C. defibrillators with shocks below 50 watt-seconds (less than 1,000 volts) are not likely to cause significant burns.

Ventricular defibrillation through the intact chest wall involves almost no risk of cardiac or intrathoracic burn.

Coronary occlusion after cardiac massage

An unusual complication following cardiac massage was reported by Tsi-Gziou Li. Direct injury of the descending branch of the left coronary artery occurred from cardiac massage with a rupture of an atheromatous plaque in a 70-year-old woman on whom a colostomy was being performed. Although cardiac activity was restored, the patient died on the second postoperative day. A recent infarct of the left ventricular wall was located distal to the occlusion of the descending branch of the left coronary artery. The coronary artery revealed a tear of the intima at the point adjacent to the atheromatous plaque. The material obstructing the lumen of the artery was a mixture of red blood cells, cholesterol crystals, calcium, and fibrin —the same material found in the plaque. This material could be traced through the tear of the vessel wall to the material occluding the artery. Fortunately, this complication appears to be rare.

Epicardial hemorrhage

Following prolonged periods of manual compression of the heart, a rather extensive epicardial hemorrhage will occasionally be encountered. The depth of the hemorrhage may not be determined unless an autopsy is performed, but it is usually not so extensive as to be incompatible with life. Apparently, a small epicardial hemorrhage does not appreciably affect the dynamics of the heart, and the blood is readily absorbed.

Myocardial damage after prolonged ventricular fibrillation

Senning reports on the use of ventricular fibrillation to facilitate intracardiac operations during extracorporeal circulation and to prevent the formation of air emboli during such procedures. He concludes that there is no evidence from ECG or histologic studies that prolonged ventricular fibrillation is responsible for any serious degree of myocardial damage if the coronary blood flow is maintained by an extracorporeal circulation. Clinically, it has been my impression that hearts defibrillated in dogs (and in patients) fail to show any remarkable degree of myocardial damage after periods of prolonged ventricular fibrillation if adequate intermittent manual compression of the heart is maintained, although a period of relative tachycardia may persist for a few days.

Repeat episode of cardiac arrest

Although a relatively infrequent experience, it is nevertheless true that a patient having experienced one cardiac arrest is more likely to experience a second one than is the average operative patient (excluding cardiac arrest associated with myocardial infarction). In my earlier series of about 1,700 cases, there were fifty patients in whom there were multiple episodes of cardiac arrest. Thirty-three of the patients had two arrests, five had three arrests, and five had four arrests. A number of these patients had Adams-Stokes disease. One patient had cardiac standstill thirty times and another twenty-three times within 24 hours, and both lived. Both of these patients were treated with the cardiac pacemaker.

Pitfalls of a cardiocentesis through the closed chest

Lahey and Eversole have suggested that before a thoracotomy is performed a needle should be inserted through the chest wall into the heart to ascertain whether or not heart pulsations are present. They argue that heart action may be active even though peripheral circulation has apparently ceased. They believe that this maneuver may help to detect the presence of a faint heartbeat that is incapable of producing a palpable peripheral pulse. Although their experience has apparently justified this procedure, I believe that such a procedure is of questionable value as a recommendation for general use. If the anesthetist is instituting artificial respiration through an endotracheal tube or by means of a simple bag method through an open mask, then the movement of the mediastinum resulting from artificial respiration may be such that the needle will also move, and a false impression will be gained that may lead to a sufficient enough delay to allow irreversible brain damage.

Cardiac tamponade from closed-chest needle puncture. One further complication of such a procedure has been described by Zoll. It consisted of a cardiac tamponade produced by needle punctures for injections of epinephrine. The patient died.

Chapter 58

COMPLICATIONS TO OTHER ORGANS AND SYSTEMS IN CARDIAC RESUSCITATION

Gastric dilatation

Diversion of air into the stomach can easily occur with pharyngeal pressures of 15 to 20 cm. of water. These pressures are commonly used during mouth-to-mouth or bag and mask resuscitation for artificial ventilation. There are several ill effects of overdistension of the stomach in addition to the likelihood of regurgitation and aspiration pneumonia. Gastric dilatation may further impair function in patients already in difficulty with hypoventilation and hypotension. An increased vagal tone and decreased venous return to the heart may occur with gastric dilatation—even to the point of being the actual cause of bradycardia, sinus arrest, or cardiac standstill. However, the gastric pressure can easily force air out of the stomach, and one should be cautioned that this itself may allow gastric secretions to enter the upper airway and even block the airway. The patient should be in a head-down position if epigastric pressure is being employed. At least one should be reasonably sure that the stomach is empty (preferably by having passed a gastric tube). Ideally, a gastric tube with suction is the safest means of preventing or handling the problem of gastric dilatation. (See also pp. 645-649.)

ENDOTRACHEAL TUBE

Unfortunately we have seen instances of the endotracheal tube being passed into the esophagus in the assumption that it was in the trachea. The time required for intubation should, in most instances, be spent giving mouth-to-mouth ventilation. Undoubtedly,

there are many advantages to the endotracheal tube if it can be passed quickly by one skilled at the technique since endotracheal intubation does decrease dead space and allows easy removal of tracheobronchial secretions. Regurgitation of gastric contents can be prevented. With inflation of an endotracheal tube cuff, only a minimal air leak, if any, will remain and ventilation can be more consistent. The use of a laryngoscope greatly facilitates the visualization of the vocal cords and the subsequent entrance into the trachea.

Gastric dilatation during artificial respiration with the bag compression method is always a possibility when endotracheal intubation is not carried out. Occasionally, tremendous dilatation may occur, but if it is suspected, it can be handled by simple pressure on the epigastrium from time to time to deflate the stomach. Its presence should always be suspected.

GASTRIC RUPTURE

Demos and Poticha reported a rupture of the stomach that occurred during combined mouth-to-mouth breathing and external cardiac resuscitation in a 67-year-old man. The tear was located along the lesser curvature. The patient survived the episode but died later of carcinoma. Presumably, the gastric tear was due to the result of forceful mouth-to-mouth breathing combined with anterior chest compression (Fig. 58-1). The tear in this patient's stomach was a longitudinal, full-thickness laceration of the lesser curvature.

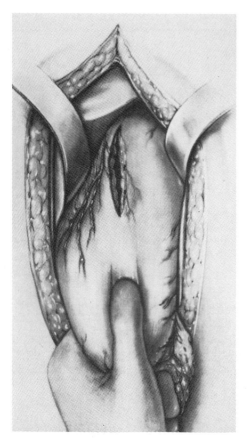

Fig. 58-1. Gastric rupture—a 5 cm. longitudinal, full-thickness tear of the gastric wall—occurring during closed-chest cardiac compression. (From Demos, N. J., and Potichk, S. M.: Surgery 55: 364, 1964.)

GASTROESOPHAGEAL LACERATIONS
WITH HEMORRHAGE

A not infrequent complication of closed-chest cardiac massage appears to be that of gastroesophageal lacerations. Lundberg and his colleagues found gastroesophageal lacerations to be the second most frequently encountered, significant complication following closed-chest cardiac massage. In fact, 10% of the patients autopsied over a 16-month period at the William Beaumont General Hospital were found to have this complication. (A total of fifty patients was autopsied following closed-chest cardiac massage during this time.)

Most commonly, the laceration is a linear one along the lesser curvature of the stomach and extends upward through the fundus and cardia into the esophagus. The gastric distension is associated with mouth-to-mouth artificial respiration, particularly when associated with external cardiac massage. Pressures as low as 120 to 150 mm. Hg will produce mucosal slits in the adult stomach.

Varying degrees of hemorrhage have been associated with this complication, but any bleeding from the nose or mouth following resuscitative efforts should alert the physician to this Mallory-Weiss type of syndrome.

RUPTURE OF THE TRANSVERSE COLON

As a result of external cardiac massage some days earlier, a perforation of the transverse colon just distal to the hepatic flexure was discovered in a 47-year-old physician. The physician collapsed while sitting in the hospital staff room. Mouth-to-mouth resuscitation and external cardiac massage were so promptly applied that the patient was awake and breathing spontaneously within 3 minutes (Tobian). Tobian postulated that the perforation of the transverse colon resulted from edema and interstitial hemorrhage of the bowel wall as well as hematoma of the mesentery and transverse colon following the initial trauma. Ultimately, this progressed to the necrosis and perforation of the bowel wall.

A hematoma of the right transverse colon following cardiac resuscitation using the closed-chest technique has also been reported (Clark).

Production of an active duodenal ulcer

Cerebral anoxia and the cerebral edema that follows may, in an occasional patient, predispose to the development of an active duodenal ulcer. Schlumberger reports such a case. The patient was a 12-year-old boy on whom an angiocardiographic study was being performed. Cyanotic heart disease was suspected, and a diagnosis of tetralogy of Fallot was entertained. Sodium thiopental (Pentothal) solution was injected intravenously under anesthesia; immediately after the injection of 35 ml. of a concentrated solution, the patient went into cardiac arrest. The heart was manually compressed and a spontaneous rhythm returned. However, cerebral damage had been severe, and the patient failed to regain consciousness. He died 4 days later after having a rather marked degree of persistent hyperthermia. Autopsy confirmed the diagnosis of tetralogy of Fallot. In addition, a large duodenal ulcer had penetrated the submucosa and a part of the smooth muscle layer. The adjacent area of tissue was edematous and was infiltrated by a small number of lymphocytes, eosinophils, and occasional neutrophils. The adrenal cortex, particularly the fascicular layer, appeared wider than normal, the cells being large and eosinophilic. Schlumberger speculates that such patients manifest Selye's general alarm syndrome, and that large amounts of corticotrophic and corticoid hormones are liberated that may lead to increased gastric secretion and to impaired healing of the erosions initially produced by the focal vascular changes.

Liver complications

Anylan and associates at Duke University Hospital have provided valuable data that may be related to this problem. They induced hypotension in dogs and then studied its effect on the liver. The anoxic environment of the liver was produced by two fundamentally different syndromes whose common denominator was a hypotension with a mean arterial pressure of 30 mm. Hg that lasted for 30 to 45 minutes. In the first group this pressure was produced by hemorrhagic hypotension, and in the second group by means of a chemical hypotension induced by the use of hexamethonium. During hemorrhagic hypotension, the effect on the liver was influenced by the constriction of the portal veins, which sometimes do not recover their normal caliber for over 6 hours. Portal venous pressures were measured, and they indicated

an increased intrahepatic vascular resistance during the hypotension. Blood volume was not decreased during chemically produced hypotension, and a better perfusion of tissues was accomplished than in the experiments with hemorrhagic hypotension.

If cardiac compression is maintained for prolonged periods of time after cardiac arrest, the degree of hypotension may permit varying degrees of liver damage. Anylan and his co-workers show a statistically significant difference in mortality and morbidity in dogs when the chemically induced hypotension is prolonged from 30 to 45 minutes. This they explain on the basis of prolongation of the relative hypoxia. They conclude in their study that the hypoxia produced by hemorrhage results in a greater mortality than that produced by a chemical ganglionic blocking agent. They also note that discernible damage, as determined by biochemical function tests and histopathologic studies, was minimal 15 to 30 days following the period of hypotension. However, in those dogs that died within the first 3 days, evidence of marked liver damage was present. Significantly enough, no important alterations in the kidney, suprarenal glands, heart, or lungs of any of the dogs were noted, nor were there elevations recorded in the blood nonprotein nitrogen or alterations in serum electrolytes. Therefore their study indicates that the liver is remarkably sensitive to the effects of hypoxia. During the resuscitative period, efforts should be made to maintain the arterial blood pressure above 40 to 50 mm. Hg.

LACERATION OF THE LIVER

Shortly after the introduction of closed-chest cardiac resuscitation, an instance of laceration of the liver by closed-chest cardiac massage was reported. Morgan, in his description of the case, states that in this first report of hepatic laceration following closed-chest cardiac massage, postmortem findings showed the abdominal cavity to contain 1,000 ml. of blood. Two large lacerations were found on the posterior surface of the

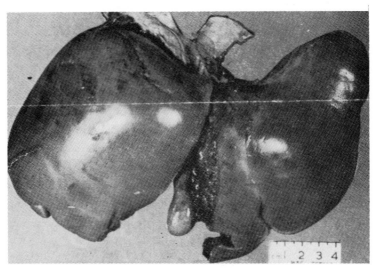

Fig. 58-2. Complete tear of the right lobe and laceration of the left lobe in the liver of a 3-year-old girl resulting from closed-chest resuscitation. (From Thaler, M. M., and Kause, V. W.: N. Engl. J. Med. **267:**500, 1962.)

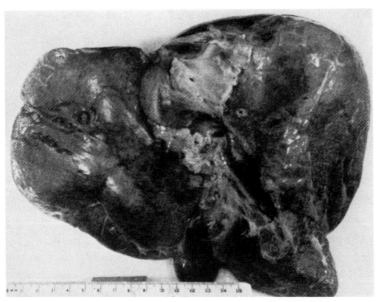

Fig. 58-3. Two lacerations of the liver from closed-chest cardiac massage in a 67-year-old man. (From Morgan, R. R.: N. Engl. J. Med. **265:**82, 1961.)

left lobe of the liver in the area closest to the thoracic vertebrae. The patient died shortly after attempts at closed-chest resuscitation.

Baringer and colleagues report an incidence of 11% in a postmortem study of forty-six patients. Two cases of multiple rupture of the liver in children, 3 years and 9 years of age, are reported by Thaler and Krause. Thaler is convinced that liver tear and rupture is the most common serious complication of external cardiac compression in infants and children, and that it results from simultaneous compression of the chest and abdomen, limiting free movement of the liver.

Numerous reports of hepatic lacerations following closed-chest cardiac compression have appeared in the literature. Several dozen of these have now been reported (Baringer, Clark, Thaler and Krause, Morgan). (See Figs. 58-2 and 58-3.)

An additional factor in the etiology of a ruptured liver following closed-chest cardiac compression may be the presence of a funnel chest. This congenital anomaly proved to be the cause of death in a patient reported by Minuck. Each time the sternum was depressed, the sharp protuberance representing the funnel chest would serve as a battering ram to compress the liver against the vertebral bodies. The patient was a 65-year-old woman who was being operated on for an astrocytoma. Although closed-chest resuscitation was successful to the extent that the patient awoke, the unrecognized hemorrhage from the liver continued, and the patient died 1 hour after the completion of the operation. More than 3,000 ml. of blood was found in the peritoneal cavity.

An apparent survival seemed likely in one of Robinson's reported cases, yet the patient died from massive intra-abdominal hemorrhage secondary to laceration of the liver.

Trauma to chest wall

Ventricular fibrillation and ventricular asystole are not infrequent complications of open-heart surgery. Following a resection of a large aneurysm of the left ventricle, two episodes of cardiac arrest were encountered in the first few hours following surgery. Because of the suspicion that exsanguinating hemorrhage was occurring, the first episode was managed by mouth-to-mouth respiration and closed-chest heart massage until the patient arrived in the operating room, at which time an open-chest approach was employed. The heart was in asystole and, following multiple blood transfusions, and manual massage, a good, strong beat and normal sinus rhythm were restored. Approximately 4 hours later, while the patient was being constantly monitored by an ECG, ventricular fibrillation suddenly occurred. Closed-chest compression and mouth-to-mouth respiration accompanied by closed-chest defibrillation were accomplished successfully. The closed-chest resuscitation was accompanied by a rupture of the sutures employed to stabilize the sternum. (The approach to the heart had been through a bilateral transverse thoracotomy.) Subsequently, on the eighth postoperative day, the patient's anterior chest wound had partially dehisced over the sternum. However, he eventually recovered with a stable sternum and chest wall.

Multiple rib fractures

Complications of multiple rib fractures are likely to occur especially in elderly patients. Since the rib cage is relatively inflexible, adjacent ribs may easily be broken at the time the chest incision is made. The broken ends present sharp edges that may lacerate the lung.

The incidence of rib fracture from external cardiac massage is probably dependent upon the skill and experience of the individual performing the resuscitation. Thirty-five percent of the fifty-seven patients studied by Jackson and Greendyke showed fractures following closed-chest resuscitation.

The incidence of fractured ribs following closed-chest cardiac massage at one large army teaching hospital was 40%. Lundberg and associates report fractured ribs in twenty of fifty patients autopsied following closed-chest cardiac massage during a 16-month period.

A 24% incidence of fractured ribs is reported in the Michael Reese series of 100 consecutive patients treated with closed-chest resuscitation. Five percent of the patients received fractured sternums.

Along with multiple rib fractures, the development of a stove-in chest has occurred with application of the closed-chest technique. Purkes and Mahabic report on a patient whose postmortem examination revealed a fractured sternum, fractures of the second, third, fourth, fifth, and sixth ribs on the left, both anteriorly and posteriorly, and fractures of the fifth and sixth ribs on the right.

FRACTURE OF THE STERNUM

Fracture of the sternum is a not uncommon complication with use of the closed-chest technique (approximately 6% in Robinson's series) Overall, fracture of the sternum occurs in approximately 2% of most series.

FRACTURE OF THE SCAPULA

A fracture of the scapula has been reported in the series recorded by Kaplan and Knott.

Vertebral fractures complicating electrical defibrillation

Compression fractures of thoracic vertebrae in psychiatric patients are well-known complications associated with some outdated methods of shock therapy. They are also reported as a sequel to closed-chest defibrilla-

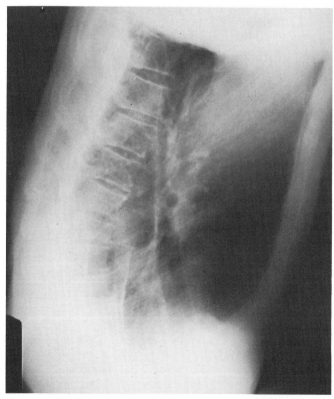

Fig. 58-4. Compression fracture of the vertebrae complicating electrical defibrillation. (Courtesy Benjamin B. Okel.)

tion. In Okel's case (Fig. 58-4), the fractures occurred between the fourth and eighth dorsal vertebrae. Earlier films did not reveal a bone or joint abnormality.

It may be that there is an overlooked complication from the rather marked generalized muscular contractions that occur with defibrillation attempts.

Closed-chest cardiac massage associated with bone marrow and pulmonary fat emboli

The incidence of fat embolization following closed-chest cardiac massage is probably at least as high as 30% to 50%. Garvey and Vak reviewed all of their autopsied cases from the department of pathology at Mount Sinai Hospital in New York City in which there had been external cardiac massage from January, 1962, to April, 1963. Ten (33%) of the patients were found to have marrow emboli plugging the lumina of small arteries of the pulmonary circulation. All of the emboli were found to have marrow elements (Fig. 58-5).

Yarnoff reports an 82% incidence of pulmonary fat embolization in eleven patients receiving external cardiac massage.

The mechanism producing the pulmonary fat emboli has been a source of some speculation. There is now some general agreement that the concussion of bones or the act of bending and compressing bones such as the rib cage may lead to microfractures within the medulla of ribs and sternum, with an increase in marrow pressure. This permits entry of fat from the marrow into the venous circulation. Significantly, pulmonary marrow emboli may occur in the absence of fractures. In fact, Jackson notes that 67% of his patients with pulmonary fat emboli showed no demonstrable fractures.

That pulmonary fat emboli are not routinely found, even as the result of a diligent search, is supported by Jackson and Greendyke, who note only one incident of minor pulmonary fat embolization in fifty control cases. In this particular case, severe fatty metamorphosis of the liver was present.

In Jackson's study, pulmonary fat emboli

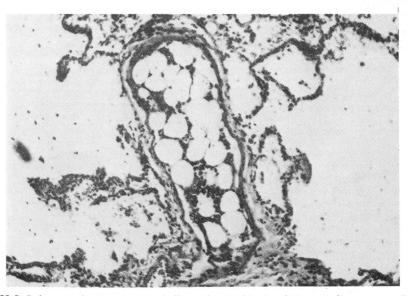

Fig. 58-5. Pulmonary bone marrow emboli associated with closed-chest cardiac massage. Lumen of pulmonary artery branch is occluded with partly fatty bone marrow. (From Garvey, J. W., and Zak, F. G.: J.A.M.A. **187:**59, 1964.)

were usually seen in the alveolar capillaries but were not infrequently observed in the larger vessels as well (Fig. 58-6).

Closed-chest cardiac compression was applied to a 61-year-old woman whose death was caused by coronary artery thrombosis and associated myocardial infarct (Winkel and Brown). Autopsy revealed red bone marrow substance in small and medium-sized vessels of the lungs. No fractures of the extremities or pelvis were present, and it was concluded that closed-chest cardiac massage was responsible for the bone marrow embolism found at autopsy. Bone marrow embolism has been reported previously in instances of trauma to the sternum. One might wonder if such embolism might not be more often detected following unsuccessful closed-chest cardiac massage. Particularly might this be suspected when one recalls the semiliquid nature of the sternal marrow and the communication of the marrow cavities

with the venous system. Himmelhoch and associates found twenty-two (42%) instances of pulmonary fat embolization out of fifty-two resuscitated patients who were autopsied.

Fat embolization is now a well-recognized complication of closed-chest resuscitation. The overall significance of pulmonary bone marrow embolism is not, however, so well known. How much do such emboli dampen an already depressed cardiorespiratory system? Is it enough to tilt the scales against a successful recovery?

Diffuse pulmonary fat and marrow emboli were found in random microscopic sections of the lungs of ten of sixteen patients treated by external cardiac massage (Lane and Merkel). (See Fig. 58-7.) Pure fat emboli were five times more frequent than bone marrow emboli in this series, and four of the patients showed embolization without demonstrable fractures of ribs or sternum.

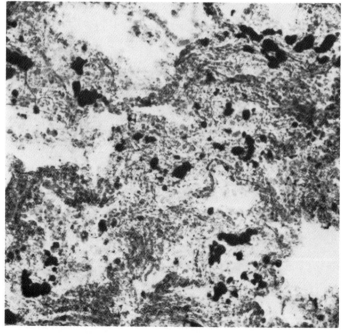

Fig. 58-6. Pulmonary fat embolism associated with multiple rib fractures sustained during closed-chest cardiac massage. (From Jackson, C. T., and Greendyke, R. M.: Surg. Gynecol. Obstet. **120:**25, 1965.)

These authors raise the question of whether emboli in the lesser circulation may not cause acute cor pulmonale responsible for some of the failures of resuscitation.

Henzel (personal communication) found Sudan fat stains of urine to be positive in three cases of external cardiac massage.

Cerebral fat emboli

Although it has been generally considered that mental deterioration following cardiac resuscitation is because of the effect of prolonged anoxia on cortical cells, another etiologic factor may, in some cases, be considered. Since closed-chest resuscitation has become widespread, a high incidence of pulmonary fat embolization has been re-ported—often above 80%. Jackson and Greendyke from the department of pathology at the University of Rochester School of Medicine in Rochester, New York, studied fifty-seven consecutive autopsies on persons known to have received external cardiac massage and fifty consecutive patients who died of natural disease processes without closed-chest resuscitation. Although they found pulmonary fat embolism in forty-six of fifty-seven patients, it is also significant that sixteen of the patients had cerebral fat emboli. In at least four of the patients, the cerebral fat emboli were thought to be clinically significant (Fig. 58-8). Fat embolization occurred particularly in vessels of the internal capsule. No cerebral fat emboli

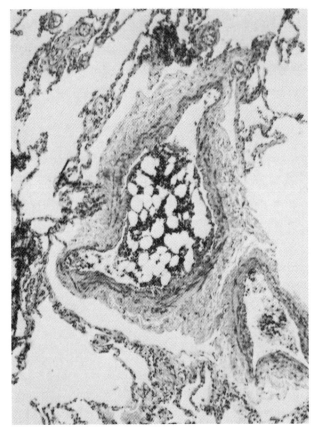

Fig. 58-7. Bone marrow fragments seen within the lumen of pulmonary vessels following external cardiac massage. (From Lane, J. H., Jr., and Merkel, W. C.: J. South. Med. Assoc., vol. 58, 1900.)

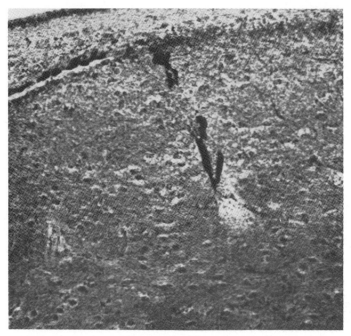

Fig. 58-8. Occlusion of capillary channels of internal capsule of the brain by fat emboli in a patient who died during closed-chest cardiac massage. (From Jackson, C. P., and Greendyke, R. M.: Surg. Gynecol. Obstet. **120**:25, 1965.)

were detected in any of the patients in the control group. Some cerebral fat embolization was observed in every instance in which more than twenty emboli per section were seen.

Jackson and Greendyke speculate that some instances of mental deterioration following closed-chest cardiac massage may be the result of cerebral fat embolization.

Postresuscitative infections

Although postresuscitative infection is of little concern with closed-chest resuscitation, it occasionally does influence the outcome of open-chest resuscitation. Since the luxury of sterile precautions (cleansing the chest and draping for the incision) can seldom be afforded in this emergency, it is logical that some concern should be expressed about the danger of empyema, pericarditis, mediastinitis, and cutaneous infection. There has been, however, a relatively low incidence of such infections following thoracotomy for cardiac massage, even when the operator is unable to use gloves or any other fundamental sterile precaution. Many infections are probably prevented by the practice of injecting penicillin and streptomycin into the thoracic cavity before closure and then inserting a rubber tube, preferably through a stab wound, in order to employ underwater drainage for several days. Occasionally, the chest may have to be tapped to remove a small collection of fluid. It is therefore important that considerations relative to a possible infection be disregarded if they are to contribute to any initial delay in instituting cardiac compression.

A case is reported from the Massachusetts General Hospital of a 43-year-old man who had undergone repeated operations for skin grafting. While the patient was being transported to the operating room, cardiac arrest occurred during anesthesia induction. An immediate thoracotomy was performed in the operating room under nonsterile condi-

Table 58-1. Blood leukocyte changes following open-cardiac massage*

	Preoperative	Postoperative			
		Day 1	Days 2 to 5	Days 6 to 10	Days 11 to 20
Number of patients	33	15	24	15	7
Highest	32,150	23,000	36,000	25,000	15,100
Lowest	6,125	7,750	5,500	5,900	7,950
Mean	12,325	15,325	16,100	13,676	11,707
Median	10,100	14,400	16,250	14,800	11,000

*From Altemeier, W. A., and Todd, J.: Studies on the incidence of infection following open chest cardiac massage for cardiac arrest, Ann. Surg. 158:596, 1963.

tions. Cardiac compression was effective, and the following morning the patient appeared well oriented and seemed to have tolerated the situation satisfactorily. On the second morning, he developed a temperature of 103° F. and was disoriented and hallucinated at intervals. He had been on streptomycin and penicillin; this was discontinued because it was feared that the hyperthermic reaction was toxic in nature. The thoracic catheter had previously been removed. On the third day chemotherapy was resumed and the temperature promptly fell to a normal range. Five days after the thoracotomy was performed, the incision site was noted to be draining. Two days later it was opened and was found to contain 150 ml. of thick, purulent material. Cultured *Bacillus subtilis* and *Pseudomonas pyocyaneus* were found. These organisms were sensitive only to bacitracin and polymyxin, which were instilled through a rubber catheter introduced into the thoracic cavity. Because of the thickness and viscosity of the draining material, streptokinase and streptodornase were used. They were mixed with 100 ml. of saline solution, injected into the catheter, and then the catheter was clamped for several hours. Following this maneuver, the thick, viscid, purulent exudate became much thinner, the volume increased to 600 ml. per day, and the patient had a sharp febrile spike, which may have been caused by absorption of the small molecular weight polypeptides following the digestion of bacterial fibrinolysin. This case illus-

trates the importance of routinely obtaining bacterial cultures and sensitivity tests.

A note of precaution to the operator—prolonged massage will frequently result in an abrasion of the skin of the back of the left hand. Minor infections can result from prolonged pressure on the hand developed because of the proximity to the rib cage during manual intermittent compression of the heart.

One case of a breast abscess having been related to the thoracotomy incision is reported.

A most provocative study on postoperative wound infections has been contributed by Altemeier and Todd. Their concern is specifically with the incidence of infection following open cardiac massage for cardiac arrest. They document statistical evidence to show how surprisingly low the infection rate is in such patients (Table 58-1). In only two instances (4.65%), from a total group of forty-three patients, did infection of the thoracotomy wound develop. (Of the forty-three patients, thirty-two were survivors who left the hospital.) Yet the opportunity for a wound infection would seem to be enhanced by the nature of the patient's condition. Three patients were being operated upon for peritonitis, one for a wound disruption, one for removal of a foreign body by bronchoscopy, and one with septicemia from a wound infection and pneumonia. Four thoracotomies were performed on nonoperative candidates (mumps, multiple frac-

Table 58-2. Related conditions predisposing to infection (17 patients)*

Diabetes	2
Azotemia	2
Malignant neoplasm	5
Peritonitis	3
Cholangitis with liver abscesses	1
Ulcerative colitis	1
Septicemia	1
Newborn infants	2
Premature infant	1

*From Altemeier, W. A., and Todd, J.: Studies on the incidence of infection following open chest cardiac massage for cardiac arrest, Ann. Surg. **158:** 596, 1963.

Table 58-3. Operative and postoperative antibiotic therapy (43 patients)*

Systemic		42
Penicillin	2	
Penicillin plus:		
Chloramphenicol	14	
Streptomycin	12	
Tetracycline	6	
Chloramphenicol and streptomycin	4	
Chloramphenicol and erythromycin	1	
Erythromycin	1	
Chloramphenicol	2	
Intrapleural		4
Penicillin alone	1	
Penicillin and streptomycin	3	
No antibiotic therapy		1

*From Altemeier, W. A., and Todd, J.: Studies on the incidence of infection following open chest cardiac massage for cardiac arrest, Ann. Surg. **158:** 596, 1963.

tures, grand mal convulsions, and drug intoxication). In addition, two patients had severe diabetes, and two patients were azotemic (see Table 58-2).

All except one of Altemeier's cases were treated with antibiotics in the postresuscitative period (Table 58-3). In only four patients were antibiotics instilled into the chest cavity. Forty-two patients were treated with antibiotics administered systemically. In addition to penicillin, streptomycin and chloramphenicol were usually used.

This study provides a new perspective for viewing of postoperative wound infections. The explanation for the failure of infections to develop in these postthoracotomy patients seems obscure and cannot be accounted for by the prophylactic antibiotic therapy.

Dissemination of pulmonary tuberculosis

In cases of cardiac arrest occurring in individuals with pulmonary tuberculosis, a point of caution should be mentioned. One case of pulmonary tuberculosis involving the left lung has been reported in which the disease spread to the opposite lung following cardiac massage. During massage, a portion of the involved lung was inadvertently compressed on several occasions, and it was considered that dissemination of the tuberculosis resulted from the resuscitative procedure.

COMPLICATION OF MOUTH-TO-MOUTH RESUSCITATION

Although the risk of infection of the resuscitator with tuberculosis during mouth-to-mouth resuscitation has been considered, no cases were known to me until the report of Heilman and Muschenheim. Primary cutaneous tuberculosis was contracted at the time of mouth-to-mouth resuscitation by a Bellevue Hospital intern. The intern had performed mouth-to-mouth respiration and closed-chest cardiac massage on a patient shortly after admission to Bellevue Hospital. Resuscitative efforts were eventually unsuccessful, and a postmortem examination revealed active tuberculosis in the right upper lobe. Previously negative P.P.D. tests became generally positive 6 weeks after the episode. Eight weeks after the initial contact, the intern noted a palpable submaxillary lymph node and several small pustules near the left nasolabial fold. Eventual cultures for acid-fast bacilli were positive. Recovery occurred after 12 months of isoniazid (INH) therapy. The authors (one having been the involved intern) strongly urge that apparatus be available on all hospital wards to reduce the necessity for mouth-to-mouth respiration. They suggest the use of rebreathing bags or endotracheal tubes.

Postmassage pulmonary edema

Pulmonary edema may be a sequel to cardiac resuscitation. The explanation may be that with either open- or closed-chest cardiac compression, retrograde venous flow into the pulmonary veins occurs with each compression. In some instances, direct trauma to the lungs is no doubt a contributing factor.

Numerous studies have attested to the increased right atrial and vena caval pressures during closed-chest pulmonary resuscitation. It seems likely that pulmonary edema complicating prolonged periods of cardiac resuscitation may be more common than has been clinically recognized.

Laceration of the lung and pneumothorax

Inadvertent laceration of portions of the left lung is quite common during cardiac massage. As a rule, no serious consequence will result, but particular care should be taken to include an underwater drainage tube to guard against subsequent tension pneumothorax. Large lacerations may be closed by a suture or two in the lung tissue itself.

Vigorous resuscitative procedures are not infrequently associated with ruptured pulmonary alveoli, especially in resuscitative attempts on infants.

TENSION PNEUMOTHORAX

Tension pneumothorax is a significant hazard of closed-chest cardiopulmonary resuscitation. If unrecognized, this complication may result in the death of the patient. Fletcher documents three such patients. The suspicion of a tension pneumothorax arose when ventilation became difficult while using the manual AMBU bag. Two of the patients had bronchial asthma with chronic obstruc-

tive pulmonary disease and may have ruptured a bleb.

In patients with cardiac arrest, a bilateral tension pneumothorax may go undetected unless an open-chest approach is employed. Gleave and Monty encountered such a case in a 48-year-old woman during surgery. Thoracotomy revealed the cause of the arrest, and direct cardiac massage produced a successful outcome. I encountered a somewhat similar case in an infant under anesthesia. A tension pneumothorax produced such an extensive shift of mediastinal structures that cardiac output was inadequate. A thoracotomy and cardiac massage produced a successful outcome.

Bronchopneumonia

Bronchopneumonia occurring after successful cardiac resuscitation is usually associated with those cases in which there is a period of cerebral edema accompanied by a delayed return of the sensorium. Chest complications, including pneumonia, become more serious with the inability of the patient to swallow, cough, or move about. By close, careful nursing care, including frequent tracheal aspirations and turning of the patient, the likelihood of this complication can be reduced.

Paralysis of the left hemidiaphragm

Paralysis of the left hemidiaphragm is a rare complication, but it has been encountered in instances where the phrenic nerve was accidentally divided or injured at the time of opening the pericardial sac.

Complications following elective cardioplegia with localized hypothermia

Freezing the myocardium with ice chips or saline slush has resulted in several instances of what is now termed "frostbitten phrenic." To avoid this complication of paralysis of the diaphragm, Hufnagel has employed a small plastic sheet that covers the phrenic nerve.

The enthusiasm for ice chip cardioplegia

or saline slush elective cardioplegia has been tempered somewhat by the work of Speicher and co-workers at the University of Pennsylvania. Patients' hearts were studied after varying periods of death following open-heart surgery in which elective cardioplegia was employed using saline slush. In the small series reported, 75% died of myocardial insufficiency as manifested clinically by progressive hypotension unrelieved by pressor drugs. Rather striking gross and microscopic findings were reported. Myocardial fibers in the subepicardial zone had a markedly coagulated appearance, with loss of all striations and breaking up of the cytoplasm into masses separated by spaces and nuclear pyknosis. The coagulated appearance of the cytoplasm suggested to the authors some type of protein denaturation. In one patient, death was ascribed to constrictive pericarditis resulting from formation of exuberant granulation tissue, dense adhesions, and diffuse thickening of both pericardial layers. In dogs, fibroblastic proliferation of the epicardium was noted. The profound hypothermia produced by saline slush applied about the heart prompted the authors to suggest that continuous exposure of the heart and pericardium to the slush should not exceed 1 hour.

Further studies of the effect of hypothermia upon the myocardium seem indicated. Almost every modality employed in the use of elective cardioplegia appears to carry with it inherent disadvantages, many of which have not been apparent, unfortunately, until some time after the method has been employed. It now appears that marked ischemia produced by prolonged hypothermia is replaced by a marked hyperemia. The hyperemia is in turn accompanied and followed by massive edema and subsequent fibroplasia.

Subclavian vein catheterization

No one should attempt a subclavian vein catheterization without a full realization of its possible complications and an ability to recognize and manage them should they occur. Most important, however, is the effi-ciency necessary to prevent these complications. Complications associated with percutaneous subclavian vein cannulation include air or catheter embolization, perforation of the right atrium with subsequent cardiac tamponade, brachial plexus or phrenic nerve injury, subclavian vein thrombosis, and (most commonly) simple and tension pneumothorax. Inadvertent arterial puncture of the subclavian artery has produced delayed massive injury and death. Cellulitis, subcutaneous emphysema, and hematoma formation also have been frequently recorded.

Knotting of the subclavian central venous catheter may occur. Erosion through the subclavian vein with subsequent extravasation of fluid is reported.

Rupture of the trachea

In particular instances of emergency intubation, I believe that there was evidence to suggest that a rupture of the trachea had taken place at passage of the endotracheal tube. Progressive emphysema of the face, chest, neck, and upper arms was observed. It was felt that this complication resulted from the forced, rapid passage of the endotracheal tube by an inexperienced operator.

Complications with the intra-arterial transfusion route

AIR EMBOLI

When whole blood, preferably aerated whole blood, is introduced into the arterial system under pressure that forces it in the direction of the heart, all precautions must be taken to assure that no air emboli reach the heart or cerebral vessels. Air entering the arterial system in such a fashion will go rapidly to the coronary arteries or to the blood vessels of the brain, and death may ensue. A simple device to prevent air emboli in such instances has been described by Wilkinson. At least an air trap should be present between the bottle of blood and the patient, and all air should be out of the distal tubing. Pumping should, of course, be discontinued before the blood has emptied completely from the bottle.

RETROPERITONEAL HEMATOMA

I know of one case in which a large retroperitoneal hematoma was formed because the needle inadvertently slipped out of the wall of the aorta into the adjacent tissue when the intra-aortic transfusion route was being used. Before any blood is pumped, care should be taken to ensure that the needle is definitely in the aorta.

GANGRENE OF EXTREMITIES

In at least six cases, gangrene and necrosis of the forearm and hand have resulted as complications of the intra-arterial transfusion route. (Transfusion was via the radial artery.) In two additional cases, ischemia of the thumb and index finger occurred. Although not frequent, this complication deserves attention.

Several factors apparently contribute to the gangrene that eventually develops. Some operators prefer to ligate the artery distal to the needle. Lippert and Furman state that the radioulnar anastomosis is not present in 2% to 5% of cases. It is believed by some that the vessel should be divided rather than ligated and left continuous in order to decrease sympathetic tone distally.

The most likely reason for the development of gangrene after radial artery transfusion seems to be that the extremity cannot withstand prolonged periods of perfusion with unoxygenated blood. Yee and his co-workers have presented a case of gangrene of the forearm and hand following the intra-arterial route.

It seems likely that the following precautions should be taken:

1. Cold blood should be avoided if possible. Cold blood may cause widespread vasospasm in the extremity.
2. Oxygenated blood is much preferred but obviously cannot always be obtained during instances of cardiac arrest.
3. It is best to make the transfusion as brief as possible.
4. If evidence of any vasospasm exists, a procaine block of the cervical sympathetic ganglia should be done.
5. Avoid ligation of the vessel, using instead the needle puncture technique.

Pneumoperitoneum

Free abdominal air under sufficient pressure to severely compromise ventilation is reported as a complication of closed-chest cardiac resuscitation (Fletcher). The mechanism in which air enters the peritoneal cavity may be severalfold. Rupture of the hollow viscus from closed-chest resuscitation could, of course, be the precipitating factor. Air extravasated from the pulmonary parenchyma to the mediastinum, following external massage, may dissect within the esophageal wall to the stomach or intestine (the air enters the peritoneal cavity through the serosal surface of the intestine or stomach).

Obviously, recognition of this complication is important; and its immediate effect can be managed simply by aspirations of the air from the abdomen or, in case of a pneumothorax, from the chest.

Accidental ventilator disconnection

A patient receiving ventilatory support, either through a tracheostomy or an endotracheal tube is usually under careful observation. Nevertheless, ventilator disconnections from tracheostomies or endotracheal tubes or failure of ventilator function may occur without immediate detection. A simple reliable alarm system, which gives an audible signal to indicate malfunction or disconnection of the ventilator, has been devised by Petty and co-workers.

Accidental electrocution of operator during ventricular defibrillation

Although hundreds of attempts at electrical cardiac defibrillation have been made during the last 27 years, I know of no instances in which injury to the operator has occurred. An anesthesiologist received a mild electrical shock while holding the patient during a defibrillation procedure, but this was a case in which the defibrillator did not employ an isolation transformer.

In one case in which a young child developed ventricular fibrillation, during the attempt at defibrillation the operator was handed a "homemade" defibrillator. When the apparatus was connected to the wall outlet and an attempt was made to defibrillate, the current was short-circuited; further attempts at defibrillation had to be carried out by using procaine. These were unsuccessful.

If an electrical defibrillation unit is used that does not employ the safety feature of an isolation transformer, the operator should take the extra precaution of wearing at least one pair of gloves, and in some instances a double pair of gloves. He should probably stand on a wooden stool, and he should make sure that his arms are well away from the patient when applying the current. In addition, all personnel should stand away from the operating table. These precautions are not necessary, however, if an isolation transformer is incorporated into the electrical defibrillator.

Self-retaining countershock electrodes have been devised (Lape and Maison) that may have some advantage in that they would protect the operator from any possible shock. I have not felt a need for self-retaining electrodes, however, since in many clinical cases it is necessary for the surgeon to be able to manipulate the electrodes at will. If the two electrodes are bound together, a problem exists that may complicate their application.

ECG pitfalls and precautions

The importance of easy recognition of extracardiac potentials should be emphasized, since they may be confused with ectopic contractions or fibrillation and thus may lead to faulty interpretation of data from the ECG monitor. Examples of such artifacts include those produced by failure to "ground" the patient, somatic muscle tremors, use of

cautery, and interference caused by the introduction of large retractors.

Several additional points merit attention. During ventricular fibrillation, if the heart is to be defibrillated with the electrical cardiac defibrillators, precautions should be taken to ensure that the ECG electrodes are disconnected from the wrists and ankles. With certain machines, it is conceivable that a burn of the skin may occur on the wrist. In addition, the current from some defibrillators will cause a "blow-out" of the electrocardiograph. The addition of an instant, automatic switch to the electrocardiograph will permit quick recovery of the ECG tracing after shock application. The result of the defibrillation attempt can thus be quickly evaluated.

One precaution in the evaluation of the ECG tracing is that an occasional tracing shows electrical activity occurring in the heart even though cardiac asystole has occurred. This has been observed on some occasions and will tend to confuse the operator unless he is aware that the electrical potential from the arrested heart may be picked up for some minutes after all apparent activity has ceased.

It is generally wise to disconnect the electrocardiograph when the electric pacemaker is in use. If the electrocardiograph is a late model, however, and does not have condensers in the input circuit, the electrical stimuli from the cardiac pacemaker will not interfere with the recording of the heart's activity by the electrocardiograph. The patient, the pacemaker, and the electrocardiograph should be commonly grounded.

Generalized clonic convulsions

Generalized clonic convulsions have been observed in many of the cases, often coming 6 to 10 hours after resuscitation. They too signal a very poor prognosis, although they are not necessarily signs of irreversible damage.

Vomiting and aspiration

Vomiting represents a potential complicating hazard, particularly in oral resuscitation of asphyxiated victims. If gastric distension is prevented by hyperextension of the head and opening of the air passages, vomiting may occur less than 50% of the time, as shown in the Norway studies.

An ever present threat in the immediate postresuscitation period is that of aspiration pneumonia from vomitus inhaled into the trachea at a time when the patient's cough reflexes are obscured. Outside the operating room and recovery area, where adequate suctioning units may not be available, the threat is probably magnified (Greenberg).

Psychiatric complications

Severe personality decomposition is occasionally seen in patients subjected to highly mechanized and anxiety-provoking emotional distress as seen in the coronary care unit, intensive care unit, recovery room, chronic dialysis facility, burn and trauma units, and so forth. Considerable concern has arisen among psychiatrists and physicians as a group in an effort to lessen the frequency of this unfortunate complication. The postcardiac resuscitation victim is no exception as he may require prolonged artificial assistance of one type or another. An endotracheal tube may prevent him from communicating easily. He may be totally unfamiliar with the purpose of the monitoring apparatus, the strange sounds, tubes, and the like. The impersonal nature of his confinement, often in a windowless room, may compound the difficulties. In addition, his psychologic problems may be compounding an acute brain syndrome provoked by an excessive period of anoxia or hypercapnia. Doubtless, the physician can aid the situation considerably by as much personal attention and as much direct communication as possible.

Most commonly, it is impossible for a patient to clearly remember the events surrounding cardiac arrest followed by successful resuscitation. A vivid account is provided, however, by a 68-year-old patient who experienced a cardiac arrest in a Canadian hospital (MacMillan and Brown). He was being monitored for a possible myocardial infarction when a ventricular premature beat fell on a T wave, provoking ventricular fibrillation. The patient was defibrillated and subsequently recovered. To him the experience was extremely vivid. He remembers looking at his watch and noting the time. Suddenly he was aware of giving a very deep sigh and that his head "flopped" over to the right. At this point he apparently lost consciousness. The patient then describes himself as leaving his body and he was able to observe it "face to face." He had a feeling of floating in space and of considerable tranquility, and he remembers thinking "so this is what happens when you die." He recalls that after traveling at great speed in space, there was a sudden sensation, almost of a sledge-hammer variety, in his left side. Having received six such shocks, he opened his eyes. He remembers recognizing the doctors and nurses and considered himself to be in complete control of his facilities.

After the experience was over he remarked to his doctor that the floating part of his sensation was so strangely beautiful that "if I go out again, don't bring me back—it's so beautiful out there."

Psychiatrists have shown increasing interest in the patterns of behavior exhibited by the patient following a successful cardiac resuscitation. Previously, there has been very little available information. Dlin and co-workers from the Department of Psychiatry and Internal Medicine at Temple University in Philadelphia consider the psychologic adaptation to the cardiac pacemaker following cardiac arrest. For example, patients who are dependent upon lifesaving devices such as the cardiac pacemaker must adjust to several basic conflicts. The patient is not prepared to make an external device an integral part of his body. When there is not time to prepare the patient emotionally, a psychiatric reaction may take place. Some patients react by denying the presence of the device. Dlin further believes that a catastrophic experience, such as cardiac arrest and pacemaker attachments, necessitates a rearrangement of the patient's concept of himself. He must shift his homeostatic balance (physical and mental) to accommodate for these changes. All such patients must make major ego-adaptive changes, and many of these patients need psychiatric support during the changes. So far, relatively few guidelines have been worked out.

The emotional adaptation of the patient following a cardiac resuscitation has been, in my experience, quite varied. The psychiatric study by Druss and Korneld on a group of ten survivors of cardiac arrest is significant. These two physicians wondered how patients might react to the unique and remarkable experience of having been "dead." Their group of ten patients was culled from sixteen successfully resuscitated patients discharged from the Columbia Presbyterian Hospital. These represented a group of eighty-five patients who had experienced cardiac arrest outside of the operating room between July, 1964, and December, 1965. Prolonged psychiatric interviews were carried out with both the patient and with his relatives. As a control, there was a study of ten additional males who had been in the intensive care unit but who had not had a cardiac arrest. Seven of the cardiac arrests occurred in association with acute myocardial infarction, one patient suffered pulmonary infarction, and two patients became involved in cardiac asystole during diagnostic procedures (either cardiac catheterization or exploratory cystoscopy).

It is of interest that nine of the ten patients with cardiac arrest had a mild to severe organic brain syndrome, which included symptoms of confusion, delusional thinking, and uncontrollable agitation. At least four defense mechanisms were elicited:

1. Denial and isolation
2. Displacement
3. Rejection
4. Hallucinatory or delusional behavior

Eight of the patients reacted by an isolation of effect and by denying that they had been afraid.

Also of interest was the finding that eight of the ten patients experienced dreams of violence and violent death. Patients were questioned about their attitude toward death. When asked what it was like to have been dead, one patient replied that there had been no pain and therefore death was believed painless. The patient stated that he did not fear death anymore because he had already experienced it. No overt alterations in patients' religious attitude were uncovered.

Persistent long-term symptoms were often present. The most common was insomnia (90%). Tenseness, anxiety, restlessness, and irritability were common. Difficulty in concentrating and a lack of memory for recent events were noted by a majority of the patients.

Several suggestions have been made by psychiatrists. For one thing, a great deal might be done to make the intensive care unit or the coronary monitoring unit a less frightening place. Increasing the degree of privacy was thought to be a helpful thing, so that patients would be less aware of the life and death struggle of other patients. Furthermore, monitoring equipment might well be placed outside the unit to reduce the frightening aspects to the patient. In addition, each patient experiencing a cardiac arrest should be talked to in some detail and given as much reassurance as possible.

Although it is a rather unusual occurrence, occasionally the patient regains consciousness during the period of cardiac massage. This "complication" certainly testifies to the adequateness of cardiac massage and seldom presents too much difficulty. Ravdin and associates, in a report on cardiac arrest in a 60-year-old woman, recorded four separate periods of cardiac arrest occurring over a 10-day period. The fourth cardiac arrest occurred while the patient was in her bed. The chest was quickly opened and the heart was found to be in ventricular fibrillation. Surprisingly enough, defibrillation was accomplished simply by manual massage. While cardiac massage was being accomplished, the patient actually regained consciousness. This required taking the patient to the operating room, where she was anesthetized with cyclopropane and the chest was closed.

In addition, I have talked with one patient who states that he was experiencing an orthopedic procedure under spinal anesthesia when suddenly he found himself looking at the overhead mirrors where he observed the surgeon's hand in his chest. The patient experienced no painful sensations at the time. He was quickly given a general anesthetic agent and remembers nothing further about the procedure. He made an uneventful recovery.

Undoubtedly, cardiac arrest, a most unfortunate and unexpected complication, evokes problems associated with the patient's relatives that require exceptional patience and understanding on the part of the physician. In a very regrettable instance, sudden cardiac arrest with ventricular fibrillation occurred immediately after intravenous injection of digitalis. The patient was a middle-aged woman in bed on a large hospital ward. A prompt diagnosis was made and a thoracotomy was instituted. The arrest occurred just at the beginning of visiting hours, and the patient's son appeared on the ward during resuscitative procedure.

The psychic trauma to the physician himself might well be mentioned. I know of one physician who was depressed so severely by the occurrence of a cardiac arrest in a young boy upon whom he was performing a tonsillectomy that he ceased performing any type of surgery.

One surgeon states that he encountered two cases of cardiac arrest in successive operative procedures! Another surgeon was called upon to attempt cardiac resuscitation three times on three different patients in a period of 3 weeks.

Several physicians stated that they encountered their first case of cardiac arrest shortly after receiving a letter asking about their experience. Dr. Hugh H. Trout, Jr., of Roanoke, Virginia, wrote: "I recently wrote you that we had not had a case of cardiac arrest during operation, and that I was sorry I had received your letter, as I was sure such would occur in the immediate future—which has happened!"

Dr. Calvin M. Smyth of Abington, Pennsylvania, wrote on March 28, 1951. He described a case of cardiac arrest and stated further: "I operated upon him the day after I received your letter and was commenting about it during the operation. I had just remarked that we had seen only one case of cardiac arrest over a period of many years. At that point I had just completed the surgery and was getting ready to sew up the abdomen. Suddenly the blood pressure, which had been maintained at 140/70 throughout the operation, dropped out of sight and the aorta stopped pulsating!" Cardiac arrest was diagnosed, and the heart was restored to a normal rhythm. The patient died some hours later, however.

Dr. John C. Burch, a past president of the Southern Surgical Association, supplied me with the interesting information that in the first operative case he was given while an intern at Bellevue Hospital in 1922, the patient had a sudden cardiac arrest. The operation was a hemorrhoidectomy.

Physicians familiar with the problems inherent in intensive care provided to many of our patients will recognize the syndrome that McKegney describes as the "intensive care syndrome."

Following prolonged cardiac massage, a 32-year-old male was finally resuscitated and eventually was able to return home despite some emotional lability. Eventually, however, the patient committed suicide by puncturing his heart with a knife (Lahdensuu).

The reader is referred to the August 2, 1969, issue of *Lancet* (p. 262) for an excellent detailed first-hand account of a physician experiencing ventricular fibrillation on his eleventh day after coronary infarction. His prodromata experiences as well as the sensations, aphasia, bruised chest, and so forth of the immediate postresuscitative period make a most interesting account.

A study done at the Massachusetts General Hospital on the effect of last rites routinely administered to Catholic patients in most hospitals is reported by Cassem and associates. In an effort to determine the anxiety-provoking aspect of last rites, they studied 30 patients. Generally speaking, anxiety is directly dependent upon the manner in which the priest administers this sacrament. Patients who are given an explanation about the routine nature of the procedure tend to respond more positively.

Chapter 59

MEDICOLEGAL ASPECTS OF CARDIAC ARREST AND RESUSCITATION*

Elwyn L. Cady, Jr.

The cross-examiner presses on:

Cross-examiner. Then what did you do?

Defendant surgeon. As we got the instruments up to the table and waited for the nurse to adjust a couple of things, I got up in position right over where I would ordinarily make the incision and, as I always do, I asked if everything was all right upstairs.

Q. Upstairs?

A. That is what we call the anesthesia level— "Is everything all right upstairs?" And as Dr. ——— [defendant anesthesiologist] checked again and as I also simultaneously noted, the skin color looked peculiar to me. He said, "We have no pulse, no blood pressure. . . . It looks like we are in real trouble."

Q. What skin area were you looking at?

A. The area that was draped, which is several square inches of skin that is not covered with drapes, where the incision is made. . . .

Q. What happened?

A. We immediately whipped the patient on his back, stripped off the drapes, jerked off the adhesive tape . . . and started external cardiac massage and, also, at the same time said, "Where is Dr. ——— [defendant personal physician of the patient]?

Add an affidavit filed by a thoracic surgeon against the defendant surgeon that "in particular, after ascertaining that his patient had suffered a cardiac arrest, he conducted and continued to conduct external cardiac compression without successful results when good medical practice required that internal cardiac compression be initiated" and the groundwork is laid for another substantial settlement for death following cardiac arrest. (*Horton v. Cedars of Lebanon Hospital Cor-*

poration, et al., Dade County, Florida, No. 68-6431, settled, 1970)

Substantial awards

Substantial monetary awards characterize cardiac arrest cases involving professional negligence. Why damages are "usually astronomical" is set forth by Sagall and Reed.* The largest jury award in any medical malpractice case at the time rendered involved a cardiac arrest. Since this is a leading case, I shall cite it throughout this chapter as *Quintal* (Case J, Table 59-1). The verdict against the hospital, Dr. Palmberg, and Dr. Thornburg was for the amount of the prayer, $400,000, and the mother was awarded $3,610.73 special damages. Federal Judge Choate in Florida made an award of $78,503.78.† A settlement for $317,000 is noted by Stetler and Moritz (*Carvanis v. Montefiore Hospital,* N. Y., 1960).‡

Justice Peters, California Supreme Court, In Bank, summarized the facts of the *Quintal* case as follows:

The case revolves around the tragic experiences of plaintiff Reginald Quintal (Reggie), who in July of 1960, when the events here involved occurred, was six years of age. Prior to July 11, 1960, Reggie was a normal, healthy child, suffer-

---

*From Sagall, E. L., and Reed, B. C.: The heart and the law, New York, 1968, The Macmillan Co., p. 158.

†*Kolesar v. United States,* 198 F. Supp. 517 (1961).

‡From Stetler, C. J., and Moritz, A. R.: Doctor and patient and the law, ed. 4, St. Louis, 1962, The C. V. Mosby Co., p. 318.

---

*References for this chapter can be found at the end of the chapter.

737

ing only from an inward deviation of the eyes. On July 10, 1960, he entered the defendant hospital for the purpose of having this condition corrected by a minor operation to be performed on July 11, 1960, by defendant Dr. Palmberg. On the morning of that day, during the course of the administration of the anesthetic by defendant Dr. Thornburg, Reggie suffered a cardiac arrest. He was resuscitated by means of an open chest heart massage. As a result of his brain being deprived of oxygen during the period his heart was stopped, he suffered severe brain damage resulting in his becoming a spastic quadriplegic, blind and mute.

Detailed facts are officially stated as follows:

In 1960, Reggie was suffering from some inward deviation of the eyes, but otherwise was normal and healthy. On May 8, 1960, he was taken to Laurel Grove Hospital in Castro Valley for an operation aimed at correcting the eye condition. The operation was performed by defendant Dr. Palmberg, an ophthalmologist, and was completed without incident. The anesthesiologist at that first operation is not a party to this case. He was an associate of defendant Dr. Thornburg. The first operation was not entirely successful in curing the deviation, and, after conservative treatment failed to cure the condition, it was decided that another operation was necessary. On July 10, 1960, Reggie was again taken to the Laurel Grove Hospital for an operation scheduled for the next morning, and estimated to take 20 minutes. Dr. Palmberg was to do the eye surgery, and Dr. Thornburg was to administer the anesthetic. The evening Reggie entered the hospital he was crying, with a running nose, was quite apprehensive, and was uncooperative. The medical record in fact shows that just before surgery he was "very apprehensive" and "very agitated." He had a temperature when he first arrived at the hospital, which increased up to midnight. The hospital records purport to show that his temperature, just before the operation, was a little under normal, but by expert testimony it was shown that there had been a correction and erasure in that record, and what the original record showed does not appear. The erasure was not explained by defendants. The records also show that it was therein noted that the preoperative medication aimed at sedating the patient was "unsatisfactory."

When Dr. Palmberg entered the operating room Reggie was already there, and Dr. Thornburg was administering the anesthetic in a normal fashion. Dr. Palmberg took no part in administering the anesthetic, but remained in the room some distance from the operating table talking to an assistant about the intended operation.

During the administration of the anesthetic, and before the process had been entirely completed, Reggie suffered a respiratory arrest followed by a cardiac arrest. This means that his breathing and heart stopped. This, of course, cut off blood and oxygen to his brain. The record shows that the brain, without damage, may be without oxygen for not more than three minutes, but that every second over the three-minute limit endangers the patient and makes brain damage more probable.

When the respiratory and cardiac arrests occurred, Dr. Thornburg called out that Reggie's heart had stopped beating. Dr. Palmberg and his assistant rushed toward the table. Dr. Thornburg let the anesthetic gases out of the anesthetic bag, filled the bag with pure oxygen, pumped the bag with one hand and with the other attempted to restore Reggie's heart action by external massage. This process was continued for 20 or 30 seconds and was then stopped to ascertain if the boy's heart had started. It had not. The process was repeated for another 20 or 30 seconds, but without success. Dr. Thornburg then asked Dr. Palmberg to open Reggie's chest in order to administer manual massage to the heart. Dr. Thornburg emphasized that this operation had to be done very quickly. Dr. Palmberg stated that he did not feel qualified to perform such an operation, and started to leave the operating room to get help. Just near the door to the operating room he encountered Dr. Beumer, a surgeon. Dr. Beumer, at Dr. Palmberg's request, entered the operating room, was quickly gloved, and was handed a scalpel. He opened Reggie's chest and began heart massage. The heart responded almost immediately, and began to beat. The beat at first was uneven and it was twice necessary to use a defibrillator (an instrument that gives electric shocks to the heart) to correct the defective heart action. Although the evidence is confusing and somewhat in conflict . . . about four minutes elapsed between the time Dr. Thornburg first noticed that the heart had stopped and the time the heart was again started by means of the open heart massage.

Cases not officially reported

A settlement of $300,000 was reported in *Medical World News,* December 4, 1964, North Shore Hospital of Manhasset paying $231,000, surgeon and anesthesiologist paying $42,500 and $26,500. Plaintiff was Alan Mitchell Grimes-Graeme of Port Washington, New York, a 10-year-old boy who sustained permanent brain damage from a cardiac arrest that occurred in the recovery room following a tonsillectomy. Negligence alleged: (1) Surgeon and anesthesiologist should have remained in the recovery room with the patient; (2) hospital was maintaining improper recovery room in equipment and personnel; and (3) R.N. was inexperienced and failed to detect cardiac arrest for several minutes.*

A verdict of $250,000 was awarded in Ohio, *Shaffer* v. *Barbeton Citizens Hospital,* No. 245574, Summit County, 1965. Plaintiff was a 40-year-old housewife who sustained partial blindness as a result of cardiac arrest during bronchography. The anesthesiologist allegedly administered four times the maximum safe dose of anesthesia.

Settlement for two million dollars was entered in *Brader* v. *Sunnyvale Medical Clinic* and *Armanini,* No. 276588, Santa Clara County, California, 1973. A 22-year-old store clerk, in preparation for an outpatient bronchogram, was given cocaine spray and a quantity was poured into the left bronchus down a catheter. An order for 1% was filled with a labeled 10% solution, the radiologist overlooking the variance from his order. The amount of $1,500,000 was contributed on behalf of the radiologist and $500,000 was on behalf of the pharmacy. No negligence was claimed with respect to resuscitation after the cardiac arrest. $100,000 of the total was allocated to the patient's parents for "premature wrongful death," there being medical opinion available that life expectancy was from 1 to 25 years only.

A compromise settlement in the amount of $130,000 was reached in one case.† Quoting from Judge George Francis' pretrial conference order:

---

*Negligence points recited to found advice "that the anesthesiologist must stay with the patient in the recovery room a reasonable length of time, if not all the time. Perhaps the surgeon, too. At least, both should be on call nearby." From Morris, C.: Resuscitation and the law. In Wecht, C. H., editor: Legal medicine annual, New York, 1969, Appleton-Century-Crofts.

†*Payette* v. *Cole,* No. LB C-22707, Superior Court of California, Los Angeles County, at Long Beach (1957).

This is an action for damages for malpractice and negligence.

Plaintiffs contend that on May 31, 1956, at about 8 A.M. defendants undertook to perform an operation on plaintiff No. 1 for removal of tonsils and adenoids; that they did it in a negligent manner, causing plaintiff No. 1 personal injuries, including rendering her unconscious ever since said date; that defendant No. 1 was a practicing physician and surgeon, holding himself out to be an eye, ear, nose and throat expert; that defendant No. 2 was a practicing physician, holding himself out to be an expert anesthesiologist; that defendant No. 3 operated the hospital where the operation was performed, and defendant No. 4 was a nurse there; that defendants No. 2 and No. 4 were the agents of the other defendants.

Plaintiff No. 1 seeks damages for personal injuries, and plaintiffs 2 and 3, her parents, seek damages for loss of services of plaintiff No. 1 and for the medical expenses of plaintiff No. 1.

All defendants deny the allegations of negligence and damage and plead unavoidable accident.

• • •

The parties agree as follows:
1. That on May 31, 1956, at about 8:43 A.M. defendants Nos. 1 and 2 began the performance of a tonsillectomy and an adenoidectomy and an operation for the removal of nasal polyps on plaintiff No. 1 and continued with the operation at defendant No. 3's hospital.
2. That defendant No. 1 was a surgeon.
3. That defendant No. 2 was the anesthetist.
4. That defendant No. 4 was a nurse at defendant No. 3's hospital.

The medicolegal theory of plaintiff's case, partially developed by depositions taken of defendants, alleged facts, as follows:

Plaintiff was a 15-year-old girl undergoing a routine T and A. As the operation proceeded, defendant No. 2 noted that the girl's color changed and she became cyanotic. He advised defendant No. 1 that something had gone wrong and he believed the girl's heart had stopped beating. Two other anesthesiologists were in the area of the operating room and were called in and confirmed defendant No. 2's diagnosis that her heart had stopped beating. At this time, defendant No. 1, as he testified, had earlier seen Dr. J. C. pass in the hallway, so defendant No. 1 ran out of the operating room and down to the doctor's change room where he found Dr. J. C. and advised him that his patient's heart had stopped and that he needed help. Defendant No. 1, in his deposition, gave only the explanation that he thought Dr.

J. C. was better qualified in this type of situation although he admitted he was the surgeon in charge at the time the emergency occurred.

Thereafter, Dr. J. C. performed a thoracotomy and cardiac massage causing the girl's heart to start beating again. However, it was too late to salvage the brain since the state of anoxia had gone on for approximately four minutes.

At the time of settlement, report of the neurologic status of the plaintiff was filed with the Court, as Exhibit "A." The following excerpts are significant:

Chief complaints. Patient in spastic paralytic state following cardiac arrest during surgery on May 31, 1956. Outside of the vital functions of circulation of blood, respiration, and metabolism— the only other motor functions demonstrable are weak attempts to swallow (reflexly), reflex blinking of eyelids, weak attempts to move lips (reflexly), reflex vocal response to discomfort, and reflex-hyperactive-general muscular twitching as a response to sudden sound and vibration. As far as can be determined the patient cannot think, see, chew, swallow to any appreciable degree, voluntarily move her head, face, eyes, body, or extremities, or exercise any control over her excretory functions.

History of present complaints. Normal, intelligent girl of 15 with no previous history of circulatory disease, neurological disease, metabolic disease, or mental disease sustained cardiac arrest while undergoing routine T and A under general anesthesia. . . . Thoracotomy and cardiac massage assisted by tracheotomy (were) performed and normal cardiac rhythm was restored in an estimated time of three to seven minutes.

• • •

Mental status. Patient is awake in the sense that her eyes are open and in a normal awake position; however, the patient appears to have no awareness of her existence; she is an organism without the ability to think; she is without a mind; there appear to be no thought processes; the delicate cells of her frontal lobes seem to be dead.

• • •

Diagnosis. Marked encephalopathy due to severe anoxia, spastic residual quadriplegia; incontinence. *Prognosis.* Poor.

• • •

Had this case been tried, one of the litigated points would have been the matter of alleged negligence in the surgeon's delay in instituting resuscitation. A case in which such a claim was not sustained was cited by Dr. Frank McArthur Barry. He states that he was involved in a lawsuit in 1952 in which he was subpoenaed by the plaintiff. It was a case of an 18-year-old girl who had had a mastoid operation under local anesthesia. Cardiac arrest subsequently occurred. Dr. Barry's office was immediately across from the operating room, and the eye, nose, and throat specialist requested that he open the chest. The suit centered around the fact that the ear, nose, and throat surgeon had not instituted the resuscitative procedure himself but had taken time to call another doctor in consultation, which was held to be a factor in the ultimate death of the individual. At the trial, the defense of the physician was based upon the fact that the cardiac arrest had occurred prior to the time that a period of training of surgeons in cardiac arrest resuscitation had been instituted in that area. The ultimate outcome in the case was in favor of the defendant.

A similar case in which claim was unsuccessfully made against a hospital was the following:

Angeline Conforto, Administratrix of the Estate of Josephine Conforto, deceased, v. Dr. V. M. Jordan, Dr. R. Wenner Machamer, and University Hospitals of Cleveland, No. 610119, Common Pleas Court of Cuyahoga County, Ohio (1952).

A 17-year-old girl entered University Hospitals of Cleveland for a mastoid operation and while Dr. Machamer, a trained anesthetist, was giving the initial anesthesia, to-wit: procaine with Adrenalin, preliminary to a shift over to a general anesthetic, her heart and lungs failed in their functioning, her heart action and breathing completely stopped for an interval of about twelve minutes and she died the following day without having regained consciousness. The cause of death was given as "cardiac arrest due to procaine sensitivity."

The anesthetic given consisted first of a local of about 30 ml. of procaine with Adrenalin, to be followed by the shift over to a general anesthetic if that proved necessary due to the expected length of the operation. About 20 ml. of the procaine had been given when the patient's blood pressure went up to 190/50 and the heartbeat disappeared entirely. Within ten minutes after her reaction, a general surgeon who happened to be in the hospital opened the chest and massaged the heart, but the interval of cardiac arrest had been too long and death ensued. In addition to opening the chest, a shocking machine (at that time the only one in the city of Cleveland and which was there at the hospital) was used, the fibrillation brought under control and coordinated action partially restored. Due, however, to the time interval which had elapsed, as above stated, the patient never regained consciousness and died the following day.

The above suit for $50,000 was filed by her mother against the two doctors and the hospital. So far as the suit involved the doctors, it was based on the claim that they had negligently failed to determine in advance that the patient was hypersensitive to procaine; so far as it referred to the hospital, the claim was that it should have had a chest surgeon immediately at hand to open the chest and massage the heart before permanent damage was done to the brain.

The director of the hospital was called for cross-examination by plaintiff's attorney and gave testimony concerning the nature of the equipment and personnel which the hospital had available and also the very rare occurrence of fatal reaction to anesthesia. His testimony was to the effect that it had never been the established practice for operating surgeons to anticipate a cardiorespiratory failure and either themselves be qualified to open the chest in an emergency or to have immediately available a surgeon who was thus qualified. His testimony showed that in only one or two instances out of 12,500 operations at the hospital had cardiac failure occurred. His conclusion was that the likelihood of its occurrence was so rare as to be negligible so far as proper hospital administration was concerned.

At the close of plaintiff's evidence, the defense counsel moved for a directed verdict on behalf of each of the defendants, which motion after oral argument was sustained by the trial court and the case dismissed. No appeal was ever taken.

As a result of this particular case, University Hospitals launched a training course which it offered to operating surgeons whose skill lay in fields other than chest or abdominal surgery, so that if cardiac arrests did occur they might be dealt with immediately even though no chest surgeon was available.

Related cases

Medicolegal situations in which cardiac resuscitation figures include the matter of competency to execute a will. Dr. Daniel C. Moore relates the following instance:

During an exploratory laparotomy for a cholecystectomy on a middle-aged white male patient under thiopental sodium (Pentothal), ether, and curare anesthesia, it was suddenly noted that the patient was pulseless. Cardiac massage was carried out and the normal rhythm of the heart was re-established. The surgery was continued and a diffuse carcinomatosis was reported. An electrocardiogram taken immediately following completion of the operation showed a normal rhythm.

In spite of rather prompt resuscitative efforts, the patient remained unconscious for 24 hours and had several convulsions. After 24 hours, however, recovery was rapid. In 4 to 5 days, he no longer appeared mentally confused. He was discharged on the fourteenth day. On the seventh day, after being told by his wife that he had cancer, the patient decided to have a will drawn up. He was considered in full control of his senses in order that he might sign the will.

A unique form of settlement was agreed upon in one case.* The basic theory of liability in this case was an error in administering morphine sulfate instead of codeine phosphate. The sequence of events was stated by the chief surgeon, Ellis Ellison, as follows:

Ross Rattet. This 2½-year-old male was admitted to Mount Sinai Hospital, accompanied by his parents, at 7:15 A.M. Friday, February 24, 1956 for a routine tonsillectomy and adenoidectomy. Routine studies consisting of hemoglobin, bleeding and clotting time were performed shortly after admission. Since the child was unable to void, a urine specimen was not obtained preoperatively. My written instructions also called for the routine preoperative hypo according to the age and weight table on the pediatric ward which was prepared by Dr. I. Greenfield, anesthesiologist. In the case of this 2½-year-old child who weighed 25 pounds, the table provided for codeine phosphate (gr. 1/10) and scopolamine (gr. 1/600). The preoperative medication was prepared and

---

Rattet v. Mt. Sinai Hospital Association, District Court, 4th Judicial District, Hennepin County, Minnesota, No. 522176 (1957).

administered at 7:20 A.M. by Miss Engh. I saw the child in the treatment room on the pediatric ward at about 7:55 A.M., and he was then taken to the operating room in his crib at 8 A.M. by the operating room orderly.

Anesthesia was started at 8:20 A.M. by Miss Ella Costello, anesthetist, who was relieved ten or fifteen minutes later by Miss Catherine Rubald. The endotracheal tube was inserted by Dr. Jacob Fischman, anesthesiologist, at about 8:50 A.M., following which a routine T and A was performed without incident. Surgery was completed at 9:10 A.M., following which, having ascertained that the child's condition appeared satisfactory, I left the operating room and went to the doctors' dressing room where I changed into my street clothes and notified the patient's parents by phone that the operation was completed and that the boy was O.K.

Miss Rubald, who was again in attendance at the completion of the anesthesia, has stated that in my absence she checked the child's blood pressure, pulse, and respirations and found them to be satisfactory, following which she removed the endotracheal tube, again checked the vital signs and then carried the child to his crib which was outside the operating room. While preparing to take the patient to the recovery room she claims that she noted that his color was not entirely satisfactory, so she carried him back into the operating room for the purpose of administering some oxygen. When she determined that the pulse was becoming weaker, she summoned Dr. Fischman who in turn summoned Dr. David Gavisier whom he had seen in the hallway outside the operating room. Dr. Gavisier was joined almost immediately by Dr. Lyle Hay, and when a diagnosis of cardiac arrest was made the two surgeons opened the chest and, finding the heart "motionless and enlarged" (ventricular diastole), instituted cardiac massage. Following only a brief period of massage, the heart began to fibrillate. The electric defibrillator was used, following which massage was again performed and a regular cardiac rhythm was restored. Drs. Hay and Gavisier have estimated the time interval from the awareness of the cardiac emergency to the restoration of the heartbeat at from three to five minutes. Miss Rubald stated that the cardiac emergency occurred at 9:20 A.M.

The patient was seen shortly after normal cardiac rhythm was restored by Dr. Berman, cardiologist. An electrocardiogram taken during the first fifteen minutes was interpreted by Dr. Berman as appearing entirely normal. The blood pressure was first obtained at a level of 40 (systole) and, following the administration of Levo-

phed in 5% glucose through a venous cutdown, was maintained at between 65 and 75 (systole) for the remainder of the afternoon.

It is to be noted that although the normal cardiac rhythm was restored without too much difficulty, the respirations remained very markedly depressed and it was necessary for Dr. Fischman to maintain respirations by "bag-breathing" the patient via an endotracheal tube until voluntary respirations became regular and effective between 1 and 2 P.M. at which time the endotracheal tube was again withdrawn. At no time was any tracheobronchial obstruction or bleeding from the operative site noted.

The extremities remained flaccid, and the pupils were very small and did not react to light for the greater part of the day. By 8:30 P.M. some spasticity was apparent in the left arm and left leg, and occasional convulsive contractions were noted in these extremities, associated with emesis of gastric secretions. By 9 P.M., the pupils were observed to react sluggishly to light, although they were still small. A sluggish corneal reflex was also evident by this time. Between 8:30 and 9:30 P.M., there was some irregularity of respiration with periods of apnea lasting four to five seconds following periods of hyperventilation. The blood pressure had become stabilized, without further Levophed, at between 85 and 95 by this time and has remained stable to date.

By February 25, 1956, A.M. the child was still comatose, but the pupils were seen to be large and reacted to light. Some spontaneous movements of the extremities were occurring. No further convulsive movements were evident, but both lower extremities were moderately spastic.

By February 25, 1956, P.M. the respiratory rate had increased to 38 to 40 per minute and some secretions were present in the trachea which could not be removed by deep pharyngeal suctioning. Since the child had remained comatose and the likelihood of a further indeterminate period of coma existed, a tracheotomy was performed at at 9 P.M. February 25, 1956. Following this procedure, the child's general condition improved a good deal and some increased responsiveness was noted.

On February 26, 1956 a gastrotomy for feeding purposes was performed by Dr. Hay and Dr. Gavisier. The patient was still comatose although exhibiting more voluntary movements than previously on this date. He had remained afebrile. Respirations, color, pulse, and blood pressure remained good. Occasional voluntary cough reflex in response to the presence of mucus in the trachea and to tracheal suctioning was present. The pupils were large and reacted to light. Movements of both lower extremities and both upper extremities could be elicited by painful stimuli.

．．．

In retrospect, certain information is available to us now that was not evident prior to the initiation of the sequence of events already described.

1. The patient arrived in the operating room asleep; however, there did not appear to be anything unusual about his color, respirations, blood pressure, or pulse.

2. The induction period of anesthesia prior to the insertion of the endotracheal tube was somewhat lengthier than usual, but at no time were the respirations markedly depressed nor the child's color unsatisfactory. Once the endotracheal tube was inserted the child's condition appeared entirely satisfactory and no contraindication to the surgery was apparent.

3. We did not learn until after the cardiac emergency had occurred in our patient that two other children had arrived in the operating room exhibiting excessive sedative effects. In neither case was an anesthetic administered since one of the cases was a minor procedure requiring no anesthetic and the other was cancelled due to the emergency occupying the T and A room at the time.

4. The occurrence of the cardiac arrest and ensuing respiratory depression occurring in my patient had caused me to suspect the possibility of an error either in the dosage of the drug administered or in the substitution of another drug. When I requested that the narcotic supply be checked, Miss Engh reported that the supply of morphine and codeine tallied correctly, but, nevertheless, following this interview she apparently sent the bottle labeled codeine to Mr. Wittich in the pharmacy. When it was recognized that the two other children had appeared excessively sedated, Mrs. D. Kaladic (head nurse) requested an analysis of the contents of the bottle labeled codeine. Mr. Wittich took the bottle to Miss Minnie Fin (chief technician) in the laboratory where an analysis revealed that the tablets contained in the bottle labeled codeine were, in actuality, morphine sulfate (presumably ¼ gr. tablets). This means that assuming the dosage was correctly calculated and administered, the child received morphine sulfate (gr. 1/10) instead of codeine phosphate (gr. 1/10).

Settlement was for $50,000 (limits of insurance coverage) *plus* care and hospitalization to be taken care of by the hospital for the rest of the child's life.

In commenting on this unusual agreement, Judge Rogers stated:

Assuming that Ross lives out his life expectancy, the total cost to Mt. Sinai Hospital for hospitalization alone will be in excess of $800,000. . . . Immediate payment by . . . (the) hospital of any jury verdict even approaching the present value of this amount of money would seriously and perhaps disastrously curtail . . . (its) services to the community. However, by spreading this total cost over Ross' lifetime, Ross will benefit from the very best of medical service available and the hospital can bear the expense.

At last report the child is presently in a Pennsylvania institution at a cost of approximately $9,000 yearly to Mt. Sinai Hospital. The hospital also pays for two trips annually for the parents to visit the child. Except for the mental deficiency resulting from anoxia, the boy is apparently quite healthy.

In an officially reported case,* negligence was alleged against a physician-anesthetist, senior visiting surgeon, resident surgeon, and nurse-anesthetist in a cardiac arrest case. A spinal anesthetic was administered for an appendectomy at about 7:50 A.M. on November 5, 1954. At about 8:10 A.M. the physician-anesthetist and senior surgeon left the operating room.

Sometime between 8:10 and 8:20 McEnaney (nurse-anesthetist) took the plaintiff's blood pressure, but "couldn't get any reading"; there was no blood pressure. She administered oxygen under pressure to the plaintiff and informed Dr. Shaw (anesthetist) of the absence of blood pressure. He directed her to give the plaintiff an injection of Neo-Synephrine, which she did. Dr. Earthrowl (resident physician) administered an "intravenous infusion." He attempted to ascertain whether the heart was beating, "but didn't hear any heart beat." Upon Dr. Pilcher's (senior visiting surgeon) arrival in the operating room, he and Dr. Earthrowl decided that plaintiff's thoracic cavity should

---

Ramsland v. Shaw, 341 Mass. 56, 166 N.E. 2d 894 (1960), followed in a similar case, *Erban v. Kay,* 342 Mass. 779, 174 N.E. 2d 667 (1961); *contra,* as against a physician-anesthetist, *Edelman v. Zeigler,* Cal. App., 44 Cal. Rptr. 114 (1965).

be opened for the purpose of massaging the heart. Such an operation was performed by Dr. Earthrowl and as a result the plaintiff's heart action and blood pressure were "restored to a normal level." The appendectomy was then performed.

The results to the plaintiff of cardiac arrest were not in dispute. Because of it, his brain failed to receive the necessary supply of oxygen and serious damage resulted. The prognosis was that the plaintiff would "have to be cared far as a dependent person as long as he lives."

The plaintiff advances several theories of negligence on the part of one or more of the defendants, and we shall consider them separately. No contention is made that there was negligence on the part of any of the defendants after the plaintiff's cardiac arrest was discovered.

The court held that directed verdicts in favor of all defendants were proper inasmuch as no case was made out on any of the five charges, to wit:

1. Negligence in choosing spinal anesthesia in view of plaintiff's history of rheumatic heart disease: *Held*, despite the reading of excerpts of White's text on heart disease in evidence under a special statute, the evidence remained in the realm of speculation.
2. Negligence in entrusting supervisory duties to the nurse-anesthetist: *Held*, there was no showing that such delegation was a departure from accepted procedures in the locality, especially since the nurse-anesthetist demonstrated 20 years' experience.
3. Failure to administer oxygen or give intravenous infusions prior to cardiac arrest: *Held*, there was no evidence that sound medical practice called for such procedures to counteract foreseeable effects of spinal anesthesia.
4. Failure to determine and record blood pressure at 5-minute intervals: *Held*, there was no showing that such omission, if a fact, in any way contributed to the injuries.
5. Negligence of nurse-anesthetist: *Held*, there was no evidence to warrant recovery against her.

Criminal proceedings

Successful defense of a wife-murder prosecution in which a "karate-chop blow" to the chest was theorized was in part predicated upon astute medicolegal consultation activity, including the following analysis based upon autopsy findings:

It is my belief that there is a very reasonable possibility that the pathological processes and findings discussed in the autopsy report could have been the result of vigorous closed-chest compression or external cardiac massage. I note that "the anterior portion of the chest is notably free of lacerations, abrasions or contusions." This is, of course, compatible with external cardiac compression.

. . .

Almost all types of injuries of the mediastinal and intrathoracic viscera have been encountered. . . . In some series as many as 24 percent of the patients had fractured ribs. Six percent of one group of cases had a fractured sternum as a complication of the closed chest resuscitation technique. (It perhaps is helpfully significant that the sternal segments are depressed inwardly.) Cardiac tamponade representing collection of blood in the pericardium is *not* uncommon.

. . .

Apparently Mrs. W. was a relatively small lady, weighing approximately 120 pounds. With a firm surface as the floor beneath her, and a very active attempt at resuscitation, the likelihood of intraabdominal or intrathoracic trauma would have been increased. Certainly a bilateral hemothorax and avulsion of the right pulmonary hilus could, in my opinion, be accounted for by closed-chest cardiac compression attempts. We have seen this on several occasions after vigorous or prolonged efforts. The collection of blood in the mediastinum is compatible.

Camps reported a case as follows:

A man was admitted to hospital for gastrectomy. The operation was successfully completed and he was returned to the ward. A short time later he collapsed from cardiac arrest. External cardiac massage was immediately carried out, without result—direct massage by opening the chest was then done. As a result, the heart restarted and severe bleeding was noticed from the abdominal drainage tube. Quite properly, it was decided to operate again and it was then found that, as a result of the pressure used in cardiac massage, there was a severe rupture of the liver, which was repaired. In spite of this he died. At the Inquest, the Coroner asked the pathologist the cause of death and the reply was that it depended upon when he died, i.e., either when the cardiac arrest occurred or after the repair of the liver. The Coroner correctly decided the cause of death was the ruptured liver.*

Legal medicine and cardiac arrest

Traditionally, legal medicine has been vitally concerned with cardiac arrest and resuscitation. "When is a person dead?" is an inquiry of the forensic pathologist[9, 10, 21, 25, 27] and, of course numerous legal rights and duties are created and extinguished upon death of an individual.[11] In this literature, cessation of cardiac activity is discussed as a sign of death, and some attention has been given to resuscitation, particularly as applied to cases of premature burial.[13, 14, 25] A case of alleged "premature autopsy" found a suit prosecuted against two general practitioners who conducted a post-mortem on the body of one Washington Irving Bishop who apparently died in a cataleptic trance.† A libel suit arose over a

newspaper's reporting of an alleged premature burial.* Belli recounts a more recent episode in which a "dead" woman "returned" to sue officials of a coroner's office.†

Now that we are able to restore cardiac function to a sizable group of people experiencing cardiac arrest, medicolegal interest is heightened in the area of malpractice litigation. It is this phase of legal medicine with which we are primarily concerned in this discussion. Of course, new medicolegal issues are in the offing with the advent of cardiac and other organ transplantation. These matters remain distinctly collateral at the moment.‡

General rules touching the practitioner and the nature of malpractice suits have been analyzed briefly elsewhere.[3] It is my purpose here to clarify some of the more specific rules of law as they become guides to conduct in the physician's management of cardiac arrest cases.§

In the common law system, which prevails in most English-speaking countries, the basic legal method is the use of decided cases as guideposts for future case decisions.

---

*From Camps, F. In Shotter, E. F., editor: Matters of life and death, London, 1970, Darton, Longman & Todd, p. 10.

†From Hamilton, A. M.: Recollections of an alienist, New York, 1916, George H. Doran Co., p. 275. See also Wilens, S. L.: My friends the doctors, New York, 1961, Atheneum, p. 36 (resuscitation at the autopsy table); Mant, A. K.: Forensic medicine; observation and interpretation, Chicago, 1960, Year Book Publishers, p. 6; Toynbee, A., Mant, A. K., Smart, N., Hinton, J., Yudkin, S., Rhode, E., Heywood, R., and Price, H. H.: Man's concern with death, New York, 1969, McGraw-Hill Book Co., Chapter 1 (premature certification of death); Kobler, J.: The reluctant surgeon, a biography of John Hunter, New York, 1960, Doubleday & Co., p. 59 (revival on dissecting table); Arnold, J. D., Zimmerman, T. F., and Martin, D. C.: Public attitudes and the diagnosis of death, **206:** J.A.M.A., 1949 (1968).

*Purdy v. Rochester Printing Co., 26 Hun. 206; 96 N.Y. 372, 48 Am. Rep. 632 (1884).

†From Belli, M. M.: 3, Modern trials, Indianapolis, 1954, The Bobbs-Merrill Co., p. 2056, sec. 358.

‡Concern is, of course, manifest over the question of when resuscitative efforts can be properly (legally and ethically) terminated. Winter, A., editor: The moment of death, a symposium, Springfield, Ill., 1969, Charles C Thomas, Publisher, p. 17; Corday, E.: Life-death in human transplantation, 55: A.B.A.J. 629 (1969).

§Additional sources may also be examined to gain a more comprehensive picture of this area of the law.[1, 8, 15, 18, 19, 22, 23, 26] Lawyers' texts are bulging with material on cardiac arrest as noted by personal communication with a distinguished advocate and sometime lecturer at the University of Kansas postgraduate programs, Lyman Field, Esq. See 13 American Jurisprudence Proof of Facts 257 (1963), Redding, J. S.: Cardiopulmonary resuscitation. In Cantor's Traumatic medicine and surgery for the attorney, service vol., Washington, 1964, Butterworth, p. 323, and Sagall, E. L.: Cardiac arrest, Lawyers' Med. J. 2:103 (1972).

*Stare decisis!** This is in contrast to the civil law method found in most countries of the world and in the state of Louisiana. Civil law technique, to a large extent, depends upon generalizations drawn up in the form of a code to which judges and lawyers turn for authority.[16] In the common law method, reference is made to the conglomeration of cases in an effort to draw up an appropriate generalization—a rule of law—that can be applied to the individual case. It should be borne in mind, therefore, that lawyers cannot in good conscience predict in advance what the legal outcome of a particular case will be with any great degree of certainty. Also, it must be remembered that each individual state administers its own variety of "tort"† law according to its own jurisprudence.

No effort is made, therefore, to state dogmatically what the law of a particular state may be on a given proposition. I can attempt, though, to elucidate several principles of law that play an important part in lawsuits stemming from cardiac arrest situations.

Cases selected for illustration have been collected in Table 59-1. After the name, or *style,* of the case, there is the legal *citation,* which indicates in what volumes of the various law reports the full opinion of the court is set out. Then follows a brief digest of the *facts* in the case. Remember that many seemingly different factual situations may point up rules of law applied generally. Finally, a condensed statement of the *holding* in the case is included. This is the principle of law on which the particular case at issue turned. Additional statements of law, termed *obiter dicta,* are often quoted by commentators, as I have done frequently here. This language, although not conclusive in any way, often gives us keys as to how future courts may handle new problems coming before them.

FAILURE TO ACT

More than one physician has reported that about all he learned from the perfunctory lectures given at his medical school was that he should not be a Good Samaritan if he wishes to avoid legal liability.* It is true that no state in this country requires a physician to undertake the care of a patient, yet the *Principles of Medical Ethics,* 1957, include the following:

> . . . In an emergency, however, he should render service to the best of his ability. . . .†

Perhaps the soundest view is that of Smith:

> I do not want the physician to believe that he assumes a heavy risk when he helps such a person in distress. Practically, the risk is almost nonexistent; the patient in such circumstances is not apt to press a claim against his benefactor, and juries are apt to be still slower to return fact findings of negligence. Yet such situations may occasionally arise, and their legal bearings have an inescapable intrinsic interest.‡

Once the physician does enter upon the patient-physician relationship, however, a

---

*"To abide by or adhere to, decided cases." (Black's Law Dictionary, ed. 4, St. Paul, 1951, West Publishing Co.)

†Having to do with private wrongs.

---

*With a few notable exceptions, American medical schools admittedly offered woefully weak instruction in legal medicine. There are many encouraging signs that this trend is now being reversed, however. See Mills, D. H.: Forensic education in medical schools: the necessity for an interdepartmental approach, **36** J. Med. Educ., 188 (1961).

†Section 5. In previous codifications, the provision was as follows: "He should, however, [always] respond to any request for his assistance in an emergency or whenever temperate public opinion expects the service."

‡From Smith, H. W.: Legal responsibility for medical malpractice. V. Further information about duty and dereliction, **116** J.A.M.A. 2757 (1941). A number of states, following California, have enacted statutes that purport to absolve physicians from liability in emergency situations. Their constitutionality remains doubtful. See Louisell, D. W., and Williams, H.: Trial of medical malpractice cases, Albany, 1960, Matthew Bender & Co., Chapter 21.

failure to act may amount to negligence. This omission to act is called "nonfeasance" and, coupled with a legal duty to perform the omitted act, amounts to "negligence."* It may well happen, then, that a failure to institute indicated resuscitation procedures will result in legal liability.

STANDARD OF CARE

When the doctor undertakes the medical management of a patient, he immediately comes under a legal duty not to injure the patient negligently (Case A, Table 59-1). It is evident that such a statement is couched in quite general terms; therefore it remains for each litigated case to give meaning to this concept as pronounced. Flexibility of the standard is emphasized by the Indiana Supreme Court:

> When one goes to a surgeon for an operation he submits himself wholly to the surgeon's professional skill and care. It then becomes the duty of the surgeon on performing the operation to exercise skill and care *commensurate with the hazards and perils that reasonably may be anticipated.* . . . Should the surgeon negligently fail to exercise such skill and care and as a proximate result of such negligence the patient is injured he may have recourse in a civil action for damage. (Case B, Table 59-1.)

Since techniques of effective cardiac resuscitation are of recent origin,† it might be well to consider a Canadian case that stresses a duty to "use very great care" when a new treatment is being employed. The patient was a 69-year-old gardener with arteriosclerosis. He injured his leg and defendant employed heat lamp treatment. Dry gangrene of the leg finally resulted. There was a conflict in the testimony as to whether the heat lamp had caused a burn. Defendant doctor gave the following testimony:

> He has been using both the Radiant lamp and the Quartz lamp since 1918. In that year in Chicago he was advised by a Dr. Wise to pro-

cure a Quartz lamp. This he did. He found this one not quite satisfactory and the following year (1919) being in New York for postgraduate work, he heard a number of doctors recommending the Quartz lamp among them a medical professor who had one and used it very much. This induced him to go to Newark where these lamps are manufactured. There on three different occasions he got information from the manufacturer as to the method of using the lamp. He has been using this kind of lamp ever since. He has made a special study of the lamp in monthly magazines. The one actually in use on the plaintiff's visit he bought a couple of years ago. He used the lamp constantly and many times during a day. He has used it mostly for goiter. He says: "I must say I have had surprising results." In Edmonton, Dr. Malcolmson, Dr. Mooney, Dr. Cruix and, he thinks, Dr. Blais and Dr. Colwill have this kind of lamp—the Quartz lamp, and there are one or two at the University. He says that in effect the Quartz lamp was excellent treatment for the plaintiff's condition.*

The Alberta Supreme Court, Appellate Division, affirmed a judgment against the doctor by a 3-2 vote. The majority opinion is quite significant in setting up a high standard of care not often entertained with such vigor. Judge Hyndman had this to say:

> The trial judge apparently came to the conclusion that there was negligence consisting merely in applying the Quartz light at all. I am not quite ready to agree that that fact alone constituted negligence. Defendant and many other medical men use this light for various diseases, such as bruises and skin troubles, with good results. What impresses me as the serious point in the matter is that great care was not exercised either at the time it was used or afterwards.
>
> It is clear that the properties of the ultra violet-ray as well as the x-ray and radium are not perfectly understood. They are to a large extent still in the experimental stage. The evidence goes to show that it is not only the heat emanating from the lamp which has effect but also the effect of the ray itself which is important, either constructively or destructively.
>
> In Taylor, Medical Jurisprudence, ed. 6, p. 99, the author says: "It would be premature to dogmatize on the subject at present; the reader is referred to the textbooks on the subject for fuller

---

*Negligence comprehends a duty plus a breach of that duty.[3]
†See Chapter 67.

*Baills v. Boulanger, 1924, 4 Dominion Law Reports 1083.

Table 59-1. Illustrative medicolegal cases

Case	Name	Citation	Facts	Legal result
A	Church v. Adler	350 Ill. App. 471, 113 N.E. 2d 327 (1953)	Patient's appendix removed along with ovaries; claims of lack of consent; error in diagnosis; infrequent visits; sterility	Dismissal reversed for plaintiff-patient since her pleadings were sufficient
B	Worster v. Caylor	231 Ind. 625, 110 N.E. 2d 337 (1953)	Surgeon accidentally perforated bowel in hernia operation at site of old wound resulting from previous gallbladder surgery	Directed verdict for surgeon affirmed, overturning decision of a lower appellate court, since doctrine of *res ipsa loquitur* did not apply
C	Watterson v. Conwell	258 Ala. 371, 61 So. 2d 690 (1952)	Recognized authority (co-author of *Fractures, Dislocations, and Sprains*) permitted orderly to complete wrapping of cast on fractured tibia and fibula; patient claimed that improper pressure of the wrap injured knee	Directed verdict for Dr. Conwell affirmed since the claim was "merest speculation"
D	Hudson v. Weiland	150 Fla. 523, 8 So. 2d 37 (1942)	Plaintiff claimed that physician was jointly liable with diathermist who had caused pain during therapy	Judgment for defendants affirmed because of an insufficiency in plaintiff's pleadings
E	Stone v. Goodman	241 App. Div. 290, 271 N.Y.S. 500 (1934)	Surgeon, intending only to repair umbilical and right oblique hernias, discovered a direct left inguinal hernia during surgery and proceeded to repair this in addition; plaintiff claimed that written consent was invalid since signed under drug influence	Verdict for patient reversed, and new trial granted surgeon since verdict was against overwhelming weight of evidence
F	McPeak v. Vanderbilt University Hospital	33 Tenn. App. 76, 229 S.W. 2d 150 (1950)	Associate professor of surgery diagnosed thrombophlebitis in veins of lower right leg of plaintiff; subsequent surgery was performed by three surgeons of the department, under direction of chief of surgery, in allegedly negligent fashion	Directed verdict for surgeons affirmed in absence of evidence indicating negligence
G	Duckworth v. Bennett	320 Pa. 47, 181 A. 558 (1935)	After 16-year-old fell on floor, examination revealed legs of equal length and no signs of hip involvement; parents requested x-rays, but none were taken until 8 weeks later when fractured femur or epiphyseal separation was revealed	Directed verdict for doctor affirmed on his own testimony and that of four other physicians called under the choice of treatment doctrine
H	Church v. Bloch	80 Cal. App. 2d 542, 182 P. 2d 241 (1947)	Negligence was claimed in obstetric care of plaintiff by doctor under contract with California Physicians Service	Nonsuit of patient was affirmed since there was lacking sufficient evidence from medical experts on essential phases of the case

	Case	Facts	Outcome
I	Olson v. Weitz — 37 Wash. 2d 70, 221 P. 2d 537 (1950)	Plaintiff suffered transverse greenstick fracture of left radius; after cast was removed, it was found necessary to perform open reduction with bone grafts; defendant doctor contended that a second fall had caused malalignment, not his negligence	A jury verdict of $15,805, reduced to $9,805 by trial court, was affirmed for plaintiff since there was sufficient evidence without expert testimony to permit jury award
J	Quintal v. Laurel Grove Hospital — 41 Cal. Rptr. 557, 397 P. 2d 161 (1964)	Detailed in the text	Settled for $255,000; two members of the court thought defendants should win; one thought original jury award should have been untouched; majority sent the case back for another trial though Chief Justice Traynor felt res ipsa loquitur inapplicable
K	Board of Medical Registration and Examination of Indiana v. Kaadt — 225 Ind. 625, 76 N.E. 2d 669 (1948)	Physician accused of gross immorality in representing that diabetics need not follow standard regimens, but rather could be cured at Diabetic Institute by consuming a particular liquid	Revocation of license upheld on the facts, thus overturning a "not guilty" verdict of lower court
L	Stammer v. Board of Regents of University of New York — 262 App. Div. 372, 29 N.Y.S. 2d 38 (1941)	Physician's license suspended by Board for 1 year for fraud and deceit in use of secret formula	Board's action overturned by court in favor of doctor; it was shown, incidentally, that at least one member of the subcommittee which conducted hearings for the board exhibited "a wholly unfair and partial attitude"
M	Reed v. Church — 175 Va. 284, 8 S.E. 2d 285 (1940)	Tryparsamide injections for syphilis resulted in optic disturbances; conflict in testimony as to whether injections were stopped after symptoms developed	Jury verdict for plaintiff affirmed since jury entitled to determine whether doctor followed medical opinion selected in a negligent manner
N	Flock v. Palumbo Fruit Co. — 63 Idaho 220, 118 P. 2d 707 (1941)	In Workmen's Compensation proceeding, contract physician held liable in not securing deep x-ray or radium therapy for patient on testimony indicating that such was proper treatment when seminoma found too extensive for surgical excision	Holding affirmed since contract physician held to same standard for failure to act as a physician acting generally
O	Rosenberg v. Feigin — 119 Cal. App. 2d 783, 260 P. 2d 143 (1953)	Physician failed to notify husband of contemplated care and treatment of wife, including an abortion	Judgment for physician affirmed since consent of wife alone sufficient, and no merit in husband's claim that his pursuit of happiness in planning for and having a family was interfered with by the doctor
P	Valdez v. Percy — 35 Cal. 2d 338, 217 P. 2d 422 (1950)	Patient signed consent for biopsy and any other surgery deemed advisable or necessary; upon strength of an incorrect tissue diagnosis, plaintiff's breast was amputated	Verdict for $7,500 on theory of negligent diagnosis affirmed since radical surgery was unnecessary in light of corrected laboratory report

Continued.

Table 59-1. Illustrative medicolegal cases—cont'd

Case	Name	Citation	Facts	Legal result
Q	Pike v. Archibald	118 Cal. App. 2d 114, 257 P. 2d 480 (1953)	Child swallowed unknown quantity of oil of wintergreen; rushed to hospital, died	Defendant's demurrer to wrongful death action sustained because of technical failures in pleading
R	Mayo v. McClung	83 Ga. App. 548, 64 S.E. 2d 330 (1951)	After original diagnosis of "strained muscle," later x-rays disclosed impacted hip fracture; 2 weeks later, fibrous union of head of femur discovered	Directed verdict for physician upheld under testimony that "medical science does not yet know how to prevent such results"
S	Edwards v. Wiggins	Ohio Com. Pl. 114 N.E. 2d 504 (1953)	After spontaneous abortion, plaintiff's sexual organs became infected; negligence claimed in failure to treat infection and employ vaginal examination to discover presence of incomplete abortion	Directed verdict for physician upheld because of failure of proof; neither circumstantial nor testimonial evidence sufficiently propounded to raise probability of negligence rather than mere possibility
T	Carbone v. Warburton	11 N.J. 418, 94 A. 2d 680 (1953); Noted, 11 NACCA Law Journal 172 (1953)	Orthopedic surgeon, carrying out débridement, left straw in compound fracture wound; tetanus followed. A general practitioner, retired 20 years, was offered as expert witness for plaintiff	Order of new trial for plaintiff affirmed since trial court wrongfully refused to permit the retired physician to testify in behalf of plaintiff
U	Huffman v. Lindquist	37 Cal. 2d 465, 234 P. 2d 34, 29 A.L.R. 2d 485 (1951)	Boy, 19 years old, suffered epidural hemorrhage in auto collision; defendant adopted conservative nonsurgical management; boy subsequently died from pulmonary embolism	Judgment of nonsuit in favor of physician affirmed since at most a mere error in diagnostic judgment involved; also, no causal relation between physician's omissions and death

information as to the action of the rays, and we have to wait for some judgments on cases. We can, however, state that much expert and scientific knowledge will be demanded from him who uses the rays and thereby causes injury, should he be called upon to compensate for such injury."

I think there might well be added to this that very great care and caution should also be taken before and after applying it.

As I said above *when a person uses a comparatively new power or force the properties of which are not fully known or understood, such as this Quartz light, it is incumbent on him to exercise very great care, if not the greatest care, possible, in its use.* Had he stood by in this instance and watched its effect and the exact time of exposure and given the case more attention afterwards when the patient complained of it I do not think he could be held guilty of negligence. But the Judge found that he was "negligent in the extreme."

The language of most malpractice cases in the United States is ordinarily not this radical. For example (Case C, Table 59-1):

There is no requirement of law that a physician should have been infallible in his diagnosis and treatment of a patient. He merely undertakes to exercise that care and skill as physicians in the same general line of practice, ordinarily exercise in such cases. In absence of an express agreement, warranting a cure, if he does exercise such care or skill he is not liable for an error in diagnosis and treatment where the proper course was pursued or where the proper course is subjected to reasonable doubt. A showing of an unfortunate result does not raise an inference of culpability.

An unreported case tried in Federal Court in Seattle, *Vaughn v. United States* (February 2, 1965), found Judge Beeks awarding $443,124 under the Federal Tort Claims Act for professional negligence of staff physicians at the U. S. Public Health Service. The *News Letter of the American Trial Lawyers Association* argued as follows:

Plaintiff, a 24-year-old employee of a masonry restoration co., sustained multiple fractures and internal injuries when he fell 112 ft. from a scaffolding at the 8th floor level of defendant's hospital on Sept. 18, 1961. He was immediately admitted to the hospital as an emergency patient in critical condition. About a month later, on Oct. 16, 1961, while still in critical condition, defendant's drs. performed surgery on plaintiff's fractured hip under general anesthesia. During the course of surgery, plaintiff experienced *cardiac arrest, and his subsequent lack of oxygen caused irreversible brain damage.*

ATLAS Member Daniel F. Sullivan, Seattle, contended the hospital's physicians were negligent in 3 respects: (1) performing surgery while plaintiff was still in critical condition when numerous medical factors, considered collectively definitely contraindicated such elective not-imperative-for-life-saving surgery on left hip; (2) *failure to obtain informed consent of plaintiff to such hip surgery as required by 42 Code of Federal Regulations, §35.15;* (3) negligence of surgical team in choice & administration of anesthesia.

Judge Beeks convincingly held that while plaintiff had failed to prove his 3d charge of negligence, he had proved the 1st two. He stated, "The Court has no hesitancy in finding that plaintiff has established by a preponderance of the credible evidence that in subjecting him to surgery on October 16 in his then existing condition the required standards of medical care were violated."

Judge Beeks also ruled that *plaintiff was not adequately informed of the risks involved in the proposed surgery while he was in a critically ill condition:* "He did not consent to risk his life for the possibility of obtaining a more functional hip."

Both sides had stipulated to damages totaling $193,124 for past & future medical & hospital expenses & future wage loss. The Ct then awarded an additional $250,000 to plaintiff for his pain & suffering & permanent disability flowing from his "vegetal existence," making a total award of $443,124. "Plaintiff is as totally and permanently disabled as a man can be and live. He could not be more so. The government contends that because he is lacking in sense responses and reasoning power he should be denied compensation for the permanent disability, but cites no authority to support this position. In effect the government says that in such circumstances a tortfeasor should pay less by reason of having reduced the victim to a mentally and physically vegetative state. The Court is not convinced that a case such as this should be an exception to the general rule, and it will not be so treated."

We submit that Judge Beeks' statement is a ringing refutation to the argument of habitual defendants that, having reduced you to a comatose condition they should not have to pay for your loss of enjoyment of life & that the more damage they do, the less they have to pay. An upside-down argument if there ever was one. Instant case is noted in *Seattle Post Intelligencer,* Feb. 3, 1965, issue.*

---

*8 News Letter of the American Trial Lawyers Association, 70-71 (1965).

SELECTION OF PROCEDURE

Akin to the principles already discussed, but usually set apart in our jurisprudence, is the problem of the choice of method to be followed in the individual case.*

On the one hand, we have a Florida court proclaiming: "It was the physician's responsibility to advise such treatment as is generally accepted by the profession as the *one most likely to cure* or relieve the particular injury from which the patient was suffering when she consulted him" (Case D, Table 59-1).

A more temperate approach was taken by a New York court (Case E, Table 59-1):

No set rule can be laid down with reference to the method to be used by a doctor in operating. When a doctor makes a diagnosis and during an operation is confronted with a situation requiring the exercise of his judgment, especially in a case of this kind where the doctor first operated on the umbilical hernia and then established the necessity to operate upon the hernia on the left side, he should not be held liable when it is not shown that he improperly exercised his judgment or that he failed to use the ordinary degree of skill. . . .

The rule requiring a physician and surgeon to use his best judgment *does not make him liable for mere error of judgment, provided he does what he thinks is the best after careful examination.* A physician and surgeon's implied engagement with his patient does not guarantee a good result, but he promises by implication to *use the skill and learning of the average physician, to exercise reasonable care, and to exert his best judgment in the effort to bring about a good result.*

Similar dictum is contained in a leading Colorado opinion† by Judge Gabbert on a failure in diagnosis:

[That the doctor] will use his best judgment in the application of his skill in deciding upon the nature of the injury and the best mode of treatment.

Recently, this rule that a physician is not responsible for an error of judgment when deciding between alternative procedures has

been followed in Tennessee in an action against Vanderbilt University Hospital (Case F, Table 59-1).

It must be borne in mind that this "error of judgment" rule can be often used strategically to win somewhat questionable cases. Thus in Case G (Table 59-1) there was an 8-week delay in taking x-ray films to discover a fractured femur or epiphyseal separation following a fall. The Supreme Court of Pennsylvania said:

We think it could not be held to be negligence or unskilled treatment for a doctor not immediately to employ the x-ray in his investigations of a patient's condition; whether this or another method of inquiry should be resorted to is a matter of judgment, and a failure to use the one or the other could not be said to be negligence. Where the most that the case discloses is an error in judgment on the surgeon's part, there is no liability . . . . Here, the doctor used his skillful fingers and trained observation to detect what was wrong. Neither court nor jury would be competent to set up an opinion counter to his, unless much more was shown than here appears. At most, all that could be said is that the defendant had made a mistake in diagnosis where the symptoms were obscure, and for this there is no liability . . . . *Where competent medical authority is divided, a physician will not be held responsible if, in the exercise of his judgment, he followed a course of treatment advocated by a considerable number of his professional brethren in good standing in his community.*

In Case H (Table 59-1), the evidence indicated that the physician was "more interested in money than in the welfare of the patient," yet there was testimony that a small, but respectable, minority of obstetricians would not attempt to turn a fetus to avoid a breech presentation nor would they take x-rays to determine the position of the fetus.

The protective character of these principles was recognized by an Ohio court in these words:

Persons engaging in a profession generally recognized by the public to be based upon scientific methods and research, careful study, long experiment, thorough testing and mature deliberations and covering an extended educational period, are

---

*See Chapter 24.

†*Bonnet v. Foote,* 47 Colo. 282, 107 P. 252, 254 (1910).

entitled to the protection of the general rule requiring only the skill and care which persons engaged in such profession are accustomed to use under the same or similar circumstances, and person so engaged using the methods and measures usually adopted by those similarly engaged are not liable for damages for resulting injuries.*

EFFECTING THE PROCEDURE

. . . . There is an obvious distinction between a claim of negligence in the choice of methods of treatment and a charge of negligence in the actual performance of the work after such choice is made. As to the first, the charge is refuted as a matter of law by showing that a respectable minority of expert physicians approved of the method selected thus taking the case from the jury. As to the second, *a charge of negligent performance, where there is any evidence tending to show such negligence, the case is for the jury,* as in other cases of negligence, whenever upon the evidence the minds of reasonable men might differ. (Case I, Table 59-1.)

It is apparent then that the physician is much more vulnerable on this matter of carrying out the selected procedure than in regard to choice of technique (Case M, Table 59-1). More and more are juries being permitted to infer negligent performance, commonly by one of three pathways:

1. *Expert testimony* comprises opinions expressed by physicians in response to hypothetical questions in the typical case. The witness is asked more or less directly whether the defendant-doctor fell below the standard of ordinary and reasonable conduct in the management of the patient. A "yes" answer by just a single expert witness is usually enough to sustain a jury verdict for the plaintiff-patient on appeal.†

2. The *"common knowledge" doctrine* is being employed with increased frequency by plaintiffs either as an adjunct to or as a sustitute for expert testimony. A legal commentator[17] cogently summarizes this matter:

---

*Willett v. Rowekamp, 58 Ohio App. 465, 16 N.E. 2d 797 (1938); affirmed, 134 Ohio St., 285, 16 N.E. 2d 457 (1938).

†See Shartel, B., and Plant, M. L.: The law of medical practice, Springfield, Ill., 1959, Charles C Thomas, Publisher, pp. 130-131.

Since juries composed of laymen are not familiar with the science of medicine and the techniques of surgery, they are incompetent to determine the standard of care or to evaluate the physician's conduct. Expert testimony is therefore required to guide the jury and assist it in understanding the significance of the facts as well as to enable it to reach an intelligent conclusion. One well-recognized exception to this rule is where the negligence is so gross that a layman could recognize it as such, or the subject matter is nontechnical and within the common knowledge of laymen. In such cases the jury is competent to arrive at a conclusion of negligence in the absence of expert testimony.

Just where to draw the line between technical and nontechnical matter is often difficult to determine. The trend of recent cases seems to be in the direction of enlarging the scope of matters which are considered to be within the realm of common knowledge. Possible reasons for this extension may be the advance of general education and a recognition of the fact that expert testimony is often difficult for the plaintiff to obtain, physicians being reluctant to testify against one another. It would seem that unless the act alleged to be negligent is clearly within the common knowledge of laymen expert testimony ought to be required, for any extension of the notion of common knowledge will result in subjecting the physician to unjustified risks never before imposed by law.

In *Quintal,* Chief Justice Traynor voted to overturn judgment for defendants on this basis alone:

There is evidence . . . that defendants were negligent in failing to make reasonable preparation for the possible occurrence of a cardiac arrest. . . . Both defendant doctors knew that cardiac arrest was an inherent risk of surgery under anesthesia. Both testified that when an arrest occurs every second counts. Both doctors had good reason to believe that a general surgeon would be readily available in the area surrounding the operating room. It may be inferred, however, that they did not confer before the operation to plan an efficient procedure for summoning such a surgeon in response to a possible emergency. Thus, defendant ophthalmologist testified that he could not remember any conversation with the anesthesiologist, although "frequently we have a conversation about the operation prior to surgery." Moreover, defendant anesthesiologist was apparently unaware of the inability of defendant ophthalmologist to perform a thoracotomy, for when the arrest occurred he did not immediately send for a general surgeon.

Instead, after it became apparent that external massage had failed, precious time elapsed while the ophthalmologist came to the table, revealed his inability to open the chest, and went to the door to get the general surgeon. More time passed while the general surgeon entered the room and put on gloves before making the incision. Although the record does not specify how much time these steps entailed, a jury could reasonably conclude from defendant ophthalmologist's testimony that the additional loss of time was enough to cause the brain damage. This time might have been saved had preparations been made for summoning the general surgeon as soon as a cardiac arrest was suspected, so that he could be ready to open the chest at the moment it became apparent that external massage had failed.

Although there is no expert testimony that the prevailing medical standard of care requires such preparation for a possible cardiac arrest, expert testimony is not required when scientific enlightenment is not necessary to show that failure to make such preparations is unreasonable. . . . On that basis alone, I would reverse the judgments notwithstanding the verdicts.

3. By application of the doctrine of *res ipsa loquitur,* a jury may be entitled to infer negligence from the fact of injury without further evidence. This doctrine is quite complex and has evolved in differing directions in the various jurisdictions. Though we cannot pursue its many ramifications here, reference to Arthur's monumental analysis[2] is encouraged. He summarizes the benefits obtained by application of the doctrine in malpractice cases:

1. The plaintiff is relieved of the necessity of securing an expert witness which is absolutely essential in malpractice cases based on want of care or skill.
2. The plaintiff has a substitute for the facts constituting the alleged acts of negligence, which are not easily accessible to him, so is freed from the duty to plead the acts of negligence of the defendant, which under the circumstances would be little more than blind guesswork.
3. The application of the doctrine calls upon the defendant, since he is the party to whom the facts are available, to speak first, thus in a manner equalizing the knowledge of the causes of the injury.
4. As a result of the use of the doctrine the plaintiff's case is in the hands of the trial judge to decide whether pleading and evidence are adequate to raise an inference of negligence sufficient to permit the jury to bring in a verdict.
5. The defendant may elect to let the case go to the jury without producing any evidence of the causes of the injury.
6. If the defendant elects to make any explanation at this stage of the trial he may either rebut the inferences, or may offer an interpretation of the facts in a manner not disadvantageous to his position. This may save undue publicity injurious to his professional career.
7. The defendant may be unable to rebut the inference of negligence in which case the doctrine holds, or, on the other hand he may establish the absence of negligence so clearly that the presumption will be overcome as a matter of law.*

That the judges have a difficult time in agreeing on the scope of this doctrine is illustrated by *Quintal* (Case J, Table 59-1). The majority opinion favored the doctrine:

The facts of the present case present a clear situation where the conditional doctrine of res ipsa applies. If the jury finds certain facts, which they are entitled to find from the evidence, then the doctrine applies. Here we have an injury which is very rare. It is an injury that could result from negligence, or could result without negligence. Is it more probable than not that it was the result of negligence? That is the question. The plaintiffs, out of the mouths of defendants and their witnesses, proved that the injury could occur as a result of negligence. There is also evidence that the injury could occur without negligence. In such circumstances the jury should be instructed that if they find certain facts to be true they should apply the inference involved in res ipsa. Here we have an injury that is a *known risk* and rarely occurs. We have the instrumentality and the procedures involved completely in the control of defendant doctors. We have the boy under an anesthetic. Certainly the facts called for an explanation. The defendants explained what they did and testified that this was due care. But there was testimony that 90 percent of the deaths resulting from cardiac arrest occurred by reason of faulty intubation. There was testimony that would justify the jury in inferring that if the operation had been

---

*From Arthur, W. R.: Res ipsa loquitur as applied in dental cases, **15** Rocky Mountain Law Review 220, 234-235, 1943.

performed within three minutes of the heart stoppage brain damage would not have resulted. We have the evidence that temperature and apprehension increase the risk. . . . Under these circumstances the jury could find that it is more probable than not that the injury was the result of negligence. That is the test.

Chief Justice Traynor, though concurring in result with the majority, felt the doctrine inapplicable:

Since the possible causes of cardiac arrests are not a matter of common knowledge . . . expert testimony is required before a conditional res ipsa loquitur instruction would be proper. Expert testimony that it is more probable than not that negligence is the cause of cardiac arrests, if believed, would permit the jury to draw an inference of negligence solely from the fact that the arrest occurred. In deciding whether an instruction on the doctrine should be given, it is therefore irrelevant that there may be facts other than the occurrence itself to suggest that the arrest was caused by negligence. Although such facts, if present, might be independent proof of negligence, they have no bearing on the question whether the jury should be permitted to draw an inference of negligence on the happening of the cardiac arrest alone. Hence reliance on evidence that the defendants may have failed properly to appreciate plaintiff's apprehension and temperature is misplaced. The only question relevant to determining whether a res ipsa loquitur instruction should be given is: Has evidence been offered by expert testimony that when cardiac arrests occur, they are more probably than not caused by negligence?

No such expert testimony appears. Plaintiffs rely on testimony of both defendant doctors that, when due care is used, cardiac arrests do not ordinarily occur. This testimony, however, fails to establish anything with respect to the question whether, among the possible causes, negligence is the more probable one when these arrests do occur. It is true that cardiac arrests do not ordinarily occur when due care is used because, as all the testimony makes clear, a cardiac arrest is a rare occurrence. As stated in Siverson v. Weber, . . . 57 Cal. 2d 834, 839, 22 Cal. Rptr. 337, 339, 372 P. 2d 97, 99, however, "The fact that a particular injury suffered by a patient as the result of an operation is something that rarely occurs does not in itself prove that the injury was probably caused by the negligence of those in charge of the operation." The record shows that plaintiffs' counsel was fully aware of this holding in the Siverson case. He could easily have framed his questions to elicit testimony as to the probability of negligence when cardiac arrests occur, but he did not do so.

Plaintiffs also rely on expert testimony "that 90 percent of the deaths occurring in patients under anesthesia are due to improper management of the airway." This testimony, however, cannot reasonably be interpreted to mean that when cardiac arrests occur, it is more probable than not that they are caused by negligence. Thus, this percentage covers deaths other than those following cardiac arrests. The expert who offered this estimate testified that deaths may occur under anesthesia from disturbances that are at least as likely to happen as cardiac arrests. He did not testify that 90 percent of *cardiac arrests* were caused by improper management of the airway. Moreover, his testimony makes clear that by "improper management" he did not mean faulty or negligent management. He defined "improper management" as any failure "to maintain the free movement of air." Although he admitted that such failures could be prevented in many instances by an anesthesiologist exercising due care, he denied that mismanagement by the anesthesiologist is necessarily involved, and could not say that it is probably the cause when cardiac arrests occur.

Defendant anesthesiologist testified that the most common cause of cardiac arrest is direct or indirect stimulation of the vagus nerve. He added that in his opinion such stimulation was the cause of this cardiac arrest. He testified further that there were several stimuli that might have been operative. This testimony however, sheds no light on whether negligence is more probably than not the cause of bringing any of these stimuli into play. Moreover, the record presents abundant uncontradicted evidence that the medical profession is in doubt as to the causes that ultimately bring about the physiological events leading to cardiac arrest. In view of such evidence, the most that can reasonably be concluded from the medical testimony with respect to the probabilities of negligence as a cause of cardiac arrest is that negligence will increase the risk of its occurrence. There is no expert testimony that when it does occur, negligence is more probably than not the cause. Accordingly, plaintiffs are not entitled to invoke the doctrine of res ipsa loquitur.

In addition, there are several other technical methods of making a prima facie case for jury consideration. These include the use of scientific literature, admissions, negligence per se, judicial notice, and reliance on basic rules of circumstantial evidence. The exact scope of these limited approaches is quite variable around the country, and even varies from case to case within a single jurisdiction.

NURSES AND OTHERS INVOLVED

With the development of closed-chest cardiac resuscitation, nurses have found their ambit of professional responsibility widened.*

Medical and nursing students, ambulance attendants, civil defense workers, firemen, policemen, and others who have a basic first-aid background can be expected to have some level of knowledge and skill in modern resuscitative techniques.

The general rules of negligence liability in emergencies should govern. Thus the "Five D's" apply (Fig. 59-1). Breach of duty (dereliction) is at the heart of the negligence suit. In the cardiac arrest situation it would require a showing that the actions of the one performing resuscitation fell below the standard of care of a reasonable person under the circumstances.[5]

Definition of the hypothetical "reasonable man" against whom the defendant is measured by judge and jury in court has flexibility. But in any event, persons with special training can be expected to live up to a standard of ordinary care that reflects their training and skill.[6]

The pivotal role of nurses in these cases is illustrated by this report of *Trotter v. Brookside Hospital, et al.*, No. 109558, Contra Costa County, California (1971):

Cardiac arrest suffered by a 26-year-old housewife sales clerk from a ghetto area, in the course of surgery for right inguinal hernia. At time of surgery, plaintiff suffered from iron deficiency anemia with a low hemoglobin count of 8.7 grams. Plaintiff contended that she was not a proper candidate for surgery under any circumstances because of the low level of hemoglobin, and that giving her a spinal anesthetic was improper in view of low level of hemoglobin and in view of her agitated state at commencement of surgery. Additionally, plaintiff alleged that the extensive brain damage she had suffered as a result of car-

diac arrest indicated that she had either been improperly monitored as to her vital signs before cardiac arrest occurred or that the resuscitative attempts were inadequate and ineffectual and that the nurse's estimate of the prolonged time lapse between detected absence of pulse and heart beats and restoration of vital signs was more correct that contradictory testimony of all doctors that vital signs were restored in less than a minute.

Plaintiff also contended that hospital was partially responsible for quadriplegic injuries suffered by plaintiff as a result of central brain damage from cardiac arrest by virtue of fact that hospital's nurses were untrained or inadequately trained in cardiac resuscitation attempts and did virtually nothing when the arrest occurred to relieve the condition, and plaintiff also alleged that the anesthesiologists were ostensible agents of the hospital and that the hospital was responsible for their conduct. Damages: $600,000 award for plaintiff against defendant-hospital and an anesthesiologist after prior settlement for $400,000 with operating surgeon, plaintiff's internist, and another anesthesiologist. After trial, court had advised jury that a partial settlement had been made with these doctors but did not indicate the amount of the settlement, and it was agreed among counsel that the trial court would deduct the $400,000 settlement from the $600,000 verdict by plaintiff against the other defendants.*

WHY RISKS OF LIABILITY IN CARDIAC ARREST CASES SHOULD BE AT A MINIMUM

A consideration of the "Three E's" (Fig. 59-1) should tend to encourage positive and prompt action and thereby reduce risks of liability.

E-1—Experimentation. Elsewhere, the entire problem of liability for experimentation in clinical medicine has been explored.[4] Two cases coming before boards dealing with revocation and suspension of licenses to practice may serve to clarify the problem briefly.

The physician (Case K, Table 59-1) was

---

*See Chapter 49.

---

*14 News Letter of the American Trial Lawyers Association, 256 (1971). Also see *Rose v. Hakim,* 335 F. Supp. 1221, 345 F. Supp. 1300 (1972), delineating negligent nursing practice, including that of a graduate unregistered nurse, in post-arrest ICU hypothermic therapy.

"A," "B," and "C"
Always **B**e **C**areful

Five "D's"
Hubert W. Smith

Plaintiff must prove:

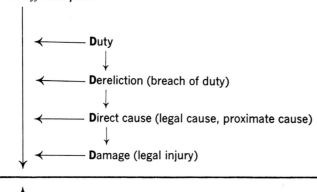

←———— **D**uty

←———— **D**ereliction (breach of duty)

←———— **D**irect cause (legal cause, proximate cause)

←———— **D**amage (legal injury)

↑ **D**efenses — contributory negligence, assumption of risk, etc.

(Defendant must prove)

Three "E's"

E-1 Experimentation
E-2 Emergency
E-3 Early action

Fig. 59-1. Mnemonic liability chart. (Adapted from Cady, E. L., Jr.: Law relating to medical practice: the doctor's diagnosis and treatment of patients. In Gradwohl, R. B. H.: Legal medicine, St. Louis, 1954, The C. V. Mosby Co.)

administering and prescribing a liquid, mostly saltpeter and vinegar, and telling over 100 patients a day that this liquid would take care of their diabetes without resort to insulin, dietary control, and other established regimens. Defendant doctor contended that to rule against him would have a crippling effect on medical science, as it would prevent the use of new remedies. The court stated:

A physician is not limited to the most generally used of several approved modes of treatment and the use of another mode known and approved by the profession is proper, but every new method of treatment should pass through an experimental stage in its development and a physician is not authorized in trying untested experiments on patients.

More analogous to an experimental use of cardiac massage in resuscitation might be a "last ditch experiment" situation (Case L, Table 59-1). In this case, decided in favor of the physician, the patient had been treated for a facial cancer with radium and x-ray to no avail, and expert opinion had been given that there was no hope for her. The Board of Regents had suspended the petitioner, holding that he had been guilty of fraud and deceit in the use of a secret formula on the patient. The court reversed this holding in these words:

> Petitioner also applied the treatment to portions of his own body to make certain that there would be no ill effects from it when applied to healthy tissue. Petitioner was consulted and he examined Mrs. Brower. The patient was informed that the treatment might do some good and that it could not do any harm and consented to its use. The treatment was thus applied under petitioner's directions and in due time a complete cure was effected. . . . The cancerous growth disappeared entirely, the sore was completely healed and there has been no reappearance. Petitioner has never submitted a bill and has never received any pay whatsoever for his services, although he made something over a hundred calls. He testified that if the formula proved satisfactory he intended to write the case up for the medical profession, and the treatment was an experiment on his part and that both he and the patient knew that. He gave the contents of the formula and made no effort to conceal the same. . . . This doctor effected a cure when the so-called orthodox methods of treatment had failed and now he has been punished for it. *It is not fraud or deceit for one already skilled in the medical art, with the consent of the patient, to attempt new methods when all other known methods of treatment have proved futile and least of all when the patient's very life has been despaired of.*
>
> Initiative and originality should not be thus effectively stifled, especially when undertaken with the patient's full knowledge and consent, and as a last resort.

It is submitted that not only is it unsound to speak of liability for experimentation as such but, further, it also constitutes negligence for the practitioner to fail to keep abreast of modern developments. These would include new methods of resuscitation, based on experimentation, when they become generally recognized. Indeed, the courts have often affirmed this positive duty.

> Due regard must be had for the advanced state of medical knowledge at the time of the treatment of any human malady, and refuge may not be taken in the practices of the medical dark ages.*

Two cases, lost on appeal by physicians, have used strong language in this regard: "A physician holds himself out as possessing the knowledge and ability necessary to the effective practice of medicine. He impliedly represents that he is keeping abreast of the literature and that he has adopted those techniques which have become standard in his line of practice." (Case M, Table 59-1.) "Physicians are required to keep abreast of and use best modern methods of treatment, and in so doing they may not unduly and narrowly restrict or confine their responsibility to the immediate place where they are practicing." (Case N, Table 59-1.)

Since any doctor who is fully prepared and competent to undertake resuscitation after cardiac arrest is practicing in line with modern developments, he should be on firm ground legally, although perchance he is unsuccessful in effecting resuscitation.

E-2—Emergency. There can be no question but that resuscitation is an emergency procedure.* Thus, as a legal matter, it is submitted that there is never any need for consent from anybody to undertake cardiac resuscitation. Cases indicating that consent of the spouse is not required in any surgery are overcoming a contrary preconception (Case O, Table 59-1). So, too, it is becoming established that broadly worded consent forms commonly used prior to surgery are not binding upon court and jury when they sit in judgment on a malpractice case. In Case P (Table 59-1) it was held that: "The consent did not foreclose inquiry into negligent conduct in determining the advisability or necessity for the operation."

When the physician encounters a case of sudden cardiac arrest in which associated findings do not show signs of an irreversible situation, then it is obvious that he must act to the best of his judgment, disregarding any effort to gain consent from relatives. The

---

Kelly v. Carroll, 36 Wash. 2d 482, 219 P. 2d 79, 19 A.L.R. 2d 1174 (1950).

---

*A "real emergency" in the classification of Shartel and Plant. See Shartel, B., and Plant, M. L.: The law of medical practice, Springfield, Ill., 1959, Charles C Thomas, Publisher, p. 16.

following case illustrates the obvious impractical aspect of consent from the relatives and is itself a measure that very likely will require the additional delay that is the margin between successful resuscitation and death.

A 32-year-old Caucasian woman was being operated upon for removal of tonsils. The operation was completed and the patient was about to be wheeled to her room when pulse and respiration ceased. Before the chest was opened and cardiac massage begun, the physician ran to where the patient's husband was waiting in order to receive consent for the emergency procedure. Three days later the patient was still unconscious and the ultimate outcome is not known.

This point that consent is not necessary is aptly summarized by the commentators:

An emergency may justify operation without consent if the emergency is critical enough. . . . A surgeon is permitted reasonable latitude in determining necessity and extent of an emergency operation. But the emergency must be one in which life or health is in imminent danger.[28] Where an emergency exists which calls for immediate action toward the preservation of life, or to prevent possible permanent impairment of the health of a patient, and it is impracticable to obtain his consent, or the consent of anyone legally capable of consenting for him, the surgeon is authorized to perform such operation as good surgery demands, without consent. Likewise, where in the course of an operation to which consent has been given, the surgeon discovers conditions not anticipated, and which, if not then corrected, would endanger the life of the patient, or cause serious impairment of health, he is justified in extending the operation accordingly, although no express consent has been given. This latitude is given to the exercise of the surgeon's discretion in such emergencies, regardless of the age, or other legal status of the patient.[12]

The "error of judgment" safeguard also enters this area of the law, as explained by this authoritative passage:

A surgeon is not liable upon an honest error in judgment in performing an operation in an emergency, or in any other case where the error would be a reasonably plausible one under the circumstances. In this connection it is noted that the cases pretty generally use language such as "in an emergency a surgeon is not bound by the ordinary rules of negligence." It would seem that the accuracy of such statements is open to some question, as the "ordinary rules of negligence" make due provision for acts done in emergencies. No doubt it would be more accurate to say that those rules are never in abeyance, and provide adequately for a determination whether the surgeon acted reasonably *under the circumstances.**

E-3—Early action. These same considerations that render consent irrelevant may likewise be used to establish an affirmative duty on the doctor to act promptly in an emergency. Just as the jury is entitled to relax application of the rules of negligence in favor of a physician who undertakes emergency action with less efficiency than he might command in more leisurely circumstances, it may also penalize the man who fails to act with reasonable haste in an emergency. In this connection it is instructive to note passages from the American Law Institute's Restatement, Second, 296 Torts†:

Emergency. (1) In determining whether conduct is negligent toward another, the fact that the actor is confronted with a sudden emergency which requires rapid decision is a factor in determining the reasonable character of his choice of action.
Comment c. *Activity requiring special training or aptitude.* In determining whether the actor is to be excused for an error of judgment in a sudden emergency, importance is to be attached to the fact that many activities require that those engaged in them shall have such natural aptitude or special training as to give them the ability to cope with those dangerous situations which are likely to arise in the course of such activities.

A hint that such a duty of "early action" is owed by the doctor can be garnered from a recent California case in which the following pleading was held proper as against a demurrer‡: "Defendants failed and re-

---

*Note, **14** Cincinnati Law Review 161 (1940).
†A restatement of this sort tries to set out in clear and definite terms what the law is or what it ought to be after a serious analysis of previous case law on the subjects.
‡"The formal mode of disputing the sufficience in law of the pleading of the other side." (Black's Law dictionary, ed. 4, St. Paul, 1951, West Publishing Co.)

fused to take prompt, necessary, usual and emergency methods which would save the life of his child. . . ." (Case Q, Table 59-1.)

PROBLEMS OF PROOF AND AVOIDANCE OF MALPRACTICE CLAIMS

Proof is defined as a "state of conviction in the mind of the trier of fact." In a jury case, it is the jurors who must be persuaded to the correctness of the position taken by plaintiff or defendant. Where a case is tried before a judge alone, then he must be convinced by the adversaries. The systematic study of proof has a number of fascinating facets as law and science interweave. Here, we can only refer to several recent cases that touch on problems of considerable interest to the practitioner. Case R (Table 59-1) deals with an unavoidable result in the treatment of a fractured hip, and the necessity for expert testimony to elucidate such a matter. Case S (Table 59-1) illustrates a failure of proof on the part of the plaintiff who developed an infection of her sexual organs following an abortion. Case T (Table 59-1) indicates how a general practitioner can be qualified to testify as to the medical conduct of a specialist. Finally, a close study of Case U (Table 59-1) illustrates a number of instructive points as concerns a conservative nonsurgical approach to acute head injuries. Regan* entered this case as *amicus curiae* and played no small part in producing a final judgment for defendants, a physician and a hospital.

Since this same authority has had perhaps more experience in "malpractice prophylaxis" than any other single individual, he is now "called to the stand" to render his expert opinion on the avoidance of malpractice claims:

Why a malpractice program? Because a malpractice insurance policy, regardless of its amount, terms, and conditions, does not compensate for:

1. The days and weeks the defendant-physicians are compelled to spend in court.
2. The damage to professional reputation in the community which is a common consequence to a malpractice suit.
3. The destruction of peace of mind which a suit, particularly for the amounts filed these days, creates.
4. The loss of public confidence inevitably attendant upon malpractice claims and suits, particularly aggravated when patients are awarded damages against physicians.

Why a malpractice program? Because no insurance policy, of itself, provides an answer to the day-by-day worry questions to which the doctor is subject. . . .

Why a malpractice program? Because a well-foundationed and efficiently administered program: (1) tends to raise medical standards; (2) improves medical public relations; (3) controls to a degree those physicians who are inclined to overcharge patients and those physicians who need special attention to keep them up to the mark; and (4) promotes the elimination of the unprincipled and unethical practitioner.

Why a malpractice program? Because a sound malpractice program fulfills all those needs and services; because there is incontestable proof that such a program decisively reduces both the meritorious malpractice claims and suits and those which are without merit; because, in short, such a program protects the individual practitioner, enhances the prestige of the profession, and contributes tremendously to the public welfare—and because unless affirmative action is taken by the medical group to stem the mounting tide of malpractice, it appears to be just a question of time until the force of the pressure of public opinion will compel governmental interference for the protection of the public.*

Briefly, the modern malpractice program emphasizes the need for (1) claims prevention, and (2) superior claims handling. Of course, if a claim ripens into a suit, then expert trial consultation is advised.[7]

•   •   •

Lest the reader gain the impression that the Horton case, with which we introduced this chapter, was indefensible, consider the

---

*Late Counsel to the Los Angeles County Medical Society and President, American Academy of Forensic Sciences.

*From Regan, L. J.: Doctor and patient and the law, ed. 3, St. Louis, 1956, The C. V. Mosby Co.

further analysis of a defense witness and his resistance to the cross-examiner's efforts to gain a concession that the affidavit of plaintiff's expert was on firm ground:

Dr. C. states in his affidavit that good medical practice would have required that direct cardiac compression be initiated through an open-chest approach in the cardiac arrest experienced by Mr. Horton. While there is still some occasional debate about the relative merits of internal cardiac compression versus external cardiac compression through the unopened chest, both methods of approach are considered to be acceptable. By *not* resorting to internal cardiac compression in [this case], one would be strained to conclude that this action was contrary to the usual, customary, and accepted approach of the physician encountering cardiac arrest in such a case today.

It is true, there are a few instances when one might argue in favor of the internal cardiac compression route as opposed to the external application of chest compression. For example, if there is strong evidence that intrathoracic bleeding is occurring associated with chest trauma, one would usually elect to open the chest. Other indications might include patients with severe chest deformities of the sternum, rib cage, or vertebrae which would make chest compression difficult. In some instances of cardiac tamponade a direct approach is best. Closed-chest cardiac compression may also be contraindicated theoretically in instances when an external defibrillator is not available and ventricular defibrillation is present, in instances of suspected tension pneumothorax, in some cases with massive air emboli, and perhaps in the third trimester of pregnancy. Some would prefer the direct approach with massive pulmonary embolism and cardiac arrest. Obviously if the chest is already opened then direct cardiac massage would appear to be indicated.

In the *vast majority* of cases, however, the closed-chest compression method is the more accepted and desirable method of restoring cerebral and myocardial circulation because it can be started within a shorter time, does not involve a thoracotomy with its resulting complications, and is effective.

After reading the material submitted. . . , it would seem that external cardiac compression was, indeed, successful in allowing for an augmented circulation. Ventricular defibrillation was promptly accomplished in association with other closed-chest resuscitation measures.

In reply to Dr. C., it is true that there are, in my opinion, situations which would prompt one to switch from external cardiac compression to internal cardiac compression. If one were having difficulty in demonstrating that closed-chest compression and artificial maintenance of circulation were being adequately achieved one would think of switching. In other words, if the patient continued to be cyanotic, if persistent attempts at ventricular defibrillation were unsuccessful, and/or if either ventricular defibrillation or asystole persisted then one would be prompted to open the chest in the hope that one might discover an etiological factor for the difficulty of resuscitation. As I see it, there were no such indications in this case.

The preponderance of evidence today indicates that closed-chest resuscitation is an entirely acceptable modality for cardiac resuscitation. In fact, Dr. ———'s [defendant surgeon] case would seem to have been the ideal candidate for closed-chest compression. Patients with vago-vagal type of asystole are the most likely to respond favorably.

Therefore, on the basis of information available to me, I see no justification at all for suggesting that Dr. ——— [defendant surgeon] not use external cardiac compression. I see no real indication for electing to perform internal cardiac compression. In fact, I believe that most physicians would be somewhat critical of the physician who used internal cardiac compression initially in a case similar to the above.

The cross-examination proceeds:

Cross-examiner. [Citation] No. 34, Doctor, is "The Treatment of Sudden Death by Open- and Closed-Chest Cardiac Massage." Would that cover the factual situation that we have in this case, where the cardiac arrest occurred in the operating room, and they were in the process of preparing to do a thoracotomy? . . .

Q. [Do you] discuss that type of situation in this, or is it limited to something else, where a man falls over in the street or something?

Witness. We don't cover that particular situation. We discuss in that article, or I do in fact, the advantages of the direct approach to cardiac massage.

Q. Which is?

A. Open chest.

Q. Go ahead.

A. And Dr. J. more or less champions the closed chest—not that we disagree, but we each stress the particular strong points of the separate approaches.

Q. What are the strong points of open-chest massage?

A. Well, in some instances, I think open chest has some advantages, and particularly in patients with pectus excavatum, or chest deformities, where they may injure the heart by pressing the chest cage against the vertebrae.

Q. Let us leave out deformity cases, because that is not relevant here. What are the other strong points?

A. The third trimester pregnancy doesn't lend itself well to closed chest. The pneumothorax patients don't do well. You have to open their chest. If you have a flail chest, from an injury, you don't have anything to really compress with, so you don't have much to go on. If you suspect intrathoracic hemorrhage, obviously it is important to open the chest and get the bleeder controlled, such as with a gunshot wound or some serious trauma.

In certain cardiac problems—very specifically, a cardiac tamponade, where you have a lot of blood or fluid in the sac or heart, you need to release that fluid, and closed-chest compression will not help that.

If one encounters a case of air embolism to the heart, I personally think you do better to open the chest and get the air out of the heart by syringe and needle.

If one has a large blood clot in the heart, pulmonary embolism, you are not going to be successful with closed chest. You are going to have to open the heart and remove the blood clot before one will achieve any success.

If one has a valvular stenosis of the aortic or mitral valve, one has to often relieve the valvular stenosis before one can get any benefit.

In some instances, the heart may not be directly under the sternum due to congenital abnormality, or some developmental defect, and it's not going to help the heart to compress the sternum, because the heart may be moved over. So you would want to open the chest in that situation.

There are a number of situations that don't lend themselves to closed-chest resuscitation.

Q. I gather from almost every one of the examples you gave—they were mostly, or all, as far as I can recall, conditions where you could not do closed-chest massage, and obviously, if you could not, internal would be better.

A. You could do it with air embolism.

Q. Let me go ahead with the question. What are the strong points of open-chest massage, where there is an election, where you could do closed under the particular physiological cirumstances that were present?

A. Well, it gives you a more direct visualization of what the heart is actually doing. That is probably the strongest point. You got your hand right on the heart, and you are looking right at the heart, and you are not relying on indirect means.

Q. Does it give better circulation of the blood throughout the body when you are using direct manipulation of the heart, as opposed to closed chest massage?

A. It depends on who is carrying out the particular technique. Some persons, probably Dr. J. can get much better output from the heart . . . using closed-chest resuscitation than many people can accommodate in using open chest. I think on the other hand, in many instances, I can get better cardiac output with open chest than perhaps I might with closed chest. . . .

Q. You have [Citation] No. 12 here which says "Cardiac Arrest Etiology." What is the first thing, or how do you recognize cardiac arrest? What are the clinical signs that present themselves that would lead a surgeon in the operating room, so to speak, to recognize that a cardiac arrest is occurring?

A. If it's in the operating room, and the surgeon has got a large vessel immediately available, either in the abdomen or chest or elsewhere, that, of course, is helpful. If there is not pulsation.

Q. I am talking about before the chest is open. . . .

A. If the patient is under anesthesia, usually respiration is being maintained, and respiratory arrest is one of the diagnostic features of sudden cessation of cardiac output. One wouldn't recognize that always under anesthesia, if the patient was being assisted.

Otherwise, absent blood pressure, absent pulse, if those are absent, the burden of proof is pretty much on the person who says that the cardiac output is being maintained, and occasionally it is. But not very often. Sometimes the color of the patient will be of some help, but in many patients it is difficult, due to skin coloration and so forth.

Q. What is it about the color that you are looking for?

A. Evidence of poor perfusion.

Q. To a layman, what would this be? What I am getting at, how does it change?

A. Sometimes it would be mottling. Sometimes it would be a cyanotic hue.

Q. Is there any recognized time lapse between the onset of cardiac arrest and the amount of time it would take for this cyanotic or mottling to manifest itself to observation?

A. That, I think, is probably less reliable than the other signs I mentioned. I would think it would be a little more variable, too. In terms of seconds, I would hesitate to give you a real precise answer on it.

Q. Could you give me a range?

A. I would estimate it to be 20 to 40 seconds, perhaps. It would only be an estimate.

Q. What other signs?

A. It may even be earlier, as a matter of fact. Absent blood pressure.

Q. We covered that, pulse, and you have covered the skin change. Any other signs now?

A. Pupillary changes would be of some help.

Q. Which way do the changes go, and what do they indicate in cardiac arrest?

A. Well, if pupils are dilating, that could be of considerable importance.

Q. What does that indicate?

A. It could indicate the cerebral blood flow is decreasing or is even stopping, or stopped.

Q. In your teaching or the handling of a cardiac arrest case, is there any recognized time period or range of time within which circulation must be restarted to avoid serious brain damage?

A. Well, under normal thermic conditions, that is, if the patient is not hyperthermic, or hypothermic, the brain usually shows some signs of irreversible damage. If the anoxia is total anoxia . . . if it is allowed to continue for, say, 4 minutes, we have found that out of 1,200 cases, only 6% survived after arrest of 4 minutes—that is, without any treatment.

Q. How long, in your experience, does it take to open the chest?

A. I think you can open the chest in 15 seconds, sometimes.

Q. That is what I was going to continue with the question. Say, assuming you want to get in as quickly as you could, and you had all the equipment available, so you did not have to wait for the proper tools to be brought up, or something like that, would your answer still be 15 seconds?

A. That would be the smallest amount of time. I think some might go in a little bit slower. I think I can get in within 15 seconds, usually.

Q. Would 15 to 30 seconds be a fair range of an accomplished thoracic surgeon to get in?

A. I think so. . . .

Q. In your present instructional program at the university, in teaching your surgery residents about the handling of a cardiac arrest as presented to him in a case where it occurred in the operating room, and all the tools and equipment were available to open the chest, and go in, what do you teach them about the election between closed-chest and open-chest resuscitation?

A. Well, we teach them that the open-chest approach should be part of the surgeon's arm, because of the ten or fifteen exceptions I gave you earlier, because it's more favorable than closed chest. Certainly, closed chest is used in a great majority of cases today.

Q. Do you teach them anything as to the period of time in which it is safe to maintain closed chest, without any necessary signs of circulation?

A. We discussed this, but more frequently it comes in under difficulty, defibrillation episodes. . . .

Q. What is taught, or what do you teach and is taught at the university medical school . . . about the length of time for which closed can be accomplished, without recognized signs, before the chest should be opened?

Counsel. What do you mean by "without recognized signs"?

Q. No blood pressure, no peripheral pulse, pupils dilated.

A. It's usually a little more complicated than that. We frequently have an ultrasonic Doppler apparatus there that can pick up blood flow that the blood pressure machines can't pick up. Sometimes that will give us a clue. Sometimes we have the electroencephalograph around. This is something new, and so is the Doppler. That gives you a clue.

Q. Let us go back before a year. Let us go back a year.

A. We almost always go 4 or 5 or 10 minutes, because you are just not able to make up your mind that things are that bad with closed chest that quick. It takes more than 2 or 3 minutes to decide that you are not doing any good with closed chest. Of course, if the heart is fibrillating, you would want to try closed-chest defibrillation. If it's not working after repeated attempts, that is another indication. It depends if the heart is in asystolia or fibrillation.

Q. If you applied closed chest without any signs for 4 or 5 or 10 minutes, there would not be any point in opening up the chest at that point, would there? Would it not be irreversible?

A. This is a fibrillating heart or asystolic?

Q. Asystolic.

A. We have had that situation with patients with pulmonary embolus, and worked and worked and didn't seem to be getting adequate circulation. I think it's almost—it's hard to believe you wouldn't be getting some evidence of a pulse or some evidence of cardiac output if you are using the technique properly. You may not be getting adequate perfusion, but you are going to be getting some perfusion.

Q. Let me just understand. If you get some perfusion, or some circulation, is this sufficient to ward off the irreversible brain damage that takes place when there is no circulation?

Counsel. Assuming that the irreversible brain damage has not already occurred?

Q. Yes.

A. Some blood is certainly a lot better than no blood. That's kind of a difficult question to quantitate.

Q. Doctor, let me ask you a question: According to what you teach at the university . . . if you are in a situation where you have a patient who is going to be operated on but has not yet been opened for a thoracotomy, he is in the operating room, and all the equipment and all the tools are available, and all the medical personnel are available, and he has a cardiac arrest—under those circumstances what do you teach there at the university about the approach to resuscitation?

A. We go with the closed-chest approach, if the chest is not opened, or the abdomen is not opened.

Q. Assuming nothing is opened.

A. We go with the closed-chest approach. Sometimes just a sharp blow to the chest will be enough to start the heart. The problem is, once you open into the chest, you have got a lot of other problems of infection, perhaps, or injury to the structures, and all kinds of things. So we would prefer to use closed chest.

Q. How long would the closed chest be maintained without any recognizable signs before you would go to internal, under those specific circumstances I have given?

A. We probably have to have EKG evidence of a flat line.

Q. Assume that you have that, that you got EKG evidence of a flat line.

A. Then we would go to our various drug approaches, using sodium bicarb, and more particularly, Adrenalin, and perhaps even later on, if we had no tone, drugs like calcium. We would probably run through our pharmacological approach first and try to get a little tone to the heart.

Q. You have done all of that. Then what is the next step in the resuscitation attempt if you still have not got any recognizable signs of circulation, no pulse, pupils still dilated?

A. Well, you have to elevate the legs, and maybe lower the head of the body, in some instances, although a lot of people disagree with that. You have to convert the heart into fibrillation, which would usually be the case, after injecting drugs; then you would begin to wonder that maybe you hadn't diagnosed the exact etiology properly, and you might consider going in.

Q. How much time would it take to administer the pharmacology aspects that you mentioned?

A. It would be variable, depending on how much you used, and what intervals. We have waited as long as 45 minutes before going into the chest, and we have waited as long as 30 minutes. . . .

There are no magic weapons that will guarantee freedom from encounters with professional liability cases. In fact, the House of Delegates of the American Medical Association concluded:

It has become apparent that problems of professional liability cannot be dealt with apart from matters of patient safety, and a mechanism to minimize liability on the part of physicians and hospitals must be directed primarily to a reduction of incidents in the course of patient care which give rise to liability or potential liability.*

Legal references

1. Alpert, M. I.: Torts—liability of a physician for malpractice, 15 University of Detroit Law Journal 97 (1952).
2. Arthur, W. R.: Res ipsa loquitur as applied in dental cases, 15 Rocky Mountain Law Review 234-235 (1943).
3. Cady, E. L., Jr.: Law relating to medical practice: the doctor's diagnosis and treatment of patients. In Gradwohl, R. B. H.: Legal medicine, St. Louis, 1954, The C. V. Mosby Co., Chapter 4.
4. Cady, E. L., Jr.: Medical malpractice: what about experimentation? 6 Ann. Western Med. Surg., 164 (1952); Medicolegal facets of clinical experimentation, 31 GP 2: 187 (1965).
5. Cady, E. L., Jr.: Law and contemporary nursing, Paterson, New Jersey, 1961, Littlefield, Adams & Co., Chapter 5.
6. Cady, E. L., Jr.: In Stephenson, H. E., Jr.: Immediate care of the acutely ill and injured, St. Louis, 1974, The C. V. Mosby Co.
7. Cady, E. L., Jr.: Technical defenses in professional liability cases, 32 Postgrad. Med. 3:A-42 (1962).
8. Elwell, J. J.: A medico-legal treatise on malpractice, medical evidence, and insanity, comprising the elements of medical jurisprudence,

---

*Preventive medicine is a medicolegal matter, too, **171** J.A.M.A. 2223 (1959).

ed. 4, New York, 1881, Baker, Vorrhis & Co., Chapters 1-3.

9. Gordon, I., Turner, R., and Price, T. W.: Medical jurisprudence, Edinburgh and London, 1953, E. & S. Livingstone, Ltd., Baltimore, The Williams & Wilkins Co., pp. 406-409.

10. Herzog, A. W.: Medical jurisprudence, Indianapolis, 1931, The Bobbs-Merrill Co., p. 32, sec. 32.

11. Jackson, P. E.: The law of cadavers, ed. 2, New York, 1950, Prentice-Hall, Inc.

12. Lott, J. N., Jr., and Gray, R. H.: Law in medical and dental practice, quoting Note, 14 Cincinnati Law Review 161 (1940), Chicago, 1942, The Foundation Press, 132, p. 142.

13. Marshall, T. K.: Premature burial, 35 Medicoleg. J. 14 (1967).

14. Marshall, T. K.: Changes after death. In Gradwohl, R. B. H.: Legal medicine (Camps ed.) Bristol, 1968, John Wright & Sons Ltd., Chapter 8.

15. McClelland, M. A.: Civil malpractice: a treatise on surgical jurisprudence, New York, 1877, Hurd & Houghton, Chapter 19.

16. Morrow, C. J.: An approach to the revision of the Louisiana Civil Code, 23 Tulane Law Review 478 (1949).

17. Note, civil liability of physicians and surgeons for malpractice, 35 Minnesota Law Review (186) 192-193 (1951).

18. Note, civil liability of a physician for non-wilful malpractice, 29 Columbia Law Review 985 (1929).

19. Note, negligence—physicians and surgeons—degree of care, 29 Yale Law Journal, 684 (1920), commenting on Krinard v. Westerman, 279 Mo. 680, 216 S.W. 938 (1919).

20. Regan, L. J.: Doctor and patient and the law, ed. 3, St. Louis, 1956, The C. V. Mosby Co., pp. 608-609.

21. Rezek, P. R.: Dying and death, 8 J. Forensic Sci. 200 (1963).

22. Sargent, F., III: Problems of negligent malpractice, 26 Virginia Law Review 919 (1940).

23. Smith, H. W.: Legal responsibility in surgical practice. In Thorek's surgical errors and safeguards, ed. 4, Philadelphia, 1943, J. B. Lippincott Co., pp. 1000-1039.

24. Smith, H. W.: Legal responsibility for medical malpractice, Chicago, 1941, American Medical Association (reprinted from J.A.M.A. March 8, May 10, May 31, June 14, June 21, July 5, 1941), p. 92.

25. Strassman, G.: Forensic thanatology. In Gradwohl, R. B. H.: Legal medicine, St. Louis, 1954, The C. V. Mosby Co., pp. 120-123.

26. Thomas, C. M.: Evidence—custom and usage among surgeons as evidence of negligence, 3 Arkansas Law Review 215 (1949).

27. Wharton, F.: Wharton, and Stille's medical jurisprudence, ed. 4, Philadelphia, 1884, Kay and Brother, Book III, p. 418, sec. 540.

28. Williams, L. T.: Surgical operations without consent, 19 Tennessee Law Review 376 (1946).

PART NINE

ELECTIVE CARDIOPLEGIA

Chapter 60

ELECTIVE CARDIAC ARREST: GENERAL CONSIDERATIONS

Since the publication of the third edition of this book, there has been much interest in the electively arrested heart. In addition to the great deal of clinical experience with cardioplegia and open-heart surgery, studies on the functional and metabolic effects of anoxic cardiac arrest, including morphological alterations and contractility studies, have been performed. Particularly has the advent of coronary artery bypass surgery increased the interest in all aspects of elective arrest. Cardioplegic solutions continue to evolve. Perhaps the latest solution for clinical use is that of the "Hamburg solution" developed by Kirsch and colleagues in Germany.

Although elective cardioplegia has been employed clinically for over a decade, it appears unlikely that the ideal cardioplegic agent or combination of agents has been found. Not only must the ideal cardioplegic agent have a prompt and complete effect, proper duration, freedom from toxicity, and a completely reliable recovery period, but it should also be easily available as a sterile, storable solution that can be injected by the aortic route or into the coronary arteries. Unfortunately, cardioplegic methods still provide only a short time for cardioplegia, and before the heart is able to function normally a period of reperfusion is necessary. Most agents are associated with various degrees of ischemic damage.

Elective cardiac arrest has been employed experimentally and clinically by use of the following:

1. Potassium citrate
2. Potassium chloride
3. Magnesium sulfate or magnesium chloride
4. Acetylcholine
5. Metacholine
6. Sealy's mixture (potassium citrate plus magnesium sulfate and neostigmine)
7. Anoxia or ischemia
8. Hypothermia
   a. Generalized
   b. Localized
      (1) Coronary perfusion with chilled blood
      (2) Cooling of the heart by external application of ice chips or saline slush
9. Induced ventricular fibrillation
10. A.C.D. solution (sodium citrate, citric acid, and dextrose)
11. Hyperbaric oxygenation with and without hypothermia
12. Perfusion with arterialized hypocalcemic blood
13. Urea
14. Prostigmin
15. Sodium citrate (Mondini-Fabris, 1954)
16. Fluoride and adenochrome (Webb)
17. Hamburg solution (Kirsch)

The exact mechanism of action of the cardioplegic agent is not always clear; a number of such agents work by binding ionized calcium, thus upsetting the calcium-potassium ratio. In addition, it has been difficult to quantitate cardioplegic agents to produce a uniform relationship between the amount of drug injected and the resulting heart action.

With all cardioplegic techniques, it appears desirable to assist the heart for a time after rhythm is reestablished. Satisfactory long-term studies on the effect of cardioplegia are not yet available.

Measures that may be helpful in decreasing the myocardial depression associated with elective arrest include the use of digitalis (prior to arrest), hypothermia, and mephentermine (Willman and associates). Generally speaking, the time factor of arrest is directly proportional to the decreased work ability of the heart following elective arrest.

Effect of various methods of cardioplegia

A number of studies concerned with histologic and functional changes following some of the methods of elective cardiac arrest have been published. One such study (Dabyork and colleagues) compares the different histologic changes in the myocardium following cardiac arrest induced by anoxia, potassium, acetylcholine, and deep hypothermia. The anoxic cardiac arrest was produced by clamping the root of the aorta. The Melrose technique of potassium arrest was used, and the Lam technique of acetylcholine arrest was employed. Hypothermia was employed by lowering the esophageal temperature to 10° C. and was maintained for 30 to 40 minutes. Best's carmine staining techniques were used for glycogen studies. Sudan 1-3 or Scharlack R stains, along with a variety of eighteen other staining techniques, was used for fat studies.

Little significant change could be noted with any of the techniques after a period of only 4 hours. Some interstitial edema and evidence of diminished glycogen content were the only changes noted. After 6 hours, however, some significant changes did appear. Anoxic and potassium arrest produced the most significant changes in the myocardium. The most pronounced pathologic changes in the myocardium were observed after potassium arrest. Glycogen content showed a considerable decrease. There was also fatty degeneration. Fiber swelling, granular degeneration, cellular infiltration, interstitial edema, interstitial hemorrhage, and fat necrosis were seen. Right ventricular dilatation appeared more commonly after potassium arrest.

Other studies of cardioplegic techniques consider the adenosine triphosphate (ATP), phosphocreatine, inorganic phosphate, and glycogen levels in biopsied heart specimens. For example, Gott and co-workers find a much more rapid fall in these levels after potassium citrate arrest than after selective hypothermic arrest. The ability of any cardioplegic technique must, among other considerations, be judged on how well it maintains energy resources of the myocardium.

In summary, various studies yield conflicting data regarding evaluation of cardioplegic agents. Methods of comparison include observations on recovery and contractility of the heart, period of pump support, oxygen consumption determination, tissue acidosis, histologic change, and, finally, overall survival results.

Altered myocardial metabolism during elective cardiac arrest

Although much information remains to be found, metabolic alterations associated with certain cardioplegic agents are partially defined. Unfortunately, some of these alterations were not known before clinical application of certain agents was begun. Focal hemorrhages and fatty degeneration after periods of ischemic arrest are known, as is focal necrosis after potassium citrate arrest. Excessive loss of myocardial glycogen and phosphocreatine (Hall and co-workers) may occur with ischemic arrest but is somewhat slowed with hypothermia. ATP levels also fall during most types of arrest.

Anaerobic metabolism rapidly replaces aerobic metabolism after ischemic arrest, although energy in the arrested heart comes primarily from residual aerobic carbohydrate metabolism, which is completed in the first 10 minutes or so after arrest.

Perhaps for some time to come, the merits will need to be weighed against the undesirable effects of induced arrest. Control of gas emboli, increased precision and rapidity in repair of defects, and diminution of blood loss are all admirable goals, provided the price in terms of complicating factors is not too high.

Biphasic recovery period

Following recovery from prolonged periods of elective cardioplegia with most techniques (such as potassium citrate, Sealy's mixture, acetylcholine, and anoxia), a biphasic type of mechanical recovery has been observed. It is not often seen with hypothermia. Redo has speculated on the nature of this observation. He presents the idea that this initial recovery may result from the washing out from the myocardium of the excess potassium that has accumulated on the outside of the cell membranes. The second observed event is a short period of arrest or decreased output that may be related to a second accumulation of potassium outside the cell membrane. This second accumulation of potassium results from cell death or injury with resultant loss of potassium following the initial cardioplegia. This second episode of cardiac arrest may be termed an "endogenous arrest" and is followed by a return of cardiac function, apparently when this accumulation of potassium is in turn also removed.

Failure of the hypothermically arrested heart to participate in the biphasic type of mechanical recovery is attributed to the fact that there is little significant cellular injury or cell deaths because of the decreased metabolic activity that takes place. Potassium that may lie outside the surface membrane is returned to the cell on rewarming when the "sodium-potassium pump" resumes its normal function.

Measurement of cardiac metabolic function

Gott and his colleagues report on a method involving myocardial rigor mortis as an indicator of cardiac metabolic function. Even though this is a relatively simple and inexpensive method of investigation, they find that the time of complete rigor mortis in hearts arrested with normothermic or moderately hypothermic methods gives a good correlation with the level of ATP. A complete state of rigor mortis of the myocardium generally occurs when the ATP level falls to approximately 15% of the original value. Employing this test in a series of arrested hearts, these investigators conclude that intermittent perfusion of a dog heart with as much as 5 ml. per kilogram of body weight every 10 minutes more than doubles the time of rigor mortis. Cooling the heart to 27° C. likewise doubles the time of rigor mortis.

It should be noted that left ventricular work loads following some types of elective arrest in the dog can be increased with predigitalization. Cooper and associates increased stroke work after potassium arrest in dogs from an average of 9.1 to 19.5 grammeters.

Prolonged cardioplegia

The perimeters of cardioplegia have not been completely established. Particularly is this true with regard to prolonged cardioplegia and its effect on subsequent cardiac function and output. Although experimental work cannot always be transferred to clinical use, various studies are available that indicate that the heart has a limited ability to tolerate the prolonged periods of elective cardioplegia under use in present methods, regardless of the technique involved. The longer the duration of arrest, the greater the adverse effect will be. In a comparison of various types of elective cardioplegia in the isolated perfused guinea pig heart made by Redo in 1962, prolonged cardioplegia with anoxic arrest shows the greatest incidence of failure. Potassium citrate, Sealy's mixture, and hypothermia seem preferable to acetylcholine, anoxia, or anticoagulant A.C.D. solution in the guinea pig heart.

Elective cardiac arrest with ventricular fibrillation

Deliberate and planned ventricular fibrillation as an adjunct to open-heart surgical procedures represents an additional means of effective cardioplegia. Senning used induced ventricular fibrillation for open-heart surgery in 1951. Glenn and co-workers at New Haven, Connecticut, have extensively employed the technique. It has provided them with a means of preventing air emboli during the open-heart procedure, facilitated the repair of the intracardiac defect, and allowed coronary artery circulation to continue throughout the procedure.

Glenn and associates have documented cardiac output studies and ventricular function curves to show that no depression occurs after this technique if an adequate cardiopulmonary bypass is accomplished (in laboratory animals with cardiopulmo-

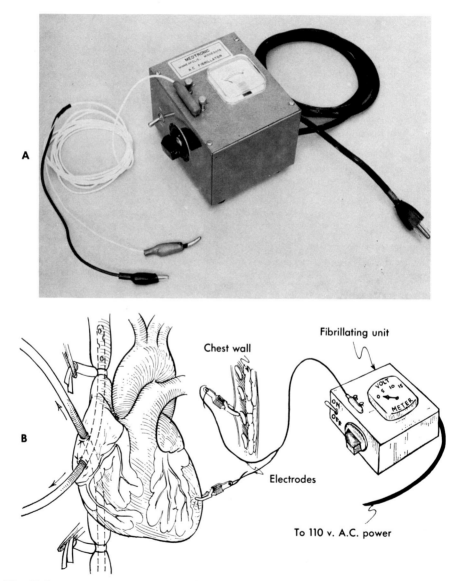

Fig. 60-1. Cardiac fibrillator for induced ventricular fibrillation. **A,** The unit. **B,** Attachment to heart. (From Levy, M. J., and Lillehei, C. W.: Surg. Forum **13:**181, 1962.)

nary bypass after 30 minutes of induced ventricular fibrillation). Clinically, they have used this method of cardioplegia for as long as 117 minutes, with an average time of 30 minutes. Glenn emphasizes the simplicity and safety of this method of cardioplegia, but cautions that this method is not without adverse effects if effective decompression of the ventricular chambers is not carried out or if coronary perfusion is inadequate.

With use of an electrical cardiac fibrillator to induce ventricular fibrillation, the management of exsanguinating hemorrhage or embolization of free mural thrombi can be facilitated. Fig. 60-1, *A,* illustrates the electrical cardiac fibrillator along with the electrodes for application to the myocardium.

Roe and associates have evaluated the effectiveness of induced ventricular fibrillation to control massive hemorrhage during closed-heart operations. The control group consisted of dogs with a left atriotomy and a normally beating heart. Other groups consisted of animals with a left atriotomy and induced ventricular fibrillation and animals with a left atriotomy and cross-clamping of the great vessels and induced ventricular fibrillation. In addition, Roe has evaluated his clinical experience with this technique in closed-heart operations on patients. In spite of clinical impressions that ventricular fibrillation significantly reduces the amount of blood lost from an accidental left atrial tear, he was unable to verify this in his experience. The blood loss in the dogs with fibrillation was approximately the same as in the control group. This, he explains, was probably the result of persistent venous return secondary to a siphonage effect, even though the ventricles were fibrillating. With cross-clamping of the great vessels, the blood loss was markedly decreased during fibrillation. In such emergencies, cross-clamping of the great vessels alone is not recommended. Myocardial distension is not well tolerated.

Advantageous use of induced ventricular fibrillation in preventing embolization is well illustrated in the case of a 13-year-old boy operated upon for removal of an intracardiac myxoma that had previously embolized the right femoral and left popliteal arteries. Prior to opening the left atrium, ventricular fibrillation was induced. Friable and gelatinous material from the tumor nearly filled the left ventricle. During removal of the tumor, fragments became dislodged and dropped to the left ventricle. In the normally beating heart, these fragments would have embolized.

In the three cases discussed by Roe, defibrillation of the deliberately induced ventricular fibrillation occurred without difficulty.

In order for ventricular fibrillation to be induced during closed-heart surgical emergencies, the cardiac fibrillator should be available and ready for immediate use. The value of the procedure results from its application without delay.

Successful repair of the torn atrial wall or removal of tumors or thrombi from the atrium should be accomplished within 3 minutes of fibrillation. Roe mentions, however, the case of a 52-year-old woman upon whom a mitral commissurotomy was being performed. Exsanguinating hemorrhage occurred, and total cessation of circulation for more than 14 minutes was required. Immediate body cooling to 32° C. was instituted and recovery was without neurologic sequelae.

Levy and Lillehei, at the forty-eighth Annual Clinical Congress of the American College of Surgeons, reported their experience with induced ventricular fibrillation in forty-five patients. Instead of the more conventional means of inducing ventricular fibrillation, fibrillary arrest was by continuous electrical stimulus applied to the myocardium (1 to 6 volts). The unit was designed to transform 110 volts (A.C., 60 cycles) into low-voltage levels of between 0.1 and 15 volts. The current was delivered to the patient by two detachable electrodes that could be sterilized. The voltage could be controlled by a rheostat (Fig. 60-1, *B*). Of the forty-five patients with induced ventricular fibrillation, forty-one survived. All were patients undergoing cardiopulmonary bypass procedure. No complications related to the arrest were described. In every case, the heart defibrillated abruptly—either when the electrical stimulus was stopped or after a defibrillating shock. The average duration of arrest was around 1 hour, with a range of from 13 to 132 minutes. Body temperature levels ranged from normothermia to 26° C.

The following advantages are cited for elective cardioplegia by induced ventricular fibrillation:

1. Possibly reverts to a normal rhythm at any time
2. Provides protracted periods of cardiac arrest
3. Reduces the risk of systemic embolization of air or clots, or both
4. Enables sutures to be placed in the neighborhood of the conduction tissue while a normal heartbeat is maintained
5. Is of special value in surgery of the interatrial septum and the mitral valve

The oxygen consumption of the myocardium has been shown to continue at a relatively high rate during ventricular fibrillation. Therefore cross-clamping of the aorta for periods exceeding 2 to 3 minutes can be harmful. Ordinarily, coronary artery circulation is maintained during open-heart surgery and ventricular fibrillation.

When ventricular fibrillation is employed as a method of elective cardioplegia during cardiopulmonary bypass and open-heart surgery, certain precautions should be kept in mind. As always, distension of either or both ventricular chambers must be prevented. Serious, and sometimes irreversible, functional derangement may occur if this precaution is not taken. When placing sutures near the bundle of His, it is important that the heart be beating.

An additional advantage of induced ventricular fibrillation as a method of choice for elective cardioplegia considers its prophylactic value toward the avoidance of air emboli. Another advantage in the use of the ventricular fibrillator is found in its employment after the accidental tearing of the patent ductus arteriosus at the time of its dissection, ligation, or division from the aorta.

Roe and co-workers measured myocardial metabolism and ventricular function before and after induced ventricular fibrillation. Unless ventricular function is consistently depressed and metabolic activities are deranged, ventricular fibrillation is allowed under ischemic conditions. If the myocardium is oxygenated during elective ventricular fibrillation, few significant metabolic disturbances are noted, and function is not appreciably interfered with.

Reis contends that the constant application of a 60 cycle alternating current to the ventricle for maintenance of ventricular fibrillation will significantly interfere with subsequent cardiac preformance. In a group of experiments, he used the repetitive application of a square wave D.C. stimulus, of 5.5 volts and 1 msec. duration at a frequency of 400 to 550 impulses per minute. Such application to the right ventricles of dogs invariably produced ventricular fibrillation. No significant alterations of the left ventricular performance were noted after periods of continuous stimulation lasting 1 hour. Evidence of anaerobic carbohydrate metabolism with a metabolic indicator of cellular hypoxia was lacking. In addition, there was less evidence of a decrease in coronary vascular resistance.

Cohn and Morrow note no significant effects on cardiac function when ventricular fibrillation is induced by a brief 7.5 volt A.C. stimulus and allowed to persist spontaneously for 1 hour. When, on the other hand, ventricular fibrillation is maintained by constant A.C. stimulation, there are significant deleterious effects on cardiac function. Coronary vascular resistance becomes elevated and myocardial oxygen consumption increases, but the increase is significantly less than in animals in which fibrillation persists without electrical stimulation. Anaerobic glycolysis ensues, leading to lactate accumulation in coronary venous blood. These workers conclude that the small alternating current used to maintain ventricular fibrillation actually impairs oxygen utilization, interferes with oxygen availability, and has a marked effect on cardiac performance.

Somewhat at variance with these findings are the studies of Lawrence and his co-workers, who found that, under experimental conditions, electrically induced ventricular fibrillation produces little or no depression of function of the healthy myocardium in the majority of instances. They believe that electrically induced ventricular fibrillation is easily the safest method currently available for producing asystole during cardiopulmonary bypass.

Fibrillatory cardioplegia is considered by Gentsch and associates to be the safest measure of cardioplegia. It is without adverse effects on ventricular function if cardiac chamber dilatation is prevented and if perfusion is adequate. Decompression of the ventricular chambers can be accomplished by left auricular sump or by direct left ventricular sump.

The pros and cons of flow-regulated versus pressure-regulated and pulsatile versus nonpulsatile coronary perfusion in elective fibrillation of the heart are discussed by Wakabayashi and associates. Thebesian shunt flow fluctuates widely during coronary perfusion. If the shunt flow increases suddenly, flow-regulated coronary perfusion, in contrast to pressure-regulated perfusion, cannot meet the flow requirements and this results in inadequate perfusion. Pressure-regulated coronary perfusion may be safe for as long as 2 hours in a fibrillating heart. Pulsatile coronary perfusion provides a more stable coronary vascular resistance than does nonpulsatile perfusion; and myocardial oxygen consumption is more stable during pulsatile perfusion than during nonpulsatile perfusion.

The effect of electively maintained ventricular fibrillation on distribution and adequacy of coronary blood flow is reported by Hottenrott and co-workers. They demonstrate that total myocardial oxygen consumption falls because oxygen delivery to the left ventricle becomes markedly reduced. This reduced left ventricular flow cannot be appreciated when only total coronary blood flow is concerned. The reduction occurs because the fibrillating stimulus impedes flow to the left ventricle and makes it ischemic. The ischemia does not occur when the non-hypertrophied ventricle fibrillates spontaneously.

More detailed information on elective fibrillation will be found in Dr. Wada's chapter (Chapter 61).

Anoxic arrest

An alternative method for induced ventricular fibrillation in the presence of massive hemorrhage is offered by Brewer and Carter. They employ anoxic arrest of the heart by compression of the superior vena cava, the pulmonary artery, and the aorta between the fingers (placed in the transverse sinus) and the anteriorially placed thumb. In their experience, arrest promptly occurs, allowing a quiet heart for precise repair of any wounds. The advantage of this method of induced cardiac arrest lies chiefly in the availability of such a technique. No equipment such as a fibrillator or defibrillator is required.

In the experience of Brewer and Carter, cardiac massage results in a rapid return of the heartbeat, assuming that there is sufficient blood available for effective coronary perfusion. Fig. 60-2 illustrates their technique for elective anoxic cardiac arrest in the treatment of massively bleeding heart wounds. After failure to control bleeding in

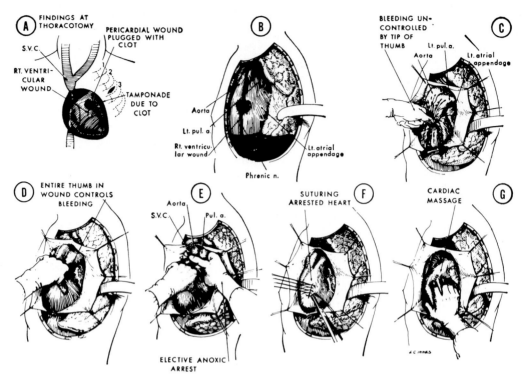

Fig. 60-2. Technique of elective cardiac arrest for the management of massively bleeding heart wounds. Arrest permits removal of the thumb from cardiac wound without excessive blood loss and subsequent suturing of the arrested heart. (From Brewer, L. A., III, and Carter, R.: J.A.M.A. **200:**1023, 1967.)

a patient with a large ventricular wound, they employed the following procedure:

1. Digital control of the hemorrhage (with the entire thumb)
2. Rapid restoration of the blood volume until the aorta is tense
3. Maximum ventilation of the lungs, allowing for maximal period of cardiac arrest
4. Elective cardiac arrest
5. Precise suturing of the cardiac wound
6. Effective cardiac resuscitation

At the Toronto General Hospital, Goldman and colleagues have been generally pleased with the immediate and long-term results of anoxic cardiac arrest as an adjunct to open-heart surgery with its provision of decreased perfusion time, a better intracardiac exposure, a quiet, bloodless field, and a flaccid heart. They have used anoxic cardiac arrest with normothermia in more than 350 patients.

Intramyocardial gas tensions recorded during experimentally produced periods of anoxic arrest by the use of an inflammable Teflon diffusion membrane and a mass spectrometer consistently demonstrated rapid lowering of the P_{O_2} levels toward zero within the first 7 minutes. A steady elevation of the P_{CO_2} levels throughout the period of anoxia was seen, which suggested that initially aerobic metabolism in the myocardium was followed by a steady rate of anaerobic metabolism (Brantigan and associates).

Reul and colleagues at Baylor College of Medicine report extensive use of ischemic cardiac arrest by aortic occlusion under normothermic conditions in aorta–coronary artery bypass grafts. After using this procedure in almost 500 patients, they conclude that normothermic ischemic arrest is a safe and simple technique readily adaptable to the procedure and that interrupted clamping of the aorta is safe up to a total period of 50 to 60 minutes. They prefer this technique to that utilizing prolonged ventricular fibrillation. It is true that dramatic decreases in P_{O_2} and increases in P_{CO_2} occur during aortic occlusion but gradually return to normal 5 to 10 minutes after occlusion. A marked respiratory metabolic acidosis is present in the coronary sinus blood after release of the clamp.

Reis and associates at the National Heart Institute also studied experimentally the effect of ischemic cardioplegia on ventricular performance. With the left ventricle contracting on a balloon, left ventricular functioning was assessed by force-velocity, systolic length-tension, and diastolic pressure-volume determinations after various periods of aortic occlusion and employing cardiopulmonary bypass. Normothermia was maintained at the onset but myocardial temperatures decreased progressively after aortic occlusion. The authors point to the adaptive mechanisms involved that protect ventricular function, such as the spontaneous cardiac hypothermia, which reduces myocardial oxygen demand, and the bronchial collateral circulation, which provides some coronary flow.

Of particular significance in the work of Brantigan and colleagues is the observation that for at least 10 minutes or so after anoxic arrest has been terminated there is a high coronary venous oxygen saturation level, which suggests a significant arteriovenous shunting with a resulting deficiency in intramyocardial oxygen. They speculate that theoretically it might be well to delay defibrillation and terminate cardiopulmonary bypass until after this initial hyperemic phase has passed.

Because of the desirability of avoiding the technical difficulty associated with direct perfusion of the coronary arteries, myocardial ischemic arrest is particularly appealing in cases of aortic valve replacement. Sanmarco and colleagues compared myocardial contractility after cardiopulmonary bypass with and without myocardial ischemia and conclude that extracorporeal circulation per se does not alter the mechanical properties of the myocardium. Ischemia of the myocardium, on the other hand, severely depressed myocardial contractility after aortic occlusion for a period of 20 minutes in the experimental animal. The healthy myocardium does compensate, however, for the ischemic insult by increasing its end-diastolic volume. Isoproterenol is an effective agent in restoring contractility.

In addition, the concern over myocardial hemorrhage from excessive perfusion pressures and late coronary ostial stenosis is obviated. Intimal dissection is avoided. One does not have to worry, as with cannulas, about proper positioning and lack of exposure. There is decreased need for suction of cardiotomy return or preventive measure against air or clot embolism. Comparing the group with anoxic arrest and those with coronary perfusion, Goldman points to no significant differences in mortality or incidence of arrhythmias although there was a saving of betwen 10 and 30 minutes and a reduction in average hospital stay for the anoxic arrest group of 3.4 days as compared with the patients undergoing coronary perfusion.

How does one estimate cardiac viability following anoxic arrest? Maginn suggests that functional and metabolic assesment of cardiac viability provides reliable information. For one thing, a ventricular surface pH greater than 7.10 is usually associated with a viable myocardium. As is known, myocardial ischemia results in a change in metabolic pathways of energy production from aerobic to anaerobic glycolysis. Tissue lactate levels rise and the functional integrity of the hydrogen ion transport system is impaired with a subsequent fall in pH.

DOES HYPERGLYCEMIA ADD PROTECTION TO THE ANOXIC MYOCARDIUM?

Scattered reports have indicated that an increased uptake of glucose during anoxia may have some preventive factor in forestalling myocardial deterioration. In order to test this possibility, Petracek and associates at Johns Hopkins studied the effect of hyperglycemia on cardiac tolerance to normothermic anoxic arrest during cardiopulmonary bypass in experimental animals. It was hoped that hyperglycemia might be an important adjunct to elective anoxic arrest during cardiac surgery by fueling anaerobic metabolism. They compared 5% dextrose in water with Ringer's lactate solution as a prime for cardiopulmonary bypass with anoxic arrest and conclude that hyperglycemia does seem to provide some protection to the anoxic myocardium, although not of an impressive degree. If the priming solution was glucose there tended to be better anatomic and functional preservation than with Ringer's lactate. Basically, however, recovery of the anoxic heart following cardiopulmonary bypass is more specifically related to the ischemic time rather than to the presence or absence of glucose in the priming solution.

IS PREISCHEMIC GLUCOSE PERFUSION OF THE HEART HELPFUL?

A number of studies including those of Prasad indicate that if a period of approximately 8 minutes of perfusion is allowed to elapse before anoxia, the myocardial cell can withstand the anoxic state more effectively and responds better to isoproterenol. Therefore, it would seem that bathing the myocardial cells in a relatively high concentration of glucose does have an effective role.

Hyperbaric oxygenation

Still another method of elective cardioplegia combines moderate hypothermia with oxygen administration at raised ambient pressures. To date, this method has been used mainly on an experimental basis (Illingworth and co-workers). Total arrest of the circulating blood flow is produced by clamping the outflow tract of the heart, including the pulmonary artery and aorta. Inflow occlusion is also produced. Prior to inflow and outflow occlusion, the tissues of the animal are exposed to a blood flow that has been oversaturated with oxygen following respiration in an atmosphere of increased oxygen tension. Illingworth and Smith have recorded that a period of 35 minutes appears to be a safe time limit in dogs. Richards and associates have extended this period to 1 hour. No neurologic or other adverse sequela has been noted in their experience.

Lower levels of hypothermia are being studied. Obviously, steps must be taken to avoid disastrous explosion if electrical defibrillation is used. Defibrillation in an atmosphere of carbon dioxide is one precaution.

Coronary perfusion with cold oxygenated blood

Schwartz and Mallick have investigated cold oxygenated blood in the perfused coronary arteries as an effective means of producing elective cardiac arrest in dogs. They are satisfied that the existing myocardial metabolic needs are adequately met with coronary perfusion by this technique and believe that it is an additional method of producing a dry, quiet operative field. Although Merritt and colleagues have again drawn attention to the ability of the magnesium ion to produce complete cardioplegia, its use as the sole agent of cardioplegia has not been widespread because of the rather marked toxic effect of magnesium. It appears to be quantitatively about five times as toxic as a similar amount of potassium. An excellent comparative study is provided by Mourtzen and Albrechtsen.

Sealy's mixture—potassium citrate, magnesium sulfate, and neostigmine—takes advantage of the synergistic effect of combining magnesium and potassium, with regard to prompt arrest and rapid return of function. Neostigmine (Prostigmin) is added for its vagal effect in slowing the heart rate in the immediate washout period and for its antifibrillary quality. The toxic effects of magnesium are minimized when potassium is also used.

Acetylcholine-induced cardiac arrest

Although some physicians do not consider it as a true cardioplegic agent, acetylcholine has enjoyed moderate popularity as such (Sealy). Lam and co-workers have had considerable experience with acetylcholine-induced arrest.

Normally, there is an optimal concentration of acetylcholine for heart contraction. When this level is exceeded, there is depression of activity, much like that which follows vagal nerve stimulation (with liberation of acetylcholine). The stimulating action of acetylcholine is less well known (Burn). Spadolini refers to acetylcholine as "the cardiac rhythm hormone." It is produced in the atria by choline acetylase and is destroyed by cholinesterase.

Burn believes that the exciting actions of acetylcholine that have been considered are not depolarizing actions. On the contrary, he believes these actions are exerted by virtue of the power of acetylcholine to increase the permeability of the atrial cell membrane to potassium ions and so to raise the resting potentials toward the equilibrium potential for potassium.

Since acetylcholine-induced arrest with small quantities of the drug can be very short termed, its use has been extensively employed for coronary arteriography. Generally speaking, it has been relatively safe. Regular sinus rhythm follows. The inhibiting effect of acetylcholine on the pacemaker and on atrioventricular conduction can be abolished by atropine sulfate.

Hypocalcemic blood

Blood made hypocalcemic from magnesium-charged cationic exchange resin (dowex-50) produces prolonged asystole with recovery and no gross evidence of damage in the dog heart (Clark and associates).

Elective cardiac arrest with adenosine triphosphate

A high-energy phosphate, adenosine triphosphate (ATP), has been utilized in elective cardiac arrest (Dodrill and colleagues). This important chemical compound is partially depleted from the heart during potassium arrest. When combined with a trace of potassium citrate, it aids as an effective cardioplegic agent. Lactic acid accumulation is slowed in the heart arrested with ATP.

Induced arrest with hypothermia

It is interesting that the human heart apparently can withstand ischemia for significantly longer periods than can the dog heart. Irreversible structural and metabolic changes affect cardiac function earlier and more severely in the canine heart. For example, anoxia lasting longer than 20 minutes in the dog heart produces a uniform decrease in left ventricular work capacity, persistent morphologic damage, and injury to myocardial restoration. This cellular damage is reflected by prolonged elevation of serum enzyme level. Even though the oxygen consumption of the empty and non-beating or fibrillating ventricle is only 20% to 25% of normal (37° C.), Dolan finds that the coronary venous acidosis and excess lactate production to be evidence of anaerobiosis. He suggests that the success of anoxic arrest in the human reflects a preservation of enzyme systems involved in normothermic anaerobiosis rather than the deceleration of lowered metabolic and enzymatic processes that occur with lowered temperatures. Increased tolerance of the anoxic heart may be provided by hemodilution perfusions because of their beneficial rheological effect on the microcirculation of the heart. A priming solution with a high glucose content may also be helpful to the anaerobic metabolic pathways of glycolysis. As mentioned elsewhere, anoxia increases glucose transport across the cell membrane and may also stimulate intracellular glucose phosphorylation, which in turn protects the glycolytic enzyme systems. Rolley and Hewitt also confirm the protective effect of glycogen and glucose upon the anoxic arrested heart as measured by cardiac function following arrest. Glucose loading prior to anoxic arrest may provide significant protection.

Using either induced ventricular fibrillation or inflow occlusion to the heart, Small and Stephenson added moderate surface cooling to a temperature of about 30° C. and were able to operate upon thirty-six consecutive cases of intracranial vascular lesions that would not otherwise have been surgically treatable because of excessive blood loss. Arrest of the circulation generally lasted 7 to 8 minutes, although a surgical arrest lasting almost 30 minutes was tolerated by one patient. In another group of patients, Small and his co-workers produced a relatively bloodless field when they markedly reduced cardiac output by rapidly pacing the heart with an intracardiac electrode in the right ventricle.

When profound hypothermia is combined with anoxic cardiac arrest, it does preserve a significant degree of cardiac function, as evidenced by data showing myocardial glycogen deposits being protected and ATP levels in the heart muscle being maintained. Even so, areas of fat necrosis and degenerative changes in the myocardium of hearts examined after anoxic arrest and deep hypothermia are seen. Studies by Rheinlander on the metabolism of the postarrested dog heart under hypothermia are revealing in that at 37° C. a depression of oxygen consumption as well as pyruvate and total fatty acid uptake by the heart takes place. At 10° C., and following 30 minutes of cardiac anoxia, there is a decrease in coronary blood flow and oxygen consumption as well as a depression of fatty acid and probably, glucose uptake by the myocardium. In essence, these studies show a considerable depres-

sion of the normal oxidative metabolic myocardial pathways 30 minutes after anoxic cardiac arrest, regardless of whether the temperature of the heart during the arrest is maintained at 37°, 30°, or 10° C.

Even though hearts can withstand periods of anoxic arrest under hypothermic conditions, hearts already damaged and hearts with a compromised circulation are less likely to survive.

Surface-induced, deep hypothermia in cardiac surgery has generally been abandoned because of the threat of ventricular fibrillation and the fear of neurologic damage. Because cardiac surgery in infants continues to provoke a high mortality rate, especially during curative procedure attempts, Mohri and associates at the University of Washington School of Medicine were prompted to induce hypothermia to between 17° and 19° C. (on dogs) by surface cooling under deep ether anesthesia and, at the same time, to maintain near-normal cardiac function. By maintaining alkalosis during cooling, they were able to maintain 100% cardiac function. Ventricular fibrillation could be avoided.

An additional problem associated with prolonged profound hypothermia (as low as 4° C.) and cardioplegia is that of considerable intravascular aggregation. The exact mechanism of the increased blood viscosity is not completely explained. Certainly it is partly due to the hemoconcentration that does occur. Low molecular weight dextran will help prevent the intravascular aggregation in profound hypothermia, but circulatory patterns for small blood vessels are not normal.

Rapid falls in body temperature do not occur in uniform patterns throughout the body. It is incorrect to assume that the temperature fall measured by readings from the esophagus and rectum reflect a similar temperature fall in the brain. Rush and his colleagues note that the difference of temperatures between the esophagus and the brain during cooling and rewarming is frequently as much as 20° C. Hypoxic acidosis during the rewarming phase is thought to originate partly during the period of hypothermia, although Rush reports that oxygen is utilized in dogs at the average rate of 0.31 ml. per kilogram of body weight per minute for the first 1½ hours of circulatory arrest, and arterial oxygen content falls to 6 vol.%. If circulatory arrest is maintained for 2 hours, metabolism continues ostensibly on an anaerobic basis.

For the reader interested in the problem of surface-induced deep hypothermia, the work of Mohri and colleagues is recommended. They have demonstrated that safe time limits of total circulatory arrest with surface hypothermia under deep ether anesthesia and respiratory alkalosis along with the use of low molecular weight dextran may be associated with neurologic injuries if carried beyond 40 minutes of circulatory occlusion at 16° to 19° C. If hydrocortisone is given the animals, the arrest may be extended another 20 minutes. An additional 30 minutes may be added if circulatory arrest is combined with hydrocortisone and selective brain cooling utilizing cold isotonic saline (3° to 4° C.) solution in addition to general deep hypothermia.

In 1969 Lillehei and associates utilized hypothermia along with partial cardiopulmonary bypass to effect total circulatory arrest in order to provide a lifesaving technique for the management of patients with ruptured mycotic aortic aneurysms, ruptured left ventricle, unusual tears in the vena cava or arch of the aorta, unusual coronary arteriovenous picture, or management of patients with infected sternotomy wounds following cardiac surgery with massive and uncontrollable hemorrhage. The procedure involves a rapid institution of partial cardiopulmonary bypass by peripheral cannulation of the femoral veins and femoral arteries and in some instances also the internal jugular vein. A low-volume oxygenator priming (10 to 15 ml. per kilogram) is in-stituted with mixtures of 5% dextrose in distilled water, balanced saline, or Rheomacrodex. Total body cooling is started coincident with the partial perfusion. After the temperature has reached the desired level the oxygenator is shut off. The arterial line is clamped and the patient's venous blood is allowed to drain into the oxygenator reservoir. With this technique, exposure reveals a bloodless, motionless field.

Elective hypothermic cardioplegia during neurosurgery

Gissen and colleagues of the Neurological Institute of New York report a fascinating application of elective circulatory arrest to facilitate the surgical treatment of basilar artery aneurysm, classically a most difficult lesion to treat. In five consecutive patients treated successfully by hemostatic control of infratentorial aneurysms, adequate exposure was provided through circulatory arrest with intermittent cardiac massage. Using generalized hypothermia (29° to 39° C.), with the vital functions carefully monitored, craniotomy and preliminary exposure of the aneurysm. Before approaching the aneurysm itself, a thoracotomy or sternotomy is done and the pericardium is opened. Applying hemostatic clips, ventricular fibrillation is applied by a 15-volt alternating current to the surface of the heart after 3 to 4 minutes and manual massage is applied to the heart for 1 minute followed by a repeated period of circulatory arrest. Some of the patients had repetitive episodes before final hemostasis was achieved. Following the first period, 250 ml. of 5% sodium bicarbonate was given and at the completion of the procedure 5 ml. of 10% calcium chloride was injected to improve myocardial tone before a single current shock was applied to the heart.

The procedure has many attractive features including the avoidance of prolonged hypothermia and occlusion of cerebral vessels. Extracorporeal bypass is not needed nor are anticoagulants used.

Hamburg solution

The cardioplegic solution used clinically at the University of Hamburg by Kirsch, Rodewald, and Kalmár is composed as follows: 2.5% magnesium-1-aspartate (159 mv. per liter); 0.3% procaine hydrochloride (11 mole per liter); 4.5% sorbitol. The Hamburg group has used this solution for elective cardiac arrest in 174 open-heart procedures under normothermic temperatures with a mild hemodilution technique. Particularly it has been used in cases in which the aorta was cross-clamped. Applying the procedure to a wide variety of pathologic conditions, the total operative mortality was 20%.

The cardioplegic solution is injected either into the aortic route or the coronary arteries after the ascending aorta is cross-clamped. Injection is made at a rate of 50 ml. over a period of 5 to 10 seconds and then more at the same rate, if needed. For aortic valve surgery, the solution is injected directly into the coronary arteries by means of a soft catheter. Generally, infants receive a total dose of approximately 30 ml. and adults 140 ml. This amounts to a dose of 1 to 2 ml. per kilogram of body weight and to about 20% of the heart weight.

After reperfusion, the heart rhythm resumes without electrical shock treatment in 64% of the patients. Contrary to simple ischemic arrest, cardioplegia with a Hamburg solution seldom is followed by arrhythmias. The first ventricular beats are usually seen after a reperfusion time of less than 1 minute. The perfusion is usually continued for 10 to 15 minutes, however. Kirsch concludes that procedures with periods of ischemia below 1 hour can be carried out with a reasonable amount of safety for the patient and that the method is superior to simple ischemic arrest. It can, in fact, compete with coronary perfusion as long as the required duration of ischemia is relatively short. If the heart is hypertrophied, coronary perfusion should probably begin after about 40 minutes of ischemia.

A 15% excessive amount of procaine is added before sterilization since this much is lost during autoclaving. Magnesium-1-aspartate was chosen instead of magnesium chloride since it seemed more easily taken into the cells. Kirsch also speculates that it may stimulate the regeneration of adenosine monophosphate from inosine phosphate via adenylsuccinate. The sorbitol in the solution serves as an osmotic carrier.

In developing the Hamburg solution it was theorized that it should be free of any component that might stimulate the breakdown of energy-rich phosphate by activation of phosphorylases. Ions and substances suitable to delay this action are desirable. Since adenosine triphosphate is used in the membrane during active transport of ions, cardioplegic solutions should not contain calcium, potassium, or sodium if avoidable. The magnesium ion, by blocking myosine as phosphorylase, may slow the decay of organic phosphate in the cell. Kirsch further theorizes that potassium citrate may have fallen into disfavor because it cannot be utilized in the Krebs cycle under anaerobic conditions and thereby an increased amount of citrate may block that system, in addition to causing calcium depletion.

In summary of this work, then, the concentration and decay rate of energy-rich phosphates determine the length of time between the beginning of ischemia and the onset of irreversible damage. Adenosine triphosphate is preserved during the first few minutes by creatine phosphate and then subsequently decays to adenosine diphosphate and adenosine monophosphate. To a large extent, these are then in turn deaminized into inosine phosphate, inosine, and inosine diphosphate. Ultimately, liberation of ammonia into the cell is probably responsible for the destruction of proteins and the production of irreversible damage. Ammonia cannot be transported into the extracellular space or to alphaketoglutaric acid or oxalacetic acid when oxygen and energy-rich phosphates are not available.

Chapter 61

ELECTRICALLY INDUCED FIBRILLATION

Juro Wada

In the nineteenth century, Provost and Batteli observed that the passage of a relatively weak electrical current through the heart provokes ventricular fibrillation and that a strong current of short duration stops fibrillation. Thereafter, many physiologic studies were made of electrical fibrillation and defibrillation. At the present time, there exists no difficulty in inducing or reversing fibrillation, and both find a wide application in cardiac surgery.

Ventricular fibrillation is induced by both D.C. and A.C. stimulus. For a long time, physiologists have known that a weak A.C. stimulus will induce fibrillation. Wiggers, Brooks, and others have shown that a D.C. monopulse stimulus given during the vulnerable period of systole will also induce ventricular fibrillation.

Vulnerable period and minimal ventricular fibrillatory threshold

The vulnerable period commences at the end of the relatively refractory period of the myocardium, or at the rising peak of the T wave of the ECG. If the electrical D.C. monopulse is applied within this period, fibrillation is easily induced. To investigate the vulnerable period, an instrument was made and tested. This instrument consisted of an R wave synchronizer, a variable delayed timer, and a stimulator. The stimulation of 1 msec. D.C. monopulse was given to the myocardium of adult mongrel dogs by bipolar electrodes placed 10 mm. apart. With the use of this instrument, a sharper localization of the vulnerable

period was obtained (Fig. 61-1). The ventricle was easily fibrillated by this method when the stimulus fell during the rise of the T wave to the end of its peak. A constant threshold current with a mean value of 13.8 ma. was found in each of twenty dogs.

Influence of acidosis and alkalosis on the threshold of fibrillation

Respiratory alkalosis was produced in dogs by inhalation of 100% oxygen and metabolic alkalosis by intravenous sodium bicarbonate. Respiratory acidosis was produced by inhalation of 10% carbon dioxide, and metabolic acidosis by hydrochloric or lactic acid. Alkalosis was then maintained at pH 7.6 and acidosis was maintained at pH 7.1. The threshold revealed no difference between alkalosis and normal. In acidosis, however, the threshold decreased markedly. A 34% decrease in the threshold with respiratory acidosis and a 32% decrease with metabolic acidosis were noted when compared with the normal (Fig. 61-2). These data correlate well with the clinical experience that acidosis sometimes induces fibrillatory arrest of the heart.

Incidental ventricular fibrillation and vulnerable period

Ventricular fibrillation has been noted to frequently follow ventricular extrasystole after cardiac operations and during cardiac catheterizations. The ECG is strikingly similar to the ECG of experimentally induced ventricular fibrillation during the vulnerable

783

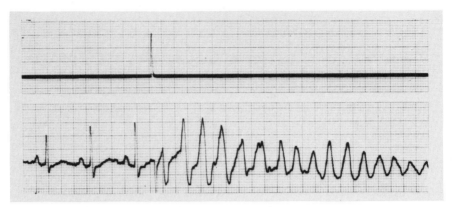

Fig. 61-1. Ventricular fibrillation in dog following D.C. monopulse shock during rise of the T wave of the ECG, or vulnerable period.

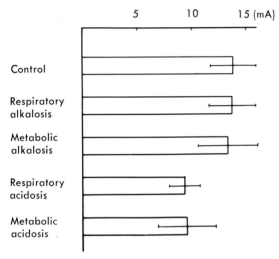

Fig. 61-2. Change of the threshold of ventricular fibrillation with alkalosis and acidosis.

period. Smirk and associates suggest that ventricular extrasystoles, which fall in a vulnerable period, sometimes induce ventricular fibrillation. Clinically, when extrasystoles develop, there is an increased incidence of ventricular fibrillation. However, if the threshold is decreased for some reason or if a pacemaker of a higher energy discharge (5 ma. or over) is used, these stimuli (given during the T wave of an extrasystole) may induce ventricular fibrillation. Arrhythmias and ventricular fibrillation may also occur with competition between pacemaker-induced beats, spontaneous idioventricular beats, and returning A-V conduction.

This understanding of the electrophysiology of the heart in the vulnerable period enabled the testing of paired and coupled pacemakers. These pacemakers induce effective contraction following postextrasystolic potentiation induced by pacemaker stimuli.

The D.C. defibrillator discharges a strong current of short duration (2 to 10 msec.). Although the shock is programmed electronically to avoid the vulnerable period, the danger of ventricular fibrillation still exists, as has been reported in the literature. In my clinical experience, one of 403 patients had tachycardia after application of D.C. shock. Extremely high energy (32 μf., 5 kv. or over) discharge occasionally produces ventricular fibrillation in dogs; however, this is not related to the cardiac cycle or the vulnerable period.

Ventricular fibrillation induced by A.C.

A.C. production of ventricular fibrillation has been known for a long while by physiologists and has particular applicability in cardiac surgery. An A.C. fibrillator has been developed that includes a variable voltage transformer with an output between 0.1 and 15 volts. Recently, my associates and I condensed the size of the instrument by using a rheostat instead of a voltage transformer. A further modification produced an automatic A.C. fibrillator having an R wave–sensitive circuit. This instrument switches on and off automatically with spontaneous return of sinus rhythm. Ventricular fibrillation is always induced with these fibrillators by passing a shock of 2 to 8 volts for 1 to 2 seconds through the myocardium.

Occasionally, ventricular fibrillation has been produced by a much weaker A.C. leaking from medical electronic apparatus during cardiac catheterization. From experiments on dogs, it was found that fibrillation can be induced by A.C. of 0.1 to 0.4 amps. Some investigators report that the fibrillatory threshold in dogs is 20 to 180 msec.

Experimental findings of electrical fibrillation of the ventricle

Coronary perfusion occurs mainly during diastole in the normal heart. During fibrillatory arrest of the heart, individual myocardial fibers act in their own independent manner, producing uncoordination and ineffectual contractions. However, the total action of the heart is similar to systole. The purpose of this experiment was to determine the coronary flow and to study myocardial metabolism during fibrillatory arrest.

During extracorporeal circulation, there was no particular difference between coronary flow in fibrillatory arrest and in normal sinus rhythm. The coronary flow in fibrillation measured approximately 6% to 10% of total perfusion volume. During arrest with induced fibrillation, oxygen contents of arterial, mixed venous, and coronary sinus blood were measured. No difference was found between sinus rhythm or fibrillatory arrest as long as the coronary perfusion was continued with extracorporeal circulation. There were slight decreases of pH and carbon dioxide tension and a slight increase of lactic acid in the blood sample of coronary return during fibrillatory arrest. This minor degree of change of blood gas and lactic acid might

be caused by the extracorporeal circulation itself. Microscopically, no myocardial damage was found. There was no depression of glycogen or lipids in myocardial cells.

Clinical applicability of electrically induced fibrillation

On the basis of the previously described experimental findings, D.C. electrically induced fibrillation of the ventricle was carried out during cardiac surgery with extracorporeal circulation. It provided a quiet operative field in which to work and it prevented air embolism. Since 1963 this method has become routine procedure in our service where more than 4,000 cardiac surgeries have been performed. In every case it was easy both to electrically produce and to control cardiac arrest. Postoperatively in selected cases no difference was found in the SGOT between the arrested and nonarrested group.

With massive hemorrhage during chest surgery, we electrically induce ventricular fibrillation, quickly repair the bleeding source, and then defibrillate the heart. This technique was satisfactorily carried out in seven patients with a fibrillatory arrest of between 2 and 7 minutes (Table 61-1). Two of the patients were arrested twice, and uncomplicated recovery followed. Roe has used this method of control for hemorrhage from the left atrium that developed during closed mitral valvuloplasty.

Stand-by use of induced fibrillation is occasionally helpful in patent ductus arteriosus (P.D.A.) surgery. When the P.D.A. is complicated by aneurysmal dilatation or calcification, the vessel wall may be torn by clamping the P.D.A. with occluding forceps for division. In such an instance, induced fibrillatory arrest for few seconds makes the clamping and division safe. After defibrillation, the cut ends of the P.D.A. can be leisurely sutured.

We have found that induced fibrillatory arrest is a more simple and practical means of producing circulatory cessation in some difficult *aortic aneurysm surgery* than is the

Table 61-1. Cases of electrically induced ventricular fibrillation used to control hemorrhage

Patient	Age (years)	Sex	Lesions	Operative procedure	Source of hemorrhage	Fibrillatory arrest	
						Approximate duration (min.)	Number of arrests
I. I.	37	M	TF with pulmonary tuberculosis	Intrapericardial A-P shunt using Teflon graft	Anastomotic site	3.5	Three
M. Y.	31	M	AI + MS	Prosthetic replacement of aortic valve and mitral valvuloplasty	Repaired aortotomy	3.0	Two
M. S.	2	F	VSD + PH	Pulmonary artery banding	Rupture of pulmonary artery	3.5	Two
K. I.	18	F	AI	Prosthetic replacement of aortic valve	Repaired aortotomy	3.5	One
E. Y.	10	F	PDA	Division of P.D.A.	Divided and sutured end of aortic site	3.5	One
S. S.	36	F	AI	Prosthetic replacement of aortic valve	Repaired aortotomy	2.0	One
H. Y.	35	F	ASI + MS	Prosthetic replacement of aortic valve and mitral valvuloplasty	Repaired aortotomy	3.5	One
T. H.	29	F	MI + TI	Prosthetic replacement of mitral and tricuspid valve	Left atrium	3.0	One

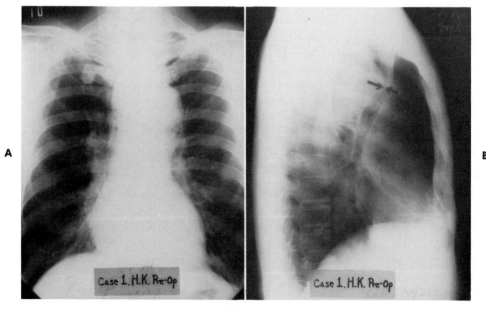

Fig. 61-3. A, P-A chest film of 59-year-old farmer. **B,** Lateral film of same patient. Arrows indicate tracheal narrowing by the tumor mass.

commonly recommended use of surface cooling or extracorporeal circulation. Two clinical experiences on aneurysmal resection with the aid of induced fibrillation are discussed in detail.

A 59-year-old male farmer, who had syphilis at age 22 and a right chest contusion at age 28, had a normal, active life until 3 months previous to admission, when he developed gradually increasing hoarseness and left chest pain. He was referred to us because of a dense tumorlike shadow in the upper mediastinum (Fig. 61-3).

His physical findings were essentially normal except for moderate emaciation, hoarseness, and distension of neck veins. Urinalysis and hematology were normal except for positive serology tests.

Plain chest film suggested a fist-sized tumor in the upper anterior mediastinum at the aortic arch level. The esophagogram indicated that the upper esophagus was shifted to the right by the tumor mass (Fig. 61-4). The bronchogram showed deviation of trachea to the right and midtracheal narrowing due to compression by the tumor mass. The aortogram was not conclusive, although the possibility of aortic arch aneurysm was not completely eliminated.

On December 16, 1965, with tentative diagnosis of upper mediastinal tumor, an intubation tube was inserted to reach beyond the tracheal compression, and G.O.F. anesthesia was started. The right anterior fourth intercostal space was entered. When an adherent tumor on the lung was dissected, a large pulsating mass overridden by the trachea and esophagus was visualized and was reconfirmed as an aneurysm by needle puncture. Pericardiotomy and careful examination revealed the aneurysm as originating from the left thorax and extending to the right thorax behind the ascending aorta. Therefore the incision was extended to the left, the sternum was transsected, and the left thorax was exposed. The root of the aneurysm was found just distal to the left subclavian artery, and its diameter was about 5 cm. The descending

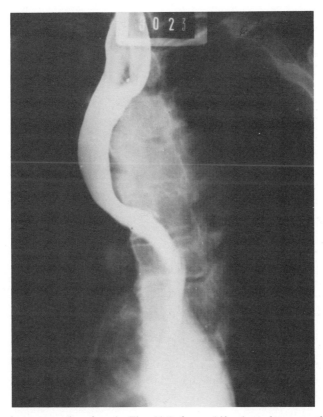

Fig. 61-4. Esophagogram of patient in Fig. 61-3 shows shift of esophagus to the right by the tumor mass.

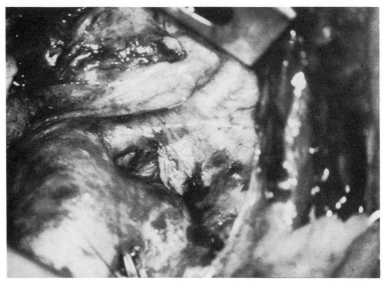

Fig. 61-5. Operative view showing left subclavian artery and root of the aneurysm originating from the descending aorta (aneurysmal dilatation extends into the right thorax behind the descending and ascending aorta).

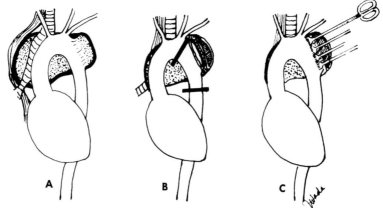

Fig. 61-6. Illustration of the operative procedure. **A,** Thoracotomy finding. **B,** Two solid bars indicate areas of occlusion. The root of the aneurysm was circumcised. **C,** Cuff of the aneurysmal opening of descending aorta was temporarily closed with multiple Allis forceps, leaving the aneurysmal sac undisturbed. D.C. debrillation followed.

aorta proximal and distal to the aneurysm was carefully dissected free from the surrounding tissue for cross-clamping. The aneurysm itself was not dissected because of dense adhesion with the surrounding structures (Fig. 61-5).

At this stage, instead of dividing surgery into two stages—performing resection of the aneurysm in the second stage under surface hypothermia or by standby pump run—use of electrically induced fibrillation was decided upon as a method of circulatory arrest.

The patient was well oxygenated; as soon as the heart was fibrillated by A.C. 6 volts, the descending aorta was cross-clamped proximal and distal to the aneurysm, and the root of the aneurysm was circumferentially incised, leaving a cuff

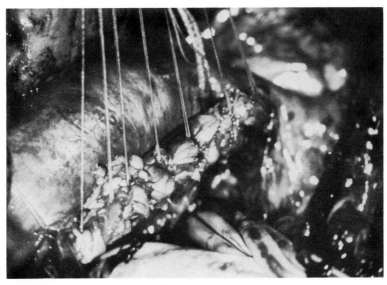

Fig. 61-7. Multiple Allis forceps were used to close aneurysmal opening of the descending aorta, which was leisurely and meticulously replaced with interrupted sutures.

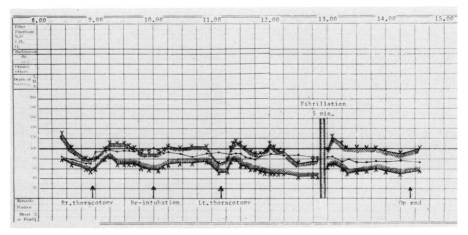

Fig. 61-8. Course of the operation.

for suturing on the aorta (Fig. 61-6). Inside, the aorta was sucked out. The intima was normal. The cuff of the aorta was quickly approximated and closed by twelve Allis forceps; the descending aorta was reconstructed temporarily (Fig. 61-7). Cross-clamps were removed and a single shock of D.C. current reinstituted active heartbeats, bringing blood pressure back to 140/90 mm. Hg. The time for continuous fibrillation was about 5 minutes (Fig. 61-8). The Allis forceps were then meticulously replaced with double row of silk

sutures. The content of the aneurysmal sac was cleaned. The chest was closed and bilateral pleural drainage tubes were connected to waterseal bottles.

Postoperatively, the patient woke up and all vital signs were satisfactory; he was connected to a respirator for 36 hours (Fig. 61-9). Increased bronchial discharge was controlled, and he became afebrile in 10 days. He was discharged from the hospital 6 weeks after the operation. At the last checkup, 2 years after the surgery, the patient was in good health (Fig. 61-10).

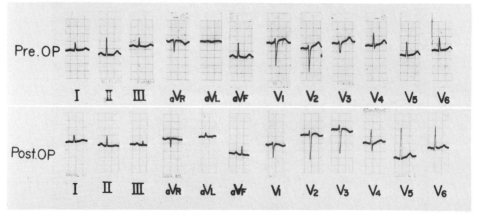

Fig. 61-9. Preoperative and postoperative ECG findings are essentially the same.

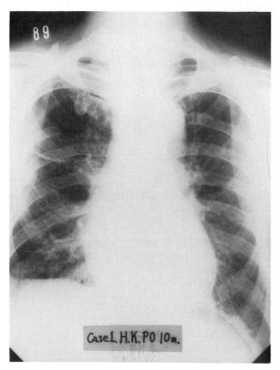

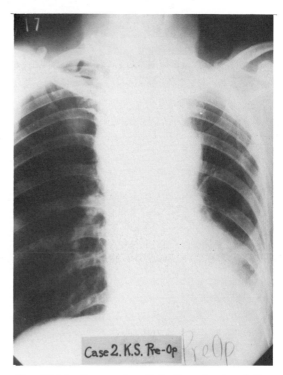

Fig. 61-10. Eleven months postoperative P-A film shows slight elevation of the right diaphragm. The patient is well and active 2 year after surgery.

Fig. 61-11. Preoperative P-A film showing left apical pleural thickening, obliteration of left costophrenic angle, and enlargement of upper mediastinal shadow.

In a second case, a 53-year-old clerk, who had a past history of syphilis at the age of 23 and left exudative pleurisy at age 25, developed tightness and neuralgic pain of the left upper chest. Six months later, he noticed a pulsating tumor on the upper sternum area and it became increasingly difficult for him to swallow.

When the patient was referred to us, he was suffering from throbbing chest pain. He was emaciated and his skin was dry. There was a pulsating, apple-sized tumor at the left sternal manubrium, which was covered by a reddened skin of no inflammatory sign. The right carotid, radial, and ulnar artery pulsations were difficult to palpate.

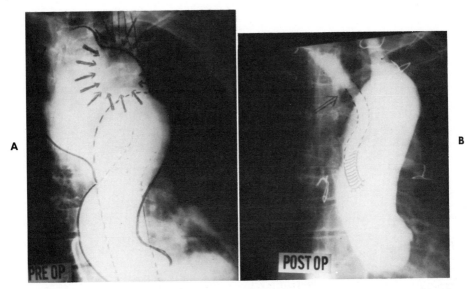

Fig. 61-12. A, Aorta, aneurysmal dilatation, left subclavian artery, and left carotid artery. Arrows indicate round bony destruction of the sternum. **B,** Position of the interposing synthetic graft between the innominate artery and the ascending aorta. Arrow indicates anastomotic site between the graft and the innominate artery.

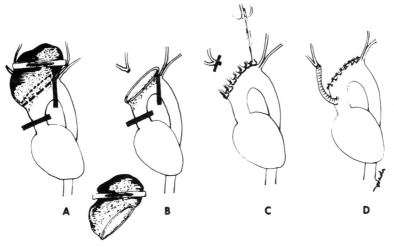

Fig. 61-13. A, Solid bar indicates sites of occlusion; dotted line indicates site of circumcision. Aneurysmal sac is to be removed, together with the anterior chest bony plate. **B,** Arch aneurysm and bony plate are removed. **C,** Aneurysmal opening of the aortic arch is temporarily approximated and closed with multiple Allis forceps. D.C. current is used to defibrillate the heart, and the distal innominate artery is clamped off. **D,** Synthetic vascular graft is used to reconstruct the resected innominate artery.

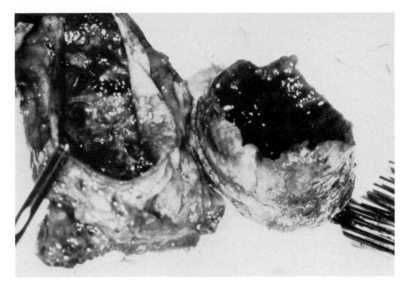

Fig. 61-14. Resected specimen. Left, aneurysmal sac attached to internal surface of the bony plate (sternum-clavicles-ribs). Right, aneurysmal sac outside the bony plate, which preoperatively had appeared as the pulsating mass in the left upper chest.

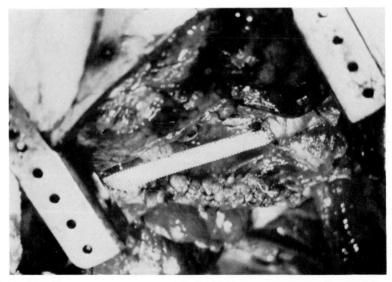

Fig. 61-15. Aneurysmorrhaphy is completed by replacing multiple Allis forceps with interrupted sutures. After sinus rhythm was obtained by D.C. debrillation, the innominate artery was reconstructed by a synthetic vascular graft.

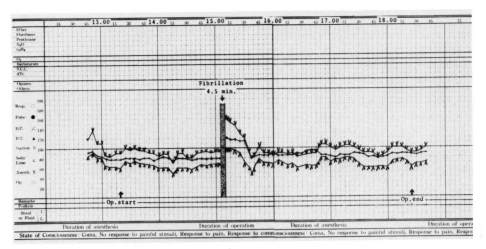

Fig. 61-16. Course of the operation.

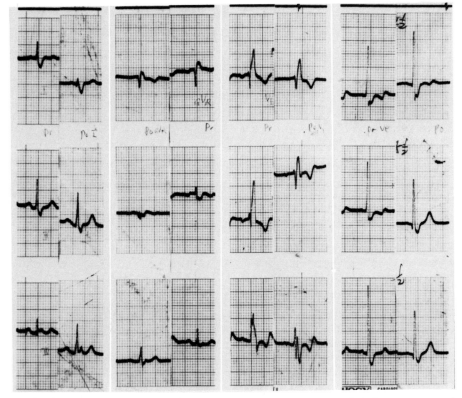

Fig. 61-17. Preoperative and postoperative ECGs. The left sides of each strip are preoperative and the right sides are postoperative ECG tracings. No gross changes are seen in the two groups.

Blood pressure in the left arm was 110/60; in the right arm, 84/70; in the legs, 160/90. No cardiac murmur was present. Hematology and urinalysis were normal, but there were strong positive serology tests. ECG showed a right axis deviation, incomplete RBBB, and L.V.H. The chest roentgenogram showed pleural thickening of the left apex, a pulsating aneurysmal shadow in the upper mediastinum, and a round bone defect 2.5 cm. in diameter in the left side of the manubrium (Fig. 61-11). The upper esophagus was shifted posteriorly. The angiogram showed a large aneurysm involving the ascending portion and the arch of the aorta. The proximal portion of the innominate artery was involved in the aneurysm, but involvement of the left carotid and subclavian arteries was not clear (Fig. 61-12).

Radical surgery of the arch aneurysm was scheduled on January 4, 1967, with a pump standby. The patient was anesthetized with G.O.F. No hypothermia was used. The left fourth intercostal space incision revealed a thick, fibrous, pleural adhesion, which was carefully dissected. A huge aneurysm of the aortic arch was densely and firmly adherent to the anterior thorax and was compressing the left subclavian and carotid arteries. The skin incision was extended to the right, and the right thorax was entered through the third intercostal space (Fig. 61-13).

Pericardiotomy revealed that the root of the ascending aorta was free from aneurysmal involvement. The aneurysm was found to originate from the distal ascending aorta and the aortic arch. The sternum was transsected. Bilateral ribs (right third and second; left fourth, third, and second) were sharply severed, along with the intercostal muscles about 3 cm. away from sternal borders; bilaterally, the clavicles and the first ribs were cut with the wire-saw. All the muscle attachments to the cranial aspect of the clavicle-sternum-clavicle were dissected. Then, the rectangular bony plate attached to the anterior third of the aneurysm floated with pulsation in the operating field. The ascending aorta was freed from surrounding structures.

A groove-tunnel was carefully created between the left carotid artery and the aneurysm around the descending aorta for cross-clamping. The base of the aneurysm was carefully dissected free from the surrounding tissues; it was about 20 cm. in its longer diameter. The lungs were ventilated. The aneurysm was circumferentially incised from its base, leaving a cuff on the arch wide enough for approximation. The aneurysm, together with the rectangular bony plate, was removed (Fig. 61-14). The interior of the aortic arch was visualized as normal. The cuff was approximated and closed

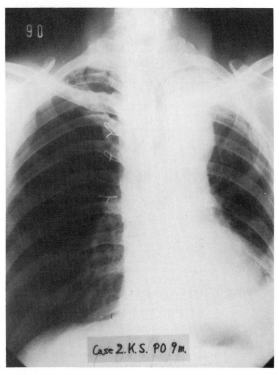

Fig. 61-18. P-A film taken 9 months postoperatively.

using multiple Allis forceps in reconstitution of the aortic arch. A single shock of D.C. current (1,000 volts, 24 watts) defibrillated the heart, and blood pressure returned to 160/100 mm. Hg in a few beats. At the same time, fresh blood collected in the right apical groove; this was found to be a backflow from the cut end of the right innominate artery, of which the proximal portion was removed together with the aneurysm. This finding indicated good blood flow to the brain through the left carotid artery. The innominate artery was cross-clamped. All vital signs were perfect, the Allis forceps were carefully and leisurely replaced by silk stitches, and the aneurysmorrhaphy was completed (Fig. 61-15). The defect of the innominate artery was reconstructed with a Teflon graft of 1 cm.^{2} × 18 cm. (between the innominate artery and the ascending aorta) in the usual fashion. After the aneurysmal sac containing the clots was removed from the rectangular bony plate, the latter was positioned in its anatomic site, and its fixation was accomplished with silk and wire sutures. After bilateral drainage tubes were inserted, the skin was closed. The time for surgery was 4 hours and 30 minutes; the time of induced fibrillation was 4.5 minutes (Fig. 61-16).

The patient was postoperatively connected to a Bennet respirator for 24 hours. The patient's recovery was excellent. Postoperative angiograms showed a well-reconstructed aortic arch and innominate artery. The pathology of the specimen showed typical meso-aortitis syphilitica (Fig. 61-17).

At the 1 year postoperative checkup, the patient showed an excellent general condition and was enjoying an active and useful life (Fig. 61-18).

Transposition of great vessels frequently requires emergency Blalock-Hanlon's procedure. Under the condition of fibrillatory arrest of the heart, the inferior and superior vena cava may be occluded. A right atriotomy is then performed, and the septal defect is created under direct vision. After completion of the technique and evacuation of trapped air, the heart is defibrillated. This method was carried out in three patients; two showed satisfactory results.

The technique of fibrillatory arrest may be used in coronary angiography. With induced fibrillatory arrest of the heart, aortic root flash of radiopaque material demonstrates in experimental animals the clear visualization of coronary arteries.

Chapter 62

CARDIAC PRESERVATION

Edward B. Diethrich

If clinical homotransplantation of the heart is ever to become a practical reality, the major problem of the simultaneous availability of compatible donors and recipients will have to be overcome. Investigators became acutely aware of this problem when the initial series of human heart transplants was performed. Many patients waited for months until a suitable donor heart was available. Others died of acute myocardial infarction or myocardial failure when an appropriate heart was not available. At the same time, numerous donor hearts were lost for a variety of reasons. In some cases no compatible recipient was available. In others, the time between death of the donor and preparation of the recipient was too brief to make appropriate arrangements or too long to provide a viable donor heart. Frequently, the donor heart was available, but was some distance from the medical center where the recipient waited. In some of these cases, the family of the neurologically deceased potential donor was agreeable to donate the heart but refused to have the body moved long distances, which would incur extra expenses and prolong arrangements for funeral services.

Various other problems regarding the availability of the donor heart have been encountered, all of which point to the need for a practical method of preserving and transporting a heart for homotransplantation purposes. When a breakthrough in the immunologic barrier of human transplantation occurs, the problems of retrieval of vital organs will become an even more pressing matter. A variety of preservation methods have been examined in both the laboratory and clinical environments but experience to date has failed to demonstrate any single technique that is both reliable and simple. This is not particularly surprising, however, since the magnitude of the problem of sustaining life of an organ with oxygen and metabolic requirements is appreciable. The current preservation techniques under investigation can be divided into one of four major categories depending upon the principle of the method involved.

1. In situ preservation
2. Preservation in an intermediate biologic host
3. Preservation by metabolic inhibition
4. Extracorporeal preservation

In situ preservation

The most common form of preservation used during the brief era of human cardiac homotransplantation was the in situ method (Barnard; Cooley). The donor is pronounced neurologically dead by an independent team and cardiac preservation is accomplished by respiratory and metabolic support in a manner resembling the care of a critically ill patient. Continuous electrocardiographic display is available to assess any rhythm disturbances that might be corrected. An intra-arterial line provides a continuous arterial pressure recording and a route for arterial blood sampling. Intravenous fluids and medications are administered as required. Oxygenation by a mechanical respirator is provided through an endotracheal tube or tracheostomy, with frequent determinations of blood gas levels. Appropriate adjustments of P_{O_2}, P_{CO_2}, and pH are made to assure a homeostatic environment. Fluid administration is sufficient to maintain an adequate renal output and frequent electrolyte determinations are obtained to assess the need for supplemental administration.

In a well-balanced in situ preservation, time is provided for examination of the donor heart prior to transplantation. This averts the disastrous situation of using a heart for transplantation which itself is diseased. This unfortunately has occurred where the hearts of young donors thought to be entirely normal were transplanted and only after the operation was completed were they found to have extensive atherosclerotic disease. Routine roentgenograms of the chest can be accomplished easily with this technique to determine cardiac size and abnormal configurations. Selective coronary arteriography, when indicated, provides a definitive picture of the coronary arteries and assures the absence of atherosclerotic disease. When necessary, the in situ preparation can be transported from one institution to another prior to transplantation.

In addition to in situ preservation of the beating heart, methods have been investigated for support after cessation of the heart beat. External cardiac massage, initially manually, and then using mechanical assisters is practical for a short period of time. The obvious limitations to this technique are temporal. Problems of transportation have also made it impractical for anything except brief preservation.

An alternative method has been investigated using an Anstadt mechanical ventricular assister applied to the heart in the in situ, open-chest position (Anstadt and Britz; Anstadt and co-workers; Skinner and co-workers). It is not impractical under some circumstances to move such a preparation even by airplane while adequately monitoring via-

bility of the preserved heart. During this preservation and transportation period, sufficient time is provided for tissue typing and cross-matching between the recipient and one or several potential donor hearts. It is quite likely, however, that all of the in situ methods of preservation at present are more sophisticated than the currently available tissue compatibility testing programs.

In this experimental method, the cadaver circulation is maintained by a mechanical ventricular assister that features a glass cup containing a Silastic diaphragm. The cup is placed over both ventricles and held in place so that the atrium is kept outside the cup by a flange at its rim and by pneumatic negative pressure applied through an opening in the apex of the cup. A pneumatic positive and negative pressure, alternating between 140 mm. Hg above and 80 mm. Hg below atmospheric pressure, is applied to the space between the glass cup and the diaphragm to produce artificial systole and diastole. Mean arterial pressure can be maintained at 80 to 100 mm. Hg by adjusting the pressure and rate of the assister. Even though cadaver circulations can be adequately maintained for several hours using this technique, its major limitation in cardiac preservation is the potential for damage to the heart itself. As an emergency measure for brief periods of preservation, it may have some future role.

Any variation of the in situ technique, although the one most reliable and commonly employed, is not without serious deficiencies. The problem of transportation of the body from one location with the inconveniences and expense to the families has been discussed. Many times, the potential donor is an accident victim who has sustained multiple injuries in addition to a fatal neurologic condition. Pulmonary injuries may make adequate oxygenation difficult. Renal or hepatic complications can create metabolic problems. Cardiac irregularities and rhythm disturbances may result from these secondary conditions as well as from the primary neurologic injury. These changes may be sudden, necessitating the immediate removal and use of the heart, even if all of the appropriate arrangements and investigations are incomplete. In spite of these limitations, in situ preservation continues to be our most practical method of sustaining viability for even many days under ideal circumstances prior to transplantation (Griepp and co-workers).

Intermediate biologic host

A natural outgrowth of the in situ preservation method is the use of an intermediate biologic host. Such an intermediate storage system would provide a method of "banking" hearts for prolonged periods of time. Several such studies have been undertaken to define the feasibility of this approach and the function of hearts preserved in such a manner (Abbott and co-workers; Carrell and Guthrie; Mann and co-workers; Sinitsyn; Tomita; Wells and co-workers). The usual experimental preparation consists of removal of the heart of one experimental animal and transplanting it to the abdomen of a recipient. Arterial and venous circulation can be established by end-to-side anastomosis between the donor ascending aorta and main pulmonary artery to the recipient abdominal aorta and inferior vena cava, respectively. This arrangement permits donor coronary perfusion to be effected by host abdominal aortic flow and donor coronary sinus effluent to be returned to the host inferior vena cava.

Heterotopic cardiac implantations of this type have been studied from both a functional and a histologic standpoint. One of the major early complications of the procedure relates to difficulties associated with immunosuppressive therapy. Pulmonary infections are among the highest in this group of postoperative problems. The results of cardiac catheterization as late as 5 to 6 weeks after implantation indicate significant functional integrity of the heart as a pump. Although episodes of acute rejection are apparent clinically during the storage period, these can be controlled with only slight impairment of the ability of the heart to function as a pump.

The ultimate answers to the practicality of this method of preservation, of course, reside in the analysis of the functional capacity of the heart once it has been transposed from the intermediate host into the final recipient. The problems of accelerated antigen-antibody reactions and the creation of hypersensitivity states may then become serious limiting factors. The technique certainly deserves further experimental study as another approach to prolonged cardiac preservation.

Metabolic inhibition

Inhibition of cardiac metabolism was one of the original methods of preserving myocardial viability during circulatory arrest for repair of congenital heart defects. Surface-induced deep hypothermia alone or in combination with systemic hypothermia using extracorporeal circulation provides very satisfactory maintenance of cardiac viability for short periods of time. Some cardiac surgical teams have employed moderate hypothermia routinely during performance of the transplantation to protect the heart during the ischemia period. This same principle can be applied to longer periods of preservation using a variety of techniques. In situ preservation, already discussed, and extracorporeal preservation, to follow, may use hypothermia as an adjunct to the method. Laboratory studies have demonstrated that the simple refrigeration of the donor heart in a balanced electrolyte solution with 10% serum at 4° C. for 8 hours allows dog hearts to return to relatively normal function after homotransplantation (Webb and Howard). The temporal limitation with all forms of refrigeration, however, has made this method of preservation an essentially impractical one for more than a few hours.

An effort has been made to extend the ischemia time by adding a metabolic inhibitor in combination with hypothermia (Nakae and colleagues). Magnesium sulfate ($MgSO_4$), a metabolic inhibitor, combined with hypothermia has achieved satisfactory preservation of rat hearts for 24 hours. The effect of this combination can be further enhanced by the addition of the osmotic agent dextran 40 to provide 48-hour preservation on occasion. The role of the metabolic inhibitor may not be entirely clear at this time but studies have demonstrated that magnesium is capable of preserving membrane permeability to potassium (Holland). Other experiments have shown that magnesium also preserves transmembrane potential of rat ventricle subjected to anoxia (Kamiyama and co-workers).

Although these are interesting studies of metabolic inhibition either with hypothermia alone or in conjunction with specific chemical agents, their practicality appears to be limited to relatively short-term preservation. Even the adjunctive benefit of hyperbaric conditions, which has been useful in kidney preservation, has added only slightly to the viable preservation period of cardiac muscle without circulation and oxygenation. Cardiac viability for prolonged periods of preservation, at least at the present time, depends upon some form of coronary arterial circulation with provisions for supply of oxygenation to the myocardial cells even if the metabolic rate has been reduced appreciably.

Extracorporeal preservation

Methods of preservation of the heart outside the cadaver have been studied rather extensively and can be divided into two major groups: (1) pump-oxygenator support and (2) preservation chamber support. The use of a heart-lung machine to preserve viability of the heart outside of the body would appear to be one of the logical avenues for investigation since temporary cardiopulmonary bypass has become so successful in the repair of cardiac lesions. The usual extracorporeal circuit entails the removal of the heart from the thoracic cavity after ligation of appropriate veins and arteries and cannulations to complete the circuit between the venous circulation, an oxygenator, heart-exchanger or refrigeration unit, and pumping head back to the arterial circulation (Bailey

and co-workers; Levitsky and others). Various oxygenators including screen, bubble, and disc have been used. Both immersion of the heart in physiologic solution and suspension with intermittent bathing have been employed. Whole blood, plasma, perfusate mixtures, and combinations of these provide about the same results in terms of functional capacity of the heart during and following the preservation period.

One of the major problems associated with evaluating these extracorporeal preservation systems is adequate testing of the functioning capacity of the myocardium to support normal circulation after the preservation period. Few studies have been designed to challenge the preserved heart by transplantation to the orthotopic position of the second animal. Some experiments have studied the functional aspects of the heart during preservation to assess work load, myocardial metabolism, and left ventricular efficiency (Pitzele and co-workers). Routinely, hearts preserved under hypothermic coronary perfusion have demonstrated unimpaired left ventricular working capacity during preservation periods up to 12 to 14 hours (Edwards and co-workers; Evans and Matsuoka; Katz; Reissmann and Van Citters). Studies indicate that minor electrolyte and water disturbances resulting from hypothermic preservation are completely reversible (Martin and co-workers). However, more severe or prolonged disturbances are undoubtedly associated with intracellular derangements that eventually lead to cellular destruction and loss of the functional capacity of the heart.

An alternative method of extracorporeal preservation using a portable preservation chamber has yielded satisfactory results for up to 44 hours of storage (Diethrich and co-workers; Robicsek and co-workers). The cardiac preservation unit is a transportable, self-contained device for monitoring a sterile heart-lung preparation in the physiologic state. The unit is 20 inches wide, 3 feet long, and 4 feet high with an approximate weight of 300 pounds. The chamber housed within

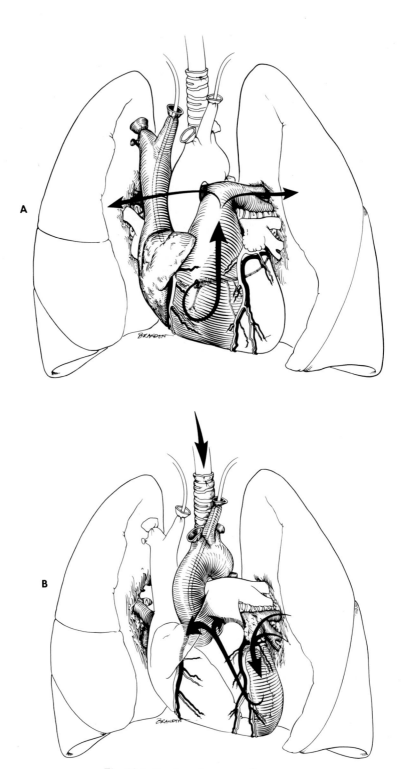

Fig. 62-1. For legend see opposite page.

the unit is an autoclavable 9 by 18 by 10 inch stainless steel vessel that allows adequate space for the enclosed heart and lungs. Immediately beneath the lid there is a tight-fitting seal of perforated aluminum covered with numerous layers of Silastic. On the back of the chamber, $1\frac{1}{2}$ inches from the top, a $\frac{1}{2}$-inch tapered nipple of stainless steel accommodates the endotracheal tube adaptor inside the tank and the respirator outside the tank. The right-hand side of the chamber houses three standard syringe tapered connectors to accommodate the pressure line needles inside and three sterile stopcocks on the outside. One stopcock is used for arterial monitoring and blood sampling when connected to the line in the subclavian artery, another is for blood or drug administration to the right heart through the azygos vein, and the remaining inlet or stopcock is used for continuous addition of fluids to the physiologic bath solution. The electrocardiogram connection is also on this side of the vessel. The left-hand side of the chamber contains the inlets and outlets for the rectangular cooling coil with four loops of $\frac{3}{8}$-inch stainless steel tubing. This cooling and heating system provides a range of temperatures as low as $13°$ C. using tap water and is capable of being adapted for supercooling gases such as Freon for profound hypothermia.

A standard operative procedure has been devised to remove the beating heart from the thoracic cavity in both the dog and the human. The pleural cavities are entered through a bilateral fourth intercostal incision extending across the sternum. Sodium heparin (2 mg. per kilogram) is administered. The superior and inferior venae cavae and

the azygos vein are isolated with double ligatures passed around each. A polyethylene catheter is introduced into the right atrium through the azygos vein for venous pressure monitoring and administration of blood, fluids, or drugs. The brachiocephalic artery, left subclavian artery, and descending thoracic aorta above the first intercostal arteries are isolated. In the human, the left common carotid is also divided. The left subclavian artery is transected and a polyethylene pressure catheter is introduced into the ascending aorta and connected to a pressure transducer for continuous arterial monitoring. Blood samples are drawn intermittently from this line during the preservation experiments.

While the arterial pressure is being monitored on an oscilloscope, the heart is isolated from the thoracic cavity by ligating first the inferior vena cava and then the descending thoracic aorta. The superior vena cava and brachiocephalic artery are ligated, trapping sufficient blood in the isolated circulation to maintain an arterial pressure above 100 mm. Hg (Fig. 62-1). An insulated braided wire, bared for 4 cm., is sutured into the left ventricular myocardium and connected to the electrocardiogram lead set for continuous monitoring of the electrical activity. The trachea is isolated and transected and a sterile cuffed intubation tube is introduced. The cuff is inflated and the tube is reconnected to a Bird respirator supplied with a mixture of 98% oxygen and 2% carbon dioxide. Then the heart and lungs are dissected free from the posterior mediastinum and removed to the awaiting preservation chamber.

The chamber is filled with a sterile physiologic solution buffered to a pH of 7.4 with

Fig. 62-1. Drawing showing catheterization of aortic arch through left subclavian artery, cannulation of right heart through azygos vein, and intubation of trachea for pulmonary ventilation. Isolated quantity of blood passes from right atrium to right ventricle, through pulmonary circulation to left atrium, and out ascending aorta from left ventricle. Then blood flows through coronary arteries and returns to the right heart through coronary sinus. **A,** Blood replacement, glucose, insulin, and steroids infused through venous catheter. **B,** Arterial sampling of blood gases, electrolytes, serum enzymes, calcium and magnesium, sugars, and BUN obtained through left subclavian artery catheter. An O_2-CO_2 mixture is administered through the trachea.

the addition of 5 gm. of calcium chloride to the 18 liter priming volume. The bath temperature is maintained between 27° and 30° C.

A variety of biochemical studies have been done during preservation of beating hearts in the chamber. Since a small amount of blood is lost with the bath and an additional 10 ml. are drawn every hour for analysis, blood is replaced by either continuous or intermittent infusion. Blood diluted with 20% Ringer's lactate is used since there is a dialyzing effect of the bath solution. Using this method, the hemoglobin and hematocrit levels are kept in a normal range. Blood urea nitrogen levels remain normal. The addition of 2 ml. of 50% dextrose every hour and 2 units of regular insulin every 4 hours maintain the blood sugar near 250 mg. per 100 ml. No alterations in sodium, potassium, or chloride volumes are observed with this method. The addition of the calcium chloride to the bath solution maintains the serum calcium levels within normal limits. Serum magnesium levels remain at low normal values, however, in spite of an addition of 3 mEq. per liter of magnesium to the bath solution.

Lactic acid values are directly proportional to the state of the myocardium. In preparations in which ischemic metabolism is present, lactic acid levels are elevated, and, under these conditions, correlated well with electrocardiographic evidence of ischemia and cardiac arrhythmias. In the preparations conducted at 30° C. with the blood pressure maintained from 80 to 100 mm. Hg, the lactic acid values are within normal range. Increase in lactic acid is observed late in some experiments when the viability of the myocardium is deteriorating.

Continuous electrocardiographic monitoring with this technique shows initial S-T depression associated with manipulation and removal of the heart to the preservation chamber. After this initial depression, however, the electrocardiogram patterns return to normal within the first hour of preservation and remain normal throughout the extent of the preservation. Occasionally, the electrocardiographic activity demonstrates classic signs of ischemia, and the postpreservation pathological studies reveal areas of myocardial infarction.

Additional studies have been conducted to determine the biochemical characteristics of both normal human and dog hearts maintained in the preservation chamber for protracted periods of time (Lindenmayer and co-workers; Sordahl and co-workers). These tests indicated a remarkable maintenance of the energy-liberating capacity of human heart mitochondria obtained from these hearts and an apparent beneficial effect of magnesium on activating NADH-linked respiration after storage. Initial measurements of mitochondrial function after incubation of the preserved heart revealed, in the presence of glutamate-malate or succinate, high respiratory rates during active phosphorylation that are comparable to those obtained in a variety of normal animal hearts.

Studies of this nature have demonstrated that a technique of extracorporeal preservation of the beating heart is not only important as a potential for ultimate cardiac transplantation, but also as a research tool that may enable a better understanding of myocardial biochemistry and cellular ultrastructure.

Continued research undoubtedly will lead to more sophisticated and satisfactory methods of both preserving and transplanting the human heart. It is important that these investigations parallel the work in other closely related fields of tissue typing and immunology in order to assure the most effective, long-term results in the human cardiac transplantation program.

Chapter 63

CARDIAC RESUSCITATION IN CARDIAC TRANSPLANTATION

Vallee L. Willman

In cardiac transplantation the consideration for resuscitation involves both the donor and the recipient. In the severely injured or ill patient that might become a donor, vigorous resuscitative efforts are frequently required to maintain human life. When cardiac arrest occurs in an individual who might well after death be a suitable donor for organs, members of the transplant team should not participate in the resuscitative efforts lest the effort be tainted by the possibility of future organ usage. The choice for or against resuscitation, or the method, should not be influenced by the possibility of use of the heart as a donor organ and resuscitation should differ in no way from accepted patterns. In most centers it is directed that the physicians caring for the patient to the point of determination of death should not be the same as those who engage in the transplantation procedure.

Once it has been determined that the patient no longer represents human life and thus becomes a donor, the physicians involved in transplantation can appropriately initiate resuscitative efforts in order to maintain the donor organ in an optimal function state. Hypotension can be treated by administering peripheral vasoconstrictors progressing to norepinephrine if required to maintain coronary perfusion and to prevent arrhythmias or cardiac arrest. Large doses of epinephrine or isoproterenol should be avoided as these can induce structural damage to the myocardium. Large amounts of base can be given

to counteract metabolic acidosis. External cardiac massage can be used to maintain circulation but the contamination associated with open-chest massage should be avoided. Should pacing be required it is attempted transcutaneously to avoid contamination or catheter damage to the heart.

When there is a discrepancy between the time when the donor heart will continue to support adequate circulation and the time when the recipient site is prepared for transplantation, the viability of the donor organ is best maintained by extracorporeal circulation rather than by extracorporeal organ perfusion. This can be by balloon assist or by venous-arterial pumping with oxygenation done in the operating room with preparations made to take the organ at the appropriate time.

Whereas resuscitation of the donor heart is directed toward preservation of myocardial integrity, resuscitation of the recipient prior to transplantation is directed toward preservation of other organ functions without concern for the ultimate effect on the heart. A recipient with failing circulation should receive the pharmacologic support that will drive the heart to the greatest extent possible without concern for the ultimate effect on the myocardium. Large amounts of isoproterenol, epinephrine, glucagon, calcium, and lidocaine are justifiable to treat specific problems. Base is infused to maintain a pH that will allow organ function. Dialysis (peritoneal or blood) might be employed to adjust fluid and electrolyte balance. Cardioversion and defibrillation should be used to treat threatening arrhythmias. Pacing, if required, can be by a transvenous electrode. If arrest, fibrillation, or extremely poor pumping function cannot be reversed, extracardiac support can be employed. External cardiac compression is suitable for short periods (1 to 2 hours) but longer periods of satisfactory support can be obtained by balloon counterpulsation if there is cardiac action by a reasonably regular mechanism or by arteriovenous pumping with oxygenation if there is arrest, fibrillation, or grossly irregular cardiac action. The latter method of support for periods up to a few hours has much to recommend it as this system will be required ultimately in the transplantation procedure. Although direct compression of the donor heart by such devices as the Anstadt cup are contraindicated because of resultant damage to the heart, in the instance of the recipient heart, this technique might have some application as also might open-chest manual cardiac compression. In these circumstances, however, meticulous aseptic technique needs be adhered to.

In clinical transplantation as it has generally been practiced there is a period of cardiac arrest and ischemia that involves resuscitation following reattachment in the recipient. In anticipation of this resuscitation, protective measures are taken to enhance success. Ischemic time is as limited as possible. The myocardium is protected by surface cooling. Some prefer to wash the blood out of the coronaries with cooled heparinized electrolyte solution. Attempts at continuous coronary perfusion have been made but are generally more troublesome than they are valuable. Care is taken to avoid the area of the A-V node and bundle of His during ex-

cision and reattachment (Hurly and co-workers).

Following implantation and restoration of coronary circulation, resuscitation of the transplanted heart is aided by extracorporeal circulation allowing for some evaluation of function prior to imposing a full work load upon it. Arrythmias are frequent with a nodal origin of the ventricular complex being common. Pacing by means of myocardial electrodes is generally considered to be the preferable management of these arrhythmias. During this period the heart is responsive to cardiotonic agents in usual doses with the usual responses for a denervated heart (Cooper and co-workers). Ventricular fibrillation is treated by countershock. Ventricular arrhythmias are treated with lidocaine and procainamide in usual doses. Pacing is employed aggressively in an attempt to regularize rhythm.

Although cardiac arrhythmias are frequent in the immediate posttransplantation period and recur with rejection episodes (Bieber and co-workers), it is unusual that ventricular fibrillation or arrest occurs except as terminal events. There is continued caution, however, in the administration of norepinephrine as there is an altered sensitivity and the usual baroreceptor damper on rate is not effective (Potter and co-workers; Willman and co-workers). There remains some controversy as to the effect of digitalis on the denervated heart and the toxic manifestation of this drug. To this time our experience suggests that it is not strikingly different from that in the normal heart. In those instances of cardiac arrest associated with anoxia or sepsis, the resuscitation of the hemografted heart differs in no important way from that of the normal innervated heart.

PART TEN

INCIDENCE AND CURRENT STATUS OF CARDIAC RESUSCITATION

Chapter 64

INCIDENCE AND RELATIVE IMPORTANCE OF CARDIAC ARREST

Since the first edition of this book (1958), a number of reports have concerned themselves with the relative frequency of cardiac arrest. It is interesting to note a study in 1962 by Stephens (division of anesthesia at the Duke University Medical Center) entitled "Cardiac Arrest is on the Decline." This careful study, although limited to one institution, does lend some general encouragement. During the period from 1950 to 1960, there were 164 operating room–related cardiac arrests occurring in 118,552 patients at the Duke University Hospital. This figure alone would hardly indicate that cardiac arrest is declining in frequency. When anesthesia was implicated, the incidence was 1:1,669. This was compared with a figure of 1:1,147 that concerned a 12-year period from 1930 to 1943. The incidence of anesthesia-related cardiac standstill was recorded as having declined from 1:1,062 in 1950 to 1:3,774 in 1959. The total number of cardiac standstills did not vary appreciably over the 10-year period. A recent report from the Peter Bent Brigham Hospital covering a 5-month period cited an incidence of one case of cardiac arrest in every thirty-seven admissions. Most of these cases represented closed-chest resuscitation attempts on the ward (Himmelhoch).

At the Miriam Hospital of Providence, Rhode Island, twenty cases of cardiac arrest during 29,716 operations were recorded during the 6-year period, 1955 to 1960. This is an incidence of one per 1,485. Five of these cases of arrest occurred outside the operating room, two in the elevator.

The incidence of sudden cardiac arrest during a 5-year period at the St. Francis Hospital of Hartford, Connecticut, has been the subject of a study by Martin (director of the anesthesia department and school of anesthesiology). A total of twenty cases of sudden cardiac arrest occurred in a series of 83,442 anesthesias. This is an incidence of one per 4,172. Nine of the cardiac arrests represented permanent survivals.

Twenty-seven cardiac arrests occurred in 63,307 surgical procedures (1:2,344) at the St. Anthony Hospital in Oklahoma City from January, 1953 to January, 1960 (Ferris and Taylor).

A review of 300 fatal cases of cardiac arrest in various South African public hospitals discloses that a considerable increase in the instance of cardiac arrest occurred between 1950 and 1960. Three reasons are suggested:

1. More operations are being performed on bad risk and moribund patients.
2. Cardiac surgery is being done on such a wide scale that ventricular fibrillation and asystole have become quite commonplace.
3. Lastly, it is believed that the anesthesiologist must still share considerable blame in that anesthesia training has, in some instances, not kept pace with the modern methods employed.

From the Illinois Research Hospital in Chicago, a cardiac arrest incidence of 1:1,200 operations is noted. Over a 4-year period, there were eleven such cases in 13,000 operations. During a 28-month period from July, 1948, to October, 1950, at the University of Minnesota Hospitals, there were 12,000 surgical operations done under anesthesia. In this group there were fourteen fatalities listed as cardiac arrests. At the New York Hospital in 1952, six cases of cardiac arrest in 10,000 operations were reported. In the Los Angeles

County Hospital, from July 1, 1946, to April 1, 1948, there were forty-six deaths in approximately 28,000 patients who were given anesthetics, or a ratio of 1:608 patients. This includes all cases of cardiac arrest.

Hosler cited a town of 60,000 population in which there were eighteen operating room cardiac arrests in a 190-bed hospital during a period of 17 months. It is interesting to note that personnel well trained in anesthesia were available at all times. Hinchey reported the occurrence of four cases of cardiac arrest within a 6-month period in a 250-bed community hospital. Bonica reported an incidence of thirteen cases from a total number of 64,400 patients who were given anesthetics during the years 1945 to 1950. Dr. Frank Lahey estimated several years ago that the Lahey Clinic had approximately two cases of cardiac arrest per operating suite per year. Cooley noted an incidence of forty-eight cases of cardiac arrest in 878 operations for pulmonic stenosis at the Johns Hopkins Hospital. This was an incidence of 1:18.

Although many hospital centers have reported an incidence of cardiac arrest as high as 1:1,000, some have had very little experience with the problem. Waltman Walters of the Mayo Clinic states that in 28 years of surgery he witnessed only two cases of cardiac arrest on his surgical service, both during exploration of the common bile duct. During his many busy years of orthopedic surgery, Dr. J. Albert Key of St. Louis had never had a patient with cardiac arrest. Dr. Potts stated in 1953 that he had never encountered a case of cardiac arrest in over 500 operations on the heart in children.

From the Grace–New Haven Hospital in New Haven, Connecticut, Turk and Glenn report that a diagnosis of cardiac arrest was made a total of forty-five times in forty-four patients during a 5-year period from December, 1948, to January, 1954. They did not state the total number of operations performed but mentioned that the incidence approximated one case of cardiac arrest for every 1,900 operations performed. At Stan-

ford University Hospital, twenty-four cases of cardiac arrest have been recorded from a total of 48,829 operations. This represents an incidence of 1:2,035 operations.

The experience of the Massachusetts General Hospital is reported by Briggs, who collected the cases of cardiac arrest at the institution. He concluded that the incidence of cardiac arrest was approximately one case in every 1,200 anesthetics administered there. About 16,000 to 18,000 anesthetics are given there each year. During the period from 1951 to 1953, there were thirty-nine cases of cardiac arrest. Eleven additional cases were found in a somewhat longer period from 1946 to 1950. From Memphis, Tennessee, Bowers was able to find but four cases of cardiac arrest from a group of 39,509 operations. An incidence of one case of cardiac arrest in every 1,200 patients subjected to anesthesia in surgery was noted by West after studying the cases occurring at St. Luke's Hospital in New York City. There were thirty cases of cardiac arrest over a period of 7 years from a group of 35,000 patients.

The Los Angeles Children's Hospital reports twenty-three cases of cardiac arrest in a 20-year period (1932 to 1952) during the course of 57,600 consecutive operations. This is an incidence of one arrest in 2,504 operations. Since fourteen of the cases occurred during the last five-year period, the incidence for this period would be one case in 1,128 operations. This is an increase of almost four times the previous 5-year period and almost twice the previous 15-year period.

The Children's Hospital of Carlton, Melbourne, Australia, reported that they had had sixteen cases of cardiac arrest. This represented an incidence of slightly over one case in 1,500 anesthetics. Of the 25,000 anesthetics administered, 7,500 were given for tonsillectomies and tooth extractions, 5,000 during minor casualty procedures, and 1,000 during minor ward procedures.

Dotter and Jackson report that the incidence of death following angiocardiography seems to be significantly increased in children.

Casten and Bardenstein have reported thirty-seven cases of cardiac arrest occurring in the 25-year period from January 1, 1930, to January 1, 1955, at the Hospital for Joint Diseases. This was an incidence of one case per 2,617 anesthetics. Seven cases occurred in children under 10 years of age (19%). It was believed that this figure was significant because children make up less than 10% of the total number of patients who were administered anesthetics at this hospital.

Although further comments on cardiac arrest and resuscitation in the pediatric patient appear throughout this book, it is important that the frequency of cardiac arrest in the pediatric patient be realized.

In a 6-year review of acute circulatory failures in the operating rooms of the University of Kansas Medical Center, Oktawiec included seventy-three cases. This was an incidence of one death in every 559 cases. (There were 40,877 cases under anesthesia from 1948 to 1953.) All of the deaths could not be attributed to cardiac arrest. Oktawiec states, however, that "cardiac arrest far exceeded the peripheral circulatory failure in incidence."

Dr. Seymour Cole has been quoted as saying the a case of cardiac arrest occurs within the area of the city of Los Angeles daily. During the first year of the University of Missouri Medical Center there was an incidence of one case per 700 anesthesias (100% were successfully resuscitated).

In summary then, it would seem that although there is considerable variation in the incidence of cardiac arrest among certain selected hospitals and among certain selected groups of patients, the general overall frequency of cardiac arrest can be expected to be relatively uniform throughout the country. Certainly it would seem, from the data available, that the magnitude of the problem becomes readily apparent. I would agree with Sealy's statement, "Sudden cardiac arrest constitutes one of the chief hazards of surgery today."

Frequency of cardiac arrest

Because of an increasing interest in the problems of cardiac arrest and resuscitation, it is frequently asked: "Is cardiac arrest actually increasing in frequency?" It is difficult to indicate statistically an increase or decrease in the incidence of cardiac arrest. It is apparent, however, that the indications for cardiac resuscitation have so enlarged, especially since the employment of closed-chest resuscitation, that resuscitation attempts are much more frequent. One finds throughout the country periodic sessions devoted to cardiac arrest in meetings of various hospital staffs, county medical societies, and state and national medical societies, including most of the specialty groups. The American Heart Association has steadfastly shown an interest. The American Board of Surgery and The American Board of Anesthesiology have included questions relating to cardiac arrest and resuscitation among those asked of prospective board diplomates. Various postgraduate courses on resuscitation are being taught. Clinical and laboratory research on cardiac arrest is being conducted at centers throughout the country. Because of the interest in the problem, one would surmise that the problem has become somewhat more acute. Some of the interest may be accounted for in an increasing awareness that cardiac asystole or ventricular fibrillation represents reversible pathology and that large numbers of patients can be successfully resuscitated.

Illustrations of cases of cardiac arrest occurring under many different conditions are noted throughout this book. Perhaps the reader will be impressed, as I am, by the obvious need for physicians to be versed in resuscitative procedure.

Incidence of cardiac arrest in the operating room

In spite of more sophisticated methods of monitoring and newer anesthetic agents and preventive measures, the incidence of cardiac arrest in the operating room continues relatively high. In fact, Jude (1970) reports fourteen such cases occurring in the operating room in a total of 17,023 operations performed over a 12-month period—an incidence of 1:1,216. Although Jude indicates that the incidence of cardiac arrest in the operating room may be higher today than 10 years ago, he suggests that perhaps, brief episodes of bradycardia or asystole may be treated by nonoperative external cardiac massage and not recorded. It is interesting that he records an incidence of 64% for ventricular fibrillation encountered in the operating room during cardiac arrest whereas a previous incidence of only 13% was recorded in the first 1,200 cases of cardiac arrest reported by us in 1953.

In Jude's series, 43% or six of fourteen patients having cardiac arrest in the operating room were successfully resuscitated and discharged. In four of the fourteen patients open-chest cardiac massage was the eventual or primary approach to resuscitation.

Although one may get the impression that resuscitation efforts are predominantly encountered on medical words and among patients with myocardial infarction, chronic lung disease, and heart failure, 30% of the cardiac arrests experienced over a 6-year period at the Hospital of the Good Samaritan Medical Center in Los Angeles were among patients directly under the care of a surgeon (Stiles).

Sex incidence of cardiac arrest

Whereas in our earlier series the distribution between male and female was often inconclusive, most hospital series show approximately two thirds of the arrest group to be males. Much of this probably stems from the fact that coronary artery disease is principally an affliction of males. Many coronary care units report three times as many males admitted as females. In the statistical study presented in the first edition of this book, a preponderance of cardiac arrest in males was noted; 38.8% were women and 61.2% were men (a ratio of 1:1.5). Of the black patients, forty-three were women and seventy-five were men, a ratio of 1:1.7. That this higher incidence in the male population may be significant is indicated from a study of the Metropolitan Life Insurance figures of the sex incidence in operations as a whole. These figures show that a slightly higher percentage of women undergo surgery than do men.

In the first decade of life, in which almost one fourth of all cardiac arrests occurs, the percentages of each sex are almost identical to those above.

Although not concerned with cardiac arrest deaths alone, but with anesthetic deaths in general, Beecher and Todd in their report on anesthetic deaths occurring during 599,000 operations reported that the male-female relationship of anesthetic deaths are just the reverse of the sexes' representation within the hospital population. They noted that males constitute 58% of all anesthetic deaths occurring in their series, although the male patient represents only 43% of a sample surgical population at any one time.

The Bureau of Medical Economic Research of the American Medical Association has released some rather significant figures. Of the number of patients in all reporting hospitals on a given day, only 46.8% of the patients in the survey were women. In nongovernmental general hospitals, 59.5% of the patients were women. The large numbers of male patients in Veterans Administration and military hospitals were responsible for greatly altering this last percentage. (In the United States women comprise 50.3% of the population.)

Most studies reported since the first edition of this book (more than 15 years ago) continue to indicate that both cardiac asystole and ventricular fibrillation are encountered almost twice as often in men as in women. In some series, the ratio is as high as 4:1 (Greenberg). Chrocca reviews twelve cases of successful resuscitation after myocardial infarction and reports that the ratio of men to women who have myocardial infarction is nearly 6:1.

Age incidence of cardiac arrest

With the extension of cardiopulmonary resuscitative efforts to the patient suddenly developing cardiac arrest and in association with a myocardial infarct, there has been an almost complete reversal in the age incidence. Today, in most large series the average patient requiring cardiopulmonary resuscitation is a male in the mid to late fifties or early sixties. The unusually high incidence of cardiac arrest in the first decade of life as seen in the operating room has been diluted down to a point of relative insignificance.

Although the somewhat surprising incidence of cardiac arrest in the first decade of life, as pointed out in the first edition of this book (Fig. 64-1), was repeatedly confirmed by other statistical studies, for example, 20% of West's cases occurred in the first decade, this related to the era before resuscitation on myocardial infarction patients.

At one time it seemed apparent that an unusually large number of cardiac arrest cases was being reported in patients during the first decade of life. After the first 1,200 cases in an early statistical study had been tabulated and a breakdown into the various decades of life had been charted, the surprising age distribution of cardiac arrest cases was even more apparent. Twenty-one percent, or more than one fifth, of the 1,200 cases of cardiac arrest took place within the first 10 years of life.

It appeared that perhaps these patients represented the large group of individuals upon whom surgery is performed for congenital heart disease. A breakdown from this aspect was carried out, and only 2% to 3% could be attributed to surgical cases of a cardiac nature. (Some time ago, a children's hospital in Australia reported thirty-two cases, none of which was related to operations upon the heart.)

Beecher and Todd reported a study of anesthetic deaths occurring in ten large teaching centers. They state:

The anesthesia death percentage is disproportionately high in the first decade of life. This indicates a great need for an attack on the anesthesia problems of infants and children.*

They do not mention the number of anesthetic deaths that were considered as cardiac arrest cases. They do speculate on why such a high death rate is present in children by stating: "Perhaps their immature

*Beecher, H. K., and Todd, D. P.: A study of the deaths associated with anesthesia and surgery, Ann. Surg. **140**:2-35, 1954.

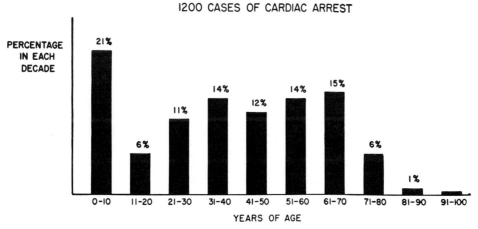

Fig. 64-1. Graph illustrating that cardiac arrest is particularly prone to occur in the first decade of life. (From Stephenson, H. E., Jr., Reid, L. C., and Hinton, J. W.: Ann. Surg. **137**: 731, 1953.)

organs are less able to withstand the stress of anesthesia than are those of healthy young adults. Doubtless, problems of ventilation are involved."

Several years ago, the Anesthetic Study Commission of the Philadelphia County Medical Society found that the relative number of preventable deaths occurring in the age group from 1 to 20 years exceeded that found in the group over 50 years of age. This was from a study of the fatalities occurring during anesthesia in that area that included cases of cardiac arrest.

A study of fifty cases of cardiac arrest from the Massachusetts General Hospital, occurring during periods from 1946 to 1950 and from 1951 to 1953, showed an age distribution considerably different than in other studies that I have noted. Seventy-six percent of the arrests occurred in patients 51 years of age or older.

Thus, with an increased shift in emphasis to the myocardial infarction patient, the previous figures have been considerably altered.

Pediatric aspects of cardiac arrest and resuscitation

The sudden, unexplained death of the infant and young child has become of increasing relative importance with the concomitant decline of infant deaths from infections and other known etiologic agents. Each year the Armed Forces Institute of Pathology receives more than 5,000 pediatric autopsy specimens. Stowens studied the material from over 700 sudden or unexpected deaths over a 4-year period while at the Armed Forces Institute of Pathology. These cases did not include children who gave any antecedent history of an infection of any kind. They were all in an apparent state of good health at the last moment preceding death. Although the pediatric material studied varied throughout the pediatric age scale, the cases of sudden or unexpected death was most common between the ages of 1 month and 6 months. The peak occurred in the fourth month. The incidence

was twice as high among boys as among girls. A distinct disease entity was found in only 15% of the 700 cases studied. In the remaining 85%, the only abnormal findings related to the lungs and consisted of generalized overexpansion of the alveoli and pulmonary edema.

In attempting to explain the age distribution of cardiac arrest, Hinton and associates offered the following:

In children, it is most important to remember that they have highly sensitive reflexes. This is pointedly demonstrated by the response of the sinus node to respiration and its influence upon cardiac rhythm; the reflexes are more readily evoked as a result. With increasing age this sensitivity gradually decreases and at the same time the incidence of cardiac arrest lessens. In the older age group, the explanation might well be lesions in the specific tissue rendering the heart increasingly vulnerable to vagal stimulation. The ventricular specific tissue is more depressed under these conditions in originating stimulus formations under the influence of anesthetic agents. At such times an undesirable reflex is not so likely nor is such a reflex readily set up; nevertheless, when it does occur, it is more serious and more obvious than the case is in the younger age periods, where more reactive ventricular specific tissue is present.[*]

In an editorial comment on these findings in the British journal *Lancet,* it was pointed out that partial explanation would be on the grounds that the margin of error for both surgery and anesthesia is slighter and more difficult to assess in the young than in the adult. It is true that a sizable number of patients included were those who had been operated upon for congenital heart disease, but these did not constitute an unduly significant number.

In 1952 I was prompted to review all operative cases in Bellevue Hospital of New York City to see if an approximation of the percentage of cases of patients 10 years of age or under needing surgery could be made. Bellevue is a 3,000-bed hospital. In 1952 there were 13,600 operations performed, of

---

[*]Hinton, J. W., Stephenson, H. E., Jr., and Reid, L. C.: Prevention of cardiac arrest, Am. Surg. **18:** 934, 1952.

which 1,100 were on patients 10 years of age or under. The percentage of operations on patients 10 years or under was 8% of the total. When compared with the instance of 21% of cases of cardiac arrest occurring in patients under 10 years of age, it was thought that this might be statistically significant.

Negovskii is of the opinion that the younger the organism, the easier is the revival of its heart. He points to the 1902 experiment of Kuliabko, who revived the heart of a child 20 hours after death and made it beat. Kountz noted that in the perfusion technique of revival of the human heart after prolonged periods of arrest following death, a more responsive heart was present in children than in adults. This is elaborated on elsewhere.

A small portion of the increased incidence of cardiac arrest in the pediatric patient results from the frequency of cardiac operations on congenitally malformed hearts. That an increased number of cardiovascular procedures would constitute a subsequent increase in cardiac arrest deaths is not justified by recalling the figure of Potts. He stated that he did not encounted a single case of cardiac arrest during the first 500 operations for congenital heart disease in infants.

Many smaller reports have testified to the disproportionate number of cardiac arrest deaths in children under 10 years of age. West reported seven from his group of thirty cardiac arrests. Interestingly enough, all of his seven cases were noted not to have had any preoperative medication.

Gross states:

Children who come to operation excited and poorly prepared may not only suffer real emotional complications, but carry a definitely higher rate of morbidity and mortality. Respiratory irregularities, aspiration of vomitus, convulsions, and cardiac arrest all occur more frequently in patients who have inadequate preparation and a stormy induction.*

---

*Gross, R. E.: The surgery of infancy and childhood, Philadelphia, 1953, W. B. Saunders Co., p. 40.

Documentation over a 10-year period of the frequency of cardiac arrest in infants and children is provided by Rockow and co-workers from the Columbia-Presbyterian Medical Center. The frequency of cardiac arrest during anesthesia in infants less than 1 year of age is significantly higher than in children 1 to 12 years of age or in adults 13 years of age and older. Similarly, the incidence of cardiac arrest for all children, including infants, is significantly higher than is the rate for adults. In infants, one cardiac arrest occurred in every 600 cases. The higher frequency of cardiac arrest in infants could not be correlated with any other factor in the total management of anesthesia.

Greenberg reports 33% of cardiac arrests occurring after operation or anesthesia to be in infants or children. Rakon reports the highest incidence to be in infants less than 1 year of age. It is apparent that the figures relative to age incidence of cardiac arrest during surgery and under anesthesia are considerably different than those pertaining to patients outside the operating and recovery rooms. These cases, which occur in such places as the medical wards, outside the hospital, or in the clinics, reflect a high incidence of sudden arrest in patients with acquired coronary artery disease.

In Altemeier's series of forty-three patients, 35% were in the first decade of life.

Incidence in good-risk versus poor-risk patients

I have been so often impressed with the frequency with which cardiac arrest is seen in the apparently healthy individual that the words of Effler and Sifers are worth quoting:

In our experience cardiac arrest has occurred more often in the good risk patient than in the so-called bad risk person who is being subjected to a surgical procedure. This is an important observation on the principal causes of cardiac cessation which have been discussed. When a poor risk patient is brought to surgery, meticuluous care is used in the selection of anesthesia agents and he is closely scrutinized during the induction and subsequent course of anesthetic administration. Usually such a patient is subjected to the least amount of trauma and blood loss and is invariably given the benefit of a high supplementary oxygen intake. It is undoubtedly the combination of careful observation and basic precautions which eliminate the causative factors of cardiac arrest in these cases. The higher mortality rate associated with the poor risk patient is explained on complications other than true cardiac arrest. It is for this reason that the tragic sequela to cardiac arrest in the so-called good risk patient must be kept in mind by all who practice surgery and anesthesiology. Until we are willing to accept the precursors of cardiac arrest as avoidable errors attributable directly to the anesthetist and surgeon there is little possibility that this dreaded accident will be eliminated from the list of operating room complications.*

It is interesting that six of the seven patients experiencing cardiac arrest at the Hospital for Joint Diseases, New York City, were considered to be in good condition, no evidence of factors that might increase the operative risk being present. This fact prompted Casten and Bardenstein to state:

This would indicate that there are intangible factors of nutrition, electrolyte and water balance, vitamin depletion, and perhaps, chronic mild degrees of respiratory acidosis which escape detection by ordinary or routine methods of clinical and laboratory examination. These conditions, commonly overlooked, may assume a degree of danger when anesthesia and surgical stress are added. In the light of experience, a more careful evaluation of risk by anesthesiologists and surgeons becomes mandatory.†

The preoperative condition of the patient will have some bearing on the incidence of cardiac arrest. However, it will play a much smaller part than would be generally supposed. From the Anesthesia Study Commission of the Philadelphia County Medical Society, a discussion of the preoperative conditions of the patient dying during anesthesia, including cases of cardiac arrest, listed 229 patients whose preoperative con-

dition had been described. One hundred seventy-three, or 58%, of the group were listed as being in good or fair condition preoperatively. Only 42% were listed as being poor preoperative risks.

In the statistical study presented in the first edition of this book, the following points were noted: (1) 415 patients had known preexisting heart disease, or only 28.7%; (2) over 24% of all 1,710 cases were in patients below 10 years of age; (3) the remaining group was quite similar to the average preoperative patients seen anywhere.

Therefore it seems apparent to us that undue attention need not be centered on the poor-risk patient. The patient with no previous history of heart disease and with almost no additional disease is perhaps just as likely to be a candidate for cardiac arrest.

Where cardiac arrest is likely to occur

A considerable percentage of all cases in which a sudden failure of the propulsive force of the heart occurs will be encountered in the operating room. It should be emphasized, however, that accidents of a cardiorespiratory nature that respond to resuscitation are not limited to the operating room. In the delivery room, asphyxia of the newborn infant requires prompt resuscitative therapy. Sudden death in the home, in industry, from inhalation of noxious gases, and other accidents represents a situation requiring knowledge of the resuscitative procedure. This knowledge may well make the difference between life and death.

In our original statistical study, cardiac arrests were encountered outside the operating room in 14.2% of cases. A prognostic relationship of those cases occurring outside the operating room as related to those within the operating room is discussed in a later chapter. It is obvious that in planning for the eventuality of cardiac arrest one must consider all areas of the hospital, including the x-ray department, the emergency room, and the wards. The largest num-

---

*Effler, D. B., and Sifers, E. C.: Cardiac arrest, Cleve. Clin. Q. 19:194-203, 1952.
†Casten, D. F., and Bardenstein, M.: Cardiac arrest in children, Bull. Hosp. Joint Dis. 16:13-21, 1955.

ber of cardiac arrests occurring outside the operating room were those on the ward or in patients' rooms. Of these, there were eighty-four. In addition, there were twenty-four in the x-ray department, eighteen in the emergency room, twelve in the bronchoscopy room, ten in the receiving room, six in the cardiac physiology laboratory, six on stretchers, six in the hall of the hospital, and five in the delivery room.

Several years ago, a physician sent us the record of a case of cardiac arrest that occurred in his office during a tonsillectomy on a 9-year-old boy. Prompt recognition of the absence of circulation and prompt application of manual systole resulted in restoration of spontaneous heart action and rapid recovery of the patient without subsequent neurologic sequelae. I am aware of successful resuscitation having occurred in the x-ray department, in the obstetric division, in the emergency room, in the cardiac physiology laboratory, and in almost every location in which cardiac arrest may be encountered (even outside of the hospital). Therefore it does not seem reasonable to confine our consideration entirely to those cases seen in the operating room. At present, success may be expected more often in the operating room; but, as the resuscitative procedure becomes a part of the armamentarium of every physician, whether he be an obstetrician, a general practitioner, an ophthalmologist, a radiologist, or otherwise, the scope of resuscitative success will enlarge.

Forty-two attempts at cardiac resusitation were reported from the Grace–New Haven Hospital. There were twenty that occurred outside the operating room, a total of over 47% of all cases; three were performed in an ambulance, two in the emergency room, two in the cardiac catheterization room, one in the x-ray room, one in the constant temperature room, one in the recovery room, and ten in patients' rooms.

During the last several years, the ability of the physician to apply resusitative measures has increased, and an accompanying rise in the indications for cardiac resuscitation has resulted. The resuscitative procedure is no longer confined to the operating room or its immediate vicinity or, for that matter, even to the limits of the hospital. As a matter of fact, 77% of a recent series of sixty-five cases was encountered on the wards (Himmelhoch).

Beck and associates added another case to this group, which we have summarized.

A 65-year-old physician suddenly collapsed as he was leaving the hospital, June 22, 1955. Earlier that day an ECG had been made which was consistent with "early posterolateral myocardial infarction." The ECG had been prompted by recent episodes of precordial distress. At the time of the physician's collapse, respirations ceased and resuscitative measures were instituted—artificial respiration, oxygen with a face mask, and needle puncture of the heart. Four minutes after his collapse, the chest was opened and the heart was found to be in ventricular fibrillation. Defibrillation was accomplished only after repeated shocks to the myocardium. The next morning the patient made a few conscious responses but did not speak. He did show marked improvement the following day—talking and moving his extremities. Improvement progressed despite periods of disorientation, confusion, and excitement. At the end of 11 days, he was discharged from the hospital, although a minor infection of the medial end of the incision was present. The infection involved the costal cartilage. We understand that the physician is again practicing medicine.

Cardiac arrest in obstetrics and gynecology

In an effort to focus attention on cardiac arrest and resuscitation by obstetricians and gynecologists, Cavanagh and co-workers reviewed their 5-years' experience. They report ten cases of cardiac arrest among 28,949 deliveries and 5,048 gynecologic operations. Four of the arrests were in obstetric patients (one in 7,207) and six were in gynecologic patients (one in 840).

Figures available on the relative incidence of arrest in obstetric patients indicate considerably less frequency than in patients involved with other operative and anesthetic procedures. In fact, Gold estimates that cardiac arrest in the obstetric patient is thirty-five to forty times less frequent than in the average patient undergoing operative or anesthetic procedures. He studied 614 maternal deaths reported in New York City from January 1, 1953, through December 31, 1958, from a total of 1,116,802 deliveries. An incidence of one fatal cardiac arrest per 79,772 deliveries resulted. Following is a breakdown of the incidence of maternal deaths in cardiac arrest from Gold's study.

62.0 maternal deaths per 100,000 live births
55.0 maternal deaths per 100,000 deliveries*
  1.4 cardiac arrests per 100,000 live births
  1.3 cardiac arrests per 100,000 deliveries*
  2.3 cardiac arrests per   100 maternal deaths

1 maternal death per   1,614 live births
1 maternal death per   1,819 deliveries*
1 cardiac arrest per 70,787 live births
1 cardiac arrest per 79,772 deliveries*
1 cardiac arrest per 44 maternal deaths†

Cardiac arrests encountered were only 2.28% of all maternal deaths. The explanation for the relatively low incidence of cardiac arrest in the obstetric patient does not seem entirely because of the favorable age group and physical status of the obstetric patient nor to the duration and type of anesthetic agent.

During a 7-year period, the Michigan Maternity Mortality Study (1950 to 1957) recorded 987 maternal deaths from direct obstetric, indirect obstetric, and nonrelated causes. Four of the surviving infants from this series were delivered following cardiac arrest of the mother after spinal anesthesia. The likelihood of delivering a live infant by cesarean section after death of the mother is moderately good. Approximately 150 successes have been recorded. In the maternal

mortality study referred to (Behney), out of seventy-two infants delivered by postmortem cesarean section, eleven survived and were discharged from the hospital. Of these children, thirty-four were stillborn and thirty-eight were alive when delivered but died shortly after birth.

The question of how long the infant can survive following cessation of all cardiac output in the mother has never been satisfactorily answered. It does seem apparent, however, that the fetus in utero is capable of withstanding a relatively anoxic environment for considerably longer times than the 4-minute period ordinarily observed in live born infants. A follow-up of eleven children who survived cesarean section after death of the mother (Behney) revealed that all children were living, well, and apparently normal from 3 to 8½ years of age.

At the one hundred and ninth annual meeting of the American Medical Association, a symposium on fatalities in the operating room was held by the Sections on Obstetrics and Gynecology. Ferguson commented on the increasing frequency of cardiac arrest during vaginal deliveries, cesarean section, and gynecologic procedures. In the 3 years prior to 1961, he stated that he had seen more cases of cardiac arrest than in all the years before. The precise explanation for this increase was not revealed.

CARDIAC ARREST FOLLOWING ARTIFICIAL RUPTURE OF THE MEMBRANES

To Dr. E. V. McKay of London, I am indebted for the report of an interesting case of cardiac arrest occurring at the time of artificial rupture of the membranes.

The patient was a 20-year-old Caucasian female in her thirty-fourth week of pregnancy. A diagnosis of anencephalic fetus had been made and artificial rupture of the membranes was elected. There was no history of previous cardiac pathology and during the rupture of the membranes the patient received self-administered trichloroethylene (Trilene) analgesia. No premedication had been thought necessary. The procedure was being carried out in the operating room. Shortly after the

---

*Live births plus fetal deaths (all periods of gestation).
†Gold, E. M.: Cardiac arrest in obstetrics, Clin. Obstet. Gynecol. **3:**114-130, 1960.

membranes had been ruptured the patient was noted to be cyanotic. Respirations had ceased and a diagnosis of cardiac arrest was made. It was estimated that probably a period of 5 minutes had passed since the onset of cardiac arrest. The pupils were widely dilated. Artificial respiration was begun and intermittent cardiac compression was carried out through the transdiaphragmatic route at a rate of 90 per minute. The heart was found to be in complete standstill and responded to cardiac massage. Intravenous administration of 1 ml. of 1:1,000 epinephrine hydrochloride by the intravenous route as well as 5 ml. of 2% procaine intravenously was carried out. In addition, atropine sulfate, 0.5 mg. (gr. 1/100) was also given. The heart was resuscitated, but the patient died within 5 hours. Autopsy did not reveal any significant findings that might have accounted for the sudden death of this patient. In commenting on the case, it was felt that the delay in instituting cardiac massage may have been accentuated by the absence of resuscitative anesthetic apparatus immediately available. Cardiac action returned temporarily after a period of 30 minutes of intermittent massage.

CARDIAC ARREST DURING
RUBIN TEST FOR PREGNANCY

As a test for tubal patency, the Rubin test is frequently done in the physician's office as a diagnostic procedure and is seldom associated with complications. There have been reported, however, four cases that were associated with the Rubin test for tubal patency. Bonica cites the case of a sudden death occurring during air insufflation of the fallopian tubes in such a test. At autopsy, the pulmonary artery and right side of the heart were found to have massive air emboli.

During the course of a combination Rubin test for pregnancy and a dilatation and curettage under cyclopropane and ether, a sudden cardiac arrest occurred in a 32-year-old female patient. A thoracotomy was immediately performed and the heart was compressed at a rapid rate of between 80 and 100 times a minute. The heart was found to be in ventricular fibrillation and was successfully defibrillated using a current of 1.5 amperes. Fibrillation was not present at the time of the thoracotomy but followed a short period of manual massage. It was estimated that approximately 4 minutes or more passed before the thoracotomy was performed. The patient's postresuscitation period was stormy. Marked hyperventilation was present during the first 16 hours. Twenty hours after the arrest, the patient showed some signs of response. Electrocardiograms appeared to be within normal limits on the first, seventh, and twentieth postoperative days. Despite antibiotics, the patient developed a subcutaneous wound infection and a thoracentesis was done to remove some remaining fluid in the chest. In spite of possible damage from the cerebral anoxia, the patient showed no mental or emotional abnormalities 6 months later. She appeared to be normal in every respect. (Reported by Johnson and Kirby.)

The problem of air embolism and cardiac resuscitation is discussed elsewhere in detail.

PULMONARY EMBOLISM BY
AMNIOTIC FLUID

A discussion of this interesting aspect of obstetrics is included elsewhere. It should be obvious that cardiac arrest may occur in patients undergoing all types of surgery or under any anesthetic technique.

Dentistry and cardiac arrest

In England each year approximately 1.3 million general anesthetics are given for dental treatment, almost all being administered in the dental chair. The overall mortality is very low, amounting to some 5 to 10 deaths in each year, or about 1 in 130,000 (Melotte).

In discussing closed-chest massage and the technique to be employed by the dentist, Melotte suggests that the dentist first identify with his fingertips the suprasternal notch between the clavicle and the xiphisternum at the decussation of the ribs. These two points mark the upper and lower ends of the sternum, over the lower third of which the dentist places the heel of one hand, locking the second over his wrists. Accurate location of the presser hand is vital to success and safety and it should be maintained in extension at the wrist so that pressure is limited to the sternum and is not spread out over the ribs. Rising on his knees so that his shoulders are directly over the patient and his arms are straight, he then uses his weight to depress momentarily the sternum at least 4 cm. in an adult, proportionately less in a child. The whole maneuver is carried out by a rocking movement, lasts about ½ second and is repeated 5 times.

The Indiana University School of Medicine and Dentistry reports the incidence of arrhythmias during 103 consecutive oral surgical procedures involving single or multiple tooth extractions performed in an outpatient clinic (Fisch and associates). All of the patients received methohexital sodium (Brevital) and halothane–nitrous oxide–oxygen anesthesia. Cardiac arrhythmias were recorded in 44 (42.7%) of the 103 procedures. In 32 instances, unifocal or multifocal ventricular premature systoles, ventricular bigeminy, ventricular tachycardia, or chaotic rhythms were documented.

Over 117 years have passed since the first report of a case of sudden death in a dental patient under anesthesia. The *Boston Medical and Surgical Journal* of 1852 editorialized on a case of sudden death under chloroform during an extraction. This, perhaps, was the first case of cardiac arrest during the extraction of teeth.

The dental profession has shown increasing interest in knowledge of resusitative procedures (Selden and Recant) and in all aspects of cardiac arrest and resuscitation. Numerous editorials on cardiac arrest and resuscitation have appeared in dental journals (Kay). Several surveys have been made to determine the number of deaths occurring under dental anesthesia. Selden and Recant report six deaths in one million general anesthetics administered for dental purposes in the city of New York during the period from 1943 to 1952.

Instruction in cardiopulmonary resuscitation is already a part of the curriculum at several dental schools. A technique for re-

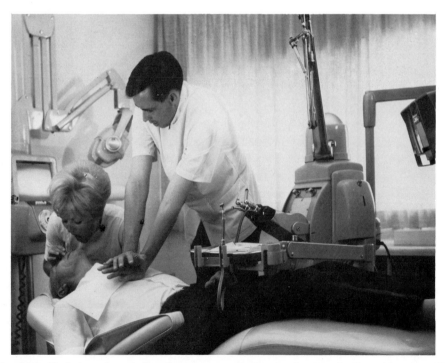

Fig. 64-2. Technique for cardiopulmonary resuscitation in the dental office. (Courtesy The American Dental Association.)

suscitation in the dental office is shown in Fig. 64-2.

American Heart Association state committees on cardiopulmonary resuscitation include members of the dental profession.

Cardiac arrest related to otorhinolaryngologic procedures

Surgery of the nose, throat, esophagus, and bronchus provides optimal conditions for vagal stimulation leading to cardiac arrest—especially when associated with hypercapnia, acidosis, and anoxia. The precise incidence of cardiac arrest in the field of otorhinolaryngology is not known. Jude and Tabbarah reviewed the records over a 10-year period at the University of Miami Jackson Memorial Hospital and were able to find only three cases of cardiac arrest occurring in this specialty. In each instance the patient was successfully resuscitated. To avoid duplication, the reader is referred to the section on vagal reflexes and their relationship to the etiology of cardiac arrest where a detailed discussion of some of the otorhinolaryngologic procedures is included.

Concerned with the sudden cardiac arrest associated with adenotonsillectomy, Boatright and co-workers directed their attention to the accompanying aspiration and subsequent aspiration pneumonia. It is their opinion that an aspirant with a pH below 2.5 is the inciting factor that precedes the rapid onset of alveolar changes leading to pulmonary edema, atelectasis, hypoxia, and subsequent cardiac arrest. Accordingly, their program embodies preventive measures to avoid the acid aspiration syndrome. In their experience, glycopyrrolate (Robinul) has been a highly satisfactory drug to accomplish this. It is an anticholinergic drug that reduces the vagal hyperactivity and dries the pharynx. The action of the drug in inhibition of gastric secretion is prolonged over that of atropine or scopolamine. In addition they give an antacid along with glycopyrrolate 1 hour prior to surgery.

Cardiac arrest in cardiac surgery

The scope of cardiac surgery has widened enormously. With open-heart surgery, surgery under hypothermia, and with "elective cardiac asystole," the problems of cardiac resuscitation are faced almost daily in most of the active cardiac surgical centers. This aspect of cardiac arrest will be discussed at length elsewhere in this book.

Knowledge of cardiac resuscitation has done much to hasten the development of cardiac surgery. By the same token, considerable understanding of the arrested heart is being contributed by the cardiac surgeon, especially in the clinical application of defibrillation, elective arrest, and support of the failing myocardium.

The neurosurgeon and cardiac arrest

Cardiac arrest is statistically somewhat more common in neurosurgical patients than in several of the other surgical specialties. The general principles of resuscitation apply here as elsewhere, except that the nature of the pathology may have a bearing upon the train of events that should be followed in resuscitation. One such example is provided by Uihlein and associates. A 36-year-old man was being prepared for surgery. Just prior to the time he was to be moved to the operating room, spontaneous respiratory efforts ceased and the pupils dilated. The chest was opened and heart action was restored following manual compression. The entire lapse of time from the onset of arrest was only 2½ minutes. Because it was believed that a second cardiac arrest could arise from compression of the brainstem on the basis of increased intracranial pressure and because it was believed that the patient's space-occupying lesion should be removed at this time, the craniotomy was begun. First, however, hypothermia to 92° F. was induced.

Venous air embolism is occasionally seen in neurosurgical patients scheduled for elective craniotomies in the head-up position. Ericsson and associates report seven such cases, five of whom were treated successfully by closed-chest resuscitation.

The problem of cardiac resuscitation may, in some instances, be complicated by the upright position, as, for example, in patients undergoing suboccipital craniectomy.

Cardiac arrest on the ward

Himmelhoch and co-workers report on sixty-five resuscitative attempts at the Peter Bent Brigham Hospital in Boston; 77% of the cases were encountered on the wards. One of the very first cases of an attempt at cardiac resuscitation was made by Tuffier and Hallion in June, 1898. This case occurred on the ward of the hospital. The patient, a 24-year-old man, suddenly became pulseless and without respirations while in bed on the fifth postoperative day. The patient's chest was opened promptly by Tuffier, and prompt manual systole was begun. Spontaneous respirations appeared, as did the pulse, but only for a short time, and the patient expired. Particularly noteworthy are Tuffier's words when he observed:

I know that this observation does not demonstrate the effectiveness of rhythmical compression of the heart. I report this for what it is worth having no other desire but to call your attention to a practice which might perhaps be of some use.*

Although the controlled environment of the operating room makes for optimal conditions in cardiac resuscitation, Tuffier's prediction is becoming increasingly true, especially with widespread use of closed-chest resuscitation. Attempts to resuscitate the individual outside the operating room have been increasing and, with the application of sound resuscitative measures, the number of successful cases should also show the same increase. When one contemplates the many sites for cardiac resuscitation in the hospi-

tal area, then it is at once apparent that the interest in the resuscitative procedure should engage the medical profession as a whole.

Cardiac arrest during urologic procedures

The first case of cardiac arrest at the University of Missouri Medical Center occurred in a middle-aged black man during the introduction of a urethral catheter (this patient was successfully resuscitated by a surgical resident). In general, there are not many specific urologic problems related to cardiac arrest. Owen fails to find any direct correlation between ureteral catheterization and the production of extrasystole. Several sudden deaths following intravenous administration of iodopyracet (Diodrast) have been reported. At a nearby hospital, there were two cases of cardiac arrest during intravenous pyelographic studies.

Schmidlapp has called attention to the possible occurrence of respiratory and cardiac arrest in performing retrograde pyelography with opaque media containing neomycin, especially in patients under ether anesthesia and in children. Although respiratory arrest after intraperitoneal and intrapleural administration of neomycin has been reported, respiratory arrest following the use of opaque media containing neomycin in retrograde pyelography has now been documented. Schmidlapp also cautions against instilling neomycin into the bladder after a prostatectomy. In another case, Schmidlapp describes respiratory and cardiac arrest in a 1-year-old girl. A thoracotomy was performed, and cardiac resuscitation was accomplished after an infusion of 6M lactate was started and 5 ml. of 20% calcium gluconate was injected into the left ventricle. The effect of neomycin involving neuromuscular blockage is potentiated by anesthesia, particularly ether. Intravenous administration of calcium or neostigmine appear to be satisfactory counteractants of this complication of neomycin.

Woodward, in presenting a report to the

---

*Tuffier, T., et Hallion, M.: De la compression rhymie du coeur dans la syncope cardiaque par embolie, Bull. Mem. Soc. Chir. Paris 24:937-939, 1898.

Urological Society of Australia, reviews the specific urologic relationship to cardiac resuscitation.

Twidwell and Garsice (department of urology at Saint Louis Hospital in Minneapolis, Minnesota) provide an excellent review of some of the aspects of cardiac arrest occurring during urologic procedures.

Cardiac arrest as seen by the radiologist

Lampe reports a case of cardiac and respiratory arrest that resulted from the injection of Conray-400 into the ascending aorta. Eighty milliliters of Conray-400 was rapidly injected at a pressure of 700 pounds per square inch. Ten seconds after the injection, the patient became apneic and convulsed. The heart restarted after multiple blows to the precordium.

An excellent review on medical emergencies in the x-ray department is presented by Ansel and Ansel from England. Directed primarily to radiologists, the report emphasizes the importance of preparedness for such an emergency. They urge that the radiographer have an alarm system with which to summon immediate assistance without having to leave the patient.

Read, in discussing the cause of death in patients undergoing cardioangiography, emphasizes the increased risk of cardioangiography over less dangerous procedures. He cites the work of Pendergrass and associates, pointing to a mortality from intravenous pyelography of less than 1:150,000. Read states that the risk with cardioangiography is ten million times greater.

Arrests have occurred during an anteriogram of the femoral artery, during angiocardiography, during intravenous urograms, also during bronchograms, choledochograms, and even myelograms. They appear to have been associated with a drug sensitivity or a reflex inhibition of the heart in most instances. Cooper suggests regular premedication with atropine prior to myelographic studies. The table should be raised slowly.

Brown and co-workers report a successful case of cardiac resuscitation that began in an x-ray dark room and in which thoracotomy was done with a pen knife. This very interesting case illustrates the need for preparedness by all physicians, as it points out that cardiac arrest may occur anywhere and under various conditions.

Warrick extensively reviews the incidence of cardiac arrest in the x-ray department. Cooper warns against circulatory disturbances, including cardiac arrest, in patients on the myelographic tilt table. Resuscitation rates in the x-ray department are below what should ideally be expected.

Cardiac arrest as seen by the ophthalmologist

Cardiac arrest is by no means rare during procedures on and about the eye. Originally, in the Cardiac Arrest Registry there were sixteen cases of cardiac arrest in patients upon whom eye operations were being performed. These patients ranged from 2 to 81 years of age. Various anesthetic agents were used, including thiopental (Pentothal), curare, ether, vinyl ether (Vinethene), ethyl chloride, and local procaine. Of the sixteen cases studied, only one survived. Of the fifteen that died, nine had hearts that were temporarily restored to a normal rhythm, only to succumb several hours after resuscitative procedure. Subsequently, additional documentation of this frequency has made cardiac arrest a familiar hazard to the ophthalmologist.

Chapter 65

GUIDELINES FOR ABANDONING EFFORTS AT CARDIAC RESUSCITATION

At what point does life end? Is it when the heart stops while the brain still has the ability to function or is it when the brain dies but the heart still beats? The answer to the question is, of course, predicated upon several conditions. For example, how does one determine brain "death." The electroencephalogram has been used increasingly to help in this determination. In spite of its reliability, however, its interpretation must be made with caution in some instances. For example, in barbiturate intoxication, recovery after as long as 72 hours of "flat" EEG tracings has been known. The American Electroencephalographic Society suggests that in determining brain death serial tracings 24 hours apart should be utilized and both tracings must be absolutely flat at maximal gain. The tracings should be made with high quality, 8-channel equipment or monitoring devices in operation during the period of recording (which should ideally last 20 to 30 minutes). To be sure there is no machine error, the electrodes should be placed also on the head of the technician.

Hamlin at Massachusetts General Hospital proposes guidelines for signaling the "point of no return" in cardiac resuscitation in an effort to avoid protoplasmic resuscitation without clinical resuscitation. He mentions the following conditions:

1. Spontaneous respirations must have ceased for 1 hour
2. Absence of reflex responses
3. EEG tracings show a flat line with no rhythm in any leads for at least 1 hour of continuous recording
4. Absence of EEG response to either auditory or somatic stimuli or to electrical stimulation

Too often the early and immediate efforts in resuscitation are directed toward the cardiac aspect rather than toward the assurance of adequate oxygenation as provided by an adequate airway, artificial respiration, and proper transport of the oxygen via the cerebral vessels. I agree with Beck and others, who believe that almost every heart can be restarted. In over 350 cases personally encountered (for consultation or otherwise), the heart resumed its spontaneous rhythm in most instances for varying periods of time. In June, 1951, on a ward, we massaged a patient's heart for 2 hours. It was not until 3 ml. of 2% barium chloride was injected into the left ventricle that the heart suddenly resumed normal tone and rhythm and a normal blood pressure was obtainable. Spontaneous respirations returned and the chest was closed. The patient suddenly expired, and at autopsy a large gastric ulcer was noted with massive hemorrhage into the gastrointestinal tract.

A remarkable case of prolonged resuscitation is described by Effler. A young man in his early twenties was brought to the hospital following an automobile accident. Cardiopuulmonary resuscitation was required and was started at approximately 9 p.m. It seemed apparent to the physician that eventual resuscitation was hopeless. It was hoped that the victim might serve as as a renal transplant donor, but the patient's wife could not be located immediately. Therefore efforts at closed-chest resuscitation continued. Finally, at about 2 a.m. the wife was located and gave autopsy permission and permission for the use of the kidneys, but at this point spontaneous cardiac action returned and the patient subsequently made a complete recovery!

As long as massage appears adequate, a good peripheral pulse is maintained, and the pupils remain constricted, efforts should be continued. If there has been an obviously long delay prior to cardiac compression, then little hope need be entertained. A number of cases have been recorded in which the patient appeared to have been severely damaged neurologically but continued to improve after several months. A remarkable degree of success at rehabilitation in such a case was achieved by Dr. Howard Rusk and Dr. Ann Whittlesey of the New York University–Bellevue Medical Center's Rehabilitation Department. Hosler cites the case of Wolf, in which massage was carried out for a period of 8 hours on a New York lawyer. The man is again practicing his profession in New York City.

Therefore it is difficult to state precisely when efforts at further resuscitation should be abandoned. If irreversible pathology appears to be present, then efforts should cease. Certainly, *under no circumstances* should they cease if one is fairly certain that anoxia is not present to the extent that would allow irreversible brain damage. If the case is diagnosed and compression is started before a 4-minute period has elapsed, then efforts at resuscitation should probably continue. If a period of 10 or 15 minutes is allowed to pass after the arrest, then it should seem obvious that future resuscitative attempts are ill advised.

After periods of prolonged intermittent cardiac compression, one may question the advisability of proceeding further. I have frequently been asked this question by physicians taking the course in cardiac arrest and resuscitation. My answer is to the effect that, if one is satisfied that there is a palpable peripheral pulse, if a systolic blood pressure of over 60 mm. Hg is being maintained, and if the pupils are remaining constricted with evidence of proper oxygenation to the body, then there is no justification for discontinuance of resuscitative efforts, including intermittent cardiac compression. If, however, it is obvious that a period of more than 4 minutes has elapsed, during which time adequate cerebral oxygenation was not being maintained, then the situation is very likely hopeless. Beck has occasionally commented on the fact, and I would agree, that if one is unable to restore a nodal rhythm to a heart in cardiac arrest the fault usually lies with some aspect of the resuscitative efforts. Either adequate pulmonary oxygenation is not being maintained, proper methods of cardiac compression are not being conducted, or proper use of pharmacologic aids is not being applied. It may be that ventricular fibrillation is present and has not been recognized. Occasionally, irreversible cardiac pathology may be present. Therefore, if one compresses the heart for a prolonged period without success, he should systematically review all the potential sources of error before deciding that further resuscitative efforts are of no avail. Prolonged heart massage for 2½ hours with complete recovery has been reported by Spencer and Bahnson.

In some instances of myocardial infarction, the remaining area of functioning myocardium has been so reduced that successful defibrillation and resuscitation cannot be accomplished.

An instance in which ventricular fibrillation persisted for 1 hour and 50 minutes is reported by Adams. The heart of an 11-year-old boy went into fibrillation just at the time of division of the patent ductus arteriosus. By electrical countershock therapy and the use of procaine hydrochloride and procainamide, successful ventricular defibrillation could not be achieved until almost 2 hours had elapsed. In spite of a prolonged period of cardiac compression, the heart was finally successfully restored to a normal sinus rhythm, and 30 minutes after the operation was completed the patient was awake and spoke in a rational manner to his mother. No complications were noted postoperatively except for evidence of an acute tubular nephritis.

Three hours of closed-chest cardiac compression were carried out for cardiac asystole and ventricular fibrillation in a 13-year-old boy (Lillehei). In spite of the prolonged period of massage, the patient appeared to have been successfully resuscitated. Neurologic deficits included some visual loss and speech difficulties. Prolonged resuscitation was continued because of the age of the patient and findings suggestive of adequate perfusion during the resuscitative attempts.

Shocket and Rosenblum report remarkable success in resuscitating a 32-year-old man in the postoperative period following total colectomy for ulcerative colitis. Despite eight attempts at conversion with D.C. electroshock, attempts at external pacing, and many of the usual pharmacologic adjuncts, no effective resuscitation could be achieved. When all electrical activity of the heart had ceased, a thoracotomy was performed. The heart was found to be weakly fibrillating and greatly dilated. Shortly after manual compression of the heart was initiated, the heart muscle tone returned and a spontaneous defibrillation occurred. The patient subsequently returned to his position as a stockbroker.

It should be emphasized that cardiac resuscitative attempts should seldom be terminated without obtaining an ECG to pinpoint the specific electrical status of the heart.

A new dimension of moral and legal implications?

Concepts change. Whereas only a short time ago fibrillation of the human ventricle was regarded as a malignant arrhythmia unresponsive to effective medical therapy, cardiac defibrillation now takes place many times a day throughout the world. As the barriers to successful resuscitation fall, the boundaries continue to be pushed further outward. Cardiac pacemakers, mechanical cardiac assist devices, hypothermia, and a host of other adjuncts make it difficult to establish rigid guidelines that are applicable not only to proper medical decision making but sometimes to ethical considerations and specific situations concerning public policy.

The new technology has created considerable confusion on such basic points as what constitutes a statutory definition of death, or more simply, when is death? Because of many considerations such as problems of insurance and survivorship, criminal responsibility, and estate inheritance, the traditionally accepted criteria for determining the point of death have been the subject of considerable scrutiny. With the advent of organ transplantations, especially transplantation of the heart, these complex questions assume even greater emphasis. Throughout the world a flurry of activity has involved not only doctors but lawyers, sociologists, forensic pathologists, theologians, philosophers, economists, and cultural anthropologists. The verbiage on the subject does not lend itself easily to condensation.

Helpful guidelines are provided by a host of groups including the Committee on Ethics of the American Heart Association, the American Encephalographic Society, and the second International Symposium on Emergency Resuscitation meeting in Norway. Additional guidelines have been provided by the English Human Tissues Act, 1961, the Declaration of Geneva (1947), the Declaration of Pope Pius XII (1957), the Canadian Model Human Tissues Act, and United States Uniform Anatomical Gift Act, first passed by the state of Kansas.

The House of Delegates of the American Medical Association at its annual meeting in June, 1973, were urged by the Connecticut delegation to place a moratorium on and discourage statutory definitions of death by individual state legislatures. The Judicial Council of the American Medical Association was asked to draw up a guiding and consensual principle acceptable to the medical profession to remedy the present situation and confusion regarding death.

The Judicial Council's report to the House of Delegates was approved to the effect that the House of Delegates adopt the position that, at present, statutory definition of death is neither desirable or necessary; that State Medical Associations urge their respective legislatures to postpone enactment of legislation defining death by statute; and that the House affirm the following statement: "Death shall be determined by the clinical judgment of the physician using the necessary available and currently accepted criteria."

How does one define the point of death. No longer is it agreed that it represents the time when the heartbeat ceases. In order to provide guidelines for the discontinuation of extraordinary life-support systems, an ad hoc committee at Harvard proposed the criterion of irreversible coma. They apparently declined to specifically define death but include the characteristics of death as being: (1) a failure to respond to even the most intense of stimuli, and unreceptivity, unresponsiveness, and total unawareness, (2) lack of spontaneous respiratory activity, (3) absence of reflexes and the presence of fixed, dilated, and nonresponsive pupils, (4) a flat isoelectroencephalogram may provide confirmatory evidence, and (5) all of the above findings should be present for a minimum period of 24 hours.

Although the *Oxford University Dictionary* and *Black's Law Dictionary* provide definitions of death, there is still no universally accepted definition.

As mentioned, much of the urgency in the problem stems from the need to formulate rules and procedures governing the donation of organs, which is largely dependent upon an adequate definition as to when life ends. From a practical standpoint, the viability of a transplanted organ exerts a strong influence. The present-day techniques of resuscitation and life-supporting mechanisms have stimulated a reappraisal of the biologic and medical foundations of life.

Various approaches are used. At the Cook County Hospital in Chicago, Collins has introduced a scoring system to provide an answer to when the patient is really dead. It is centered on brain electrical activity, heartbeat, reflex reactions to stimuli, blood circulation in capillaries, and self-sustained breathing.

The state of Kansas adopted the first Uniform Anatomical Gift Act in the United States (1968). It was later amended to conform to the Uniform Anatomical Gift Act as drawn by the Joint Commission of Uniform State Laws. The bill was as follows:

(A) A person will be considered medically and legally dead if, in the opinion of the physician (based on ordinary standards of medical practice) there is absence of spontaneous respiratory and cardiac function and, because of the disease or condition which directly or indirectly caused these functions to cease, or because of the passage of time since these functions ceased, attempts at resuscitation are considered hopeless, and, in this event, death will have occurred at the time these functions ceased, or (B) a person will be considered medically and legally dead if, in the opinion of the physician (based on ordinary standards of medical practice) there is the absence of spontaneous brain function; and if (based on ordinary standards of medical practice) during reasonable attempt to either maintain or restore spontaneous circulatory or respiratory function in the absence of aforesaid brain function, it appears that further attempts at resuscitation or supportive maintenance will not succeed, death will have occurred at the time when these conditions first coincide. Death is to be pronounced before artificial means of supporting respiratory or circulatory function have terminated and before any vital organ is removed for purposes of transplantation. (C) These alternate definitions of death are to be utilized for all purposes in the state, including the trials of civil and criminal cases, any law to the contrary not withstanding.

The American Heart Association's Committee on Ethics noted that in cases of severe, overt brain trauma or cases of a very rapidly deteriorating donor, the usual 24-hour duration of a flat EEG was unnecessary in order to certify irreversible coma.

Black's Law Dictionary (fourth revised edition) defines death as "the cessation of life; the ceasing to exist; defined by physicians as the total stoppage of the circulation of the blood, and cessation of the vital functions consequent thereon, such as respiration, pulsation, etc."

As an adjunct in the determination of brain death, isotope angiography with a scintillation camera for visualization of cerebral arteries and venous sinuses appears promising (Goodman and associates). An isotope angiogram showing no evidence of cerebral vasculature may provide a simple, rapid, and accurate indication of brain death.

With the growing tendency to define death in connection with irreversible cessation of cerebral function, Corday points to a fear that this concept is designed to take care of the special interests of heart transplantation and may disregard important implications.

It is interesting that several countries leave the determination of the time of death to the judgment of the physician and impose no specific criteria on them. For example, in New South Wales and Australia, a qualified practitioner may permit the removal of organs for transplant when he is satisfied himself that "life is extinct." In Sweden, Finland, and Denmark, organs may be removed in the absence of specific consent by either the donor or his relatives so long as neither has explicitly refused such consent. This apparently is true also in Czechoslovakia.

Crafoord considers irreversible brain death to have occurred in those patients who demonstrate failure of dye to enter the skull after repeated injections during a 10- to 15-minute period.

Crafoord, in presenting the Gold Medal Address at the tenth International Congress on Diseases of the Chest, centered his attention on cerebral death when asked to define a dying patient. He reminds us that as long as conscious or unconscious brain function persists, the patient is dying, but when there is no further brain activity, we no longer have a dying patient—we have a corpse. The need for a new definition of death does not concern Crafoord; he emphasizes that in every human being who dies, it is the irreversible brain damage that gradually stops

the life of all other cell systems and this occurs regardless of whether the brain damage has occurred prior to cessation of circulation and gas exchange, or whether it arises as a result of primary inhibition of pulmonary and cardiac function.

It is important to remember that the presence of a flat or isoelectric EEG does not, in itself, constitute conclusive evidence of brain death since conditions such as extreme hypothermia or central nervous system depression from drug overdose (especially barbiturates and meprobamate) may temporarily produce a flat EEG. As with so many rules of medicine, there are exceptions. In 1953 we were able to show for the first time, on the basis of a large number of resuscitation attempts (1200), that return of cerebral function is seldom possible after a period of more than 4 minutes of complete anoxia. Even so, there are notable exceptions, some completely unexplained.

While it is virtually impossible to pinpoint the "moment" of death in view of the advances provided by the technology of resuscitation, it does seem that it is logical to assume that death occurs when vital functions come to an irreversible end and that the determination of death will continue to be a clinical assessment by the physician. Perhaps Simpson is right that death takes place when all hope of a sustained existence is finally abandoned.

How often is cardiac resuscitation ill-advised?

This is a difficult question to answer as one must be intimately associated with all aspects of each case. It is true, however, that many chronically ill and near-terminal patients receive half-hearted resuscitative efforts as their last event. Stiles attempted to evaluate this over a 6-year period and judged that only 8% of 305 calls for resuscitation were ill-advised. In such instances the primary diagnosis was malignancy, most with widespread metastasis.

Chapter 66

CARDIAC RESUSCITATION:
WHAT IS BEING ACCOMPLISHED?

What is being accomplished in cardiac resuscitation? Has the tremendous amount of energy and effort been of sufficient value to warrant continuation of efforts? Already there are generally reliable statistics. As an overall figure in 1974, it would appear that approximately 13% of all cardiac resuscitative efforts attempted in the hospital will be successful to the extent that the patient will be discharged. This figure of 13% success will, of course, vary to a degree, depending upon the patient mix, the sophistication of cardiac arrest efforts within the hospital, and the presence of an effective cardiac resuscitation committee.

Other questions that may be answered today are those relating to proper candidates for resuscitation and complications of resuscitation and their avoidance. Figures are now available to indicate the long-term survival rate of patients having been successfully resuscitated. Information concerning the frequency of serious cerebral damage is also now available.

Twenty-seven years have passed since the first successful electrical defibrillation of the human heart. Since that time there has been a steady increment to the physician's armamentarium. In the early 1950s cardiac resuscitation teams were organized, mobile cardiac resuscitation units were devised, and formal instruction in the art and science of resuscitation was begun. With the widespread use of the A.C. defibrillators, resuscitative efforts moved outside the operating room to the occasional resuscitation on the ward, in the emergency room, and elsewhere. With the advent of closed-chest defibrillation, resurgence of interest in mouth-to-mouth artificial ventilation, and the demonstrated value of closed-chest external cardiac compression, cardiac resuscitation efforts received their greatest impetus. Sophisticated monitoring systems and the segregation of high risk individuals into intensive care and coronary care units soon followed, along with a marked improvement in the pharmacologic approach to cardiac arrhythmias and their prevention or treatment. As a logical sequence, resuscitative efforts moved out of the hospital with the training of large numbers of paramedical personnel and some lay groups.

Successful resuscitation in the operating room continues to be considerably higher than that in most areas of the hospital. Of 17,000 surgical patients in Jackson Memorial Hospital (Jude), there were fourteen cardiac arrests and six of the patients left the hospital alive: a successful resuscitation rate of 43%. Drye reports 100%.

Whether closed-chest or direct manual cardiac compression is attempted, it has become obvious that a physician's first effort at cardiac resuscitation is usually most ineffective, regardless of his specialty. This inability has been noted even among experienced surgeons, including chest surgeons. The value of practice by the physician is to be highly regarded, and, whether this occurs in the animal laboratory on dogs or by the use of a manikin or other aids, it appears that much benefit will result. However, the dog heart, as a rule, is of a different size than the average human heart, and, although the anatomy is generally the same, the limitations from practice on dogs leave something to be desired. It has been the practice at some hospitals to allow the intern or the assistant resident to massage the heart of any patient with cardiac arrest for a short period of time in order that additional experience can be gained. Such a plan seemingly pays dividends. Experimentally, Lape and Maison verified the beneficial effect of practice in maintaining an adequate mean arterial pressure in the animal laboratory. They were able to maintain an arterial pressure of not less than 80 mm. Hg for 20 minutes at a compression rate of 25 times per minute. The average mean arterial pressure that they were able to obtain by such compression was 97 mm. Hg. They note a direct correlation between the amount of practice and the effectiveness of the cardiac compression. The first successful closed-chest resuscitation outside the operating room at the University of Missouri Medical Center was accomplished by a medical student who had spent the previous summer doing laboratory experiments on this problem.

Reliable survival figures on open-chest resuscitation first became available through the study of Cardiac Arrest Registry data. The prognostic aspects of cardiac arrest have subsequently been broken down into separate items as they lend importance to particular points of interest. It is obvious that success requires attention to a multitude of details.

Overall survival rate

A number of early reports on closed-chest resuscitation were concerned with survival figures. Baringer and co-workers attempted closed-chest resuscitation on eighty-four unselected cases of circulatory arrest at the Massachusetts General Hospital. Four patients subsequently left the hospital. Of the eighty-four patients, fifteen recovered consciousness and twenty-three survived for over 3 hours. Defibrillation was successfully achieved in ten out of eighteen cases, and effective spontaneous heartbeats were resumed in only thirty-six of the eighty-four patients. Of those who were successfully re-

suscitated, all four were those with circulatory arrests. One of the four patients who survived ultimately had a thoracotomy and internal defibrillation following the initial external cardiac massage. Weale and Rothwell-Jackson, after a review of published survival figures for closed-chest resuscitation, wonder if the results with closed-chest resuscitation entirely deserve the statements of some authors that open-chest cardiac massage is seldom warranted. Jude, Kouwenhoven, and Knickerbocker's series with a favorable response in 60% of 118 patients reveals also that 24% were long-term survivals with adequately functioning central nervous systems. Himmelhoch and co-workers report four (6%) survivals in sixty-five cases from the Peter Bent Brigham Hospital.

Because the application of resuscitative technique has become so widespread outside the operating room, it is difficult to evaluate survival figures for closed-chest resuscitation. Few large series have been reported.

Iung and Wade collected the cases of cardiac arrest occurring at the Hurley Hospital in Flint, Michigan, from January, 1959, to July, 1961. There was a 28% survival rate in twenty-five patients treated by the thoracotomy approach. Fifty percent of fourteen patients survived following the closed-chest method.

If cardiac arrest occurs in an otherwise healthy person during a well-controlled situation in the operating room and a diagnosis is made within the first 2 or 3 minutes, the patient almost always should be resuscitated without any subsequent neurologic sequelae. Unfortunately, such an ideal situation seldom occurs. Complicating factors entering into the diagnosis and treatment have resulted in an overall survival rate considerably lower than what appears to be possible. In the first large group of cardiac arrest reports that was collected from doctors in many parts of the world, an overall survival rate of 29% was established. *This represents a permanent survival rate and does not include cases in which the heart was resuscitated but in which the patient subsequently died.* The survival rate of 29% includes patients in all decades of life, both in and out of the operating room (a total of 497 patients). Mortality figures include cases occurring under many types of environmental situations and from many parts of the world, in army and veterans' hospitals, in private, city, and teaching hospitals. A variety of resuscitative techniques have been used, depending on the locality concerned.

Using open-chest technique, thirty-two (74%) of Altemeier's series of forty-three patients survived and were discharged from the hospital. These were all cases who had initially survived longer than 72 hours after closure of the thoracotomy incision.

From a group of more than fifty hospitals, the experience with 5,076 cases of cardiac arrest is reported in Table 66-1. The survival rate, based on the number of patients discharged from the hospital, is 16% or 819 patients.

Pierce, in a report on cardiac arrests and deaths associated with anesthesia in a large community hospital, compares a 1957 study with one conducted from 1963 to 1965. Not only does he note a distressing increase in the rate of cardiac arrests associated with anesthesia but he also reports a lowered resuscitation rate. Seventy-five percent of the patients experiencing cardiac arrest in the operating room in 1957 were successfully resuscitated as compared with 50% in the 1963 to 1965 period. This decreased survival occurred in spite of a period of increased emphasis on attention to cardiac resuscitation, newer techniques of resuscitation, a more rational use of pressor agents, agents to counteract metabolic acidosis, and more intensive postresuscitative management including the use of mannitol and general hypothermia. Pierce states that there was no question as to the competency of the individuals who applied the closed-chest technique; these same individuals had experienced success in nonsurgical, nonanesthetized patients. He further states that lack of success could

not be attributed to slowness, inefficiency, or inaccuracy of diagnosis.

From Albany, New York, Medical Center Hospital comes a report of cardiopulmonary resuscitations covering the period from January 1, 1963, through December 31, 1963. The procedure was carried out fifty-nine times in forty-eight patients. Forty of the forty-eight patients died in the hospital. Eight (17%) were discharged from the hospital. One of these eight continued to show evidence of moderate anoxic brain damage. Of these eight, four died within the first year following discharge.

The distressingly low survival rate following cardiac syncope outside of the operating room would probably be because of the severe preexistent heart disease.

A long-term survival rate of 12% (nine of seventy-eight arrests) was achieved at the Sinai Hospital, Baltimore, from July, 1965, to April, 1966. This 500-bed hospital had earlier reported a 5% survival. The improvement in resuscitative results is attributed to an increased awareness of the role of resuscitation among both the attending staff and house staff, to the institution of a training program for nursing personnel (allowing nurses to start resuscitative efforts while awaiting the arrival of a physician), and to the value received from holding critique sessions within 24 hours of each arrest.

A long-term survival rate of 11% occurred in Roser's series from Emanuel Hospital, Portland, Oregon. This study from a 450-bed general hospital includes ninety-eight patients seen between March, 1964, and September, 1966.

The Central Middlesex Hospital in London had twenty-two long-term survivors in their first 100 cases of cardiac resuscitation. Almost 50% of these patients had experienced myocardial infarction. This group demonstrates only a 9% long-term survival.

Neufeld's report from Mercy Hospital, Toledo, Ohio, covers a 1-year record (1965) during which ninety-three patients were ex-

Table 66-1. Survival following closed-chest resuscitation

Physician and hospital reporting	Number of arrests	Discharge from hospital	Physician and hospital reporting	Number of arrests	Discharge from hospital
Ayers, W. R. and others Albany Medical College Albany, New York	48	8	Hofkin, G. A. Sinai Hospital Baltimore (Followed Nachlas' report from same hospital)	78	9
Baringer, J. R. and others Massachusetts General Hospital Boston	84	4	Holmdahl, M. University Hospital Upsala, Sweden	51	15
Benfield, J. R. and others University of Wisconsin Hospital Madison, Wisconsin	84	10	Iung, O. S., and Wade, F. V. Hurley Hospital Flint, Michigan	14	7
Benson, D. W., Jude, J. R., and Kouwenhoven, W. B. Johns Hopkins Hospital Baltimore	197	47	Jeresaty, R. M. and others St. Francis Hospital Hartford, Conn.	237	52
Bizzarri, D. and others New York Medical College Metropolitan Medical Center New York	100	21	Johansson, B. W. Malmo, Sweden	65	13
			Johnson, A. L. and others Royal Victoria Hospital Montreal Children's Hospital Montreal	552	82
Chazan, J. A. Beth Israel Hospital Boston	22	2	Johnson, J. D. Latter Day Saints Hospital Salt Lake City	51	18
Chow, E. A. Southern Pacific Memorial Hospital San Francisco	68	3	Jordan, D. and others University Hospital Columbus, Ohio	100	3
Columbia-Presbyterian Medical Center New York	85	16	Jude, J. R. and others Johns Hopkins Hospital Baltimore	304	73
Cotlar, A. M. and others Chouty Hospital New Orelans	73	25	Kaplan, B. M. and others Michael Reese Hospital Chicago	100	6
Day, H. W. Bethany Hospital Kansas City, Kansas	24*	13	Kern, E. University Hospitals Paris	3	0
Fornace, A. J. Riverview Osteopathic Hospital Norristown, Pennsylvania	11	5	Keszler, H. Prague	12	3
Grace, W. J. and others St. Vincent's Hospital New York	108	15	Klassen, G. A. and others Royal Victoria Hospital Montreal Children's Hospital Montreal	126	17
Greenberg, H. B. Touro Infirmary New Orleans	4	3	Lawen, P. University Hospital Hamburg	4	3
Himmelhoch, S. R. and others Peter Bent Brigham Hospital Boston	65	4	Lawrence, R. M. and others University Hospitals Rochester, N. Y.	111	15
Ho, S. K., and Quattlebaum, F. Bethesda Lutheran Hospital St. Paul, Minnesota nate, J.	119	20	Lillehei, C. W. and others University of Minnesota Hospital Minneapolis	200	33

*All in coronary care unit.

Table 66-1. Survival following closed-chest resuscitation—cont'd

Physician and hospital reporting	Number of arrests	Discharge from hospital	Physician and hospital reporting	Number of arrests	Discharge from hospital
Mayer, H. Bellevue Hospital New York	3	3	Safar, P. Baltimore City Hospital Baltimore	150	5
Medford, F. E. Memorial Hospital Charleston, W. Va.	56	10	Safar, P. Presbyterian-University Hospital Pittsburgh	100	11
Middlesex Hospital London	100	22	Sandoval, R. G. Muhlenberg Hospital Plainfield, N. J.	26	12
Minuck, M. St. Boniface General Hospital St. Boniface, Manitoba	63	5	Semple, H. C. and others Victoria Infirmary Glasgow	24	8
Nachlas, M. M. and others Sinai Hospital Baltimore	60	3	Shipman, K. H. and others Presbyterian Hospital Denver	49	12
Negovskii, V. Moscow	31	5	Spanknebel, G. L. Memorial Hospital Worcester, Mass.	37	7
Neufeld, O. Mercy Hospital Toledo, Ohio	93	17	Stoch, E. Royal Melbourne Hospital Melbourne, Australia	59	8
Poulsen, H. University Hospital Aarhus, Denmark	5	1	Stribling, W. D. Hall County Hospital Gainesville, Ga.	12	5
Rivkin, L. M. University of California Medical Center San Francisco	70	15	Sykes, M. K. Hammersmith Hospital London	251	34
Robinson, H. J. and others Bryn Mawr Hospital Bryn Mawr, Pa.	39	18	University Hospital New York University	196	14
Roser, L. A. Emanuel Hospital Portland	98	10	University of Pennsylvania Philadelphia	103	6
Ruben, I. L. Montefiore Hospital New York	117	17	Weingarten, C. H. Boston	25	1
Ruszen, R. L. and others Carraway Methodist Hospital Birmingham, Ala.	56	10	Wilder, R. J. Baltimore	153	15
			Total	5,076	819 (16%)

posed to closed-chest resuscitative measures. Eighteen percent were long-term survivors.

From December, 1959, to November, 1963, there were thirty-three successfully resuscitated patients out of a group of approximately 200 cases seen on the thoracic surgical service of Dr. C. Walton Lillehei at the University of Minnesota Hospital (an incidence of approximately 16.5%).

Survival rates reported in the literature have varied from figures much lower than this to some that are considerably higher. Shortly before his death, Dr. Frank Lahey of the Lahey Clinic reported a recovery rate in the last thirteen cases at his clinic of 76.9%, with all patients showing negative EEGs (open-chest massage was used). Others have noted a 100% survival rate in

Table 66-2. Additional survival rates following closed-chest resuscitation

Physician and hospital reporting	Number of arrests	Discharge from hospital	Physician and hospital reporting	Number of arrests	Discharge from hospital
Brown, C. S., and Scott A. A. Toronto General Hospital Toronto, Ontario	184	19	Linko, E. and others (1967) Tampere Central Hospital Tampere, Finland	100	27
Clarkson, E. H. (1969) Southern Baptist Hospital New Orleans	76	8	Minuck, M., and Perkins, R. St. Boniface General Hospital St. Boniface, Manitoba	293	27
Copplestone, J. F. (1969) Department of Health Wellington, New Zealand (ambulance resuscitation)	130	5	Peschin, A. and others (1969) George Washington University Hospital Washington, D. C.	734	28
Galzsche, H. and others University Hospital Aarkus, Denmark (all with heart disease)	405	26	Sandoe, E., and others (1969) University Hospital of Copenhagen Copenhagen	164	41
Greenfield, I. (1964) Mount Sinai Hospital Minneapolis	360	10	Smith, H. J. and others (1965) McGill University Montreal	254	40
Hansen, P. F., and Sandoe, E. (1966) Rigshospitalet Copenhagen	47	16	Stannard, M., and Sloman, G. (1969) Royal Melbourne Hospital Victoria, Australia (coronary care unit)	28	9
Hollingsworth, J. H. (1969) University of Virginia Hospital Charlottesville, Va.	368	30	Stemmler, E. J. (1965) University of Pennsylvania Hospital Philadelphia	103	5
Hubbell, R. W., and Okel, B. B. DeKalb General Hospital Decatur, Ga. (general hospital)	104	18	Stiles, Q. R. and others (1971) Hospital of the Good Samaritan Medical Center Los Angeles	305	44
Jeresaty, R. M., and others (1969) St. Francis Hospital Hartford, Conn. (community hospital)	237	52	Swanson, L. W. (1970) St. Joseph Mercy Hospital Mason City, Iowa (community hospital)	91	43
Jude, J. R. and others (1970) University of Miami School of Medicine Miami (operating room arrests)	14	6	Tai, A. R. Hamilton Civic Hospital Hamilton, Ontario	98	5
Jung, M. A. and others (1968) Toronto Western Hospital Toronto	100	20	Tufts University Medical College Boston	150	20
Lemire, J. G., and Johnson, A. L. (1972) Royal Victoria Hospital Montreal	1,204	230	Turner, Glenn (1971) St. John's Hospital Springfield, Mo. (coronary care unit)	169	43
			Total	5,718	755 (13%)

their own small series of three or four cases. At the Grace–New Haven Hospital, Turk and Glenn noted a rate of 16.7% permanently successful resuscitation attempts out of a group of forty-two patients. This covered a 5-year period, from December, 1948, to January, 1954.

Briggs states that there were seven recoveries in the first nine cases of cardiac arrest at the Massachusetts General Hospital in 1954, an almost 80% recovery rate. White reported a 90% mortality in ten cases (1909).

Bost, in 1923, reported sixteen survivals out of a total of seventy-five patients. In 1941 Bailey reported only six survivals out of a personal experience with forty-one cases. (This was the largest personal experience at that time.)

A more detailed breakdown of early series appeared in the first and second editions of this book. Survival figures have exhibited wide variation.

Many of the variables involved in successful cardiac resuscitation will be discussed under separate headings in this chapter. Table 66-2 enumerates survival following closed-chest resuscitation for hospitals whose data were largely unavailable to us at the time of the printing of the third edition. This composite picture consists of community hospitals, teaching hospitals, a few situations limited only to coronary care units, and several series which have been on a continuation basis for a number of years. A total of almost 6,000 arrests compares with slightly over 5,000 reported in the last edition. The overall resuscitation rate has dropped slightly. Nevertheless, encouraging reports, such as that from Corday, lend hope of improvement. Corday and his group at the Institute of Medical Research–Cedars of Lebanon Hospital were able to report a 67% survival rate following asystole or ventricular fibrillation in the coronary care unit.

In evaluating various comparative statistical figures on cardiac resuscitation attempts, one should be cautioned not to compare series that are not representative of comparable types of patients in comparable situations. Ideally, a cardiac resuscitation committee should be able to record and evaluate all resuscitation attempts occurring within the hospital for a given period of time. Unfortunately, transient episodes of ventricular fibrillation may go unrecorded in the operating room, in the cardiac catheterization laboratory, or even in the coronary care units. Generally the results are better in these areas than on the general surgical and medical wards.

Prognosis in coronary care units

The United States Public Health Service through their heart disease control program (Flynn and Fox) summarize the experience of seven coronary care units in which 1,528 patients were treated. Of the patients, 11.8% experienced ventricular fibrillation or ventricular standstill. There was a hospital survival rate of 32.8% of those experiencing cardiac arrest in the coronary care unit. Obviously, as with all statistical analyses of this sort, only generalizations can be made since standards, staff, and equipment in coronary care units will vary a great deal and the type of patients admitted may differ. Some coronary care units may admit patients much more rapidly than others.

Trends in resuscitation survival

To date there has been no sizable series of patients who received external cardiac massage to equal or surpass the outstanding 70% survival rate reported in the initial study of Kouwenhoven, Jude, and Knickerbocker.

Most significant are those comparative evaluations done over a period of years within the same hospital by an effective cardiac resuscitation committee. The beneficial effect of widespread monitoring devices, adequately trained personnel, proper emphasis by a cardiac resuscitation committee, and rapid dissemination of new information and techniques will usually reflect a gradually improving picture of successful resuscitation. Over a 7-year period at the Hospital of Good Samaritan Medical Center in Los Angeles, there was a marked improvement in the success rate. For example, in 1964 no patients survived cardiac arrest, but in 1970, 27% were successfully resuscitated and discharged from the hospital. At the St. Boniface General Hospital in Manitoba the percentage of permanent survivors increased from 6.2% in 1964 to 11% in 1967. The largest such series is reported from the Royal Victoria Hospital in Montreal and concerns 1,204 patients with cardiac arrest as seen over an entire decade. Survivors discharged from the hospital increased from 13.5% in 1960 to 22.4% in 1970.

In viewing the reported statistics of successful resuscitations one has the nagging suspicion that these may be somewhat higher than is actually the case around the country. I suspect that the successful case is more likely to be remembered and recorded than its counterpart. Despite an effective cardiac resuscitation team and reporting system, many cases are never fully reported. For example, the Toronto General Hospital reports that there were 328 calls for the cardiac arrest team during a 1-year period, from November, 1968, through October, 1969, but that only 184 reports were received. In other words, only about 56% of the arrests for which the team was called are reported with sufficient information to be of any value.

Cardiac resuscitation in a community hospital

An analysis of reported results of external cardiac resuscitative efforts in community hospitals does not indicate a great deal of variation from the university teaching hospital or the large city-county type of hospital. For details of these programs the reader is referred to some representative reports such as those of Hubbell and Okel, Ho and Quattlebaum, Swanson, and Jeresaty and co-workers, even though the patient mix is somewhat different in each hospital and

there is often a different composition of the cardiac resuscitation team because there may be fewer hospital staff officers and fellows available. There was a 22% long-term survivorship in the report of Jeresaty and colleagues (which included cardiopulmonary resuscitation efforts outside the operating rooms) in a 654-bed community hospital.

In a 318-bed general hospital in Mason City, Iowa, during three successive years there was a 37%, 40%, and 48% success rate in temporary resuscitation and a 26% rate of successful discharge from the hospital the third year (Swanson). During a 32-month period at the 300-bed Bethesda Lutheran Hospital in St. Paul, Minnesota, a well-organized cardiac resuscitation team functioned (without a residency program). Seventeen percent of 119 patients were discharged alive following cardiac resuscitation. No permanent central nervous system impairment was encountered.

Results of nighttime cardiac resuscitation

Almost without exception hospitals report that they have their poorest results in cardiopulmonary resuscitation attempts between 7 P.M. and 7 A.M. At the St. Francis Hospital, Hartford, Connecticut, success rates were almost halved during the night shift. Out of a total of 110 resuscitations performed on 98 patients, there were no permanent survivors from resuscitation attempts that occurred between 11 P.M. and 8 A.M. There were also no permanent survivors in a 3-year cardiopulmonary resuscitation experience at the University of Virginia among 368 patients with cardiac arrest occurring between 11 P.M. and 7 A.M. who were located on general wards in the hospital. For some reason there seems not only to be a poor resuscitation rate but fewer resuscitation attempts are made on the nursing shift on duty between 11 P.M and 7 A.M. One must suspect that there may be less surveillance of the patient at that time.

It is interesting to consider the data provided by Kerzner and Lown who monitored

78 patients during hospital convalescence from myocardial infarction and compared the incidence of ventricular premature beats during waking and sleeping hours. Fifteen percent of these patients had a paroxysm of ventricular tachycardia or salvos of ventricular premature beats. Of particular interest is the fact that major arrhythmias were recorded only while the patient was asleep.

The effectiveness of ambulance attendants in cardiac defibrillation

Rose and Press estimate that about 70% of the patients who die from acute myocardial infarction (approximately 1,000 each day in the United States) do so before they reach the hospital. Of those dying outside the hospital it is estimated that approximately 40% die within the first 15 minutes. Another 30% of the nonhospital deaths occur from 15 minutes to 2 hours after the onset. Obviously the question arises repeatedly, can ambulance attendants be effectively trained to provide lifesaving cardiac defibrillation with the mobile coronary care unit? Two years ago, Grace estimated there were twenty-six mobile coronary care units, or "heartmobiles" in the United States. Some of the better known early mobile coronary care units include Grace's unit at St. Vincent's Hospital in New York City; the Ohio State University Hospital Unit in Columbus, Ohio; units in Miami and Jacksonville, Florida, Los Angeles, Montgomery County, Maryland; Seattle; and the University of Missouri at Columbia.

Experience of the Oregon coronary ambulance project, organized in 1969, is described by Rose and Press. Fortunately, the Oregon Board of Medical Examiners ruled in January, 1969, that the use in ambulances of a portable external electrical defibrillator by trained ambulance attendants in cases of emergency would be allowed under the Medical Practice Act. This would be considered an emergency procedure rather than the practice of medicine, much in the manner of artificial, mechanically aided pulmonary resuscitation. Thus it was that in the state of

Oregon trained ambulance attendants began using cardiac defibrillation equipment without the presence of either physicians or nurses. The ambulance attendants are intensively trained. This training includes recording and reading of electrocardiograms, experience in the coronary care units, and intensive drilling in the recognition of arrhythmias. Initially twenty registered nurses from coronary care units volunteered to ride in the ambulance to provide additional supervision and to give added confidence to the ambulance attendant. Monitoring leads incorporated into the defibrillator paddles saved time and obviated the need to apply "blind" defibrillation. An effective method of record keeping was also incorporated into the program.

From September 1, 1969, through December 31, 1970, cardiopulmonary resuscitation or defibrillation or both were performed at the scene or in the ambulance in fourteen cases. In four of these cases ventricular fibrillation was present prior to the arrival of the ambulance and the patient was being given cardiopulmonary resuscitation by others when the ambulance arrived. All four of these patients were defibrillated, and three regained consciousness and survived. During transportation to the hospital an additional four additional patients developed ventricular fibrillation, two of whom were successfully resuscitated and eventually left the hospital. Of the three patients who developed cardiac asystole en route to the hospital, two survived and were discharged. From this pilot study alone it would seem that highly motivated and well-trained allied health personnel can achieve a high degree of accuracy in interpretation of electrocardiograms, and can detect abnormalities including ventricular fibrillation so that successful defibrillation can result.

The mobile coronary care unit in Seattle, Washington, at Harbor View Medical Center was developed in conjunction with the Seattle Fire Department. Of a group of 3,058 ambulance runs in 18 months, 11% of the patients had ventricular fibrillation on arrival of the ambulance. Of the 324 patients found to have ventricular fibrillation at the time of arrival of the mobile coronary care unit, 36% were resuscitated and taken to the hospital for coronary care. Overall, there was a 13% long-term success over the 18-month period in that 42 patients were resuscitated from ventricular fibrillation and eventually returned to work or their family. Incidentally, a breakdown of the cost effectiveness of the program revealed that there was a cost of approximately $3,000 per each life definitely saved (Conn).

Respiratory and cardiac resuscitation as the first aid measure administered by ambulance drivers during a 1-year period was analyzed by the Advisory Committee in New Zealand. External cardiac resuscitation was applied in 130 cases. There was only a 3.8% survival rate, however.

Resuscitation time

The total time devoted to resuscitation of the patient is inversely related to the degree of success in the majority of situations. For example, the mean resuscitation time was 45 minutes in 140 failures at the St. Francis Hospital in Hartford, Connecticut. It was only 10 minutes in the fifty-two long-term survivors. None of the patients survived when more than 30 minutes of continuous cardiopulmonary resuscitation was required.

Ventricular asystole

When cardiac standstill or ventricular asystole occurs, either early or late, after a myocardial infarction, the prognosis is considerably more serious than if ventricular fibrillation occurs. Perhaps this is a reflection of the severe myocardial damage, shock, and cardiac failure that is associated.

Time factor

Next in priority to the preventive aspect of cardiac arrest comes the vital importance of the *time factor*. Here lies the crux of successful resuscitation. Beyond the need for active resuscitative measures, the need for consciousness of the urgency of the situation must play a part in any of our thoughts relative to cardiac arrest. If the percentage of permanent survivals is to be increased and if neurologic complications are to be reduced, then every possible source of delay in beginning immediate manual systole must be eliminated.

From the first 1,200 cases of cardiac arrest analyzed in the first edition of this book, it became apparent that 94% of the successful and permanently resuscitated cases were massaged within 4 minutes (Fig. 66-1). In other words, cerebral circulation must be artificially augmented within this time period or else permanent irreversibility will occur. Thus for the first time statistically significant data became available to support previous clinical impressions regarding the matter of cerebral anoxia and reversibility.

The importance of reducing the time from discovery of the arrest to starting resuscitation is further emphasized by Brown and Scott. Of those who initially survived in their group of 184 patients, 90% had resuscitation initiated within the first 2 minutes. Furthermore, of those patients who left the hospital alive, 94% had resuscitation begun within the first 2 minutes. There was only one survivor whose resuscitation procedure was initiated after 5 minutes.

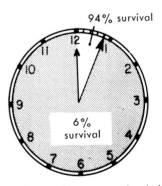

Fig. 66-1. Unless cardiac compression is instituted within a 4-minute period, only an occasional patient will survive. Therefore the crux of successful resuscitation revolves around immediate recognition of cardiac arrest and institution of artificial respiration and circulation.

That cardiac arrest is a 3- to 4-minute emergency seems certain. The severity of the neurologic complications is in direct proportion to the degree of anoxia that follows circulatory failure. Regardless of statements in the literature to the effect that some patients may survive a period of more than 4 minutes, my studies fail to substantiate this. Such figures are entirely out of line with clinical experience. One author editorialized: "If the interval was between five and fifteen minutes between cardiac arrest and massage, the recovery rate fell to 33%." A 33% recovery rate with this degree of anoxia is not possible under present conditions.

With widespread use of closed-chest resuscitation, an appreciable delay in restoring cerebral circulation may be avoided in many instances, especially outside the operating operating room.

Environment at time of cardiac arrest

It is natural to expect that the rate of survival in patients who suffer cardiac arrest outside the controlled environment of the operating room would be considerably less than in those who experience cardiac arrest in the operating room. Not only are the elements necessary for prompt diagnosis missing but also the personnel is often not trained in surgery. In spite of these handicaps, 21.1%, or forty-four of the 209 cases reported as having occurred outside the operating room, were listed as having permanently survived cardiac arrest.

From the series of Turk and Glenn, over 40% of the successful results occurred in resuscitation attempts outside the operating room.

Prognosis as related to age

The suggestion is often made that the young heart may more frequently be resuscitated and the young patient may more often be permanently revived than an older patient in whom an increased likelihood of underlying cardiac pathology is prevalent.

This proved to be a false assumption, as demonstrated in the large statistical study presented in the first edition of this book. The permanent survival group was exceedingly low in the first decade of life. In this group, only 17% of the female patients and 27% of the male patients survived.

Prognosis in dental cases

Closed-chest resuscitation is receiving increased attention in dental journals and at professional meetings.

So far, few survivals from cardiac arrest occurring during dental procedures have been reported. It is believed that this fact is one of circumstance only and is mentioned simply in passing. I would be interested to learn of successful resuscitations.

Survival under spinal anesthesia

One study reports 170 cases of cardiac arrest occurring in patients under spinal anesthesia. Sixty-four were permanently resuscitated. This represents a figure of 37.6% —considerably higher than the overall survival figures.

Survival periods after cardiac arrest

Although there are some notable exceptions to the following figures, I have noted in previous editions of this book a study showing that, of those patients whose hearts were restored to spontaneous contraction but who were not in the 29% permanently surviving group, the majority died within the first several hours after resuscitation attempts. In the first 6 hours, 64.2% died, and a total of 85.7% died within the first 24 hours. Only 4.2% of the total deaths came after a 6-day period. Therefore it can be predicted with a reasonable degree of certainly that, in those instances where cerebral damage has occurred, the majority will die within the first 24 to 36 hours.

Prognosis in patients with congenital heart lesions

Cardiac resuscitation efforts are almost daily occurrences during cardiac surgery in hospitals about the country. It is interesting to note the early work of Kountz.

Kountz noted a marked difference in the resuscitation of the hearts that he attempted to revive by perfusion methods. Hearts that had succumbed to diseases of the heart itself were difficult to revive, with one exception, this being congenitally defective hearts, which in his experience were relatively easy to revive. Since the same result was noted in a case of emphysema in which chronic anoxemia had been a pronounced factor, it was speculated that, perhaps, lowered oxygen tension of time might be a circumstance favorable to revival.

Prognosis in patients with A-V heart block

Martt reports that three fourths of the patients with complete atrial ventricular heart block who had experienced Adams-Stokes attacks were dead within 18 months following the initial hospital diagnosis.

Prognosis in patients with dilated, fixed pupils

Despite the generally acknowledged belief that dilated, fixed pupils represent irreversible damage in the patient with cardiac arrest, numerous cases have been documented in which fixed, dilated pupils persisted for as long as 45 minutes, followed by subsequent complete recovery without neurologic sequelae.

Prognostic aid from funduscopic examination

Kevorkian, who has concerned himself with a study of the eyegrounds in death and in circulatory failure, suggests that the presence of moving segments in the eyegrounds may indicate probable recovery following resuscitation of the heart. If stationary segments are visualized, irreversible neurologic damage may be expected. Eyeground examination should be included in the immediate postresuscitative examination.

Cheyne-Stokes respiration

Periodic Cheyne-Stokes respiration frequently may be observed following cardiac resuscitation. In my experience, this signifies an extremely poor prognosis.

Cardiac resuscitation without permanent survival

When speaking of survival figures, it is always important to differentiate between cardiac resuscitation (which refers solely to restoration of the normal heartbeat) and total or permanent survival of the patient. Resuscitation of the heart itself usually offers little difficulty if adequate knowledge of cardiac resuscitation is available. In almost every heart we massaged in one series of fifty-nine cases of cardiac arrest, it was possible to restore some sort of spontaneous and rhythmic activity to the heart—at least for a period of several hours. Beck has often stated that almost every heart can be resuscitated. Unless obvious irreversible pathology is present, one should certainly reexamine his methods of resuscitation if he is unable to restore a normal rhythm to a heart that has suddenly ceased beating. For example, pericardial tamponade may be unrecognized in closed-chest resuscitation.

The large statistical study presented in the first edition reveals that the heart was restarted in 56% of the cases. Since this figure is almost twice that quoted for overall permanent survival rates in this period, it should seem obvious that, provided more prompt diagnosis and treatment are available, a marked increase in the overall survival figures can be anticipated.

Partial resuscitation

Out of a total of forty-two patients in whom resuscitation was attempted, only 38.1%, or sixteen patients, were partially resuscitated as reported from the Grace–New Haven Hospital. In nineteen, or 45.2% of the patients, no cardiac function whatsoever could be restored. This is considerably higher than has been the experience of most. In fact, we had only two cases of the fifty-nine encountered in which some degree of cardiac rhythm could not be restored. With closed-chest technique, it is less easily determined whether this is true.

Long-term survival

There is now good evidence to indicate that patients who are resuscitated after ventricular fibrillation following an acute myocardial infarction and who are subsequently able to leave the hospital have an excellent chance of surviving. Geddes and co-workers record a 78% survival for mean period of 9 months in a group of fifty patients who had ventricular fibrillation following myocardial infarction. In a group of thirty-six patients, thirty-two of whom had cardiac arrest caused by acute myocardial infarction, 73% survived for a mean period of 16 months (Norris). This New Zealand study showed that male survivors under the age of 60 years who have been followed for more than 3 months have been improved to the extent that three fourths are back at work.

The Royal Infirmary of Edinburgh (Lawrie) reports an 88% survival after 1 year among fifty-three patients with an episode of ventricular fibrillation associated with an acute myocardial infarction. There was, in fact, a 93% 1-year survival in those who fibrillated but whose myocardial infarction was not associated with cardiac failure and hypotension. If the latter was present, the survival fell to 77%.

There were no significant changes in the mental status of any of the twenty-six survivors studied in a group of 193 patients treated for cardiac arrest (Minuck). Persistent severe physical disability was uncommon, with 70% returning to gainful employment.

That patients may expect to live out a normal lifetime following cardiac arrest in many ways seems increasingly likely. There are now a number of cases on record of individuals who survived for extended periods of time following episodes of cardiac arrest.

One such patient is known to have lived a normal life for 18 years after cardiac arrest and resuscitation occurred in 1926 during a gallbladder operation. The successful case of electrical cardiac defibrillation (the first in literature, which Beck reported in 1947) on a 14-year-old boy was followed for 21 years; a mention by Hosler indicates that the boy was living a normal life. I have talked with several patients who have thoracotomy scars from previous cardiac arrests and they seem to be living normal lives. A member of the teaching staff at our hospital is active 7 years after resuscitation.

Survival following required cardiopulmonary resuscitation associated with myocardial infarction is compatible with long-term survival. In fact, 89% of twenty-seven long-term survivors with myocardial infarction were still alive for periods, as long as 3 years in the St. Francis Hospital series at Hartford, Connecticut.

In contradiction to this, a group of thirteen late deaths was observed from among twenty-five patients discharged after cardiac arrest caused by acute myocardial infarction treated at the University Clinic in Copenhagen. Almost half these patients died of recurrent cardiac arrest and for this reason Sandoe raises the possibility that the late mortality in this group may be decreased by continuous administration of antiarrhythmic drugs.

There is some disagreement regarding the value of long-term treatment with antiarrhythmic drugs for persons surviving primary ventricular fibrillation occurring as a complication of acute myocardial infarction. Sudden death that could be attributed to an arrhythmia did not occur in any patient surviving successful primary ventricular defibrillation (Stannard and Sloman). Ventricular fibrillation occurred twenty-eight times in 350 patients suffering primary ventricular fibrillation while in a coronary care unit at the Royal Melbourne Hospital in Australia. Nine, or approximately one third of these patients survived to leave the hospital. Known survival up to 4½ years occurred with all the men under the age of 65 returning to work. None of the survivors are invalids. In most series, three fourths of the survivors are still alive 1 year after discharge and one half at the end of 3 years.

Congenital deafness and prolonged Q-T interval

The prognosis for successful resuscitation is particularly favorable in the patient with syncopal attacks and sudden cardiac arrest who also has congenital deafness and the syndrome of associated prolonged Q-T interval. Provided prompt recognition of the arrest occurs, these hearts can be quickly restored to an effective beat.

Reoperation after resuscitation from cardiac arrest

The question may arise, "What are the possibilities of a repeat episode of cardiac arrest during a repeat operative procedure?" In my experience, this repetition has been exceedingly rare. Such was also the experience of Howland and associates. Forty-two subsequent operations after cardiac resuscitative procedures were observed. No repeat episodes of cardiac arrest occurred, although there was one death resulting from exsanguination at the time of partial hepatectomy. The decision to continue with an operation once cardiac arrest has occurred is naturally dependent upon a number of considerations. In many instances, a decision is dictated by the stage of the operation associated with the arrest.

Should reoperation after cardiac arrest be necessary, one might first try to estimate the possible myocardial damage that occurred from the anoxia of arrest as well as the possible myocardial damage resulting from the resuscitative procedure itself. Since it is true that structural damage to the myocardium has been reported in a number of pathologic studies, Howen and co-workers suggest that reoperation for elective procedures be considered analogous to the man-

agement of patients with varying degrees of myocardial ischemia subsequent to coronary occlusion episodes. The patients resuscitated after a brief period of vagal arrest by closed-chest massage probably represent cases with little myocardial damage. Certainly, all patients needing reoperation after resuscitation require thorough evaluation to avoid any of the predisposing factors relating to the first arrest. Particularly, steps should be taken to minimize a reflex cardiac arrest. These preventive measures are discussed in Chapter 3.

Decisions relating to reoperation may be related to rules used for elective procedures on patients following episodes of coronary occlusion. If considerable depression of cardiovascular function has occurred from the cardiac resuscitative efforts or if cerebral instability is present, then elective surgery should be delayed until such time as a more normal status has returned. If ECG tracings indicate injury currents or if transaminase levels have been elevated following resuscitation, an operation might best be delayed for 3 months. For patients whose hearts have been restarted with a minimum of trauma to the myocardium, it would seem reasonable to perform surgery within a matter of several weeks. In the instances of reoperation by Howland and co-workers, a particular effort was made to avoid hypoxia. Reemphasis is made for establishment of a patent airway, adequate ventilation, careful administration of muscular relaxants, avoidance of substandard oxygenation and anesthetic mixtures, and adequate removal of carbon dioxide. Other instances of reoperation after resuscitation have been reported (Eerola and Taulaniemi).

Continuation of operation after cardiac resuscitation

Cardiac arrest encountered during a surgical procedure may evoke a question of judgment regarding the wisdom of continuing with the operative procedure once resuscitation has occurred. I have encountered cardiac arrest on induction of anesthesia in several instances and have elected to continue with the procedure once the heart action is restored. These cases usually involve procedures of an emergency or semiemergency nature in which a second opportunity might not be provided. In other instances, a stage in the operative procedure that requires completion may have been reached. In general, however, it is my opinion that cardiac arrest should signal the completion of any operative procedure planned for the particular day and that the patient should be returned to his room to be reevaluated.

Prognosis following myocardial infarction and cardiac arrest

Jude, from his study of more than thirty patients who experienced sudden death from myocardial infarction, states that he believes the patient should have a 10% to 20% chance of surviving—provided ventricular fibrillation is present. Those whose hearts stop in asystole experience a survival rate of practically zero, however. It is, perhaps, too early to estimate the salvage rate from cardiac arrest and subsequent resuscitation in patients with myocardial infarction. Particularly difficult to treat is that group of patients who develop a malignant arrhythmia 1 to 3 weeks after the initial infarct. Sealy reports that he has always been able to get a temporary return of cardiac action, only to have ventricular fibrillation recur.

In an excellent review of this subject, Robinson and Sloman report their results of resuscitaion in fifty-three patients with proved myocardial infarction. Long-term survival was accomplished in eleven of fifty-three patients (20%). In thirty-two patients, cardiac arrest developed during ECG monitoring.

What happens to the patient who survives ventricular fibrillation complicating a myocardial infarction? One answer is provided by Geddes, Adgey, and Pantridge from the Royal Victoria Hospital in Belfast, Ireland. From a follow-up study of fifty patients who survived ventricular fibrillation complicating ischemic heart disease, they note that the long-term prognosis regarding survival appears similar to that of patients whose myocardial infarction was not complicated by ventricular fibrillation. Thirty-nine (78%) of the fifty survivors are still alive. The number of episodes of ventricular fibrillation in the immediate postinfarction period did not appear to influence long-term survival. In fact, three patients survived ventricular fibrillation. Two of these patients survived thirty and thirty-three episodes, respectively. Sixteen percent of the patients had three or more distinct episodes. Sixty-one percent of the patients studied by Pantridge have been able to return to work.

The chances of successful cardiac resuscitation in the myocardial infarction patient are brightest in those experiencing arrest within 24 hours after the onset of the infarction.

Robinson and Sloman divide myocardial infarction patients into the following three categories:

Mild—those patients exhibiting no evidence of shock or of cardiac failure apart from a transient rise in jugular venous pressure

Severe—patients with definite evidence of circulatory embarrassment including hypotension and manifestations of cardiac failure

Cardiogenic shock—those patients exhibiting the clinical criteria for the diagnosis of severe shock such as a systolic blood pressure below 80 mm. Hg, pallor or cyanosis, a cold sweating skin, oliguria, and failure of improvement in the patient's condition within half an hour after the relief of pain and the administration of oxygen.*

Of particular interest is the fact that the successful long-term survivals were largely from the first classification, that is, those with mild infarctions. Eight of the eleven patients were in the first category. Also of interest is the fact that the success of resuscitation was much greater in those patients whose hearts were found to be in fibrillation than in those whose hearts were in asystole. In fact, in none of the patients in the second categories were

*Robinson, J. S., and Sloman, G.: Resuscitation from cardiac arrest after acute myocardial infarction, Med. J. Aust. 1:578-582, 1965.

there any long-term survivals. Likewise, no survivals were found in the nine patients classified as experiencing cardiogenic shock.

Thirty-three percent of the patients resuscitated after myocardial infarction by Robinson's group represent long-term survival after ventricular fibrillation. The prognosis in cardiac arrest after myocardial infarction appears to be considerably brighter if the arrest mechanism is that of ventricular fibrillation.

Robinson and Sloman describe two patients with asystole who had inferior infarction and complete atrioventricular block. An externally applied electrical pacemaker did allow for a temporary return of ventricular activity, but both patients subsequently died.

One hundred consecutive cases of cardiac arrest, utilizing the closed-chest massage technique, were studied over an 11-month period at Michael Reese Hospital in Chicago. Six percent of these patients were successfully resuscitated to the extent that they eventually left the hospital with their prearrest neurologic status. Only two of the six patients were alive as of July 1, 1963. All 100 cases were confirmed circulatory arrests as monitored by the oscilloscope or ECG. As distinguished from series heavily weighted toward the surgical side, this series includes only two incidences of resuscitation in the operating or recovery room. Eighty-four percent of these patients had significant myocardial pathology prior to circulatory arrest. Thirty-two patients experienced acute myocardial infarction. Of the six patients successfully resuscitated, only two were not in the intensive care unit. One patient developed cardiac asystole while undergoing pericardiocentesis. A second successful resuscitation was associated with the administration of a large dose of quinidine. Other successful resuscitations have occurred either in the cardiac catheterization laboratory, the operating room, the emergency room, or the intensive care unit.

Hyperpyrexia

Marked elevation of the patient's temperature following cardiac resuscitation indicates a poor prognosis. If associated with a comatose patient, it invariably indicates a degree of irreversible brain damage that is often incompatible with life. Efforts should be made to lower the temperature, nevertheless. Sponging the patient with alcohol, applying ice-water bags to the axilla and groin, and other means of lowering the body temperature should be employed in the hope that the pathology is on the basis of cerebral edema rather than irreversible brain damage. Ideally, of course, a cooling blanket should be used (see discussion of hypothermia).

There was recovery of one patient with a hyperpyrexia of 105° F. In another patient, who subsequently died, the highest elevation reached 108° F.

Respiratory paralysis

Spontaneous respiration may be absent for a considerable period of time with subsequent complete recovery. Although this is obviously a most ominous finding, the loss of spontaneous respiration does not in itself accord to irreversible brain damage.

Preexisting heart disease

The presence of preexisting cardiac pathology has been assumed to be associated with a poor prognosis or a poor survival rate in cardiac resuscitation. According to Stilwell and Mueller: "The preexistence of cardiac disease may subject the patient to cardiac arrhythmias, congestive failure, and cardiac arrest. Such patients tolerate hypoxia very poorly and the successful resuscitation of such a patient is very unlikely." This fact was not borne out in the series reported in previous editions. Instead, the percentage of patients with successful recovery following cardiac arrest is as high in the group with known cardiac disease as in the supposedly normal group of patients.

It should be emphasized from the outset that the possibility of resuscitation does not necessarily have a direct relationship to the etiology of the arrest. The initiating cause of cardiac standstill has little to do with the failure of spontaneous beats to occur on massage. This confusion has led to many difficulties in the handling of cardiac arrest. As is pointed out elsewhere in this book, the ventricular specific tissue is the least vulnerable to oxygen lack on the basis of forming adequate stimuli. According to the statistical study reported in the three previous editions, about 24% of the cases of cardiac arrest were found to have preexisting cardiac pathology that included previous coronary occlusion episodes, hypertensive cardiovascular disease, diabetic arteriosclerotic disease, congenital heart lesions, and others. Of this group, 130 patients, or 31%, experienced permanent survival. This value is very nearly the same as the overall survival rate. Also interesting is the fact that cardiac contractions were restored in 53% of the total cases.

Converse notes that patients classified preoperatively as being in an abnormal cardiac state do somewhat better from the viewpoint of cardiac arrhythmias than those patients who are considered to have normal hearts. The reasons for this are just as obscure as the reasons why patients who have abnormal cardiac rhythms before the induction of anesthesia sometimes assume normal ECG patterns once anesthesia is established. From the University of Minnesota, Miller reports fourteen such cases; in each instance, the patient had previous cardiac pathology.

Miscellaneous factors

Because of the changeover of hospital house officers in July of each year, there is a period of time in which some of the house physicians, especially interns, may be inexperienced in cardiopulmonary resuscitative techniques. That a corresponding dip in resuscitative success does occur has been documented by Roser.

Causes of failure in cardiac resuscitation

The causes of failure to successfully resuscitate the human heart may be listed under the following general headings:
1. Inexcusable delay in instituting proper resuscitative measures
2. Inadequate knowledge of resuscitation, including postresuscitative care, and failure to establish ventilation
3. Reluctance to apply the available knowledge
4. Inadequate equipment for proper resuscitation
5. Premature discontinuance of resuscitative efforts

Physicians today must be prepared to face the realities of cardiac resuscitation. Out of 300 fatal cases of cardiac arrest in South Africa, for example, almost one third were associated with totally inadequate attempts at resuscitation.

Equipment necessary for proper resuscitation is still relatively simple and should be available in all hospitals. Even so, almost 50% of thirty-one fatal cases of ventricular fibrillation recently described were associated with absence of an electrical defibrillator. If the survival rates are to be dramatically improved, it will be necessary for nurses staffing the various coronary care units to be fully trained in the electrocardiographic recognition of arrhythmic complications and to be able to institute resuscitative efforts, including the application of the electrical defibrillator.

It must be admitted that attempts at cardiac resuscitation are not likely to be highly successful in moribund patients or those suffering from chronic pulmonary and cardiac disease.

Injudicious use of variously injected drugs is sometimes responsible for failure of cardiac resuscitation. Also, failure to establish adequate artificial respiration is frequently a cause. Improper postresuscitative management may be cited in a similar category.

All too often, an unsuccessful resuscitative attempt represents the first such cardiac arrest encountered by a particular physician. Since cardiac arrest is a relatively infrequent experience for any particular physician, it is therefore imperative that he be able to treat his first case with maximum efficiency —without waiting to gain any degree of personal experience.

Unfortunately, attempts at resuscitation

are often rendered inefficient by the startling suddenness and absence of antecedent warning with which arrest is announced. To those unaccustomed to emergencies, this may entail a demoralizing effect on the operator even though he is well aware of the proper resuscitative measures that must be employed quickly.

The Anesthesia Study Commission of the Philadelphia County Medical Society cited some of the following errors in resuscitation among 307 fatalities listed as having occurred in patients under anesthesia. Although not concerned with cardiac arrest, their suggestions are relevant as applied to cardiac resuscitation. The commission reported that one of the main reasons was the use of inefficient methods of maintaining respiratory function when it was depressed or paralyzed. Stimulants, vasopressor drugs, and analeptics were too frequently used when rhythmic inflation of the lungs with oxygen alone was indicated.

The extremely low survival rate of patients with sudden arrest of the heart during eye procedures and the depressingly low survival rate of cases occurring in the x-ray department are good examples of failure resulting from the general reasons cited above.

The following situations combined with cardiac resuscitative efforts have proved to have especially poor survival rates. Considerable improvement must occur in these areas if resuscitative efforts are to significantly improve.

1. Resuscitation after arrest in patients with cardiogenic shock
2. Arrest after ventricular rupture
3. Asystole following a myocardial infarction
4. Persistent hypotension after resuscitation
5. Recurrent arrest after myocardial infarction

PART ELEVEN

EPILOGUE

Chapter 67

THE PAST: HISTORICAL VIEWS CONCERNING CARDIAC ARREST AND RESUSCITATION

Werner Overbeck

Translated by Carl H. Ide

The history of surgical operations dates back to antiquity. Records regarding attempts of resuscitation in cardiac arrest, however, cannot be found. The reason for this is that ancient as well as medieval physicians were of the opinion that the heart was the seat of the life spirit; therefore if the heart became diseased, it would be fatal. A theory of the qualities of the pulse had, indeed, been developed in antiquity. The quality of the pulse, however, was not related to diseases of the heart but to general resistance and energy of life of the invalid (Neuburger). These opinions were also held in the teachings of Galen (A.D. 138-201) and were decisive for European medical thinking up to early modern times. William Harvey (1578-1657), too, adhered to this theory when, in his address to the king in *Exercitatio anatomica de motu cordis et sanguinis in animalibus* (1628), he said:

The heart of the animal is the foundation of his life, his most important organ, the sun of his microcosm; on his heart, his entire activity depends, from his heart his entire vivacity and strength emanate.

Thus wounds of the heart were considered to be absolutely fatal by Hippocrates (460-370 B.C.) and many others up to the beginning of modern times (Neuburger and Pagel).

If one thinks of only *one* essential feature of cardiac arrest, it is the absence of heart sounds. However, the assertion of Harvey that heart sounds exist was dismissed mockingly in a letter to Harvey from an Italian physician, who wrote that in Rome one probably does not have as perceptive ears as in London to hear those sounds.

For a systematic investigation and description of the diseases of the heart, the discovery of the circulation of the blood by Harvey, the comparison of symptoms of diseases with autopsy findings by Morgagni of Padua (1682-1771), and, finally, the invention of the stethoscope by Laennec and his teachings on auscultation (1815-1820) were essential. The exact experimental research with animals was particularly established by François Magendie (1783-1855) in Paris.

Experimental research with animals

Through his keen perception, Andreas Vesalius became the pioneer of new medical thought. In his work we find the first experiments to bring about the resuscitation of the quiescent hearts of pigs and dogs. In *Librum VII,* Chapter 19, he wrote:

In order to revive the animal to some extent, one must attempt to open the trunk of the arteria aspera. Into it a cannula of thin or thick caliber should be introduced. One blows into it so that the lung is raised as if the animal is inhaling. Through light blowing of air into the animal in vivo, the lung expands as much as the lung cavity permits. The heart regains strength and changes through the variation of its movements. When the lung is inflated once and again, one may examine the movements of the heart through inspection and palpation and one feels and can see at the same time the trunk of the arteria magna which passes to the back, either in the cavity of the chest or close to the vertebrae lumbrorum. Nothing appears more distinctly than the rhythm of the heart and the artery. After one has observed it for a time, one must again blow into the lung. Through this bit of artistry—I have seen none in all of anatomy that has afforded me greater joy—cognizance of the variations of beats may be gained. When the lung, however, is flaccidly collapsed for some time, one can see a vigorously undulating, rapid, but weak and wormlike beat or movement of the heart and of the arteries. When one blows into the lung, though, the beat then becomes strong and rapid and shows curious irregularities.

Twenty years later, Harvey mentioned these observations by Vesalius in his anatomical lectures and made his own observations during vivisection. He was also the first to point out the synchronized movements between the auricles and ventricles. He noted correctly that the movements of the auricles precede those of the ventricles.

Harvey observed that a resuscitated heart seems to respond to the movement of the auricles, first relatively fast, and later, in the dying heart, once again, slowly. His experiment on a pigeon he described essentially as follows:

In an experiment which was performed on a pigeon after the heart, including the auricles, had stopped beating movements, I laid my finger moistened and warmed with sputum on the heart. When through this stimulation it had, so to speak, raised its vitality, I saw the heart and its auricles move, contract and relax, and, so to speak, it was as if it were called back from death to life.

The experiments of Vesalius were repeated by Robert Hooke (1635-1703) and nearly 100 years later in 1755 by John Hunter (1718-1793). Hunter recognized the importance of the oxygenated blood for the activity of the heart and built, in this respect, foundations for a successful resuscitation, as he dismissed emetics and phlebotomy as a means

of resuscitation and in place of them recommended air insufflation into the trachea. The first establishments of lifesaving associations can be traced back to him (Killian and Dönhardt). The discovery of oxygen by Lavoisier (1743-1794) coincides with this time. Spallanzani (1729-1799) was indeed able to apply the findings of Lavoisier and prove that death of animals who suffer from lack of air is not caused by cessation of circulation alone, as was assumed up to then, but is referable to phenomena in the CNS caused by lack of oxygen (Castiglioni). Donley stated that in the seventeenth century the Swiss physician Johann Jakob Wepfer (1620-1695) described the effect of several substances on the hearts of dead animals. In his work entitled *Circutae aquaticae historia et noxae* (published in Basel in 1679) Wepfer stated that he was successful in keeping the heart in motion for a short time. The Frenchman Bichat (1771-1802) published his treatise *Sur la vie et la mort* in 1800, which, in addition to studies of physiologic aspects of life and death, also contained views on attempts at resuscitation of the heart. Bichat explained in detail the necessity of maintenance of the circulation, and, more importantly, the coronary circulation. Indeed, he would have had but one more small step, namely, to think of the fact that it is possible to partially maintain this coronary circulation through manual compression.

Approximately 100 years later the German surgeon R. Haecker published an attempt of resuscitation in an extensive study on surgery of the heart.

In an anesthetized rabbit, the heart was exposed under low atmospheric pressure. Sterile olive oil was injected into the pericardium to the point of turgidity. After obtaining normal atmospheric pressure, the lungs collapsed and a progressing weakness and slowing down of the heart beat ensued. After restoration of the low atmospheric pressure, the heart recovered. Having performed this maneuver several times with the same result, he reversed the conditions of the experiment. Under normal atmospheric pressure, the pericardium was filled to the point of turgidity.

After a while, the heart stopped. When the low atmospheric pressure was restored, it started beating again and the animal recovered completely. The experiment was repeated obtaining the same result.

The introduction of the chloroform narcosis carried with it cases of sudden death. This produced a definte stimulus for the investigation of possibilities of resuscitation of the heart. At the end of the year 1848 it became clear to Sibson that death caused by chloroform usually occurs rapidly in man and is referable to paralysis of the heart. In 1858 John Snow (1813-1858) described fifty cases of death by chloroform. He too attributed sudden heart failure as the cause of death in forty of these patients.

Moritz Schiff, a Frankfort physiologist, was first a student of Magendie; then he worked in Florence. As a result of frequent use of anesthesia on animals, he concluded:

The use of chloroform as an anesthetic is to be rejected as dangerous. Ether should be preferred. No case of unforeseen death has yet been reported

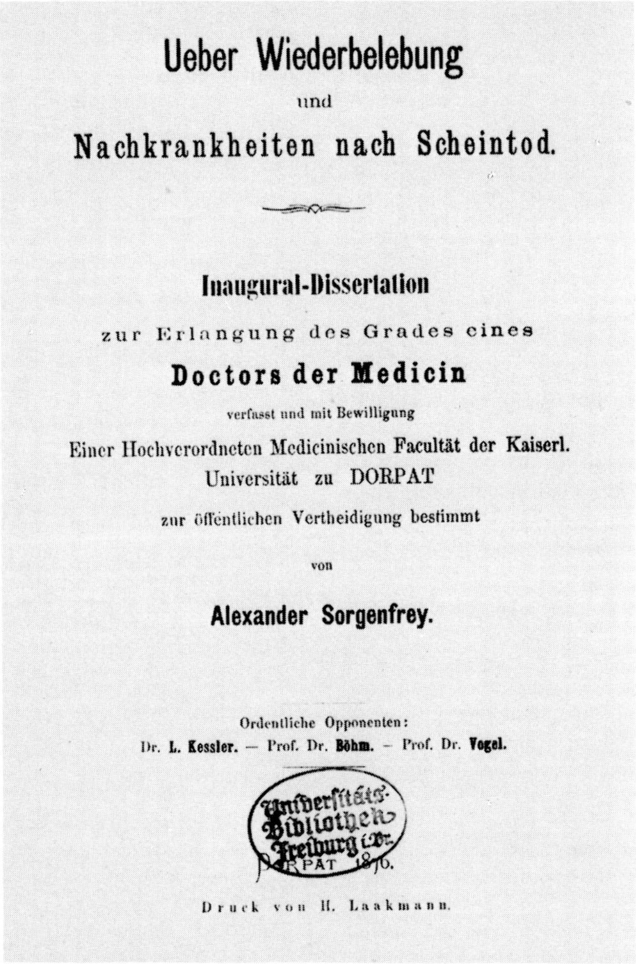

Ueber Wiederbelebung

und

Nachkrankheiten nach Scheintod.

Inaugural-Dissertation

zur Erlangung des Grades eines

Doctors der Medicin

verfasst und mit Bewilligung

Einer Hochverordneten Medicinischen Facultät der Kaiserl. Universität zu DORPAT

zur öffentlichen Vertheidigung bestimmt

von

Alexander Sorgenfrey.

Ordentliche Opponenten:

Dr. L. Kessler. — Prof. Dr. Böhm. – Prof. Dr. Vogel.

Druck von H. Laakmann.

Fig. 67-1. Translation: Concerning resuscitation and complications after apparent death, inaugural dissertation written for the purpose of obtaining the degree of Doctor of Medicine and with the permission of a highly appointed medical faculty of the Imperial University in Dorpat approved for public defense, by Alexander Sorgenfrey. Appointed examiners: Dr. L. Kessler, Prof. Dr. Böhm, Prof. Dr. Vogel, Dorpat, 1876. Printed by H. Laakmann.

with it, when the attention of the surgeon was sufficiently directed to the respiration (Schiff, 1896).

These thoughts of Schiff received little attention, and chloroform remained highly regarded. T. G. Hake mentioned Schiff's method of resuscitation of a heart in cardiac arrest in *Practitioner* (Vol. 70, 1874). Schiff himself had not put forth any important publication. In the meantime, two dissertations were published in Dorpat, one by Mickwitz in the fall of 1874, the other by Sorgenfrey 2 years later (Fig. 67-1). Schiff's method can be found in the pertinent literature before and after the turn of the century (Velich; Cackowic; Green). The publications of Mickwitz and Sorgenfrey almost fell into oblivion.

What actually is the difference between the method of Schiff and that of Mickwitz and Sorgenfrey? Schiff ascertained that the blood pressure drops under the influence of chloroform. He believed this to be caused by a paralysis of the peripheral vascular nerves. Schiff successfully employed two methods to again raise the blood pressure: compression of the abdominal aorta, and injection of 8% sodium chloride solution into the veins. When cardiac arrest had already occurred, he used artificial circulation, as he called it. In 1895 he described his method as follows:

Should, for example, the effect of chloroform induce the heart to be flaccid and quiet due to distension by blood, neither artificial respiration nor air aspiration, nor a galvanic current can cause the heart to beat again in a rigid thorax. If, however, one opens the thorax, while one slowly blows air into the lungs, makes methodical compressions with the hand around the heart in order to express the blood, simultaneously closes the abdominal aorta through the pressure in the beginning in order to further direct the artificial circulation toward the head, and if one endeavors not to overburden the coronary circulation through the manual pressure, then the heart can sometimes show new movements after 11½ minutes. As soon as a manometer in the carotid artery shows a strong blood pressure, one releases the abdominal aorta and continues the artificial circulation. Soon, one may interrupt the artificial circulation for a

time, repeat it less and less often, for the circulation of the animal recovers. If the pneumothorax is merely one-sided, then the artificial respiration may be ended. The dog is resuscitated, newly animated. As a rule, the animals are killed after several hours. They never reached the point of independent movement, since cramps prevented them.

Schiff also observed that the heart may be affected with "small unceasing and disconnected fibrillating contractions." This ventricular fibrillation was first more exactly described by Hoffa and Ludwig in 1850. Levy could prove that cardiac death during chloroform anesthesia is referable to ventricular fibrillation, and that under light chloroform anesthesia a nervous irritation or an injection of epinephrine may lead, through irregular ventricular beats, to ventricular fibrillation and cardiac death.

Because of a different motivation than Schiff's, the young physician Louis Mickwitz performed resuscitation experiments on cats in Dorpat in 1874. He was to examine the effect of alkalies and alkaline earths in animal experiments, but he repeatedly lost the experimental animals while determining the lethal dose of the potassium salts. For resuscitation of the animals, he usually used a bellows. When he did not have any at hand, he compressed the thorax of the experimental animal manually, and after 1 minute the heart began to beat again. The blood pressure rose and soon spontaneous respiration returned. Through this "remarkable discovery," Mickwitz was led to develop his "compression of the thorax," combined with artificial respiration, into a method. He described his method as follows:

The most practical way in carrying it out, is, for instance, to stand on the left side of the animal, compressing the lower aperture of the thorax by clasping the rib arches with the corresponding hand and simultaneously exercising a moderate amount of pressure in the direction of the spinal column and towards the head of the animal. In the meantime, the right hand compresses rhythmically the thorax in the area of the heart. In this manner, one can allow a secure and firm pressure to affect the mobile heart, which can now no longer slide caudally and thus can be compressed between the hands with the use of moderate force. In intervals of 15-20 seconds, five to six consecutive compressions are made each time, whereby one must see to it that they coincide with the passive expiration. If the compressions are continued for a satisfactory amount of time, then one will succeed in reviving the heart, sooner or later (maximum time 36 minutes), if the dose of the poison was not too great and the animal was strong enough. Suddenly, it starts to beat regularly, the blood pressure which had fallen almost to zero, usually reaches medium pressure in a short time.

The respiration usually resumes a few minutes (at one time after 22 minutes) after the heart starts beating, in the beginning slowly, approximately 3-6 times per minute, later more frequently. After a time, reflex sensitivity returns, first upon touch to the cornea, later to the rest of the body.

The activity of the heart did not resume when 8 minutes had passed after the arrest, and compression of the thorax was started at that time.

Two years later a doctoral candidate of Professor Boehm of Dorpat began anew with these experiments (Sorgenfrey). During these experiments, a tracheal cannula was connected to a bellows and an artifical respiration carried out (30 air inflations and 30 compressions of the thorax per minute). The effect of the enforced circulation was proved by an incision into the carotid artery, from which the blood spurted with varying heights with every compression of the thorax. At this time, Sorgenfrey gave expression to the hope that the resuscitation method could be employed in first aid stations and hospitals if tracheotomy could be avoided by introduction of a catheter into the air passages. But, despite the fact that Boehm publicized the experiments performed by him and his associates in 1878, the method of external heart massage found little application in man. As late as 1890, Holtz, in connection with death by chloroform, wrote:

We are powerless against paralysis of the circulation, while asphyxia can be treated through artificial respiration as long as the heart keeps beating.

For further research in respect to resuscitation of the heart, the experiments that Langendorff in 1895 was able to institute with a special method in a surviving heart of a mammal were of importance. Martin, Arnaud, Hedon, and Gilis used retrograde perfusion for flow through the coronary arteries with closure of the aortic valves. Even 40 years prior to this, the London surgeon J. E. Erichsen (1818-1896) did the opposite. He ligated the coronary arteries of dogs and rabbits and found that the animals were dead within at most 10 minutes. He concluded from this that every illness that influences the coronary circulation may lead to sudden death. Hallers' (1708-1777) theory that the heart is stimulated by the blood entering its cavities was refuted through Langendorff, who undertook experiments dealing with its flow through the coronaries in an isolated mammalian heart. Aside from the blood infusion, Ringer's solution was also used (Rusche).

Schiff's resuscitation attempts were repeated by Tuffier and Hallion in France in 1898, and in the same year Tuffier succeeded for the first time with this method in obtaining temporary return of the heartbeat and the respiratory movement in a patient (Boureau).

F. S. Locke of London attracted a great deal of attention in 1901 when, during the Fifth International Congress of Physiologists in Turin, he demonstrated an isolated rabbit heart which he allowed to beat uninterruptedly for approximately 7 hours. The result could be attributed to the infusion of a Ringer's solution modified by the addition of 0.1% glucose and heated to 35° C. and the administration of oxygen.

Kuliabko saw this inspiring experiment and was motivated by it to make his own endeavors. He was successful in maintaining the heartbeat for several hours in isolated chicken and pigeon hearts after Locke's method. He was especially interested to find out how long after death the hearts of humans and animals who had died of disease were capable of movement. A rabbit heart was induced to beat after being kept in the refrigerator for 44 hours and kept on beating for another 3 hours. Of ten isolated hearts of children, which he perfused postmortem with a modified Locke's solution, only three showed no contractions at all. The remaining ones could be induced to contract in isolated parts up to 10 to 30 hours after death.

The ability of survival of the mammalian heart at low temperatures was then investigated by Velich in Prague in 1903. He was able to resuscitate dog hearts that had been frozen for 24 hours. To be exact, it resulted only in pulsations of the auricles and weak vibrations of the ventricles.

Prus in Lemberg, on the basis of his experiments, postulated that resuscitation is possible upon death by chloroform, but not upon death by electrical current. Therefore he strongly advised against use of electrical current for resuscitation in man.

Prevost, who could show that electrical discharges would produce isolated contractions of the ventricles, arrived at different results. In more extensive work, he developed a theory of defibrillation together with Batelli. A certain amount of electrical discharge could transform cardiac fibrillation to normal contractions.

Heart massage originating from the abdominal area is based on animal experiments by Bourcart, which he published in 1903. Through a glass tubing that was introduced into the larynx, he performed artificial respiration. After a median upper-abdominal laparotomy, he could put his hand under the diaphragm and massage the quiescent heart. He did not know that 1 year prior to this (1902) in England two people were resuscitated with the subdiaphragmatic method of heart massage.

In 1904 a monograph by Maurice d'Halluin appeared: *Resurrection due Coeur*, with the parts *La vie du coeur isolée* and *Le massage du coeur*. d'Halluin was of the opinion that the fibrillations were the cause of the failures of heart massage in cardiac arrest. Just as the physiologist Hering, he too succeeded in bringing the heart to a standstill

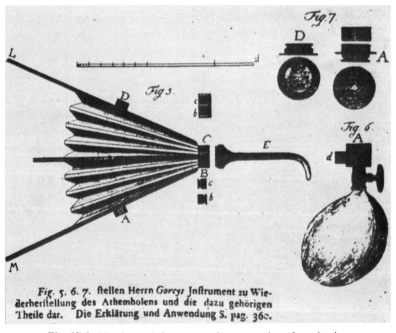

Fig. 5. 6. 7. ſtellen Herrn *Gorcys* Jnſtrument zu Wiederherſtellung des Athemholens und die dazu gehörigen Theile dar. Die Erklärung und Anwendung S. pag. 360.

Fig. 67-2. Mr. Gorcey's instrument for restoration of respiration.

by injecting potassium chloride solution. Only then was heart massage begun.

J. A. Gunn and P. A. Martin then showed renewed evidence of the existence of a supplementary or residual circulation through cardiac massage. They injected a dye into the right ventricle which, after manual compression of the heart, appeared first in the lung and later in the peripheral arteries.

Resuscitation in man

In 1848 Gorré of Boulogne reported to the Paris Academy on a death by chloroform and stated that all means of resuscitation known to the European physicians in general were applied, particularly, massage of the temples and the precordial region, pouring of cool water on the face, tickling of the pharynx with a feather, and blowing of air into the air passages. The blowing in of air was already judged to be equal to other methods and was found to be especially useful. These air insufflations, though, had been done in the beginning of the nineteenth century with tubes that were introduced into the trachea.

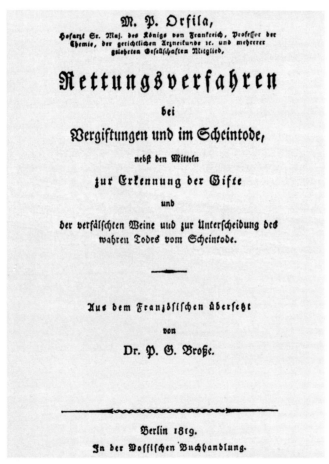

Fig. 67-3. Translation: M. P. Orfila, court physician of His Majesty the King of France, Professor of Chemistry and of Forensic Medicine and member of several scientific societies, First-aid methods in cases of poisoning and in apparent death, with means of identification of poisons and adulterated wines and of differentiation of true from apparent death. Translated from the French by Dr. P. G. Brosse, Berlin, 1819. In Vossis' Book Store.

In his *Handbook of National Science of Medicine for Theologists,* published in 1817, Masius, professor of medicine in Rostock, gives advice for resuscitation of persons seemingly dead. Aside from mouth-to-mouth respiration, artificial respiration with the respirator after Gorcy was recommended. This machine had been described by Hufeland in the *Latest Annales of French Medicine* in 1791. Through the combination of two bellows, atmospheric air as well as air from the lung could be sucked out. Fresh air, in turn, could be directed into the lung and used air removed to the outside (Cuveland and Cuveland) (Fig. 67-2).

The French toxicologist Orfila published a book in 1818 entitled *First-Aid Methods in Cases of Poisoning and in Apparent Death* (Fig. 67-3). Here, we find references for the endotracheal intubation with Chaussier's tube. Orfila preferred this method of insufflation to mouth-to-mouth respiration, which is also described. Having knowledge of the experiments at the Dorpat Physiologic Institute, Braatz, in 1884, recommended the artificial respiration according to Schüller and compression of the thorax. In 1871 Steiner recommended electropuncture of the heart with galvanic current. He did not report personal experiences with cardiac arrest in human beings; merely six animals had been revived with this method.

Professor P. Niehans, at the end of the 1880s, made the first attempt to cause the quiescent heart in man to beat again using the direct heart massage of Schiff. Zesas, who had assisted Niehans during the operation, did not record this incident until 1903.

A 40-year-old man was operated for a goiter. Before the start of the operation, cardiac arrest. After unsuccessful attempts with artificial respiration, a resection of the ribs was carried out and the heart exposed. The heart, indeed, became firmer after massage, fibrillated; normal contractions, though, no longer occurred.

A similar case is reported by Tuffier (Boureau). In 1900 Maag in Denmark and Aglinzeff in St. Petersburg performed direct heart massage on patients, one of whom was revived for 1 hour.

According to the literature available to us, in 1901 Kristian Igelsrud (Tromsö, Norway) was the first to be successful (Fig. 67-4). It was not until 1904 that this case was published by W. W. Keen in the *Philadelphia Therapeutic Gazette.* Toward the end of anesthetization during an operation for carcinoma of the uterus, cardiac and pulmonary arrest occurred. The third and fourth ribs on the left were resected and the pericardium opened. After compression of the heart for 1 minute, the heartbeat returned. The patient recuperated completely (Green). Kristian Igelsrud (whose name was changed back to the original Norse spelling of Egilsrud in 1909 [Nils Ytreberg, Tromsö Bys Historie, p. 374]) was born in Eidsvold, Norway, in 1867. After finishing his studies of medicine at the University of Christiania

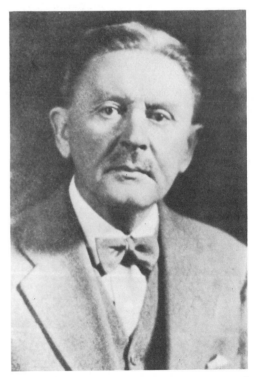

Fig. 67-4. Kristian Igelsrud. (Courtesy Johan S. Egilsrud, New York City.)

(now Oslo), he continued his studies under Dr. Sanger in Leipzig and also in Berlin and Vienna, specializing in surgery. In 1899 he was appointed chief surgeon of the State Hospital, Tromsö, Norway. During the summer of 1901, having just returned from Berlin where he had observed an unsuccessful attempt at resuscitation by massaging the heart, Igelsrud performed the first successful resuscitation operation in the presence of Professor Keen of Philadelphia, who happened to be visiting the hospital. Professor Keen then reported the operation to the medical journals and urged Igelsrud to come to America. It was not until 1916 that he finally moved to Minneapolis, where he practiced surgery until his death, from cancer, in 1940.

Several attempts were undertaken in the following years. If the left pleural cavity was opened at the same time, the patients usually succumbed due to the burden of the additional pneumothorax. Laparotomy with incision of the diaphragm as approach to the heart, suggested by Mauclaire in 1901, was still unsuccessfully applied by Poirier.

Sir William Arbuthnot Lane (1856-1943) was able to massage the heart via the diaphragm when cardiac arrest occurred during an operation of the colon. The third successful case in the world literature was contributed by Gray in 1902.

In 1918 Bost of Washington described a variation of Mauclaire's suggested transdiaphragmatic method. He succeeded in resuscitating a patient, who, nevertheless, died without having regained consciousness after 3 days.

While direct heart massage attracted great attention, indirect massage through compression of the thorax received little notice in the world literature up to the middle of this century.

The first application of compression of the thorax was probably performed by John Hovard (1736-1790). Hovard himself abandoned his method, since he had the misfortune of breaking several ribs of a rather important person during a demonstration in front of police inspectors (Negovskii). In Europe, however, this method of resuscitation was later revived. König of Göttingen compressed the thorax in the region of the heart during a chloroform syncope. Through a change of the method, in 1891 his assistant Maass succeeded in resuscitating two patients with a serious chloroform syncope.

The first case concerned a 9-year-old boy. He was to be operated on for a palatine fissure. During deepening of the narcosis, cardiac arrest occurred. Immediately, the tongue was pulled forward and with the frequency of the respiration, approximately 30 to 40 times per minute, the region of the heart was compressed. The beginning cyanosis disappeared and the wide pupils constricted rapidly. The pulse of the radial or carotid artery, however, was not palpable. If the pressure on the chest was discontinued, the patient at first breathed almost normally; soon, though, the pupils dilated maximally. Pressure in the area of the heart repeatedly caused a constriction of the pupils and, after a more prolonged application, even a light reddening of the cheeks and lips. Only the pulse failed to return. Finally, a tracheotomy was performed to keep the airway open. After half an hour his condition grew worse. According to previous experiences, the patient had to be regarded as lost.

Maass then describes the critical phase as follows:

Initially, I worked on for 3-4 minutes in the same manner and, thereby, had the impression that the in- and outflow of air grew progressively less. The indication for an attempt with Sylvester's method, therefore, became apparent. So that the effect on the heart would be least weakened, I exerted the expiratory pressure more forcefully. Even though the respiration was very deep, the pupils stayed maximally dilated. When I stopped, the previously and spontaneously present respiratory movements ceased. With the wide, totally non-reactive pupils, soft globes, the quite candid deathly pallor of the face, the absence of respiration and pulse, I now had to regard the patient as dead. In spite of this, I returned immediately to the direct compression over the region of the heart and, indeed, in my excitement, applied it very rapidly and forcefully. The pupils again became rather quickly constricted, and with the continuation in the rapid tempo they became almost smaller than before; the few gasping respiratory movements, too, returned within the pause. The more rapid compressions were continued with a few short pauses for another half hour; here a change took place, in that next, the spontaneous respiratory movements became apparently more energetic within the pauses, then, though, became distinctively more numerous. The last of these, always followed by maximally dilated pupils, was finally, constantly, accompanied by a gradually more distinct movement of flexion in all joints of the upper extremities, raising of the shoulders, and wide gaping of the mouth. No sign of any heart action, however, was demonstrable, as yet, through repeated palpation of the carotid artery and auscultation during the pauses. During the compression, the carotid artery was not observed. When approximately 50 minutes after the beginning of the syncope had elapsed, peculiar movements occurred in the region of the heart, which were thought to be twitches of the intercostal musculature, since absolutely no heart sounds could be heard.

Only after at least an hour had passed since the beginning, I thought I felt a fluttering movement of the carotids. Then, as I continued the resuscitation attempts, in a short time, color rushed into the hitherto pale bluish cheeks and lips. After an interruption, the patient was breathing very quietly and a quick superficial pulse was distinctly palpable in the carotid artery. The pupils soon dilated again, though not maximally. It appeared, then, twice, as if the respiration became poorer; therefore, several additional compressions were done which might not have been necessary. Following this, any threatening symptoms no longer occurred.

The patient, having a rather low body temperature, was placed in bed with warm water bottles. The facial coloration heightened. The radial pulse returned only after a long time—1½ to 2 hours. The pupils stayed widely dilated all afternoon, but reacted to light. The boy slept until the next morning and could only be brought to defend himself against strong slapping of his cheeks. He did not give answers. Complete recovery took place very slowly. Initially, he took only a liquid diet; he could not manage solid food. For 8 to 10 days he was strikingly stuporous; then, however, slowly he regained his former, certainly not very high, intelligence. The patient was discharged, completely well, with an obturator (plate for closure of the cleft palate).

The method of Maass was published in France, and in 1893 his method was demonstrated by König and Maass at the Surgical Congress in Berlin. In 1903 Sick described a case of cardiac arrest in a 15-year-old boy. In 1936 Bruns recommended Maass-König's method as manual respiratory and heart massage.

Among the forty cases of resuscitation with cardiac arrest described by Green at the beginning of the century, seven were treated by compression of the closed chest. Crile of Cleveland had developed this method. He used rhythmical compressions of the anterior wall of the chest, together with artificial respiration. He put to use the then-known effect of epinephrine upon the muscles of the vascular system by infusion of epinephrine solutions. Here, too, for the first time reference was made to wrapping of the legs and compression of the abdomen in order to fill the remaining circulatory system with blood. (See also Pike, Guthrie and Stewart, Stephenson and Hinton.)

In his book *Anemia and Resuscitation,* Crile, 1914, wrote regarding the problem of artificial circulation:

First born in spirit was the thought that, when any part of the body, especially the thorax and the abdomen, is put under pressure, the valves of the heart and the veins cannot but cause the blood of the veins to flow toward the heart, and the blood in the arteries to flow toward the periphery. Now the action of the heart is understood. If one exercises a series of rhythmic compressions on the thorax and the abdomen instead of a single regional pressure, the entire circulation can be put into motion; that is, the person who exerts the rhythmic compressions causes an external pseudo-cardiac movement. The author was able, personally, to produce on a recently deceased person, a total circulation which caused a pulse in the radial artery and bleeding of the peripheral vessels; even a measurable blood pressure (registered by a sphygmomanometer) could be recorded through the combined effect of a tightly blown up rubber suit, which covered the lower extremities and the abdomen and the strong, rhythmical pressure through the hands, placed broadly on both sides of the thorax.

Indeed, it was possible to arbitrarily redden or

blanch the face. Without doubt, such an excellent method like Schafer's owes its success as much to the artificial circulation as to the artificial respiration. This aspect one seems to have neglected.

Kouvenhoven and his associates at Johns Hopkins Hospital in Baltimore are credited with applying closed-chest cardiac massage for the first time on a large number of patients and for having again made it popular. By 1962, it had been used successfully 222 times in 179 patients (Frey, Jude, and Safar). In August 1961 the indirect cardiac massage was recommended at the International Symposium on Emergency Resuscitation in Stavanger (Maggio and Way).

An important historical event in the field of resuscitation was the first successful defibrillation in man in 1947 (Beck). Since Batelli's experiments, numerous scientists worked on the problem of cardiac defibrillation. Important preliminary studies for its success had been performed by Hooker and Wiggers in the United States. In 1940 the latter recommended the use of a series of shocks with alternating current (Hooker, 1930, 1932; Wiggers, 1930, 1940).

In 1952 Zoll in Boston was able to obtain a response of the heart to an electrical stimulus in two patients with Adams-Stokes syndrome, in one for 25 minutes, in the other for 5 days.

The progress in cardiac surgery and the desire to operate on the opened and bloodless heart led to the necessity of putting the heart to rest and later causing it to beat again. To trace all the related techniques to their origin would exceed the framework of this contribution; therefore, only the most important ones are mentioned. The inhibiting action of potassium upon the activity of the heart muscle had been known since the end of the nineteenth century. Sydney Ringer had shown that with the administration of an excessive amount of potassium the heart comes to a standstill in diastole. Until 1955, potassium chloride had always been used in experiments. Melrose in England introduced

potassium citrate for elective cardiac arrest in 1955; his method had been generally accepted for a time (Melrose). In the same year, Lillehei in America accomplished anoxemic cardiac arrest by compressing the aorta with a tourniquet. From 1955 to 1957, Lam employed the effect of acetylcholine successfully in eighty operations.

More recently, hypothermic arrest of the heart led to promising results. With long interruption of the coronary circulation, however, artificial normothermic perfusion is presently preferred.

A physician may at any time be called upon to attempt resuscitation of the heart. Knowledge concerning cardiac resuscitation has, meanwhile, become extensive; the literature is vast. In 1953 the rate of success of resuscitation in 1,200 collected cases was recorded as 25% for the first 1,000 (Stephenson and Hinton). Since many attempts are in progress to familiarize an ever growing number of physicians with techniques of resuscitation, it is hoped that greater success will be achieved in the future.

Historical review

1543 Andreas Vesalius' (1514-1564) anatomical work *De humani corporis fabrica libri septem* is printed in Basel. Description of rekindling of the extinguishing activity of the heart in animals.

1628 Publication of William Harvey's (1578-1657) pioneer writing concerning the circulation of the blood, in which he describes the resuscitation of a pigeon.

1665-1666 Robert Hooke (1635-1703), a British botanist, repeats and confirms the experiments of Vesalius.

1679 Johann Jakob Wepfer (1620-1695) publishes his work *Circutae acquaticae historia et noxae,* in which he describes resuscitation attempts on a pharmacologic basis.

1755 John Hunter (1728-1793), a Scottish surgeon, performs experiments dealing with resuscitation in animals.

1800 Publication of the treatise *Sur la vie et la mort* by Xavier Bichat (1771-1802) in Paris. Robert Hooke's experiments repeated.

1842 E. Erichsen (1818-1896), a London surgeon, finds that ligature of the coronary arteries in dogs causes death.

1847 Sir James Simpson (1811-1870) of Edinburgh uses chloroform for the first time during a delivery.

1848 First cases of death by chloroform reported in Europe and America.

1850 The German physiologists M. Hoffa and Carl Ludwig (1816-1895) describe cardiac fibrillation for the first time.

1858 London physician John Snow (1813-1858), the first anesthesiologist, describes fifty cases of death by chloroform. Forty of these cases are attributed to cardiac failure.

1871 F. Steiner, assistant of Billroth of Vienna, recommends electropuncture of the heart for resuscitation.

1874 T. G. Hake publishes in England Moritz Schiff's (1823-1896) method of resuscitation in animal experiments (open-chest cardiac massage). Dissertation by Louis Mickwitz published in Dorpat, with a description of a method of resuscitation in animals (closed-chest cardiac massage).

1876 Dissertation of Alexander Sorgenfrey is published in Dorpat. He further develops Mickwitz's method.

1878 Publication of the work of R. Boehm of Dorpat, *Concerning Resuscitation after Poisoning and Asphyxiation*, in which he presents evidence for the artificial circulation of the blood with external heart massage.

1880 H. N. Martin (1848-1896), an American physiologist, together with Applegard, develops a method causing the mammalian heart to beat in situ.

1880-1884 Sidney Ringer (1835-1919) in London studies the action of the blood salts on the activity of the heart and makes up the Ringer's solution.

End of 1880s Swiss surgeon P. Niehans, performs for the first time the direct heart massage; he was not successful.

1891 Maass, assistant physician in the Göttingen Surgical Clinic, is able to resuscitate two patients with cardiac arrest in incidents involving anesthesia with a modification of König's method.

1893 Demonstration of the indirect cardiac massage by König and Maass at the Surgical Congress in Berlin.

1895 Experiments on the isolated mammalian heart by O. Langendorff.

1898 Moritz Schiff's resuscitation experiments are repeated by Tuffier and Hallion in France. T. Tuffier (1857-1929) succeeds for the first time in achieving temporary return of the heartbeat and respiration with the direct heart massage in a case of sudden cardiac arrest of a patient. Direct heart massage as a means of resuscitation in man is also attempted by the surgeons Gallet, de Liege, and Michaux in France.

1899 German surgeon Wehr reports a new method for opening the chest as an approach to the heart.

1900 Prus in Lemberg performs resuscitation experiments on dogs with the direct heart massage. F. Batelli in Geneva repeats Prus' experiments and discovers a method of defibrillation with alternating current.

1900 Unsuccessful attempts of resuscitation in man with direct heart massage by Prus in Lemberg, Maag in Denmark, and Aglinzeff in St. Petersburg.

1901 Fifth International Congress of Physiologists in Turin, at which J. Locke of London maintains the heartbeat of a rabbit for approximately 7 hours. Kristian Igelsrud, Norway, succeeds with the first complete resuscitation of a patient using direct heart massage. French surgeon Mauclaire recommends the transdiaphragmatic approach for direct heart massage, which soon thereafter is applied by his colleague, Poirier.

1901-1903 The physiologist Kuliabko of St. Petersburg succeeds in inducing isolated bird and mammalian hearts, finally also children's hearts postmortem, to beat.

1902 Two patients are resuscitated with the direct heart massage by Sir W. A. Lane (1856-1943) and Gray in England. Lane mentions at the same time the subdiaphragmatic method.

1903 Alois Velich, Privatdozent in Prague, repeats the experiments of Kuliabko. M. Bourcart in Geneva performs resuscitation experiments on dogs with the subdiaphragmatic method of the direct heart massage.

1904 Publication of the book *Resurrection du coeur* by Maurice d'Halluin of France, who discusses the topic of cardiac resuscitation thoroughly for that time.

1907 German surgeon R. Haecker publishes his voluminous work on heart surgery, which contains a resuscitation attempt on rabbits.

1911-1914 Substantial contributions on cardiac fibrillation by British physiologist A. G. Levy.

1914 In the United States, Crile publishes the book *Anemia and Resuscitation* in which he describes a method of indirect cardiac massage.

1915 J. A. Gunn and P. A. Martin, two British scientists, offer additional proof of the auxiliary circulation during heart massage by injecting a dye into the right ventricle and tracing its path.

1918 The surgeon Bost of Washington, D. C., describes a new technique of heart massage that represents a variation of the transdiaphragmatic method.

1947 First successful electrical defibrillation in man by the American surgeon Beck.

1952 P. M. Zoll in Boston is able to induce heartbeats in two patients with Adams-Stokes syndrome through electrical stimulation of the thorax.

1953 Stephenson and Hinton, United States, collect 1,200 cases of cardiac resuscitation of the English-speaking world.

1955 D. G. Melrose, United States, publishes his work on elective cardiac arrest with potassium citrate.

1957 C. R. Lam, United States, publishes his successful experiments dealing with elective cardiac arrest caused by acetylcholine.

1958-1960 In the Johns Hopkins Hospital in Baltimore, Jude, Kouvenhoven, and Knickerbocker develop the method of external cardiac massage.

Historical references

Aglinzeff, K. D.: Noch ein Wiederbelebungsversuch nach Prus–Maag, Centralbl. Chir. (Leipzig) 28:20, 1900.

Beck, C. S., et al.: Ventricular fibrillation of long duration abolished by electric shock (Herzflimmern von langer Dauer, welches durch Elektroschock unterbrochen wurde), J.A.M.A. 135:985, 1947.

Bichat, X.: Physiologische Untersuchungen über den Tod (1800), Übersetzung von Rudolf Boehm, Leipzig, 1911, J. A. Barth.

Boehm, R.: Über Wiederbelebung nach Vergiftungen und Asphyxie, Arch. Exp. Path. Pharmakol. 8:68, 1878.

Bost, T. C.: A new technique of heart massage (Eine neue Technik der Herzmassage), Lancet 2:552, 1918.

Bourcart, M.: De la réanimation par le massage sousdiaphragmatique du coeur en cas de mort par le chloroforme (Von der Wiederbelebung durch subdiaphragmatische Herzmassage bei Chloroformtodesfällen), Rev. Méd. Suisse Romande 23:42, 1903.

Boureau, M.: Le massage du coeur mis a nu (Die Massage am freigelegten Herzen), Rev. Chir. (Paris) 26:526, 1902.

Braatz, E.: Ueber die Wiederbelebungsversuche bei Chloroformtod, insbesondere über die dabei angewendete Electricität, Wien. Med. Bl. 7:967, 1004, 1036, 1884.

Bruns, O.: Über die beste manuelle Beatmungsmethode und ihre notwendige Ergänzung durch Herzmassage, Münch. Med. Wochenschr. 2:45, 1936.

Cackowic, M. V.: Über direkte Massage des Herzens als Mittel zur Wiederbelebung, Arch. Klin. Chir. 88:917, 1907.

Castiglioni, A.: A history of medicine, New York, 1946, Alfred A. Knopf, Inc.

Clairmont, P., Denk, W., and Haberer, H. V.: Lehrbuch der Chirurgie, Wien, 1930, E. Ranzi.

Crile, G. W.: Anemia and resuscitation, New York, 1914, Appleton-Century.

Cuveland, H., and Cuveland, E.: "Von der Hülfe bei plötzlichen Lebensgefahren." Zugleich ein Beitrag zur Anamnese der Mund-zu-Mund-Beatmung, Deutsch. Ärztebl. 37:1906, 1967.

Donley, J. E.: John James Wepfer, a renaissance student of apoplexy, Bull. Hopkins Hosp. 20:1, 1909.

Effler, D. B., et al: Elective cardiac arrest for open-heart surgery (Elektiver Herzstillstand für die Chirurgie am geöffneten Herzen), Surg. Gynecol. Obstet. 105:407, 1957.

Frey, R., Jude, J., and Safar, P.: Die äussere Herzwiederbelebung, Deutsch. Med. Wochenschr. 87:857, 1962.

Gray, H. M. W.: Subdiaphragmatic transperitoneal massage of the heart as a means of resuscitation (Subdiaphragmatische transperitoneale Herzmassage als Wiederbelebungsmittel), Lancet 2:506, 1905.

Green, R. E.: Heart massage as a means of restoration in cases of apparent sudden death, with synopsis of forty cases (Herzmassage als Mittel zur Wiederbelebung bei plötzlichen Todesfällen, mit einer Sammlung von vierzig Fällen), Lancet 2:1708, 1906.

Gunn, J. A., and Martin, P. A.: Intrapericardial medication and massage in treatment of arrest of the heart (Intrapericardiale Medikation und Massage bei der Behandlung des Herzstillstandes), J. Pharmacol. Exp. Ther. 7:31, 1915.

Haecker, R.: Experimentelle Studien zur Pathologie und Chirurgie des Herzens, Arch. Klin. Chir. (Berlin) 84:1035, 1907.

d'Halluin, M.: Résurrection du coeur, La vie du coeur isolé, Le massage du coeur, 1904, Lille.

d'Halluin, M.: Moyen de combattre les trémulation fibrillaires engendrées par le massage du coeur (Ein Mittel um die durch die Herzmassage hervogerufenen fibrillären Zuckungen abzustellen), Zbl. Physiol. 18:837, 1904.

Harvey, W.: Lectures on the whole of anatomy (an annotated translation of Prelectiones Anatomiae Universalis by C. P. O'Malley, F. N. L.

Poynter, K. F. Russell), Berkeley, 1961, University of California Press.

Harvey, W.: Movement of the heart and blood in animals (translation by K. J. Franklin), Oxford, 1957.

Hoffa, M., and Ludwig, C.: Einige neue Versuche über Herzbewegung, Z. Rationelle Med. 9:107, 1850.

Holtz, H.: Über das Verhalten der Pulswelle in der Äther- und Chloroformnarkose, Beitr. Klin. Chir. Tübingen 7:43, 1890.

Hooker, R.: Chemical factors in ventricular fibrillation, Am. J. Physiol. 92:639, 1930.

Hooker, R.: Factors in ventricular fibrillation, Am. J. Physiol. 99:279, 1932.

Hübotter, F.: Biographisches Lexikon hervorragender Ärzte, Berlin Wien, 1934.

Killian, H., and Dönhardt, A.: Wiederbelebung, Stuttgart, 1955, Georg Thieme Verlag.

Kouvenhoven, W. B., Jude, J. R., and Knickerbocker, G. G.: Closed-chest cardiac massage (Die Herzmassage beim geschlossenen Thorax), J.A.M.A. 173:1064, 1960.

Kuliabko, A.: Versuche am isolierten Vogelherzen, Zbl. Physiol. 15:588, 1901.

Kuliabko, A.: Studien über die Wiederbelebung des Herzens, Arch. Physiol. 90:461, 1902.

Kuliabko, A.: Weitere Studien über die Wiederbelebung des Herzens, Arch. Physiol. 97:539, 1903.

Lam, C. R., et al.: Clinical experiences with induced cardiac arrest during intracardiac surgical procedures (Klinische Erfahrungen mit willkürlich herbeigeführtem Herzstillstand während intracardialen chirurgischen Eingriffen), Ann. Surg. 146:439, 1957.

Langendorff, O.: Untersuchungen am überlebenden Säugetierherzen, Arch. Physiol. 61:291, 1895.

Levy, A. G.: Sudden death under light chloroformanaesthesia (Plötzlicher Tod unter leichter Chloroformanaesthesie), J. Physiol. 42:111, 1911.

Levy, A. G.: The exciting causes of ventricular fibrillation in animals under chloroform anaesthesia (Die erregenden Ursachen des Kammerflimmerns bei Tieren in Chloroformnarkose), Heart 4:319, 1912-1913.

Levy, A. G.: The genesis of ventricular extrasystoles under chloroform; with special reference to consecutive ventricular fibrillation (Die Entstehung ventriculaerer Extrasystolen unter Chloroform; mit besonderer Beachtung des nachfolgenden Kammerflimmerns), Heart 5:299, 1913-1914.

Locke, F. S.: The action of Ringer's fluid and of dextrose on the isolated rabbit heart (Die Wirkung der Ringerlösung und der Dextrose auf das isolierte Kaninchenherz), Zentralbl. Physiol. 15:490, 1901.

Maag: Ein Versuch der Wiederbelebung (ad modum Prus) eines in Chloroformnarkose gestorbenen Mannes, Centralbl. Chir. (Leipzig) 28:20, 1901.

Maass: Die Methode der Wiederbelebung bei Herztod nach Chloroformeinathmung, Berl. Klin. Wochenschr. 12:265, 1892.

Maggio, G., and Way, W.: Ein Fall von äusserer Herzmassage bei Herzinfarkt, Anaesthesist 12: 353, 1963.

Malgaigne: Rapport sur divers cas de mort attribués au chloroforme, et sur dangers que peut présenter l'inhalation de cet agent (Bericht über verschiedene Todesfälle durch Chloroform, und über die Gefahren, welche die Inhalation dieses Mittels hervorrufen kann), Gaz. Med. France 27:895-914, 1848.

Mauclaire, M.: La chloroformisation, l'éthérisation et la cocainisation lombaire, Gaz. Hôp. 140: 1345, 1901.

Mayer, S.: Ueber die direkte Reizung des Säugethierherzens, Centralbl. Chir. (Leipzig) 3:53, 1875.

Melrose, D. G., et al.: Elective cardiac arrest, Lancet 2:21, 1955.

Mickwitz, L.: Vergleichende Untersuchungen über die physiologische Wirkung der Salze der Alcalien und alcalischen Erden (dissertation), Dorpat, 1874.

Negovski, W.: Zur Wiederbelebung des Organismus, Anaesthesist 12:277, 1963.

Neuburger and Pagel: Handbuch der Geschichte der Medizin, Jena, 1905.

Neuburger, M.: Die Entwicklung der Lehre von den Herzkrankheiten, Wien. Med. Wochenschr. 78:78, 1928.

Orfila, M.: Rettungsverfahren bei Vergiftungen und im Scheintode. Übersetzung von P. G. Brosse, Vossische Buchhandlung Berlin 1819 zitiert bei 62 Rettungsverfahren für vergiftete und asphyktische Personen. Übersetzung von J. F. John. Vossische Buchhandlung Berlin 1831.

Prévost, J. L.: Contribution à l'étude des trémulation fibrillaires du coeur electrisé (Ein Beitrag zum Studium der fibrillären Zuckungen des elektrisierten Herzens), Rev. Méd. Suisse Rom. 545: 1898.

Prévost, J. L., and Batelli, F.: Quelques effets de décharges électriques sur le coeur de mammifères (Einige Wirkungen elektrischer Entladungen auf das Herz der Säugetiere), J. Physiol. Expér. 2:40, 1900.

Prévost, J. L., and Batelli, F.: Influence de l'alimentation sur le rétablissement de fonction du coeur (Der Einfluss der Ernährung auf die Wiederherstellung der Herzfunktion), Zentralbl. Physiol. 15:482, 1901.

Prus, J.: Über die Wiederbelebung in Todesfällen in Folge von Erstickung, Chloroformvergiftung und elektrischem Schlage, Wien. Klin. Wochenschr. 21:486, 1900; Centralbl. Chir. (Leipzig) 27:1002, 1900.

Ringer, S.: Concerning the influence exerted by each of the constituents of the blood on the contraction of the ventricle (Über den Einfluss der einzelnen Bestandteile des Blutes auf die Kontraktion der Ventrikel), J. Physiol. 3: 380, 1880-1882.

Ringer, S.: A further contribution regarding the influence of the different constituents of the blood on the contraction of the heart (Ein weiterer Beitrag betreffend den Einfluss der verschiedenen Blutbestandteile auf die Kontraktion des Herzens), J. Physiol. 4:29, 1884.

Safar, P.: Closed-chest cardiac massage (Herzmassage am geschlossenen Thorax), Acta Anaesthesiol. Scand. (1961) S. 125

Schiff, M.: Gesammelte Beiträge zur Physiologie, Lausanne, 1896.

Schmid, M.: Beiträge zur Geschichte der Theorien von den Kreislaufkrankheiten nach Entdeckung des Blutreislaufs (dissertation), München, 1953.

Schwiete, W. M.: Wiederbelebung vor 150 Jahren, Deutsch. Med. Wochenschr. 37:1689, 1967.

Sibson, F.: On the death from chloroform (Über den Chloroformtod), London Med. Gaz. 42:108, 1848.

Sick, P.: Zur operativen Herzmassage, Centralbl. Chir. (Leipzig) 30:981, 1903.

Singer and Underwood: A short history of medicine, Oxford, 1962.

Snow, J.: Chloroform and other anesthetics, London, 1858, John and Churchill.

Sorgenfrey, A.: Ueber die Wiederbelebung und Nachkrankheitenu nach Scheintod (dissertation), Dorpat, 1876.

Sprengel, W.: Geschichte der Chirurgischen Operationen, Halle, 1899.

Steiner, F.: Ueber die Electropunctur des Herzens als Wiederbelebungsmittel in der Chloroformsynkope, Arch. Klin. Chir. 12:741, 1871.

Stephenson, H. E., Jr.: Cardiac arrest and resuscitation, Saint Louis, 1964, The C. V. Mosby Co.

Stephenson, H. E., Jr., and Hinton, J. W.: Use of

intra-aortic and intracardiac transfusions in cardiac arrest (Die Anwendung von intraaortalen und intracardialen Transfusionen bei Herzstillstand), J.A.M.A. 152:500, 1953.

Sudhoff, K.: Kurzes Handbuch der Geschichte der Medizin, Berlin, 1922.

Tillmanns, H.: Lehrbuch der allgemeinen Chirurgie, Leipzig, 1904.

Velich, A.: Kritische und experimentelle Studien über die Wiederbelebung von tierischen und menschlichen Leichen entnommenen Herzen, München. Med. Wochenschr. 33:1421, 1903.

Vesalius, A.: De Humani Corporis Fabrica, Basel, 1555.

Wehr: Über eine neue Methode der Brustkorberöffmung zur Freilegung des Herzens. Ber.üb. Verhandl. d. deutschen Gesellsch. f. Chirurgie, Beilage, Centralbl. Chir. (Leipzig) 26:74, 1899.

Wiggers, C. J.: Studies of ventricular fibrillation caused by electric shock (Studien über das durch elektrischen Schock erzeugte Herzflimmern), Am. J. Physiol. 92:223, 1930.

Wiggers, C. J.: The mechanism and nature of ventricular fiibrillation (Mechanismus und Natur des Herzflimmerns), Am. Heart J. 20:399, 1940.

Wiggers, C. J.: The physiologic basis for cardiac resuscitation from ventricular fibrillation—method for serial defibrillation (Die physiologische Basis für die Wiederbelebung des Herzens bei Herzflimmern—Methode zur serienweisen Defibrillation), Am. Heart J. 20:413, 1940.

Willius, F. A., and Dry, F. J.: A history of the heart and the circulation, Philadelphia, 1948, W. B. Saunders Co.

Wunderlich, C. A.: Geschichte der Medizin, Stuttgart, 1859.

Zenker, R., Heberer, G., and Borst, H. G.: Eingriffe am Herzen unter Sicht, Deutsch. Med. Wochenschr. 84:577, 1959.

Zesas, D. G.: Zur Frage der Herzmassage beim Chloroformkollaps, Wien Med. Wochenschr. 54: 1498, 1904.

Zoll, P. M.: Resuscitation of the heart in ventricular standstill by external electric stimulation (Wiederbelebung des Herzens bei Stillstand der Ventricel durch äussere elektrische Stimulierung), N. Engl. J. Med. 247:768, 1952.

Zoll, P. M.: Badische Medicinalordnung von 1807.

Chapter 68

A LOOK TOWARD THE FUTURE

Since by far the largest group of patients requiring cardiopulmonary resuscitation involves those with acute myocardial infarctions, it is entirely logical that a preponderance of effort has been made in this direction. Obviously, mobile coronary care units will increase in their effectiveness. Doubtless their number will rapidly increase. With further identification of important risk factors, our detection of these patients seems increasingly likely. Instruction of the patient and particularly of the family seems a logical extension of this effort as well as even the possibility of self-administration of prophylactic medication.

Soffer suggests that every patient with coronary heart disease carry a "wallet history" containing information about previous cardiac history, medications, and perhaps even a copy of his electrocardiogram.

Already there are signs that some inroad is being made to salvage a portion of the 365,000 "coronary deaths" that occur outside the hospital in the United States alone. Hospital and community programs are rapidly becoming increasingly sophisticated and effective in the ability to reach these patients.

In view of the strides that are being made with experimental ventricular defibrillation by an automatic and completely implanted system, it seems likely that such a system can be developed for use in some particularly high risk groups.

The increasing use of electromagnetic tape recorders for continuous recording of the electrocardiogram in detecting previously uninvestigated arrhythmias seems clearly to be a "worthwhile wave of the future." Monitoring the individual for a period of time and under varying circumstances allows the physician to select a drug that will give some protection to the patient for it seems clear that the patient prone to some dysrhythmias has a life span potential that is statistically diminished.

Inherited abnormalities of myocardial repolarization have come under increasing scrutiny, particularly since the realization that approximately 1% of all children with congenital deafness also inherit a prolongation of the Q-T interval with a predisposition to syncopal attacks and sudden deaths. The exact cause of the prolonged Q-T interval still remains a mystery. With increased attention to this problem the chances of unravelling the cellular events governing electrical activity of the heart increases.

Some strides have been made in ventricular support of the heart refractory to the immediate measures necessary for cardiopulmonary resuscitation. Certainly this represents an area of logical extension of cardiopulmonary resuscitative efforts, and we hopefully anticipate significant advances that can be applied on a clinical basis.

Any program to effectively diminish the incidence of sudden cardiac deaths must include education of the victim that will stimulate a call for help at the first onset of any sign of trouble.

At the time of the preparation of the third edition of this book, approximately 130 persons had received heart transplants. Now, more than 5 years later the figure is still less than 240. What have we learned from cardiac transplantation? In these hearts with their neural connections abolished, much information on the humoral influences and their effect upon either the stabilization or the upsetting of the electrical activity of the heart may be provided. Contractile properties of cardiac muscle and action of drugs on the heart have been studied. Attention has been focused on the ethics of human experimentation.

It would seem most obvious that in the months and years ahead the patient and the physician will insist that every hospital have an adequate program for training its staff and that the quality control of resuscitation efforts be maintained at a high level. We would hope that hospital accreditation will insist on effective and functioning cardiac resuscitation committees responsible for disseminating all new advances in the area of resuscitation, maintaining resuscitation equipment in proper repair, and providing up-to-the-minute data on all resuscitative efforts as well as providing a continued evaluation of the quality of resuscitative efforts.

Since the possibilities of successful resuscitation are diminished during the evening and at night hours in a hospital, it is imperative that the hospital emergency facilities be upgraded to permit successful resuscitation 24 hours a day.

With more sophisticated equipment continuingly being developed, management of the patient inevitably benefits. For example, there is an obvious advantage in defibrillators in which the paddles oscilloscope after the defibrillatory shock.

The increased tempo of research activity aimed at an improved understanding of underlying mechanisms triggering cardiac arrest is encouraging. The physician's ability to identify and predict high risk candidates for sudden death is improving.

The future will likely see an increased interest in psychologic determinants of sudden death.

It is hoped that in the future hospital administrators and staff will attach greater significance to the risk of malfunction of life-support equipment. A greater appreciation of the common electrical hazards to

which patients are exposed and the proper utilization and care of medical electronic equipment is obviously going to produce increased dividends for the patient.

As chairman of the Inner Society Commission of Heart Disease Resources, Green and his committee point to common inadequacies in the maintenance of life-support equipment in a group of eleven major Detroit hospitals. They spot-checked cardiac monitors, electrocardiograms, defibrillators, cardioverters, pacemakers, cardiac catheterization equipment, resuscitation carts, and other such emergency equipment. Seventy-one cardiac monitors representing nine different brands were checked and inadequacies included difficult-to-use controls and difficult-to-repair assemblies, defects in the power cord, weight-meter malfunctions, cathode tube malfunction, excessive current leakage (in twenty-four of seventy-one monitors), a current spike or sudden increase in current when the monitor was switched on or off, faulty internal wiring connections, and defective internal components. Power cord defects, malfunction in control knobs, inaccurate markers, inaccurate paper speed, unacceptably low or high frequency cut off and excessive leakage of current (thirty-three of forty-four) were examples of defects found in forty-four electrocardiographs representing nine different brands. Nine different brands of defibrillators were examined and such defects were encountered as a difficult-to-find power switch as well as an unnecessarily complex connector for the patient cable, a fragile connector, loosely fittting connectors that could be pulled out accidentally, several bent or defective paddles, machines that lacked automatic discharge, units with unnecessarily high component densities, and an exposed high voltage capacitor. Four out of nine A.C. defibrillators were out of calibration and two were unsafe to turn on. Surprisingly, five out of eleven emergency rooms visited had no defibrillators at all. In several hospitals the nurse responsible for defibrillation actually did not know the internal from the external paddle electrodes and often the internal paddles were unsterile! External paddles were often bent, corroded, pitted, or otherwise in unacceptable condition. Some of the hospitals had no resuscitation team. Resuscitation carts were often littered with unnecessary spare parts, dried-up tubes of electrode paste, and rolls of tape and other redundant equipment. Amazingly enough, the investigative team found examples where the pacing catheter tips were electrically exposed in all nine brands of pacemakers studied. In eighteen of forty-seven units tested, output amplitude was thought to be out of calibration. In eighteen, the pacemaker rate was actually quite different from the rate seen on the dial. In spite of the great advances in cardiac pacemakers, several hospitals actually had no facilities for endocardial pacing.

As predicted in previous editions, a great deal has subsequently been learned about the blood supply to critical regions of the heart such as within the small sinus node arteries supplying the conduction areas. As increasing attention centers on these crucial regions, the overall significance of the microcirculation affecting the conduction system may be determined. Better nerve-mapping probes are being developed as an aid in heart surgery.

Continued attention is being directed toward risk factors associated with coronary artery disease and sudden death—hypercholesterolemia, hypertension, hyperglycemia, and excessive cigarette smoking. In some studies, over three fourths of the men suffering instantaneous death could be categorized as having two or more of these risk factors. Efforts directed at further identification of risk factors as well as alleviating them would seem to be obviously productive. Clearly, if the incidence of sudden death is to be reduced, success must be obtained in getting the victim of the myocardial infarction to the hospital sooner. While the median elapsed time between onset of acute symptoms and hospital admission is now about 8 hours, only about 15% of the patients reach the hospital within 4 hours. Why? Presumably because of lack of information regarding the significance of their symptoms, misinterpretation of symptoms, or denial of the importance of their symptoms. The unavailability of medical attention ranks relatively low as a major source of delay. Will the self-administration of antiarrhythmic drugs such as atropine or lidocaine at the onset of a heart attack prove of value?

The development of an effective prophylactic antiarrhythmic drug free of toxicity and side reactions would be a truly significant advance.

The search for the ideal antiarrhythmic drug continues; in fact there is still some disagreement as to what qualifications the ideal antiarrhythmic agent should have. We must continue to look hopefully to the pharmacologists and physiologists in their search for these new drugs. Interdisciplinary research is needed now more than ever.

Electrophysiologists have contributed significantly to our understanding of the electrical stability of the heart. There are obviously still many unanswered questions about the cardiac conduction system. For example, little is known of the normal development of the cardiac conduction system of the human. Despite the many years that necropsy studies have been performed there is still a paucity of information concerning the conduction system, its blood supply, and possible contribution to the demise of the patient in cases of sudden unexplained death. Although much more information is now available on the biochemical and metabolic events taking place at the cellular level during periods of anoxia in the myocardium, it appears that only a beginning has been made.

During the remainder of the 1970s it seems logical that we will see increasing attention directed toward providing immediate care of the individual with an acute cardiac problem. No doubt there will be a proliferation of life-support stations at many key places outside the hospital, as at airports and in factories.

Finally, even though cardiopulmonary resuscitation efforts are prompt and appear technically correct, some patients experiencing sudden cessation of cardiac output suffer severe neurologic deficits. The explanation has often been obscure and indicates factors other than simply the time factor may be involved.

During periods of transient cardiac arrest, a series of events appear to be triggered producing significant inadequacies of the microcirculation that persist even after CPR is initiated. From Norway, Hartveit and Halleraker have documented the aggregation of formed elements of the blood in the microcirculation of the kidneys and lungs in patients after external cardiac massage. By contrast, these findings were absent in a similar group not receiving CPR. Anaerobic glycolysis occurring in the brain and producing lactic acid locally has a devastating effect on the microcirculation through microemboli and thrombi formation with aggregation and sludging of formed blood elements.

Amazingly, dogs whose brains are made bloodless by elevated cerebrospinal fluid pressures can tolerate up to 25 minutes of complete anoxia with subsequent recovery (Neely and Youmans). The damaging effect on the enzymatic system from sludged microcirculation is reflected in adenosine triphosphatase levels determined by sequential cerebral biopsies (Sealy and co-workers). Along with considerable indications of intravascular coagulation in some patients subjected to cardiac resuscitation and with provocative evidence of some causative factors, efforts toward a recovery of the patency of the microcirculation may prove fruitful in CPR. Because of specific antisludging and lysosome membrane stabilization properties, steroids and low molecular weight dextran seem of promise. Both drugs not only act to decrease cerebral edema with its adverse effect on perfusion but reduce platelet adhesiveness.

Despite only gradual gains here and minimal gains there, a feeling of optimism persists that we may be embarking upon a higher ground of success in combatting the problem of sudden death. Certainly, a feeling of futility is no longer justified.

STANDARDS FOR CARDIOPULMONARY RESUSCITATION (CPR) AND EMERGENCY CARDIAC CARE (ECC)

At the National Conference on Standards for Cardiopulmonary Resuscitation (CPR) and Emergency Cardiac Care (ECC) held in May 1973, standards for CPR and ECC were developed and recommended. They relate to (1) recommended principles and techniques for basic and advanced life support, (2) CPR training and certification according to American Heart Association standards, (3) training of medical and allied health personnel, (4) the role of the American National Red Cross and other agencies in training the lay public, (5) the role of life support units in stratified systems of emergency cardiac care, and (6) medico-legal aspects of CPR and ECC. The complete conference proceedings will be published by the National Academy of Sciences.

PART I. INTRODUCTION

These standards have been developed as a working guide for the proper training and performance of cardiopulmonary resuscitation and emergency cardiac care. They have been prepared by leading authorities and

Reprinted by permission of the American Heart Association, Inc., 44 East 23rd Street, New York, New York 10010.

represent a consensus of many qualified persons from a variety of disciplines. However, the performance of cardiopulmonary resuscitation and emergency cardiac care is an art that is constantly changing and developing as the benefits of continuing experience and research become available, and the standards should serve to implement changes as required. They are in no way intended to limit new concepts or advances. Deviations from these standards may occur in certain situations not contemplated by the standards or where a trained clinician has a sound basis for his actions.

The American Heart Association and the National Academy of Sciences–National Research Council cosponsored a National Conference on Standards for Cardiopulmonary Resuscitation (CPR) and Emergency Cardiac Care (ECC) in Washington, DC, May 16-18, 1973. This Conference was conducted because of the changes that have occurred during the past several years. In May 1966, the National Academy of Sciences–National Research Council sponsored a Conference on Cardiopulmonary Resuscitation that recommended the training of medical, allied health, and professional paramedical personnel in cardiopulmonary resuscitation according to the standards of the American Heart

867

Association.[8, 10] Those recommendations resulted in widespread acceptance of cardiopulmonary resuscitation and training in the technique.

Since the 1966 meeting, cardiopulmonary resuscitation has become a part of the broader field of emergency cardiac care. This development has been influenced by the efforts and activities of many groups. Outstanding contributions have been made by the American Heart Association through its training materials and programs,[1-7] by the decisions of National Academy of Sciences–National Research Council committees and their publications,[8-15] by the reports of the Inter-Society Commission on Heart Disease Resources,[16-22] and by the recommendations and evaluations of government agencies,[23-29] professional medical societies,[30-34] private groups,[35-39] and individuals.[40, 41] These programs have been assisted financially and organizationally by federal agencies such as Regional Medical Programs, Health Services and Mental Health Administration, National Heart and Lung Institute, Department of Transportation, and by numerous state and local governing bodies, professional organizations, and rescue groups.

As a result of these activities, it has become increasingly apparent that a broad national program of life support measures is required to bring the benefits of cardiopulmonary resuscitation and emergency cardiac care to all segments of the public. This can be accomplished only by intensive public and professional programs.

These programs must

1. Provide education to increase awareness of the risk factors that may lead to heart attack, early warning signs and recognition of heart attack, and what to do in a cardiopulmonary emergency.

2. Eliminate patient and physician denial and reduce the time interval between onset of symptoms and the delivery of life support through the emergency medical care system.

3. Assure adequate training of large segments of the public in basic life support measures.

4. Generate integrated, community-wide stratified programs of emergency cardiac care as part of comprehensive emergency medical services.

5. Guarantee the availability and accessibility of an emergency care system for effective stabilization and treatment of emergency patients at the scene and during transportation by well-trained emergency medical technicians and other ambulance and rescue personnel.

6. Provide adequate life support units throughout all communities.

7. Standardize the roles of hospital staff and the adequacy of equipment and facilities in hospital emergency departments.

The Conference, accepting as a model program one that embodied all the above attributes, has created standards with this statement that will assist in promoting a national program of life support measures. Recommendations of the Conference are as follows:

1. Basic life support CPR training programs must be extended to the general public, starting with specific need groups such as policemen, firemen, lifeguards, rescue workers, high-risk-industry workers, and families of cardiac patients, and then expanded to include training of school children and other segments of the general public. The American National Red Cross, medical organizations, and other agencies concerned with lifesaving will participate in these programs.

2. Training in cardiopulmonary resuscitation and emergency cardiac care must be according to the standards of the American Heart Association. The association will continue to review, revise, and up-date the standards on the basis of scientific information and experience.

3. Certification of competency at various levels of life support must be based on nationally standardized curricula that include both written and performance tests.

4. Delivery of basic and advanced life support by highly trained personnel must be required for all life support units and hospitals on an integrated, stratified, community-wide basis.

5. These goals must be implemented by legislation and medicolegal action where needed, to ensure the delivery of effective cardiopulmonary resuscitation and emergency cardiac care to the entire population.

General considerations

It has been estimated that about one million persons in the United States experience acute myocardial infarction each year.

More than 650,000 die annually of ischemic heart disease. About 350,000 of these deaths occur outside the hospital, usually within two hours after the onset of symptoms. Thus, sudden death from heart attack is the most important medical emergency today. It seems probable that a large number of these deaths can be prevented by prompt, appropriate treatment. In addition, many victims who die as a result of such accidental causes as drowning, electrocution, suffocation, drug intoxication, or automobile accidents could be saved by the prompt and proper application of cardiopulmonary resuscitation and emergency cardiac care. This can best be assured by the victim's entry into an organized and effective system of emergency cardiac care.

Emergency cardiac care (ECC) is an integral part of a total, community-wide comprehensive system of emergency medical services (EMS) and should be integrated into the total system response capability for all types of life-threatening situations. The system must provide proper identification and appropriate action for all medical emergencies. However, the standards presented here concern themselves only with the principles and concepts of emergency cardiac care.

Emergency cardiac care

In this statement, emergency cardiac care includes all the following elements:

1. Recognizing early warning signs of heart attacks, preventing complications, reassuring the victim, and moving him to a life support unit without delay.
2. Providing immediate basic life support at the scene, when needed.
3. Providing advanced life support as quickly as possible.
4. Transferring the stabilized victim for continued cardiac care.

Emergency transportation alone, *without life support,* does not constitute emergency cardiac care. Although transportation is an important aspect, the major emphasis of ECC is life support through stabilization of the victim *at the scene* of the life-threatening emergency. Stabilization must be maintained during transport of the victim to the site of continuing cardiac care.

Within the definition of emergency cardiac care there are two other important concepts that must be clarified—basic life support and advanced life support.

Basic Life Support is an emergency first aid procedure that consists of the recognition of airway obstruction, respiratory arrest and cardiac arrest, and the proper application of cardiopulmonary resuscitation (CPR). CPR consists of opening and maintaining a patent airway, providing artificial ventilation by means of rescue breathing, and providing artificial circulation by means of external cardiac compression.

Advanced Life Support is basic life support plus use of adjunctive equipment, intravenous fluid lifeline (infusion), drug administration, defibrillation, stabilization of the victim by cardiac monitoring, control of arrhythmias, and postresuscitation care. Also it includes establishing necessary communication to assure continuing care, and maintaining monitoring and life support until the victim has been transported and admitted to a continuing care facility. Advanced life support requires the general supervision and direction of a physician who assumes responsibility for the unit. It must have adequate communications on a 24-hour-per-day basis. This may necessitate appropriate legislation or standing orders for implementation.

To be effective, emergency cardiac care should be an integrated part of a total community-wide emergency care and communication system. It is to be based on local community needs and resources and be consistent with state and national policies. The success of such a community-wide system requires multijurisdictional participation and planning to ensure operational, as well as equipment, compatibility within that system and between adjacent systems. The initial planning of a community-wide system should be under the direction of a local community advisory council on emergency services charged with the responsibility of assessing community needs and resources, defining priorities, and planning to meet those needs. Critical evaluation of operating policies, procedures, statistics, and case reports must be a continuing responsibility of state or local governments or the council. Such an evaluation should provide the basis for modification and evolution of the system.

It is well recognized that the emergency cardiac care segment of a community-wide emergency system is best provided through a stratified system of coronary care.[19] This stratified system has three levels:

> Level 1: Emergency Life Support Units
> (a) Life Support Units
> (1) Basic
> (2) Advanced
> (b) Mobile Life Support Units
> (1) Basic
> (2) Advanced
> Level 2: Coronary Care Units
> Intermediate Care Units
> Level 3: Regional Reference Centers.

The standards recommended within this statement are concerned only with the first level, *emergency life support units.* Components such as public education, professional education, and emergency medical communication are essential parts of the total emergency system.

Public education. The greatest risk of death from heart attack lies in the first two hours after onset. The potential victim must first be educated to recognize the usual manifestations of heart attack—persistent chest-shoulder-arm pain, sweating, nausea-vomiting, palpitation, fatigue. He then must know how to gain access to the emergency medical system. The fastest way for an emergency medical team to respond is through the use of a universal emergency telephone number, such as 911. Once this number is established, it must be promoted through an educational program so that it will be used.

Each individual should have a well-formulated plan of action for use in an emergency. This plan will be based on the plan of action optimal for his own community. In some cases, this means that a physician

should be called first, and, if he is not immediately available, the victim should proceed without delay to an emergency department or a facility with life support capability.

When symptoms suggest an acute heart attack, the Conference recommends that a mobile life support unit be summoned to reduce the elapsed time from the onset of symptoms to entry into an emergency medical services (EMS) system.

Professional education. Physicians must be aware of the emergency medical system in their own communities. Their actions should reflect the knowledge that most cardiac fatalities occur outside the hospital, and that every effort must be made to reduce the delay between the initial symptoms and the victim's entry into an effective emergency care system. The physician should be aware of possible delays and avoid them.

Physician competence in CPR must be assured, and he should formulate a plan of action for emergency cardiac situations occurring in his office, in patients' homes, and elsewhere in the community.

Emergency medical communications. Emergency medical communications is a vital element that must be integrated into any system of emergency medical services for it to function effectively. An adequate communication network for an ECC response is but one facet of total emergency medical services, but the communications system that supports emergency cardiac care also should support emergency medical service as a whole.

The communications system will help preserve life and minimize morbidity at the scene, during transit, and in the hospital emergency department. There should be careful coordination of equipment and frequencies, including subcarriers for telemetry, to facilitate both compatibility of subsystems at their interface and effective regionalization in the future.

Agreements for sharing communication channels and other forms of coordination are necessary. Emergency medical communications should be integrated into the emergency system and coordinated with such other agencies as fire, police, highway patrol, Coast Guard, and Military Assistance to Safety and Traffic.

The emergency medical system should provide for central receipt of all emergency calls and central dispatching of all elements of that system, depending on the nature of the emergency, geographic location, capability of the rescuing units, and other emergencies in progress. The central emergency medical communication center must have full knowledge of emergency care systems, their composition, their disposition, and all activities, as well as medical capabilities and census of each hospital in the area. The central dispatchers also must be issued medical guidelines to help them determine the appropriate medical facility to care for each medical emergency.

Personnel of the central dispatching agency should receive special training in methods of rapid and complete questioning to determine the medical problem. They must be able to distinguish quickly the medical requirements for each type of emergency situation and follow the medical guidelines as to the most appropriate available receiving facility. In some communities, multilingual dispatchers will be required.

The communication network should be able to link each of the following to each other by means of two-way voice communications via the telephone, radio, or other means: the rescuer at the scene, the rescue vehicle, all hospitals that might receive the victim, and advisory medical personnel. Telephone-to-radio circuit interconnection, or telephone patch, should be considered as one means of extending the EMS communication system, including remote consultation, to any person or facility within reach of a telephone.

In many instances, two-way communication may be augmented by electrocardiogram telemetry. Telemetry methods and telemetry techniques must be standardized within health care delivery regions to assure that all systems within a region are compatible.

It is vital that the rescuer be able to communicate directly with the EMS physician or specially designated nurse who can advise him regarding definitive medical theory. The communications network should ensure that the receiving station or hospital is notified of the impending arrival of the victim, the nature of his problem, and his general medical condition.

Conference recommendations. Conference participants reported that the present rules and regulations of the Federal Communications Commission (FCC) frustrate the achievement of a comprehensive communication system. Adequate emergency medical service communication channels are as vital to the public as the communication channels used by police and fire services. The Conference Committees recommend that the FCC establish an emergency medical radio service that would provide sufficient spectrum space and adequate protection from interference by other services. Furthermore, the frequencies should be freely available for a variety of emergency medical applications, eg, medical voice supervision, continuous and intermittent telemetry, and relay from fixed and mobile transmitters. This freedom is necessary to ensure the growth of effective emergency medical service programs.

Role of the American Heart Association

In 1963, the American Heart Association established a Committee on Cardiopulmonary Resuscitation. This was expanded in 1971 to a Committee on Cardiopulmonary Resuscitation and Emergency Cardiac Care. The activities of this Committee have established for it a multiplicity of continuing roles in these areas. The Conference recognizes that these roles concern basic life support, advanced life support, and all aspects of emergency cardiac care, and that they have evolved into the following Committee charges:

1. To establish and revise standard concepts and techniques periodically for basic and advanced life support as related to cardiopulmonary resuscitation and stratified emergency cardiac care.

2. To establish standards for training and retraining in basic and advanced life support.

3. To establish standards for training aids and materials.

4. To develop and distribute training materials.

5. To collaborate with other national medical and allied health organizations in establishing and promoting training programs in basic and advanced life support for medical and allied health groups.

6. To train and certify instructor-trainers and instructors for various organizations such as American National Red Cross, YMCA, Medical Self Help, fire and rescue departments, police departments, ambulance emergency medical technicians, lifeguards, Scouts, Department of Defense, and other interested groups, which then will be responsible for CPR instruction of key personnel and trainees for their various groups at the community level according to the American Heart Association training standards.

7. To act as a catalyst at both the local and national levels to motivate and stimulate the development of regional planning councils, which are required for the development of stratified emergency cardiac care systems.

8. To develop and implement a simultaneous, coordinated, large-scale public education program at the national and local levels in the areas of CPR, early warning signs, and risk factors, as related to development and use of stratified emergency cardiac care systems. To help meet the needs of public response, it is planned that these programs will be coordinated with the American National Red Cross and other first aid and medical agencies.

9. To direct intensive professional education efforts to physicians to increase their awareness of the necessity for early entry of patients into (a) monitored cardiac care systems and (b) precoronary care areas.

10. To promulgate criteria at a national level to aid in decisions regarding when basic life support should not be instituted, when advanced life support should not be instituted, and when basic or advanced life support may be terminated.

11. To evolve practical guidelines for developing stratified cardiac care systems that are capable of implementation at the community level.

12. To disseminate criteria for American Heart Association affiliates and chapters to certify persons in basic and advanced life support according to nationally standardized course content and testing.

13. To disseminate such information to the medical community as (a) to date, there has not been a successful legal action against a person who has given CPR in good faith, (b) in general, medical practice acts exempt nonphysicians who are acting in an emergency situation, and (c) through the use of the CPR techniques where recommended, a large number of cardiac arrest victims have been successfully resuscitated at locations outside of hospitals and many long-term survivors have returned to full and productive lives.

14. To assist in the creation of effective "Good Samaritan" coverage for physicians, nurses, professional allied health personnel, and nonmedical personnel performing basic or advanced life support in good faith either inside or outside any life support unit.

PART II. BASIC LIFE SUPPORT

Basic life support is an emergency first aid procedure that consists of recognizing respiratory and cardiac arrest and starting the proper application of cardiopulmonary resuscitation to maintain life until a victim recovers sufficiently to be transported or until advanced life support is available. This includes the A-B-C steps of cardiopulmonary resuscitation:

A. Airway   artificial
B. Breathing   ventilation   cardiopulmonary
                                   resuscitation
C. Circulation   artificial
                   circulation

These steps always should be started as quickly as possible. They are performed in the order shown above (also shown in Fig. 1, Life Support Decision Tree) except in special circumstances such as: (a) in monitored patients or (b) in witnessed cardiac arrests. When cardiac arrest occurs in the monitored patient and trained personnel and defibrillators are available immediately, a precordial thump and/or advanced life support procedures should be instituted without delay. In a witnessed cardiac arrest, the A-B-C sequence should include use of a precordial thump. (See "Precordial Thump," page 881.)

There must be a maximum sense of urgency in starting basic life support. The outstanding advantage of CPR is that it permits the earliest possible treatment of respiratory arrest or cardiac arrest by properly trained

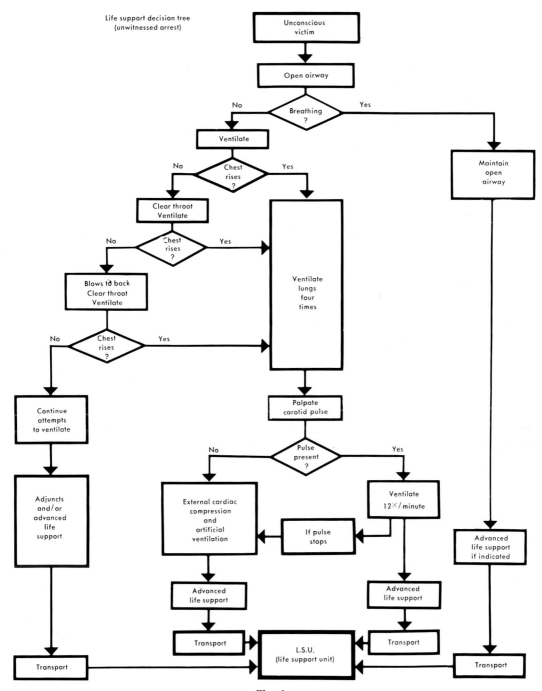

Fig. 1

persons. Optimally, only seconds should intervene between recognizing the need and starting treatment.

Indications for basic life support are:

1. Respiratory arrest and
2. Cardiac arrest. Cardiac arrest can result from:
   (a) cardiovascular collapse (electromechanical dissociation)
   (b) ventricular fibrillation, or
   (c) ventricular standstill (asystole).

In cases of collapsed or unconscious persons, the adequacy or absence of breathing and circulation must be determined immediately. If breathing alone is inadequate or absent, rescue breathing may be all that is necessary. If circulation is also absent, artificial circulation must be started in combination with rescue breathing. The methods of recognizing adequacy or absence of breathing or circulation and the recommended techniques for performing artificial ventilation and artificial circulation are presented below. Their proper stepwise sequence is detailed in the Life Support Decision Tree (Fig. 1).

Artificial ventilation

Opening the airway and restoring breathing are the basic steps of artificial ventilation. The steps can be performed quickly under almost any circumstance and without adjunctive equipment or help from another person. They constitute emergency first aid for airway obstruction and respiratory inadequacy or arrest.

Respiratory inadequacy may result from an obstruction of the airway or from respiratory failure. An obstructed airway is sometimes difficult to recognize until the airway is opened. At other times, a partially obstructed airway is recognized by labored breathing or excessive respiratory efforts, often involving accessory muscles of respiration, and by soft tissue retractions of the intercostal, supraclavicular, and suprasternal spaces. Respiratory failure is characterized by minimal or absent respiratory effort, failure of the chest or upper abdomen to move, and inability to detect air movement through the nose or mouth.

Airway. The most important factor for successful resuscitation is immediate opening of the airway. This can be accomplished easily and quickly by tilting the victim's head backward as far as possible. Sometimes this simple maneuver is all that is required for breathing to resume spontaneously. To perform the head tilt, the victim must be lying on his back. The rescuer places one hand beneath the victim's neck and the other hand on his forehead. He then lifts the neck with one hand and tilts the head backward by pressure with his other hand on the forehead. This maneuver extends the neck and lifts the tongue away from the back of the throat. Anatomical obstruction of the airway caused by the tongue dropping against the back of the throat thereby is relieved. The head must be maintained in this position at all times. (See Fig. 2.)

The head tilt method is effective in most cases. If head tilt is unsuccessful in opening the air passage adequately, additional forward displacement of the lower jaw—jaw thrust—may be required. This can be accomplished by a triple airway maneuver in which the rescuer places his fingers behind the angles of the victim's jaw and (1) forcefully displaces the mandible forward while (2) tilting the head backward and (3) using his thumbs to retract the lower lip to allow breathing through the mouth as well as through the nose. The jaw thrust is per-

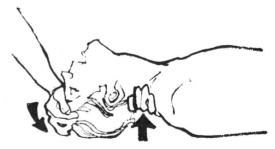

Fig. 2. Head tilt method of opening airway.

formed best from a position at the top of the victim's head.

However, if the victim does not resume spontaneous breathing, the rescuer must move to the victim's side to perform mouth-to-mouth or mouth-to-nose ventilation. Several variations of the jaw thrust may be used. When using jaw thrust for mouth-to-mouth ventilation, the rescuer must keep the victim's mouth open with his thumbs and seal the nose by placing his cheek against it. However, this is more difficult to teach and practice on manikins, and more difficult and tiring to perform on victims than the head tilt method. For mouth-to-nose ventilation with jaw thrust, the rescuer uses his cheek to seal the victim's mouth and does not retract the lower lip with his thumbs. Such special details of performance and the problems associated with manikin practice limit use of jaw thrust techniques to specially trained personnel.

Breathing. If the victim does not promptly resume adequate spontaneous breathing after the airway is opened, artificial ventilation, sometimes called rescue breathing, must be started. Mouth-to-mouth breathing and mouth-to-nose breathing are both types of artificial ventilation.

To perform mouth-to-mouth ventilation, the rescuer uses his hand behind the victim's neck to maintain the head in a position of maximum backward tilt. He pinches the victim's nostrils together with the thumb and index finger of his other hand, which also continues to exert pressure on the forehead to maintain the backward head tilt. The rescuer then opens his mouth widely, takes a deep breath, makes a tight seal with his mouth around the victim's mouth and blows into the victim's mouth. He then removes his mouth and allows the victim to exhale passively, watching the victim's chest fall. This cycle is repeated *once every five seconds* as long as respiratory inadequacy persists.

Adequate ventilation is ensured on every breath by the rescuer

1. Seeing the chest rise and fall

2. Feeling in his own airway the resistance and compliance of the victim's lungs as they expand

3. Hearing and feeling the air escape during exhalation. The initial ventilatory maneuver should be *four quick, full, breaths* without allowing time for full lung deflation between breaths. (See Fig. 3.)

In some cases, mouth-to-nose ventilation is more effective than mouth-to-mouth ventilation. The former is recommended when it is impossible to open the victim's mouth, when it is impossible to ventilate through his mouth, when the victim's mouth is seriously

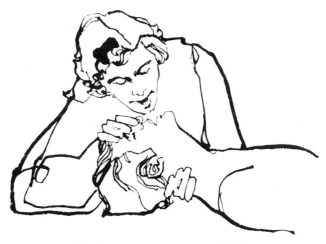

Fig. 3. Mouth-to-mouth resuscitation.

injured, when it is difficult to achieve a tight seal around his mouth, and when, for some other reason, the rescuer prefers the nasal route.

For the mouth-to-nose technique, the rescuer keeps the victim's head tilted back with one hand on the forehead and uses the other hand to lift the victim's lower jaw. This seals the lips. The rescuer then takes a deep breath, seals his lips around the victim's nose and blows in until he feels the lungs expand. The rescuer removes his mouth and the victim is allowed to exhale passively. The rescuer can see the chest fall when the victim exhales. When mouth-to-nose ventilation is used, it may be necessary to open the victim's mouth or separate his lips to allow the air to escape during exhalation because the soft palate may cause nasopharyngeal obstruction. This cycle should be repeated approximately every five seconds.

Direct mouth-to-stoma artificial ventilation should be used for persons who have had a laryngectomy. They have a permanent stoma that connects their trachea directly to the skin. It is recognized as an opening at the front of the base of the neck. Neither head tilt nor jaw thrust maneuvers are required for mouth-to-stoma resuscitation. For a patient with a temporary tracheostomy tube in his airway, it is usually necessary for the rescuer to seal the victim's mouth and nose with his hand or a tightly fitting face mask to prevent leakage of air when the rescuer blows into the tracheostomy tube. This problem can be prevented if the tracheostomy tube is provided with an inflatable cuff.

No adjuncts are required for effective rescue breathing; so artificial ventilation should never be delayed to obtain or apply adjunctive devices.

Infants and children. Opening the airway and performing artificial ventilation are essentially the same for children as for adults. There are some differences, however. For infants and small children, the rescuer covers both the mouth and nose of the child with his mouth and uses small breaths with less volume to inflate the lungs *once every three seconds.* The neck of an infant is so pliable that forceful backward tilting of the head may obstruct breathing passages. Therefore, the tilted position should not be exaggerated.

Accident cases. In accident cases, it is imperative that caution be used to avoid extension of the neck when there is a possibility of neck fracture. A fractured neck should be suspected in diving or automobile accidents when the victim has lacerations of the face and forehead. If a fracture is suspected, all forward, backward, lateral, or turning movement should be avoided. To open the airway, a modification of the jaw thrust maneuver described above should be used. In this variation, the rescuer places his hands on either side of the victim's head so the head is maintained in a fixed, neutral position without the head extended. The index fingers should then be used to displace the mandible forward without tilting the head backward or turning it to either side (modified jaw thrust). If required, artificial ventilation usually can be provided in this position. If this is unsuccessful, the head should be tilted back very slightly and another attempt made to ventilate, using the modified jaw thrust maneuver.

Foreign bodies. The rescuer should not look for foreign bodies in the upper airway unless their presence is known or strongly suspected. The first effort to ventilate the lungs will determine whether an airway obstruction is present. If the first attempts to ventilate are unsuccessful despite properly opening the airway and providing an airtight seal around the mouth, an attempt should be made immediately to clear the airway with the fingers. The victim should be rolled onto his side, with the rescuer's knee placed under his shoulder. The victim's mouth then is forced open with the thumb and index crossed-finger technique. The rescuer runs his index finger or index and middle fingers down the inside of the victims cheek toward the base of the tongue, deep into his throat. The rescuer's fingers are moved across the back of the victim's throat with a sweeping motion. Repeated attempts may be required. Where skilled, advanced life support personnel and equipment are available, direct laryngoscopy may permit the foreign body to be removed.

Larger foreign bodies frequently can be extricated by these finger maneuvers. If the rescuer is unable to dislodge the foreign body, or if it is impacted below the epiglottis, the victim should be rolled onto his side toward the rescuer, who then delivers sharp blows with the heel of his hand between the victim's shoulder blades. Further attempts at clearing the airway then should be made. If unsuccessful, there should be repeated efforts at mouth-to-mouth resuscitation, blows to the back, and probing the upper airway with the fingers. A small child having airway obstruction should be quickly picked up and inverted over the arm of the rescuer while the blows are being delivered between the child's shoulder blades.

If all of these maneuvers fail, emergency cricothyroid puncture and insertion of a 6 mm tube have been recommended for adults. However, this requires appropriate instruments and training and must be regarded as an advanced life support technique.

Gastric distension. Artificial ventilation frequently causes distension of the stomach. This occurs most often in children, but it is not uncommon in adults. It is most likely to occur when excessive pressures are used for inflation or if the airway is obstructed. Slight gastric distension may be disregarded. However, marked distension of the stomach may be dangerous because it promotes regurgitation, and it reduces lung volume by elevating the diaphragm. Several cases of gastric rupture resulting from overdistension have been reported. Obvious gross distension should be relieved whenever possible. In the unconscious victim, this can be accomplished without adjuncts by using one hand to exert moderate pressure over the victim's epigastrium between the umbilicus and the rib cage. To prevent aspiration of gastric contents during this maneuver, the victim's head and shoulders should be turned to one side.

Artificial circulation (external cardiac compression)

When sudden, unexpected cardiac arrest occurs, all of the A-B-C's of basic life support are required in rapid succession. This includes both artificial ventilation and artificial circulation (external cardiac compression). Cardiac arrest is recognized by pulselessness in large arteries in an unconscious victim having a death-like appearance and absent breathing. The status of the carotid pulse should be checked as quickly as possible when cardiac arrest is suspected. In an unwitnessed cardiac arrest, the rescuer first opens the airway and quickly ventilates the lungs four times. He then maintains the head tilt with one hand on the forehead, and with the tips of the index and middle fingers of the other hand, gently locates the victim's larynx and slides his fingers laterally into the groove between the trachea and the muscles at the side of the neck where the carotid pulse can be felt. The pulse area must be felt gently, not compressed.

There are a number of reasons for recommending palpation of the carotid pulse rather than other pulses. First, the rescuer already is at the victim's head to perform artificial ventilation and the carotid pulse is in the same area. Second, the neck area generally is accessible immediately, without removal of any clothing. Third, the carotid arteries are central and sometimes these pulses will persist when more peripheral pulses are no longer palpable. Trainees should practice palpation of the carotid pulse during classes. In hospital situations, palpation of the femoral artery is an acceptable option to use instead of the carotid artery. It is not practical to feel the carotid pulse in infants and small children. Instead, the rescuer's hand should be placed gently over the precordium to feel the apical beat.

Absence or questionable presence of the pulse is the indication for starting artificial circulation by means of external cardiac compression. External cardiac compression consists of the rhythmic application of pressure over the lower one half of the sternum, but *not over the xiphoid process*. The heart lies slightly to the left of the middle of the chest between the lower sternum and the spine. Intermittent pressure applied to the sternum compresses the heart and produces a pulsatile artificial circulation. During cardiac arrest, properly performed external cardiac compression can produce systolic blood pressure peaks of over 100 mm Hg, but the diastolic pressure is zero and the mean pressure seldom exceeds 40 mm Hg in the carotid arteries. The carotid artery blood flow resulting from external cardiac compression on a cardiac arrest victim usually is only one quarter to one third of normal.

External cardiac compression always must be accompanied by artificial ventilation. Compression of the sternum produces some ventilation, but the volumes are insufficient for adequate oxygenation of the blood. Therefore, artificial ventilation is *always* required when external cardiac compression is used.

Technique for external cardiac compression. The patient always must be in the horizontal position when external cardiac compression is performed since, during cardiac arrest, there is no blood flow to the brain when the body is in the vertical position, even during properly performed external cardiac compression. It is imperative, therefore, to get the cardiac arrest victim into a horizontal position as quickly as possible in situations where he is vertical, such as in a dental chair, trapped in a vehicle, stricken on a telephone pole, while in a stadium seat, or in any similar situation. Elevation of the lower extremities, while keeping the rest of the body horizontal, may promote venous return and augment artificial circulation during external cardiac compression.

Effective external cardiac compression requires sufficient pressure to depress an adult's lower sternum a minimum of 1½ to 2 inches. For external cardiac compression to be effec-

tive, the victim must be on a firm surface. This may be the ground, floor, or a spineboard on a wheeled litter. If the victim is in bed, a board, preferably the full width of the bed, should be placed under his back. However, chest compression must not be delayed while this support is awaited.

The rescuer positions himself close to the victim's side and places the long axis of the heel of one hand parallel to and over the long axis of the lower one half of the sternum. Great care must be exercised not to place the hand over the lower tip of the sternum (xiphoid process) that extends downward over the upper abdomen. To avoid this, the rescuer feels the tip of the xiphoid and places the heel of his hand on the lower one half of the sternum about 1 to 1½ inches away from the tip of the xiphoid and toward the victim's head. He then places the other hand on top of the first one (and may interlock the fingers), brings his shoulders directly over the victim's sternum, keeps his arms straight, and exerts pressure almost vertically downward to depress the lower sternum a minimum of 1½ to 2 inches. The compressions must be regular, smooth, and uninterrupted. Relaxation must immediately follow compression and be of equal duration. The heel of the rescuer's hand should not be removed from the chest during relaxation but pressure on the sternum should be completely released so that it returns to its normal resting position between compressions. (See Fig. 4.)

Since artificial circulation always must be combined with artificial ventilation, it is preferable to have two rescuers. One rescuer positions himself at the victim's side and performs external cardiac compression while the other one remains at the victim's head, keeping it tilted back, and continues rescue breathing. *The compression rate for two rescuers is 60 per minute.* When performed without interruption, this rate can maintain adequate blood flow and pressure and will allow cardiac refill. This rate is practical because it avoids fatigue, facilitates timing on

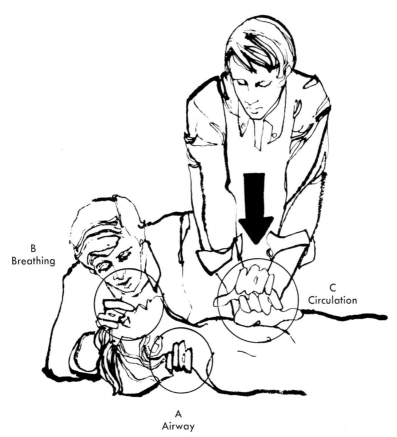

B
Breathing

C
Circulation

A
Airway

Fig. 4. Two-rescuer cardiopulmonary resuscitation.
- 5 chest compressions
  —Rate of 60/minute
  —No pause for ventilation
- 1 lung inflation
  —After each 5 compressions
  —Interposed between compressions

the basis of one compression per second, and allows optimum ventilation and circulation to be achieved by quickly interposing one inflation after each five chest compressions without any pause in compressions (5:1 ratio). The rate of 60 compressions per minute allows breaths to be interposed without any pauses. Interposing the breaths without any pauses in compression is important, since any interruption in cardiac compression results in a drop in blood flow and blood pressure to zero. (See Fig. 4.)

Two rescuers can perform CPR best when they are on opposite sides of the victim. They can then switch positions when necessary without any significant interruption in the 5:1 rhythm. This is accomplished by the rescuer who is performing artificial ventilation moving to the side of the victim's chest immediately after he has inflated the lungs. He places his hands in the air next to those of the other rescuer who continues to perform external cardiac compression. As soon as the other hands are properly placed, the rescuer performing chest compression removes his hands (usually after the third or fourth in the series of compressions) and the other rescuer then continues with the series of compressions. The rescuer who had been compressing then moves to the victim's head and interposes the next breath.

If the victim's trachea has been intubated,

lung inflation is easier and compression rates up to 80 per minute can be used since breaths can be either interposed or superimposed following endotracheal intubation.

When there is only one rescuer, he must perform both artificial ventilation and artificial circulation using a 15:2 ratio. This consists of *two very quick lung inflations after each 15 chest compressions* (Fig. 5). Because of the interruptions for lung inflation, the single rescuer must perform each series of 15 chest compressions at the faster rate of *80 compressions per minute* in order to achieve an actual compression rate of 60 per minute. The two full lung inflations must be delivered in rapid succession, within a period of five to six seconds, without allowing full exhalation between the breaths. If time

for full exhalation were allowed, the additional time required would reduce the number of compressions and ventilations that could be achieved in a one-minute period.

Infants and children. With a few exceptions, the cardiac compression technique is similar for children. For small children, only the heel of one hand is used, and, for infants, only the tips of the index and middle fingers are used. The ventricles of infants and small children *lie higher in the chest* and the external pressure should be exerted over the midsternum. The danger of lacerating the liver is greater in children because of the pliability of the chest and the higher position of the liver under the lower sternum and xiphoid. Infants require one half to three fourths of an inch compression of the ster-

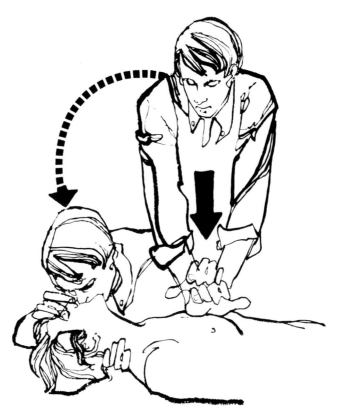

Fig. 5. One-rescuer cardiopulmonary resuscitation.
- 15 chest compressions (rate of 80/ minute)
- 2 quick lung inflations

num; young children require three fourths to 1½ inches. The compression rate should be 80 to 100 per minute with breaths delivered as quickly as possible after each five compressions.

In infants and small children, backward tilt of the head lifts the back. A firm support beneath the back is therefore required for external cardiac compression and can be provided by the rescuer slipping one hand beneath the child's back while using the other hand to compress the chest. A folded blanket or other adjunct can also be used beneath the shoulders to provide support. For small infants, an alternate method is to encircle the chest with the hands and compress the midsternum with both thumbs.

Checking effectiveness of CPR. The reaction of the pupils should be checked periodically during cardiopulmonary resuscitation, since this provides the best indication of delivery of oxygenated blood to the victim's brain. Pupils that constrict when exposed to light indicate adequate oxygenation and blood flow to the brain. If the pupils remain widely dilated and do not react to light, serious brain damage is imminent or has occurred. Dilated but reactive pupils are less ominous. Normal pupillary reactions may be altered in the aged and frequently are altered, in any individual, by the administration of drugs.

The carotid pulse should be palpated periodically during CPR in order to check the effectiveness of external cardiac compression or the return of a spontaneous effective heartbeat. This should be done after the first minute of CPR and every few minutes thereafter, when additional rescuers are present and interruptions can be minimized. It should be checked particularly at the time of change of rescuers.

Precordial thump

Continuing research and clinical experience have delineated a role for the precordial thump, but only in specific types of cardiac arrest cases. Recognizing both its limitations and usefulness, the Conference recommends the precordial thump as a basic maneuver to be used by all levels of rescuers following the detection of pulselessness in adults in these cases:

1. Witnessed cardiac arrest (basic life support)
2. Monitored patient (advanced life support)
3. Pacing known atrioventricular block (advanced life support).

The effectiveness of the precordial thump in the unmonitored patient or in an unwitnessed cardiac arrest has not been determined. Since the myocardium frequently may be anoxic in these situations a specific recommendation for precordial thump cannot be made for them. At this time the precordial thump is not recommended for use on children.

In cases where the primary cause of cardiac arrest is not hypoxia, such as in a witnessed cardiac arrest or in a monitored patient, a single precordial thump may be effective in restarting circulation and may reverse certain dysrhythmias if performed within the first minute after arrest. In those situations, an initial thump on the midsternum using the fist may be the first maneuver performed following the determination of pulselessness.

Such a blow generates a small electrical stimulus in a heart that is reactive. The thump may be effective in restoring a beat in cases of ventricular asystole due to block, and in reversing ventricular tachycardia, or ventricular fibrillation of recent onset. When necessary it may be possible to use the fist as a pacemaker in some cases of heart block. When a series of chest thumps are used for this purpose, the pulse should be palpated before each thump.

The precordial thump is not useful for anoxic asystole and cannot be depended upon to convert an established ventricular fibrillation, nor is it useful for electromechanical dissociation associated with exsanguination. It should not be used for a ventricular tachycardia that is providing adequate circulation.

The precordial thump should be used to

provide a stimulus to a potentially reactive heart. However, it is not a substitute for effective external cardiac compression.

There are also hazards associated with the precordial thump. In cases of an anoxic heart that is still beating, the low voltage stimulus may induce ventricular fibrillation. In addition, persons who do not restrict themselves to the recommended single blow may delay starting effective CPR.

In delivering the precordial thump, these rules should be followed:

1. Deliver a sharp, quick single blow over the midportion of the sternum, hitting with the bottom, fleshy portion of the fist struck from 8 to 12 inches over the chest. (See Fig. 6.)

2. Deliver the thump within the first minute after cardiac arrest.

3. If there is no immediate response, begin basic life support at once.

The precordial thump is integrated into the basic pattern of CPR differently, depending upon the circumstances surrounding the cardiac arrest. The techniques for using the thump in cases of witnessed arrest or an arrest of a monitored patient are given below.

Technique for witnessed cardiac arrest

1. Tilt the head to open the airway and simultaneously palpate the carotid pulse.

2. If the pulse is absent, give a precordial thump.

3. If the victim is not breathing, give four quick, full lung inflations.

4. If pulse and breathing are not immediately restored, begin one-rescuer or two-rescuer CPR.

Technique for monitored patient. (For use with patients who have sudden ventricular fibrillation [VF], asystole, or ventricular tachycardia [VT] without pulse.)

1. Give a single precordial thump.

2. Quickly check the monitor for cardiac rhythm and simultaneously check carotid pulse.

3. If there is ventricular fibrillation or ventricular tachycardia without a pulse, counter-shock as soon as possible.

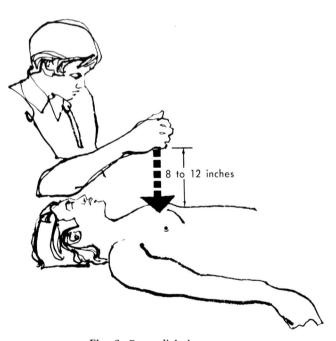

8 to 12 inches

Fig. 6. Precordial thump.

4. If the pulse is absent, tilt the head, give four quick, full lung inflations.

5. Check the carotid pulse again.

6. If the pulse is absent, begin one-rescuer or two-rescuer CPR.

It must be emphasized strongly that no time should be lost in waiting to assess the results of the precordial thump or by delivering repeated precordial thumps.

Pitfalls in performance of CPR

When CPR is performed improperly or inadequately, artificial ventilation and artificial circulation may be ineffective in providing basic life support. Enumerated below are important points to remember in performing external cardiac compression and artificial ventilation.

1. Do not interrupt CPR for more than five seconds for any reason, except in the following circumstances.

(a) Under emergency conditions, endotracheal intubation usually cannot be accomplished in five seconds. However, it is an advanced life support measure and should be performed only by those who are well trained and well practiced in the technique and *only* after the victim has been properly positioned and all preparations made. Even under these circumstances, interruptions in CPR for endotracheal intubation should never exceed 15 seconds.

(b) When moving a victim up or down a stairway, it is difficult to continue effective CPR. Under these circumstances, it is best to perform effective CPR at the head or foot of the stairs, then interrupt CPR at a given signal and move quickly to the next level where effective CPR is resumed. Such interruptions usually should not exceed 15 seconds.

2. Do not move the patient to a more convenient site until he has been stabilized and is ready for transportation or until arrangements have been made for uninterrupted CPR during movement.

3. Never compress the xiphoid process at the tip of the sternum. The xiphoid extends downward over the abdomen. Pressure on it may cause laceration of the liver, which can lead to severe internal bleeding.

4. Between compressions, the heel of the hand must completely release its pressure but should remain in constant contact with the chest wall over the lower one half of the sternum.

5. The rescuer's fingers should not rest on the victim's ribs during compression. Interlocking the fingers of the two hands may help avoid this. Pressure with fingers on the ribs or lateral pressure increases the possibility of rib fractures and costochondral separation.

6. Sudden or jerking movements should be avoided when compressing the chest. The compression should be smooth, regular and uninterrupted (50% of the cycle should be compression and 50% should be relaxation). Quick jabs increase the possibility of injury and produce quick jets of flow; they do not enhance stroke volume or mean flow and pressure.

7. Do not maintain continuous pressure on the abdomen to decompress the stomach while performing external cardiac compression. This may trap the liver and could cause it to rupture.

8. The shoulders of the rescuer should be directly over the victim's sternum. The elbows should be straight. Pressure is applied vertically downward on the lower sternum. This provides a maximally effective thrust, minimal fatigue for the rescuer, and reduced hazard of complications for the victim. When the victim is on the ground or floor, the rescuer can kneel or stand at his side. When he is on a bed or high-wheeled litter, the rescuer must be on a step or chair or kneeling on the bed or litter. With a low-wheeled litter, the rescuer can stand at the victim's side. Problems arise with the use of low-wheeled litters in ambulances. Special arrangements must be made for proper positioning of the rescuer based on the design of the ambulance.

9. The lower sternum of an adult must be

depressed 1½ to 2 inches by external cardiac compression. Lesser amounts of compression are ineffectual since even properly performed cardiac compression provides only about one quarter to one third of the normal blood flow.

10. While complications may result from improperly performed external cardiac compression and precordial thumps, even properly performed external cardiac compression may cause rib fractures in some patients. Other complications that may occur with properly performed CPR include fracture of the sternum, costochondral separation, pneumothorax, hemothorax, lung contusions, lacerations of the liver, and fat emboli. These complications can be minimized by careful attention to details of performance. It must be remembered, however, that during cardiac arrest, effective cardiopulmonary resuscitation is required even if it results in complications, since the alternative to effective CPR is death.

Special resuscitation situations

Drowning. Extensive research has delineated the events and mechanisms of drowning and the detailed physiological variations between fresh water and sea water submersion. However, basic life support resuscitation procedures following drowning are the same as basic life support principles presented above, and CPR should be performed as quickly as possible. There are a few special considerations, given below:

1. When attempting to rescue a drowning victim, the rescuer should get to him as quickly as possible, preferably with some conveyance, such as a boat or surfboard. If a conveyance is not available, a flotation device should be carried by the rescuer. The rescuer always must exercise care not to endanger himself while trying to aid a drowning person.

2. External cardiac compression should never be attempted in the water because it is impossible to perform it there effectively.

3. Mouth-to-mouth or mouth-to-nose ventilation may be performed in the water, al-though it is difficult and often impossible in deep water unless the rescuer has some type of flotation device to support the victim's head.

4. Artificial ventilation always should be started as soon as possible, even before the victim is moved out of the water, into a boat or onto a surfboard. As soon as the rescuer can stand in shallow water he should begin artificial ventilation.

5. In cases of suspected neck injury, the victim must be floated onto a back support before being removed from the water. If artificial respiration is required, the routine head tilt or jaw thrust maneuvers should not be used. Artificial ventilation should be accomplished with the head maintained in a neutral position and using a modified jaw thrust maneuver (as described under "Accident Cases," page 876).

6. When removed from the water, the victim should have standard artificial ventilation or cardiopulmonary resuscitation performed according to the standards previously described.

7. Drowning victims swallow large volumes of water and their stomachs usually become distended. This impairs ventilation and circulation and should be alleviated as soon as possible. To relieve the distension, the victim may be turned on his side and his upper abdomen compressed or he may be turned over quickly into the prone position and lifted with the rescuer's hands under the stomach to force water out. This is referred to as "breaking" the victim.

8. There should be no delay in moving the victim to a life support unit where advanced life support capabilities are available. Every submersion victim, even one who requires only minimal resuscitation, should be transferred to a medical facility for follow-up care.

Electric shock. Electric shock may induce a variety of phenomena ranging from the benign to the lethal. The outcome depends largely upon the amplitude and duration of contact with the current. Other than burns of varying severity and injuries due to falls, the possible emergency events to be recognized include:

1. Tetany of the musculature of breathing, which is usually confined to the duration of the shock but may produce secondary cardiac arrest if the tetanizing shock is of a prolonged duration.

2. Prolonged paralysis of respiration, which may result from a massive convulsive phenomenon and may last for minutes after the shock current has terminated.

3. Ventricular fibrillation or other serious cardiac arrhythmias (such as runs of premature ventricular contractions or ventricular tachycardia that may progress to ventricular fibrillation) produced by low voltage currents (110 to 220 v) sustained for several seconds.

The prognosis for victims of electric shocks is not predictable easily since the amplitude and duration of the charge usually are not known. Failure of either respiration or circulation is likely to result.

After safely clearing the victim from an energized object, the rescuer should determine his cardiopulmonary status immediately. If spontaneous respiration or circulation is absent, the technique of cardiopulmonary resuscitation outlined in this statement should be initiated.

In cases where electric shock occurs on a public utility pole, a precordial thump should be delivered and mouth-to-mouth ventilation started at once. The victim must *then* be lowered to the ground as quickly as possible. CPR is only effective when performed on a victim in the horizontal position.

Beginning and terminating basic life support

CPR is most effective when started immediately after cardiac arrest. If cardiac arrest has persisted for more than ten minutes, cardiopulmonary resuscitation is unlikely to restore the victim to his prearrest central nervous system status. If there is any question of the exact duration of the arrest, the victim should be given the benefit of the doubt and resuscitation started.

Basic life support is not indicated for a victim who is known to be in the terminal stages of an incurable condition. When resuscitation is indicated and started in the absence of a physician, it should be continued until one of the following occurs:

1. Effective spontaneous circulation and ventilation have been restored.

2. Resuscitation efforts have been transferred to another responsible person who continues basic life support.

3. A physician assumes responsibility.

4. The victim is transferred to properly trained and designated professional medical or allied health personnel charged with responsibilities for emergency medical services.

5. The rescuer is exhausted and unable to continue resuscitation.

The decision to stop resuscitative efforts is a medical one. (See sections on "Advanced Life Support" and "Medicolegal Considerations.")

Training and certification in basic life support

Artificial ventilation only. Every effort should be made to teach artificial ventilation to all members of the general public. Training the entire population should be accomplished through American National Red Cross courses, as well as through schools, YMCA's, clubs, local groups, and medical, paramedical and rescue organizations. All school children should be required to have annual training in artificial ventilation beginning in the fifth grade, and a major national effort should be mounted to achieve this objective in the shortest possible time.

The Conference further recommends that training should be provided by courses conducted by trained and certified instructors according to the technique described above and in accordance with the training standards of the American Heart Association. For optimum results, training should include such media as lectures, demonstrations, posters, slides, and movies. Actual practice on training manikins is required to assure efficiency of performance. Acceptable manikins must simulate obstruction of the airway when the head is not tilted back maximally, allow mouth-to-mouth and mouth-to-nose ventilation, and simulate rise of the chest when the lungs are inflated. Training should be to a level of demonstrated proficiency in mouth-to-mouth and mouth-to-nose resuscitation on adult manikins and mouth-to-mouth-and-nose on infant manikins.

Basic life support. CPR is an emergency procedure that requires special training both to recognize cardiopulmonary arrest and to perform artificial ventilation and artificial circulation. In order to ensure the widest possible benefits of its application, programs should be started to train the general public in basic life support according to the recommended American Heart Association standards. Initially, groups with the greatest need such as policemen, firemen, rescue workers, lifeguards, high-risk industry workers, and families of cardiac patients may receive preference, but the goal should be to train the general public, starting with school children at the eighth grade level.

Basic life support training of the public should be under the auspices of the American National Red Cross, the YMCA, and comparable volunteer and public service agencies concerned with saving lives. Training programs must adhere to the standards of the American Heart Association. These agencies should participate in training CPR instructors to teach basic life support and in certifying allied health personnel and nonmedical groups, public specialty groups, school children, and other segments of the population according to the training and performance standards of the American Heart Association as recommended by the National Research Council.

In addition to lectures, demonstrations, and films, actual practice and demonstration of proficiency in both the ventilatory and the circulatory components of cardiopulmonary resuscitation are required on training manikins. CPR cannot be taught or practiced on conscious or unconscious human subjects.

Manikins used in CPR training programs must provide (a) airway obstruction when the neck is flexed, (b) effective chest movement as a result of proper lung ventilation via mouth or nose, and (c) adequate movement of the sternum as a result of properly applied external cardiac compression against resistance. In addition, it is desirable for training devices to provide a simulated carotid pulse and an objective means (lights, gauges, strip chart) by which the student or instructor can determine adequacy of lung inflation and chest compression and mistakes in hand position. Palpation of the actual carotid pulse should also be practiced on other trainees.

To simplify instruction in basic life support, initial training should cover the recommended A-B-C sequence used for an unwitnessed cardiac arrest. When the trainee understands and can perform this effectively, further instruction should include use of precordial thump for witnessed cardiac arrest and for monitored patients.

Certification in CPR. The purpose of certification is, as far as possible, to maintain adherence to uniform national standards established or recognized by the American Heart Association. Certification will be accomplished through the use of national cognitive (written or oral) and performance examinations. Receipt of certification will be contingent on satisfactory completion of such examinations and will indicate that the person certified was found to be qualified at the time of examination to perform and/or teach those, and only those, emergency techniques indicated by the certifying individual or agency. The process of training, certification, and recertification is intended to develop and maintain a mechanism for emergency cardiac care and resuscitation that is both broadly available and uniformly effective, in a manner most consistent with the public interest and safety. Certification does not imply that the American Heart Association or any designated certifying individual or agency either warrants or assumes responsibility for the performance of individuals subsequent to their certification.

An initial course leading to certification in CPR should be for small groups and should include didactic presentations and sufficient supervised, intensive manikin practice for every student to become proficient in detecting breathlessness and pulselessness and in performing the sequential steps of rescue breathing and external cardiac compression. Both one-rescuer and two-rescuer CPR should be practiced.

Periodic recertification or refresher courses that include retesting on manikins are required for all personnel, including instructors. The exact frequency for such recertification may need to be regulated on the basis of the professional skill and experience of particular groups. At present, suggested requirements for nonmedical groups are recertification one year from the initial course and then at least every three years thereafter, or more frequently where indicated.

CPR instructors. CPR instructors should be highly motivated individuals who represent special or organized groups in the community in which they will provide CPR training, have a background in or the capability for teaching, have an interest in or a role in the delivery of CPR, have completed an initial CPR course, and have successfully completed the CPR instructor's course according to American Heart Association standards and have a valid instructor's certificate.

Certification of instructors will indicate that the recipient has passed the examination for instructor certification as defined elsewhere in this statement, and it will authorize the holder to conduct CPR courses according to standards of the American Heart Association. Certification of instructors is not intended to imply that the American Heart Association or any other certifying agency warrants or assumes responsibility for the performance of individuals trained by such certified instructors.

Certification of instructors is valid for a specified time and must be renewed periodically. If instructors are actively engaged in CPR instruction or performance and are familiar with new techniques, they may be recertified after review by local certifying authorities. If they are not actively engaged in training, they should attend a recertification course as detailed above.

Conference recommendations. The Conference recommends that CPR training be given to all eighth grade pupils and that it be repeated each year through high school. Additional pilot studies are required to determine the effectiveness of newer training methods.

The Conference mandates that CPR courses be required as part of the curriculum of all medical, dental, nursing, osteopathic, respiratory therapy, and other allied health schools. In order to implement this, the Association of American Medical Colleges should be made aware of this requirement so that all schools include instruction in basic life support and require a demonstration of proficiency in performance of this technique as part of their curricula.

The Conference recommends that every hospital with acute care facilities must assign to a specific committee the responsibilities for providing CPR teams on a 24-hour-per-day basis and that they be capable of performing CPR and all aspects of emergency life support. The CPR or emergency life support team should consist of nurses, technicians, respiratory therapists, house staff, and on-call attending staff. Wherever possible, the CPR hospital committee should be composed of, at least, a surgeon, a cardiologist, an anesthesiologist, an in-service nurse, and an administrator. The committee should be responsible for providing a written plan of action (protocol), CPR training and practice sessions, and a record of CPR occurrences available for periodic audit and review.

The Conference recommends that all nurses and physicians, including house staff, should be competent in all phases of CPR. To accomplish this, it is recommended that all hospitals require that, for annual staff reappointment, all physicians must either:

1. Demonstrate proficiency in basic life support through participation in actual resuscitation efforts or in teaching CPR to others, or

2. Agree to attend an approved training or retraining course offered by the hospital or their local heart association.

All hospital medical and nursing emergency department personnel must be trained and certified in basic and advanced life support, and all allied health personnel must be trained in basic life support.

The Conference further recommends that all hospitals and all state boards of health, divisions of hospital licensing, change their rules to conform to the above requirements and that they be included in the standards for hospital accreditation by the Joint Commission on Accreditation of Hospitals and as a stated policy of the American Hospital Association.

PART III. ADVANCED LIFE SUPPORT

As used in this statement, advanced life support consists of the following elements:

1. Basic life support.

2. Using adjunctive equipment and special techniques, such as endotracheal intubation and open chest internal cardiac compression.

3. Cardiac monitoring for dysrhythmia recognition and control.

4. Defibrillating.

5. Establishing and maintaining an intravenous infusion lifeline.

6. Employing definitive therapy, including drug administration (a) to correct acidosis and (b) to aid in establishing and maintaining an effective cardiac rhythm and circulation.

7. Stabilization of the patient's condition.

In some cases, advanced life support includes transportation that has (a) communication to ensure continuity of care and (b) the capability of constant monitoring and life support until the patient has been transported and admitted to a continuing care facility.

Advanced life support may be provided either by nonmobile life support units or by mobile life support units. Each unit must be staffed with highly trained personnel and specialized equipment in order to deliver the quality of care demanded by the criteria listed above. Each of these elements of advanced life support includes various components as described below.

Basic life support

All approaches to advanced life support must include a well-established basic life support capability, as described in Part II, "Basic Life Support," and illustrated in . . . Fig. 1, Life Support Decision Tree.

Adjunctive equipment and special techniques

Adjunctive equipment is not essential for cardiopulmonary resuscitation. It may be used when it becomes available, but only by specialized personnel who have had adequate training with the specific devices to be used. Basic life support should not be delayed while awaiting equipment, nor should use of equipment result in diverting attention or effort from basic resuscitative measures. When considering adjunctive equipment, it must be remembered that personnel must be trained to a level of demonstrated proficiency in the use of adjunctive equipment, even equipment of a relatively simple nature. In addition, adjunctive equipment must be tested periodically for satisfactory performance according to prescribed regulations. Adequate records of such tests also must be maintained.

Adjuncts for airway and ventilation

Oxygen. Supplemental oxygen should be used as soon as it becomes available. Rescue breathing (exhaled air ventilation) will deliver about 16% to 17% oxygen to the patient. Ideally, this will produce an alveolar oxygen tension of 80 torr. However, because of the low cardiac output (large arteriovenous O_2 gradient) associated with external cardiac compression and the presence of intrapulmonary shunting and ventilation-perfusion abnormalities, marked discrepancies will occur between the alveolar and arterial oxygen tension and hypoxemia may ensue. Hypoxemia leads to anaerobic metabolism and metabolic acidosis, which frequently impair the beneficial effects of chemical and electrical therapy.

Because of this, the Conference recommends that supplemental oxygen always be used when bag-valve-mask or bag-valve-tube systems are used. This will enhance myocardial and cerebral oxygenation that is essential for successful resuscitation.

Oropharyngeal airway. Oropharyngeal airways should be used whenever a bag-valve-mask system or automatic breathing device with mask is used, but only if done by an individual properly trained in their use. Airways should be used only on deeply unconscious persons. If introduced into a conscious or stuporous person, they may promote vomiting or laryngospasm. Care is required in the placement of the airway because incorrect insertion can displace the tongue back into the pharynx and produce airway obstruction. Oropharyngeal airways should be available in infant, child, and adult sizes. Nasopharyngeal airways also may be used for adults. As with all adjunctive equipment, explicit training and practice is required for their use.

S-tube. Numerous S-tube airway adjuncts are available. They range from simple tubes with mouth-pieces and bite blocks to more elaborate devices with valves. Despite many different designs, they share certain limitations.

S-tubes

1. Do not provide as effective an airway seal as direct mouth-to-mouth or mouth-to-mask ventilation.

2. Do not reduce potential transmission of infection.

3. Require training for safe and effective use.

4. Induce vomiting if used improperly.

5. Require the single rescuer to move to the victim's head and reposition the S-tube to inflate the lungs between chest compressions.

S-tubes do offer useful features, such as

1. Overcoming aesthetic problems of direct mouth-to-mouth contact.

2. Assisting in maintaining a patent airway.

3. Keeping the mouth open.

However, it is generally found that direct mouth-to-mouth or mouth-to-mask ventilation provide more effective artificial ventilation.

Masks. Well-fitting masks have proven to be an effective, simple adjunct available for use in artificial ventilation by medical, allied health, and nonmedical personnel. Manikin practice with masks should be required for all personnel who are likely to use a mask for mouth-to-mask ventilation. The mask may be a standard anesthesia mask or a folding pocket mask and should have the following characteristics: transparent material, well-sealing cuff, headstraps, oxygen insufflation inlet, 15 mm/22 mm coupling size, and availability in one average size for adults and additional sizes for infants and children. The mask is most effectively used when the rescuer positions himself at the top of the patient's head and uses the jaw thrust maneuver, as described on page 874.

Bellows devices. Bellows devices are *ineffectual* for providing artificial ventilation. The Conference condemns all ventilation bellows that have been made commercially available. All of them suffer a common design flaw so that even professional rescuers cannot provide adequate lung ventilation when applying downward or sideward compression with a bellows. *Bellows devices should not be used for resuscitation.*

Bag-valve-mask devices. When bag-valve-mask units are used, they usually provide less ventilatory volume than mouth-to-mouth or mouth-to-mask ventilation because of the difficulty in providing a leakproof seal to the face while maintaining an open airway. For this reason, the manually-operated, self-inflating bag-valve-mask units can be used effectively only by well-trained and experienced medical personnel, such as anesthesiologists.

Extensive specialized training and demonstrated continuing proficiency is required with the bag-valve-mask device. The rescuer must position himself at the top of the victim's head. He then must maintain the head in extension, keep the lower jaw elevated, and secure an optimum mask fit with one hand while using the other hand to squeeze the bag. Attempts have been made to achieve effective ventilation with these devices by using two rescuers, one to hold the mask and one to squeeze the bag, but this is an awkward procedure.

Because of this difficulty in using the bag-valve-mask unit, the Conference recommends that these devices be used only when the patient has a cuffed endotracheal tube or a cuffed esophageal obturator airway inserted. Either of these tubes will ensure delivery of an adequate volume of oxygen-enriched atmosphere and will prevent gastric insufflation and aspiration of stomach contents. When an endotracheal tube or esophageal obturator airway is used the rescuer may position himself at the victim's side. When a mask is used, the rescuer always should position himself at the top of the victim's head and not at his side.

An adequate bag-valve-mask unit should fulfill these criteria:

1. Self-refilling, *but without sponge rubber inside*—because of difficulty in cleaning, disinfecting, eliminating ethylene oxide, and fragmentation.

2. Non-jam valve system at 15 liters/minute oxygen inlet flow.

3. Transparent, plastic face mask with an air-filled or contoured, resilient cuff.

4. No pop-off valve, except pediatric models.

5. Standard 15 mm/22 mm fittings.

6. System for delivery of high concentrations of oxygen through an ancillary oxygen inlet at the back of the bag or via an oxygen reservoir.

7. True nonbreathing valve.

8. Oropharyngeal airway.

9. Satisfactory for practice on manikins.

10. Satisfactory performance under all common environmental conditions and extremes of temperature.

11. Available in adult and pediatric sizes.

Esophageal obturator airway. The esophageal obturator airway is a recent innovation in the management of cardiac arrest patients. It appears to be a useful airway adjunct, but its future role remains to be determined. The airway consists of a cuffed endotracheal tube mounted through a face mask and modified with a soft plastic obturator blocking the distal orifice and multiple openings in the upper one third of the tube at the level of the pharynx. It is passed into the esophagus. The mask then is seated on the face and the cuff inflated. When mouth-to-tube or bag-valve-tube ventilation is performed, the air is discharged through the pharyngeal openings in the tube and passes down the trachea since the esophagus is blocked. This prevents gastric distension and regurgitation during resuscitation. The esophageal obturator airway should only be inserted in patients who are not breathing or who are deeply unconscious.

The potential advantages of the esophageal obturator airway are that no visualization is required for introduction and that it can be introduced more easily and quickly than an endotracheal tube. In a large series of cardiac arrest cases, the airway has been shown to be used successfully without injury to the esophagus when used by professional allied health personnel who had been trained in its use on intubation manikins and unconscious patients.[41] However, the potential for damage to the esophagus is ever present unless use of the airway is restricted to adequately trained individuals.

Removal of the esophageal airway frequently is followed by immediate regurgitation. In order to cope with this, the airway should not be removed until the patient is conscious and breathing or has a return of reflexes. When it is to be removed, the patient should be turned on his side and adequate suction should be available. It is also possible to pass a nasogastric tube around the esophageal tube and decompress the stomach prior to removing the esophageal tube. A standard cuffed endotracheal tube can be introduced into the trachea prior to removal of the esophageal tube.

Endotracheal intubation. Oxygenation of the lungs by exhaled-air methods or by simple airway adjuncts should always precede attempts at tracheal intubation. Adequate lung inflations interposed between external cardiac compressions require high pharyngeal pressures. These pressures promote gastric distension, which elevates the diaphragm and interferes with adequate lung inflation. This distension promotes regurgitation, with the potential hazard of aspiration of gastric contents into the lungs. Therefore, the trachea should be intubated as soon as practical by trained personnel. This isolates the airway, keeps it patent, prevents aspiration, and assures the delivery of a high concentration of oxygen to the lungs. With a cuffed endotracheal tube (or esophageal obturator airway), it is easier to provide adequate ventilation since it is not necessary to interpose breaths as with direct mouth-to-mouth, mouth-to-mask, or bag-valve-mask techniques. It then becomes possible to use a faster, uninterrupted chest compression rate of 80 per minute and provide better artificial circulation.

Because of the difficulties, delays, and complications in properly placing an endotracheal tube, its use should be restricted to medical personnel and professional allied health personnel who are highly trained and either use endotracheal intubation frequently or are retrained frequently in this technique.

The indications for endotracheal intubation include:

1. Cardiac arrest

Table 1. Recommended sizes for endotracheal tubes and suction catheters*

Age	Endotracheal tube (internal diameter)	Suction catheters
Newborn	3.0 mm	6 Fr.
6 months	3.5 mm	8 Fr.
18 months	4.0 mm	8 Fr.
3 years	4.5 mm	8 Fr.
5 years	5.0 mm	10 Fr.
6 years	5.5 mm	10 Fr.
8 years	6.0 mm	10 Fr.
12 years	6.5 mm	10 Fr.
16 years	7.0 mm	10 Fr.
Adult (female)	8.0-8.5 mm	12 Fr.
Adult (male)	8.5-9.0 mm	14 Fr.

*One size larger and one size smaller should be allowed for individual variations.

2. Respiratory arrest

3. Inability of rescuer to ventilate the unconscious patient with conventional methods.

4. Inability of the patient to protect his own airway (coma, areflexia), or

5. Prolonged artificial ventilation.

The Conference recommends that all emergency department training programs and equivalent programs give satisfactory training to all professional personnel in the safe and effective introduction of endotracheal tubes.

Endotracheal tubes should be available in various sizes. They should have standard 15 mm/22 mm fittings, be provided with a stylet, be cuffed for adults and older children, and be uncuffed for infants and small children. The recommended sizes for endotracheal tubes are given in Table 1.

Oxygen-powered mechanical breathing devices

CONVENTIONAL PRESSURE-CYCLED AUTO-MATIC RESUSCITATORS (IPPB respirators, positive-negative pressure resuscitators, resuscitators-inhalators) should not be used in conjunction with external cardiac compression because effective external cardiac compression prematurely triggers termination of the inflation cycle so inadequate ventilation results. These devices are complex, difficult to use, more costly, and relatively less effective, even for artificial ventilation alone, than oxygen-powered ventilation devices that are manually triggered (time-cycled).

MANUALLY TRIGGERED (TIME-CYCLED) DEVICES are easier to use effectively. They have high instantaneous flow rates that allow them to be used for artificial ventilation alone. The devices also allow breaths to be interposed between compressions during CPR. Most will function as inhalators too, for patients who are breathing spontaneously but require oxygen.

Manually triggered, oxygen-powered resuscitators should be able to

1. Provide instantaneous flow rates of 100 liters/minute or more and an inspiratory pressure safety release valve that opens at 50 cm of water, although it is recognized that this high instantaneous flow rate usually will result in gastric distension unless a cuffed endotracheal tube or cuffed esophageal obturator airway is used.

2. Provide 100% oxygen.

3. Operate satsifactorily under environmental conditions, including all temperature extremes found in North America.

They also should have the following minimum design criteria:

1. A standard 15 mm/22 mm coupling for mask, endotracheal tube, esophageal airway, and tracheostomy tubes.

2. A rugged, breakage-resistant mechanical design that is compact and easy to hold.

3. A trigger positioned so that both hands of the rescuer can remain on the mask to hold it in position while supporting and tilting the head and keeping the jaw elevated.

Suction devices. Portable and installed suction equipment should be available for resuscitation emergencies. The portable unit should provide vacuum and flow adequate for pharyngeal suction. It should be fitted with large-bore, non-kinking suction tubing and semirigid pharyngeal suction tips. There should be multiple sterile suction catheters of various sizes for suctioning via endotracheal or tracheostomy tubes, a nonbreakable

collection bottle, and a supply of water for rinsing the tubes and catheters.

The installed suction unit should be powerful enough to provide an air-flow of over 30 liters/minute at the end of the delivery tube and a vacuum of over 300 mm Hg when the tube is clamped. The amount of suction should be controllable for use on children and intubated patients.

There should be an additional set of rigid pharyngeal suction tips (tonsil suction tips) and sterile curved tracheal suction catheters of various sizes. For tracheal suction, a Y- or T-piece, or a lateral opening, should be between the suction tube and suction source for on-off control. The suction yoke, collection bottle, water for rinsing, and suction tube should be readily accessible to the attendant at the head of the litter. The tube should reach the airway of any patient, regardless of his position. Suction apparatus must be designed for easy cleaning and decontamination.

Nasogastric tube for gastric decompression. It is preferable to insert a nasogastric tube after the airway has been isolated by endotracheal intubation. However, if gastric distension interferes with adequate ventilation, a nasogastric tube may be inserted at an earlier time by trained medical, nursing, or authorized allied health personnel. External cardiac compression should not be interrupted during this procedure.

Adjuncts for artificial circulation

Bedboard. Cardiopulmonary resuscitation should be performed at the site where the victim was found, whether inside or outside the hospital. If the cardiac arrest occurs in a hospital bed, a firm support should be provided beneath the patient's back when CPR is performed. A simple serving tray or support of comparable size is useful but not best. To provide proper support, a bedboard that extends from the shoulders to the waist and across the full width of the bed should be available. Spineboards should be used for ambulance services and mobile life support units. Spineboards also are useful for extricating and immobilizing victims. They may be used directly on the floor of the emergency vehicle or on a wheeled litter.

Manual chest compressors. Simple, hinged, manually operated mechanical chest compressors can be used for effective external cardiac compression. They should provide an adjustable stroke of 1½ to 2 inches and be able to be applied with interruptions in manual CPR of no longer than five seconds each. These compressors are inexpensive and make it easier for an individual to provide prolonged, effective external cardiac compression.

Automatic chest compressors. Optimum management of persons with cardiac arrest is obtained when the definitive therapy required to restore spontaneous circulation and to stabilize the victim is available at the site of the arrest, prior to any transportation that may be necessary. When this is not possible, the use of an automatic mechanical device provides the most consistently effective cardiopulmonary resuscitation during transportation or prolonged resuscitation. When such devices are used, external cardiac compression always must be started with the manual method first. Physicians and other medical personnel who will be using the automatic equipment must have careful and extensive training and manikin practice in the manual method, the mechanical method, and the proper technique for changing from one to the other without interrupting CPR for more than 5 to 10 seconds at any one time. A well-trained and coordinated team of persons is necessary to use the compressor.

These devices eliminate the operator fatigue that causes variations in cardiac output, and they provide simultaneous ventilation with high oxygen concentrations. While these devices afford more regular and uninterrupted CPR, they have the following limitations:

1. They are relatively heavy and difficult to move because of their associated oxygen tanks and components.

2. They may be difficult to use without accidentally displacing the plunger while moving a victim up and down stairs or on a steep incline.

3. The use of commercially available models is limited to adults.

Compressor-ventilators should be employed only with a cuffed endotracheal tube, esophageal airway, or, if used with a mask, only by well-trained and experienced personnel. Their performances should be comparable to that recommended for the manual method.

Internal cardiac compression

Internal cardiac compression is indicated in certain conditions where external cardiac compression may be ineffective. These circumstances include penetrating wounds of the heart and other internal thoracic injuries, cardiac tamponade, tension pneumothorax with mediastinal displacement, chest or spinal deformities, and severe emphysema causing barrel-type chest. If it is suspected or can be determined that any of these conditions is present, or, if closed chest cardiac compression does not appear to establish sufficiently effective artificial circulation, open chest internal cardiac compression may be performed in conjunction with artificial ventilation.

Open chest cardiac compression should only be performed by a physician with the necessary skill, equipment, and facilities. In this procedure, a thoracotomy is performed through the left fifth intercostal space and the pericardial sac is opened to allow direct manual cardiac compression.

Cases of crushed chest or flail chest may require only effective artificial ventilation. If there is cardiac arrest so that artificial circulation also is required outside of a hospital, external cardiac compression may be used with the recognition that, while it may compound internal injuries, it represents the only alternative to certain death.

If a tension pneumothorax is suspected in an emergency situation, a large bore needle may be inserted on the side of the pneumothorax through the second intercostal space

2 inches from the midline. If the diagnosis is confirmed, this should be replaced with a chest tube and valve or an underwater seal drainage as soon as possible.

In trauma cases, especially chest trauma, it may be very difficult to detect evidence of circulatory activity. Special efforts, including palpation of femoral and carotid pulses and auscultation for heart sounds, may be required to determine the cardiac status. Individuals who deal frequently with serious trauma cases should be trained thoroughly in CPR and its possible complications.

Cardiac monitoring

Electrocardiographic (ECG) monitoring should be established immediately on all patients who present symptoms of suspected heart attack or sudden collapse.

Most sudden deaths following acute myocardial infarction are due to electrical derangement of the rhythm of the heart (dysrhythmias). Susceptibility to electrical derangement is greatest immediately following and several hours after myocardial damage or severe ischemia. It is during this critical and unstable period that patients should be under continuous and critical monitoring.

Although rhythm changes may occur abruptly without warning, potentially lethal situations usually can be prevented by early detection and prompt treatment.

Each person providing advanced life support must have adequate training and testing to establish his capability of dysrhythmia detection and treatment. Once trained, his competency must be reenforced and examined continually. This can be accomplished through regularly scheduled assignment to hospital patient care, such as in the emergency department, coronary care unit, intensive care unit, or operating room.

ECG monitoring is a vital step in the prevention of cardiac arrest in patients with acute myocardial infarction. Personnel providing advanced life support must be familiar with monitoring equipment, including its problems and artifacts. They also must be capable of recognizing, at a minimum, the following electrocardiographic dysrhythmias:

1. Cardiac standstill (ventricular asystole).
2. Bradycardia (rate of less than 60 per minute).
3. The difference between supraventricular and ventricular rhythms.
4. Premature ventricular contractions (frequency, multifocal, and R on T).
5. Ventricular tachycardia.
6. Ventricular fibrillation.
7. Atrioventricular blocks of all degrees.
8. Atrial fibrillation and flutter.

In addition to recognizing these dysrhythmias, all personnel must be familiar with the potential dangers inherent in each waveform and with the therapeutic regimen that is required when any one of them is present.

In situations in which the initial emergency problem is a cardiac arrest, CPR steps and techniques outlined under "Basic Life Support" should be initiated. As quickly as possible thereafter, ECG electrodes should be applied. For this purpose, a monitor-defibrillator with combination ECG electrode-defibrillator paddles is recommended. These ECG electrode-defibrillator paddles are applied to the chest and an immediate determination of the cardiac rhythm may be made.

If ventricular fibrillation is present, defibrillation should be immediate. (See section on "Defibrillation.")

If there is a relatively regular ECG rhythm, pulse and blood pressure should be checked immediately to determine if electromechanical dissociation is present.

If the rhythm and circulation are satisfactory, oxygen should be administered, an intravenous lifeline established, and regular ECG electrodes applied for continuous monitoring.

Drugs, as indicated in the section on "Drugs and Definitive Therapy," should be used to maintain a stable cardiac rhythm and adequate circulation.

Monitoring and supportive therapy should be continued in situations where communications must be established to transfer the patient.

Defibrillation

Defibrillation produces a simultaneous depolarization of all muscle fascicles of the heart, after which a spontaneous beat may resume if the myocardium is oxygenated and not acidotic. Direct current defibrillator shocks should be delivered as soon as possible when the heart is known to be in ventricular fibrillation. Countershocks also are indicated on an emergency basis in the presence of ventricular tachycardia without a peripheral pulse. It has not been demonstrated that defibrillation is useful in cases of ventricular asystole, although it is sometimes used when it is impossible to be sure whether the heart is in a fine ventricular fibrillation or true ventricular standstill.

For defibrillation, the standard electrode position always should be used: one electrode just to the right of the upper sternum below the clavicle and the other electrode just to the left of the cardiac apex or left nipple. Standard electrode paste may be used but saline-soaked four by four gauze sponges are also excellent conductors. The sponges may be applied rapidly and external cardiac compression may be resumed after defibrillation without the problem of hand slippage on the chest that occurs when electrode paste is used.

A single defibrillator shock does not produce serious functional damage to the myocardium; so there is no reason to withhold it in the unconscious, pulseless adult patient when a direct current defibrillator is available even though the patient is unmonitored. In these circumstances, unmonitored defibrillation with a single shock may be performed by medical or properly trained and authorized allied medical personnel. It must be emphasized that this single shock must not delay the prompt application of basic life support measures in any way. *Unmonitored defibrillation is not recommended for children.*

In instances of apparent cardiac arrest secondary to hypoxemia, eg, drug overdose, CPR for a period of two minutes is recommended, with reevaluation prior to the delivery of an unmonitored defibrillator shock.

The optimum amount of electrical energy has not been established and there are no conclusive data concerning the ideal defibrillator output waveform. The output delivered into a 50-ohm load should range from 0 to at least 250 watt-seconds, preferably 300 watt-seconds for the conventional Lown waveform.[22] This range will provide adequate energy for the majority of patients. The energy requirements of defibrillators with other waveforms may vary from this range. In emergency situations, it has been customary to deliver a maximum shock of 400 joules (watt-seconds) for cases of ventricular fibrillation. However, lower settings frequently are effective in converting ventricular fibrillation and ventricular tachycardia and produce less myocardial damage. The damage resulting from defibrillator shocks is directly proportional to the energy used, and maximal settings, when not required, may further impair an already damaged myocardium. The energy level delivered through a 50-ohm load should be indicated on the front panel of the defibrillator. All defibrillators, particularly those that register stored energy, should be checked at regular, frequent intervals with suitable test equipment to determine the delivered energy. Breakdown and defects develop in units that are used frequently at high energy levels. Well-organized, detailed, and recorded preventive maintenance should be performed regularly also.

Establishing and maintaining intravenous infusion

It is essential to provide an intravenous route for the intermittent or continuous rapid administration of drugs and fluids that may be required to reestablish or support a stable cardiac rhythm and adequate circulation. This route must be established as early as possible and must be a routine part of advanced life support.

Drugs and definitive therapy

Drug administration and other forms of definitive therapy are required for most patients who receive cardiopulmonary resuscitation or emergency cardiac care. Tracheal intubation by trained personnel and the early administration of high concentrations of oxygen are of major importance in reducing hypoxemia during the cardiorespiratory emergency. While the dangers of hypoxemia are easily demonstrated experimentally and clinically, there is no evidence that lung damage occurs with high concentrations of oxygen if it is used for periods of less than 24 hours.

Drug administration is of critical importance in emergency cardiac care. Drugs usually are administered intravenously during the cardiopulmonary resuscitation emergency to ensure their delivery into the cardiovascular system as artificial circulation is provided. A cutdown or long-term intravenous route should be established as early as possible. Intracardiac injections are sometimes used, but this route is usually limited to epinephrine early in the cardiac arrest and before an intravenous infusion has become available.

For purposes of these Conference recommendations, drugs are divided into two categories: essential and useful.

Essential drugs
    Sodium bicarbonate
    Epinephrine
    Atropine sulfate
    Lidocaine
    Morphine sulfate
    Calcium chloride
    (Oxygen is also considered an essential
      drug.)

Sodium bicarbonate. Sodium bicarbonate is necessary to combat metabolic acidosis. It is administered intravenously in an initial dose of 1 mEq/kg by either bolus injection or continuous infusion over a ten-minute period. Once effective spontaneous circulation is restored, further administration of sodium bicarbonate usually is not indicated and may be harmful.

The available dosage forms for sodium bicarbonate are:
1. Prefilled syringe:
     50 ml of 8.4% sol. (50 mEq)
     50 ml of 7.5% sol. (44.6 mEq)
2. Ampules:
     50 ml of 8.4% solution (50 mEq)
     50 ml of 7.5% solution (44.6 mEq)
3. Bottles:
     500 ml of 5% solution (297.5 mEq)

The dosage of 1 mEq/kg should be used regardless of dosage form.

Where ventricular fibrillation is present, defibrillation should be attempted immediately. Then sodium bicarbonate should be administered. If an effective circulation is not restored after defibrillation and the initial dose of bicarbonate, a repeat dose of 1 mEq/kg should be given. It is recommended that, in hospitalized patients, further administration of sodium bicarbonate be governed by arterial blood gas and pH measurement.

Effective ventilation must accompany sodium bicarbonate administration to remove carbon dioxide in the arterial blood. Where blood gases and pH determinations are not available, one half of the initial dose may be administered at ten-minute intervals. Metabolic alkalosis and hyperosmolality from excessive therapy must be avoided. Catecholamines may be given simultaneously or in rapid succession with sodium bicarbonate, but generally they should not be added to continuous infusions of the bicarbonate since this may cause inactivation of the catecholamines.

Sodium bicarbonate should not be used alone in cases of cardiac standstill or cases of persistent ventricular fibrillation. In these instances, repeated doses of epinephrine and sodium bicarbonate should be administered while continuing effective external cardiac compression and artificial ventilation. The combined use of epinephrine and sodium bicarbonate may result in a cardiac standstill converting into a ventricular fibrillation, which then can be defibrillated. Use of both drugs during ventricular fibrillation improves the status of the myocardium and enhances the effectiveness of the defibrillation.

Epinephrine. Although epinephrine can be shown experimentally to produce ventricular fibrillation, its actions in restoring electrical activity in asystole and in enhancing defibrillation in ventricular fibrillation are well documented also. Epinephrine increases myocardial contractility, elevates perfusion pressure, lowers defibrillation threshold, and, in some instances, restores myocardial contractility in electromechanical dissociation. A dose of 0.5 ml of a 1:1,000 solution diluted to 10 ml, or 5 ml of a 1:10,000 solution, should be administered intravenously every five minutes during a resuscitation effort. Intracardiac administration may be utilized by personnel well trained in the technique if there has not been sufficient time to establish an intravenous route.

Atropine sulfate. Atropine sulfate reduces vagal tone, enhances atrioventricular conduction, and accelerates the cardiac rate in cases of sinus bradycardia. It is most useful in preventing arrest in profound sinus bradycardia secondary to myocardial infarction, particularly where hypotension is present. When there is profound bradycardia, acceleration of the heart rate to the normal rate of 60 to 80 beats per minute probably improves cardiac output and may reduce the incidence of ventricular fibrillation secondary to ectopic electrical activity.

Atropine sulfate is indicated for the treatment of sinus bradycardia with a pulse of less than 60 beats per minute when accompanied by premature ventricular contractions or systolic blood pressure of less than 90 mm Hg. It is also indicated for high degree atrioventricular block when accompanied by bradycardia. It is of no value in ventricular ectopic bradycardia in the absence of atrial activity. The recommended dose is 0.5 mg administered intravenously as a bolus, and repeated at five-minute intervals until a pulse rate greater than 60 is achieved. The total dose of atropine sulfate should not exceed 2 mg except in cases of third degree atrioventricular block, where larger doses may be required.

Lidocaine. Lidocaine raises the fibrillation threshold and exerts its antidysrhythmic effect by increasing the electrical stimulation threshold of the ventricle during diastole. In usual therapeutic doses, there is no significant change in myocardial contractility, systemic arterial pressure, or absolute refractory period. This drug is particularly effective in depressing irritability where successful defibrillation repeatedly reverts to ventricular fibrillation. It also is particularly effective in the control of multifocal premature ventricular beats and episodes of ventricular tachycardia. Fifty to 100 mg should be administered slowly as a bolus intravenously and may be repeated if necessary. It may be followed by a continuous infusion of 1 to 3 mg/minute, usually not exceeding 4 mg/minute. Lidocaine, as 500 mg in 500 ml of 5% dextrose in water, provides a solution of 1 mg/ml for infusion. Lidocaine is of no value in asystole.

Morphine sulfate. Morphine sulfate is not indicated in cardiopulmonary resuscitation emergencies, but it is important in cases of myocardial infarction to relieve pain and in the treatment of pulmonary edema. For pain relief in acute myocardial infarction, 1 ml of morphine sulfate (15 mg) should be diluted to 5 ml (3 mg/ml). Of this solution, 1 ml (3 mg) to 1.5 ml (4.5 mg) should be given intravenously every 5 to 30 minutes as required. Experience has indicated that the titration of small doses at frequent intervals provides the desired effect and avoids significant respiratory depression.

Calcium chloride. Calcium chloride increases myocardial contractility, prolongs systole, and enhances ventricular excitability. Sinus impulse formation can be suppressed, and sudden death following a rapid intravenous injection of calcium chloride has been described, particularly in fully digitalized patients. Calcium chloride is useful in profound cardiovascular collapse (electromechanical dissociation). It may be useful in restoring an electrical rhythm in instances of asystole and may enhance electrical defibrillation.

The absolute dose of calcium required in cardiac arrest emergencies is difficult to determine and may vary widely. The usual recommended dose of calcium chloride is 2.5 ml to 5 ml of a 10% solution (3.4 to 6.8 mEq Ca^{++}). Where required, this amount should be injected intravenously as a bolus at intervals of ten minutes. Calcium gluconate provides less ionizable calcium per unit volume. If it is used, the dose should be 10 ml of a 10% solution (4.8 mEq). Calcium can also be administered as calcium gluceptate. The dose of this drug is 5 ml (4.5 mEq).

Repeated large doses of calcium may elevate calcium blood levels with a detrimental effect. Calcium must not be administered together with sodium bicarbonate since this mixture results in formation of a precipitate.

Alternate drug routes. When prompt establishment of an intravenous lifeline is not possible, epinephrine (1 to 2 mg/10 ml sterile distilled water) or lidocaine (50 to 100 mg/10 ml sterile distilled water) can be effective when instilled directly into the tracheobronchial tree via an endotracheal tube. The endotracheal administration of other drugs for cardiopulmonary resuscitation has not yet been established.

Intramuscular atropine sulfate (2 mg) or lidocaine (300 mg) is effective in establishing therapeutic and prophylactic blood levels for dysrhythmia control, but this route requires the presence of adequate spontaneous circulation.

Useful drugs
   Vasoactive drugs
      Levarterenol
      Metaraminol
   Isoproterenol
   Propranolol
   Corticosteroids

Vasoactive drugs (levarterenol, metaraminol). The use of potent peripheral vasoconstrictors has been challenged by some authorities because of the possibility of reducing cerebral, cardiac, and renal blood flow. The choice of a vasoconstrictor or a positive inotropic agent remains controversial in the treatment of cardiac arrest and the immediate post-resuscitation period. However, during cardiac compression and the post-resuscitation period, blood pressure must be supported where low blood pressure and inadequate cerebral and renal perfusion give evidence of shock.

The selection of therapy is dictated by the patient's clinical state. In peripheral vascular collapse, manifested clinically by hypotension and the absence of significant peripheral vasoconstriction, intravenous levarterenol (Levophed) bitartrate in high concentrations of 16 μg/ml of metaraminol bitartrate (Aramine) in concentrations of 0.4 mg/ml of dextrose in water should be titrated intravenously. Metaraminol can be given intravenously as a bolus in a dose of 2 to 5 mg every five to ten minutes. Continuous administration is required to maintain a satisfactory blood pressure and adequate urinary output. These drugs are potent vasoconstrictors and have a positive inotropic effect on the myocardium. They are especially useful where systemic peripheral resistance is low.

Isoproterenol. For patients with profound bradycardia demonstrated to be the result of complete heart block, isoproterenol (Isuprel) hydrochloride is the drug of choice for immediate treatment. It should be infused in amounts of 2 to 20 μg/minute (1 to 10 ml of a solution of 1 mg in 500 ml of 5% glucose in water) and adjusted to increase heart rate to approximately 60 beats per minute. It is useful also for profound sinus bradycardia refractory to atropine.

Propranolol. The antiarrhythmic properties of the beta adrenergic blocking agents have proven useful in instances of repetitive ventricular tachycardia or repetitive ventricular fibrillation where maintenance of a rhythmic heartbeat cannot be achieved with lidocaine. The usual dose of propranolol is 1 mg intravenously. This may be repeated to a total of 3 mg under careful monitoring. Caution is required in patients with chronic obstructive pulmonary disease and cardiac failure.

Corticosteroids. Present evidence favors the use of pharmacological doses of synthetic corticosteroids (5 mg/kg of methylprednisolone sodium succinate or 1 mg/kg of dexamethasone phosphate) for prompt treatment of cardiogenic shock or shock lung occurring as complications of cardiac arrest. Where cerebral edema is suspected following cardiac arrest methylprednisolone sodium succinate in doses of 60 to 100 mg every six hours may be beneficial. When pulmonary complications such as a postaspiration pneumonitis is pres-

ent, dexamethasone phosphate may be used in doses of 4 to 8 mg every six hours.

Postcardiac arrest drug treatment. In addition to corticosteroids, potent diuretic agents, hypothermia, and controlled hyperventilation may be useful for the prevention or attenuation of cerebral edema which may follow successful resuscitation. Potent diuretic agents (furosemide and ethacrynic acid) in doses of 40 to 200 mg may help to promote diuresis. Hyperosmolality may be aggravated by these agents.

Drug dosage for infants and children. The recommended drug dosages for infants and small children are listed in Table 2.

Stabilization of patient's condition for transportation

Successful treatment is directly related to the rapidity with which a functional spon-

Table 2. Commonly used drugs for infants and children

Drug	Suggested dose	Remarks
Epinephrine	Intracardiac—0.3 to 2 ml diluted 1:10,000 (0.1 ml/kg)	
Calcium chloride (10%)	I.V.—maximum dose of 1 ml/5 kg Intracardiac—1 ml/kg diluted 1:1 with saline	Use caution in digitalized children
Sodium bicarbonate	I.V.—1 ml (0.9 mEq)/kg diluted 1:1 with sterile water	Repeat dose after pH obtained and base deficit calculated
Levarterenol (Levophed) bitartrate	Infants: I.V.—1 mg in 500 ml of 5% D/W* Children: I.V.—2 mg/500 ml of 5% D/W	Titrate to desired effect Not to be used in endotoxic shock or renal shut-down
Metaraminol (Aaramine) bitartrate	I.V.—25 mg/100 ml of 5% D/W	Titrate to desired effect
Mephentermine (Wyamine) sulfate	I.V.—0.05 mg	
Lidocaine (Xylocaine)	Infants: I.V.—0.5 mg/kg Children: I.V.—5 mg and repeat until desired effect I.V. Drip—6 mg/kg/4 hrs (100 mg in 500 ml of 5% D/W)	Not to exceed 100 mg/hr
Isoproterenol (Isuprel) hydrochloride	I.V. Drip—1 to 5 mg/500 ml of 5% D/W	Titrate to desired effect

*Dextrose in water.

taneous rhythm can be restored. In cases of cardiac emergency outside the hospital, it is now clear that restoring adequate, spontaneous circulation at the scene is more likely to result in the victim's survival than the most skillfully continued basic life support mesaures during transportation. Every effort must be made to treat and stabilize the patient at the scene, since it is difficult to perform CPR effectively during transportation. Once the patient is stabilized, it is reasonable to transfer him to a life support unit.

Stabilization involves:

1. Assuring effective ventilation, either spontaneous or assisted.

2. Maintaining a stable cardiac rhythm and effective circulation, utilizing drugs as indicated.

3. Maintaining a functioning ECG monitor and an intravenous lifeline.

4. Establishing and maintaining communications necessary for consultation, transportation, and admission to a continuing care facility.

Termination of basic or advanced life support

The decision to terminate resuscitative efforts is a medical one (also see "Medicolegal Considerations") and depends upon an assessment by a physician of the cerebral and cardiovascular status of the patient. The best criteria of adequate cerebral circulation are the reaction of the pupils, the level of consciousness, movement, and spontaneous respiration. Deep unconsciousness, absence of spontaneous respiration, and pupils that are fixed and dilated for 15 to 30 minutes usually are indicative of cerebral death and further resuscitative efforts are generally futile. Cardiac death is likely when there is continuing absence of ventricular electrocardiographic activity after 10 minutes or more of adequate cardiopulmonary support including appropriate drug therapy. In children, or in unusual circumstances, eg, when the arrest is associated with hypothermia, resuscitative efforts should be continued for longer periods since recovery has been seen even after prolonged unconsciousness.

PART IV. LIFE SUPPORT UNITS

A life support unit (LSU) is an integral part of a stratified system for cardiac care that is strategically located, properly identified, and has specific capability of rendering life support to patients with cardiopulmonary emergencies. Life support units can be either basic or advanced units. *Basic life support units* exist wherever there are individuals trained in CPR techniques and should be found at all patient care stations of hospitals, medical and dental offices, factories, public office buildings, and within homes and schools. *Advanced life support units,* in addition, must be able to monitor cardiac rhythms and treat cardiac dysrhythmias.

The Conference has set minimum standards for advanced life support units.

Standards for LSU's
STRUCTURE AND ACCESS

The advanced life support unit must have accessible approaches and be clearly identified by conspicuous markers indicating the availability of emergency cardiac care. It must be equipped to communicate with appropriate emergency agencies as well as to provide basic and advanced life support. The logical sites for life support units are where cardiopulmonary emergencies reasonably can be anticipated, such as in hospitals and all areas where many people congregate.

IN HOSPITALS

There should be triage for early symptoms and signs of heart attack in the hospital. The emergency department may be used to screen, monitor, and treat persons who arrive either on their own or by referral.

Every general hospital with acute care facilities should provide in its emergency department an advanced life support station so that any patient who has symptoms suspicious of myocardial infarction or other cardiopulmonary emergency will be placed immediately on monitoring and surveillance until a definite decision is made regarding his management. Cardiac monitoring always should precede any administrative details or medical history-taking.

If there is strong suspicion that the patient has an acute myocardial infarction, he should be transferred to a coronary care unit. It cannot be overemphasized that a patient with a history compatible with acute myocardial infarction should not be discharged from the emergency area merely because the initial electrocardiogram is normal. When the diagnosis is in doubt, it is always advisable to continue observation and monitoring. During transfer to the CCU by trained personnel, a patient should be connected to a battery-operated monitor-defibrillator and should be accompanied by appropriate drugs for administration en route if necessary.

OUT OF HOSPITALS

Sports arenas, convention centers, stadiums, civic auditoriums. Areas where large numbers of people congregate, such as sports arenas, convention halls, stadiums, and auditoriums, should provide life support units. Once such a unit is established, it must be identified and a diagram of its location should be printed in the program and pre-program fliers and mailers.

The LSU should be located in a place with a high degree of visibility, such as near entrances or adjacent to exhibits that are known to be popular. Consideration should be given to proximity to major pedestrian traffic arteries and accessibility to all individuals. All personnel employed by the facility should know of the existence and location of the life support unit.

The unit should be identified by a sign reading "Emergency Life Support Unit," rather than "Emergency Aid Station," to emphasize the function of the unit. At the entry or registration area, a large sign should be provided to define the method of access to the LSU or to define what action to take if a life-threatening emergency occurs.

Where the physical layout lends itself to use of small mobile transport units, such as modified mobile carts, consideration should be given to a complete mobile system integrated with the LSU or with multiple LSU's.

The plan of action for an LSU in a public facility must include integration into the total emergency medical system.

Industrial plants and office building complexes. In areas where a large number of people work, steps comparable to those for public facilities must be taken. A plan of action should be formulated as part of the total emergency medical system, including rapid access to the life support unit. In large complexes, LSU's are essential.

Areas with large in-transit populations. Airports and major railway terminals should provide similar LSU facilities with appropriate identification and easy access for travelers suffering life-threatening emergencies.

In addition, special provisions should be made for passengers aboard commercial aircraft. Airlines should provide passenger-carrying aircraft with standard kits of drugs (refer to "Essential Drugs" and "Useful Drugs") and syringes that can be made available to doctors with proper identification for in-flight treatment of cardiopulmonary emergencies. Oxygen, in cylinders with reducing valves capable of delivering up to 15 liters/minute for a period of 60 minutes (two E cylinders), should be available also. The cylinders, valves, and delivery equipment should be stored so that the oxygen may be delivered quickly to passengers anywhere in the aircraft.

The Conference recommends that the American Medical Association and all airlines request physicians to make their presence and availability known to the flight personnel prior to departure of the aircraft.

Capabilities of advanced life support units

An advanced life support unit must have certain capabilities with regard to availability, communication, and components. Advanced life support capability is to be provided within the confines of the LSU and to the entire physical complex which it serves, during the times required.

A faultless system of communication is essential to the effective delivery of advanced life support to persons in its area. This is to be correlated with responsible agencies (eg, security, administration) to ensure an effective flow of action for response.

The third capability an LSU must have concerns staff and equipment. Expert personnel, with all necessary equipment, must be available at all times in order to provide *advanced* life support by

1. Identifying patients with cardiopulmonary emergencies promptly.

2. Instituting immediate monitoring and establishing intravenous lifeline prior to obtaining a detailed medical and administrative history.

3. Providing continued surveillance until a professional decision on management is made.

In out-of-hospital LSU's, each unit must have the ability to stabilize the patient's condition prior to transfer to a continuing care facility. This necessitates providing a trained team with the appropriate portable equipment. The area's emergency medical system should allow personnel and equipment exchange to the transfer vehicle, effectively converting it to a mobile intensive care unit (MICU) to provide continuity of care until hospital admission is complete. In areas where MICU's are available, it is not necessary for the LSU team to leave its immediate vicinity. Basic life support always should be available, even when the life support unit team is occupied with transfer.

Personnel. Persons capable of providing the quality and degree of care necessary for an LSU to operate in a rapid, efficient, and professional manner are essential. These units may be staffed by qualified physicians, by specially trained nurses responding to standing orders, or by specifically trained allied health personnel who are authorized to perform this service. Each person staffing an LSU should be governed by a clear, written policy that defines his area of responsibility.

A physician knowledgeable and skilled in the management of basic and advanced cardiopulmonary emergencies must assume the medical responsibility for the unit. This responsibility includes direct or remote supervision under the physician's continuous or intermittent direction. Any physician who assumes responsibility for a patient in a LSU must be qualified to perform and administer advanced life support.

Nursing personnel must be familiar with and experienced in basic and advanced life support and must be able to direct lifesaving measures as well as provide a supporting role. In this regard, they should be familiar with the use of voice and ECG telemetry equipment if their station is so equipped.

Specialized continuing education programs for all LSU personnel are required to maintain an optimal level of proficiency and to acquaint personnel with new techniques and methods.

Emergency Medical Technicians (EMT's) must be trained at least to the level required for the training of ambulance personnel and others responsible for the prehospital phase of emergency cardiac care. Training programs must be hospital-affiliated and provide direct patient contact and care. A well-defined program additionally must include assisting in the care of the critically ill and injured patient, discussing cases, evaluating activities, and updating skills and knowledge on a regular basis. It is necessary that allied health personnel maintain their skills by continued periodic participation in hospital patient care and by demonstrating their proficiency on a set schedule. They must be able to function effectively without the physical presence of a physician or nurse, and, where provided, be totally competent to operate all equipment, including that necessary for communications and telemetry. Specialized continuing education programs for all LSU personnel are required to maintain an optimal level of proficiency and to acquaint personnel with new techniques and methods.

Equipment and drugs. The basic equipment and drugs necessary for an adequate advanced life support unit include those concerned with maintaining the airway and providing artificial ventilation and circulation.

Respiratory management. For airway management and artificial ventilation, the following equipment is necessary for all life support units:

Oxygen supply (two E cylinders) with reducing valves capable of delivering 15 liters/minute and with mask and reservoir bag
  Oxygen reserve (two E cylinders)
  Mask for mouth-to-mask ventilation
  Oropharyngeal airways
  S-tube (optional)
Laryngoscope with blades (curved and straight, for adult, child, and infant) and extra batteries and bulbs
Assorted adult-size (cuffed) and child-size (uncuffed) endotracheal tubes with stylet and 15 mm/22 mm adaptors
Syringe with clamp or plastic two-way or three-way valve for endotracheal tube cuffs
Acceptable bag-valve-mask, with provisions for 100% oxygen ventilation or a manually triggered (time-cycled) oxygen powered resuscitator
Suction (preferably portable), with catheters—sizes 6 to 16—and Yankauer-type suction tips
  Nasogastric tube
  Esophageal obturator airway (optional)
  Cricothyrotomy set

Circulatory management. To provide adequate management of the circulatory system, the following equipment is essential for all advanced life support units:

Portable defibrillator-monitor with ECG electrode-defibrillator paddles or portable DC defibrillator and portable ECG monitor
Portable ECG machine, direct writing, with connection to monitor
  Venous infusion sets (micro and regular)
  Indwelling venous catheters (regular and special units):
    Catheter outside needle (sizes 14 to 22)
    Catheter inside needle (sizes 14 to 22)
    Central venous pressure catheters
Intravenous solutions (5% dextrose in water, lactated Ringer's)
  Cutdown set
  Sterile gloves
  Urinary catheters

Assorted syringes and needles, stopcocks, venous extension tubes
  Intracardiac needles
  Tourniquets, adhesive, disposable razor, and similar items
  Thoracotomy tray

Essential drugs. All life support units must have these drugs available:

Sodium bicarbonate (prefilled syringes, 50 ml ampules, or 500 ml 5% bottles)
  Epinephrine (prefilled syringes)
  Atropine sulfate (prefilled syringes)
  Lidocaine (Xylocaine [prefilled syringe])
  Morphine sulfate
  Calcium chloride

Useful drugs. These drugs are recommended for hospital and nonhospital life support units:

  Aminophylline
  Dexamethasone (Decadron)
  Dextrose 50% (Ion-o-trate Dextrose 50%)
  Digoxin (Lanoxin)
  Diphenhydramine hydrochloride (Benadryl)
  Ethacrynic acid
  Furosemide (Lasix)
  Isoproterenol (Isuprel) hydrochloride
  Lanatoside C (Cedilanid)
  Meperidine (Demerol) hydrochloride
  Metaraminol bitartrate (Aramine)
  Methylprednisolone sodium succinate (Solu-Medrol)
  Nalorphine (n-allylnormorphine) hydrochloride
  Levarterenol (Levophed) bitartrate
  Phenylephrine (Neo-Synephrine) hydrochloride
  Potassium chloride
  Propranolol hydrochloride (Inderal)
  Procainamide hydrochloride (Pronestyl)
  Quinidine
  Succinylcholine chloride
  Tubocurarine chloride

Referral. Each life support unit must have an established policy for referral. This policy should be based on the knowledge of the medical capabilities for critical care in the vicinity and the ability of the individual LSU to communicate and consult with these facilities at all times. The patient should be referred to the most appropriate hospital. The LSU assumes full patient responsibility until safe transfer has been effected.

When the continuing care facility (hospital) provides both a coronary care unit and an emergency department, provisions should be made for the cardiac patient to enter the CCU directly, bypassing the emergency department. In some instances, however, further stabilization and specialized treatment may be necessary in the emergency department before transfer to the CCU.

Records. A system of records must be developed and maintained throughout the course of each use of an LSU. The design must be such that a copy can be immediately available for the continuing care facility that assumes the eventual responsibility for the patient. There also must be a copy available for the long-term records of the LSU.

Communications. At a minimum, the LSU must be able to communicate directly with the agency or persons who are bringing the patient to the unit and with the facility to which they transfer the patient for continuing care. It is recommended that the LSU also be in contact with the central coordinating and dispatching authority.

Standards for mobile LSU's

A mobile life support unit is a vehicle that has all the components, personnel, and capabilities of the LSU. Mobile life support units also can be categorized as basic or advanced, depending on the kind of life support they are equipped to provide. At a minimum, all ambulances should be capable of basic life support. Advanced mobile life support units should be able to rapidly transport necessary equipment and skilled personnel to a patient with a cardiopulmonary emergency and to render basic and advanced life support. This advanced mobile LSU may or may not transport the patient to a definitive care area. If not, it should be able to provide its life support capability in the form of personnel and portable equipment to some other transporting vehicle to effect safe transport after the patient has been stabilized.

Structure. Mobile life support must be a part of a well-defined, community-wide plan for providing emergency medical services.

The plan must integrate the mobile LSU's into an emergency cardiac care system containing fire departments, rescue teams, and ambulances, so that basic life support can be provided within four minutes from the emergency call. There should be a sufficient number and sufficient placement of mobile life support units to assure advanced life support to the patient within ten minutes or less.

Vehicle design for LSU's should be in relation to their role in the plan.[11] These vehicles may be only for transportation of equipment and personnel, or they may be for transportation of equipment, personnel, and patients. It is also necessary to provide central control, coordination, and a dispatching agency, with dispatchers trained in identifying the type of emergency and its precise geographic location.

All mobile LSU's must have sufficient trained personnel to provide two rescuers to remain with and administer to the needs of the patient throughout the emergency and until he is delivered to a continuing care facility.

Capabilities. The mobile LSU's must be strategically deployed and have the capability for recognition, emergency treatment, and stabilization of cardiac patients. It is important that the patient be stabilized quickly at the site where the cardiopulmonary emergency occurred. Continuous monitoring of the patient by rescue personnel from the time of arrival of the mobile unit to the delivery of the patient to a LSU is a necessity. Communication with the base station, unit, and physician are desirable.

A mobile life support unit has some requirements that are different from those of a regular LSU. The mobile unit must possess the ability to develop and maintain appropriate, portable lifelines that will support ventilation and circulation continuously so that the patient may be transferred to the vehicle.

The training required for operation of regular life support units also must be augmented for personnel serving in the mobile life support unit. Training is needed in the areas of field operation of communications and telemetric equipment, vehicular guidance and defensive driving, local geography and traffic control, and how to interact with other agencies in situations such as establishing security and crowd control.

Components. There are no differences between the components required for a mobile LSU and those for other LSU's regarding personnel, equipment, drugs, and records.

Additional mandatory features of the mobile LSU are specialized training of personnel, equipment that is portable and self-contained, special vehicle design, and a communications network.

Communications. At a minimum, two-way voice communications with the central coordinating and dispatching authority and with the continuing care unit to which the patient will be delivered is necessary initially. The unit therefore must possess the capability of communicating with one or more continuing care facilities in order to give:

1. Notification of patient's expected time of arrival.

2. Notification of patient's condition.

3. Confirmation of acceptance by facility for continuing care.

4. Consultation regarding care.

As a later phase, there can be augmentation with physician's consultation and, when appropriate, ECG telemetry offers the advantage of remote monitoring and rhythm consultation, provided that medical consultation is on-line and a part of the system.

PART V. MEDICOLEGAL CONSIDERATIONS AND RECOMMENDATIONS

The Conference wishes to make clear that, unless otherwise provided, nothing in these standards is intended to limit or inhibit persons, either inside or outside of health care facilities, from providing emergency medical treatment. Emergency care should always be provided in life-threatening situations. In addition, unless otherwise indicated, these standards are universally applicable. In cases involving techniques of basic and advanced life support, minimum requirements for appropriate action have been defined. In areas of policy, recommendations have been made, and it is intended that these recommendations will become reflective of actual practice.

It is appreciated that full implementation of these standards will place an enormous burden on the personnel and facilities of agencies, organizations, and institutions that are or will be involved in emergency care, as well as those agencies, organizations, and institutions responsible for training and certification. Since it may be unrealistic to expect immediate compliance with these standards in some circumstances, a reasonable time for implementation should be allowed.

Initiation and termination of resuscitation efforts

Physicians. Physicians have an obligation to initiate CPR in any instance in which it is medically indicated. When the victim of cardiac arrest is not the patient of the physician, a unique relationship is created that may be described as the Good Samaritan–victim relationship.

The physician should continue basic life support measures until one of the following occurs:

1. The patient's personal physician takes charge,

2. He has reasonable assurance that the victim will continue to receive properly performed basic and/or advanced life support by properly trained and designated professional personnel, or

3. The patient recovers or is pronounced dead.

Nonphysicians. Nonphysicians should initiate CPR according to the standards of the American Heart Association and to the best of their knowledge and capability in cases they recognize as cardiac arrest. They should not be held liable for failure to initiate CPR if such decision is consistent with current standards.

The nonphysician who initiates basic or

advanced life support should continue his resuscitation efforts until one of the following occurs:

1. Effective spontaneous circulation and ventilation have been restored,
2. Resuscitation efforts have been transferred to another responsible person who continues basic life support,
3. A physician or a physician-directed individual or team assumes responsibility,
4. The victim is transferred to properly trained and designated professional medical or allied health personnel charged with responsibilities for emergency medical services, or
5. The rescuer is exhausted and unable to continue resuscitation.

Orders not to resuscitate

The purpose of cardiopulmonary resuscitation is the prevention of sudden, unexpected death. Cardiopulmonary resuscitation is not indicated in certain situations, such as in cases of terminal irreversible illness where death is not unexpected or where prolonged cardiac arrest dictates the futility of resuscitation efforts. Resuscitation in these circumstances may represent a positive violation of an individual's right to die with dignity. When CPR is considered to be contraindicated for hospital patients, it is appropriate to indicate this in the patient's progress notes. It also is appropriate to indicate this on the physician's order sheet for the benefit of nurses and other personnel who may be called upon to initiate or participate in cardiopulmonary resuscitation.

Conference recommendations for advanced life support

1. Every hospital must have a written plan and a mechanism for advanced life support consistent with available personnel, equipment, and facilities, and available throughout the installation on a 24-hour-per-day basis. This plan should be tested regularly and should be reviewed annually by the responsible hospital CPR/ECC committee.
2. Lack of CPR certification should not,

per se, prevent administration of advanced life support by properly trained medical, nursing, and allied health personnel in an emergency situation.

Conference recommendations on necessary legislative action

1. It is recommended that state legislation be clarified to allow professional allied health personnel who are rendering emergency care outside of the hospital and are certified in advanced life support to function with maximum effectiveness. Such legislation must provide specifically that individuals certified in advanced life support be permitted to function when a physician is not present, provided, however, that such certified person is under the general supervision of a physician. General supervision is defined as direct or remote supervision by continuous or intermittent communication with a licensed physician to assure physician involvement in decisions requiring such involvement. This requirement for supervision by a physician shall not be interpreted to mean that such life-saving procedures as cardiac defibrillation, appropriate drug therapy, and other measures should ever be withheld when the circumstances demand such action according to the training standards for emergency medical technicians functioning in this capacity.
2. It is recommended that all hospital and other acute care facility staff and employees who are involved in direct patient care in any capacity must be certified in basic life support and should have knowledge of and be involved in the CPR plan of that facility.
3. It is recommended that all county, state, and national medical organizations make serious and concerted efforts to *(a)* clarify the Medical Practice Act in their state in terms of its application to persons rendering basic and advanced life support and *(b)* establish an official mechanism to approve CPR courses given in accordance with American Heart Association standards and

by instructors certified according to American Heart Association standards.

4. It is recommended that national certification be established to ensure that those trained in basic life support and advanced life support have had appropriate training according to American Heart Association standards and are proficient in the application of that training.

5. It is recommended that qualified immunity (ie, for acts done in good faith and not involving gross negligence or willful, wanton, or reckless misconduct) be provided for those certified in basic or advanced life support.

6. It is recommended that a declaration of the immunity provided by common law for lay persons who either have not been certified or have not been trained in basic life support should be prepared with publicized widely.

7. It is recommended that immunity from civil liability for certified instructors and associations that are involved in instruction in accordance with the American Heart Association standards should be provided.

8. It is recommended that all policemen, firemen, and other first-line responders be trained and certified in basic life support as a necessary and indispensable job requirement. All professional emergency department personnel should have adequate training and certification in basic and advanced life support.

9. It must be established and properly promulgated that policemen and any law enforcement official, or any individual functioning in a similar capacity, have an affirmative obligation *(a)* to defer to a person more qualified than themselves in the delivery of basic life support and *(b)* not to interfere in an ongoing effort at stabilization of an individual receiving basic life support until a reasonable, mutually agreeable decision is made by that individual and the rescuer that transportation or other appropriate measures in the delivery of care be initiated.

Conference recommendations on implementation of standards

To assure maximum effectiveness, the Conference recommends that its standards, as contained in this statement, be adopted and implemented by the following agencies and organizations:

1. The Joint Commission on Accreditation of Hospitals, insofar as they apply to hospitals.

2. State regulatory bodies for promulgation of standards and recommendations.

3. Professional medical and allied health associations, for the purpose of issuing statements jointly or individually for maximum dissemination of these standards, to ensure uniformity in their application and to protect both those who act in accordance with them and the emergency victim.

4. The American Heart Association, in taking all necessary steps to disseminate these standards broadly, including appropriate programs, training materials, and publications, and by seeking support for such dissemination from appropriate foundations, federal agencies, medical organizations, and other sources.

5. The American National Red Cross and other life-saving agencies, charged with the responsibility of providing adequate training to nonprofessional rescuers and the general public.

6. All government health care services and facilities.

7. Other responsible agencies and organizations, including medical, dental, and nursing schools; airlines; industry; and sports centers.

It is further recommended that this statement be given the widest possible publication, republication, and distribution in its complete form, or in its individual parts, provided proper procedures are followed.

References
AMERICAN HEART ASSOCIATION (AHA)

1. *Emergency Resuscitation Team Manual: A Hospital Plan*. New York: AHA, 1968. (EM-439)

2. *Emergency Measures in Cardiopulmonary Resuscitation* (Revised). New York: AHA, 1969. (EM376A)
3. *Definitive Therapy in Cardiopulmonary Resuscitation* (Revised). New York: AHA, 1971. (EM377A)
4. *Cardiopulmonary Resuscitation: A Manual for Instructors.* New York: AHA, 1967. (EM-408)
5. *Training of Ambulance Personnel in Cardiopulmonary Resuscitation.* New York: AHA, 1965. (EM386A)
6. *The Dentist's Role in Cardiopulmonary Resuscitation.* New York: AHA, 1968. (EM-407A)
7. *Training of Lifeguards in Cardiopulmonary Resuscitation.* New York: AHA, 1970. (EM-438A)

NATIONAL ACADEMY OF SCIENCES–NATIONAL RESEARCH COUNCIL (NAS–NRC)

8. Cardiopulmonary Resuscitation: Statement by the Ad Hoc Committee on Cardiopulmonary Resuscitation of the Division of Medical Sciences, National Academy of Sciences–National Research Council. *JAMA,* 198:372-379, 1966.
9. "Accidental Death and Disability: The Neglected Disease of Modern Society," Committee on Trauma and Committee on Shock, Division of Medical Sciences. Washington, DC: NAS-NRC, September 1966.
10. *Cardiopulmonary Resuscitation: Conference Proceedings,* May 23, 1966. Washington, DC: NAS-NRC, 1967. (Publication 1494)
11. "Medical Requirements for Ambulance Design and Equipment." Committee on Emergency Medical Services, Division of Medical Sciences, Washington, DC: NAS-NRC, September 1968. (Publication USGPO 1970 0-381-725)
12. "Ambulance Design Criteria." Committee on Ambulance Design Criteria of the Highway Research Board, Division of Engineering. Washington, DC: NAS-NRC, June 1969.
13. *Training of Ambulance Personnel and Others Responsible for Emergency Care of the Sick and Injured at the Scene and During Transportation.* Committee on Emergency Medical Services, Division of Medical Sciences. Washington, DC: NAS-NRC, March 1968. (Publication USGPO 1970 0-381-726)
14. "Advanced Training Program for Emergency Medical Technician-Ambulance." Committee on Emergency Medical Services, Division of Medical Sciences. Washington, DC: NAS-NRC, September 1970.

15. "Roles and Resources of Federal Agencies in Support of Comprehensive Emergency Medical Services." Division of Medical Sciences, Washington, DC: NAS-NRC, March 1972.

INTER-SOCIETY COMMISSION FOR HEART DISEASE RESOURCES

16. Cardiovascular disease—Acute care. *Circulation* 43:A97-A133, January 1971.
17. Resources for the management of emergencies in hypertension. *Circulation* 43:A157-A160, March 1971.
18. Resources for the acute care of peripheral vascular diseases. *Circulation* 43:A161-A169, April 1971.
19. Resources for the optimal care of patients with acute myocardial infarction. *Circulation* 43:A171-A183, May 1971.
20. Resources for the optimal care of acute respiratory failure. *Circulation* 43:A185-A195, June 1971.
21. Electronic equipment in critical care areas. Part II. The electrical environment. *Circulation* 44:A237-A246, October 1971.
22. Critical performance criteria-defibrillators. Instrumentation Study Group. *Circulation* 47:A359-A361, June 1973.

OTHER GOVERNMENT AGENCIES

23. US Department of Transportation, National Highway Safety Bureau. "Basic Training Program for Emergency Medical Technician-Ambulance: Concepts and Recommendations," 1969. (Publication USGPO 1970 0-372-388)
24. US Department of Transportation, National Highway Safety Bureau. "Basic Training Program for Emergency Medical Technician-Ambulance: Course Guide and Course Coordinator Orientation Program," 1969. (Publication USGPO 1970 0-372-389)
25. US Department of Transportation, National Highway Safety Bureau. "Basic Training Program for Emergency Medical Technician-Ambulance: Instructor's Lesson Plans," 1969. (Publication USGPO, Catalogue No. TD 2.208:EM 3/3, 1969)
26. US Department of Transportation, National Highway Traffic Safety Administration. "Communications-Guidelines for Emergency Medical Services." Washington: Government Printing Office, 1972.
27. US Department of Health, Education, and Welfare, Health Services and Mental Health Administration. "Emergency Medical Services Communication Systems," August 1972. (DHEW Publication No. HSM 73-2003)
28. US Department of Health, Education, and

Welfare. Public Health Service. "Compendium of State Statutes on the Regulation of Ambulance Services, Operation of Emergency Vehicles, and Good Samaritan Laws." Health Services and Mental Health Administration, Division of Emergency Health Services (Revised), 1969. (Publication USGPO 1969 0-353-618)

29. US Department of Health, Education, and Welfare. Public Health Service. "Emergency Health Services Selected Bibliography." Health Services and Mental Health Administration, Division of Emergency Health Services, 1970. (Publication USGPO 1970 0-354-043)

PROFESSIONAL MEDICAL SOCIETIES

30. American College of Surgeons Committee on Trauma. A curriculum for training emergency medical technicians. *Bull Am Coll Surgeons* 54:273-276, 1969.

31. American College of Surgeons. Committee on Trauma. Essential equipment for ambulances. *Bull Am Coll Surgeons* 55:7-13, 1970.

32. American Academy of Orthopaedic Surgeons. Emergency Care and Transportation of the Sick and Injured, by the Committee on Injuries. Chicago: AAOS, 1971.

33. American Medical Association. Commission on Emergency Medical Services. Developing Emergency Medical Services: Guidelines for Community Councils. Chicago: AMA, 1973.

34. American Society of Anesthesiologists. Community-wide emergency medical services: Recommendations by the Committee on Acute Medicine of the American Society of Anesthesiologists. *JAMA* 204:595-602, 1968.

PRIVATE GROUPS

35. Manually operated resuscitators. *Health Devices* 1:13-17, April 1971.

36. Inspection of defibrillators. *Health Devices* 1:109-113, August 1971.

37. Battery-operated defibrillator/monitors. *Health Devices* 2:87-103, February 1973.

38. Line-operated synchronized defibrillators. *Health Devices* 2:117-129, March 1973.

39. External Cardiac compressors. *Health Devices* 2:136-151, April 1973.

INDIVIDUALS

40. Yu PN: Pre-hospital care of acute myocardial infarction. *Circulation* 45:189-204, 1972.

41. Don Michael TA, Gordon AS: Esophageal obturator airway: A new adjunct for artificial ventilation. Proceedings, National Conference on Standards for CPR and ECC, NAS-NRC, Washington, DC, to be published.

Sources of references

A. American Heart Association, Committee on Cardiopulmonary Resuscitation and Emergency Cardiac Care, 44 E 23rd St, New York 10010. Also available from affiliates. (References 1-8, 39)

B. Division of Medical Sciences, National Academy of Sciences-National Research Council, 2101 Constitution Ave, Washington, DC 20418. (References 8-9, 11, 14-15)

C. Information Clearinghouse, Division of Emergency Health Services, Health Services and Mental Health Administration, 5600 Fishers Lane, Rockville, MD 20852. (References 9, 13-14, 27)

D. American Medical Association, Commission on Emergency Medical Services, 535 N Dearborn St, Chicago 60610. (References 8-9, 33)

E. Printing and Publishing Office, National Academy of Sciences, 2101 Constitution Ave, Washington, DC 20418. (Reference 10)

F. Superintendent of Documents, US Government Printing Office, Washington, DC 20402. (References 11-13, 23-26, 28-29)

G. Inter-Society Commission for Heart Disease Resources, 44 E 23rd St, New York 10010. (References 16-22)

H. American College of Surgeons, 55 E Erie St, Chicago 60611. (References 30-31)

I. American Academy of Orthopaedic Surgeons, 430 N Michigan Ave, Chicago 60611. (Reference 32)

J. American Society of Anesthesiologists, Committee on Acute Medicine, 515 Busse Hwy, Park Ridge, IL 60068. (Reference 34)

K. Emergency Care Research Institute, 913 Walnut St, Philadelphia 19107. (References 35-39)

BIBLIOGRAPHY*

Books†

Abramson, H.: Resuscitation of the newborn infant and related emergency procedures, ed. 3, St. Louis, 1973, The C. V. Mosby Co.

Ambulance attendant's training manual, Harrisburg, 1964, Pennsylvania Department of Health, Chapter 2.

Ambulance attendant's training manual, Philadelphia, 1965, American College of Surgeons.

Bartko, D.: Experimental brain hypoxia, Baltimore, 1971, University Park Press.

Bencini, A., and Parola, P.: L'arresto circolatorio

As with the previous three editions of this book, we are again printing an almost completely new bibliography. The large volume of new contributions to the literature makes it impractical to retain many references from previous editions. For the reader interested in source material, it may be necessary to refer to the earlier editions, especially the third.

†Two International Symposia on Emergency Resuscitation have been held. The first was held in Stavanger, Norway, in 1961 and the second in Oslo, Norway, in 1967. The proceedings of the second International Symposium, as organized by the Norwegian Association of Anaesthesiologists of the World Federation, are available.

An excellent new monograph on cardiorespiratory resuscitation by Gilston and Resnekov is of particular value in its considerations of the respiratory problems of cardiac resuscitation.

The publication of numerous books dealing primarily with cardiopulmonary resuscitation reflects the widespread interest in the subject within recent years. The books listed represent the majority of such efforts. Some are manuals on the subject; some are concerned only with a particular facet of cardiopulmonary resuscitation. Others are written for paramedical readers as well as for the physician with only superficial knowledge of the subject. At least three books are of considerable historical interest and are already in the category of "rare books," as copies are most difficult to obtain.

improvviso, Pavia, Italy, 1957, Casa Editrice Renzo Cortina.

Bendixen, H. H., et al.: Respiratory care, St. Louis, 1965, The C. V. Mosby Co.

Boba, A.: Death in the operating room, Springfield, Ill., 1965, Charles C Thomas, Publisher.

Boerema, J., et al., editors: Clinical application of hyperbaric oxygen, New York, 1964, Elsevier Publishing Co.

Braun, P., and Rosenberg, S.: Cardiopulmonary resuscitation (teaching manual), Trenton, N. J., 1964, New Jersey State Department of Health.

Brest, A. N.: Heart substitutes, mechanical and transplant, Springfield, Ill., 1966, Charles C Thomas, Publisher.

Brooks, C. McC, et al.: Excitability of the heart, New York, 1955, Grune & Stratton, Inc.

Brooks, D. K.: Resuscitation, Baltimore, 1967, The Williams & Wilkins Co.

Caccamo, L. P., et al.: Resuscitation—a programmed course, Philadelphia, 1968, F. A. Davis Co.

Cardiac pacing and cardioversion, Symposium presented by The American College of Cardiology and Presbyterian–University of Pennsylvania Medical Center, Philadelphia, 1967, Charles Press.

Cardiopulmonary resuscitation—a manual for instructors, New York, 1967, American Heart Association.

Chung, E. K., editor: Principles of cardiac arrhythmias, Baltimore, 1971, The Williams & Wilkins Co.

Committee on Cardiopulmonary Resuscitation: Definitive therapy in cardiopulmonary resuscitation, New York, 1965, 1971, American Heart Association.

Committee on Cardiopulmonary Resuscitation: Emergency measures in cardiopulmonary resuscitation, New York, 1965, 1969, American Heart Association.

Corday, E., et al.: Vasopressor treatment of cardiogenic shock. In Mills, L. C., and Moyer, J. H., editors: Shock and hypertension: pathogenesis and treatment, New York, 1965, Grune & Stratton, Inc.

Crile, G.: An autobiography, Philadelphia, 1947, J. B. Lippincott Co.

Crile, G. W.: Blood pressure in surgery: an experimental and clinical research, Philadelphia, 1903, J. B. Lippincott Co.

Crile, G. W.: Anemia and resuscitation, New York, 1914, D. Appleton & Co.

d'Halluin, M.: Résurrection du coeur. La vie du coeur isolé. Le massage du coeur, Paris, 1904, Place de l'École de Medicine, Vigot Frères, Editeurs.

Don Michael, T. A.: Cardiac arrest and resuscitation, Abadan, 1965, IORC Printing Services.

Dorozynski, A.: The man they wouldn't let die, New York, 1965, The MacMillan Co.

Emergency Resuscitation Team Manual: A hospital plan, New York, 1968, American Heart Association.

Feldman, S., and Ellis, H.: Principles of resuscitation, Oxford, 1967, Blackwell Scientific Publications.

Flagg, P. J.: The art of resuscitation, New York, 1944, Reinhold Publishing Corp.

Fredericks, L. E.: Anesthesia for open heart surgery, Springfield, Ill., 1966, Charles C Thomas, Publisher.

Friedberg, C. K.: Diseases of the heart, ed. 3, Philadelphia, 1966, W. B. Saunders Co.

Gaevskaya, M. S.: Biochemistry of the brain during the process of dying and resuscitation, New York, 1964, Consultants Bureau.

Gastaut, H., et al., editors: Cerebral anoxia and the electroencephalogram, Springfield, Ill., 1961, Charles C Thomas, Publisher.

Gilston, A., et al.: Cardiopulmonary resuscitation, Philadelphia, 1971, F. A. Davis, Co.

Gordon, A. S.: Cardiopulmonary Resuscitation Conference Proceedings, Washington, D. C., 1967, National Research Council.

Griffith, G. C.: The therapy of cardiogenic shock. In Likoff, W., and Moyer, J. H., editors: Coronary heart disease, New York, 1963, Grune & Stratton, Inc.

Gurvich, A. M.: Elektricheskaia aktivnost' umiraiushchego i ozhiviushchego mozga [Electrical activity in the dying and resuscitated brain], Leningrad, 1966, Klin. Med.

Gurvich, N. L.: Fibrilliatsiia i defibrilliatsiia serdtsa [Fibrillation and defibrillation of the heart], Moscow, 1957, Medgiz, p. 250.

Guthrie, C. C.: Blood-vessel surgery and its applications, New York, 1912, Longmans, Green & Co.

Guthrie, C. C.: Blood vessel surgery and its applications (a reprint edited by Harbinson, S. P., and Fisher, B.), Pittsburgh, 1959, University of Pittsburgh Press.

Holt, G. W.: The vagi in medicine and surgery, Springfield, Ill., 1968, Charles C Thomas, Publisher.

Hosler, R. M.: A manual on cardiac resuscitation, Springfield, Ill., 1954, Charles C Thomas, Publisher.

Hosler, R. M.: A manual on cardiac resuscitation, ed. 2, Springfield, Ill., 1958, Charles C Thomas, Publisher.

Hurst, J. W.: Cardiac resuscitation, Springfield, Ill., 1960, Charles C Thomas, Publisher.

James, T. N.: Anatomy of the coronary arteries, New York, 1961, Harper & Row, Publishers.

James, L. S., et al.: Birth asphyxia and resuscitation. In Conn, H. F., editor: Current therapy, Philadelphia, 1969, W. B. Saunders Co.

Joki, E.: Exercise and cardiac death, Basel, 1971, S. Karger AG.

Jude, J. R., and Elam, J. O.: Fundamentals of cardiopulmonary resuscitation, Philadelphia, 1965, F. A. Davis Co.

Jude, J. R., Scherles, L., and Farr, M. E.: Cardiopulmonary resuscitation, Baltimore, 1966, Heart Association of Maryland.

Kantrowitz, A.: An intracorporeal auxiliary ventricle. In Levine, S. N., editor: Advances in biomedical engineering and medical physics, New York, 1968, John Wiley & Sons, Inc.

Kelman, G. R.: Applied cardiovascular physiology, London, 1971, Butterworth & Co. (Publishers) Ltd.

Killian, H., and Donhardt, A.: Resuscitation, Hamburg, Germany, 1955, Ganzleinen.

Kilpatrick, D. G., et al.: A current distribution electrode system for defibrillation, Philadelphia, 1961, IRE National Convention Board.

Levine, H. D.: Cardiac emergencies and related disorders—their mechanism and management, New York, 1960, Landsberger Medical Books, Inc.

Manual of water safety and life-saving, Melbourne, 1968, Royal Life-Saving Society of Australia.

Marinescu, V., et al.: Resuscitarea respiratorie si cardiaca, Rome, 1963, Editura Academiei Republicii Populare Romine.

Master, A. M., et al.: Cardiac emergencies and heart failure, Philadelphia, 1952, Lea & Febiger.

Mechanical devices to assist the failing heart, Washington, D. C., 1966, National Academy of Sciences–National Research Council.

Meltzer, L. E., et al.: Intensive coronary care, Philadelphia, 1970, Charles Press.

Milstein, B. B.: Cardiac arrest and resuscitation, Chicago, 1963, Year Book Medical Publishers, Inc.

Modell, J. H.: The pathophysiology and treatment

of drowning and near-drowning, Springfield, Ill., 1971, Charles C Thomas, Publisher.

Natof, H. E., and Sadove, M. S.: Cardiovascular collapse in the operating room, Philadelphia, 1958, J. B. Lippincott Co.

Negovskii, V. A.: Pathophysiologie und Therapie der Agonie und des klinischen Todes, Translated by Kirsch, R., Berlin, 1959, Akademie-Verlag.

Negovskii, V. A.: Ozhivlenie organizma i iskusstvennaia gipotermiia [Resuscitation of the organism and artificial hypothermia], Moscow, 1960, Medgiz.

Negovskii, V. A.: Resuscitation and artificial hypothermia, New York, 1962, Consultants Bureau.

Negovskii, V. A., editor: Osnovy reanimatologii [Foundations of reanimatology (resuscitology)], Moscow, 1966, Klin. Med.

Negovskii, V. A.: Nepriamoi massazh serdtsa i ekspiratornoe iskusstvennoe dykhanie [Indirect heart massage and expiratory artificial respiration], Moscow, 1966, Sovetskaia Rossiia.

Negovskii, V. A.: Fibrillation and defibrillation of the heart, Moscow, 1967, Medgiz.

Negovskii, V. A.: Current problems in reanimatology, Moscow, 1971, Izdatelstvo "Meditsina."

Nielsen, K. C.: Experimental studies on the involvement of adrenergic mechanisms in the development of ventricular fibrillation during induced hypothermia, Lund, Sweden, 1968, Studentlitteratur.

Norris, W., et al.: A nurse's guide to anaesthetics, resuscitation and intensive care, Glasgow, 1969, Glasgow University Press.

Pearson, J. W.: Historical and experimental approaches to modern resuscitation, Springfield, Ill., 1965, Charles C Thomas, Publisher.

Penin, H., and Kaufer, C., chairmen: Der Hirntod (symposium), Stuttgart, 1969, Georg Thieme Verlag KG.

Persky, L.: In situ preservation of the kidney, Urology, Deerfield, Ill., 1971, Travenol Laboratories, Inc.

Safar, P., editor: Resuscitation—controversial aspects (an international symposium in Vienna), Berlin, 1963, Springer-Verlag.

Safar, P.: Resuscitation of the unconscious victim, Springfield, Ill., 1959, Charles C Thomas, Publisher.

Safar, P.: Cardiopulmonary resuscitation, 1968, World Federation of Societies of Anaesthesiologists.

Scheidt, S., et al.: Physiologic effects of intraaortic balloon pumping: report of a cooperative clinical trial, John A. Hartford Foundation, Inc., 1972.

Scherf, D., and Schott, A.: Extrasystoles and allied arrhythmias, New York, 1953, Grune & Stratton, Inc.

Schultz, L. S., et al.: The Minnesota system for cardiorespiratory assistance, Minneapolis, 1972, University of Minnesota Press.

Segal, B. L., and Kilpatrick, D. G.: Engineering in the practice of medicine, Baltimore, 1967, The Williams & Wilkins Co.

Shaw, G., Smith, G., and Thomson, T. J.: Resuscitation and cardiac pacing, London, 1964, Cassell & Company Ltd.

Sherman, M.: Review of research grants supported by the National Heart and Lung Institute, 1949 to 1970, Bethesda, Md., 1970, National Institutes of Health.

Shires, A. T.: Care of the trauma patient, New York, 1966, McGraw-Hill Book Co.

Siddons, H., and Sowton, E.: Cardiac pacemakers, Springfield, Ill., 1967, Charles C Thomas, Publisher.

Stauch, M.: Arrest of circulation and resuscitation, Stuttgart, 1967, Flexible Textbooks.

Stephenson, H. E., Jr.: Cardiac arrest and resuscitation, eds. 1, 2, and 3, St. Louis, 1958, 1964, 1969, The C. V. Mosby Co.

Stock, J. P. P.: Diagnosis and treatment of cardiac arrhythmias, New York, 1969, Appleton-Century-Crofts.

Surawicz, B., and Pellegrino, E. D.: Sudden cardiac death, New York, 1964, Grune & Stratton, Inc.

Training of ambulance personnel in cardiopulmonary resuscitation, New York, 1965, American Heart Association.

Whipple, G. H., et al.: Acute coronary care, Boston, 1972, Little, Brown and Co.

White, B. B.: Therapy in acute coronary care, Chicago, 1971, Year Book Medical Publishers, Inc.

Whittenberger, J. L., editor: Artificial respiration: theory and applications, New York, 1962, Harper & Row, Publishers.

Ya Khabarova, A.: The afferent innervation of the heart, New York, 1961, Consultants Bureau.

Zolotokrylina, E. S.: Patofiziologicheskie obosnovaniia profilaktiki i lecheniia terminal'nykh sostoianii, razvivshikhsia vsledstvie ostroi krovopoteri i shoka. [The pathophysiological foundations for the prevention and treatment of terminal states which developed following acute exsanguination and shock.] In Foundations of reanimatology, Moscow, 1966, Akademie-Verlag, pp. 252-284.

Films

KEY TO LIBRARIES

OA   Motion Picture Library

American Academy of Orthopaedic Surgeons
29 East Madison Street
Chicago, Illinois 60602

ACS   Motion Picture Library
American College of Surgeons
55 East Erie Street
Chicago, Illinois 60611

AHA   44 East 23rd Street
New York, New York 10010

AMA   Medical-Health Film Library
American Medical Association
535 North Dearborn Street
Chicago, Illinois 60610

D&G   Surgical Film Library
Davis & Geck
Division of American Cyanamid Company
1 Caspar Street
Danbury, Connecticut 06810

EFL   Eaton Medical Film Library
Eaton Laboratories Division
The Norwich Pharmacal Company
Norwich, New York 13815

MEND   Office of the National Coordinator
Medical Education for National Defense
2300 East Street, N.W.
Washington, D. C. 20390

PHS   Public Health Service Audiovisual Facility
Communicable Disease Center
Atlanta, Georgia 30333

SG   Surgeon General
Personnel and Training Division
Attn.: Chief Training Doctrine Branch
Department of the Army, Main Navy Building
Washington, D. C. 20025

TITLES

A chance to save a life (Boy Scouts of America)
1969, 14 minutes, sound, color
Airway obstruction: cause and prevention (James O. Elam, David G. Green)
1962, 12 minutes, sound, color   AMA 8
Anatomy and technique of elective tracheotomy (G. Jan Beekhuis)
1964, 23 minutes, sound   ACS 101
Back pressure arm lift method of artificial respiration
1952, 9 minutes, sound   AMA 1088
Bedside tracheotomy (Benson B. Roe)
1964, 12 minutes, sound   ACS 022
Breath of life (Archer Gordon)
1965, 16 minutes, 16 mm., color   AHA
Breathing for others, part I (Stewart Hardy Films for British Admiralty)

1963, 14 minutes, 16 mm., color   AHA
Cardiac arrest (John Beard)
1958, 16 minutes, sound, color   AMA 1049
Cardiac arrest (Egbert H. Fell, Lowell F. Peterson, Newton Chun)
1955, 17 minutes, sound   D&G CS 526
Cardiac monitoring in the prevention and treatment of catastrophic circulatory arrest (Denton A. Cooley)
1960, 15 minutes, sound   ACS 033
Closed-chest cardiac massage, part III
11 minutes, 16 mm., color   EFL EM 366
External cardiac massage (James R. Jude)
1961, 22 minutes, sound   ACS 088
External cardiac massage (James R. Jude, William B. Kouwenhoven, G. Guy Knickerbocker)
1961, 22 minutes, sound, color   AMA 219
Extract from Vickers film on treatment of myocardial infarction with a hyperbaric bed at Westminster Hospital, London, England, The Bethlehem Corporation, Hyperbaric Oxygen Therapy Division, Bethlehem, Pa., 1968.
Initial examination and therapy (Emergency care of the injured patient in the emergency department, part I) (Walter F. Ballinger, II)
1967, 18 minutes, sound, color   MEND
Innovations in transfusion therapy (Carl W. Walter)
1963, 29 minutes, sound   ACS 120
Intermittent positive pressure breathing (Theodore H. Noehren)
1960, 31 minutes, sound, color   AMA 198
Introduction to respiratory and cardiac resuscitation (Peter Safar)
1961, 35 minutes, color   SG
Organization of cardiac resuscitation (John R. Derrick, Thomas D. Kirksey)
1965, 17 minutes, sound   ACS 408
Nurse's role in cardiopulmonary resuscitation
1966, 25 minutes, color   AHA
Parenteral fluid therapy (Harry Weisberg)
1964, 15 minutes, sound   ACS 402
Physicochemical principles in the treatment of shock (William Schumer)
1966, 50 minutes, sound   ACS 495
Prescription for life (Archer S. Gordon)
1966, 50 minutes, sound, color   ACS 537
Principles of artificial respiration (James L. Whittenberger, Benjamin A. Ferris, Jr., Jere Mead)
1957, 27 minutes, sound, color   AMA 158
Pulse of life (Archer S. Gordon, Allen B. Dobkin, James O. Elam, James R. Jude, Peter Safar)
1962, 27 minutes, sound, color   AMA 113
(16-minute version available through Pyramid Films, Box 1048, Santa Monica, California)

Rescue breathing (Lewis and Marguerite S. Herman)
  1958, 21 minutes, sound   PHS, MIS 376
Resuscitation care of the severely wounded (Curtis P. Artz)
  1957, 35 minutes, sound   ACS 213
Resuscitation for cardiac arrest (Claude S. Beck)
  1956, 18 minutes, sound   ACS 211
Save that life (Scott Peters Enterprises)
  7 minutes, sound, color
Seconds count, part II (Stewart Hardy Films for British Admirality)
  1963, 15 minutes, 16 mm., color   AHA
Shock (Lloyd D. MacLean)
  1965, 29 minutes, sound, color   D&G CS 969
Simple method for tracheal suction and bronchoscopy (David E. Thomas)
  1963, 12 minutes, sound   ACS 226
Specific problems (Emergency care of the injured patient in the emergency department, part II) (Walter F. Ballinger, II)
  1967, 23 minutes, sound, color   MEND
That they may live (University of Saskatchewan College of Medicine)
  1959, 19 minutes, sound, color PHS MIS 562
To save a life
  16 minutes, 16 mm., color   American Gas Assoc. Film Serv. 420 Lexington Ave. New York, New York 10017
Training manikin, part IV (Stewart Hardy Films for British Admiralty)
  1963, 9 minutes, color   AHA
Water rescue (James Elam)
  1961, 12 minutes, 16 mm., color   1540 Broadway New York, New York 10036
What happens next? . . . Code 4: organizing a hospital resuscitation program (Smith, Kline & French Laboratories)
  1965, 14 minutes, sound   AMA 39
Why blood volume? (Jacob Fine)
  1964, 25 minutes, sound   ACS 343

SLIDES

Cardiopulmonary resuscitation for dentists
  1966, 35 mm., color   AHA
Cardiopulmonary resuscitation, the nurse's role
  1965, 35 mm., 15 color slides   AHA
Definitive therapy
  1965, 35 mm., 35 color slides   AHA
Emergency measures
  1965, 35 mm., 35 color slides   AHA
Training of ambulance personnel in cardiopulmonary resuscitation
  1965, 35 mm., 23 color slides   AHA

Additional references*

Abbott, C. P., et al.: A technique for heart transplantation in the rat, Arch. Surg. 89:645, 1964.
Abel, R. M., et al.: Renal dysfunction following open-heart operations, Arch. Surg. 108:175-177, 1974.
Aber, C. P., et al.: Cardiac monitoring in a regional hospital, Br. Med. J. 1:209-212, 1969.
Aberg, H.: Atrial fibrillation. III. A study of the fibrillatory waves using a new technique, Acta Soc. Med. Upsal. 4:17-27, 1969.
Aberg, H., and Cullhed, I.: Direct current countershock complications, Acta Med. Scand. 183:415-421, 1968.
Aberg, H., and Cullhed, I.: Direct current conversion of atrial fibrillation—long-term results, Acta Med. Scand. 184:433-440, 1968.
Abildskov, J. A., et al.: False complete bilateral bundle branch block, J. Electrocardiol. 4:58-61, 1971.
Abrams, L. D.: Induction pacing, Ann. N. Y. Acad. Sci. 167:964-967, 1969.
Abrams, L. D., et al.: A surgical approach to the management of heart-block using an inductive coupled artificial pacemaker, Lancet 1:1372-1378, 1960.
Abuaud, R., et al.: Cardiac arrest, Rev. Med. Chil. 94:631-636, 1966.
Achilli, M., et al.: Resuscitation after serious bilateral thoracic-pulmonary injuries, Acta Anaesthesiol. (Padova) 20:817-823, 1969.
Acosta, C.: Glossopharyngeal neuralgia associated with cardiac arrest. Case report, J. Neurosurg. 32:706-707, 1970.
Acute care medicine internship first of its kind to be offered, Bull. Am. Coll. Surg. 56:3-4, 1971.
Adachi, M.: The effect of various cardioplegic procedures on myocardial oxygen consumption in normo- and hypothermia, Tohoku J. Exp. Med. 94:177-185, 1968.
Adams, C. W.: Treatment of cardiac arrest, J. Tenn. Med. Assoc. 64:411-414, 1971.
Adebahr, G.: Histological findings in the heart in attempted resuscitation, Dtsch. Z. Ges. Gerichtl. Med. 57:205-211, 1966.
Adgey, A. A., et al.: Incidence, significance, and management of early bradyarrhythmia complicating acute myocardial infarction, Lancet 2:1097-1101, 1968.

*Please note that almost all the references in the fourth edition of CARDIAC ARREST AND RESUSCITATION are entirely new to this edition. Space does not permit listing of references included in the first, second, and third editions. It is suggested that the reader refer to the previous editions for this information.

Adgey, A. A., et al.: Management of ventricular fibrillation outside hospital, Lancet 1:1169-1171, 1969.

Adgey, A. A., et al.: Mobile coronary team saves lives outside hospital, Mod. Med. 37:124, 1969.

Advanced training program for emergency medical technicians—ambulance, U. S. Department of Health, Education, and Welfare. Pub. HSM 72-2007, Washington, D. C., 1968.

After the "definition of irreversible coma," N. Engl. J. Med. 281:1070-1071, 1969.

Agostinis, G.: Non-cardiogenic ventricular fibrillation in a hospitalized patient with peripheral vascular disease with grave humoral imbalance. Resuscitation without sequels, Acta Anaesthesiol. (Padova) 20:201-214, 1969.

Ahlgren, E. W.: Guidelines to management of some respiratory problems, Clin. Anesth. 3:198-209, 1968.

Ahnefeld, F. W.: Resuscitation in cardiac arrest, Verh. Dtsch. Ges. Inn. Med. 74:279-287, 1968.

Ahnefeld, F. W., et al.: Methods of resuscitation and transportation problems in emergency situations in medical practices, Internist (Berlin) 11:41-46, 1970.

Ahuja, S. P., et al.: Mode of onset of ventricular arrhythmias, Acta Cardiol. (Brux.) 23:399-407, 1968.

Albano, A., et al.: Rhythmic percussion of the precordium with the closed fist as the first procedure in therapy of cardiac arrest, Minerva Med. 58:2659-2665, 1967.

Albert, M. L., et al.: Paraplegia secondary to hypotension and cardiac arrest in a patient who has had previous thoracic surgery, Neurology (Minneap.) 19:915-918, 1969.

Aldrete, J. A., et al.: Possible predictive tests for malignant hyperthermia during anesthesia, J.A.M.A. 215:1465-1469, 1971.

Alegre, J. M., et al.: Perforation of myocardium by pacemaker catheter, J.A.M.A. 212: 481-482, 1970.

Aleksandrow, W., et al.: Late results of patients after resuscitation during cardiac arrest, Pol. Tyg. Lek. 26:342-344, 1971.

Alexander, S.: Treatment of arrhythmias associated with acute myocardial infarction, Med. Clin. North Am. 53:315-326, 1969.

Alksne, J. F.: Brain death as seen by the neurosurgeon, Laval Med. 41:180-182, 1970.

Allen, J. D., et al.: Effects of bretylium on experimental cardiac dysrhythmias, Am. J. Cardiol. 29:641-649, 1972.

Allen, P., et al.: The results of demand pacing in cardiac arrhythmias, Ann. Thorac. Surg. 8:146-151, 1969.

Allensworth, D. C., et al.: Persistent atrial standstill in a family with myocardial disease, Am. J. Med. 47:775-784, 1969.

Allison, S. P.: Insulin and cardiogenic shock, Br. Med. J. 1:760, 1969.

al-Naaman, Y. D., et al.: Cardiac arrest between prophylaxis and treatment, J. Cardiovasc. Surg. (Torino) 12:161-162, 1971.

Altschuld, R. A., et al.: Metabolism of the ischaemic myocardium, Heart Bull. 19:109-113, 1970.

Amador, E., et al.: Sudden death during disulfiram-alcohol reaction, Q. J. Stud. Alcohol 28: 649-654, 1967.

American Heart Association: Cardiopulmonary resuscitation. A manual for instructors, New York, 1967, The Association.

American Heart Association: The dentist's role in cardiopulmonary resuscitation, New York, 1968, The Association.

American Heart Association: Emergency resuscitation team manual: a hospital plan, New York, 1968, The Association.

American Heart Association: The nurse's role in cardiopulmonary resuscitation, New York, 1965, The Association.

American Heart Association: Rescue breathing, New York, 1970, The Association.

Anaesthesia accidents, Ned. Tijdschr. Geneeskd. 118:2147-2148, 1968.

Andersen, N., et al.: The prophylactic antiarrhythmic effect on quinidine in myocardial infarction, Acta Med. Scand. 184:171-176, 1968.

Anderson, R., et al.: Relation between metabolic acidosis and cardiac dysrhythmias in acute myocardial infarction, Br. Heart J. 30:493-496, 1968.

Anderson, R. M., et al.: Incison for cardiac pacemaker pouch, Surgery 66:809-810, 1969.

Anderson, S. T., et al.: Lignocaine in the management of ventricular arrhythmias, Med. J. Aust. 1:208-211, 1969.

Andjus, R. K., and Smith, A. U.: Reanimation of adult rats from body temperatures between 0° C. and +2° C., J. Physiol. (Lond.) 128: 446-473, 1955.

Andree, R. A., and Pilchik, E. E.: When death is inexorable, Science 169:717, 1970.

Andrews, M. C.: Cardiovascular collapse and cardiac arrest in the early puerperium, Am. J. Obstet. Gynecol. 108:18-21, 1970.

Angelakos, E. T., et al.: Effect of catecholamine infusions on lethal hypothermic temperatures in dogs, J. Appl. Physiol. 26:194-196, 1969.

Anstadt, G. L., and Britz, W. E.: Continued studies in prolonged circulatory support by direct mechanical ventricular assitance, Trans. Am. Soc. Artif. Intern. Organs 14:297-303, 1968.

Anstadt, G. L., Schiff, P., and Baue, A. E.: Prolonged circulatory support by direct mechanical ventricular assistance, Trans. Am. Soc. Artif. Intern. Organs 12:72-78, 1966.

Anthony, C. L., Jr., et al.: Management of cardiac and respiratory arrest in children, Clin. Pediatr. (Phila.) 8:647-654, 1969.

Anthony, P. P., et al.: Gastric mucosal lacerations after cardiac resuscitation, Br. Heart J. 31: 72-75, 1969.

Antipov, B. V.: The heart conduction system during temporary anemization and the administration of cardioplegic substances, Eksp. Khir. Anesthesziol. 13:70-74, 1968.

Aochi, O., et al.: Clinical investigation of isoproterenol—with special reference to its application in cardiac emergencies, Jap. J. Anesthesiol. 17:247-256, 1968.

Apnea-alarm mattress insures safe sleep for premature infant, J.A.M.A. 210:1183, 1969.

Arbeit, S. R., et al.: Dangers in interpreting the electrocardiogram from the oscilloscope monitor, J.A.M.A. 211:453-456, 1970.

Arbeit, S. R., et al.: Controlling the electrocution hazard in the hospital, J.A.M.A. 220: 1581-1584, 1972.

Arfel, G.: Problèmes électroencéphalographiques de la mort, Paris, 1970, Masson.

Ariano, M.: Cardiac electrostimulation in emergency conditions, Acta Anaesthiol. (Padova) 19(Suppl. 4):49-68, 1968.

Arioso, G., et al.: Problems of anesthesia and resuscitation on board merchant ships during navigation, Ann. Med. Nav. (Roma) 76:9-70, 1971.

Arnott, W. M.: Potassium-glucose-insulin, Am. Heart J. 77:845-846, 1969.

Arnulf, G., et al.: Cardiac arrest in ventricular fibrillation after circulatory reestablishment in the coronary arteries, J. Cardiovasc. Surg. (Torino) 12:174-176, 1971.

Aronow, S., et al.: Ventricular fibrillation associated with an electrically operated bed. N. Engl. J. Med. 281:31-32, 1969.

Aronson, A. L., et al.: Heart block and pacing electrodes, N. Engl. J. Med. 282:873, 1970.

Arthure, H.: Laparoscopy hazard, Br. Med. J. 4: 492-493, 1970.

Artificial heart pace slows, Med. World News 10: 18-19, 1969.

Artificial hearts—how close are we? Mod. Med. 37:44-52, 1969.

Ascheulova, E. N., et al.: The dynamics of oxygen consumption of the myocardium in experiments involving cardiac arrest with artificial circulation and normal and hypothermia, Patol. Fiziol. Eksp. Ter. 11:37-41, 1967.

Askansas, Z., et al.: Cardiologic resuscitation, Pol. Arch. Med. Wewn. 40:675-682, 1968.

Askgaard, B.: Cardiac arrest. Distribution and therapeutic results in 160 cases, Ugeskr. Laeger 131:1752-1757, 1969.

Asknas, Z., et al.: Intensive care and reanimation, Z. Gesamte Inn. Med. (Suppl.) 24:40-44, 1969.

Athanasiou, D. J.: Orthostatically-induced asystolic heart attacks, Munch. Med. Wochenschr. 108:1227-1233, 1966.

Attai, L. A., et al.: Intracorporeal cadaver organ preservation by mechanical ventricular assistance, Surg. Forum 19:202-204, 1968.

Aurousseau, M.: Research and new trends in resuscitation units, Bull. Inst. Natl. Sante Rech. Med. 25:757-762, 1970.

Austin, W. H., et al.: Metabolic acidosis in myocardial infarction, J. Maine Med. Assoc. 60: 17, 1969.

Automatic detection and defibrillation of lethal arrhythmias—a new concept, J.A.M.A. 213:615, 1970.

Avenhaus, H.: Drug therapy of patients with atrioventricular block and following pacemaker implantation, Med. Klin. 63:2113-2118, 1968.

Averill, K. H.: To start a heart, Emergency Med. 3:29-32, 1971.

Azzolina, G.: The function of the practitioner in cardiac arrest, Friuli Med. 21:1175-1182, 1966.

Baba, K.: Use of immediate hypothermia for the prevention of cerebral damage following resuscitation in cardiac arrest, Jap. J. Anesthesiol. 20: 252-258, 1971.

Babies "iced" for heart operations, Med. World News 9:28-30, 1968.

Bacalzo, L. V., Jr., et al.: Preferential cerebral hypothermia. Tromethamine and dextran 40 and tolerance to circulatory arrest of 90 to 120 minutes, Arch. Surg. 103:393-397, 1971.

Bacaner, M., et al.: Effect of bretylium tosylate on ventricular fibrillation threshold, Arch. Intern. Med. 124:95-100, 1969.

Bacaner, M.: Experimental and clinical effects of bretylium tosylate on ventricular firbrillation, arrhythmias, and heart block, Geriatrics 26: 132-148, 1971.

Bacaner, M. B., and Schrienemachers, D.: Bretylium tosylate for suppression of ventricular fibrillation after experimental myocardial infarction, Nature (Lond.) 220:494-496, 1968.

Bacazio, L. V., Jr., et al.: Resuscitation after unexpected circulatory arrest: tolerance to cerebral ischemia provided by cold carotid perfusion, Biomed. Sci. Instrum. 5:75-78, 1969.

Bacon, W. T., et al.: A small community hospital can have a coronary care unit, Med. Surg. Rev. 6:4-10, 1970.

Badger, G. F., et al.: Myocardial infarctions in the practices of a group of private physicians. 3. Causes of death among patients who have survived a myocardial infarction, J. Chronic Dis. 21:467-471, 1968.

Badger, G. F., et al.: Myocardial infarction in the practices of a group of private physicians. 4. Factors related to the longevity of patients with myocardial infarction during the first five years, J. Chronic Dis. 21:473-482, 1968.

Baffes, T. G., et al.: Adaptation of cardiac catheterization techniques for insertion of intravascular cardiac pacemakers, Ill. Med. J. 137:616-621, 1970.

Bagchi, N., et al.: Antagonism to ouabain induced ventricular fibrillation, action of reserpine, propanolol, INPEA, and quinidine, Jap. J. Pharmacol. 19:620-621, 1969.

Bailey, L. L., et al.: Experimental technique for perfusion of the canine donor heart in vitro, Arch. Surg. 100:129-131, 1970.

Bailey, R. R.: Precordial thumping, Lancet 2: 569, 1970.

Baima-Bollone, P. L.: Medicolegal findings and considerations of the so-called "intracardiac injection" of adrenaline, Minerva Med. 87:1-13, 1967.

Bain, B.: Pacemakers and the people who need them, Am. J. Nurs. 71:1582-1585, 1971.

Baird, W. M.: An animal model for the evaluation of drugs in the treatment of acute circulatory arrest, U. Mich. Med. Cent. J. 35:23-26, 1969.

Baker, S. P., et al.: An evaluation of the hazard created by natural death at the wheel, N. Engl. J. Med. 238:405-409, 1970.

Balagot, R. C., et al.: Comparative evaluation of some DC cardiac defibrillators, Am. Heart J. 77:489-497, 1969.

Balcon, R.: Direct current shock in the treatment of cardiac infarction, Curr. Med. Drugs 8:3-9, 1967.

Baldini, M. G., et al.: Mobile conorary care—a controversial innovation, N. Engl. J. Med. 281: 905-907, 1969.

Balliuzek, V. F., et al.: A sterile room for resuscitation of patients after homologous heart transplantation, Eksp. Khir. Anesteziol. 15:84-87, 1970.

Balloon does inside job on heart, Med. World News 9:19, 1968.

Balslov, J. T., et al.: Treatment of cardiac arrest in 200 patients with special reference to results and complications, Nord. Med. 79:243-249, 1968.

Baquero, O., et al.: Cardiac arrest and the dentist, Rev. Fed. Odont. Colombia 17:53-55, 1967.

Baraka, A., et al.: Cardiac arrest during IPPV in a newborn with tracheoesophageal fistula, Anesthesiology 32:564-565, 1970.

Barber, R. E., et al.: A prospective study in patients with irreversible brain damage, N. Engl. J. Med. 283:1478-1484, 1970.

Barnard, C. N.: The operation. A human cardiac transplant: an interim report of a successful operation performed at Groote Schuur Hospital, Capetown, S. Afr. Med. J. 41:2815-2816, 1967.

Barrera, F., et al.: Interrelations of cardiac necrosis, acute hypotension, and ventricular fibrillation, Am. Heart J. 75:421-424, 1968.

Barrett, J. S., et al.: Ventricular arrhythmias associated with use of diazepam for cardioversion, J.A.M.A. 214:1323-1324, 1970.

Barrie, H.: Neonatal resuscitation, Acta. Anaesth. Scand. (Suppl.) 25:389+, 1966.

Barrier, G.: Resuscitation of newborn infants in the delivery room, Bull. Fed. Soc. Gynecol. Obstet. Lang. Fr. 21:372-373, 1969.

Bass, M.: Sudden sniffing death, J.A.M.A. 212: 2075-2079, 1970.

Baue, A. E., et al.: Mechanical ventricular assistance in man, Circulation 37 (Suppl.) 2:33-36, 1968.

Bay, G.: Disturbances of consciousness. Syncope, Adams-Stokes syndrome, Tidsskr. Nor. Laegerforen. 87(Suppl):1758-1761, 1967.

Bay, V., et al.: Successes and failures of resuscitation, Bruns Beitr. Klin. Chir. 214:481-490, 1967.

Bayley, T. J.: Long-term ventricular pacing in treatment of sinoatrial block, Br. Med. J. 3: 456-458, 1971.

Beach, T. P., et al.: Circulatory collapse following succinylcholine: report of a patient with diffuse lower motor neuron disease, Anesth. Analg. (Cleve.) 50:431-437, 1971.

Becelli, S., et al.: Incidence and reversibility of ventricular fibrillation in a first-aid service, Policlinico (Med.) 76:130-146, 1969.

Beck, C. S.: The Last Great Northwest of surgery, Ohio Med. J. 64:335-340, 1968.

Beck, C. S.: Reminiscences of cardiac resuscitation, Rev. Surg. 27:77-86, 1970.

Beck, W., et al.: Hemodynamic studies in two long-term survivors of heart transplantation, J. Thorac. Cardiovasc. Surg. 62:315-320, 1971.

Beckwith, B. M., et al.: The sudden death syndrome of infancy, Hosp. Pract. 2:42-52, 1967.

Behrman, R. E., et al.: Treatment of the asphyxiated newborn infant, J. Pediatr. 74:981-988, 1969.

Beller, B. M., et al.: Refractory supraventricular

arrhythmias in the elderly, J.A.M.A. 215:589-594, 1971.

Bellet, S., et al.: Intramuscular lidocaine in the therapy of ventricular arrhythmias, Am. J. Cardiol. 27:291-293, 1971.

Belsey, R. H.: Cardiac arrest and resuscitation, Br. J. Plast. Surg. 21:133-139, 1968.

Belzer, F. O., and Kountz, S. L.: Preservation and transplantation of human cadaver kidneys: A two-year experience, Ann. Surg. 172:394-404, 1970.

Belzer, F. O., et al.: Preservation and transplantation of human cadaver kidneys, Transplantation 14:363, 1972.

Benchimol, A., et al.: Hemodynamic consequences of atrial and ventricular pacing in patients with normal and abnormal hearts, Am. J. Med. 39:911-912, 1965.

Bender, F.: Treatment of tachycardiac arrhythmias and arterial hypertension with verapamil, Arzneim. Forsch. 20(Suppl. 9a):1310+, 1970.

Benfield, J. R.: Cardiopulmonary resuscitation at University of Wisconsin, Arch. Surg. 96:664-670, 1968.

Bengtsson, M., et al.: A psychiatric-psychological investigation of patients who had survived circulatory arrest, Acta Psychiatr. Scand. 45:327-346, 1969.

Bennett, D. R., et al.: Prolonged "survival" with flat EEG following cardiac arrest, Electroencephalogr. Clin. Neurophysiol. 30:94, 1971.

Bennett, M. A., and Pentecost, B. L.: Warning of cardiac arrest due to ventricular fibrillation and tachycardia, Lancet 1:1351-1352, 1972.

Bennett, W. M., et al.: A practical guide to drug usage in adult patients with impaired renal function, J.A.M.A. 214:1468-1475, 1970.

Benson, D. M.: Emergency treatment of cardiac arrhythmias, J.A.M.A. 215:1157-1158, 1971.

Berant, M., and Gassner, S.: The Valsalva maneuver and unexplained sudden death in asthma, Clin. Pediatr. 8:732-734, 1969.

Berconsky, I., et al.: Treatment of auriculoventricular block using a pacemaker, Prensa Med. Argent. 56:333-338, 1969.

Beregovich, J., et al.: Artificial pacing in complicated myocardial infarct, Mod. Med. 37:133, 1969.

Beregovich, J., et al.: Management of acute myocardial infarction complicated by advanced atrioventricular block. Role of artificial pacing, Am. J. Cardiol. 23:54-65, 1969.

Beregovich, J., et al.: Hemodynamic effects of isoproterenol in cardiac surgery, J. Thorac. Cardiovasc. Surg. 62:957-964, 1971.

Berger, E. N., et al.: Effect of hypoxia and of the adrenal cortex hormones on the emergence of acetylcholine heart arrest, Patol. Fiziol. Eksp. Ter. 12:31-33, 1968.

Berger, R. L.: Current status of pulmonary embolectomy, Heart Bull. 19:12-15, 1970.

Berglund, E., et al.: Haemodynamic measurements prior to ventricular fibrillation or asystole following experimental coronary occlusion, Thorax 24:626-628, 1969.

Bergman, A. B., et al., editors: Sudden infant death syndrome: Proceedings of the second International Conference on Causes of Sudden Death in Infants, Seattle, 1970, University of Washington Press.

Bergman, F., et al.: The connection between myocardial infarction and gallstones in an autopsy series, Acta Pathol. Microbiol. Scand. 73:559-564, 1968.

Bergman, J. A., and Aazon, R. K.: Subclavian catheters in cardiac arrest, J.A.M.A. 217:210, 1971.

Berkovits, B. V., et al.: Bifocal demand pacemaker, Circulation 40(Suppl. 3):44, 1969.

Bernard, R., et al.: Role of temporary pacing in cardiac resuscitation, Acta Cardiol. (Brux.) 25:144-156, 1970.

Bernard, R., and Thys, J. P.: Tracheal and bronchial electrocardiographic derivations in cardiopulmonary resuscitation, Acta Cardiol. (Brux.) 25:396-403, 1970.

Bernhard, W. F.: Biventricular bypass: physiologic studies during induced ventricular failure and fibrillation, J. Thorac. Cardiovasc. Surg. 62:859-868, 1971.

Bernreiter, M.: Permanent transvenous pacing in a patient with drug-resistant ventricular arrhythmias, J. Kans. Med. Soc. 70:240-243, 1969.

Bernreiter, M.: Reducing mortality in myocardial infarction, Geriatrics 23:138-144, 1968.

Bernreiter, M.: Prolonged Q-T, ventricular premature contractions, and sudden death, Mo. Med. 67:104-105, 1970.

Bernsmeier, A.: Electrotherapy of cardiac arrhythmias, Munch. Med. Wochenschr. 110:1977-1981, 1968.

Bernstein, W. H., et al.: Postmyocardial infarction ventricular septal perforation complicated by bacterial endocarditis, Am. J. Cardiol. 24:432-453, 1969.

Berry, Y. B.: Recognition and management of airway obstruction, J.A.M.A. 209:1722, 1969.

Bersano, E., et al.: Left atrial infarction, Dis. Chest 54:249-250, 1968.

Bertrand, C. A., et al.: Disturbances of cardiac rhythm during anesthesia and surgery, J.A.M.A. 216:1615-1617, 1971.

Bertrand, H.: Presentation of a folding resuscita-

tion stretcher, Anesth. Analg. (Paris) **24**:361-366, 1967.

Bès, A., et al.: Hemodynamic and metabolic studies in "coma dépassé." A search for a biological test of death of the brain. In: Cerebral blood flow. International symposium on the clinical applications of isotope clearance measurement of blood flow, Berlin, 1969, pp. 213-215.

Bessert, I., et al.: On the numerical relation between reanimation patients, patients with dissociated brain death, and potential organ donors in a reanimation center, Electroencephalogr. Clin. Neurophysiol. **29**:210-211, 1970.

Besterman, E.: Cardiac resuscitation, Nurs. Times **65**:396-398, 1969.

Betleri, I., et al.: Successful resuscitation after postoperative cardiac arrest, Zentralbl. Chir. **91**:1931-1933, 1966.

Bevilacqua, C.: Medico-legal problems related to resuscitation methods, Acta Anesthesiol. (Padova) **21**:95-105, 1970.

Bhatia, M. L., et al.: Potassium- and digitalis-induced complete heart block, J. Indian Med. Assoc. **53**:26-28, 1969.

Biazrov, S., et al.: Use of the defibrillator after prolonged direct heart massage, Klin. Med. (Mosk.) **47**:119-120, 1969.

Bidwai, P. S., et al.: Cardiac arrest following two-step exercise electrocardiogram, Indian Heart J. **21**:241-243, 1969.

Bieber, C. P., et al.: Pathology of the conduction system in cardiac rejection, Circulation **34**:567, 1969.

Bilbro, R. H.: Syncope after prostatic massage, N. Engl. J. Med. **282**:167-168, 1970.

Bilgutay, A. M., et al.: Vagal tuning, J. Thorac. Cardiovasc. Surg. **56**:71-82, 1968.

Bilgutay, A. M., et al.: Augmented ventilation by synchronous phrenic nerve stimulation, Trans. Am. Soc. Artif. Intern. Organs **16**:213-219, 1970.

Bilitch, M.: Ventricular fibrillation and pacing, Ann. N. Y. Acad. Sci. **167**:934-940, 1969.

Binet, L., and Strumza, M. V.: La réanimation après anoxie, Presse Med. **7**:121-124, 1951.

Bing, R. J.: What is cardiac failure, Am. J. Cardiol. **22**:2-6, 1968.

Bing, R. J., et al.: Myocardial infarction—basic clinical and therapeutic considerations, Mich. Med. **67**:19-23, 1968.

Binnie, C. D., et al.: Electroencephalographic prediction of fatal anoxic brain damage after resuscitation from cardiac arrest, Br. Med. J. **4**:265-268, 1970.

Binnie, C. D., et al.: EEG prediction of outcome after resuscitation from cardiac or respiratory arrest, Electroencephalogr. Clin. Neurophysiol. **29**:105, 1970.

Birch, A. A., Jr., et al.: Changes in serum potassium response to succinylcholine following trauma, J.A.M.A. **210**:490-493, 1969.

Birkhan, J., et al.: Exercises in resuscitation, Harefuah **78**:241-244, 1970.

Birks, W., et al.: Heart arrest and resuscitation, Chirurg **40**:157-162, 1969.

Bjerkelund, C. J., and Orning, O. M.: An evaluation of D.C. shock treatment of atrial arrhythmias, Acta Med. Scand. **184**:481-491, 1968.

Bjerkelund, C. J., and Orning, O. M.: Efficacy of anticoagulant therapy in preventing embolism related to D.C. electrical conversion of atrial fibrillation, Am. J. Cardiol. **23**:208-216, 1969.

Blachly, P. H.: Electroconvulsive treatment compared with electrocardioversion: a source of ideas, Compr. Psychiatry **9**:13-30, 1969.

Blackstone, E. H., et al.: Perfusion-induced myocardial injury, J. Thorac. Cardiovasc. Surg. **56**:689-698, 1968.

Blair, E., et al.: Gram-negative bacteremic shock: mechanisms and management, J.A.M.A. **207**:333-336, 1969.

Bleifeld, W., et al.: Quinidine for prophylaxis of arrhythmias in acute myocardial infarction, N. Engl. J. Med. **286**:667, 1972.

Blichert-Toft, M., et al.: Plasma cortisol and 17-ketosteroids in urine in relation to cardiac arrest, Ugeskr. Laeger **129**:759-760, 1967.

Blocking out death in heart surgery, Med. World News **10**:16, 1969.

Bloem, T. J.: A patient with a recent myocardial infarct and many complications, Ned. Tijdschr. Geneeskd. **112**:1590-1593, 1968.

Blondeau, M., et al.: Disorders of rhythm and auriculo-ventricular conduction in recent myocardial infarct, Arch. Mal. Coeur **60**:1733-1751, 1967.

Bloodwell, R. D., et al.: Cardiac valve replacement without coronary perfusion. In Brewer, L. A., III, editor: Prostatic heart valves, Springfield, Ill., 1969, Charles C Thomas, Publisher, pp. 397-418.

Bloomfield, D. K., et al.: Survival in acute myocardial infarction before and after the establishment of a coronary care unit, Chest **57**:224-229, 1970.

Bloomfield, S. S., et al.: Quinidine for prophylaxis of arrhythmias in acute myocardial infarction, N. Engl. J. Med. **285**:979-986, 1971.

Bluestone, R., et al.: Long-term endocardiac pacing for heart block, Lancet **2**:307-311, 1965.

Boal, B. H., et al.: Complication of intracardiac electrical pacing—knotting together of temporary and permanent electrodes, N. Engl. J. Med. **280**:650-651, 1969.

Boatright, C. F., et al.: Sudden cardiac arrest in adenotonsillectomy, Trans. Am. Acad. Ophthalmol. Otolaryngol. **74**:1139-1145, 1970.

Boba, A.: Fatal postanesthetic complications in two muscular dystrophic patients, J. Pediatr. Surg. **5**:71-75, 1970.

Body, G., et al.: A simplified cardiac resuscitation trolley for ward use, Lancet **2**:955-956, 1968.

Boley, S. J., et al.: Potassium vasoactivity—a biphasic effect, Surgery **67**:350-354, 1970.

Bondoli, A., et al.: Changes in pulmonary alveoli beta-lipoprotein levels following fresh water drowning and cardiac resuscitation, Minerva Anestesiol. **36**:315-319, 1970.

Bonhoeffer, K.: The oxygen consumption of normal and hypothermic dog hearts before and during different forms of induced cardiac arrest, Bibl. Cardiol. **18**:1-73, 1967.

Booth, B. H., et al.: Electrocardiographic changes during human anaphylaxis, J.A.M.A. **26**:627-631, 1970.

Borchgrevink, C. F.: Low molecular weight dextran in acute myocardial infarction, Geriatrics **24**:138-144, 1969.

Bordel-Blanco, E., et al.: Use of haemocel for restoring the blood volume in the resuscitation of severely injured patients, Rev. Esp. Anestesiol. Reanim. **17**:771-774, 1970.

Borja, A. R., and Hinshaw, J. R.: A safe way to perform infraclavicular subclavian vein catheterization, Surg. Gynecol. Obstet. **130**:673-676, 1970.

Borman, J. B., et al.: External-internal defibrillation. An experimental and clinical appraisal, J. Thorac. Cardiovasc. Surg. **62**:98-102, 1971.

Bornemann, C., and Scherf, D.: Paroxysmal ventricular tachycardia abolished by a blow on the precordium, Dis. Chest. **56**:83-84, 1969.

Borney, G., et al.: Use of lidocaine in an unusual case of ventricular fibrillation, Minerva Med. **62**:2844-2848, 1971.

Bostem, F. H., et al.: Interest of electrophysiology in reanimation and resuscitation, Electroencephalogr. Clin. Neurophysiol. **27**:647-648, 1969.

Bouchat, J., et al.: Retinal ischemia, anaphylactic shock and cardiac arrest, Bull. Mem. Soc. Fr. Ophthalmol. **82**:202-207, 1969.

Bourdais, A., et al.: Colibacillus septicemia and bacteremia in resuscitation. Apropos of 20 cases, Lyon Med. **225**:815-829, 1971.

Bournique, R.: Collection of information on electrical accidents and their medical consequences. In International Symposium on Electrical Acci-

dents, Proceedings of the Medical Section, Geneva, 1962, International Occupational Safety and Health Information Centre, pp. 19-25.

Bouvrain, Y.: Reflections apropos of 51 cases of ventricular tachycardia in acute myocardial infarct, Arch. Mal. Coeur **60**:1815-1818, 1967.

Bouvrain, Y., et al.: Activity of the cardiac resuscitation unit of the Hospital Lariboisiere, Presse Med. **76**:1393-1396, 1968.

Bouvrain, Y., et al.: Sudden death caused by unexpected ventricular fibrillation in acute myocardial infarct, Arch. Mal. Coeur **61**:1235-1251, 1968.

Bower, M. G., et al.: Hemodynamic effects of glucagon, Arch. Surg. **101**:411-416, 1970.

Boyd, D. R., et al.: The resuscitation and initial management of the severely injured, J. Occup. Med. **12**:262-266, 1970.

Boz'ev, A. A.: Effect of the duration of complete cessation of blood circulation on restoration of vital functions in resuscitation with the heart lung machine, Biull. Eksp. Biol. Med. **70**:23-26, 1970.

Brachetti, D.: Heart arrest, G. Clin. Med. **51**:254-259, 1970.

Bradlow, B. A.: Supraventricular paroxysmal tachycardia interrupted by repeated episodes of total cardiac standstill with syncopal attacks, Chest **58**:122-128, 1970.

Braimbridge, M. V., et al.: External DC defibrillation during open heart surgery, Thorax **26**:455-456, 1971.

Brandolini, G., et al.: Importance of the gastrointestinal motility in resuscitation, Acta Anaesthesiol. (Padova) **20**:595-602, 1969.

Brant, B., et al.: Vasodepressor factor in declamp shock production, Surg. Forum **19**:22-23, 1968.

Brantigan, J. W., et al.: Intramyocardial gas tensions during anoxic cardiac arrest, Surg. Forum **21**:152-153, 1970.

Brantigan, J. W., et al.: Intramyocardial gas tensions in the canine heart during anoxic cardiac arrest, Surg. Gynecol. Obstet. **134**:67-80, 1972.

Braunwald, E.: The sympathetic nervous system in heart failure, Hosp. Pract. **5**:31-39, 1970.

Braunwald, E., and Sobel, B. E.: Treatment of paroxysmal supraventricular tachycardia by electrical stimulation of the carotid-sinus nerves, N. Engl. J. Med. **281**:885-887, 1969.

Braunwald, E., et al.: Effective closure of the mitral valve without atrial systole, Circulation **33**:404-409, 1966.

Braunwald, E., et al.: Mechanisms of contraction of the normal and failing heart, N. Engl. J. Med. **277**:794-800, 853-863, 910-920, 962-1021, 1967.

Braunwald, E., et al.: Mechanism of action of

digitalis glycosides, Mod. Concepts Cardiovasc. Dis. **37**:129-134, 1968.

Braunwald, N. S., et al.: Carotid sinus nerve stimulation for the treatment of intractable angina pectoris: surgical technique, Ann. Surg. **172**:870-876, 1970.

Breall, W. S.: Tinkering with cardiac output, Med. World News **10**:4, 1969.

Breckenridge, C. G., and Hoff, H. E.: Ischemic and anoxic dissolution of the supramedullary control of respiration, Am. J. Physiol. **175**:449-457, 1953.

Breckenridge, I. M., et al.: Potassium intake and balance after intrathoracic operations, J. Thorac. Cardiovasc. Surg. **63**:305-311, 1972.

Bregman, D., et al.: Clinical experience with the unidirectional dual-chambered intra-aortic balloon assist, Circulation **43** and **44** (Suppl. 1): 82, 1971.

Bregman, D.: Technic of circulatory assistance, N. Engl. J. Med. **285**:1261, 1971.

Brendel, W., et al.: Electrolyte changes in deep hypothermia. II. Remarks on the clinical and biological survival time, Pfluegers Arch. **228**: 220-239, 1966.

Brendel, W., et al.: Clinical death in hypothermia, Z. Ges. Exp. Med. **146**:189-205, 1968.

Brendler, S. J., et al.: Patient recovery from severe midbrain lesions, Mod. Med. **38**:82, 1970.

Brendler, S. J., et al.: Recovery from decerebration, Brain **93**:381-392, 1970.

Brewer, L. A., III, et al.: Management of cardiac and intrapericardial vascular injuries. Role of thoracotomy and elective cardiac arrest, Bull. Soc. Int. Chir. **28**:241-250, 1969.

Brikker, V. N., et al.: On the mechanism of death in myocardial infarct, Kardiologiia **7**:33-38, 1967.

Britton, K. E., et al.: Acute renal failure, Br. Med. J. **4**:168, 1971 (letter to editor).

Brock, M., et al.: Cerebral blood flow and cerebral death, Acta Neurochir. (Wien) **20**:195-209, 1969.

Brooks, D. H., et al.: Cinematographic studies of the interior of the actively contracting heart, Ann. Surg. **167**:786-790, 1968.

Brooks, D. K.: Resuscitation, London, 1967, Edward Arnold (Publishers) Ltd., p. 3.

Brooks, H., et al.: Sotalol-induced beta blockade in cardiac patients, Circulation **42**:99-110, 1970.

Brooks, N.: Antiarrhythmic prophylaxis in acute myocardial infarction, N. Engl. J. Med. **284**: 852, 1971.

Bross, W., et al.: Clinical aspects of cardiac arrest, J. Cardiovasc. Surg. (Torino) **12**:185-187, 1971.

Brown, A. W., and Brierley, J. B.: Electronmicroscopic changes during hypoxia, Br. J. Exp. Path. **49**:87-94, 1968.

Brown, B. G., et al.: Diastolic augmentation by intra-aortic balloon; circulatory hemodynamics and treatment of severe, acute left ventricular failure in dogs, J. Thorac. Cardiovasc. Surg. **53**:789, 1967.

Brown, C. S., and Scott, A. A.: Cardiopulmonary resuscitation: a review of 184 cases and some applications for future improvements, Can. Anaesth. Soc. J. **17**:565-573, 1970.

Brown, L. B., et al.: Social effects of myocardial infarction in men under 50 years of age: review after one to eight years, Med. J. Aust. **2**:125-128, 1969.

Brown, N. K., et al.: The preservation of life, J.A.M.A. **211**:76-81, 1970.

Brown, R. W., et al.: The natural history of A-V conduction defects in acute myocardial infarction, Am. Heart J. **78**:460-466, 1969.

Bruce, D. L., and Wingard, D. W.: Anesthesia and the immune response, Anesthesiology **34**: 271-282, 1971.

Bruce, R. A., and Kluge, W.: Defibrillatory treatment of exertional cardiac arrest in coronary disease, J.A.M.A. **216**:653-658, 1971.

Brunner, D., et al.: Prevention of recurrent myocardial infarction by physical exercise, Isr. J. Med. Sci. **5**:783-785, 1969.

Buchanan, J., et al.: Effect of direct-current countershock on atrial flutter with complete heart block in a case of staphylococcal septicemia, Postgrad. Med. J. **44**:811-813, 1968.

Buckberg, G. D., et al.: Pulmonary changes following hemorrhagic shock and resuscitation in baboons, J. Thorac. Cardiovasc. Surg. **59**:450-460, 1970.

Buckley, J. J., et al.: Prevention of ventricular fibrillation during hypothermia with bretylium tosylate, Anesth. Analg. (Cleve.) **50**:587-593, 1971.

Buckley, M. J., et al.: The cardiovascular effects of antiarrhythmic agents, Heart Bull. **17**:104-108, 1968.

Budow, J., et al.: Pulmonary edema following direct current cardioversion of atrial arrhythmias, J.A.M.A. **218**:1083-1085, 1971.

Büky, B.: Effect of magnesium on ventricular fibrillation due to hypothermia, Br. J. Anaesth. **42**:886-888, 1970.

Bullock, J. D., et al.: Degree of carotid sinus sensitivity revealed by carotid massage, Mod. Med. **40**:56, 1972.

Burack, B., et al.: Transesophageal cardiac pacing, Am. J. Cardiol. **23**:469-472, 1969.

Burch, G. E., and Giles, T. D.: Study of the

effectiveness of the coronary care unit, South. Med. J. 64:435-440, 1971.

Burchett, G. D.: Efficacy of intravenous polarizing solutions: the effect of intracellular potassium concentration and transmembrane potential in clinical patients, J. Am. Osteopath. Assoc. 68: 174-179, 1968.

Burck, H. C.: On the morphology of the kidneys in acute kidney failure and in acute death, Klin. Wochenschr. 45:1208-1216, 1967.

Burgess, D. M.: Cardiac arrest and bone cement, Br. J. Med. 3:588, 1970.

Burgess, M. J., et al.: Time course of vulnerability to fibrillation after experimental coronary occlusion, Am. J. Cardiol. 27:617-621, 1971.

Burns-Cox, C. J.: Sugar intake and myocardial infarction, Br. Heart J. 31:485-490, 1969.

Burnside, J., et al.: Coronary artery rupture by a mitral valve prosthesis after closed chest massage, Ann. Thorac. Surg. 9:267-271, 1970.

Bush, H. L., et al.: Improved technic for cervical cardiac homotransplantation in the dog, J. Thorac. Cardiovasc. Surg. 62:68-75, 1971.

Butner, A. N., et al.: Clinical trial of phase-shift balloon pumping in cardiogenic shock: results in 29 patients, Surg. Forum 20:199, 1969.

Butt, M. P., et al.: Pulmonary function after resuscitation from near-drowning, Anesthesiology 32:275-277, 1970.

Büyüköztürk, K.: Principles of heart-lung reanimation therapy, Tip. Fak. Mecm. 32:747-759, 1969.

Cafferky, E. A., et al.: Congenital aneurysm of the coronary artery with myocardial infarction, Am. J. Med. Sci. 257:320-327, 1969.

Cagliani, P., et al.: Case of cardiocirculatory arrest caused by potassium depletion. Examination of resuscitation problems and clinical physiopathology, Minerva Cardioangiol. 18:512-524, 1970.

Calinog, T. A., et al.: Operative assessment of ventricular aneurysm and adynamic myocardium, J. Thorac. Cardiovasc. Surg. 60:710-718, 1970.

Callard, G. M., et al.: Acute resuscitation in the intensive care unit, Med. Clin. North Am. 55: 1157-1170, 1971.

Calvanese, J.: On a cardiac arrest case. Defibrillation recorded solely by external cardiac massage, Anesth. Analg. (Paris) 24:53-59, 1967.

Camillo, O. S.: Clinics and therapy of shock in myocardial infarct, Cardiol. Prat. 20:359-365, 1969.

Cammilli, L., et al.: Remote heart stimulation by radio frequency for permanent rhythm control in the Morgagni-Adams-Stokes syndrome, Surgery 52:765-776, 1962.

Cantwell, J. D., et al.: Cardiac complications while jogging, J.A.M.A. 210:130-131, 1969.

Caponnetto, S., et al.: Permanent atrial arrest in a subject with fascio-scapulo-humeral muscular dystrophy, Boll. Soc. Ital. Cardiol. 14:232-240, 1969.

Caponnetto, S., et al.: Persistent atrial standstill in a patient affected with facioscapulohumeral dystrophy, Cardiology 53:341-350, 1968.

Capron, A. M., and Kass, L. R.: A statutory definition of standards for determining human death; an appraisal and a proposal, University of Pennsylvania Law Review 121:87-118, 1972.

Carbonera, D., et al.: Complications of closed-chest heart massage, Acta. Anaesth. (Padova) 19:1217-1226, 1968.

Carden, E., and Bernstein, M.: Investigation of the nine most commonly used resuscitator bags, J.A.M.A. 212:589-592, 1970.

Cardiac arrest, Lancet 2:262-264, 1969.

Cardiac arrest: Etiopathogenesis, symptoms and therapy, Policlinico (Prat.) 77:1255-1257, 1970.

Cardiac arrest: multiple etiology, N. Y. J. Med. 69:3153-3154, 1969.

Cardiac arrythmia during oral surgery, J.A.M.A. 209:1225, 1969.

Cardiac infarct prognosis poor if plasma FFA high, Mod. Med. 38:177, 1970.

Cardiac insufficiency in the newborn infant, Rev. Port. Pediatr. Pueric. 31:163-180, 1968.

Cardiac pulsator keeps cadaver heart alive, Hosp. Tribune 3:3, 1969.

Carmerini, F.: Disadvantages and risks of cardioversion, Minerva Cardioangiol. 14:739-749, 1966.

Carmerini, F., et al.: Emergency endocardic stimulation in the treatment of cardiac arrest, Cardiol. Prat. 20:75-86, 1969.

Caroli, G., et al.: Analytical examination of the various monitoring systems and considerations on their clinical use, Minerva Anestesiol. 35: 1041-1044, 1969.

Carotid reflex during neck dissection, Modern Med. 38:194, 1970.

Carral y de Teresa, R.: Panoramic changes due to recent acquisition in the different medical specialties. V. Treatment of cardiac arrhythmias, Gac. Med. Mex. 95:893-896, 1965.

Carrell, A.: The surgery of blood vessels, Bull. Johns Hopkins Hosp. 18:18, 1907.

Carrell, A., and Guthrie, C. C.: The transplantation of veins and organs, Am. Med. 10:1101, 1905.

Carstens, P. H.: Pulmonary bone marrow embolism following external cardiac massage, Acta Path. Microbiol. Scand. 76:510-514, 1969.

Cartier, F., et al.: Circulatory arrest following

asphyxia. Value of external cardiac massage, Sem. Ther. **43**:40-44, 1967.

Carveth, S. W.: Cardiac resuscitation program at the Nebraska football stadium, Dis. Chest **53**:8-11, 1967.

Carveth, C. W., et al.: "The spectator's heart." Nebr. Med. J. **55**:610-613, 1970.

Casamayor del Cacho, M., et al.: Heart rhythm disorders due to potassium depletion. Two observations of ventricular fibrillation, Rev. Esp. Cardiol. **23**:404-419, 1970.

Cassem, N. H., et al.: How coronary patients respond to last rites, Postgrad. Med. **45**:147-152, 1969.

Castellani, L., et al.: Responsibilities and possibilities of the resuscitative-anesthetist in the improvement of the operative prognosis and postoperative sequels in geriatric orthopedic traumatology and surgery, Atti. Accad. Fisiocr. Siena (Med. Fis.) **17**:106-120, 1960.

Castellanos, A., Jr.: Pacemaker-induced cardiac rhythm disturbances, Ann. N. Y. Acad. Sci. **167**:903-910, 1969.

Castellanos, A., Jr.: Diagnosis of left anterior hemiblock and left posterior hemiblock in the presence of inferior wall myocardial infarction, Bull. N. Y. Acad. Med. **47**:923-930, 1971.

Castellanos, A., Jr., et al.: Cardioversion of drug-related arrhythmias, Acta Cardiol. [Brux.] **22**:444-458, 1967.

Castellanos, A., Jr., et al.: Mechanisms of digitalis-induced ventricular fibrillation, Dis. Chest **54**:53-56, 1968.

Castellanos, A., Jr., et al.: Mechanisms of slow ventricular tachycardias in acute myocardial infarction, Dis. Chest **56**:470-475, 1969.

Castelli, E., et al.: Cardiocirculatory arrest in resuscitation: case reports, Boll. Soc. Ital. Cardiol. **15**:649-657, 1970.

Castelli, S., et al.: Cerebral ischemic crises due to cardiac inhibition in children, Riv. Clin. Pediatr. **80**:592-594, 1967.

Cattao, A. D.: Prognosis of heart arrest, Minerva Anestesiol. **34**:1249-1257, 1968.

Cavallini, T., et al.: Anesthesia in cardioversion, Atti. Accad. Fisiocr. Siena (Med. Fis.) **15**:637-649, 1966.

Celis, A., et al.: Experimental lymphography in cardiac arrest, electrical ventricular fibrillation and deep hypothermia, Acta Radiol. (Diagn.) (Stockh.) **10**:465-475, 1970.

Celis, A., et al.: Lymphatic flow and cardiac recovery in ventricular arrest and fibrillation, determined by the most common methods in surgery and heart transplantation. Cir. Cir. **37**:10-36, 1969.

Center, S., et al.: Synchronous and standby cardiac pacing, Mod. Med. **36**:116-117, 1968.

Cerri, A., et al.: On a case of ventricular fibrillation during myocardial infarct treated with cardioversion, Boll. Soc. Ital. Cardiol. **12**:351-354, 1967.

Chadda, K. D., et al.: Magnesium in cardiac arrhythmia, N. Engl. J. Med. **287**:1102, 1972.

Chamberlain, D. A., et al.: Defective adaptor delays resuscitation, Lancet **1**:188, 1970.

Chandler, B. M., et al.: Association of depressed myofibrillar adenosine triphosphatase and reduced contractility in experimental heart failure, Circ. Res. **21**:717-725, 1967.

Chardack, W. M., et al.: A transistorized self-contained implantable pacemaker for the long-term correction of complete heart block, Surgery **48**:643-654, 1960.

Chardack, W. M., et al.: Five years' clinical experience with an implantable pacemaker: An appraisal, Surgery **58**:915-922, 1965.

Chardack, W. M., et al.: Pacing and ventricular fibrillation, Ann. N. Y. Acad. Sci. **167**:919-933, 1969.

Charms, B. L., et al.: Intracardiac defibrillation, Clin. Res. **19**:307, 1971.

Chartrand, C., et al.: Atrial pacing in the postoperative management of cardiac homotransplantation, Ann. Thorac. Surg. **8**:152-160, 1969.

Chatterjee, S., et al.: Evaluation of intra-aortic balloon counterpulsation, J. Thorac. Cardiovasc. Surg. **61**:405-410, 1971.

Chatterjee, S. N.: Management of cardiac arrest, J. Indian Med. Assoc. **53**:348-349, 1969.

Chawla, N. P., et al.: The use of an implanted demand pacemaker in bradyarrhythmias, Arch. Intern. Med. **124**:593-599, 1969.

Chayet, N. L.: Is it safe to save a life? Emergency Med. **3**:239, 1971.

Chazan, J. A., et al.: The acidosis of cardiac arrest, N. Engl. J. Med. **278**:360, 1968.

Cheng, T. O.: Thumps and zaps for pseudo-arrhythmias, N. Engl. J. Med. **286**:1111, 1972.

Cherniakhoyshif, F. R., et al.: Apparatus for resuscitation and treatment in acute oxygen insufficiency, Nov. Med. Priborostr. **2**:150-156, 1970.

Cherian, G., et al.: DC cardioversion. Late onset of ventricular fibrillation and its control with temporary endocardial pacing, J. Assoc. Physicians India **19**:359-362, 1971.

Chernoff, H. M.: Coronary artery disease and left anterior hemiblock, Conn. Med. **35**:44-45, 1971.

Cherry, G., et al.: The relationship to ventricular fibrillation of early tissue sodium and potassium shifts and coronary vein potassium levels in experimental myocardial infarction, J. Thorac. Cardiovasc. Surg. **61:**587-598, 1971.

Chest thumps and the heartbeat, N. Engl. J. Med. **284:**392-393, 1971.

Cheung, P. L.: Cardioversion for chronic atrial fibrillation, Nurs. Times **64:**1590-1591, 1968.

Chiba, S., et al.: Ventricular fibrillation induced by saxitoxin into the AV node artery and its prevention by phenoxybenzamine, Tohoku J. Exp. Med. **99:**103-104, 1969.

Chiche, P.: Emergencies and emergency care in cardiology, Coeur Med. Interne **7:**413-423, 1968.

Chiebus, H., et al.: Sudden arrest of circulation—causes and results of treatment, Kardiol. Pol. **12:**97-102, 1969.

Chikamori, J.: Morphologic studies on ultrastructural changes of myocardial cell in humans and dogs with induced anoxic cardiac arrest, Jap. Circ. J. **32:**1743-1766, 1968.

Chilling truth about cold swim, Med. World News **10:**29, 1969.

Choffat. P., et al.: Thoraco-abdominal injuries imputable to transthoracic heart massage, Anesth. Analg. (Paris) **28:**385-392, 1971.

Chopra, M. P., et al.: Lignocaine therapy after acute myocardial infarct, Br. Med. J. **1:**213-216, 1969.

Chrobok, H.: Remarks on reversible left branchblock in acute coronary insufficiency and fresh cardiac infarct, Przegl. Lek. **26:**719-720, 1970.

Chulia Campos, V., et al.: Use of haemocel in resuscitation of persons drowned in seawater, Rev. Esp. Anestesiol. Reanim. **17:**779-783, 1970.

Church, G.: Low cost coronary care unit equipment, J.A.M.A. **206:**2523, 1968.

Church, G., et al.: Intensive coronary care—a practical system for a small hospital with a house staff, N. Engl. J. Med. **281:**1155-1159, 1969.

Chusid, E. L., et al.: Treatment of hypoxemia, J.A.M.A. **214:**889-894, 1970.

Ciafalo, F. R., et al.: Effects of alpha-methyl-meta-tyrosine on ouabain-induced ventricular arrhythmia in the rabbit, Proc. West. Pharmacol. Soc. **11:**105, 1968.

Cihak, R. J.: Sudden heart failure in a 30-year-old woman, J.A.M.A. **211:**489-491, 1970.

Citro, A., et al.: Reanimation in a case of repeated heart arrest, Acta Anaesthesiol. [Padova] **18:**341-352, 1967.

Clark, J. E., and Caedo, R. E.: Fluid and electrolyte management in renal failure, Am. Fam. Physician **2:**125, 1972.

Clark, R. B.: Resuscitation of the newborn as it relates to number and training of available personnel, South. Med. J. **64:**1481-1484, 1971.

Clark, R. B., et al.: Experiences with chemical resuscitation of the newborn, J. Int. Anesth. Res. Soc. **47:**285-289, 1968.

Clarkson, E. H.: Cardiopulmonary resuscitation programs in general hospitals, Hosp. Management **107:**7306, 1969.

Clauss, R. H., et al.: Assisted circulation. I. The arterial counterpulsator, J. Thorac. Cardiovasc. Surg. **41:**447, 1961.

Clauss, R. H., et al.: Assisted circulation by counterpulsation with an intraaortic balloon. Methods and effects, Engl. Med. Biol. **4:**44, 1962.

Clauss, R. H., et al.: Pharmacologic assistance to the failing circulation, Surg. Gynecol. Obstet. **126:**611-631, 1968.

Cleveland, J. C.: Complete recovery after cardiac arrest for three hours, N. Engl. J. Med. **284:** 334-335, 1971.

Cliche, P.: Emergencies and emergency care in cardiology, Coeur Med. Interne **7:**413-423, 1968.

Cloche, R., et al.: Morphology and evolution of the EEG in acute cerebral anoxia (42 cases), Electroencephalogr. Clin. Neurophysiol. **25:**89, 1968.

Cloutier, C. T., et al.: The effect of hemodilutional resuscitation on serum protein levels in humans in hemorrhagic shock, J. Trauma **9:**514-521, 1969.

Cobb, F. R., et al.: Cardiac inotropic and coronary vascular responses to countershock, Circ. Res. **23:**731-742, 1968.

Cobb, L. A., et al.: Early experience in the management of sudden death with a mobile intensive coronary care unit, Circulation (Suppl. 3) **3-**144, 1970.

Cobb, L. A.: Personal communication, 1970.

Cockburn, R., et al.: The effect on pentobarbital anesthesia on resuscitation and brain damage in fetal rhesus monkeys asphyxiated on delivery, J. Pediatr. **75:**281-291, 1969.

Cohn, J. N.: Treatment of shock following myocardial infarction, Calif. Med. **111:**66-68, 1969.

Cohn, J. N.: Therapy of shock caused by myocardial infarction, Heart Bull. **19:**49-51, 1970.

Cohn, L. H., et al.: Emergency coronary artery bypass, Surgery **10:**821-829, 1971.

Col, J. J., et al.: Incidence and mortality of intraventricular conduction defects in acute myocardial infarction, Am. J. Cardiol. **29:**344-350, 1972.

Colin, J. M.: Cardiac arrest, J. Med. Bordeaux **143:**1949-1954, 1966.

Collan, R., et al.: Cardiac arrest caused by rapid elimination of nitrous oxide from cerebral ventricles after electroencephalography, Can. Anaesth. Soc. J. 16:519-524, 1969.

Collins, J. A., et al.: The surgical intensive care unit, Surgery 66:614-619, 1969.

Collins, J. A., et al.: Acid-base status of seriously wounded combat casualties. II. Resuscitation with stored blood, Ann. Surg. 173:6-18, 1971.

Coltart, D. J., et al.: Primary oxalosis of the heart, Br. Heart J. 33:315-319, 1971.

Columbo, L., et al.: The use of levulose in resuscitation, Acta Anaesthesiol. (Padova) 20 (Suppl. 2):79-90, 1969.

Comer, E. O.: Cardiac resuscitation, J. La. State Med. Soc. 121:9-14, 1969.

Computerized monitoring for small hospitals, Med. World News 10:23, 1969.

Congdon, E. E., et al.: Efficacy of glucagon therapy in heart failure, J. Am. Osteopath. Assoc. 69:1114-1117, 1970.

Connolly, H. A., Jr.: Cardiac massage as a life saver after severe hemorrhage, J. Med. Soc. N.J. 66:623-624, 1969.

Conrad, J. K., et al.: Transvenous pacing in two patients with repetitive ventricular arrhythmias, Arch. Intern. Med. 122:507-511, 1968.

Constantineanu, M.: A-V heart block in myocardial infarction, Am. J. Cardiol. 26:549-550, 1970.

Cooke, R., et al.: Multiple-purpose crib for neonatal intensive care, Pediatrics 42:928-933, 1968.

Cooley, D. A., et al.: Transplantation of the human heart, J.A.M.A. 205:479, 1968.

Cooley, D. A., et al.: Ischemic contracture of the heart: "stone heart," Am. J. Cardiol. 29:575-577, 1972.

Cooper, E. S., et al.: Cardiac arrhythmias, cerebral function, and stroke, Curr. Concepts Cerebrovasc. Dis. Stroke 5:53-57, 1970.

Cooper, J. K., et al.: Mobile coronary care—a controversial innovation, N. Engl. J. Med. 281:906-908, 1969.

Cooper, T., and Dempsey, P. J.: Assisted circulation. II. Methods of mechanical circulatory assistance, Mod. Concepts Cardiovasc. Dis. 37:101, 1968.

Cooper, T., et al.: Drug responses of the transplanted heart, Dis. Chest 45:284, 1964.

Cooper, T., et al.: Beta-adrenergic receptor blockade in cardiac therapy, Heart Bull. 17:113-115, 1968.

Copperman, I. J.: The fist as an external cardiac pacemaker, Lancet, 2:611, 1970.

Copplestone, J. F.: Effectiveness of respiratory and cardiac resuscitation as a first aid measure, N. Z. Med. J. 70:302-305, 1969.

Coran, A. G., et al.: The effect of crystalloid resuscitation in hemorrhagic shock on acid-base balance: a comparison between normal saline and Ringer's lactate solutions, Surgery 69:874-880, 1971.

Corato, R., et al.: Resuscitation of the patient with electrical injury, Acta Anaesthesiol. (Padova) 21:249-254, 1970.

Corbascio, A. N., et al.: 2,4,7-triamino-O-tolylpteridine [WR 3090] and propanolol. A comparative study of their anti-arrhythmic actions, Proc. West. Pharmacol. Soc. 11:107-109, 1968.

Corbitt, J. D., Jr., et al.: Muscle changes of the anterior chest wall secondary to electrical countershock, Am. J. Clin. Path. 51:107-112, 1969.

Corday, E.: Pressor agents in cardiogenic shock: pro and con, Am. J. Cardiol. 23:900-911, 1969.

Corday, E., et al.: Reevaluation of the treatment of shock secondary to cardiac infarction, Dis. Chest 56:200-209, 1969.

Corday, E., et al.: Physiologic principles in the application of circulatory assist for the failing heart; intraaortic balloon circulatory assist and venoarterial phased partial bypass, Am. J. Cardiol. 26:595, 1970.

Cordier, M.: Electrocution in the operating room, Anesth. Analg. (Paris) 28:285-292, 1971.

Corliss, R. J., et al.: Electrical conversion of arrhythmias, Wis. Med. J. 65:234-239, 1966.

Corliss, R. J., et al.: Hemodynamic effects after conversion of arrhythmias, J. Clin. Invest. 47:1774-1786, 1968.

Corne, R. A., and Mathewson, F. A.: Congenital complete atrioventricular heart block, Am. J. Cardiol. 29:412-415, 1972.

Cornii, A., et al.: Ventricular fibrillation in acute myocardial infarct. Apropos of 7 cases with recovery, Acta. Clin. Belg. 24:236-250, 1969.

The coronary care unit—pro and con, Am. J. Cardiol. 32:597-602, 1968.

Coronary disease mortality rate is highest first day, Mod. Med. 37:145, 1969.

Corrigan, G. E.: Fatal air embolism after Yoga breathing exercises, J.A.M.A. 210:1923, 1969.

Coskey, R. L.: Cardiopulmonary resuscitation, J.A.M.A. 217:79-80, 1971.

Council for International Organizations of Medical Sciences: Conference of heart transplantation organized with the assistance of WHO and UNESCO, Geneva, 1968.

Couture, F., et al.: 46 episodes of cardiac resuscitation, Laval Med. 39:109-112, 1968.

Crafoord, C. C.: Cerebral death and the transplantation era, Dis. Chest 55:141-145, 1969.

Crampton, R. S.: EEG evaluation of lidocaine convulsions, J.A.M.A. 205:179, 1968.

Cremonini, G.: Resuscitation and intensive care

departments in modern hospitals. Unit premises: hygienic problems and microclimate, Acta Anaesthesiol. (Padova) 21:69-79, 1970.

Criscitiello, M. G.: Therapy of A-V block, N. Engl. J. Med. 279:1289, 1968.

Cronin, R. F. P., et al.: Shock following myocardial infarction: a clinical survey of 140 cases, Can. Med. Assoc. J. 93:57, 1965.

Cronk, J. D.: Phenol with glucagon in cardiotherapy, N. Engl. J. Med. 284:219-220, 1971.

Cropper, C. F.: Heart-lung resuscitation, Nurs. Times 65:1095-1097, 1969.

Cross, E. B., et al.: The coronary care unit; concept, status, and needs, Med. Ann. D.C. 36:599-605 passim 1967.

Crow, H. J., et al.: Serial electrophysiologic studies in a case of 3-month survival with flat EEG following cardiac arrest, Electroencephalogr. Clin. Neurophysiol. 27:332-333, 1969.

Csapo, G.: Atrial arrhythmia caused by ventricular extrasystole, Orv. Hetil. 112:255-257, 1971.

Csapo, G., et al.: Ventricular fibrillation after heart valve replacement, Verh. Dtsch. Ges. Kreislaufforsch. 36:101-104, 1970.

Csiky, M.: Role of potassium ions in experimental ventricular fibrillation during hypothermia, Acta Chir. Acad. Sci. Hung. 10:85-92, 1969.

Cucchi, L., et al.: Endogenous infection in patients resuscitated in the intensive care unit, G. Ital. Mal. Torace. 23:291-292 passim, 1969.

Cullum, P. A., et al.: The warm ischaemic time of the canine heart, Cardiovasc. Res. 4:67-72, 1970.

Cunescu, V.: Electrocardiographic changes of cerebral origin, Med. Interna (Bucur.) 21:699-713, 1969.

Curran, W. J.: Legal and medical death—Kansas takes the first step, N. Engl. J. Med. 284:260-261, 1971.

Curry, J. J., et al.: Myocardial infarction with ventricular fibrillation during pregnancy, treated by direct current defibrillation with fetal survival, Chest 58:82-84, 1970.

Cutler, B. S., et al.: Application of the "G-suit" to control of hemorrhage in massive trauma, Ann. Surg. 171:511-514, 1971.

Czyzewska, F., et al.: Electrocardiographic changes after successful cardiac resuscitation by heart massage through the diaphragm, Pol. Tyg. Lek. 24:174-175, 1969.

Dack, S., et al.: Heart block with Stokes-Adams syndrome: indications for and results of pacing, Ann. N. Y. Acad. Sci. 167:519-533, 1969.

Damia, G. V., et al.: Possibilities of recovery after external cardiac massage of long duration, Minerva Anestesiol. 36:350-352, 1970.

Dammann, J. F., Jr., et al.: Assessment of continuous monitoring in the critically ill patient, Dis. Chest 55:240-244, 1969.

Danielson, K. S., et al.: Evaluation of dextrose, insulin, and potassium on ventricular irritability in acute myocardial infarction, J. Thorac. Cardiovasc. Surg. 60:653-660, 1970.

Danon, M.: Resuscitation of the newborn, J. Am. Osteopath. Assoc. 69:1-9, 1970.

Danzig, R.: Practical experiences in a coronary care unit, Geriatrics 24:95-101, 1969.

Datey, K. K.: Intensive coronary care unit, Indian Heart J. 21:1-3, 1969.

Datey, K. K.: The coronary care unit in a non-teaching hospital. Ill. Med. J. 136:60-61, 1969.

Datey, K. K., et al.: Intensive cardiac care unit in the management of acute myocardial infarction, J. Assoc. Physicians India 16:123-130, 1968.

Datey, K. K., et al.: 100 patients of acute myocardial infarction treated in an intensive coronary care unit, J. Indian Med. Assoc. 52:405-509, 1969.

Dato, A., et al.: A simple apparatus to help in cardiocirculation, Minerva Cardioangiol. 17:995-998, 1969.

Davidson, J.: The treatment of the cardiac arrest emergency, Br. J. Anaesthiol. 42:553-556, 1970.

Davis, E. Y.: Posterior thump-version, N. Engl. J. Med. 284:919, 1971.

Day, H. W.: An intensive coronary care area, Dis. Chest 44:423, 1963.

Day, H. W.: Acute coronary care—a five year report, Am. J. Cardiol. 21:252-257, 1968.

Day, H. W.: The coronary care unit, Heart Bull. 18:41-44, 1969.

Day, H. W.: History of coronary care units, Am. J. Cardiol. 30:405-408, 1972.

Deaths related to cardiac catheterization, Mod. Med. 36:81, 1968.

DeBakey, M. E., et al.: Orthotopic cardiac prosthesis: preliminary experiments in animals with biventricular artificial heart, Cardiovasc. Res. Cent. Bull. 7:127-142, 1969.

Dechene, J. P.: Recent acquisitions in resuscitation: intensive care, Laval Med. 41:1088-1092, 1970.

Defabianis, E.: Cardiocirculatory reanimation in dental practice, Minerva Stomatol. 18:83-89, 1969.

Degani, A.: Pathogenesis of cardiac arrest, Fracastoro 61:698-703, 1968.

Degerli, U., et al.: Cardiac arrest, its treatment and results, Turk. Tip. Cemiy. Mecm. 33:531-541, 1967.

Degonde, J., et al.: Recent techniques of electrical reanimation of the heart and the EEG, Electroencephalogr. Clin. Neurophysiol. **25**:88, 1968.

Delamonica, E. A.: Suppression-burst in a case of cardiac arrest, Dis. Nerv. Syst. **30**:618-621, 1969.

Delahaye, J. P., et al.: Cardiovascular emergencies, J. Med. Lyon **47**:1028-1040, 1966.

Delaye, J., et al.: Mortality and cardiac arrest in myocardial infarct in the acute phase. Causes; mechanisms; premonitory signs. Apropos 137 personal cases, Rev. Lyon Med. **17**:83-93, 1968.

Delfino, U., et al.: Indications for amino acids in resuscitation, Minerva Anestesiol. **37**:129-133, 1971.

DeLuca, F. M., et al.: Changes in some plasmatic enzymes after external transthoracic electric shock in cardiac arrhythmias, Atti. Accad. Fisiocr. Siena (Med. Fis.) **15**:213-222, 1966.

DeLuca, F. M., et al.: The transvenous intracavitary electrode catheter in cardiac stimulation, Atti. Accad. Fisiocr. Siena (Med. Fis.) **15**: 213-222, 1966.

Dembo, D. H.: The nurse's role in cardiopulmonary resuscitation, Md. State Med. J. **17**: 89-90, 1968.

Denborough, M. A., et al.: Arrhythmias and late sudden death after myocardial infarction, Lancet **1**:386-388, 1968.

Dennison, A. D., Jr.: Ominous arrhythmias following myocardial infarction, Tex. Med. **63**: 58-62, 1967.

Denniston, R. H., and Davis, T. E.: An arrhythmia monitor for use in an automatic standby defibrillator, Proc. 24th Ann. Conf. Engin. Med. Biol. **13**:217, 1971.

Denniston, R. H., et al.: Automatic standby defibrillator, J. Assoc. Adv. Med. Instrum. **5**:110, 1971.

Dental cardiopulmonary emergency procedures, J. Am. Dent. Assoc. **75**:806-807, 1967.

Deraney, M. F.: Glucagon? One answer to cardiogenic shock, Am. J. Med. Sci. **261**:149-154, 1971.

Dery, R.: The anesthetist-resuscitator in the treatment of "status asthmaticus," Laval Med. **40**: 238-242, 1969.

Desai, J. R., et al.: Successful cardiac resuscitation by external cardiac massage and mouth-to-mouth breathing, J. Indian Med. Assoc. **52**: 391-392, 1969.

Deshpande, S. Y., et al.: Ventricular tachycardia and fibrillation due to carotid sinus stimulation, R. I. Med. J. **51**:622-624, 1968.

Desruelles, J., et al.: Myocardial conduction disorders at the initial phase of myocardial in-

farct (apropos of 270 monitored patients), Arch. Mal. Coeur **64**:605-606, 1971.

Dessertenne, F., et al.: Ventricular fibrillation and twisted peaks, Presse Med. **77**:193-196, 1969.

Devlin, J. G., et al.: Hyperinsulinism with hypoglycemia following acute myocardial infarction, Metabolism **17**:999-1004, 1968.

Devorss, J., et al.: Repetitive ventricular tachyarrhythmia: result of pacemaker failure, J.A.M.A. **220**:1494, 1972.

Dewar, H. A., et al.: A year's experience with a mobile coronary resuscitation unit, Br. Med. J. **4**:226-229, 1969.

Dewar, H. A., et al.: Deaths from ischaemic heart disease outside hospital and experience with a mobile resuscitation unit, Br. Heart J. **31**:389, 1969.

Dhurandhar, R. W., et al.: Bretylium tosylate in the management of refractory ventricular fibrillation, Can. Med. Assoc. J. **105**:161-165 passim, 1971.

Dhurandhar, R. W., et al.: Primary ventricular fibrillation complicating acute myocardial infarction, Am. J. Cardiol. **27**:347-351, 1971.

Diamond, G., et al.: Haemodynamic effects of glucagon during acute myocardial infarction with left ventricular failure in man, Br. Heart J. **33**:290-295, 1971.

Dickinson, C. J., and Secker-Walker, R. H.: Longitudinal distribution of blood in rabbits in relation to the heart, with observations on the contributions of different organs, Circ. Res. **27**: 851-861, 1970.

Diebold, J., et al.: A recent case of death during an asthma crisis, Arch. Anat. Pathol. (Paris) **16**:70, 1968.

Diederich, K. W., et al.: Quantitative comparative studies on the changing nature of the ventricular fibrillation threshold by antifibrillatory substances, Z. Kreislaufforsch. **59**:736-743, 1970.

Diehl, H. S.: Structure and function: why did the heart stop? Dis. Chest. **56**:370-372, 1969.

Dieminger, H. J., et al.: Resuscitation of a newborn weighing 6130 g. by external heart massage following acute heart arrest, Zentralbl. Gynaek. **91**:982-984, 1969.

Diethelm, G.: Cardiac resuscitation: a review of methods and assessment of results, Med. J. Aust. **2**:269-273, 1969.

Dieter, R. A., et al.: Hypokalemia following hemodilution cardiopulmonary bypass, Ann. Surg. **171**:17-23, 1970.

Diethrich, E. B., et al.: Serum enzyme and electrocardiographic changes immediately following myocardial revascularization, Ann. Thorac. Surg. **5**:195-203, 1968.

Diethrich, E. B., et al.: Extracorporeal preservation of the beating heart, J. Assoc. Adv. Med. Instrum. **3:**6, 237-241, 1969.

Dietzman, R. H., et al.: Treatment of cardiogenic shock. IV: The use of phenoxybenzamine and chlorpromazine, Am. Heart J. **75:**136-138, 1968.

Dietzman, R. H., et al.: Low output syndrome, J. Thorac. Cardiovasc. Surg. **57:**138-149, 1969.

Dietzman, R. H., et al.: Corticosteroids as effective vasodilators in the treatment of low output syndrome, Chest **57:**440-453, 1970.

Dietzman, R. H., et al.: Corticosteroid treatment of low-output syndrome, Mod. Med. **38:**161, 1970.

Discussion on emergency measures in cardiopulmonary resuscitation, Acta Anaesth. Scand. (Suppl.) **29:**101+, 1968.

Dixon, T. C.: Cardiac arrest: experience and results in emergency treatment outside the operating theatre, Med. J. Aust. **1:**754-759, 1970.

Dixon, T. C., et al.: A report of 342 cases of prolonged endotracheal intubation, Med. J. Aust. **2:**529-533, 1968.

Dizzy? Look for a hidden arrhythmia, Med. World News **10:**16-17, 1969.

Dobson, M., et al.: Attitudes and long-term adjustment of patients surviving cardiac arrest, Br. Med. J. **3:**207-212, 1971.

Doctor's race to deliver a living heart, Med. World News **10:**56-62, 1969.

Dodinot, B. P., et al.: Clinical experience with atrial-synchronous pacing, Ann. N.Y. Acad. Sci. **167:**1038-1054, 1969.

Dohmen, M.: Cardiac arrest in children, Minn. Med. **51:**1559-1562, 1968.

Dohmen, M., et al.: On the clinical evaluation of cerebral anoxia in acute heart-blood circulation arrest, Zentralbl. Chir. **92:**3007, 1967.

Dolata, W., et al.: High-energy myocardial phosphates during resuscitation, Pol. Med. J. **9:**1183-1188, 1970.

Dolgin, M.: Treatment of cardiac failure with glucagon, Am. Heart J. **79:**843-844, 1970.

Domanig, E., et al.: Initial experiences with a prolonged ischaemic cardiac arrest, Thoraxchirurgie **17:**75-82, 1969.

Domenichelli, B., et al.: External heart massage in recurrent ventricular fibrillation, Chir. Patol. Sper. **17:**467-482, 1969.

Donaldson, P., et al.: Electrical cardioversion of atrial fibrillation, Can. Med. Assoc. J. **100:**370-373, 1969.

Don Michael, T. A., et al.: "Mouth-to-lung airway" for cardiac resuscitation, Lancet **2:**1329, 1968.

Doring, H. J., et al.: Significance of right ventricular load in the occurrence of epinephrine-chloroform- (or epinephrine-fluothane-) induced

ventricular fibrillation, Pfluegers Arch. **307:**R23-24, 1969.

Dorney, E. R.: Home evaluation of permanently implanted pacemakers, South. Med. J. **64:**784-790, 1971.

Dorra, M.: Closed chest cardiac resuscitation. Results. Indications. Technics, Sem. Ther. **41:**147-153, 1965.

Doty, D. B., et al.: The distribution of body fluids following hemorrhage and resuscitation in combat casualties, Surg. Gynecol. Obstet. **130:**453-458, 1970.

Douglas, A. H.: Akinesia and dyskinesia in myocardial infarction, J.A.M.A. **205:**252, 1968.

Douglas, A. H.: Control of tachycardia by procainamide, J.A.M.A. **101:**728, 1969.

Dowdy, E. G., and Fabian, L. W.: Ventricular arrhythmias induced by succinylcholine in digitalized patients: a preliminary report, Anesth. Analg. **42:**501-513, 1963.

Downes, J. J.: Resuscitation and intensive care of the newborn infant, Int. Anesthesiol. Clin. **6:**911-953, 1968.

Drabkova, J., et al.: Contribution of resuscitation methods to the complex therapy of eclampsia in pregnancy and labor, Cesk. Gynekol. **35:**476-477, 1970.

Drachman, D. A.: Ophthalmoplegia plus. The neurodegenerative disorders associated with progressive external ophthalmoplegia, Arch. Neurol. **18:**654-674, 1968.

Dreifus, L. S., et al.: Ventricular fibrillation. A possible mechanism of sudden death in patients and Wolff-Parkinson-White syndrome, Circulation **43:**520-527, 1971.

Dressler, W.: Disturbances of rhythm underlying Adams-Stokes seizures, Ann. N. Y. Acad. Sci. **167:**941-949, 1969.

Druss, R. G., et al.: The survivors of cardiac arrest, J.A.M.A. **201:**291-296, 1967.

Duggan, J. J., et al.: Handling the threat of fatal coronary disease, J.A.M.A. **214:**1329, 1970.

Duke, M.: A simple flow chart for use in cardiac arrest, J.A.M.A. **202:**143-145, 1967.

Dulfano, M. J.: Deactivated pacemakers, N. Engl. J. Med. **280:**672-673, 1969.

Dunbar, R. W., et al.: The effect of mepivacaine, bupivacaine, and lidocaine on digitalis-induced ventricular arrhythmias, Anesth. Analg. (Cleve.) **49:**761-766, 1970.

Dunkman, W., et al.: Clinical and hemodynamic results of intraaortic balloon pumping and surgery for cardiogenic shock, Circulation **46:**465, 1972.

Dunn, J. M., et al.: Hypothermia combined with positive pressure ventilation in resuscitation of the asphyxiated neonate, Am. J. Obstet. Gynecol. **104**:58-67, 1969.

Dunne, J. T., et al.: The effect of magnesium sulfate on anoxia and resuscitation in the neonate, Am. J. Obstet. Gynecol. **109**:369-374, 1971.

Dupont, B., et al.: The long-term prognosis for patients resuscitated after cardiac arrest. A follow-up study, Am. Heart J. **78**:444-449, 1969.

Durbin, F. C., et al.: Cardiac arrest and bone cement, Br. Med. J. **4**:176, 1970.

Dusinberre, R. K. Y.: Statutory definition of death, N. Engl. J. Med. **286**:549, 1972.

Dutta, S. N., et al.: Possible myocardial adaptation to acute coronary occlusion. Relation to catecholamines, Arch. Int. Pharmacodyn. Ther. **185**:5-12, 1970.

Duziak, A.: Successful cardiac resuscitation using conservative methods, Wiad. Lek. **22**:819-821, 1969.

Dyk, T., et al.: Bidirectional tachycardia in a case of recurrent paroxysmal tachycardia with ventricular fibrillation, Cardiology **52**:132-137, 1968.

Dykes, J. R., et al.: Insulin secretion in cardiogenic shock, Br. Med. J. **2**:490, 1969.

Dykes, M. H., et al.: Sudden cessation of cardiac output during spinal fusion, Anesth. Analg. (Cleve.) **49**:596-599, 1970.

Dysrhythmias related to cardiac trauma, Chest **61**:30-31, 1972.

Dzhavadian, N. S., et al.: Direct mechanical massage of the heart, Zh. Eksp. Klin. Med. **7**:101-111, 1967.

Dziedzic, H.: Ventricular fibrillation during electrocardiographic potassium test, Pol. Tyg. Lek. **23**:1862-1863, 1968.

Early warning system for heart, Med. World News **10**:15-16, 1969.

Earnest, D. L., et al.: Danger of rectal examination in patients with acute myocardial infarction—fact or fiction? N. Engl. J. Med. **281**:238-241, 1969.

Eastwood, G. L.: ECG abnormalities associated with barium enema, J.A.M.A. **219**:719-722, 1972.

Ebaid, M., et al.: Complicated intraventricular communication caused by tricuspid insufficiency after bacterial endocarditis, Arq. Brasil Cardiol. **23**:337-344, 1970.

Ebert, P. A.: Relationship of myocardial potassium content and atrial fibrillation, Circulation **41-42 (Suppl. II)**:6-8, 1970.

Ebert, P. A., et al.: Persistent hypokalemia following open heart surgery, Circulation **31-32 (Suppl. I)**:137-143, 1965.

Ebert, P. A., et al.: The anti-arrhythmic effects

of cardiac denervation, Ann. Surg. **168**:728-735, 1968.

Ecker, R. R., et al.: Late effects of anoxic arrest on cardiac contractility, Surg. Forum **20**:158-159, 1969.

Edmark, K. W., et al.: DC defibrillator failure, J. Thorac. Cardiovasc. Surg. **55**:741-745, 1968.

Edmonds-Seal, J.: Acid-base studies after cardiac arrest, Acta Anesthesiol. Scand. (Suppl.) **23**:235+, 1966.

Edwards, J. E., et al.: Pathology of the failing heart, Prog. Cardiovasc. Dis. **13**:1-23, 1970.

Edwards, W. S., et al.: Coronary blood flow and myocardial metabolism in hypothermia, Ann. Surg. **139**:275, 1954.

Effect of glucagon on heart, N. Engl. J. Med. **279**:434, 1968.

Effert, S., et al.: Emergency pacing techniques, Ann. N. Y. Acad. Sci. **167**:614-621, 1969.

Effert, S., et al.: On technical progress in monitoring systems for heart patients, Dtsch. Med. Wochenschr. **94**:768-773, 1969.

Egdahl, R. H.: Symposium on biomedical engineering and surgery, Am. J. Surg. **114**:2-3, 1967.

Ehrström, J., et al.: Hypothermia in the resuscitation of severely asphyctic newborn infants, Ann. Clin. Res. **1**:40-49, 1969.

Eichna, L. W.: The treatment of cardiogenic shock. 3. The use of isocproterenol in cardiogenic shock, Am. Heart J. **74**:48-52, 1967.

Elam, J. O., et al.: Artificial respiration by mouth-to-mouth method, N. Engl. J. Med. **250**:749, 1954.

el Etr, A. A.: The management of cardiac arrest, Surg. Clin. North Am. **48**:17-28, 1968.

Elias, E. G., et al.: Cardiac arrest: contraindication for surgery? N. Y. State J. Med. **71**:684-686, 1971.

Ellis, F. H.: Surgery for chronic asynergy of the left ventricle, Surgery **70**:801-808, 1971.

elSherif, N.: Supraventricular tachycardia with AV block, Br. Heart J. **32**:46-56, 1970.

Emminger, E., et al.: The time factor in reanimation, Munch. Med. Wochenschr. **112**:2275-2278, 1970.

Emrys-Roberts, M.: Death and resuscitation, Br. Med. J. **4**:364-365, 1969.

Engle, M. A.: Treatment of the failing heart, Pediatr. Clin. North Am. **11**:247-267, 1964.

Ersek, R. A., et al.: Spontaneous rupture of a false left ventricular aneurysm following myocardial infarction, Am. Heart J. **77**:677-680, 1969.

Escher, D. J. W., et al.: Emergency treatment of cardiac arrhythmias, J.A.M.A. **214**:2028-2034, 1970.

Espiritu, E. T., et al.: Effects of alpha and beta adrenergic blockade on the capability of the heart after myocardial infarction, Surg. Forum 19:151-153, 1968.

Essential equipment for ambulances, Res. Staff Phys. 17:1s-12s, 1971.

Eustace, B. R., et al.: Successful resuscitation after cardiac arrest due to haemorrhage, case report, Br. J. Anaesth. 40:629-631, 1968.

Evans, C., et al.: Near drowning, Br. Med. J. 1: 47, 1971.

Evans, C. L., and Matsuoka, Y.: Effect of various mechanical conditions on gaseous metabolism and efficiency of mammalian heart, J. Physiol. 49:378, 1915.

Evans, D., et al.: The effects of closed-chest venoarterial bypass with oxygenation on cardiopulmonary hemodynamics, J. Thorac. Cardiovasc. Surg. 62:76-83, 1971.

Evans, J. A.: Personal communication, 1969.

Evers, W., et al.: Anesthesiologist's role in modern cardiopulmonary resuscitation, N. Y. State J. Med. 70:2003-2006, 1970.

Ewy, G. A.: Ventricular arrhythmias following acute myocardial infarction, Southwest. Med. 52:75-85, 1971.

Eydan, R.: Diagnosis of reanimation. Syndrome of subphrenic retroperitoneal irritation, Anesth. Analg. (Paris) 28:273-284, 1971.

Fagin, I. D., et al.: Mortality from myocardial infarction before and after establishment of a coronary care unit, J. Am. Geriatr. Soc. 16: 908-918, 1968.

Faivre, P. G., et al.: Electric treatment and prevention of cardiac arrest. 5-year record, Brux. Med. 49:14-24, 1969.

Falicki, Z., et al.: Psychic disturbances as a result of cardiac arrest, Pol. Med. J. 8:200-206, 1969.

Falkowski, S.: Delirium following resuscitation with mild psycho-organic sequelae, Psychiatr. Pol. 5:359-361, 1971.

Falsetti, H. I., et al.: Technique of compression in closed-chest cardiac massage, J.A.M.A. 200: 793-795, 1967.

Fancher, D. C., et al.: Cardiopulmonary resuscitation on the street, Wis. Med. J. 69:235-236, 1969.

Fano, A., et al.: Complete heart block with Stokes-Adams attack from transient ventricular fibrillation, Jap. Heart J. 10:369-371, 1969.

Fantera, A.: Special clinical aspects of corticoid therapy in high doses of anesthesia and resuscitation, Acta Anaesthesiol. (Padova) 20(Suppl. 1):97+, 1969.

Fatteh, A.: Lifesaving fist punches, J.A.M.A. 216:145, 1971.

Faucon, G., et al.: Fibrillation and cardiac metabolic level, J. Physiol. (Paris) 62(Suppl.3): 373, 1970.

Fava, E., et al.: In vitro sensitivity and in vivo resistance of some microbial strains in resuscitation, G. Ital. Chemioter. 16:38-49, 1969.

Favaloro, R.: Heart arrest. Cardiorespiratory resuscitation, Prensa Med. Argent. 57:1141-1144, 1970.

Fazzini, P. F., et al.: Atrioventricular block in acute myocardial infarction, Acta Cardiol. (Brux.) 25:517-525, 1970.

Fearon, R. E.: Coronary shock, Conn. Med. 31: 609-614, 1967.

Fearon, R. E., et al.: Demand pacing in carotid sinus syncope, Am. Heart J. 81:581, 1971.

Feeley, E. M.: The new graduate in cardiopulmonary resuscitation, Am. J. Nurs. 70:1304-1307, 1970.

Fehmers, M. C. O., et al.: Intramuscularly and orally administered lidocaine in the treatment of ventricular arrhythmias in acute myocardial infarction, Am. J. Cardiol. 29:514-519, 1972.

Fel'd, B. N.: Significance of excitation dispersion of different areas of the heart for the development of extrasystole and ventricular fibrillation in experimental myocardial infarct, Kardiologiia 11:55-62, 1971.

Feldman, A. E., et al.: Repetitive ventricular fibrillation in myocardial infarction refractory to bretylium tosylate subsequently controlled by ventricular pacing, Am. J. Cardiol. 27:227-230, 1971.

Feldman, H., and Hillman, H.: A clinical description of death in rats and the effect of various conditions on the time until cessation of ventricular contraction following section between the brain and spinal cord, Br. J. Exp. Pathol. 50:158-164, 1969.

Feldman, R. A., et al.: Lactate accumulation in primate spinal cord during circulatory arrest, J. Neurosurg. 34:618-620, 1971.

Feller, J. F., and Horisberger, B.: Control of physical and cerebral faculties following resuscitation for circulatory arrest, Helv. Chir. Acta 36:155-160, 1969.

Fendler, J. P., et al.: Pheochromocytoma and problems of resuscitation, Coeur Med. Interne 10:101-105, 1971.

Feola, M., et al.: Intra-aortic balloon pumping (IABP) at different levels of experimental acute left ventricular failure, Chest 59:68-76, 1971.

Feola, M., et al.: Assisted circulation: experimental intra-aortic balloon pumping, Artificial Heart Program Conference Proceedings, Washington, D. C., 1969, p. 637.

Fernandez, J. P., et al.: Rapid active external

rewarming in accidental hypothermia, J.A.M.A. **212**:153-155, 1970.

Fernandez-Herlihy, L.: Heart block in polymyositis, N. Engl. J. Med. **284**:1101, 1971.

Ferrer, J. M.: Fatal air embolism via subclavian vein, N. Engl. J. Med. **282**:688, 1970.

Ferris, C. D., et al.: A study of parameters involved in alternating-current defibrillation, Med. Biol. Eng. **7**:17-29, 1969.

Ferris, L. P., et al.: Effect of electric shock on the heart, Electr. Eng. **55**:498-515, 1936.

Fibrillation preventable by two drugs, Med. Trib. **13**:14, July 26, 1972.

Fiehring, H.: Electrotherapy of cardiac arrest, Z. Gesamte Inn. Med. **24** (Suppl.):37-39, 1969.

The fifth death of Lev Dandau, Med. World News **10**:49, 1969.

Fillmore, S. J., et al.: Serial blood gas studies during cardiopulmonary resuscitation, Ann. Intern. Med. **72**:465-469, 1970.

Filtering out brain damage, Med. World News **11**:29, 1970.

Finkle, A. L.: Recent concepts of diagnosis, therapy and research in uremia, J. Am. Med. Wom. Assoc. **15**:149, 1960.

Finkle, A. L., and Smith, D. R.: Parameters of renal functional capacity In reversible hydroureteronephrosis in dogs. V. Effects of 7 to 10 days of ureteral constriction on RBF-Kr, C-In, TcH$_2$O, CPAH, osmolality and sodium reabsorption, Invest. Urol. **8**:299-310, 1970.

Finster, M.: Resuscitation of the newborn, Acta Anaesthesiol. Scand. (Suppl.) **37**:86+, 1969.

Fisch, C.: Pacemaker electrocardiography, J. Indiana Med. Assoc. **62**:1316, 1969.

Fisch, C.: Myocardial infarction: A-V block, J. Indiana Med. Assoc. **63**:908, 1970.

Fisch, C.: Atropine in A-V block: a paradoxic response, J. Indiana State Med. Assoc. **64**:39, 1971.

Fisch, C., et al.: Cardiac arrhythmias during oral surgery with halothane-nitrous-oxide-oxygen anesthesia, J.A.M.A. **208**:1839-1842, 1969.

Fischer, J. E., et al.: Steroid therapy of severe fat embolism, Surg. Forum **21**:480-482, 1970.

FitzGibbon, G. M., et al.: Successful surgical treatment of postinfarction external cardiac rupture, J. Thorac. Cardiovasc. Surg. **63**:622-630, 1972.

Flanagan, J. P., et al.: Air embolus—a lethal complication of subclavian venipuncture, N. Engl. J. Med. **281**:488-489, 1969.

Fleming, W. H., et al.: Synchronized counterpulsation in the management of ventricular fibrillation following coronary artery ligation, J. Thorac. Cardiovasc. Surg. **56**:253-257, 1968.

Fleming, W. H., et al.: Comparative study of arterio-arterial and intra-aortic balloon counterpulsation in the therapy of cardiogenic shock, J. Thorac. Cardiovasc. Surg. **60**:818-828, 1970.

Fletcher, G. F.: Hazardous complications of "closed chest" cardiopulmonary resuscitation, Am. Heart J. **77**:431-432, 1969.

Florent, C., et al.: Emergency cardiorespiratory resuscitation. Study of 69 cases, Anesth. Analg. (Paris) **27**:541-592, 1970.

Floris, V., et al.: Histopathologic contribution to the study of anoxic encephalopathy in the adult, Acta Neurol. (Napoli) **22**:250-273, 1967.

Fluck, D. C.: Intensive care for acute myocardial infarction, Guys Hosp. Rep. **116**:107-114, 1967.

Fluck, D. C.: One hundred patients of acute myocardial infarction treated in an intensive coronary care unit, J. Indiana Med. Assoc. **52**:405-409, 1969.

Flynn, J. T.: Arrhythmias related to coffee and tea, J.A.M.A. **211**:663, 1970.

Flynn, J. T., et al.: Human tolerance to electric countershock, N. Y. State J. Med. **69**:253-264, 1969.

Foley, W. J.: Open cardiac massage, Surg. Gynecol. Obstet. **128**:827-828, 1969.

Folkman, M. J., and Watkins, E.: An artificial conduction system for the management of experimental complete heart block, Surg. Forum Proc. **8**:331-334, 1957.

Folli, G., et al.: Aptitude to exercise in patients with previous myocardial infarct, Acta Cardiol. (Brux.) **23**:273-287, 1968.

Folling, M.: Resuscitation in a medical reception department, Tidsskr. Nor. Laegeforen. **91**:1386-1388, 1971.

Fonkalsrud, E. W.: Airway problems, Ariz. Med. **26**:149-151, 1969.

Forbes, M. B., et al.: Long-term transvenous cardiac pacing, Mod. Med. **36**:120, 1968.

Foresman, R. A., and Tyers, G. F.: Repairing the chronically implanted cardiac pacemaker without surgery, Surg. Forum **19**:105-107, 1968.

Foster, G. L., et al.: The effects of oxygen breathing in patients with acute myocardial infarction, Cardiovasc. Res. **3**:179-189, 1969.

Fouchard, J., et al.: Ventricular fibrillation in advanced cardiopathy: possibilities and limits of resuscitation, Coeur Med. Interne **9**:105-113, 1970.

Fowler, N. O., editor: Treatment of cardiac arrhythmias, Mod. Treat. **7**:1-237, 1970.

Fowler, N. O., et al.: Syncope and cerebral dysfunction caused by bradycardia without atrioventricular block, Am. Heart J. **80**:303-312, 1970.

Fox, A. C.: High-energy phosphate compounds and LDH isoenzymes in the hypertrophied right ventricle. In Alpert, N., editor: Cardiac hypertrophy, New York, 1971, Academic Press, Inc., pp. 203-212.

Francesconi, F.: Considerations on a case of intraoperative cardiac arrest, Acta Anaesthesiol. (Padova) 19:1227-1229, 1968.

Francis, C. K., et al.: Interruption of aberrant conduction of atrioventricular junctional tachycardia by cough, N. Engl. J. Med. 286:357-388, 1972.

Francisco, J. T.: Smothering in infancy: its relationship to the "crib death syndrome," South. Med. J. 63:1110-1114, 1970.

Franco, S. C.: Electric shock and cardiopulmonary resuscitation, Arch. Environ. Health 19:261-264, 1969.

Frank, H. A., et al.: Surgical aspects of long-term electrical stimulation of the heart, J. Thorac. Cardiovasc. Surg. 57:17-30, 1969.

Fred, H. L., et al.: Selection of patients for pulmonary embolectomy, Dis. Chest 56:139-142, 1969.

Free fatty acids and heart-attacks, Lancet 1:843-844, 1971.

Freeman, D. J.: Experiences with a "Cook Book" operated coronary care unit in a 145-bed general hospital, Wis. Med. J. 68:191-194, 1969.

Frey, H., et al.: Metabolic effects of long-term glucagon infusion, Acta Endocrinol. (Suppl.) (Kbh.) 155:198, 1971.

Friberg, O.: On the treatment of complications in dental work, Odontol. Foren. T. 31:297-307, 1967.

Friedberg, C. K.: Diseases of the heart, vol. 1, ed. 3, Philadelphia, 1966, W. B. Saunders Co., p. 801.

Friedberg, C. K.: Current status of treatment of shock complicating acute myocardial infarction, J. Trauma 9:141-142, 1969.

Friedberg, C. K.: Syncope: pathological physiology: differential diagnosis and treatment, Mod. Concepts Cardiovasc. Dis. 40:61-63, 1971.

Frieden, J.: Answers to questions of the electrocardiogram in extracardiac disease, Hosp. Med. 5:120-138, 1969.

Friesen, W. G.: Atrial pacing to control heart rate and rhythm in acute cardiac conditions, Can. Med. Assoc. J. 104:900-904 passim, 1971.

Friesen, W. G., et al.: A hemodynamic comparison of atrial and ventricular pacing in postoperative cardiac surgical patients, J. Thorac. Cardiovasc. Surg. 55:271-279, 1968.

Frommer, P. L.: The myocardial infarction research program of the National Heart Institute, Am. J. Cardiol. 22:108-110, 1968.

Frost, P. M.: Cardiac arrest and bone cement, Br. Med. J. 3:524, 1970.

Fry, J.: Acute myocardial infarction. The pre-hospital phase, Schweiz Med. Wochenschr. 98:1210-1212, 1968.

Fryda, R. J., et al.: Postoperative complete heart block in children, Br. Heart J. 33:456-462, 1971.

Funiciello, A. M., et al.: Circulatory arrest in infants. Review of the most important therapeutic measures in the light of personal experience, Acta Chir. Ital. 26:409-422, 1970.

Furman, S., and Schwedel, J. B.: An intracardiac pacemaker for Stokes-Adams seizures, N. Engl. J. Med. 261:943-948, 1959.

Furman, S., et al.: Choice of cardiac pacemaker, Ann. N. Y. Acad. Sci. 167:557-570, 1969.

Furman, S., et al.: Electronic analysis for pacemaker failure, Ann. Thorac. Surg. 8:57-65, 1969.

Furman, S., et al.: Principles and techniques of cardiac pacing, New York, 1970, Harper & Row, Publishers.

Furman, S., et al.: Transtelephone pacemaker clinic, J. Thorac. Cardiovasc. Surg. 61:827-834, 1971.

Gabriele, O. F.: Pacing via coronary sinus, N. Engl. J. Med. 280:219, 1969.

Gadboys, H. R., et al.: Long-term follow-up of patients with cardiac pacemakers, Am. J. Cardiol. 21:55-59, 1968.

Galdo, A., and Cabrera, A.: Blood transfusion in anesthesia and neurosurgic resuscitation, Rev. Esp. Otoneurooftalmol. Neurocir. 28:223-228, 1969-1970.

Galdston, R., et al.: On borrowed time: observations on children with implanted cardiac pacemakers and their families, Am. J. Psychiatry 126:104-108, 1969.

Galetti, P.: Report of a year of resuscitation activities, Minerva Med. 59:3837-3844, 1968.

Galha, V. D., et al.: Demand pacing for transient heart block associated with changes in posture, J.A.M.A. 216:1340-1342, 1971.

Gall, F.: Intrapericardial aortic injury, heart arrest and successful resuscitation, Thoraxchirurgie 15:301-303, 1967.

Gallivan, G. J., et al.: Ischemic electrocardiographic changes after truncal vagotomy, J.A.M.A. 211:798-801, 1970.

Gallo, E., et al.: Influence of counterpulsation on experimental acute cardiac failure, J. Thorac. Cardiovasc. Surg. 52:745, 1966.

Ganelina, I. E., et al.: Case of multiple occurrence of clinical death against a background of ventricular fibrillation and ventricular tachycardia, Klin. Med. (Mosk.) 49:118-121, 1971.

Garcia, F., et al.: First aid equipment for patients with heart arrest, Rev. Esp. Anestesiol Reanim. 17:136-140, 1970.

Gaspar, H., et al.: Cardiac arrhythmias in acute

myocardial infarction, Dis. Chest **53:**775-778, 1968.

Gasparetto, A.: Current possibilities and limitations of resuscitation, Acta Anaesthesiol. (Padova) **20:**1035-1043, 1969.

Gasparetto, A.: Resuscitation and intensive care departments in modern hospitals: Facilities and equipment, Acta Anaesthesiol. (Padova) **21:**80-86, 1970.

Gauger, G. E.: What do "fixed, dilated pupils" mean? N. Engl. J. Med. **284:**1105, 1971.

Gault, J. H., et al.: Fatal familial cardiac arrhythmias, Am. J. Cardiol. **29:**548-553, 1972.

Gaultier, M., et al.: Cardiac reanimation in poisoning, Sem. Ther. **43:**190-194, 1967.

Gavrilescu, S., et al.: Hemodynamic effect of glucagon in patients with chronic complete heart block, Cor Vasa **13:**85-91, 1971.

Gazes, P. C.: Treatment of acute myocardial infarction. 2. Ventricular ectopic arrhythmias, Postgrad. Med. **48:**168-172, 1970.

Geddes, J. S.: Instant intensive care for myocardial infarction, Nurs. Times **64:**1614-1616, 1969.

Geddes, L. A., et al.: Strength-duration curves for ventricular defibrillation in dogs, Circ. Res. **27:**551-560, 1970.

Geiger, J. P., and Gielchinsky, I.: Acute pulmonary insufficiency. Treatment in Vietnam casualties, Arch. Surg. **102:**400-405, 1971.

Geis, W. P., et al.: Extrapericardial (mediastinal) cardiac tamponade, Arch. Surg. **100:**305-306, 1970.

Geissler, W., et al.: Pathophysiology and clinical course of cardiac arrest, Z. Gesamte. Inn. Med. **24** (Suppl.):24-28, 1969.

Genis, E. D.: Peculiarities in neurosecretory function of the hypothalamus in clinical death and resuscitation, Fiziol. Zh. **14:**30-36, 1968.

Georgopoulos, A., et al.: The antifibrillatory effects of antazoline, Bull. Soc. Int. Chir. **28:**326-331, 1969.

Gerami, S.: Personal communication, December, 1972.

Geraud, J., et al.: Cerebral arteriovenous oxygen differences. Reappraisal of their signification for evaluation of brain function. In: Research on the cerebral circulation, Springfield, Ill., 1969, Charles C Thomas, Publisher, pp. 209-222.

Gerbershagen, H. U., et al.: Cardiac arrest following high spinal anesthesia, Anaesthesist **20:**192-193, 1971.

Gersony, W. M., et al.: Ventricular fibrillation masked by the implanted unipolar pacemaker, Dis. Chest **55:**503-505, 1969.

Gerst, P. H., et al.: Increased susceptibility of the heart to ventricular fibrillation during metabolic acidosis, Circ. Res. **19:**63-70, 1966.

Gerstenbrad, F., et al.: Acute brain stem syndrome as a complication after heart surgery, Bruns Beitr. Klin. Chir. **216:**210-222, 1968.

Gerya, Y. F., et al.: In Negovskii, V. A., editor: Acute problems in resuscitation and hypothermia, New York, 1965, Consultants Bureau, p. 60.

Gettes, L. S., et al.: Effect of changes in potassium and calcium concentrations on diastolic threshold and strength-interval relationships of the human heart, Ann. N. Y. Acad. Sci. **167:**693-705, 1969.

Ghidoni, J. J., et al.: Massive subendocardial damage accompanying prolonged ventricular fibrillation, Am. J. Pathol. **56:**15-29, 1969.

Giardina, B., et al.: Indications and results of therapy with gentamicin sulfate in prolonged resuscitation, G. Ital. Chemioter. **16:**408-411, 1969.

Gibbs, J. R.: Resuscitation of drowned children, Br. Med. J. **2:**470-471, 1971.

Giedwoyn, J. O.: Pacemaker failure following external defibrillation, Circulation **44:**293, 1971.

Gilbert, R. P.: Hematocrit after acute myocardial infarction, Am. Heart J. **77:**713, 1969.

Gillardeau, G.: Cardiac insufficiency during resuscitation, J. Med. Bordeaux **143:**1939-1946, 1966.

Gilles, F. H.: Hypotensive brain stem necrosis. Selective symmetrical necrosis of tegmental neuronal aggregates following cardiac arrest, Arch. Pathol. **88:**32-41, 1969.

Gilles, F. H., and Nag, D.: Vulnerability of human spinal cord in transient cardiac arrest, Neurology (Minneap.) **21:**833-839, 1971.

Gissen, A. J., et al.: Elective circulatory arrest during neurosurgery for basilar artery aneurysms, J.A.M.A. **207:**1315-1318, 1969.

Give man the right to die, British M.D. says, J.A.M.A. **210:**657, 1969.

Glass, B. A., et al.: Excision of myocardial infarcts, Arch. Surg. **97:**940-946, 1968.

Glenn, W. W. L., et al.: Heart block in children. Treatment with a radiofrequency pacemaker, J. Thorac. Cardiovasc. Surg. **58:**361-373, 1969.

Glenn, W. W. L., et al.: Remote stimulation of the heart by radiofrequency transmission. Clinical application to a patient with Stokes-Adams syndrome, N. Engl. J. Med. **261:**948-951, 1959.

Glucagon may help in cardiovascular distress, J.A.M.A. **210:**1001, 1969.

Glucose, insulin may reduce heart surgery arrhythmias, J.A.M.A. **207:**1626, 1969.

Gode, G. R.: Paraplegia and cardiac arrest: case reports, Can. Anaesth. Soc. J. **17:**452-455, 1970.

Goetz, R. H., et al.: Unidirectional intraaortic balloon pumping in cardiogenic shock and intractable left ventricular failure, Am. J. Cardiol. 29:213-222, 1972.

Goldberg, L. I.: The treatment of cardiogenic shock. VI. Search for an ideal drug, Am. Heart J. 75:416-420, 1968.

Golden, R. J.: Minimal risk of quinidine-induced ventricular fibrillation, J.A.M.A. 211:2162, 1970.

Goldfarb, D., et al.: Cardiovascular responses to diastolic augmentation in the intact canine circulation and after ligation of the anterior descending coronary artery, J. Thorac. Cardiovasc. Surg. 55:243, 1968.

Goldman, B. S., et al.: Implantable transvenous cardiac pacemakers: indications, complications, and management, J. Am. Geriatr. Soc. 18:905-915, 1970.

Goldman, B. S., et al.: Functional and metabolic effects of anoxic cardiac arrest, Ann. Thorac. Surg. 11:122-132, 1971.

Goldstein, J. H., et al.: A simple cardiac monitor for ophthalmic surgery, Arch. Ophthalmol. 86:97-99, 1971.

Goodman, J. M., et al.: Determination of brain death by isotope angiography, J.A.M.A. 209:1868-1872, 1969.

Goodman, M. J., et al.: Complete bundle-branch block complicating acute myocardial infarction, N. Engl. J. Med. 282:237-240, 1970.

Gordon, T., et al.: Premature mortality from coronary heart disease, J.A.M.A. 215:1617-1625, 1971.

Gotsman, M. S., et al.: Acute myocardial infarction—an ideal concept of progressive coronary care, S. Afr. Med. J. 42:829-832, 1968.

Gott, B. H.: Arrhythmia problems and athletic participation, J.A.M.A. 211:502, 1970.

Gott, V. L., et al.: Myocardial rigor mortis as an indication of cardiac metabolic function, Surg. Forum 13:172-174, 1962.

Gotzsche, H., et al.: Cardiac arrest in heart disease, Acta Anaesthesiol. Scand. (Suppl.) 29:217-230, 1968.

Gould, L., et al.: Cardiac arrest during endrophonium administration, Am. Heart J. 81:437-438, 1971.

Gould, L., et al.: Potential hazard of two functioning pacemakers, Chest 62:109-110, 1972.

Gourin, A., et al.: Total cardiopulmonary bypass, myocardial contractility, and the administration of protamine sulfate, J. Thorac. Cardiovasc. Surg. 61:160-166, 1971.

Grace, W. J.: Terror in the coronary care unit, Am. J. Cardiol. 22:746, 1968.

Grace, W. J.: The use of monitoring devices in acute myocardial infarction, Adv. Cardiopulm. Dis. 4:91-105, 1969.

Grace, W. J.: The mobile coronary care unit and the intermediate coronary care unit in the total systems approach to coronary care, Chest 58:363-368, 1970.

Grace, W. J., et al.: The mobile coronary care unit, Dis. Chest 55:452-455, 1969.

Grace, W. J., et al.: The first hour in acute myocardial infarction, Chest 58:279, 1970.

Grace, W. J., et al.: Acute myocardial infarction: the course of the illness following discharge from the coronary care unit, Chest 59:15-17, 1971.

Graham, L. E.: Patients' perceptions in the CCU, Am. J. Nurs. 69:1921-1922, 1969.

Grahl-Madsen, R., and Nielsen, J. S.: Temporary intracardiac pacemaker treatment, Ugeskr. Laeger 129:1302-1305, 1967.

Grande, A., et al.: Clinical and haemodynamic features of a case of idiopathic dilatation of the right ventricle, Panminerva Med. 10:65-70, 1968.

Grandjean, T.: The diagnosis and treatment of cardiac arrest in myocardial infarct by modern technical means, Praxis 55:499-503, 1968.

Granoff, D. M., et al.: Cardiorespiratory arrest following aspiration of chloral hydrate, Am. J. Dis. Child. 122:170-171, 1971.

Green, R., Jr., et al.: Sudden unexpected death in three generations, Arch. Intern. Med. 124:359-363, 1969.

Greenburg, A. G., et al.: The hemodynamic effects of tromethamine in hypercarbia and asphyxia, Ann. Thorac. Surg. 8:320-326, 1969.

Greenberg, H. B., and Hyman, A. L.: Cardioversion for drug-resistant supraventricular tachycardia with heart failure, South. Med. J. 61:253-255, 1968.

Greene, W. Q., et al.: Factors affecting adjustment of heart patient to pacemaker, Mod. Med. 37:96, 1969.

Greenfield, I.: Emergency red. A plan for hospital personnel in the treatment of cardiac and respiratory emergencies, Minn. Med. 47:745-747, 1964.

Greenough, K.: Iatrogenic cardiac invalidism: can the coronary care unit be responsible? J. Rehabil. 34:16-17, 1968.

Gregory, J. J., et al.: Resuscitation of the severely ill patient with acute myocardial infarction, Am. J. Cardiol. 20:836-841, 1967.

Gregory, J. J., et al.: The management of sinus bradycardia, nodal rhythm and heart block for the prevention of cardiac arrest in acute myocardial infarction, Prog. Cardiovasc. Dis. 10:505-517, 1968.

Griepp, R. B., et al.: Acute rejection of the allografted human heart, Ann. Thorac. Surg. **12:** 113-126, 1971.

Griepp, R. B., et al.: Determinants of operative risk in human heart transplantation, Am. J. Surg. **122:**192-198, 1971.

Griepp, R. B., et al.: Hemodynamic performance of the transplanted human heart, Surgery **70:** 88-96, 1971.

Griffith, G. C.: Coronary care unit in the 1970's, Chest **59:**548-551, 1971.

Grinberg, V. A., et al.: Cardiac arrest during anesthesia, Klin. Khir. **7:**48, 1970.

Grinnan, G. L. B., et al.: Cardiopulmonary homotransplantation, J. Thorac. Cardiovasc. Surg. **60:**609-635, 1970.

Grivaux, M., et al.: Lactic acidosis in resuscitation, Ann. Med. Interne (Paris) **122:**105-112, 1971.

Gros, C., et al.: Critères cliniques et arteriographiques des comas dépassés en neuro-chirurgie, Ann. Anesthesiol. Franç. **11:**163-171, 1970.

Grosfeld, J. L., et al.: Monitoring venous pH and gas tensions, Arch. Surg. **100:**584-588, 1970.

Gross, J. B., and Hoff, H. E.: Vagal activity and cardiac arrest in chloral hydrate narcosis, Cardiovasc. Res. Center Bull. **6:**85-98, 1968.

Grossman, J. I., and Rubin, I. L.: Cardiopulmonary resuscitation, Am. Heart J. **78:**569-572, 709-714, 1969.

Grossman, J. I., et al.: Lidocaine in cardiac arrhythmias, Arch. Intern. Med. **121:**396-401, 1968.

Gueron, M., and Weizman, S.: Cathecholamines and myocardial damage in scorpion sting, Am. Heart J. **75:**715-717, 1968.

Groveman, J., et al.: Rhinoplethysmography, pulse monitoring at the nasal septum, Anesth. Analg. **45:**63-68, 1966.

Guliaev, G. V., et al.: On cardiovascular collapse in inhalation anesthesia during operations on the spinal cord and spine, Vopr. Nierokhir. **31:** 33-37, 1967.

Gulotta, C. J.: Fundamental concepts in the coronary care unit, J. La. State Med. Soc. **121:** 6-8, 1969.

Gunn, C. G., et al.: Edema of the brain following circulatory arrest, J. Surg. Res. **2:**141-143, 1962.

Gurevich, M. A., et al.: Intravital diagnosis of lesion of the papillary muscles in myocardial infarct, Klin. Med. [Mosk.] **46:**129-133, 1968.

Gurubatham, A. I., et al.: Cardiac arrest: 221 defibrillations, Med. J. Aust. **2:**760-761, 1969.

Gurvich, N. L., et al.: ECG changes in prolonged clinical death and subsequent resuscitation of the organism, Biull. Eksp. Biol. Med. **71:** 9-12, 1971.

Gurvich, N. L., and Yuniev, G. S.: Restoration of heart rhythm during fibrillation by a condenser discharge, Am. Rev. Soviet Med. **4:**252-256, 1947.

Gurvich, N. L., and Yuniev, G. S.: Restoration of regular rhythm in the mammalian fibrillating heart, Am. Rev. Soviet Med. **3:**236-239, 1946.

Gurvitch, A. M.: Rhythmic bursts in the medullary reticular formation and their connection with agonal respiration during hypoxia and the post-hypoxic period, Electroencephalogr. Clin. Neurophysiol. **21:**355-364, 1966.

Gurvitch, A. M.: Sur les possibilités du prognostic précoce de la restauration des fonctions nerveuses après l'arrêt circulatoire, Agressologie **7:** 61-78, 1966.

Guthrie, C. C.: Refractory period in heart, Am. J. Physiol. **81:**483-484, 1927.

Gutierrez Goicoecha, J. M.: Resistance of the myocardium in anoxia, Rev. Esp. Anestesiol. Reanim. **18:**5-25, 1971.

Gutierrez, M. R., et al.: Significance of T wave interruption by premature beats as a cause of sudden death, Can. Med. Assoc. J. **98:**144-149, 1968.

Hackett, T. P., et al.: The coronary-care unit—an appraisal of its psychologic hazards, N. Engl. J. Med. **279:**1365-1370, 1968.

Haese, W. H., et al.: Peculiar focal myocardial degeneration and fatal ventricular arrhythmias in a child, N. Engl. J. Med. **287:**180-181, 1972.

Hagen, J., et al.: A program for preparedness in anesthetic and emergency techniques in the oral surgery office, J. Oral Surg. **29:**166-170, 1971.

Haiderer, O., et al.: Assisted circulation: a comparison of three methods of circulatory bypass of the left heart, Dis. Chest **54:**44-49, 1968.

Halder, R., et al.: Phentolamine in heart block, Br. Med. J. **4:**307, 1971.

Hall, J. I., et al.: Factors affecting cardioversion of atrial arrhythmias with special reference to quinidine, Br. Heart J. **30:**84-90, 1968.

Halmagyi, M.: A simple device for the differential diagnosis of cardiac arrest, Acta Anaesthesiol. Scand. (Suppl.) **24:**273+, 1966.

Hamby, W. M.: Renal regulation of sodium excretion, Med. Clin. North Am. **55:**1509, 1971.

Hampton, J. R., et al.: Drugs for the prevention of myocardial infarction, Am. J. Med. Sci. **258:** 1-6, 1969.

Han, J.: Ventricular vulnerability during acute coronary occlusion, Am. J. Cardiol. **24:**857-864, 1969.

Han, J., et al.: Temporal dispersion of recovery excitability in atrium and ventricle as a function of heart rate, Am. Heart J. **71:**481-487, 1966.

Hanaoka, W., et al.: Prognosis of myocardial infarction with special reference to arrhythmias, Jap. Circ. J. **31**:1599-1600, 1967.

Hanegreefs, G.: Heart arrest, Rev. Belge Med. Dent. **22**:433-438, 1967.

Hankiewicz, M.: Arresting coronary circulation during open-heart surgery, Pol. Tyg. Lek. **25**: 1881-1884, 1970.

Harada, M., et al.: Case of appalic syndrome from cardiac arrest, Brain Nerve (Tokyo) **22**: 733-739, 1970.

Harden, A.: EEG studies following resuscitation after cardiac arrest in 60 babies, Electroencephalogr. Clin. Neurophysiol. **27**:333, 1969.

Harman, M. A., et al.: Surgical intervention in chronic postinfarction cardiac failure, Circulation **39**(Suppl.):91-97, 1969.

Harris, A.: Pacing after acute myocardial infarction, Postgrad. Med. J. **47**:16-22, 1971.

Harris, P., et al., editors: Calcium and the heart, New York, 1971, Academic Press, Inc.

Harris, T. M., et al.: Monitoring inspired oxygen pressures during mechanical ventilation, J.A.M.A. **206**:2885-2887, 1968.

Harris, W. S., et al.: Hyper-reactivity to atropine in Down's syndrome, N. Engl. J. Med. **279**: 407-409, 1968.

Harrison, D. C.: Beta adrenergic blockade, Am. J. Cardiol. **29**:432-435, 1972.

Harthorne, J. W., et al.: Epicardial versus endocardial pacemakers, Ann. Thorac. Surg. **6**: 417-423, 1968.

Harti, O., et al.: Auricular tachycardia with AV-block—a rare rhythmus disorder, Wein. Med. Wochenschr. **121**:273-275, 1971.

Hartveit, F., and Halleraker, B.: Intravascular changes in kidneys and lungs after external cardiac massage: a preliminary report, J. Pathol. **102**:54-58, 1970.

Hasan, S., et al.: Near drowning in humans. A report of 36 patients, Chest **59**:191-197, 1971.

Hasbrouck, J. D.: Morphine anesthesia for open-heart surgery, Ann. Thorac. Surg. **10**:364-369, 1970.

Hastreiter, A. R.: Atrial flutter, J. Pediatr. **74**: 1006, 1969.

Hauser, J. B., et al.: Esophageal perforation during vagotomy, Arch. Surg. **101**:466-468, 1970.

Hayashi, H.: Coronary care unit in Japan, Isr. Med. Sci. **5**:777-779, 1969.

The heart: a historic plaything? Med. World News **10**:49, 1969.

Heart arrest in hypothermia needs longer observation time, Lakartidningen **68**:11-15, 1971.

Heart rate may provide key to sudden death control, J.A.M.A. **214**:1975-1976, 1970.

Heart to heart, J.A.M.A. **211**:1690, 1970.

Heikkila, J.: Acute mitral incompetence in myocardial infarction. Clinical recognition, Geriatrics **24**:150-166, 1969.

Heilbrunn, A., et al.: Cardiac arrest. The use of drugs in resuscitation. An experimental study, J. Kans. Med. Soc. **68**:344-349, 1967.

Heimbecker, R. O.: Surgery for massive myocardial infarction, Prog. Cardiovasc. Dis. **11**: 338-350, 1969.

Helal, S. M.: Ethacrynic acid diuretic effect in 50 patients, J. Egypt. Med. Assoc. **51**:857-863, 1968.

Hellmuth, G. A.: Cardiac flutter and fibrillation, Adv. Cardiopulm. Dis. **3**:324-364, 1966.

Henderson, M.: Carotid sinus reflex during radical neck dissection, South. Med. J. **62**:1195-1197, 1969.

Hendrix, G. H.: Intravenous use of diazepam in cardioversion, South. Med. J. **62**:483-484,1969.

Henney, R. P., et al.: Prevention of hypokalemic cardiac arrhythmias associated with cardiopulmonary bypass and hemodilution, Surg. Forum **21**:145-155, 1970.

Henson, D. W., et al.: Myocardial lesions following open-heart surgery, Arch. Pathol. **88**:423-430, 1969.

Henson, R. A., et al.: Areflexic paraplegia, Q. J. Med. **35**:205, 1967.

Herbert, W. H.: The effect of ventricular action currents on the sinoatrial node, J. Electrocardiol. **3**:121-126, 1970.

Hermansen, K.: Antifibrillatory effect of some beta-adrenergic receptor blocking agents determined by a new test procedure in mice, Acta Pharmacol. Toxicol. (Kbh.) **26**:17-27, 1970.

Hernandez-Richter, H. J., et al.: Chance of survival in internal and external heart massage at the scene of accident, Munch. Med. Wochenschr. **111**:373-375, 1969.

Hershberg, P. I.: First aid therapy: a new concept in the treatment of myocardial infarction, Med. Times **96**:575-591, 1968.

Hewitt, R. L., et al.: Army heart pump for postsystolic augmentation, Arch. Surg. **99**:88-91, 1969.

Hill, J. D., et al.: Experimental and clinical experiences with prolonged oxygenation and assisted circulation, Ann. Surg. **170**:448-459, 1969.

Hillman, H.: Facteures biochimiques intervenant sur le potential de repos des cellules nerveuses des mammiferes, Biol. Med. (Paris) **53**:333-346, 1964.

Hillman, H.: Treatment after exposure to cold, Lancet **7714**:1257, 1971.

Hillman, H., and Aldridge, T.: Towards a legal

definition of death, Solicitors J. **110**:323-326, 1972.

Hillman, H., et al.: The clinical history of cardiac arrest and recovery of anaesthetised rats, and their reproduction, Resuscitation **1**:51-60, 1972.

Hilty-Tammivaara, R., et al.: Exercise-released ventricular fibrillation in hypertrophic subaortic stenosis treated with propanolol, Acta Med. Scand. **187**:317-322, 1970.

Himeno, K.: Mechanism of the ventricular fibrillation following intravenous adrenaline administration under halothane anesthesia, J. Kumamoto Med. Soc. **45**:69-93, 1971.

Hirsch, H.: EEG and reanimation, Electroencephalogr. Clin. Neurophysiol. **27**:629, 1969.

Hirshowitz, B., et al.: Survival after cardiac arrest in a case of severe burn. Isr. J. Med. Sci. **3**:553-557, 1967.

Ho, S. K.: Cardiac resuscitation in a community hospital, Minn. Med. **50**:1925-1928, 1967.

Hochberg, H., et al.: Automatic electrocardiographic monitoring in the coronary care unit, Angiology **20**:200-206, 1969.

Hochberg, H., et al.: Coronary care unit monitored by automated ECG, Mod. Med. **38**:136, 1970.

Hochberg, H. M., et al.: Monitoring of electrocardiograms in a coronary care unit by digital computer, J.A.M.A. **207**:2421-2424, 1969.

Hockaday, J. M., et al.: Electroencephalographic changes in acute cerebral anoxia from cardiac or respiratory arrest, Electroencephalogr. Clin. Neurophysiol. **18**:575-586, 1965.

Hoffer, R. E., et al.: Acute anterior descending coronary artery ligation, ventricular ligation, ventricular fibrillation, and ventricular assistance, Arch. Surg. **98**:703-708, 1969.

Hoffer, R. E.: Mechanical ventricular assistance for circulatory support in acute coronary artery occlusion in the pig: the Anstadt cup, Dis. Chest, **53**:502-506, 1968.

Hoffman, D.: On extrathoracic heart massage in newborns, Dtsch. Gesundh. **23**:453-455, 1968.

Hoffman, N. O.: Poisoning with dibenzepin (Deprex) resulting in ventricular fibrillation, Ugeskr. Laeger **132**:1877-1879, 1970.

Hoffman, S. A., et al.: Postoperative ventricular arrhythmias caused by isoproterenol. J. Thorac. Cardiovasc. Surg. **58**:664-667, 1969.

Hoffmann, M., et al.: EEG changes following temporary cardiac arrest and open cardiac massage, Electroencephalogr. Clin. Neurophysiol. **28**:326, 1970.

Hofkin, G. A.: Survival after cardiopulmonary resuscitation, J.A.M.A. **202**:652-654. 1967.

Hoflehner, G., et al.: Contribution to the problem of acute circulatory arrest, Wien. Med. Wochenschr. **118**:624-627, 1968.

Hohmann, G.: Heart arrest following neuroleptoanalgesia, Anaesthesist **15**:286, 1966.

Holder, B. J.: Cardiopulmonary resuscitation. Implications and responsibilities for the occupational health nurse, Occup. Health Nurs. **18**:13-15, 1970.

Holland, W. C.: Action of anesthetic agents on loss of potassium from isolated guinea pig auricles, J. Pharmacol. Exp. Ther. **111**:1-8, 1954.

Hollenberg, N. K., et al.: Acute renal failure due to nephrotoxins. Renal hemodynamics and angiographic studies in man, N. Engl. J. Med. **282**:1329, 1970.

Hollingsworth, J. H.: Results of cardiopulmonary resuscitation, a 3-year university hospital experience, Ann. Intern. Med. **71**:459-466, 1969.

Holmdahl, M. H., et al.: Experiences with heart-lung resuscitation in coronary infarction, Acta Anaesthiol. Scand. **11**:129-137, 1967.

Holmes, J. C.: Cardiac resuscitation, Mod. Treat. **7**:209-227, 1970.

Holscher, B.: Electron microscope studies of evaluation of membrane active cardioplegic agents for the resuscitation of the artificially arrested heart, Thoraxchirurgie **14**:193-200, 1966.

Holscher, B.: Histologic and biochemical studies on magnesium-Novocamide induced heart arrest in normothermal perfusion of rabbits with Haemacel-diluted autologous blood, Z. Kreislaufforsch. **55**:126-134, 1966.

Hood, F. R., Jr.: Experience with permanent cardiac pacemakers in Alaska, Alaska Med. **13**:20-21, 1971.

Hooker, D. R., et al.: The effect of alternating electrical currents on the heart, Am. J. Physiol. **103**:444-454, 1933.

Hooper, A. C.: Complications of experimental external cardiac massage, Ir. J. Med. Sci. **3**:435, 1970.

Horatz, K., et al.: Resuscitation in circulatory arrest, Munch. Med. Wochenschr. **108**:577-582, 1966.

Hosek, P.: Therapeutic experience in poisonings at the resuscitation department of the Kladno hospital, Cas. Lek. Cesk. **110**:135-136, 1971.

Hoshino, M.: Experimental and clinical studies on induced cardiac arrest, with special reference to electrical ventricular fibrillation, Jap. Circ. J. **35**:657-676, 1971.

Hossli, G.: Clinical measures in circulatory standstill, Praxis **58**:475-480, 1969.

Howat, D. D.: Vascular and respiratory emergencies, Ann. R. Coll. Surg. Engl. **47**:162-175, 1970.

Hoyer, S., and Wawersik, J.: Untersuchungen der Hirndurchblutung und des Hirnstoffwechsels beim Decerebrationssyndrom, Langenbecks Arch. Chir. **322:**602-605, 1968.

Huang, S., et al.: Cardiac involvement in pseudo-xanthoma elasticum, Am. Heart J. **74:**680-686, 1967.

Hubbell, R. W., and Okel, B. B.: The value of a cardiac resuscitation program in a community hospital, J. Med. Assoc. Ga. **58:**112-116, 1969.

Hubner, P. J. B., et al.: Shortcomings of mechanical cardiac monitoring, Mod. Med. **37:**127, 1969.

Huguenard, P., et al.: Resuscitation of nonsurgical head injury cases, Laval Med. **42:**552-558, 1971.

Hukuhara, T., and Nakayama, S.: Further studies on the effects of the transection of the brain stem upon the respiratory movements. Jap. J. Physiol. **9:**43-48, 1959.

Hulleman, A.: Suicide due to consumption of bananas. Death of a bilaterally nephrectomized female patient due to hyperkalemia after consumption of bananas, Dtsch. Med. Wochenschr. **94:**1765-1767, 1969.

Hultgren, H. N., et al.: Pulmonary edema, Mod. Concepts Cardiovasc. Dis. **37:**1-6, 1969.

Hunsaker, M. R.: A-V heart block in myocardial infarction, Am. J. Cardiol. **23:**911-912, 1969.

Hunt, D., et al.: Bundle branch block in acute myocardial infarction, Br. Med. J. **1:**85-88, 1969.

Hunt, D., et al.: Enzyme changes after DC cardioversion, Mod. Med. **37:**137, 1969.

Hunt, N. C., et al.: Conversion of supraventricular tachycardias with atrial stimulation, Circulation **38:**1060-1065, 1968.

Hunt, W. H., III., et al.: Ventricular tachycardia vs. rapid atrial fibrillation and W-P-W syndrome, N. Engl. J. Med. **281:**1246-1247, 1969.

Hunter, S. W., et al.: A bipolar myocardial electrode for complete heart block, J. Lancet **79:**506-508, 1959.

Hurley, E. J., et al.: Stokes-Adams attacks in transplanted hearts, Surg. Forum **16:**218-219, 1965.

Hurst, J. W., et al.: Cardiac arrhythmias: evolving concepts, Mod. Concepts Cardiovasc. Dis. **37:**73-78, 1968.

Hurst, J. W., et al.: The atrial kick and cardiac pacing, N. Engl. J. Med. **282:**624-625, 1970.

Hurwitz, R. A.: Effect of glucagon on dogs with acute and chronic heart block, Am. Heart J. **81:**644-649, 1971.

Hussar, A. E.: Sudden unexpected deaths, J.A.M.A. **210:**1764, 1969.

Hussar, A. E., et al.: Myocardial infarction and fatal coronary insufficiency during electroconvulsive therapy, J.A.M.A. **204:**1004-1007, 1968.

Hussman, L. H., et al.: Electroencephalographic or biologic survival, J.A.M.A. **207:**153, 1969.

Husveti, S., et al.: Janos Balassa, pioneer of cardiac resuscitation, Anaesthesia **24:**113-115, 1969.

Hutchinson, J. E., III, et al.: Emergency treatment of cardiac arrest in CHD with coronary bypass graft, J.A.M.A. **216:**1645, 1971.

Hyams, L., et al.: The epidemiology of myocardial infarction at two age-levels, Am. J. Epidemiol. **90:**93-102, 1969.

Hyland, J., et al.: Cardiac arrest and bone cement, Br. Med. J. **4:**176-177, 1970.

Hypoxic heartache, N. Engl. J. Med. **279:**829-830, 1968.

Iisalo, E., et al.: Potassium, glucose, and insulin in the treatment of acute myocardial infarction, Curr. Ther. Res. **11:**209-215, 1969.

Ikram, H., et al.: Atrial function following cardioversion, Am. Heart J. **74:**729-730, 1967.

Ikram, H.: Propanolol in persistent ventricular fibrillation complicating acute myocardial infarction, Am. Heart J. **75:**795-798, 1968.

Impending death affects emotions of dying patient, Mod. Med. **37:**100, 1969.

Improved tracheostomy tube has 'sausage' cuff, J.A.M.A. **211:**759, 1970.

Inkovaara, J., et al.: Long-term prognosis after ventricular fibrillation in acute myocardial infarction, Duodecim **87:**1046-1052, 1971.

Instant blood analysis for trauma, Med. World News **11:**18-20, 1970.

Inter-society Commission for Heart Disease Resources, Study Group on Coronary Artery Disease: Resources for the optimal care of a patient with acute myocardial infarction, Circulation **43:**A171-183, 1971.

Isaacs, J. H., et al.: Right pneumonectomy complicated by cardiac arrest in pregnancy, Ill. Med. J. **135:**586-587, 1969.

Ishida, M.: Experimental studies on circulatory arrest during deep hypothermia. Effect of Cytochrome C and prednisolone on tissue respiration of the vital organs, Arch. Jap. Chir. **37:**304-307, 1968.

Isselhard, W.: Measures for improving the recovery of the heart following anaerobiosis, Langenbecks Arch. Chir. **319:**665-688, 1967.

Iukhin, L. S.: A case of cardiac arrest during induction anaesthesia in a patient with a thermal burn, Eskp. Khir. Anestheziol. **11:**87-88, 1966.

Iwahata, D.: Comparative study on the 2 methods of induced cardiac arrest: with special reference to their effects on myocardial metabolism, Jap. Circ. J. **35:**281-293, 1971.

Iyengar, S. R. K., et al.: An experimental study of subendocardial hemorrhagic necrosis after anoxic cardiac arrest, Ann. Thorac. Surg. **13:** 214-222, 1972.

Jackson, M. M.: Nursing in the coronary care unit, U. Mich. Med. Center J. **34:**202-205, 1968.

Jacobey, J. A., et al.: Clinical experience with counterpulsation in coronary artery disease. J. Thorac. Cardiovasc. Surg. **56:**846-857, 1968.

Jain, P. D.: Successful resuscitation following cardiac arrest, J. Indian. Med. Assoc. **54:**563-565, 1970.

Jain, S. C., et al.: Elective countershock treatment with an intracardiac electrode in resistant cases of atrial arrhythmias, Sixth World Congress of Cardiology, London, 1970, p. 174.

James, L. S., et al.: Respiratory physiology of the fetus and newborn, N. Engl. J. Med. **271:**271, 1352, 1964.

James, T. N.: QT prolongation and sudden death, Mod. Concepts Cardiovasc. Dis. **38:**35-39, 1969.

James, T. N.: Changing concepts in electrocardiography, Mod. Concepts Cardiovasc. Dis. **39:** 129-132, 1970.

Jaron, D.: Support of the circulation by in-series mechanical assistance, Proc. 1972 Int. Conf. Cybernetics and Society, Washington, D. C., 1972, pp. 3-10.

Jaron, D., et al.: Measurement of ventricular load phase angle as an operating criterion for in series assist devices: hemodynamic studies utilizing intra-aortic balloon pumping, Trans. Am. Soc. Artif. Intern. Organs **16:**466-471, 1970.

Jeffrey, F. E., et al.: Increased tolerance of patients with circulatory congestion due to orthostatic stress, Mitt. Dtsch. Pharm. Ges. **39:**323-332, 1969.

Jelenko, C., III, et al.: The hot line: a unique ambulance-emergency room communication system, J. Trauma **8:**1102-1104, 1968.

Jenkins, A. M., et al.: Resuscitation room survey, Scott. Med. J. **14:**29-35, 1969.

Jennings, G. H., and Newton, M. A.: Persistent paraplegia after repeated cardiac arrests, Br. Med. J. **3:**572-573, 1969.

Jeresaty, R. M., et al.: Postinfarction interventricular septal defects. Report of two cases with long survival, one with surgical repair, Am. Heart J. **74:**543-550, 1967.

Jeresaty, R. M., et al.: Experience with external cardiac resuscitation in a community hospital, Conn. Med. **32:**193-200, 1968.

Jeresaty, R. M., et al.: External cardiac resuscitation in a community hospital. A three-year experience, Arch. Intern. Med. **124:**588-592, 1969.

Jeresaty, R. M., et al.: Sinoatrial arrest due to lidocaine in a patient receiving quinidine, Chest **61:**683-686, 1972.

Jernigan, W. R., et al.: Use of the internal jugular vein for placement of central venous catheter, Surg. Gynecol. Obstet. **130:**520-524, 1970.

Jestadt, R., et al.: On repeated electric defibrillation in ventricular fibrillation and flutter following myocardial infarct, Med. Welt **14:**863-864 passim, 1968.

Jewitt, D. E., et al.: Right atrial electrocardiogram in the analysis of arrhythmias following acute myocardial infarction, Br. Heart J. **30:** 97-104, 1968.

Jewitt, D. E., et al.: Free noradrenaline and adrenaline excretion in relation to the development of cardiac arrhythmias and heart failure in patients with acute myocardial infarction, J. Physiol. (Lond.) **202:**24P-25P, 1969.

Jewitt, D. E., et al.: Incidence and management of supraventricular arrhythmias after acute myocardial infarction, Am. Heart J. **77:**920-923, 1969.

Jobba, G., et al.: Liver rupture caused by external heart massage, Orv. Hetil. **112:**986-987, 1971.

Johanson, W. G., et al.: Acute myocardial infarction complicated by complete heart block. Use of the transvenous pacemaker with observations on a new demand pacemaker, J. Lancet **87:** 393-396, 1967.

Johansson, B. W., et al.: Longevity in complete heart block, Ann. N. Y. Acad. Sci. **167:**1031-1037, 1969.

Johns, G.: Cardiac arrest following induction with propanidid, Br. J. Anaesth. **42:**74-77, 1970.

Johnson, A. L., et al.: Results of cardiac resuscitation in 552 patients, Am. J. Cardiol. **20:**831-835, 1967.

Johnson, A. S., et al.: Substernal cardiac massage and assistance, Surgery **63:**800-805, 1968.

Johnson, J. D.: A plan of action in cardiac arrest, J.A.M.A. **186:**468-473, 1963.

Johnson, J., and Castle, C. H.: Cardiopulmonary resuscitation training. A plan for providing it in a large geographic region, Rocky Mt. Med. J. **68:**11-15, 1971.

Johnson, J. D., et al.: Hypocalcemia and cardiac arrhythmias, Am. J. Dis. Child. **115:**373-376, 1968.

Johnson, M. S.: Nurses' guide to central venous pressure monitoring, Milit. Med. **135:**100-106, 1970.

Johnson, R., et al.: Cardiorespiratory resuscitation, Union Med. Can. **96:**673-676, 1967.

Johnson, V., and Eiseman, B.: Reinforcement of ventilation with electrophrenic pacing of the paralyzed diaphragm, J. Thorac. Cardiovasc. Surg. **62**:651-657, 1971.

Joki, E., et al.: Sudden cardiac death of pilot in flight, Cardiology **52**:235-239, 1968.

Joly, J. B.: Research in resuscitation. Applied research and applications of the research, Bull. Inst. Natl. Sante Rech. Med. **25**:777-782, 1970.

Jones, G. R.: Deaths from asthma, Br. Med. J. **2**: 698, 1968.

Jones, L. W., and Weil, M. H.: Water creatinine and sodium excretion following circulatory shock with renal failure, Am. J. Med. **51**:314, 1971.

Jones, S. R., et al.: Sudden death in sickle-cell trait, N. Engl. J. Med. **282**:323-325, 1970.

Jorgensen, E. O.: The EEG after circulatory and respiratory arrest, Acta Neurol. Scand. **46** (**Suppl. 43**):279+, 1970.

Jorgensen, E. O.: The EEG following circulatory and respiratory arrest, Electroencephalogr. Clin. Neurophysiol. **30**:273, 1971.

Joshi, V. V.: Effects of burns on the heart, J.A.M.A. **211**:2130-2133, 1970.

Jouvet, M.: Diagnostic électro-sous-corticographique de la mort du système nerveux central au cours de certains comas, Electroencephalogr. Clin. Neurophysiol. **11**:805-808, 1959.

Jude, J. R., and Nagel, E. L.: Cardiopulmonary resuscitation 1970, Mod. Concepts Cardiovasc. Dis. **39**:133-139, 1970.

Jude, J. R., and Tabbarah, H. J.: Otolaryngological aspects of cardiac arrest, Ann. Otol. Rhinol. Laryngol. **79**:889-894, 1970.

Jude, J. R., et al.: Cardiac resuscitation in the operating room: current status, Ann. Surg. **171**: 948-955, 1970.

Julian, D. G., et al.: Disturbances of rate, rhythm and conduction in acute myocardial infarction, Am. J. Med. **37**:915-927, 1964.

Julian, D. G., et al.: Closed-chest cardiac resuscitation at the end of the 18th century, Br. Heart J. **32**:555, 1970.

Jullien, J. L.: The state of sudden apparent death associated with myocardial infarct. The possibility of reanimation, Coeur Med. Interne **7**: 443-449, 1968.

Jung, M. A., et al.: Value of a cardiac arrest team in a university hospital, Can. Med. Assoc. J. **98**:74-78, 1968.

Just a mild sore throat and then, sudden death, Med. World News **8**:82, 1967.

K+ replacement following bypass, Med. World News **24**:21, 1970.

Kachatrian, S. A.: Effect of insulin and glucose on the adenosine triphosphate-adenosine triphosphatase system in resuscitation, Z. Eksp. Klin. Med. **7**:13-21, 1967.

Kadlic, T.: Problem of cerebral death in resuscitation, Rozhl. Chir. **49**:569-574, 1970.

Kahn, A. H.: Cardiac pacing in acute myocardial infarction complicated by complete heart block, Am. Heart J. **81**:723, 1971.

Kahn, D. R., et al.: Cardioversion after mitral valve operations, Circulation **35-36**(**Suppl. 1**): 82-85, 1967.

Kahn, D. R., et al.: Effect of anticoagulants on the transplanted heart, J. Thorac. Cardiovasc. Surg. **60**:616-635, 1970.

Kahn, D. R., et al.: Long-term function after human heart transplantation, J.A.M.A. **218**: 1699, 1971.

Kaindl, F., et al.: The evaluation of myocardial function following long-term ischemic heart arrest, Wein. Z. Inn. Med. **50**:231-235, 1969.

Kaiser, G. C.: Implantable pacemakers: detection and management of malfunction, Heart Bull. **18**:51-54, 1969.

Kaiser, G. C., et al.: Bradycardia treated by pacemakers, Mod. Med. **37**:164, 1969.

Kaiser, G. C., et al.: Surgical treatment of bradycardia, Arch. Surg. **98**:612-619, 1969.

Kaiser, G. A., et al.: Specialized cardiac conduction system. Improved electrophysiologic identification technique at surgery, Arch. Surg. **101**: 673-676, 1970.

Kalff, G., et al.: Successful resuscitation after afibrinogenemia and cardiac arrest, Geburtsh. Frauenheilk. **27**:408-413, 1967.

Kamiyama, T. M., et al.: Preservation of the anoxic heart with a metabolic inhibitor and hypothermia, Arch. Surg. **100**:596-600, 1970.

Kantrowitz, A., and Kantrowitz, A.: Experimental augmentation of coronary flow by retardation of the arterial pressure pulse, Surgery **34**:678, 1953.

Kantrowitz, A., et al.: Experimental and clinical experience with a new implantable cardiac pacemaker, Circulation **24**:967-968, 1961.

Kantrowitz, A., et al.: A clinical experience with an implanted mechanical auxiliary ventricle, J.A.M.A. **197**:525, 1966.

Kantrowitz, A., et al.: Initial clinical experience with intraaortic balloon pumping in cardiogenic shock, J.A.M.A. **203**:113-118, 1968a.

Kantrowitz, A., et al.: Clinical experience with cardiac assistance by means of intraaortic phase-shift balloon pumping, Trans. Am. Soc. Artif. Intern. Organs **14**:344, 1968b.

Kantrowitz, A., et al.: Technique of femoral artery cannulation for phase-shift balloon pumping, J. Thorac. Cardiovasc. Surg. **56**:219, 1968c.

Kantrowitz, A., et al.: A permanent mechanical auxiliary ventricle: experimental and clinical experience, J. Cardiovasc. Surg. (Torino) **9**: 1-16, 1968d.

Kantrowitz, A., et al.: Mechanical intraaortic cardiac assistance in cardiogenic shock. Hemodynamic effects, Arch. Surg. **97**:1000-1004, 1968.

Kantrowitz, A., et al.: Phase-shift balloon pumping in cardiogenic shock, Prog. Cardiovasc. Dis. **12**:293, 1969.

Kantrowitz, A., et al.: Phase-shift balloon pumping in medically refractory cardiogenic shock, Arch. Surg. **99**:739-743, 1969.

Kantrowitz, A., et al.: Current status of the intraaortic balloon pump and initial clinical experience with an aortic patch mechanical auxiliary ventricle, Transplant. Proc. **3**:1459, 1971.

Kantrowitz, A., et al.: Initial clinical experience with a new permanent mechanical auxiliary ventricle: the dynamic aortic patch, Trans. Am. Soc. Artif. Intern. Organs **18**:159, 1972.

Kaplan, M. A., and Cohen, K. L.: Ventricular fibrillation in the Wolff-Parkinson-White syndrome, Am. J. Cardiol. **24**:259-264, 1969.

Kassanoff, I., et al.: Stadium coronary care, J.A.M.A. **221**:397-400, 1972.

Katz, A. M.: Control of the myocardial contractile system, Heart Bull. **18**:75-78, 1969.

Katz, A. M., and Tada, M.: The "stone heart": a challenge to the biochemist, Am. J. Cardiol. **29**:578-579, 1972.

Katz, A. M., et al.: Mechanical and biochemical correlates of cardiac conduction, Mod. Concepts Cardiovasc. Dis. **40**:45-48, 1971.

Katz, L. N:. Analysis of several factors regulating the performance of the heart, Physiol. Rev. **35**:91, 1955.

Käufer, C.: Spontaneous reversible cardiac arrest, Dtsch. Med. Wochenschr. **96**:2147, 1970.

Kaumann, A. J., et al.: Prevention of ventricular fibrillation induced by coronary ligation, J. Pharmacol. Exp. Ther. **164**:326-332, 1968.

Kaverina, K. P.: Characteristics of transfusion therapy in resuscitation of patients with massive hemorrhage, Probl. Gematol. Pereliv. Krovi **15**:13-17, 1970.

Kay, J. H., et al.: Left ventricular excision, exclusion, or plication for akinetic areas of the heart, J. Thorac. Cardiovasc. Surg. **59**:139-146, 1970.

Kearns, J. B., et al.: Ventricular fibrillation during hypothermia, J. Physiol. (Lond.) **203**:51P-53P, 1969.

Keatinge, W. R.: Survival in cold water, Oxford, 1969, Blackwell & Co. (Publishers) Ltd., p. 5.

Keaveny, T. V., et al.: Renal vasomotor responses in the agonal period, Angiology **22**:77, 1971.

Keen, G., et al.: The effects of circulatory arrest during profound hypothermia upon human myo-cardial fine structure, Cardiovasc. Res. **4**:348-354, 1970.

Keep, V. R.: Dental clearance followed by cardiac arrest, Aust. Dent. J. **13**:342-344, 1968.

Kelley, N., et al.: Cardiopulmonary resuscitation and C.S., Hosp. Management **110**:45-48, 1970.

Kelly, D. T., et al.: Electrical pacing of the heart with observations on the single and paired electrical stimuli during acute reversible experimental heart failure in the anaesthetized dog, S. Afr. Med. J. **42**:432-437, 1968.

Kelly, J.: Pregnancy following mitral valve reconstruction: cardiac arrest for 30 minutes with complete recovery, Proc. R. Soc. Med. **61**:680, 1968.

Kenigsberg, K., et al.: Reflex bradycardia after tracheoesophageal fistula repair, Surgery **71**:125-129, 1972.

Kennedy, J. H.: Assisted circulation: an extended concept of cardiopulmonary resuscitation, J. Thorac. Cardiovasc. Surg. **57**:688-701, 1969.

Kennedy, J. H.: Current status of research in artificial support to circulation, Chest **60**:519-521, 1971.

Kennedy, J. H., et al.: A subminiature implantable self-powered cardiac pacemaker, experimental observations, Ann. Thorac. Surg. **2**:576-584, 1966.

Kennedy, J. H., et al.: Criteria for selection of patients for mechanical circulatory support, Am. J. Cardiol. **27**:33-40, 1971.

Kent, G. T., et al.: High incidence of unsuspected diabetes cases, Mod. Med. **37**:123, 1969.

Kerkiacharian, A.: Heart arrest and closed chest massage. A case in a young infant during a femoral osteotomy, Rev. Med. Moyen Orient. **24**:542-544, 1967.

Kernohan, R. J., et al.: Mobile intensive care in myocardial infarction, Br. Med. J. (Suppl.) **3**:178-180, 1968.

Kettner, W., et al.: Fatal contrast media accident following Visotrast 290 in a patient with heart disease, Z. Aerztl. Fortbild. (Jena) **65**:157-159, 1971.

Kezdi, P., et al.: Aortic flow velocity and acceleration as an index of ventricular performance during myocardial infarction, Am. J. Med. Sci. **257**:61-71, 1969.

Khalimova, K. M., et al.: Characteristics of the changes in afferent impulsation in cardiac nerves in experimental myocardial infarct complicated by ventricular fibrillation, Kardiologiia **10**:68-75, 1970.

Khook, K. A., et al.: The use of heart massage under conditions of a military hospital, Voen. Med. Zh. **9**:60-61, 1969.

Killip, T.: Arrhythmia, sudden death and coronary artery disease, Am. J. Cardiol. **22:**614-616, 1971.

Killip, T., et al.: Percutaneous techniques for introducing flexible electrodes for intracardiac pacing, Ann. N. Y. Acad. Sci. **167:**597-603, 1969.

Kimball, J. T.: Aggressive management of acute myocardial infarction, J. Iowa Med. Soc. **59:**207-210, 1969.

Kimball, J. T.: The current status of synchronized and unsynchronized precordial electric shock, Geriatrics **26:**111-118, 1971.

King, G. R., et al.: Microwave oven a danger to implanted pacemaker, Mod. Med. **38:**124, 1970.

King, R. B., et al.: Case of recovery from drowning and prolonged anoxia, Med. J. Aust. **1:**919, 1964.

King, S. B., III, et al.: Premature atrial contractions—a look at those aberrantly conducted, Rocky Mt. Med. **68:**60-62, 1971.

Kirklin, J. W.: Personal communication, September, 1971.

Kirimli, B.: Organization of cardiopulmonary resuscitation training programs, Laval Med. **40:**265-268, 1969.

Kirimli, B., and Safar, P.: Arterial versus venous transfusion in cardiac arrest from exsanguination, Anesth. Analg. (Cleve.) **44:**819-830, 1965.

Kirimli, B., et al.: Drugs in cardiopulmonary resuscitation, Acta Anaesthesiol. Scand. (Suppl.) **23:**255+, 1966.

Kirimli, B., et al.: Cardiac arrest from exsanguination in dogs. Evaluation of resuscitation methods, Acta Anaesthiol. Scand. (Suppl.) **29:**183+, 1968.

Kirimli, B., et al.: Resuscitation from cardiac arrest due to exsanguination, Surg. Gynecol. Obstet. **129:**89-97, 1969.

Kirimli, B., et al.: Evaluation of sodium bicarbonate and epinephrine in cardiopulmonary resuscitation, Anesth. Analg. (Cleve.) **48:**649-658, 1969.

Kirimli, B., et al.: Pattern of dying from exsanguinating hemorrhage in dogs, J. Trauma **10:**393-404, 1970.

Kirsch, U.: Determination of fibrillation threshold of guinea pig heart in spontaneous respiration by means of an intracardiac electrode, Arzneim. Forsch. **19:**225-258, 1969.

Kirsch, U., et al.: Induced ischemic arrest, J. Thorac. Cardiovasc. Surg. **63:**121-128, 1972.

Kirsh, M. M., et al.: Human cardiac transplantation, J. Extra-corporeal Techn. **3:**6-7, 1970.

Kishon, Y., et al.: Diagnosis and investigation of arrhythmias with proximity electrodes, Mayo Clin. Proc. **44:**515-524, 1969.

Kiss, Z. S., et al.: Electrical cardiac pacing in patients without heart block, Aust. Ann. Med. **19:**220-225, 1970.

Klebanoff, G., et al.: Temporary suspension of animation using total body perfusion and hypothermia: a preliminary report, Cryobiology **6:**121-125, 1969.

Kleiger, R. E., et al.: Cardioversion of paroxysmal arrhythmias, J.A.M.A. **213:**107-113, 1970.

Kleine, J. W., et al.: Resuscitation wall-chart, Arch. Chir. Neerl. **22:**283-287, 1970.

Klets, R. L., et al.: Ventricular fibrillation as a complication of electroimpulse therapy of cardiac arrhythmia, Kardiologiia **10:**117-121, 1970.

Klionsky, B.: Role of hyperkalaemia in experimental fetal asphyxia, Arch. Dis. Child. **43:**747, 1968.

Klupp, H., et al.: Liberation of potassium from muscles under the influence of muscle relaxants, Arch. Int. Pharmacodyn. Ther. **98:**340, 1954.

Knapp, R. D., Jr.: Lidocaine and myocardial infarction, J.A.M.A. **206:**647-648, 1968.

Knappe, J., et al.: Heart arrest in myocardial infarction, its treatment with transfer electric stimulation, Z. Gesamte Inn. Med. **23:**68-72, 1968.

Knappe, J., et al.: The transient electrostimulation of the heart in total atrioventricular block, Dtsch. Gesundheitsw. **23:**584-587, 1968.

Koch-Weser, J., et al.: Antiarrhythmic prophylaxis with procainamide in acute myocardial infarction, N. Engl. J. Med. **281:**1253-1260, 1969.

Koch-Weser, J., et al.: Arrhythmias after infarction reduced by procainamide, Mod. Med. **38:**181, 1970.

Koga, Y., et al.: Resuscitation and preservation of canine cadaver hearts, Trans. Am. Soc. Artif. Intern. Organs **14:**140-145, 1968.

Kolar, J., et al.: Influence of cardiostimulation on mortality in acute myocardial infarct complicated by complete A-V block and disturbances of intraventricular conduction, Cas. Lek. Cesk. **110:**385-390, 1971.

Kolesov, E. V., et al.: Ensuring the safety of cardiologic tests with temporary heart arrest, Vestn. Khir. **97:**55-59, 1966.

Kolff, W. J.: The artificial heart: research, development, or invention? Dis. Chest. **56:**314-329, 1969.

Kolff, W. J.: Experiences with air embolism, J. Extra-corporeal Techn. **3:**8-9, 1970.

Kolff, W. J.: Replacing the forever failing heart, Chest **57:**299-301, 1970.

Konda, Y., et al.: On the effect of cardiac arrest on the microvibration (MV) over the body surface, J. Physiol. Soc. Jap. **32:**284-285, 1970.

Kones, R. J.: Glucagon in heart block, South. Med. J. **64:**459-461, 1971.

Konttinen, A., et al.: Origin of elevated serum enzyme activities after direct-current counter-shock, N. Engl. J. Med. 281:231-234, 1969.

Kopriva, C. J., and Lowenstein, E.: An anesthetic accident: cardiovascular collapse from liquid halothane delivery, Anesthesiology 30:246-247, 1969.

Körner, M.: Heart rhythm disorders as fore-runners of cardiac and circulatory arrest, H.N.O. 19:188-189, 1971.

Korolev, B. A., et al.: Cardiac arrest in mitral commissurotomy and its effect on the outcome of surgery, Vestn. Khir. 105:118-123, 1970.

Kossakiewicz, J., and Dyaczynska, A.: Adaptation of hospital admission rooms to resuscitation pur-poses, Wiad. Lek. 24:897-898, 1971.

Kostuk, W. J., and Beanlands, D. S.: Complete heart block associated with acute myocardial infarction, Am. J. Cardiol. 26:380-384, 1970.

Kouwenhoven, W. B.: The development of the defibrillator, Ann. Intern. Med. 71:449-458, 1969.

Kouwenhoven, W. B., et al.: Closed-chest cardiac massage, J.A.M.A. 173:1064-1067, 1960.

Kowal, J. S., et al.: Cardiac resuscitation pro-gram, Hospitals 44:77-80, 1970.

Krakauer, J. S., et al.: Clinical management ancillary to phase-shift balloon pumping in cardiogenic shock: preliminary comments, Am. J. Cardiol. 27:123, 1971.

Krall, J. I., et al.: Treatment of ventricular arrhythmias with bretylium tosylate, Am. Heart J. 81:288, 1971.

Kramer, R. S., et al.: Effect of profound hypo-thermia on preservation of cerebral ATP con-tent during circulatory arrest, J. Thorac. Car-diovasc. Surg. 56:699-709, 1968.

Kramer, S. G., et al.: Intensive care unit flow sheet, Surgery 67:590-592, 1970.

Kraska, T., et al.: Aortic flow rate in dogs during ventricular heterotopy, Pol. Med. J. 9:464-467, 1970.

Krause, E. G.: Biochemical changes in heart arrest, Z. Gesamte Inn. Med. 24(Suppl.):19-24, 1969.

Krause, E. G., et al.: On the activity of phos-phorylase, the rate of glycolysis and the be-havior of phosphocreatines and orthophosphates in the myocardium of the guinea pig in circula-tory arrest, Acta Biol. Med. Ger. 16:595-605, 1966.

Kravitz, A. E., and Killip, T.: Cardiopulmonary resuscitation: Status report, N. Engl. J. Med. 286:1000, 1972.

Kravitz, H.: Resuscitation and treatment following submersion, Ill. Med. J. 135:690-691, 1969.

Kreitmeyer, H. J.: Functional circulatory arrest in traffic accidents, Med. Klin. 58:1495-1497, 1963.

Kreuscher, H.: "Mainz" resuscitation table, An-aesthesist 19:410-411, 1970.

Krikle, D. M.: Phentolamine in heart block, Br. Med. J. 4:558, 1970.

Kringelbach, J., et al.: Extended Q-T Interval and cardiac syncope (Ward's syndrome), Nord. Med. 85:91-92, Jan. 71.

Krosch, H., et al.: Acute cardiac arrest in nephro-genic cardiopathies, Z. Gesamte Inn. Med. 24(Suppl.):28-30, 1969.

Kubicki, S.: The role of EEG in resuscitation, Electroencephalogr. Clin. Neurophysiol. 27:623, 1969.

Kubik, M. M., et al.: Survival after 195 defibrilla-tions, Br. Med. J. 4:432, 1969.

Kubler, W.: Effective heart ischemia duration in relation to the energy starting position of the myocardium, the form of cardioplegia, and the temperature, Langenbecks Arch. Klin. Chir. 319:648-660, 1967.

Kubler, W., et al.: The energy metabolism of the heart during ischemia and during post-ischemic regeneration with and without artificial cardiac arrest, Br. J. Surg. 56:630, 1969.

Kubo, T., et al.: Interaction between extracellular sodium and the excitatory effect of acetylcholine on the nonpacemaker potential arrested by propanolol in the isolated rabbit's atria, Jap. J. Pharmacol. 19:621-623, 1969.

Kugelberg, J.: Ventricular defibrillation with square-waves, Acta Chir. Scand. (Suppl.) 356:123-128, 1966.

Kugelberg, J.: Ventricular defibrillation. A new aspect, Acta Chir. Scand. (Suppl.) 372:1-93, 1967.

Kugelberg, J.: Atrial defibrillation. A new aspect, Scand. J. Thorac. Cardiovasc. Surg. 2:203-208, 1968.

Kugler, J., et al.: EEG and electrical inactivity in emergencies, Munch. Med. Wochenschr. 110:2843-2890, 1968.

Kuhlgatz, G., et al.: Clinical studies and morpho-logic findings following resuscitation attempts [defibrillation and heart massage], Anaesthesist 16:238-243, 1967.

Kuhn, L. A.: Treatment of cardiogenic shock. I. The nature of cardiogenic shock, Am. Heart J. 74:578-581, 1967.

Kuhn, L. A., et al.: Effects of isoproterenol on hemodynamic alterations, myocardial metab-olism, and coronary flow in experimental acute myocardial infarction with shock, Am. Heart J. 77:772-783, 1969.

Kuller, L. K.: Preventive care to reduce sudden heart deaths, Mod. Med. 38:169, 1970.

Kumar, S., et al.: Influence of hypoxia and coronary ligation on cardiac arrest in dogs anaesthetized with pentobarbitone, Br. J. Anaesth. 41:307-310, 1969.

Kuner, J., and Goldman, A.: Prolonged nasotracheal intubation in adults versus tracheostomy, Dis. Chest. 51:270-274, 1967.

Kurien, V. A., et al.: The role of free fatty acids in the production of ventricular arrhythmias after acute coronary artery occlusion, Eur. J. Clin. Invest. 1:225-241, 1971.

Kurihara, Y., et al.: Very rare cardiac arrest due to succinylcholine shock—a successfully treated case, J. Jap. Med. Assoc. 63:752-753, 1970.

Kurtz, D., et al.: Intérêt de l'EEG dans les suites d'arrêt cardiaque réversible, Acta Neurol. Belge 70:213-228, 1970.

Kurtz, D., et al.: Prognostic value of the EEG following reversible cardiac arrest. From 90 cases, Electroencephalogr. Clin. Neurophysiol. 29:530-531, 1970.

Kuruvila, E. C., and Beven, E. G.: Arteriovenous shunts and fistulas for hemodialysis, Surg. Clin. North Am. 51:1219, 1971.

Kwast, H. A.: "Endocardial thump," N. Engl. J. Med. 284:795, 1971.

Laddu, R.: Antiarrhythmic activity of 1-[di2,6-xylylmethoxy]-3-[isopropylamino] propanolol-2-hydrochloride [BS-7977-d] in the dog heart lung preparation, Eur. J. Pharmacol. 9:129-135, 1970.

Lagergren, H., and Johansson, L.: Intracardiac stimulation for complete heart block, Acta Chir. Scand. 125:562-566, 1963.

Lahdensuu, M., and Rokkanen, P.: Resuscitation in a case of severe thoraco-abdominal injury, Ann. Chir Gynaecol. Fenn. 58:247-248, 1969.

Lajos, T. Z., et al.: Surgery for acute myocardial infarction, Ann. Thorac. Surg. 8:452-457, 1969.

Lal, H. B.: A study of myocardial infarction. V. Therapeutic trials, Indian J. Med. Res. 56 (Suppl.):1107-1115, 1968.

Lal, H. B., et al.: Some observations on the alteration of the adhesiveness of human blood platelets after infusion with low molecular weight dextran, J. Assoc. Physicians India 16:523-527, 1968.

Lal, S., et al.: Oxygen administration after myocardial infarction, Lancet 1:381, 1969.

L'Allemand, H., et al.: Respiratory arrest—heart arrest—death, Langenbecks Arch. Chir. 325:1092-1101, 1969.

Lambert, C. J., et al.: Emergency myocardial revascularization for impending myocardial infarctions, Chest 61:479-480, 1972.

Lang, T. W., et al.: Dynamics of potassium flux in cardiac arrhythmias, Am. J. Cardiol. 29:199-207, 1972.

Langendorf, R.: Terminology and classification of disturbances of A-V conduction, Bull. N. Y. Acad. Med. 47:877-884, 1971.

Langhorne, W. H.: The coronary care unit, a year's experience in a community hospital, J.A.M.A. 201:662-665, 1967.

Langhorne, W. H.: Coronary care unit revisited, Chest 57:550-553, 1970.

Langley, R. B., et al.: Acute coronary care in small hospital, Isr. J. Med. Sci. 5:780-782, 1969.

Langsjoen, P. H., et al.: The treatment of myocardial infarction with low molecular weight dextran, Am. Heart J. 76:28-34, 1968.

Larard, D. G.: Cardiac arrest following induction with propanidid, Br. J. Anaesth. 42:652, 1970.

Lareng, L., et al.: Multiple cardiac arrest during severe drug poisoning with deep hypothermia, Cah. Anesthesiol. 17:349-367, 1969.

Lareng, L., et al.: What respirators must be used in postoperative respiratory resuscitation? Cah. Anesthesiol 19:221-224, 1971.

Larsen, H. R.: Heart arrest in asthmatics after the use of aerosol sprays, Ugeskr. Laeger 132:2277-2278, 1970.

Lasky, I. I.: Pacemaker failure from automobile accident, J.A.M.A. 211:1700, 1970.

Lassers, B. W.: Artificial pacing in the management of complete heart block complicating acute myocardial infarction, Br. Med. J. 2:142-146, 1968.

Lassers, B. W.: First-year follow-up after recovery from acute myocardial infarction with complete heart-block, Lancet 1:1172-1174, 1969.

Lassner, J.: Preoperative heart arrest under neuroleptanesthesia, Cah. Anesthesiol. 15:403-406, 1967,

Latarjet, J.: Use of a coronary vasodilator in treatment of tetanus, Lyon Med. 223:211-213, 1970.

Lau, F. Y., et al.: Protection of implanted pacemakers from excessive electrical energy of D. C. shock, Am. J. Cardiol. 23:244-249, 1969.

Lawin, P., et al.: Three cases of heart arrest due to induction of neuroleptic analgesia, Type II, in patients pretreated with vasodilator drugs, Anaesthesist 15:19-20, 1966.

Lawrie, D. M.: Ventricular fibrillation in acute myocardial infarction, Am. Heart J. 78:424-425, 1969.

Lawrie, D. M.: Long-term survival after ventricular fibrillation complicating acute myocardial infarction, Lancet 2:1085-1087, 1969.

Lawrie, D. M.: Ventricular fibrillation in acute myocardial infarction. Am. Heart J. 78:424-426, 1969.

Lawrie, D. M.: Survival after ventricular fibrillation, Mod. Med. 38:131, 1970.

Lawrie, D. M., et al.: Ventricular fibrillation complicating acute myocardial infarction, Lancet 2:523-528, 1968.

Laws, H. L., et al.: The case for the combined intensive care unit, Surg. Gynecol. Obstet. 131: 523-524, 1970.

Lebis, J.: Heart arrest during an anesthesia by Propanidide, Anesth. Analg. (Paris) 25:677-678, 1968.

Lebowitz, W. B.: Electrical conversion of arrhythmias under diazepam sedation, Conn. Med. 33:173-174, 1969.

Ledwich, J. R., et al.: Idiopathic recurrent ventricular fibrillation, Am. J. Cardiol. 24:255-258, 1969.

Lee, W. R.: Deaths from electric shock in 1962 and 1963, Br. Med. J. 2:616-619, 1968.

Lee, W. R., et al.: An experimental comparison in dogs of expired air and oxygen ventilation during external cardiac massage, Br. J. Anaesth. 43:38-50, 1971.

Legchilo, A. N.: Direct heart massage in right-sided thoracotomy, Vestn. Khir. 98:106-108, 1967.

Leigh, M. D., et al.: Bradycardia following intravenous administration of succinylcholine chloride to infants and children, Anesthesiology 18: 698-700, 1957.

Leinbach, R. C., et al.: Effects of intra-aortic balloon pumping on coronary flow and metabolism in man, Circulation 41-42 (Suppl. III): 76, 1970.

Lemberg, L., et al.: Cardiac drugs in the coronary care unit, Chest 59:289-296, 1971.

Lemberg, L., et al.: Pacing on demand in AV block, J.A.M.A. 191:106-108, 1965.

Lemire, J. G., and Johnson, A. L.: Is cardiac resuscitation worthwhile? N. Engl. J. Med. 286:970-973, 1972.

Leonard, C. T., and Hillman, H.: The degree of recovery, and the biochemical changes in the brains of rats during cooling and recovery from hypothermic cardiac arrest, Resuscitation, 2: 1973.

Leone, M., et al.: Spontaneous cardiac arrest in gynecological surgery, Quad. Clin. Ostet. Ginec. 22:361-374, 1967.

L'Epee, P., et al.: Liver rupture of unexpected cause, Med. Leg. Domm. Corpor. (Paris) 2: 187, 1969.

Letac, B., et al.: Hemodynamic study of external cardiac massage, Presse Med. 78:1735-1738, 1970.

Letac, R., et al.: Experimental trial of a simple method for total ventricular assistance, Bord. Med. 4:1189-1191, 1971.

Levander-Lindgren, M., et al.: Mechanically induced ventricular systoles during external massage and thumping of the chest, Scand. J. Thorac. Cardiovasc. Surg. 4:219-224, 1970.

Levin, P. D., et al.: Patient and pacemaker survival after pacemaker implantation, Chest 58: 4-7, 1970.

Levinsky, W. J., et al.: Fatal air embolism during insertion of CVP monitoring apparatus, J.A.M.A. 209:1721, 1969.

Levitsky, S., et al.: A functional evaluation of the preserved heart, J. Thorac. Cardiovasc. Surg. 60:675-736, 1970.

Levitsky, S., et al.: Normothermic myocardial anoxia, Ann. Thorac. Surg. 11:229-237, 1971.

Levowitz, B. S., et al.: Vascular responses to potassium ion, Surg. Gynecol. Obstet. 129:979-988, 1969.

Lewandowski, J., and Spiechowicz, J.: Results of resuscitation carried out in a department of surgery, Pol. Przegl. Chir. 43:713-718, 1971.

Lewandowski, K., et al.: Successful resuscitation after cardiac arrest due to a penetrating wound of the heart, Br. J. Anaesth. 41:712-714, 1969.

Lewis, J. F., et al.: Automatic monitoring in the postoperative recovery room, Surg. Gynecol. Obstet. 130:333-341, 1970.

Lewman, L. V., et al.: Congenital tumor of atrioventricular node with complete heart block and sudden death, Am. J. Cardiol. 29:554-557, 1972.

Leyton, R. A., et al.: The ultrastructure of the failing heart, Am. J. Med. Sci. 258:304-327, 1969.

Lichteln, P., et al.: Infarction and cardiac wall aneurysm in juvenile sportsmen, Schweiz. Med. Wochenschr. 98:1097-1105, 1968.

Lichti, E. L., et al.: Cardiac massage efficacy monitored by Doppler ultrasonic flowmeter, Mo. Med. 68:317-320, 1971.

Liddicoat, J. E., et al.: Cardiac preservation, Rev. Surg. 27:447-449, 1970.

Lieberman, A.: Syncope after prostatic massage, N. Engl. J. Med. 282:515, 1970.

Lieberman, A.: The case of the Zapista from Durango, J. Indiana State Med. Assoc. 63: 904-907, 1970.

Life after death, Br. Med. J. 4:693-694, 1967.

Lillehei, C. W., et al.: Management of catastrophic cardiac problems, Mod. Med. 38:140, 1970.

Lillehei, C. W., et al.: Partial cardiopulmonary bypass, hypothermia, and total circulatory arrest. A lifesaving technique for ruptured mycotic aortic aneurysms, ruptured left ventricle, and other complicated cardiac pathology, J. Thorac. Cardiovasc. Surg. 58:530-544, 1969.

Lillehei, R. C.: Pressor agents in cardiogenic

shock: pro and con, Am. J. Cardiol. **23**:900-911, 1969.

Lindenmayer, G. E., et al.: Re-evaluation of oxidative phosphorylation in cardiac mitochondria from normal animals and animals in heart failure, Circ. Res. **23**:439-450, 1968.

Linko, E., et al.: Resuscitation in cardiac arrest, Acta Med. Scand. **182**:611-620, 1967.

Linn, B. S., et al.: Cardiac arrest among geriatric patients, Br. Med. J. **2**:25-27, 1970.

Lipp, H., et al.: Recurrent ventricular tachyarrhythmias in a patient with a prolonged Q-T interval, Med. J. Aust, **1**:1296-1299, 1970.

Lippestad, C. T., et al.: Sinus arrest in proximal right coronary artery occlusion, Am. Heart J. **74**:551-556, 1967.

Lippestad, C. T., et al.: Production of sinus arrest by lignocaine, Br. Med. J. **1**:537, 1971.

Lister, J. W., et al.: The hemodynamic effect of slowing the heart rate by paired or coupled stimulation of the atria, Am. Heart J. **73**:362-368, 1967.

Lister, J. W., et al.: Treatment of supraventricular tachycardias by rapid atrial stimulation, Circulation **38**:1044-1059, 1968.

Lister, J. W., et al.: Electrical stimulation of the atria in patients with an intact AV conduction system, Ann. N. Y. Acad. Sci. **167**:785-806, 1969.

Liu, C. K., et al.: Transient and delayed hypokalemia and ventricular arrhythmia in patients undergoing open-heart surgery, Clin. Res. **14**:161, 1966.

Liu, C. K., et al.: Cardiac problems, Int. Anesthesiol. Clin. **5**:645, 1967.

Lochner, W., et al.: Metabolism of the artificially arrested heart and of the gas-perfused heart, Am. J. Cardiol. **22**:299-311, 1968.

Lockey, E., et al.: Potassium and open-heart surgery, Lancet **1**:671-675, 1966.

Logic, J. R., et al.: Idioventricular tachycardia complicating experimental myocardial infarction, Dis. Chest **56**:477-480, 1969.

Long, G. J., et al.: A danger—insecure positioning of anesthetic vaporizers, Med. J. Aust. **1**:1108, 1969.

Lonnum, I.: Hazards connected with emptying of the colon. A case of sinus arrest with cardiac standstill following enema, J. Oslo City Hosp. **17**:182-220, 1967.

Lopez, J. F., et al.: Slowing the heart rate by artificial electrical stimulation with pulses of long duration in the dog, Circulation **28**:759, 1963.

Lotto, A.: Report on one year of clinical activity of the coronary unit of the resuscitation department of the Policlinico Universitario of Milan, Boll. Soc. Ital. Cardiol. **15**:434-446, 1970.

Lowenstein, E., et al.: Cardiovascular response to large doses of intravenous morphine in man, N. Engl. J. Med. **281**:1389-1393, 1969.

Lowery, B. D,. et al.: Electrolyte solutions in resuscitation in human hemorrhagic shock, Surg. Gynecol. Obstet. **133**:273-284, 1971.

Lown, B.: Are mobile coronary care units the answer? Hosp. Pract. **4**:1-2, 1969.

Lown, B.: Cardioversion, Calif. Med. **110**:441-444, 1969.

Lown, B.: Cardioversion, J. Med. Assoc. Ga. **58**:320-322, 1969.

Lown, B.: Cardioversion, J. Iowa Med. Soc. **59**:430-433, 1969.

Lown, B.: Cardioversion. J. Kans. Med. Soc. **70**:328-330, 1969.

Lown, B.: Cardioversion. J. Okla. Med. Assoc. **62**:285-288, 1969.

Lown, B.: Cardioversion. S. D. J. Med. **22**:21-23, 1969.

Lown, B.: Approaches to sudden death from coronary heart disease, Circulation **44**:130-142, 1971.

Lown, B., and Kosowsky, B. D.: Artificial cardiac pacemakers, N. Engl. J. Med. **283**:907-916, 971-977, 1023-1031, 1970.

Lown, B., and Selzer, A.: The coronary care unit, Am. J. Cardiol. **22**:597-602, 1969.

Lown, B., and Vassaux, C.: Lidocaine in acute myocardial infarction, Am. Heart J. **76**:586-587, 1968.

Lown, B., et al.: New method for terminating cardiac arrhythmias. Use of synchronized capacitor discharge, J.A.M.A. **182**:548-555, 1962.

Lown, B., et al.: Unresolved problems in coronary care, Am. J. Cardiol. **20**:494-508, 1967.

Lown, B., et al.: Role of intensive care centers in the treatment of myocardial infarct, Presse Med. **75**:1767-1772, 1967.

Lown, B., et al.: Coronary and precoronary care, Am. J. Med. **46**:705-724, 1969.

Lubell, D. L.: Cardiac pacing from the esophagus, Am. J. Cardiol. **27**:641-644, 1971.

Lucas, B. G.: Prevention and management of heart arrest, Rev. Bras. Anest. **19**:86-89, 1969.

Ludewig, R. M., et al.: Effect of external counterpressure on venous bleeding, Surgery **66**:515-520, 1969.

Luger, G. W., et al.: Recurrent ventricular fibrillation after myocardial infarct treated with propanolol (Inderal), Ned. Tijdschr. Geneeskd. **115**:799-801, 1971.

Lukasik, S.: Some clinical aspects of fibrillation and ventricular arrest, Przegl. Lek. **25**:817-818, 1969.

Lumsden, T.: Observation on the respiratory centres, J. Physiol. 57:354-367, 1923.

Lundsgaard-Hansen, P.: Surgical aspects of cardiac metabolism, Surg. Gynecol. Obstet. 122:1095-1108, 1966.

Lundsgaard-Hansen, P.: Surgery and basic research: induced heart arrest, Schweiz. Med. Wochenschr. 96:839-845, 1966.

Lyon, L. J., et al.: Temporary control of ventricular arrhythmias by drug-induced sinus tachycardia, Arch. Intern. Med. 123:436-438, 1969.

McAlpine, F. S.: Cardiopulmonary resuscitation: the anesthesiologist's role, Med. Clin. North Am. 53:385-396, 1969.

McCall, M. M.: Cardiac arrest and resuscitation, Coll. Works Cardiopulm. Dis. 15:84-95, 1969.

McCarthy, C.: Survival after "cardiac arrest" in ischaemic heart disease: a long-term followup, Ir. J. Med. Sci. 7:545-549, 1968.

McCarthy, C., et al.: Prognosis of atrial arrhythmias treated by electrical countershock therapy, Br. Heart J. 31:496-500, 1969.

McCarthy, J.: Cardiac arrest, Nurs. Times 66:1178, 1970.

McCord, C. W., et al.: Preservation of cation exchange mechanism in the revived dog cadaver heart, Surg. Forum 20:143-145, 1969.

McDonahay, D. R., et al.: Clinical experiences with permanent demand pacemakers, Mayo Clin. Proc. 46:44-51, 1971.

McFarlane, J., et al.: Ventricular defibrillation with single and multiple half sinusoidal pulses of current, Cardiovasc. Res. 5:286-292, 1971.

McGinn, J. T.: Indomethacin for pericarditis, N. Engl. J. Med. 279:436, 1968.

McGraw, W. C.: Cardiopulmonary resuscitation in the elderly patient, Am. Geriatr. Soc. 17:159-162, 1969.

McHenry, M. M.: Cardiac monitoring in a community hospital, Calif. Med. 108:179-187, 1968.

McHenry, P. L., et al.: Right precordial QRS pattern due to left anterior hemiblock, Am. Heart J. 81:498-502, 1971.

McIlwain, H., and Rodnight, R.: Practical neurochemistry, London, 1962, J. & A. Churchill, Ltd., p. 177.

McKegney, F. P.: The intensive care syndrome, Conn. Med. 30:633-636, 1966.

McLaughlin, J. S.: Cardiogenic factor in shock, South. Med. J. 61:767-771, 1968.

McLean, K. H., et al.: A coronary care unit: results of the first year of operation, Med. J. Aust. 1:471-476, 1968.

McNamee, B. T., et al.: Long-term prognosis following ventricular fibrillation in acute ischaemic heart disease, Br. Med. J. 4:204-206, 1970.

McTaggart, D., et al.: Coronary care in a provincial hospital, Med. J. Aust. 1:965-967, 1969.

McWilliams, V.: Some thoughts on resuscitation, Nurs. Times 65:366, 1969.

Macaulay, M. B., et al.: Syncope in myxoedema due to transient ventricular fibrillation, Postgrad. Med. J. 47:361-363, 1971.

MacConaill, M.: Critical potassium concentration for the persistence of ventricular fibrillation, Rev. Can. Biol. 27:361-363, 1968.

MacFarlane, J. K., et al.: Effects of left heart bypass in experimental cardiogenic shock, J. Thorac. Cardiovasc. Surg. 57:214-224, 1969.

MacGregor, J. K., et al.: Serious complications and sudden death in the Pickwickian syndrome, Johns Hopkins Med. J. 126:279-295, 1970.

Macieira-Coelho, E., et al.: Atrial activity following conversion of experimental atrial fibrillation by direct current shock, Acta Cardiol. (Brux.) 23:439-453, 1968.

Mackay, R. S., and Leeds, S. E.: Physiological effects of condenser discharges with application to tissue stimulation and ventricular defibrillation, J. Appl. Physiol. 6:67-75, 1953.

Mackenzie, J. W., et al.: Clinical use of the micromodule pacemaker receiver, Surgery 59:944-949, 1966.

MacMillan, R. L., and Brown, K. W.: Cardiac arrest remembered, Can. Med. Assoc. J. 104:889-890, 1971.

Magidson, O.: Resection of postmyocardial infarction ventricular aneurysms for cardiac arrhythmias, Dis. Chest 56:211-220, 1970.

Maginn, R. R.: Estimation of cardiac viability following arrest, Surg. Forum 19:153-155, 1968.

Maher, P. H.: First annual report on the results of intensive coronary care at the Greenwich Hospital Association, Conn. Med. 33:177-180, 1969.

Majid, P. A., et al.: Autonomic control of insulin secretion and the treatment of heart failure, Br. Med. J. 4:328-334, 1970.

Making sure breath isn't wasted, Emergency Med. 1:21-23+, 1969.

Maksimov, D. G., et al.: On ECG changes during extinction of cardiac activity, Fiziol. Zh. S.S.S.R. 54:942-946, 1968.

Malach, M.: Digitalis for congestive heart failure with heart block in acute myocardial infarction, Am. Heart J. 76:18-20, 1968.

Malach, M., et al.: Lidocaine for ventricular arrhythmias in acute myocardial infarction, Am. J. Med. Sci. 257:52-60, 1969.

Malaplate, M., et al.: Diazepam (Valium) in anesthesia-resuscitation, Laval Med. 42:124-128, 1971.

Malek, P., et al.: Effect of mercury derivatives of

fluorescein on the fibrillation threshold in experimental myocardial infarction, Experientia
27:273, 1971.

Malin, L.: Technical trends in instrumental resuscitation. Problems of its use in first aid. Apparatus, technics, and related problems in
respiratory and cardiocirculatory resuscitation,
Arcisped. S. Anna Ferrara **22:**393-462, 1969.

Malm, O. J.: Treatment of acidosis and electrolyte disturbances in asphyxia and cardiac arrest,
Acta Anaesthesiol. Scand. (Suppl.) **29:**165+,
1968.

Maloof, J. A., et al.: Hemodynamics in closed
chest compression—report of a case, Ala. J.
Med. Sci. **6:**106-110, 1969.

Malovichko, A., et al.: Use of tetraolean in resuscitation, Farm. Zh. **26:**90-91, 1971.

Manchester, J. H., et al.: Reversion of atrial
fibrillation following hyperkalemia, Chest **58:**
398-402, 1970.

Mandal, A. K., et al.: Potassium and cardiac
surgery, Ann. Thorac. Surg. **7:**428-437, 1969.

Manieri, L., et al.: Cardiac arrest during fluo-
thane-ether anesthesia, Acta Anaesthesiol. (Padova) **18:**235-238, 1967.

Man-made hearts go into gear, Med. World News
10:34-35, 1969.

Mann, D.: The efficiency of isoprenaline in acute
cardiac and circulatory arrest, Z. Gesamte Inn.
Med. **24**(Suppl.):48-50, 1969.

Mann, F. C., et al.: Transplantation of the intact
mammalian heart, Arch. Surg. **26:**219, 1933.

Manni, C., et al.: Death and resuscitation in
drowning, Minerva Anesthesiol. **36:**381-478,
1970.

Manning, G. W., et al.: Vagus stimulation and
the production of myocardial damage, Can.
Med. Assoc. J. **37:**314-318, 1937.

Marchand, P.: Cardiac arrest and resuscitation,
S. Afr. Med. J. **38:**479-484, 1964.

Marchand, P., et al.: Long-pulse stimuli for cardiac pacing, Ann. N. Y. Acad. Sci. **167:**706-
717, 1969.

Margolis, J.: Complete heart block: procrastination suggested in using pacemaker, J.A.M.A.
212:1524-1525, 1970.

Marinescu, V., et al.: Some peculiar aspects in
the treatment of cardiac arrest, J. Cardiovasc.
Surg. (Torino) **12:**181-184, 1971.

Marinescu, V., et al.: The treatment of cardiac
asystole with cardiac electric stimulators, Med.
Interna (Bucur.) **19:**967-975, 1967.

Maroon, J. C., et al.: Detection of minute venous
air emboli with ultrasound, Surg. Gynecol.
Obstet. **127:**1236-1238, 1968.

Marriott, H. J. L.: Management of cardiac dys-

rhythmias complicating acute myocardial infarction, Geriatrics **23:**147-156, 1968.

Marriott, H. J. L.: Arrhythmias in myocardial infarction, Chest **57:**575-576, 1970.

Marriott, H. J. L.: Constant monitoring for cardiac dysrhythmias and blocks, Mod. Concepts
Cardiovasc. Dis. **39:**103-108, 1970.

Martin, A.: Disorders of cardiac rhythm and conduction: their diagnosis and management, Chicago Med. Sch. Q. **28:**145-178, 1969.

Martin, D. R., et al.: Primary cause of unsuccessful liver and heart preservation: cold sensitivity
of the ATPase system, Ann. Surg. **175:**111-117,
1972.

Martincik, J., et al.: Pregnancy cardiopathy as
cause of death, Zentralbl. Gynaekol. **92:**1677-
1680, 1970.

Martino, R. A., et al.: Myocardial function
after electrically-induced ventricular fibrillation,
Am. J. Cardiol. **24:**537-543, 1969.

Martinoli, E.: Ventricular tachycardia caused by
a pacemaker, Minerva Med. **61:**5420-5424, 1970.

Marty, A. T., et al.: High oncotic pressure effects
of dextrans, Arch. Surg. **101:**421-424, 1970.

Maslov, V. I.: Treatment of brain disorders following the occurrence of clinical death, Khirurgiia (Mosk.) **41:**103-107, 1965.

Massion, W. H., et al.: Effect of biventricular
massage on barbiturate-induced circulatory arrest, J. Thorac. Cardiovasc. Surg. **63:**230-234,
1972.

Maternal deaths due to cardiac arrest after spinal
anesthesia, Ohio Med. J. **65:**264-266, 1969.

Mathews, E. C., et al.: Q-T prolongation and
ventricular arhythmias with and without deafness in the same family, Am. J. Cardiol. **29:**702-
711, 1972.

Mathivat, A.: External electric shock in the treatment of fibrillation and auricular flutter, Sem.
Ther. **44:**342-344, 1968.

Mattern, W. D., et al.: Oliguric acute renal failure and malignant hypertension, Am. J. Med.
52:187, 1972.

Mattila, M. A.: Artificial ventilation during cardiopulmonary resuscitation, Duodecin **85:**753-
757, 1969.

Mattioli, G., et al.: Control of ventricular fibrillation by means of coupled electrical stimulation (clinical case), Boll. Soc. Ital. Cardiol.
12:449-452, 1967.

Maurer, W., et al.: Cardiac arrest outside the
clinic. Report of cases of closed and additional
successful open heart massage at the Zah-
narztlichen Institute, Schweiz. Med. Wochenschr. **96:**466-468, 1966.

Max resuscitation trolley, Biomed. Eng. **4:**30,
1969.

Mayer, E. T.: Distribution pattern of cerebral cortex damages following heart arrest and circulatory collapse, Verh. Dtsch. Ges. Pathol. 51:371-376, 1967.

Maynard, D., et al.: Device for continuous monitoring of cerebral activity in resuscitated patients, Br. Med. J. 4:545-546, 1969.

Mayo MD picks up the beat, Med. World News 10:346, 1969.

Mazchenko, N. S.: Heart arrest following administration of Lysthenon, Vestn. Khir. 105:124-125, 1970.

Mazur, L.: Two cardiac arrests during laryngectomy, Otolaryngol. Pol. 22:733-735, 1968.

Mazze, R. I., et al.: Hyperkalemia and cardiovascular collapse following administration of succinylcholine to the traumatized patient, Anesthesiology 31:540-548, 1969.

Mazzel, E. S.: Stopping of the heart in internal medicine, Prensa Med. Argent. 54:93-97, 1967.

Meijler, F. L., et al.: Paired stimulation of the heart, Acta Cardiol. (Brux.) 23:1-22, 1968.

Meitus, M.: Fetal electrocardiography and cardioversion with direct current countershock, Dis. Chest 48:324, 965.

Melotte, G.: Cardio-respiratory arrest during dental anesthesia. A concise routine of treatment, Practitioner 203:211-215, 1969.

Merle D'Aubigné, R., et al.: Peroperative electrocution and cardiac resuscitation, Cah. Anesthiol. 16:245-253, 1968.

Messinger, W. J., and Mirkinson, A. M.: Permanent atrial standstill. Eight-year observation of a patient, Arch. Intern. Med. 124:211-214, 1969.

Meyer, J. S., et al.: Cerebral autoregulation and "dysautoregulation" and their relation to cerebral vascular symptoms, Curr. Concepts Cerebrovasc. Dis. 6:1-5, 1971.

Meyer, O., et al.: Heart arrest in neuroleptoanalgesia, Anaesthesist 17:24-26, 1968.

Meyer, P., et al.: Syncopal crisis in the course of attacks of paroxysmal tachycardia caused by total cardiac pauses and by ventricular fibrillation, Arch. Mal. Coeur 64:289-295, 1971.

Michael, A.: Resuscitation: various results during the past decades, Lyon Med. 221:1129-1132, 1969.

Michelinakis, E., et al.: Circulatory arrest and bone cement, Br. Med. J. 3:639, 1971.

Michenfelder, J. D., et al.: Air embolism during neurosurgery, J.A.M.A. 206:1353-1358, 1969.

Michie, D. D.: Use of active notch filtration with electrically-induced cardiac asystole to establish zero blood flow for in vivo flowmeter calibration, Angiology 22:244-250, 1971.

Middleton, G. W.: Beach rescue trolley, Br. Med. J. 1:231, 1970.

Milhaud, A., et al.: Use of lignocain in the treatment of the hyperexcitability syndrome of recent myocardial infarct, Arch. Mal. Coeur 62:1474-1484, 1969.

Miller, A., et al.: Use of oxygen inhalation in evaluation of respiratory acidosis in patients with apparent metabolic alkalosis, Am. J. Med. 45:513-519, 1968.

Miller, D. S., et al.: Quinidine-induced recurrent ventricular fibrillation: treated with transvenous pacemaker, South. Med. J. 64:597-601, 1971.

Miller, H. J.: Paroxysmal atrial tachysystole with exit block, J. Electrocardial. 4:80-82, 1971.

Miller, J. R., et al.: Neurological sequelae of systemic circulatory arrest, Neurology (Minneap.) 18:181, 1968.

Miller, R. D., et al.: Pneumothorax during infant resuscitation, J.A.M.A. 210:1090-1091, 1969.

Milligan, J. E., et al.: The effect of pretreatment with hyperbaric oxygen on the response to anoxia and survival on resuscitation in newborn rabbits, Am. J. Obstet. Gynecol. 103:504-510, 1969.

Milliken, J. A.: Recurrent ventricular fibrillation treated by multiple countershocks, Can. Med. Assoc. J. 100:295-297, 1969.

Milliken, R. A.: An explosion hazard due to an imperfect design, Arch. Surg. 105:125-127, 1972.

Miloschewsky, D., et al.: Cardiovascular collapse following induction with propanidid, Br. J. Anaesth. 42:833, 1970.

Minuck, M., and Perkins, R.: Long-term study of patients successfully resuscitated following cardiac arrest, Can. Med. Assoc. J. 100:1126-1128, 1969.

Minuck, M., et al.: Long-term study of patients successfully resuscitated following cardiac arrest, Anesth. Analg. (Cleve.) 49:115-118, 1970.

Mironova, I. P., et al.: On the problem of complications during therapy of cardiac defibrillation using thiopental anesthesia, Ter. Arkh. 39:117-118, 1967.

Mirowski, M., et al.: Standby automatic defibrillator—an approach to prevention of sudden coronary death, Arch. Intern. Med. 126:158-161, 1970.

Mirowski, M., et al.: Automatic defibrillation, J.A.M.A. 217:946, 1971.

Mirowski, M., et al.: Prevention of sudden coronary death through automatic detection and treatment of ventricular fibrillation using a single intravascular catheter system, Circulation 44:11-124, 1971.

Mirowski, M., et al.: Ventricular defibrillation

through a single intravascular catheter electrode system, Clin. Res. **19**:328, 1971.

Mirowski, M., et al.: Transvenous automatic defibrillator—preliminary clinical tests of its defibrillating subsystem, Trans. Am. Soc. Artif. Intern. Organs **18**:520-524, 1972.

Mise, J., et al.: Management of life prolongation at the terminal stage and its discontinuation, Naika **23**:839-844, 1969.

Mitsui, T., et al.: Optimal heart rate in cardiac pacing in coronary sclerosis and non-sclerosis, Ann. N. Y. Acad. Sci. **167**:745-755, 1969.

Mittra, B.: Effects of potassium, glucose and insulin therapy on cardiac arrest after myocardial infarction, Ir. J. Med. Sci. **7**:373-385, 1968.

Miturzynska-Stryjecka, H., and Widmoskaba-Czekajska, T.: Disturbances of acid-base equilibrium and blood oxygenation during cardiac arrest and resuscitation, Pol. Tyg. Lek. **27**:50, 1972.

Miyashita, H., et al.: Present status of coronary care units, Saishin. Igaku. **23**:91-97, 1968.

Mizuguchi, K., et al.: Cardiac arrest induced by succinylcholine, Jap. J. Anesthiol. **17**:672-676, 1968.

Mobin-Uddin, K., et al.: Experimental prevention of myocardial infarction by bronchial collateral circulation, J.A.M.A. **208**:301-306, 1969.

Moffitt, E. A., et al.: Postoperative care in open-heart surgery, J.A.M.A. **199**:129-131, 1967.

Mohri, H., et al.: The challenge of prolonged suspended animation, Surg. Forum **18**:216-218, 1967.

Mohri, H., et al.: Challenge of prolonged suspended animation a method of surface-induced deep hypothermia, Ann. Surg. **168**:779-787, 1968.

Mollaret, P., and Goulon, M.: Le come dépassé (memoire preliminaire), Rev. Neurol. (Paris) **101**:3-15, 1959.

Montemurro, G., et al.: On a case of cardiac arrest during atrial fibrillation, Boll. Soc. Ital. Cardiol. **13**:837-833, 1968.

Morales, A. R., et al.: Cardiac surgery and myocardial necrosis, Arch. Pathol. **83**:71-79, 1967.

Morely, A., et al.: Resuscitation and the nurse. Measures she can take, Nurs. Times **66**:814-815, 1970.

Morely, A., et al.: The nurse and the machine-dependent patient, Nurs. Times **66**:849-852, 1970.

Morikawa, M., et al.: Ventricular fibrillation ascribed to intravenous atropine during nitrous oxide-halothane anesthesia, Jap. J. Anesthiol. **17**:479-481, 1968.

Morin, J. E., et al.: A safe technique for battery change in Cordis pacemaker, J. Thorac. Cardiovasc. Surg. **59**:721-722, 1970.

Morisot, P., et al.: On a case of cardiac arrest during surgery, caused by mediastinal emphysema in a patient under controlled artificial respiration, Anesth. Analg. (Paris) **24**:43-51, 1967.

Morris, A., et al.: Epithelial inclusion cysts of the heart, Arch. Pathol. **77**:36-40, 1965.

Morris, J. F., et al.: Comparative study of two hand-held respirators, J.A.M.A. **211**:802-803, 1970.

Morrow, A. G., et al.: Experimental evaluation of a radioisotope-powered cardiac pacemaker, J. Thorac. Cardiovasc. Surg. **60**:836-841, 1970.

Morrow, D. H., et al.: Cardiac asystole following intravenous administration of aqueous penicillin, Anesth. Analg. (Cleve.) **48**:55-57, 1969.

Mortality Study Committee: Case number 202-286. Related to surgery and anesthesia, Manit. Med. Rev. **50**:18, 1970.

Mortara, F., et al.: Contribution of the floating catheter during respiratory resuscitation of patients with chronic pulmonary diseases, Maroc Med. **49**:402-410, 1969.

Moss, A. J.: Oxygenation of the heart, Hosp. Pract. **6**:104-111, 1971.

Moss, G. S., et al.: Emergency treatment of hemorrhagic shock, Const. Surg. **1**:43-47, 1971.

Mossad, B.: Anesthesia in complete heart block, J. Egypt Med. Assoc. **52**:434-441, 1969.

Most, A. S., et al.: Myocardial infarction surveillance in a metropolitan community, J.A.M.A. **208**:2433-2438, 1969.

Motté, G.: Ventricular fibrillation, Ann. Cardiol. Angeiol. (Paris) **18**:45-55, 1969.

Motté, G., et al.: Ventricular fibrillation occurring on the public street (apropos of a case treated with success), Bull. Soc. Med. Hop. Paris **119**:941-948, 1968.

Motté, G., et al.: Treatment of rhythm disorders and cardiac arrest, Presse Med. **78**:229-332, 1970.

Moulder, P. V., et al.: Pressure-derivative loop for left ventricular resuscitation, Arch. Surg. **96**:323-327, 1968.

Moulijn, A. C., et al.: Cardiac arrest in the surgical treatment of coronary artery disease, J. Cardiovasc. Surg. (Torino)**12**:172-173, 1971.

Moulopoulos, S. D., et al.: Diastolic balloon pumping (with carbon dioxide) in the aorta—a mechanical assistance to the failing circulation, Am. Heart J. **63**:699,1962.

Mounsey, P.: Intensive coronary care. Arrhythmias after acute myocardial infarction, Am. J. Cardiol. **20**:475-483, 1967.

Mower, M. M., et al.: Endomyocardial effects of

intraventricular countershock, Clin. Res. **19:** 330, 1971.

Mower, M. M., et al.: Low energy levels for intra-ventricular defibrillation, Clin. Res. **19:** 330, 1971.

Mower, M. M., et al.: The effects of intra-atrial and intra-ventricular countershock on the surrounding myocardium, Circulation **44:**11-203, 1971.

Mower, M. M., et al.: Assessment of various models of acetylcholine induced atrial fibrillation for study of intra-atrial cardioversion Clin. Res. **20:**388, 1972.

Mower, M. M., et al.: Ventricular defibrillation with a single intravascular catheter system having distal electrode in left pulmonary artery and proximal electrode in right ventricle or right atrium, Clin. Res. **20:**389, 1972.

Mrosovsky, N.: Lowered body temperature, learning and behaviour. In Fisher, K. C., et al., editors: Mammalian hibernation, Edinburgh, 1967, Oliver & Boyd, Ltd., pp. 152-175.

Mueller, H., et al.: The effects of intra-aortic counterpulsation on cardiac performance and metabolism in shock associated with acute myocardial infarction, J. Clin. Invest. **50:**1885-1900, 1971.

Muggia, A. L., et al.: Complete heart block with thyrotoxic myocarditis, N. Engl. J. Med. **283:** 1099-1100, 1970.

Mulder, D. G., et al.: Epicardial pacemaker implantation for complete heart block, Ann. Thorac. Surg. **6:**424-430, 1968.

Mulder, J. A.: A successful resuscitation? Ned. Tidjschr. Geneeskd. **114:**1774-1777, 1970.

Mullanney, P. J.: Acute immersion syndrome, Postgrad. Med. **48:**89-91, 1970.

Muller, H. R., et al.: Long term results after reanimation by transthoracic cardiac massage (EEG and EMG observations), Rev. Neurol. (Paris) **117:**515-516, 1967.

Mundth, E. D., et al.: Circulatory assistance and emergency direct coronary-artery surgery for shock complicating acute myocardial infarction, N. Engl. J. Med. **283:**1382-1384, 1970.

Mundth, E. D., et al.: Evaluation of methods for myocardial protection during extended periods of aortic cross-clamping and hypoxic cardiac arrest, Bull. Soc. Int. Chir. **29:**227-235, 1970.

Mundth, E. D., et al.: Myocardial revascularization for the treatment of cardiogenic shock complicating acute myocardial infarction, Surgery **70:**78-87, 1971.

Muntoni, E., et al.: Total hemodilution and anoxic arrest as the procedure of choice in open heart surgery, Arch. Chir. Torac. Cardiovasc. **26:**1-7, 1970.

Murnaghan, M. F.: Comparative effectiveness of lignocaine, quinidine, propanolol and procainamide as antifibrillatory agents, Br. J. Pharmacol. **40:**149P, 1970.

Murnaghan, M. F.: Sensitization by low temperature of the isolated perfused heart to induced ventricular fibrillation, Pfluegers Arch. **325:**125-138, 1971.

Murphy, K. F., et al.: Mask vs. intubation in resuscitation, Ann. Intern. Med. **73:**338-339, 1970.

Myers, M. B., and Cherry, G.: Ventricular fibrillation area thresholds in the dog and pig, J. Thorac. Cardiovasc. Surg. **59:**401-412, 1969.

Mykyta, L. J., et al.: A system of emergency resuscitation in a general hospital, Med. J. Aust. **1:**1352, 1971.

Myocardial contraction in normal and failing hearts, Med. J. Aust. **2:**55, 1970.

Nachlas, M. M., and Siedband, M. P.: The influence of diastolic augmentation on infarct size following coronary artery ligation, J. Thorac. Cardiovasc. Surg. **53:**698, 1967.

Nachnani, G. H., et al.: Systolic murmurs induced by pacemaker catheters, Arch. Intern. Med. **124:**202-205, 1969.

Naess, K.: Nasal obstruction as a cause of sudden death, J.A.M.A. **206:**2742, 1968.

Nahum, L. H.: When to use a transvenous catheter pacemaker, Conn. Med. **34:**393-394, 1970.

Najafi, H., et al.: Postmyocardial infarction left ventricular aneurysm, Arch. Surg. **98:**766-770, 1969.

Najafi, H., et al.: Left ventricular hemorrhagic necrosis, Ann. Thorac. Surg. **7:**550-561, 1969.

Najafi, H., et al.: Acute coronary insufficiency and life-threatening cardiac arrhythmias eight months after triple heart valve replacement, Surg. Clin. North Am. **50:**119-127, 1970.

Najafi, H., et al.: Emergency left ventricular aneurysmectomy for dying patients, Ann. Thorac. Surg. **10:**327-333, 1970.

Nakae, S., et al.: Extended survival of the normothermic anoxic heart with metabolic inhibitors, Ann. Thorac. Surg. **3:**37-42, 1967.

Nakagawa, A.: Comparative studies on the methods of deliberately induced cardiac arrest with special reference to the left ventricular function curve, J. Kumamoto Med. Soc. **42:**1-40, 1968.

Nakamaru, Y., and Schwartz, A.: The influence of hydrogen ion concentration on calcium binding and release by skeletal muscle sarcoplasmic reticulum, J. Gen. Physiol. **59:**22-32, 1972.

Nakhjaven, F. K., et al.: Experimental myocardial infarction in dogs. Description of a closed chest technique, Circulation **38:**777-782, 1968.

Naney, A. P.: Diazepam for cardioversion, J.A.M.A. 215:487, 1971.

Nargiello, E., et al.: Cardiac arrest with recovery following hypothermia, J. Med. Soc. N. J. 59:292-295, 1962.

Narula, O. S., et al.: Localization of A-V conduction defects in man by recording of the bundle of His electrogram, Am. J. Cardiol. 25:228-238, 1970.

Narula, O. S., et al.: Atroventricular block. Localization and classification by His bundle recordings, Am. J. Med. 50:146-165, 1971.

Narula, O. S., et al.: Significance of first degree A-V block, Circulation 43:772-774, 1971.

Nathan, D. A., et al.: Synchronization of ventricle with atrium in complete heart block by a self-contained implantable pacer. Experimental data, Circulation 26:767, 1962.

Nava, A., et al.: Paroxysmal tachycardia and ventricular fibrillation in patients with a regularly operating pacemaker, Folia Cardiol. (Milano) 28:157-170, 1969.

Neaverson, M. A., et al.: Sudden unexpected death, Med. J. Aust. 2:667-669, 1967.

Neeling, A. de: Quinidine syncope and death, Ned. Tijdschr. Geneeskd. 112:233-237, 1968.

Negovskii, V. A.: Quelques problèmes de reanimation experimentale et clinique, Probl. Reanim. 5:189-209, 1968.

Negovskii, V. A.: Aspects metaboliques et toxemiques de l'irreversibilite de la mort clinique, Agressologie 9:393-400, 1968.

Negovskii, V. A.: The second step in resuscitation—the treatment of the "post-resuscitation disease," Resuscitation 1:1-8, 1972.

Negovskii, V. A., et al.: O Reanimatsil v travmatologiki, Ortop. Travmatol. Protez. 27:3-11, 1966.

Negovskii, V. A., et al.: Primenenia tham'a dlia bor'by s atsidozom v terminal'nykh sostoianiiakh, vyzannykh kropotere, Ortop. Travmatol. Protez. 27:30-35, 1966.

Negovskii, V. A., et al.: Utilisation d'une impulsion electrique unique pour arrêter les hemorragies par atonic uterine, Sem. Ther. 42:53-54, 1966.

Negovskii, V. A., et al.: Arterial versus venous transfusion in cardiac arrest from exsanguination: further studies in dogs, Anesth. Analg. (Cleve.) 51:251-257, 1972.

Neligan, M. A., et al.: Experience with the Abrams-Lucas inductively coupled cardiac pacemaker, Ir. J. Med. Sci. 140:53-59, 1971.

Nelson, R. M., et al.: Differential atrial arrhythmias in cardiac surgical patients, J. Thorac. Cardiovasc. Surg. 58:581-587, 1969.

Nesmith, M. A., Jr.: A case of lightning stroke, J. Fla. Med. Assoc. 58:36-37, 1971.

Neville, J., et al.: An implantable demand pacemaker, Clin. Res. 14:256, 1966.

Neville, W. E., et al.: Microcirculation of the transplanted heart, J. Thorac. Cardiovasc. Surg. 58:625-637, 1969.

Nevins, M. A.: Drug-pacemaker interactions, J. Thorac. Cardiovasc. Surg. 61:610-616, 1971.

Nevins, M. A.: Ventricular arrhythmias and diazepam, J.A.M.A. 215:643, 1971.

Nevins, M. A., et al.: Failure of demand pacemaker sensing due to electrode fracture, Chest 59:110-113, 1971.

New anti-arrhythmic agent (disopyramide) tested for safety, efficacy, J.A.M.A. 213:697-698, 1970.

New concept holds promise as life saver, Am. Heart 19:1-2, 1969.

Ngai, S. H., et al.: Physiologic aspects of anesthesiology, N. Engl. J. Med 282:541-554, 1970.

Niazi, S. A., and Lewis, F. J.: Tolerance of adult rats to profound hypothermia and simultaneous cardiac arrest, Surgery 36:25-32, 1954.

Niazi, S. A., and Lewis, F. J.: Profound hypothermia in the dog, Surg. Gynecol. Obstet. 102:98-106, 1956a.

Niazi, S. A., and Lewis, F. J.: Profound hypothermia in the monkey with recovery after long periods of standstill, J. Appl. Physiol. 10:137-138, 1956b.

Niazi, S. A., and Lewis, F. J.: Profound hypothermia in man, Ann. Surg. 147:264-266, 1958.

Nielsen, K. C.: Possible relation between the degree of cardiac adrenergic innervation and the resistance to hypothermic ventricular fibrillation in young cats, Acta Physiol. Scand 76:1-9, 1969.

Nielsen, K. C., and Owman, C.: Effect of reserpine on the spontaneous ventricular fibrillation development during induced deep hypothermia in cats, Arch. Int. Pharmacodyn. Ther. 175:412-421, 1968.

Nielsen, K. C., and Owman, C.: Control of spontaneous ventricular fibrillation during induced hypothermia in cats by acute cardiac sympathectomy, Acta Physiol. Scand. 76:73-81, 1969.

Niles, N. R.: Structure and function: why did the heart stop? Dis. Chest 56:370-371, 1969.

Nimura, Y., et al.: Analysis of a cardiac cycle of the left side of the heart in cases of left ventricular overloading or damage with the ultrasonic Doppler method, Am. Heart J. 75:49-65, 1968.

Nixon, P. G., et al.: Left ventricular diastolic pressure in cardiogenic shock treated by dextrose infusion and adrenaline, Lancet **1:**1230-1232, 1968.

Nobel, B. G.: Hints and kinks from Poor Richard's Clinical Almanac, N. C. Med. J. **30:**314-319, 1969.

Nobel, J. J.: Emergency respiratory support units, J.A.M.A. **210:**1284, 1969.

Nobel, J. J.: "Handy devices" criticized, Emergency Med. **2:**7, 1970.

Nobel, J. J., and Rauch, R. M.: Emergency resuscitation and life support vehicle, Med. Res. Eng. **7:**11-16, 1968.

Noehren, T. H., et al.: A ventilation unit for special intensive care of patients with respiratory failure, J.A.M.A. **203:**125-127, 1968.

Nolan, S. P.: John Hunter and cardiopulmonary resuscitation, Surgery **66:**611-613, 1969.

Nord, H. J., et al.: Treatment of congestive heart failure with glucagon, Ann. Intern. Med. **72:**649-653, 1970.

Norman, J. C., et al.: Surgical treatment of Adams-Stokes syndrome using long-term inductive coupled coil pacemaking, Ann. Surg. **159:**344-361, 1964.

Norman, J. C., et al.: Implantable nuclear-powered cardiac pacemaker, N. Engl. J. Med. **283:**1203-1206, 1970.

Norris, R. M.: Acute coronary care, N. Z. Med. J. **67:**470-476, 1968.

Norris, R. M.: Bradyarrhythmia after myocardial infarction, Lancet **1:**313-314, 1969.

Norris, R. M.: Long-term survival after cardiac arrest, N. Z. Med. J. **69:**144-146, 1969.

Norton, L., et al.: Gastric secretory response to pressure on vagal nuclei, Am. J. Surg. **123:**13-18, 1972.

Novey, H. S.: Alarming reaction after intravenous administration of 30 ml. of epinephrine, J.A.M.A. **207:**2435-2436, 1969.

Nowicki, J.: Induced cardiac arrest during open heart surgery, J. Cardiovasc. Surg. (Torino) **12:**157-160, 1971.

Nusbaum, M., et al.: Technic for permanent implantation of atrial pacemaker, Surgery **68:**916-918, 1970.

Obel, P. I., and Marchand, P.: Successful treatment of vagotomy of 2 patients with peptic ulcer and Stokes-Adams (vasovagal) syncope, Am. J. Cardiol. **28:**731-734, 1971.

O'Brien, F.: The attack on heart attacks, Washington U. Mag. **40:**4-12, 1970.

O'Connell, T. G.: An appraisal of cardiac pacemaking, Ir. J. Med. Sci. **8:**123-131, 1969.

O'Higgins, J. W., et al.: The effect of helium inhalation on asphyxia in dogs, J. Thorac. Cardiovasc. Surg. **61:**870-874, 1971.

Ohler, R. L.: The coronary care unit. Data-

phone as a means of providing 24-hour physician coverage, J. Maine Med. Assoc. **60:**162-164, 1969.

Ohresser, P.: Resuscitation of the myasthenic patient after thymectomy, Ann. Chir. **25:**531-532, 1971.

Ohresser, P., et al.: Technic and current results in the treatment of heart disease, Mars. Med. **105:**613-615, 1968.

Okel, B. B.: Vertebral fracture from cardioversion shock, J.A.M.A. **203:**369, 1968.

Okros, S.: Ultrastructural changes of myofibrils following acute heart failure "paralysis cordis," Acta Med. Leg. Soc. (Liege) **20:**197-198, 1967.

Oliver, M. F., et al.: Relation between serum-free acute myocardial arrhythmias and death after acute myocardial infarction, Lancet **1:**710-714, 1968.

Olivieri, B., et al.: On a case of cardiac arrest resolved by intracardiac injection of Alupent, Minerva Cardioangiol. **14:**493-498, 1966.

O'Neill, J. A., Jr., et al.: Endocrine gland gastric secretory changes induced by increased intracranial pressure, Am. J. Surg. **123:**19-25, 1972.

Open cannulation of subclavian vein is recommended, Mod. Med. **38:**130-131, 1970.

Orellane, L. E., et al.: Continuous measurement of potassium and sodium losses of the myocardium during a heart arrest by coronary perfusion with low sodium, calcium-free procaine containing oxygen saturated cardioplegic solutions, Arch. Kreislaufforsch. **53:**264-307, 1967.

Osborn, J. J., et al.: Respiratory causes of "sudden unexplained arrhythmia," in postthoracotomy patients, Surgery **69:**24-28, 1971.

The other end of the stick, J.A.M.A. **210:**896, 1969.

Otteni, J. C., et al.: Complications of tracheotomy: sudden death, Ann. Chir. Thorac. Cardiovasc. **6:**1171-1172, 1967.

Otteni, J. C., et al.: Continuous monitoring of the peripheral circulation with digital photoplethysmography. Its importance in anesthesia-resuscitation, Cah. Anesthesiol. **18:**735-742 passim, 1970.

Otteni, J. C., et al.: Intra-arterial blood pressure in continuous measurement by microcatheter. Indication, technic, results, Anesth. Analg. (Paris) **28:**167-182, 1971.

Overbeck, W., et al.: Historical considerations on cardiac arrest and resuscitation, Thoraxchirurgie **17:**177-184, 1969.

Oye, I., et al.: Glucagon in heart arrest, Tidsskr. Nor. Laegeforen. **91:**670, 1971 .

Pacelli, L., et al.: Resuscitation in cardiocirculatory arrest, Minerva Anestesiol. 34:1261-1270, 1968.

Pacemaker surveillance, Chest 61:204-205, 1972.

Pacifico, A. D., et al.: Equilibration of radio-potassium (K^{42}) in patients undergoing open intracardiac operations, Surgery, 69:93-96, 1971.

Paduart, P., et al.: Resuscitation in status asthmaticus, Acta Clin. Belg. 24:255-275, 1969.

Page, D. L., et al.: Myocardial changes associated with cardiogenic shock, N. Engl. J. Med. 285:134-137, 1971.

Page, I. H.: A note on harvesting human organs, Mod. Med. 38:87-88, 1970.

Paine, R.: The nervous system and the heart, Mo. Med. 62:663-667, 1965.

Pairolero, P. C., et al.: Experimental left ventricular akinesis, J. Thorac. Cardiovasc. Surg. 60:683-693, 1970.

Palich, W. E., et al.: Cardiopulmonary resuscitation of dogs: principles and practice, J. Am. Vet. Med. Assoc. 151:1719-1732, 1967.

Palohelmo, J. A.: Prolonged continuous intravenous lignocaine in myocardial infarction, Lancet 1:734-735, 1969.

Pampiglione, G., and Harden, A.: Prognostic value of neurophysiological studies in the first hours that follow resuscitation, Rev. Neurol. [Paris] 117:523-524, 1967.

Pampiglione, G., and Harden, A.: Prognostic value of neurophysiological studies in the first hours following resuscitation: a review of 120 children after cardiac arrest, Electroencephalogr. Clin. Neurophysiol. 25:91, 1968.

Pampiglione, G., and Harden, A.: Resuscitation after cardiocirculatory arrest. Prognostic evaluation of early electroencephalographic findings, Lancet 1:1261-1265, 1968.

Pannacchia, S.: Problems of anesthesia and resuscitation on board ships, Ann. Med. Nav. (Roma) 76:118-120, 1971.

Pantridge, J. F.: Cardiac arrest after myocardial infarction, Lancet 1:807-808, 1966.

Pantridge, J. F.: Bradycardia in myocardial infarction, Lancet 2:1393, 1969.

Pantridge, J. F.: The mobile coronary care unit, Hosp. Pract. 4:64-73, 1969.

Pantridge, J. F.: Mobile coronary care, Chest 58:229-234, 1970.

Pantridge, J. F., and Geddes, J. S.: A mobile intensive-care unit in the management of myocardial infarction, Lancet 2:271-273, 1967.

Pantridge, J. F., et al.: Pre-hospital coronary care, Am. J. Cardiol. 24:666-673, 1969.

Pantridge, J. F., et al.: Resuscitation ambulances, Lancet 1:250, 1970.

Pantridge, J. F., et al.: Acute phase of myocardial infarction, Lancet 2:501, 1971.

Papadopoulos, C.: Arrhythmias in myocardial infarction, Md. Med. J. 18:9305, 1969.

Pappas, G., et al.: Fractured intracardiac transvenous pacemaker. Am. Heart J. 78:807-810, 1969.

Paprocki, M., et al.: Morphologic and clinical analysis of central nervous system lesions in cases of cardiac arrest, Pol. Tyg. Lek. 22:1248-1251, 1967.

Parameshvara, V.: Intensive coronary care unit, J. Indian Med. Assoc. 50:309-312, 1968.

Parker, B. M., et al.: Extended use of cardiac pacemakers, Chest 59:244-245, 1971.

Parker, D. P., et al.: Demonstration of the supernormal period in the intact human heart as a result of pacemaker failure, Chest 59:461-446, 1971.

Parker, J. C., and Smith, E. E. Effects of xanthine oxidase inhibition in cardiac arrest, Surgery 71:339-344, 1972.

Parker, J. O.: Ventricular fibrillation complicating internal mammary artery opacification, Am. J. Cardiol. 25:376, 1970.

Parker, W. S.: Resuscitation ambulances, Lancet 1:415, 1970.

Parkinson, P. I., et al.: Survival after 204 defibrillations, Br. Med. J. 3:175, 1969.

Parmley, W. W., et al.: Glucagon: a new agent in cardiac therapy, Am. J. Cardiol. 27:298-303, 1971.

Paroxysmal tachycardia and bundle-branch block: unusual response to carotid sinus massage, J.A.M.A. 215:1157, 1971.

Parsonnet, V.: Types of pacemakers. J.A.M.A. 207:367, 1969.

Parsonnet, V., et al.: Clinical use of an implantable standby pacemaker, J.A.M.A. 196:784-786, 1966.

Parsons, D. W.: Cardiac arrest and bone cement, Br. Med. J. 3:710, 1970.

Partington, T., et al.: Rupture of the ventricular septum from myocardial infarction. Haemodynamic response to surgical treatment, Thorax 24:118-123, 1969.

Pasengrau, D. G., et al.: Hemodynamic effects of ventricular defibrillation, J. Clin. Invest. 49:282-297, 1970.

Pashchuk, A., et al.: Resuscitation in patients with severe combined injuries and uncompensated shock, Ortop. Travmatol Protez. 31:83-85, 1970.

Patient monitoring cut down to size, Med. World News 10:18, 1969.

Pattay, J.: Respiratory and cardiac resuscitation,

Schweiz. Monatsschr. Zahnheilkd. **78**:878-883, 1969.

Patterson, R. H., et al.: Filter to prevent cerebral damage during experimental cardiopulmonary bypass, Surg. Gynecol. Obstet. **132**:71-74, 1971.

Patton, R. D., et al.: Large doses of procainamide for paroxysmal ventricular tachycardia, J.A.M.A. **209**:1221-1222, 1969.

Patton, R. D., et al.: Bundle of His electrograms: a new method for analyzing arrhythmias, Am. J. Cardiol. **26**:324-327, 1970.

Patton, R. D., et al.: Pacemakers for digitalis-associated bradyarrhythmias, Chest **57**:194-196, 1970.

Paul, O.: Management of arrhythmias complicating myocardial infarction, Northwest Med. **67**:740-745, 1968.

Paulley, J. W.: Mortality among widowers, Br. Med. J. **2**:52-53, 1969.

Paulussen, F., et al.: Fine structural investigation of the myocardium during special cardioplegia with ischemia and depression of energy requirements, Verh. Dtsch. Ges. Pathol. **52**:504-510, 1968.

Paulussen, F., et al.: The fine structure of the myocardium during ischemia with depression of the energy requirement by special cardioplegia, Klin. Wochenschr. **46**:165-171, 1968.

Payne, J. P.: On the resuscitation of the apparently dead, Ann. R. Coll. Surg. Engl. **45**:98-107, 1969.

Peal, S.: Some psychologic observations of patients with myocardial infarction. A pilot study, Psychiatr. Commun. **10**:1-20, 1968.

Pearson, J. D., et al.: Cardiac arrest and arrhythmias due to self-poisoning with imipramine, Anaesthesia **24**:69-71, 1969.

Pedroni, A.: Morgagni-Adam-Stokes crisis in a patient with bradycardiac inferior nodal rhythm, Boll. Soc. Med. Chir. Cremona **25**:53-61, 1969.

Peleska, B.: Electric impulse therapy in cardiac tachyarrhythmias, IEEE Trans. Biomed. Eng. **16**:123-131, 1969.

Pellegrini, G., et al.: Coronary arteriography in cardiac arrest, Panminerva Med. **9**:585-590, 1967.

Pellegrini, G., et al.: Coronary arteriography with induced cardiac arrest. Clinical experimentation, Minerva Cardioangiol. **14**:727-731, 1966.

Pelligra, R., et al.: Anti-G suit as a therapeutic device, Aerosp. Med. **41**:943-946, 1970.

Peltola, P.: The effect of aldosterone on sodium and potassium metabolism in congestive cardiac failure, Ann. Clin. Res. **1**:286-290, 1969.

Pennington, J. E., et al.: Chest thump for reverting ventricular tachycardia, N. Engl. J. Med. **283**:1192-1195, 1970.

Pentecost, B. L., et al.: Bradyarrhythmia complicating myocardial infarction, Lancet **2**:1300-1301, 1968.

Perera, G. A.: Paroxysmal arrhythmias and migraine, J.A.M.A. **215**:488, 1971.

Peretz, D. I.: Advanced heart block during acute myocardial infarction treated with an electrode pacing catheter, Can. Med. Assoc. J. **96**:451-456, 1967.

Peretz, D. I.: Cardiac pacing in the management of advanced heart block during acute myocardial infarction, Am. Heart. J. **75**:845-846, 1968.

Perot, G. J., et al.: Anesthesia-resuscitation problems in patients with sickle cell anemia, Med. Trop. (Mars.) **29**:377-381, 1961.

Peschin, A., et al.: A five-year review of 734 cardiopulmonary arrests, South. Med. J. **63**:506-510, 1970.

Péter, V.: Basic questions of resuscitation, Fogorv. Sz. **63**:105-155, 1970.

Petracek, M. R., et al.: Effect of hyperglycemia on cardiac tolerance to normothermic anoxic arrest during cardiopulmonary bypass in dogs, Ann. Surg. **172**:1069-1075, 1970.

Petrovsky, B. V., et al.: Problems of artificial hearts and their experimental study, J. Thorac. Cardiovasc. Surg. **57**:431-441, 1969.

Petterino, E.: Clinical and organizational aspects of resuscitation. Minerva Med. **59**:5618-5628, 1968.

Petty, T. L., and Neff, T. A.: Letter to the editor: Renal function in respiratory failure, J.A.M.A. **217**:82, 1971.

Petty, T. L., et al.: A simple ventilator warning device, Inhalation Ther. **14**:67-68, 1969.

Petty, T. L., et al.: Essentials of an intensive care respiratory unit, Chest **59**:554-556, 1971.

Pevzner, M. A., et al.: Electrochemical determination of oxygen in the myocardium in controlled heart arrest with artificial circulation, Eksp. Khir. Anesthesiol. **11**:98, 1966.

Phillips, B., et al.: A comparison of central venous and arterial gas values in the critically ill, Ann. Intern. Med. **70**:745-749, 1969.

Phillips, H., et al.: Cardiovascular effects of implanted acrylic bone cement, Br. Med. J. **3**:460-461, 1971.

Phillips, J., and Ichinose, H.: Clinical and pathologic studies in the hereditary syndrome of a long QT interval, syncopal spells and sudden death, Chest **58**:236-243, 1970.

Phillips, S. J., and Butner, A. N.: Percutaneous transvenous cardiac pacing initiated at bedside: results in 40 cases, J. Thorac. Cardiovasc. Surg. **59**:855-858, 1970.

Picard, J. M., et al.: Resuscitation of electric burn patients, Therapie 26:361-369, 1971.

Picard, P., et al.: Eight years' experience with the use of modified fluid gelatin for resuscitation, Bibl. Haematol. 33:522-524, 1969.

Pierce, W. S., et al.: The development and experimental evaluation of an implantable left ventricular bypass pump, Surgery 66:1034-1043, 1969.

Pifarré, R., et al.: Helium in the prevention of ventricular fibrillation. Dis. Chest 56:135-138, 1969.

Pifarré, R., et al.: Myocardial revascularization by transmyocardial acupuncture, N. Engl. J. Med. 58:424-431, 1969.

Pifarré, R., et al.: Oxygen lung toxicity after hyperbaric oxygenation for acute myocardial infarction, Ann. Thorac. Surg. 10:300-308, 1970.

Pifarré, R., et al.: Effect of oxygen and helium mixtures on ventricular fibrillation, J. Thorac. Cardiovasc. Surg. 60:648-652, 1970.

Pike, F. H., et al.: Studies in resuscitation. II. The reflex excitability of the brain and spinal cord after cerebral anaemia, Am. J. Physiol. 21:359-371, 1908.

Pilapil, V. R.: Cardiopulmonary resuscitation in the pediatric patient, Milit. Med. 134:1510-1515, 1969.

Pitt, B., and Ross, R. S.: Beta adrenergic blockade in cardiovascular therapy, Mod. Concepts Cardiovasc. Dis. 38:47-54, 1969.

Pitzele, S., et al.: Functional evaluation of the heart after storage under hypothermic coronary perfusion, Surgery, 70:4, 569-577, 1971.

Plum, F.: Brain histology in anoxic encephalopathy after short period of apnea, J.A.M.A. 214:1895, 1970.

Poche, R., et al.: The effect of oxygen deficiency on the fine structure of the myocardium, Beitr. Pathol. 136:58-95, 1967.

Polo, M., et al.: Brief considerations on complications of local anesthetics (apropos of 3 treated cases), Acta Anaesthesiol. [Padova] 19(Suppl. 4):254+, 1968.

Pool, P. E.: Energy stores and energy utilization in the myocardium in hypertrophy and heart failure. In Alpert, N., editor: Cardiac hypertrophy, New York, 1971, Academic Press, Inc., pp. 539-547.

Poole, E.: EEG and survival, Br. Med. J. 2:157-161, 1970.

Poole, E. W.: Observations on periodic and evoked phenomena in a case of presumed cardiac arrest, Electroencephalogr. Clin. Neurophysiol. 25:509, 1969.

Pomfret, D., et al.: Dangerous complication of temporary floating pacing electrodes, N. Engl. J. Med. 280:651-652, 1969.

Popescu, P. N., et al.: Tachyarrhythmias caused by acute myocardial infarct, Med. Interna (Bucur.) 22:1443-1450, 1970.

Popova, L. M.: A clinico-morphologic analysis of decerebrate rigidity arising following resuscitation, Zh. Nevropatol. Psikhiatr. 70:1776-1784, 1970.

Popova, L. M., et al.: Analysis of the lethal outcomes in cerebral insult under conditions of respiratory resuscitation, Klin. Med. (Mosk.) 48:61-70, 1970.

Portnoi, V. F., et al.: Cerebral electrical activity in resuscitation by the artificial circulation method following long-term cardiac arrest, Patol. Fiziol. Eksp. Ter. 14:12-17, 1970.

Potassium, glucose, and insulin treatment for acute myocardial infarction, Lancet 2:1355-1360, 1969.

Potter, L. T., et al.: Synthesis, binding, release and metabolism of norepinephrine in normal and transplanted dog hearts, Circ. Res. 26:468, 1965.

Powell, J. N., et al.: Cardiac arrest associated with bone cement, Br. Med. J. 3:326, 1970.

Powell, W., et al.: Effects of intra-aortic balloon counterpulsation on cardiac performance, oxygen consumption, and coronary blood flow in dogs, Circ. Res. 26:753, 1970.

Powers, S. R., Jr., et al.: Monitoring, J. Trauma 10:1025-1040, 1970.

Practical care of the acute coronary patient, Lond. Clin. Med. J. 9:7-9, 1968.

Prasad, K., et al.: Cesium in the prevention of cardiac arrhythmias induced by coronary ligation, Surg. Forum 21:166-167, 1970.

Prior, P. F.: EEG findings in dying and resuscitated adult patients, Electroencephalogr. Clin. Neurophysiol. 27:333, 1969.

Prior, P. F., et al.: An attempt to assess the prognostic value of the EEG after cardiac arrest, Electroencephalogr. Clin. Neurophysiol. 24:593, 1968.

Priscu, R., et al.: Cardiac syncope in infants, Pediatria (Bucur.) 20:99-112, 1971.

Proctor, E., et al.: Survival in dogs after eight hours' ventricular fibrillation using total supportive perfusion by pump-oxygenator and peripheral cannulation, Guys Hosp. Rep. 118:65-74, 1969.

Proctor, E., et al.: Total circulatory support by peripheral cannulation and pump oxygenation during 8 hours of ventricular fibrillation in dog, J. Thorac. Cardiovasc. Surg. 57:702-707, 1969.

Proctor, H. J., et al.: Changes in lung compliance

in experimental hemorrhagic shock and resuscitation, Ann. Surg. **169:**82-92, 1969.

Pryor, R.: The clinical significance of left intraventricular blocks, Bull. N. Y. Acad. Med. **47:**973-986, 1971.

A punch in time and a percussive beat, Emergency Med. **3:**29, 1971.

Puri, P. S., et al.: Effect of drugs on myocardial contractility in the intact dog and in experimental myocardial infarction. Basis for their use in cardiogenic shock, Am. J. Cardiol. **21:**886-892, 1968.

Puri, P. S., et al.: Effects on myocardial contractility, hemodynamics and cardiac metabolism of a new beta-adrenergic blocking drug, Sotalol, Dis. Chest **55:**235-239, 1969.

Pyfer, H. R., et al.: Cardiac arrest during exercise training, J.A.M.A. **210:**101-102, 1969.

Quan, K. C.: Prolonged external cardiac massage, Pa. Med. **72:**62-67, 1969.

Quinidine use after fibrillation electroconversion, Mod. Med. **40:**68-69, 1972.

Rab, S. M.: Traumatic myocardial infarction, Br. J. Clin. Pract. **23:**172-173, 1969.

Radford, M. D., et al.: Long-term results of DC reversion of atrial fibrillation, Br. Heart. J. **30:**91-96, 1968.

Radushkevich, V. P., et al.: Radioisotope scanning of the liver in the recovery period after resuscitation of the organism, Khirurgiia (Mosk.) **46:**105-109, 1970.

Ragaza, E. P., et al.: Intermittent complete heart block associated with swallowing as a complication of acute myocardial infarction, Am. Heart J. **79:**386-400, 1970.

Rance, C. P.: Cardiac arrest after intravenous frusemide, Lancet **1:**1265-1266, 1969.

Randall, W. C.: The role of the autonomic nervous system in cardiac control, Heart Bull. **19:**16-21, 1970.

Ranganathan, N., et al.: Electrocardiographic clues in diagnosing syncope, Postgrad. Med. **49:**128-131, 1971.

Rassman, W., et al.: An implantable intrathoracic total and partial circulatory support system, J. Thorac. Cardiovasc. Surg. **56:**858-867, 1968.

Rastelli, G. C., et al.: Experimental study and clinical appraisal of external defibrillation with the thorax open, J. Thorac. Cardiovasc. Surg. **55:**116-122, 1968.

Rastelli, G. C., et al.: Transthoracic cannulation of the left atrium for circulatory assist, J. Thorac. Cardiovasc. Surg. **56:**879-885, 1968.

Rastogi, S. K., et al.: Cardiac emergencies, J. Indian Med. Assoc. **53:**77-83, 1969.

Ratliff, J. L., et al.: Intraventricular cardiac massage, J.A.M.A. **215:**117, 1971.

Ravagnan, R., et al.: The effectiveness of external cardiac massage, Minerva Anestesiol. **32:**533-534, 1966.

Ray, C. G., et al.: Studies in the sudden infant death syndrome in King County, Washington, J.A.M.A. **211:**619-623, 1970.

Reagan, L. B., et al.: Ventricular defibrillation in a patient with probable acute coronary occlusion, Surgery **39:**482-486, 1956.

Real replacement for morphine? Med. World News **10:**22, 1969.

Redakycyjny, A.: An analysis of the results of resuscitation management and its critical moments, Pol. Arch. Med. Wewn. **45:**613-616, 1970.

Redding, J. S.: Abdominal compression in cardiopulmonary resuscitation, Anesth. Analg. (Cleve.) **50:**668-675, 1971.

Redding, J. S., et al.: Metabolic acidosis: a factor in cardiac resuscitation, South. Med. J. **60:**926-932, 1967.

Redding, J. S., et al.: Problems in the management of drowning victims, Md. Med. J. **19:**58-61, 1970.

Regan, T. J., et al.: Myocardial K^+ loss after countershock and the relation to ventricular arrhythmias after nontoxic doses of acetyl strophanthidin, Am. Heart J. **77:**367-371, 1969.

Reich, M. P., et al.: Tissue oxygenation following resuscitation with crystalloid solution following experimental acute blood loss, Surgery **69:**928-931, 1971.

Reichenback, D. D., and Benditt, E. P.: Myocardial degeneration, Arch. Pathol. **85:**189-199, 1968.

Reidemeister, J. C., et al.: Electrocardiographic findings following cardioplegia caused by extracellular sodium and calcium deprivation and novocaine administration, Thoraxchirurgie **14:**602-609, 1966.

Reidemeister, J. C., et al.: Clinical results with cardioplegia using extracellular sodium and calcium withdrawal and procaine administration, Langenbecks Arch. Klin. Chir. **319:** 701-707, 1967.

Reidemeister, J. C., et al.: Clinical experiences in Bretschneider's cardioplegia, Thoraxchirurgie **19:**104-118, 1971.

Reidenberg, M. M.: Renal function and drug action, Philadelphia, 1971, W. B. Saunders Co.

Reier, C. E., et al.: Conscious analgesia and amnesia for cardioversion, J.A.M.A. **210:**2052-2054, 1969.

Reinhardt, D. F., et al.: Cardiac arrhythmias and aerosol "sniffing," Arch. Environ. Health **22:**265-279, 1971.

Reintoft, M.: Cardiac arrest with unchanged ECG

activity—pump failure or mechanical asystole, Nord. Med. **84**:1326-1328, 1970.

Reis, R. L., et al.: Hemodynamic effects of amniotic fluid embolism, Surg. Gynecol. Obstet. **129**:45-48, 1969.

Reis, R. L., et al.: Left ventricular function after ischemic cardioplegia, Arch. Surg. **99**:815-820, 1969.

Reis, R. L., et al.: The effects of epicardiectomy on the performance of the acutely ischemic left ventricle, J. Thorac. Cardiovasc. Surg. **56**:647-657, 1969.

Reissmann, K. A. R., and Van Citters, R. L.: Oxygen consumption and mechanical efficiency of the hypothermic heart, J. Appl. Physiol. **9**:427, 1956.

Rell, R. H., et al.: Severe hypothermia as a result of barbiturate overdose complicated by cardiac arrest, Lancet **1**:392-394, 1968.

Renal transplantation from cadavers, Br. Med. J. **3**:251, 1972 (editorial).

Replogle, R. L.: Circulatory effects of blood viscosity, Heart Bull. **18**:47-49, 1969.

Resnekov, L.: Jogging and coronary artery disease, J.A.M.A. **210**:126, 1969.

Resnekov, L.: Electroconversion of cardiac dysrhythmias, Am. Heart. J. **79**:581-586, 1970

Resnekov, L., et al.: Complications in 220 patients with cardiac dysrhythmias treated by phased direct current shock and indications for electroconversion, Br. Heart J. **29**:926-936, 1967.

Resnekov, L., et al.: Appraisal of electroconversion in treatment of cardiac dysrhythmias, Br. Heart J. **30**:786-811, 1968.

Resnekov, L., et al.: Ventricular defibrillation by monophasic trapezoidal-shaped double-pulses of low electrical energy, Cardiovasc. Res. **2**:261-264, 1968.

Resuscitation after cardiac arrest, Nurs. Times **63**:1295, 1967.

Resuscitation and survival in motor vehicle accidents, J. Trauma **9**:356, 1969.

Resuscitation of the newborn, Indian J. Pediatr. **36**:13-15, 1969.

Reul, G. J., et al.: Safety of ischemic cardiac arrest in distal coronary artery bypass, J. Thorac. Cardiovasc. Surg. **62**:511-521, 1972.

Richman, S. M.: The control of idioventricular rhythm in acute myocardial infarction by transvenous intracardiac pacing, Conn. Med. **33**:252-254, 1969.

Richmond, D. R., et al.: Electrical pacing for heart block complicating acute myocardial infarction, Med. J. Aust. **1**:476-480, 1968.

The riddle of lethal fever during anesthesia, Med. World News **11**:21, 1970.

Riga, C.: Resuscitation and intensive care depart-

ments in modern hospital, Acta Anaesthesiol. (Padova) **21**:49-61, 1970.

Riker, W. L.: Cardiac arrest in infants and children, Pediatr. Clin. North Am. **16**:661-669, 1969.

Rittenhouse, E. A., et al.: Studies of carbohydrate metabolism and serum electrolytes during surface-induced deep hypothermia with prolonged circulatory occlusion, Surgery **67**:995-1005, 1970.

Rittenhouse, E. A., et al.: Circulatory dynamics during surface-induced deep hypothermia and after cardiac arrest for one hour, J. Thorac. Cardiovasc. Surg. **61**:359-369, 1971.

Rittmeyer, P.: Intensive therapy in drowning, Hefte Unfallheilkd. **99**:54-58, 1969.

Rivera, A., Jr., et al.: Brain glycogen in the recovering asphyxiated monkey, Exp. Neurol. **26**:309-315, 1970.

Rivers, J. F., et al.: Drowning: its clinical sequelae and management, Br. Med. J. **2**:157-161, 1970.

Rizzotti, G.: Resuscitation and intensive care departments in modern hospitals. Unit premises: placement and structural characteristics, Acta Anaesthesiol. (Padova) **21**:62-68, 1970.

Roberts, B. W.: Chest thumps and the heart beat, N. Engl. J. Med. **284**:392-393, 1971.

Roberts, S., et al.: Airborne intensive care unit, Ann. Surg. **172**:325-333, 1970.

Roberts, W. C.: Pathology of acute myocardial infarction, Hosp. Pract. **6**:89-105, 1971.

Robertson, P. A.: A functional emergency cart, Am. J. Nurs. **70**:1684-1686, 1970.

Robicsek, F., et al.: The maintenance of function of the donor heart in the extracorporeal stage and during transplantation, Ann. Thorac. Surg. **6**:330-342, 1968.

Robicsek, F., et al.: Myocardial protection during open-heart surgery, Ann. Thorac. Surg. **10**:340-353, 1970.

Robinson, J. S.: Coronary care unit versus hospital mortality in acute myocardial infarction, Isr. J. Med. Sci. **5**:772-776, 1969.

Robinson, J. S.: Cardio-respiratory arrest during dental anesthesia, Br. Dent. J. **128**:323-335, 1970.

Rochet, E., et al.: Cardiorespiratory syncope under anesthesia in a pregnant woman. Successful resuscitation followed by a cesarean section, Lyon Med. **217**:1615-1620, 1967.

Roe, B. B.: Internal-external defibrillation in the presence of pericardial symphysis, Ann. Thorac. Surg. **13**:188-189, 1972.

Roelandt, J., et al.: Parasystolic ventricular tachycardia. Observations on differential stimulus threshold as possible mechanism for exit block, Br. Heart J. **33**:505-512, 1971.

Rogel, S., et al.: Increased excitability of the heart induced by electrical stimulation in the absolute refractory period, Chest **6**:578-582, 1971.

Rogers, J. A.: Equipment of the coronary care unit, J. La. State Med. Soc. **121**:4-5, 1969.

Rogers, L. A.: Complications of tracheostomy, South Med. J. **62**:1496-1500, 1969.

Rogers, P. D., and Hillman, H.: Increased recovery of rats respiration following profound hypothermia, J. Appl. Physiol. **29**:58-63, 1970a.

Rogers, P. D., and Hillman, H.: Increased recovery of anesthetised hypothermic rats by intracarotid infusions and abdominal pumping, Nature (Lond.) **228**:1314-1315, 1970b.

Rogers, P. D., and Hillman, H.: Biochemical changes in the blood during hypothermic cardiac arrest and recovery of rats, Resuscitation, **1**:25-29, 1972.

Romanova, N. P., et al.: State of the hypothalamo-hypophyseal neurosecretory system in terminal states caused by mechanical asphyxia in the period of restoration of vital functions (experimental study), Sud. Med. Ekspert. **13**:20-23, 1970.

Rösch, W., et al.: Asystolic heart arrest in achalasia, Dtsch. Med. Wochenschr. **94**:2191-2194, 1969.

Rose, L. B., et al.: Cardiac defibrillation by ambulance attendants, J.A.M.A. **219**:63-68, 1972.

Rose, W. H.: Cardiopulmonary resuscitation, J. Miss. Med. Assoc. **9**:118-120, 1968.

Rosen, K. M.: Transient and persistent atrial standstill with His bundle lesions. Electrophysiologic and pathologic correlations, Circulation **44**:220-236, 1971.

Rosen, Z.: Resuscitation in the Bible, Harefuah **79**:27-28, 1970.

Rosenberg, A. S., et al.: Emergency cardiac pacing in hyperkalemia, Arch. Intern. Med. **126**:658-659, 1970.

Rosenblatt, G., et al.: A sleep regimen for acute myocardial infarction, Lancet **1**:1040, 1968.

Rosenheim, S. H.: Sickle-cell trait and sudden death, N. Engl. J. Med. **283**:1229-1230, 1970.

Rosensweig, J., et al.: Treatment of acute myocardial infarction by counterpulsation, J. Thorac. Cardiovasc. Surg. **59**:243-250, 1970.

Rosoff, S. D., and Schwab, R. S.: The EEG in establishing brain death. A 10-year report with criteria and legal safeguards in the 50 states. Presented at American Electroencephalographic Society, June, 1967.

Ross, A., et al.: External ophthalmoplegia and complete heart block, N. Engl. J. Med. **280**:313-315, 1969.

Ross, R. S.: Electrical hazards for cardiac patients, N. Engl. J. Med. **281**:390, 1969.

Ross, R. S.: Hypotension and the shock syndrome in myocardial infarction, J. Iowa Med. Soc. **59**:847-849, 1969.

Rosselot, E., et al.: Trifascicular block treated by artificial pacing, Am. J. Cardiol. **26**:6-11, 1970.

Rosselot, E., et al.: Venoarterial pulsatile circulatory assist in the treatment of resistant ventricular fibrillation, Am. J. Cardiol. **27**:46-50, 1971.

Rossi, N. P.: Surgically treatable complications of myocardial infarction, Surgery **65**:118-126, 1969.

Rossi, P., et al.: Immediate and remote results of treatment of 170 episodes of cardiac arrest, Cuore Circ. **54**:229-246, 1970.

Roth, F., et al.: Dangerous increase in serum potassium following succinylcholine administration, Anaesthesist **20**:35-38, 1971.

Rothfeld, E. L., et al.: Paired pacing after coronary artery ligation, Am. J. Cardiol. **23**:224-228, 1969.

Rothfeld, E. L., et al.: Antiarrhythmic drugs in the prevention of ventricular arrhythmias related to paired pacing, Am. J. Cardiol. **26**:52-55, 1970.

Rothwell-Jackson, R. L.: The adjuvant use of pressor amines during cardiac massage, Br. J. Surg. **55**:545-550, 1968.

Rovelli, F.: Cardiac arrest, Cardiol. Prat. **18**:1-6, 1967.

Rovelli, F.: Endocardiac stimulation in heart arrest and in the treatment of Morgagni-Adams-Stokes disease, Cardiol. Prat. **18**:37-50, 1967.

Rozin, L. B.: Cardiac arrest in the surgical treatment of burn patients, Eksp. Khir. Anesteziol. **12**:101, 1967.

Rozin, L. B., et al.: Determining the risk of heart arrest during surgery of burns, Eksp. Khir. Anesteziol. **15**:3-6, 1970.

Ruban, G. E.: A case of death due to reflex heart arrest after a hammer blow on the chest, Sud. Med. Ekspert. **10**:52, 1967.

Rubeiz, G. A., et al.: Successful use of external cardioversion in the treatment of ventricular fibrillation caused by quinidine, Am. J. Cardiol. **16**:118-121, 1965.

Rubenfire, M., et al.: Mechanically-induced cardiac arrhythmia following open heart surgery, Chest **59**:335-338, 1971.

Rubin, G. J.: Applications of electrocardiology in canine medicine and practice, J. Am. Vet. Med. Assoc. **153**:17-39, 1968.

Rubin, R. T.: Atropine, ECT, and cardiac arrest, Am. J. Psychiatry **124**:863-864, 1967.

Rufty, A. J., Jr., et al.: The problem of shock in acute myocardial infarction, J. La. State Med. Soc. **121**:21-24, 1969.

Ruiz, U., et al.: Assisted circulation by synchronous pulsation of extramural pressure, J. Thorac. Cardiovasc. Surg. **56**:832-845 passim, 1968.

Rush, B. F., et al.: More liberal use of a plasma expander, N. Engl. J. Med. **280**:1202-1205, 1969.

Ryan, A. H., et al.: Control of spasms by asphyxiation, Am. J. Physiol. **22**:440-444, 1908.

Ryden, L., et al.: The effect of lignocaine on the stimulation threshold and conduction disturbances in patients treated with pacemaker, Cardiovasc. Res. **3**:415-418, 1969.

Rzepecki, W.: Resuscitation in cases of cardiac arrest in lung surgery, Kardiol. Pol. **11**:131-136, 1968.

Sabah, A. H.: Blindness after cardiac arrest, Postgrad. Med. J. **44**:513-516, 1968.

Sabel, G. H.: Advantages of face mask for cardiac arrest, N. Engl. J. Med. **287**:724, 1972.

Sabena, V.: Nosology of resuscitation and intensive care centers, Acta Anaesthesiol. (Padova) **21**:106-109, 1970.

Sack, K., et al.: Artificial postmortem fat embolism, Zentralbl. Allg. Pathol. **111**:24-31, 1968.

Safar, P.: Recognition and management of airway obstruction, J.A.M.A. **208**:1009-1011, 1969.

Safar, P., et al.: Ambulance design and equipment for mobile intensive care, Arch. Surg. **102**:163-171, 1971.

Sahebjami, H.: Myocardial infarction and cardiac rupture, South. Med. J. **62**:1058-1063, 1969.

Sakakibara, S., et al.: Coronary care unit, Jap. J. Thorac. Surg. **21**:70-71, 1968.

Salalykin, V. I., et al.: Experience with restoration of cardiac activity in neurosurgical patients, Vopr. Neirokhir. **30**:51-54, 1966.

Salehi, E., et al.: Possibilities of complications in neuroleptoanalgesia, Acta Anesth. Scand. (Suppl.) **23**:18-21, 1966.

Salomon, H.: Hospital electrical hazards revisited, N. Engl. J. Med. **287**:146-147, 1972.

Saltiel, J., et al.: Reversibility of left ventricular dysfunction following aorto-coronary by-pass grafts, Am. J. Roentgenol. Radium Ther. Nucl. Med. **110**:739-746, 1970.

Samet, P.: Indications for cardiac pacing in acute myocardial infarction, J. Fla. Med. Assoc. **55**:1079-1080, 1968.

Samet, P., et al.: Localization of the site of block in patients with complete heart block, J. Fla. Med. Assoc. **57**:20-22, 1970.

Sandoe, E., et al.: Long-term prognosis in patients resuscitated from cardiac arrest, Isr. J. Med. Sci. **5**:769-771, 1969.

Sanmarco, M. E., et al.: Myocardial contractility following cardiopulmonary bypass with and without myocardial ischemia, Ann. Thorac. Surg. **8**:237-251, 1969.

Sarachek, N. S., and Leonard, J. L.: Familial heart block and sinus bradycardia, Am. J. Cardiol. **29**:451-458, 1972.

Sarin, C. L., et al.: Effects of extracorporeal circulation on left ventricular function with and without anoxic arrest, J. Thorac. Cardiovasc. Surg. **56**:395-400, 1968.

Sataline, L., et al.: Hypercalcemia, heart-block, and hyperthyroidism, J.A.M.A. **213**:1342, 1970.

Sato, G., et al.: Further experience with electrical stimulation of the phrenic nerve: electrically-induced fatigue, Surgery **68**:817-826, 1970.

Sato, M. P.: Emergency treatment of acute cardiac arrest, Sanfujin Jissai **18**:487-495, 1969.

Saury, A., et al.: Apropos of two cardiovascular accidents in women due to coitus, Ann. Med. Leg. (Paris) **46**:473-474, 1966.

Sawyer, H. P., Jr.: Resuscitation in the delivery room, Trans. N. Engl. Obstet. Gynecol. Soc. **21**:57-69, 1967.

Scanlon, P. J., et al.: Right bundle-branch block associated with left superior or inferior intraventricular block. Clinical setting, prognosis, and relation to complete heart block, Circulation **42**:1123-1133, 1970.

Scardi, S., et al.: Recurrent paroxysmal ventricular tachycardia, Minerva Med. **61**:5879-5883, 1970.

Scatter, P., et al.: Heart function in postoperative artificial respiration, Thoraxchirurgie **14**:422-427, 1966.

Schaldach, M., and Kirsch, V.: In vivo electrochemical power generation, Trans. Am. Soc. Artif. Intern. Organs **16**:184-192, 1970.

Schamroth, L., et al.: Concealed interpolated A-V junctional extrasystoles and A-V junctional parasystole, Am. J. Cardiol. **27**:703-707, 1971.

Schartum, S.: Ventricular arrest caused by the Valsalva maneuver in a patient with Adams-Stokes attacks accompany defecation, Acta Med. Scand. **184**:65-68, 1968.

Schaumberg, H. H., et al.: Heart block in polymyositis, N. Engl. J. Med. **284**:480-481, 1971.

Schechter, D. C.: Role of the humane societies in the history of resuscitation, Surg. Gynecol. Obstet. **129**:811-815, 1969.

Schechter, D. C., et al.: History of sphygmology and of heart block, Dis. Ches. **55**(Suppl. 1):535-579, 1969.

Schechter, D. C., et al.: Early experience with

resuscitation by means of electricity, Surgery **69:**360-372, 1971.

Scheidt, S., et al.: Shock after acute myocardial infarction, Am. J. Cardiol. **26:**556, 1970.

Scheinman, M. M., et al.: Clinical significance of changes in serum magnesium in patients undergoing cardiopulmonary bypass, J. Thorac. Cardiovasc. Surg. **61:**135-140, 1971.

Scheinman, M. M., et al.: Critical assessment of use of central venous oxygen saturation as a mirror of mixed venous oxygen in severely ill cardiac patients, Circulation **40:**165-172, 1969.

Scheinin, T. M., et al.: Effects of quinidine and digitalis on the incidence of ventricular fibrillation after direct current discharges in the dog, Ann. Med. Exp. Biol. Fenn. **45:**384-388, 1967.

Scheppokat, K. D., et al.: Comparison of asynchronous and demand pacing, Ann. N. Y. Acad. Sci. **167:**968-980, 1969.

Scher, A. M.: Excitation of the heart, Heart Bull. **18:**21-24, 1969.

Scherf, D.: Concerning paroxysmal tachycardia, Dis. Chest **56:**465-466, 1969.

Schilt, W., et al.: Temporary non-surgical intra-arterial cardiac assistance, Trans. Am. Soc. Artif. Intern. Organs **13:**322, 1967.

Schimert, G., et al.: Surgical help for failing heart is encouraging, Mod. Med. **38:**147, 1970.

Schlepper, M., et al.: Pacemaker-induced reciprocal rhythm, Chest **58:**392-395, 1970.

Schlesinger, Z., et al.: Ventricular aneurysmectomy for severe rhythm disturbances, J. Thorac. Cardiovasc. Surg. **61:**602-604, 1971.

Schleusing, G., et al.: Heart arrest in experimental metabolic acidosis, Z. Gesamte. Inn. Med. **24**(Suppl.):4548, 1969.

Schlömerich, P.: Intensive care in heart arrest, Hefte Unfallheilkd. **99:**11-21, 1969.

Schlosser, V.: Experimental studies on the determination of instant cardiac sufficiency following total ischemia in normothermia and hypothermia, Bruns Beitr. Klin. Chir. **215:**194-231, 1967.

Schlosser, V.: Experimental studies on the evaluation of therapeutic results in acute spontaneous heart arrest, Hefte Unfallheilkd. **99:**27-30, 1969.

Schluger, J., et al.: Use of pacemaker therapy in heart blocks analyzed, Mod. Med. **38:**74, 1970.

Schmidt, A. P.: Complete heart block due to inflammatory lesion of conduction system, Mayo Clin. Proc. **44:**169-175, 1969.

Schneider, M., et al.: Heart circulatory arrest and its therapeutic consequences, Dtsch. Gesundheitsw. **22:**685-674, 1967.

Schoen, H. R.: Comparative animal experiment

studies of the prolongation of the revival time of the heart and the whole organ in normothermia by pharmacologic pretreatment, Arch. Kreislaufforsch. **57:**1-54, 1968.

Schon, G., et al.: Relationship of blood substitutes to pulmonary changes and volemia, Ann. Surg. **173:**504-510, 1971.

Schonfelder, M.: Morphological findings in the myocardium following reanimation, Anaesthesist **15:**381-389, 1966.

Schreiner, G. E., and Teehan, B. P.: Dialysis of poisons and drugs; annual review, Trans. Am. Soc. Artif. Intern. Organs **17:**513, 1971.

Schrogie, J. J.: Training in cardiopulmonary resuscitation, U. S. Public Health Rep. **80:**69-74, 1965.

Schuder, J. C.: Completely implanted defibrillator, J.A.M.A. **214:**1123, 1970.

Schuder, J. C., and Stoeckle, H.: A micromodule pacemaker receiver for direct attachment to the ventricle, Trans. Am. Soc. Artif. Intern. Organs **8:**344-351, 1962.

Schuder, J. C., et al.: Experimental ventricular defibrillation with an automatic and completely implanted system, Trans. Am. Soc. Artif. Intern. Organs **16:**207-212, 1970.

Schuder, J. C., et al.: Transthoracic ventricular defibrillation in the dog with unidirectional rectangular double pulses, Cardiovasc. Res. **4:**497-501, 1970.

Schuder, J. C., et al.: High power solid state pulse generator for an automatic and completely implantable ventricular defibrillator, Proc. Annu. Conf. Eng. in Med. Biol. **12:**86, 1970

Schuder, J. C., et al.: Ventricular defibrillation using bipolar catheter and truncated exponential stimuli. Proc. Annu. Conf. Eng. in Med. Biol. **13:**35, 1971.

Schuder, J. C., et al.: Ventricular defibrillation with catheter having distal electrode in right ventricle and proximal electrode in superior vena cava, Circulation **44:**11-99, 1971.

Schuder, J. C., et al.: Relationship between duration of ventricular fibrillation and effectiveness of therapeutic shock, Proc. Annu. Conf. Eng. in Med. Biol. **14:**229, 1972.

Schuder, J. C., et al.: A multielectrode-time sequential laboratory defibrillator for the study of implanted electrode systems, Trans. Am. Soc. Artif. Intern. Organs **18:**514-519, 1972.

Schuder, J. C., et al.: Ventricular defibrillation in the dog with a bielectrode intravascular catheter (submitted for publication).

Schultze, H. U.: Contrast media accident endangering life after injection of 1 ml. of Visotrast 370, Radiol. Diagn. (Berl.) **11:**137-139, 1970.

Schumann, H. D., et al.: Experience with the treatment of acute cardiac arrest, Zentralbl. Chir. 94:134-152, 1969.

Schuster, H. P., et al.: Intensive therapy and prognosis of acute heart arrest, Klin. Wochenschr. 47:4-16, 1969.

Schuurmans Stekhoven, W.: The decerebration drama, Ned. Tijdschr. Geneeskd. 113:761-762, 1969.

Schwab, R. S., et al.: EEG as an aid in determining death in the presence of cardiac activity (ethical, legal and medical aspects), Electroencephalogr. Clin. Neurophysiol. 15:147-148, 1963.

Schwartz, A.: Calcium and the sarcoplasmic reticulum. In Harris, P., and Opie, L. H., editors: Calcium and the heart, New York, 1971, Academic Press, Inc., pp. 66-92.

Schwartz, L. S., et al.: Sudden death in syncope with aortic stenosis, Mod. Med. 37:116, 1969.

Schweitzer, F.: Electrotherapy of the heart and its aftercare, Wien. Med. Wochenschr. 118:592-595, 1968.

Schylla, G., et al.: Complications of tracheotomy and prolonged resuscitation in patients of an internal intensive care unit, Med. Welt 51:2183-2192, 1970.

Scott, M. E., and Patterson, G. C.: Cardiac output after direct current conversion of atrial fibrillation, Br. Heart J. 31:87-90, 1969.

Scott, M. E., et al.: Management of complete heart block complicating acute myocardial infarction, Lancet 2:1382-1385, 1967.

Scott, M. E., et al.: The long-term prognosis of atrial fibrillation following direct-current conversion, Ulster Med. J. 37:155-161, 1968.

Scott, M. E., et al.: The value of direct current conversion of atrial fibrillation, Am. Heart J. 75:579-581, 1968.

Sealy, W. C., et al.: Identification and division of the bundle of Kent for premature ventricular excitation and supraventricular tachycardia, Surgery 68:1009-1017, 1970.

Seelye, E. R., et al.: Metabolic effects of deep hypothermia and circulatory arrest in infants during cardiac surgery, Br. J. Anaesth. 43:449-459, 1971.

Seller, R. H., et al.: Magnesium and digitalis toxicity, Heart Bull. 18:30-35, 1969.

Selye, H., et al.: Sensitization by corn oil for the production of cardiac necroses by various steroids and sodium salts, Am. J. Cardiol. 23:719-722, 1969.

Selzer, A., et al.: Quinidine syncope, Circulation 30:17, 1964.

Semple, T., et al.: Physical stimulation of the heart, Br. Med. J. 1:224-225, 1968.

Serres, E. J., et al.: Open chest pulsatile left-heart bypass without anticoagulation, Arch. Surg. 101:18-21, 1970.

Seshwar, K. P.: Correlation of serum glutamic oxaloacetic transaminase levels and arrhythmias in acute myocardial infarction, N. Y. State J. Med. 69:1041-1045, 1969.

Severe accidental hyperthermia, Lancet 7740:237, 1972.

Sforza, I.: Preventive sedation and emergency therapy of cardiac arrest in ambulatory stomatological surgery, Arcisped. S. Anna Ferrara 20:175-188, 1967.

Shaban, I. V.: Possibility of spontaneous restoration of bioelectric heart activity after its prolonged cessation in the course of dying, Dokl. Akad. Nauk S.S.S.R. 189:685-687, 1969.

Shaban, I. V.: Relationship between automatism, conduction, and excitation of the human heart in the process of dying, Kardiologiia 10:140-142, 1970.

Shafer, R.: The patients are better off in a hyperbaric bed, Hosp. Management 107:58-59, 1969.

Shahaway, M. E.: Arrhythmias and the varieties of sleep, N. Engl. J. Med. 282:815, 1970.

Shahrrestani, E., et al.: Avoidance and treatment of complications of myelography, Z. Orthop. 108:139-148, 1970.

Shalit, M. N., et al.: Single sign of brain death unlikely, Mod. Med. 38:123, 1970.

Shanahan, E. A., et al.: Effect of modified preoperative and postoperative potassium supplementation on the incidence of postoperative ventricular arrhythmias, J. Thorac. Cardiovasc. Surg. 57:413-421, 1969.

Shanoff, H. M.: Diuretics in cardiac edema—1969, Can. Med. Assoc. J. 101:66-70, 1969.

Shapiro, W., et al.: Alterations in cardiac function immediately following electrical conversion of atrial fibrillation to normal sinus rhythm, Circulation 38:1074-1084, 1968.

Sharma, B., et al.: Insulin secretion in heart failure, Br. Med. J. 1:396-399, 1970.

Sharma, P. L.: Effect of pancuronium bromide, a new steroidal neuromuscular blocking agent on halothane-adrenaline-evoked ventricular arrhythmias in dog, Indian J. Med. Res. 58:1736-1741, 1970.

Sharma, P. L., et al.: Mechanism of action of adrenergic beta-receptor blocking agents in the prevention of cyclopropane adrenaline-evoked ventricular arrhythmias in the dog, Indian J. Med. Res. 56:1256-1264, 1968.

Sharma, P. L., et al.: Effect of succinylcholine, gallamine and d-tubocurarine on adrenaline-evoked ventricular arrhythmias in dogs under halothane-nitrous oxide anesthesia, Indian J. Med. Res. 56:1272-1281, 1968.

Sharnoff, J. G.: Prevention of sudden cardiopulmonary arrest in the perioperative period with prophylactic heparin, Lancet 2:292-293, 1969.

Sharnoff, J. G., et al.: Some implications in the successful heparin prophylaxis of sudden cardiopulmonary arrest by thrombosis and embolism, Am. Heart J. 80:848-850, 1970.

Sharp, W. V., et al.: A bioelectric polyurethane elastomere for intravascular replacement, Trans. Am. Soc. Artif. Intern. Organs 12:179, 1966.

Sharp, W. V., et al.: Pulmonary embolectomy. A lesson in aggressive persistence, Vasc. Surg. 3:18-24, 1969.

Shea, M. A., and Bernstein, E. F.: An evaluation of the Baylor left Ventricular Bypass device in the treatment of cardiocirculatory failure, Ann. Surg. 174:177-193, 1971.

Shelly, W. M., et al.: Cuffed tubes as a cause of tracheal stenosis, J. Thorac. Cardiovasc. Surg. 57:623-627, 1969.

Shenasky, J. H., et al.: The renal hemodynamic and functional aspects of external counterpressure, Surg. Gynecol. Obstet. 134:253-258, 1972.

Shenkin, H. N., et al.: Air embolism from exposure of posterior cranial fossa in prone position, J.A.M.A. 210:726, 1969.

Shikunova, L. G.: Partial replacement of the blood in the treatment of patients with terminal states and in the postresuscitation period, Zh. Eksp. Klin. Med. 8:83-87, 1968.

Shillingford, J., et al.: Treatment of bradycardia and hypotension syndrome in patients with acute myocardial infarction, Am. Heart J. 75:843-844, 1968.

Shim, C., et al.: Transient cardiac arrhythmia during tracheal suction, Mod. Med. 38:127, 1970.

Shimanuki, H., et al.: Succinylcholine-induced cardiac arrest in a case of severe thermal burns, Jap. J. Anesthesiol. 18:321-327, 1969.

Shimomura, K., et al.: Ventricular fibrillation initiated by low sodium and potassium solution. I. Experiment in isolated frog heart, Jap. Heart J. 10:535-544, 1969.

Shinohara, Y.: Ventricular fibrillation threshold in experimental coronary occlusion: comparative studies on the effect of G-I-K solution and some new antiarrhythmic agents, Jap. Circ. J. 32:1269-1282, 1968.

Shires, D. B.: Rupture of the right ventricle, J.A.M.A. 203:888-890, 1968.

Shirok, Y., et al.: Method of resuscitation. 3. Effect of an emergency resuscitating agent directly injected into the myocardium, Jap. J. Anesthesiol. 20:56-61, 1971.

Shoemaker, W. C., et al.: The dilemma of vasopressors and vasodilators in the therapy of shock, Surg. Gynecol. Obstet. 132:51-57, 1971.

Shofer, O. E.: Cardiac arrest in the x-ray patient, Radiography 36:139-140, 1970.

Shubin, H., et al.: Objective index of haemodynamic status for quantification of severity and prognosis of shock complicating myocardial infarction, Cardiovasc. Res. 2:329-337, 1968.

Shumakov, V. I., et al.: Implanted artificial heart ventricle, Grudn. Khir. 10:31-37, 1968.

Shumakov, V. I., et al.: Restoration of heart rhythm in ventricular fibrillation using different methods of assisted circulation, Kardiologiia 11:116-120, 1971.

Sidorenko, G. I., et al.: Some problems of the equipping of hospital wards for infarct patients, Kardiologiia 7:111-114, 1967.

Siegel, D. G., et al.: A critique of studies of long-term survivorship of patients with a myocardial infarction, Am. J. Public Health 58:1348-1354, 1968.

Siegel, J. H., et al.: Myocardial failure, vascular tone, and oxygen transport in septic shock in a human being, Surg. Forum 17:5-6, 1966.

Siemsen, A. W., et al.: Limited-care hemodialysis, Trans. Am. Soc. Artif. Intern. Organs 18:70, 1972

Siemssen, S. O., et al.: Prolonged deep hypothermia with induced circulatory arrest for the extirpation of an angiofibroma in the rhinopharynx, Ugeskr. Laeger 129:586-600, 1967.

Siggers, D. C., et al.: Long-term use of implanted pacemakers in the control of complete heart block, Guys Hosp. Rep. 119:322-328, 1970.

Sigler, L. H.: Sudden death due to cardiac rupture in myocardial ischemia and infarction. Causes, mechanism, and possible prevention, N. Y. J. Med. 69:794-799, 1969.

Silvera, J. S. da: Cardio-respiratory resuscitation in dental practice, Rev. Port. Estamatol. Cir. Maxilofac. 11:153-199, 1970.

Simmons, R. L., et al.: Postresuscitative blood volumes in combat casualties, Surg. Gynecol. Obstet. 128:1193-1201, 1969.

Simone, M.: Poly- and pluri-valent resuscitation departments, Acta Anaesthesiol. (Padova) 21:110-114, 1970.

Sinclair-Smith, B. C.: Electrical reversion of cardiac arrhythmias, South. Med. J. 65:289-294, 1972.

Singer, R. B.: Mortality in 966 life insurance applicants with bundle branch block or wide QRS, Trans. Assoc. Life Ins. Med. Dir. Am. 52:94-114, 1969.

Singh, V. K.: Nature of ventricular fibrillation during hypothermia, Indian Heart J. 20:393-396, 1968.

Single phone call mobilizes hospital in cardiac emergencies, J.A.M.A. 209:857, 1969.

Sinitsyn, N.: Peresadke Serdtsa Kat novi metod experimental noe, Biology 1, Meditsine, 1948, Copy photostat of Dispatch N. 763, Army Medical Library, Washington, D. C.

Siska, K., et al.: Protection of the myocardium during ischaemic asystole with intracoronary administration of ATP, J. Cardiovasc. Surg. (Torino) 10:274-281, 1969.

Skinner, D. B., et al.: Applications of mechanical ventricular assistance, Ann. Surg. 166:500-511, 1967.

Skinner, D. B., et al.: Acute circulatory support by mechanical ventricular assistance following myocardial infarction, J. Thorac. Cardiovasc. Surg. 54:785-794, 1967.

Skinner, D. B., et al.: Mechanical ventricular assistance in human beings, Ann. Thorac. Surg. 5:131-140, 1968.

Skinner, D. B., et al.: Preservation and transplantation of dog organs maintained in vivo for 24 hours by mechanical ventricular assistance, J. Surg. Res. 10:253, 1970.

Skinner, D. B., et al.: Resuscitation following prolonged cardiac arrest, Ann. Thorac. Surg. 11:201-209, 1971.

Skuratovskii, A. S., et al.: Device for artificial respiration in pressure chamber under higher gas pressure during reanimation after the death from rapid decompression, Fiziol. Zh. 17:276-277, 1971.

Slama, R., et al.: The syndrome, "QT lengthening and syncope due to torsion of the points," Laval Med. 42:353-366, 1971.

Sleet, R. A.: Report of 24 cases of myocardial infarction treated at home, Br. Med. J. 4:875-877, 1969.

Slijepchevic, S., et al.: The role of oxygenation in the etiology of posthypercapnic ventricular fibrillation, Med. Ann. D. C. 38:597-599, passim, 1969.

Slin'ko, A. G.: Prolonged effectiveness of external cardiac massage in heart arrest, Vestn. Khir. 98:89-90, 1967.

Slodki, S. J.: Limits of cardioversion, Adv. Cardiopulm. Dis. 4:54-60, 1969.

Sloman, G., et al.: Coronary care unit: a review of 300 patients monitored since 1963, Am. Heart J. 75:140-143, 1968.

Slowing heart rate by vagal stimulation, Mod. Med. 37:190-192, 1969.

Smailis, A. I.: Our experience with the use of electric defibrillation of the heart, Sov. Med. 29:149, 1966.

Smith, J., et al.: Need for oxygen enrichment in myocardial infarction, shock, and following

cardiac arrest, Acta Anaesthesiol. Scand. (Suppl.) 29:127-145, 1968.

Smith, M., et al.: Cardiac arrhythmias, increased intracranial pressure and the autonomic nervous system, Chest 61:126-133, 1972.

Smith, R. B., et al.: Cardiac arrest following succinylcholine in patients with central nervous system injuries, Anesthesiology 33:558-560, 1970.

Smith, R. B.: Hyperkalemia following succinylcholine administration in neurological disorders, Can. Anaesth. Soc. J. 18:199, 1971.

Smith, R. E., et al.: Resuscitation of the newborn, J. Miss. Med. Assoc. 11:417-422, 1970.

Smith, T. W., et al.: Late recovery of conduction following surgically induced atrioventricular block, Ann. Thorac. Surg. 9:372-377, 1970.

Smith, W. G.: A coronary-care unit in a general medical ward, Lancet 2:397-399, 1968.

Smolarek, Z.: Repeated arrest of blood circulation treated with external heart massage, Wiad. Lek. 23:1507-1509, 1970.

Smyth, N. P.: Collective review of cardiac pacemaking, Ann. Thorac. Surg. 8:167-190, 1969.

Smyth, N. P., et al.: Experimental heart block in the dog. An improved method, J. Thorac. Cardiovasc. Surg. 59:201-205, 1970.

Snook, R.: Resuscitation at road accidents, Br. Med. J. 4:438-450, 1969.

Snyder, C., et al.: Isolation of sodium as a cause of ventricular fibrillation, Invest. Radiol. 6:245-248, 1971.

Sodi-Pallares, et al.: A therapeutic approach at cellular level in cardiovascular disorders, Geriatrics 21:107-116, 1966.

Sodi-Pallares, D., et al.: Entropy and cardiology, Geriatrics 21:138-142, 1966.

Sodi-Pallares, D., et al.: Complete surgical period of the cardiac patient. The role of the internist-cardiologist, Geriatrics 22:115-124, 1967.

Sodi-Pallares, D., et al.: Polarizing solution in myocardial infarction, Am. J. Cardiol. 21:275-276, 1968.

Sodi-Pallares, D., et al.: Potassium, glucose, and insulin in myocardial infarction, Lancet 1:1315-1316, 1969.

Sodium bicarbonate proves a lifesaver in near-drownings, Med. World News 10:20-21, 1969.

Soffer, A.: Ways and means of conduction, Dis. Chest 55:93-97, 1969.

Soffer, A.: Colloquy on a new beta blocking drug, Dis. Chest 55:182-183, 1969.

Soffer, A.: Only one third reach the hospital, Dis. Chest 55:272-273, 1969.

Soffer, A.: Intensive cardiac care and digitalis glycosides, Dis. Chest 55:321-322, 1969.

Soffer, A.: The chest physician and intensive care, Chest 59:554-557, 1971.

Sokolianskii, I. F., et al.: Some indices of functional state of the organism in drowning and resuscitation, Fiziol. Zh. 16:326-329, 1970.

Somogyi, E., et al.: Data regarding the morphology of electroshocks experimentally applied to the heart, Zacchia 3:389-404, 1967.

Sondergaard, T., et al.: Clinical experience with cardioplegia according to Bretschneider, Langenbecks Arch. Klin. Chir. 319:661-665, 1967.

Sonnenblick, E. H., et al.: Oxygen consumption of the heart: physiologic principles and clinical implications, Mod. Concepts Cardiovasc. Dis. 40:9-16, 1971.

Sordahl, L. A., et al.: The possible relationship between ultrastructure and biochemical state of heart mitochondria, Arch. Biochem. Biophys. 132:404-415, 1969.

Sordahl, L. A., et al.: Respiratory activity of mitochondria from isolated human and dog hearts maintained in a portable preservation chamber, J. Mol. Cell. Cardiol. 1:379-388, 1970.

Soroff, H. S., et al.: Physiologic support of heart action, N. Engl. J. Med. 280:693-704, 1969.

Sowton, E., et al.: Physiologic changes in threshold, Ann. N. Y. Acad. Sci. 167:679-685, 1969.

Spain, D. M., et al.: Sudden death from coronary heart disease, Chest 58:107-110, 1970.

Spann, J. F., et al.: Recent advances in the understanding of congestive heart failure, Mod. Concepts Cardiovasc. Dis. 39:79-84, 1970.

Spath, G.: Intensive medicine. Acute circulatory arrest and reanimation, Munch. Med. Wochenschr. 113:867-874, 1971.

Spencer, E. R., Jr.: Cardiopulmonary resuscitation: status report, N. Engl. J. Med. 286:1000-1001, 1972.

Spieckermann, P. G., et al.: Preischemic stress and resuscitation time of the heart, Verh. Dtsch. Ges. Kreislaufforsch. 35:358-364, 1969.

Spinal chill to stem paralysis, Med. World News 29:15, 1970.

Spivack, A. P., et al.: The arrhythmia trainer, J.A.M.A. 202:299-301, 1967.

Spracklen, F. H., et al.: Late ventricular dysrhythmias after myocardial infarction, Br. Med. J. 4:364-366, 1968.

Spritzer, R. C., et al.: Electrocardiographic follow-up of patients with demand pacemakers, Am. Heart J. 80:367-375, 1970.

Spritzer, R. C., et al.: Serious arrhythmias during labor and delivery in women with heart disease, J.A.M.A. 211:1005-1007, 1970.

Stadelmann, G., et al.: Metabolic changes in the myocardium under the conditions of experi-

mental ventricular fibrillation during extracorporeal circulation in the dog, Thoraxchirurgie 15:447-456, 1967.

Stadnik, J., et al.: Resuscitation by direct heart massage, Wiad. Lek. 20:1461-1463, 1967.

Staewen, W. S., et al.: A laboratory prototype for automatic ventricular defibrillation, Proc. Annu. Conf. Eng. in Med. Biol. 12:118, 1970.

Stahl, W. M., and Stone, A. M.: Prophylactic diuresis with ethacrynic acid for prevention of postoperative renal failure, Ann. Surg. 172:361, 1970.

Stanley, T. H.: Initial studies of the left heart bypass as a long-term cardiac assist device, Surgery 65:649-658, 1969.

Stannard, M., and Rigo, S. J.: Resuscitation from cardiac arrest in the presence of acute pulmonary oedema, Med. J. Aust. 2:990-991, 1967.

Stannard, M., and Sloman, G.: Ventricular fibrillation in acute myocardial infarction: prognosis following successful resuscitation, Am. Heart J. 77:573, 1969.

Stannard, M., et al.: Propranolol with atropine to treat myocardial infarct, Mod. Med. 36:87, 1968.

S-T charts coronary future in the healthy, Med. World News 11:4, 1970.

Stead, E. A., Jr.: Myocardial infarction—the first fifteen minutes, Med. Times 96:665-666, 1968.

Stein, E. H., et al.: Brief psychotherapy of psychiatric reactions to physical illness, Am. J. Psychiatry 125:1040-1047, 1969.

Stein, H., et al.: Successful prolonged resuscitation after open heart surgery, Thorax 26:449-454, 1971.

Stein, M., et al.: Arrhythmias and left ventricular efficiency following infarction and infarctectomy, Arch. Surg. 99:802-808, 1969.

Steinke, W. E., and Curry, J. J.: "Subclavian steal" syndrome in acute myocardial infarction masquerading as dissecting aneurysm of the aorta, Am. J. Cardiol. 22:436-439, 1968.

Stephens, R. L., and Carveth, S. W.: Management of cardiac arrest: a planned resuscitation program, Nebr. Med. J. 15:468, 1968.

Stephenson, H. E., Jr.: The teaching of emergency medical care in medical schools in the U. S. and Canada, Bull. Am. Coll. Surg. 56:9, 1971.

Stephenson, S. E., Jr., et al.: Physiologic P-wave cardiac stimulation, J. Thorac. Cardiovasc. Surg. 38:604-609, 1959.

Stern, M. P., et al.: Complete heart block complicating hyperthyroidism, J.A.M.A. 212:2117-2119, 1970.

Stevovic, M., et al.: Case of acute cardiac arrest during anesthesia and surgical intervention with favorable outcome, Vojnosanit. Pregl. **26**:244-245, 1969.

Stewart, W. K., et al.: Cardiac arrest trolley, Scott. Med. J. **14**:180-183, 1969.

Stiles, C. M., et al.: The use of diazepam as premedication for cardioversion, J. Kans. Med. Soc. **69**:277-278, 1968.

Stiles, Q. R., et al.: Cardiopulmonary arrest. Evaluation of an active resuscitation program, Am. J. Surg. **122**:282-287, 1971.

Stinson, E. B., et al.: Cardiac transplantation in man. VIII. Survival and function, J. Thorac. Cardiovasc. Surg. **60**:303-321, 1970.

Stinson, E. B., et al.: Hemodynamic observations after orthotopic transplantation of the canine heart, J. Thorac. Cardiovasc. Surg. **63**:344-352, 1972.

Stock, E.: Prognosis of myocardial infarction in a coronary care unit, Med. J. Aust. **2**:377, 1967.

Stock, E.: Frusemide after recent myocardial infarction, Med. J. Aust. **57**:480-481, 1970.

Stock, R. J.: Clinical significance of intraventricular block in acute myocardial infarction, Bull. N. Y. Acad. Med. **47**:987-996, 1971.

Stock, R. J., et al.: Observations on heart block during continuous electrocardiographic monitoring in myocardial infarction, Circulation **38**:993-1005, 1968.

Stoeckle, H., et al.: Incidence of arrhythmias in the dog following transthoracic ventricular defibrillation with unidirectional rectangular stimuli, Circ. Res. **23**:343-348, 1968.

Stoianov, K., et al.: Safe term for induced circulatory arrest in normothermia and hypothermia, Khirurgiia [Sofiia] **19**:258-263, 1966.

Stojanovic, K. V., et al.: Cardiac arrest, J. Cardiovasc. Surg. (Torino) **12**:177-180, 1971.

Stolfi, J. E.: Pre-hospital emergency care of the heart attack patient, Emergency Med. Today **1**:8, 1972.

Stolfi, J. E.: Collapsible airway for mouth-to-mouth resuscitation, J.A.M.A. **216**:678, 1971.

Stoll, W.: Intracardiac injection within the scope of resuscitation of newborn infants, Gynaecology **167**:382-385, 1969.

Stopczyk, M., et al.: Clinical trials of application of paired-pulse stimulation to heart in failure after cardiac surgery, Pol. Med. J. **8**:1042-1048, 1969.

Stout, C.: Coronary thrombosis without coronary athersclerosis, Am. J. Cardiol. **24**:564-569, 1969.

St. Petery, J., and Victorica, B. E.: Ventricular fibrillation caused by arsenic poisoning, Am. J. Dis. Child. **120**:367-371, 1971.

Strassman, G., et al.: Brain lesions, especially lenticular nucleus softening in heroin addicts,

barbiturate poisoning, late death after hanging and heart arrest during anesthesia, Beitr. Gerichtl. Med. **25**:236-242, 1969.

Strauer, B. E.: The influence of glucagon on myocardial mechanics of papillary muscles obtained from patients with chronic congestive heart failure, Naunyn Schmiedebergs Arch. Pharmacol. **270**:90-93, 1971.

Streisand, R. L., et al.: Respiratory and metabolic alkalosis and myocardial contractility, J. Thorac. Cardiovasc. Surg. **62**:432-436, 1971.

Strimer, R., et al.: Epidemiologic features of 1,134 sudden, unexpected infant deaths, J.A.M.A. **209**:1493-1497, 1969.

Subclavian route for monitoring venous pressure, Mod. Med. **37**:117, 1969.

Sudden death risk from ventricular premature systoles, Mod. Med. **37**:102, 1969.

Sudden unexpected death, J.A.M.A. **209**:1358, 1969.

Sugg, W. L., et al.: Reduction of extent of myocardial infarction by counterpulsation, Ann. Thorac. Surg. **7**:310-316, 1969.

Sugg, W. L., et al.: Cardiac assistance (counterpulsation) in ten patients, Ann. Thorac. Surg. **9**:1-12, 1970.

Sugimoto, T., et al.: Factors determining vulnerability to ventricular fibrillation induced by 60-cps alternating current, Circ. Res. **21**:601-608, 1967.

Sujansky, E., et al.: A dynamic aortic patch as a permanent mechanical auxiliary ventricle: experimental studies, Surgery **66**:875-882, 1969.

Summers, D. N., et al.: Intra-aortic balloon pumping; hemodynamic and metabolic effects during cardiogenic shock in patients with triple coronary artery obstructive disease, Arch. Surg. **99**:733-738, 1969.

Super ICU means super resident training, Hosp. Physician **6**:68-71+, 1970.

Sur, R. N., et al.: Effect of betamethasone on strophosid induced ventricular fibrillation in guinea-pigs, Indian J. Exp. Biol. **8**:334-335, 1970.

Surawicz, B.: Ventricular fibrillation, Am. J. Cardiol. **28**:268-290, 1971.

Sustaita, H., et al.: Penetrating wounds of the heart, Chest **57**:340-343, 1970.

Sutton, R., et al.: Heart-block following acute myocardial infarction. Treatment with demand and fixed-rate pacemakers, Lancet **2**:645-648, 1968.

Sutton, R., et al.: The conduction system in acute myocardial infarction complicated by heart block, Circulation **38**:987-992, 1968.

Sutton, R. B., et al.: Pulmonary edema following

direct current cardioversion, Chest **57**:191-194, 1970.

Sutton, W. A., et al.: Significant determinants of successful reversion of fibrillation by a new DC defibrillator, Am. Heart J. **79**:630-639, 1970.

Suwa, K., et al.: Arterial-alveolar carbon dioxide gradient after cardiac resuscitation in the dog, Anaesthesiology **30**:37-42, 1969.

Swanson, L. W.: Community hospital experience with emergency cardiac resuscitation, J. Iowa Med. Soc. **60**:569-570, 1970.

Syrovatko, F. A., et al.: Outcome of resuscitation and subsequent state of health in women who sustained clinical death during labor complications, Akush. Ginekol. (Mosk.) **46**:55-58, 1970.

Szalaj, W., et al.: A case of hypokalemia with cardiac arrest during diabetic coma, Pol. Tyg. Lek. **24**:180-181, 1969.

Szanto, K., et al.: Dehydrobenzperidol and A-V block. Clinical case study of 2 heart arrests, Anaesthesist **17**:331-332, 1968.

Szekely, P., et al.: Direct current shock and digitalis, Br. Heart J. **31**:91-96, 1969.

Szekely, P., et al.: Antidysrhythmic drugs and direct current shock, Mod. Med. **38**:194-195, 1970.

Szmydt, W., et al.: Preliminary experiences in cardiologic resuscitation, Pol. Tyg. Lek. **23**: 1096-1098, 1968.

Szymdt, W., et al.: Antiarrhythmic drugs in prevention of recurrent ventricular fibrillation, Pol. Tyg. Lek. **26**:99-101, 1971.

Szreter, T.: Circulatory arrest in open heart surgery under hypothermia, Pol. Przegl. Chir. **39**:990-993, 1967.

T & A death rate 1 in 16,000, J.A.M.A. **210**: 1003, 1969.

Tacker, W. A., et al.: Defibrillation without A-V block using capacitor discharge with added inductance, Circ. Res. **22**:633-638, 1968.

Taddeucci, E., et al.: On cardiac arrest, Cardiol. Prat. **19**:325-329, 1968.

Tahernia, A. C.: Managing cardiac arrest in infants and children, Postgrad. Med. J. **47**: 204-209, 1970.

Tai, A. R.: Cardiopulmonary resuscitation in a general hospital, G. P. **36**:118-123, 1967.

Takahashi, T.: DC defibrillation of atrial fibrillation and its hemodynamic effects, Jap. Circ. J. **33**:251-273, 1969.

Takeuchi, K.: Standards for determining death. Cerebral death from the standpoint of the neurosurgeon, Surg. Ther. (Osaka) **20**:433-444, 1969.

Talpins, N. L., et al.: Counterpulsation and intra-aortic balloon pumping in cardiogenic shock:

circulatory dynamics, Arch. Surg. **97**:991-999, 1968.

Tam, W., et al.: The autoperfusing heart-lung preparation. A vehicle for the preservation of the resuscitated cadaver heart, Coll. Works Cardiopulm. Dis. **15**:9-16, 1969.

Tanaka, S., et al.: Cardiovascular responses of the failing dog heart to counterpulsation, J. Thorac. Surg. **58**:112, 1969.

Tansy, M. F., et al.: A vagosympathetic pathway capable of influencing common bile duct motility in the dog, Surg. Gynecol. Obstet. **133**: 225-236, 1971.

Tarjan, P. P., et al.: Cardiac pacemakers and microwave ovens, J.A.M.A. **214**:1328, 1970.

Taussig, H. B.: "Death" from lightning and the possibility of living again, Am. Sci. **57**:306-312, 1969.

Tawa, N.: Pathoanatomical studies on the acute cardiac death with special references to the brain, Jap. J. Leg. Med. **21**:137-163, 1967.

Taylor, L. F.: A statutory definition of death in Kansas, J.A.M.A. **215**:296, 1971.

Taylor, R. F.: Resuscitation following circulatory arrest, Manit. Med. Rev. **48**:108-109, 1968.

Taylor, R. R.: Myocardial potassium and ventricular arrhythmias following perfusion of ischaemic myocardium, Aust. N. Z. J. Med. **1**:114-120, 1971.

Taylor, R. S.: The significance of left intraventricular pressure during early resuscitation after temporary total myocardial ischaemia, Br. Surg. J. **56**:631, 1969.

Taylor, S. H.: Insulin and heart failure, Br. Heart J. **33**:329-333, 1971.

Taylor, S. H., et al.: Prevention of dysrhythmias after coronaries, Mod. Med. **38**:103, 1970.

Tchen, K. T.: The influenza epidemic, Br. Med. J. **1**:429-430, 1970.

Teaching the heart to take it easy, Med. World News **10**:16-17, 1969.

Telivuo, L., et al.: Comparison of alkalizing agents in resuscitation of the heart after ventricular fibrillation, Ann. Chir. Gynaecol. Fenn. **57**:221-224, 1968.

Tenckhoff, H., and Curtis, F. K.: Experience with maintenance peritoneal dialysis in the home, Trans. Am. Soc. Artif. Intern. Organs **16**:90, 1970.

Testolin, R.: Resuscitation and intensive care departments in modern hospitals, Acta Anaesthesiol. (Padova) **21**:87-94, 1970.

Theisen, K., et al.: Recurring heart arrest in bronchial adenoma, Internist (Berlin) **11**:152-156, 1970.

Theiss, E.: Successful reanimation—also in a small hospital? Chirurg **41**:427-429, 1970.

Thevenet, A., et al.: Circulatory arrest in deep hypothermia in surgery of the aortic arch branches, Ann. Chir. Thorac. Cardiovasc. 7: 69-71, 1968.

Thevenet, A., et al.: The use of a myocardial electrode inserted percutaneously for control of complete atrioventricular block by artificial pacemaker, Dis. Chest 34:621-631, 1958.

Thind, G. S., et al.: Direct current cardioversion in digitalized patients with mitral valve disease, Arch. Intern. Med. 123:156-159, 1969.

Thomas, E. T.: Circulatory collapse following succinylcholine: report of a case, Anesth. Analg. (Cleve.) 48:333-337, 1969.

Thomas, M.: Emergency treatment of patients with acute myocardial infarction, Acta Anaesthesiol. Scand. (Suppl.) 29:230+, 1968.

Thomas, T. V.: Emergency evacuation of acute pericardial tamponade, Ann. Thorac. Surg. 10: 566-570, 1970.

Thomford, N. R., et al.: Sudden hyperpyrexia during general anesthesia, Surgery 66:850-855, 1969.

Thompson, P.: Reduction of complications of hemodialysis with internal arteriovenous fistulas between radial artery and cephalic vein (radiocephalic shunt), Adv. Surg. 3:2, 1972.

Thorne, M. G.: Hiccup and heart block, Br. Heart J. 31:397-399, 1969.

Thurston, J. G.: The Westminster Hospital coronary unit—experiences with 260 patients admitted consecutively with diagnosis of acute myocardial infarction, Postgrad. Med. J. 45: 163-169, 1969.

Thys, J. P., et al.: Resuscitation in poisoning caused by narcotics and psychotropic drugs, Acta Clin. Belg. 24:149-164, 1969.

Tibblin, S., et al.: Dissociation of the hyperglycemic and vascular effects of glucagon, Surgery 67:816-825, 1970.

Tice, D. A.: Effects of paired electrical stimulation on myocardial performance in experimental heart failure, Surg. Forum 18:126-127, 1967.

Tice, D. A., et al.: Surgical treatment of postmyocardial infarction scars (ventricular aneurysms), Am. Heart J. 80:282-286, 1970.

Timmis, G. C., et al.: Heart block in the aged. Is the patient too old to be permanently paced? Chest 60:113-114, 1971.

Tobey, R. E.: Paraplegia, succinylcholine and cardiac arrest, Anesthesiology 32:359-364, 1970.

Tolmie, J. D., et al.: Succinylcholine danger in the burned patient, Anesthesiology 28:467-470, 1967.

Tolova, S. V.: Effect of prolonged arrest of circulation on some indices of the external respiration and the structure of the respiratory act during the recovery period following clinical death, Izv. Akad. Nauk S.S.S.R. [Biol.] 5:756-760, 1966.

Tolova, S. V., et al: Time periods of restoration of respiratory center function in dogs after sudden heart arrest and reanimation with complete artificial blood circulation, Biull. Eksp. Biol. Med. 70:13-16, 1970.

Tomecek, J., et al.: Phase-shift cardiac assistance with a valve balloon: experimental results, Trans. Am. Soc. Artif. Intern. Organs 15:406, 1969.

Tomita, F.: Heart homotransplantation in the rat, Sapporo Med. J. 30:165, 1966.

Tonner, H. D.: Reanimation and management of drowned persons, Z. Allgemeinmed. 47:1059-1063, 1971.

Torpey, D., et al.: Preoperative resuscitation and preparation of the traumatized patient, Int. Anesthesiol. Clin. 6:1041-2019, 1968.

Torresani, J., et al.: Clinical experience in transvenous and myocardial pacing, Ann. N. Y. Acad. Sci. 167:995-1007, 1969.

Touche, M., et al.: Reversible or avoidable ventricular fibrillation, Ann. Cardiol. Angeiol. (Paris) 19:163-171, 1970.

Towers, M. K.: Cardiac arrest, Practitioner 204: 252-261, 1970.

Towne, G. E., et al.: Pole-top cardiopulmonary resuscitation, J. Occup. Med. 13:398-401, 1971.

Towne, W. D., et al.: Intractable ventricular fibrillation associated with profound accidental hypothermia—successful treatment with partial cardiopulmonary bypass, N. Engl. J. Med. 287: 1135-1136, 1972.

Traber, D. L., et al.: A detailed study of the cardiopulmonary response to ketamine and its blockade by atropine, South. Med. J. 63:1077-1081, 1970.

Training of ambulance personnel and others responsible for emergency care of the sick and injured at the scene and during transportation. U. S. Department of Health, Education, and Welfare, Emergency Health Series C-4, Public Health Pub. 107/C-4.

Trajano, L. F.: Treatment of myocardial infarction in a coronary care unit, Minn. Med. 52: 743-745, 1969.

Transplant hearts take the strain, Med. World News 48:13-14, 1970.

Tranum, B. L., et al.: Case report: successful treatment of ventricular tachycardia associated with thiordazine (Mellaril), South. Med. J. 62: 357-358, 1969.

Tregubov, G. S., et al.: Resuscitation of a 76-year-old patient during adenomectomy, Urol. Nefrol. (Mosk.) 32:51, 1967.

Treister, B., et al.: Atrial flutter, J. Pediatr. **74**: 1005-1006, 1969.

Trenckmann, H.: Mechanical and pharmacotherapeutic measures in acute cardiac arrest, Z. Gesamte Inn. Med. 24(Suppl.):30-37, 1969.

Trethewie, E. R.: Bradyarrhythmia complicating myocardial infarction, Lancet **1**:577, 1969.

Trethewie, E. R.: Electrocution at high power with suggestions for a protective relay, Med. J. Aust. **1**:1003-1006, 1970.

Trinkle, J. K., et al.: Mechanical support of the circulation: a new approach, Arch. Surg. **101**: 740-743, 1970.

Trinkle, J. K., et al.: Circulatory arrest during deep hypothermia induced by peritoneal dialysis, Arch. Surg. **103**:648-650, 1971.

Trubina, I. E.: Acid-base equilibrium in resuscitation using extracorporeal circulation following prolonged clinical death, Patol. Fiziol. Eksp. Ter. **15**:57-59, 1971.

Tsiv'ian, IaL, and Kuznetsov, D. I.: Double cardiac arrest due to administration of listenon, Khirurgiia (Mosk.) **44**:109-110, 1968.

Turkel, R. A., et al.: The use of diazepam in cardioversion, South. Med. J. **62**:61-64, 1969.

Turner, M., et al.: Suppression of electrical activity. Pathophysiologic implications, Electroencephalogr. Clin. Neurophysiol. **28**:518, 1970.

Tuveri, A., et al.: Late ventricular fibrillation following cardiac electroshock, Boll. Soc. Ital. Cardiol. **14**:219-224, 1969.

Tuveri, A., et al.: Preliminary observations on the therapy of some grave complications of recent myocardial infarct, Atti. Accad. Fisiocr. Siena (Med. Fis.) **16**:571-575, 1967.

Tyberg, J., et al.: Effectiveness of intra-aortic balloon counterpulsation in the experimental low output state, Am. Heart J. **80**:89, 1970.

Tyers, G. F., and Wolfson, S. K., Jr.: Automatic external cardiac massage, Arch. Surg. **98**:771-775, 1969.

Ueda, H., et al.: The current status of ischemic heart disease and myocardial infarction in Japan, Jap. Heart J. **10**:1-10, 1969.

Uldall, P. R., and Kerr, D. N. S.: Post-traumatic acute renal failure, Br. J. Anaesth. **44**:283, 1972.

Unger, P.: Arrhythmias complicating acute myocardial infarction. Presented at annual meeting of Ontario Medical Association, Toronto, May, 1968.

Urbaszek, W., et al.: Studies on the action mechanism in electric double stimulation of the heart, Z. Gesamte Inn. Med. **23**:385-392, 1968.

Urschel, C., et al.: Alteration of mechanical performance of the ventricle by intraaortic balloon counterpulsation, Am. J. Cardiol. **25**:546, 1970.

Valli, B.: Sinusal cardiac arrest. Presentation of a case treated with external cardiac massage for 50 minutes before complete resumption of cardiac activity, Acta Anaesthesiol. (Padova) **19**(Suppl. 9):526+, 1968.

Vána, S.: Effect of a stroke to the heart region on the electric heart activity shortly after heart arrest, Vnitri. Lek. **15**:858-863, 1969.

Vanremoortere, E., et al.: Fibrillation threshold curves and antiarrhythmic drugs, Arch. Int. Pharmacodyn. Ther. **176**:476-479, 1968.

Vanremoortere, E. C.: Vulnerability of premature beats to A.C. stimuli of long duration, Acta Cardiol (Brux.) **26**:121-149, 1971.

Varriale, P., et al.: Clinical evaluation of furosemide in congestive heart failure, J. Kans. Med. Soc. **71**:189-191, passim, 1970.

Vassaux, C., et al.: Cardioversion of supraventricular tachycardias, Circulation **39**:791-802, 1969.

Vaughn, C. C., et al.: Cardiovascular effects of glucagon following cardiac surgery, Surgery **67**: 204-211, 1970.

Veghelyi, P. V.: Ethics of intensive treatment, Anaesthesist **19**:468-472, 1970.

Venere, G., et al.: Immediate and late results of the treatment of interatrial communications in hypothermia, Atti. Soc. Ital. Cardiol. **2**:41-42, 1968.

Venn, P. H.: External cardiac massage, Lancet **2**: 931, 1961.

Verhonick, P. J.: The nurse monitor in the patient-care system, S. Med. Bull. **56**:24-26, 1968.

Vermeersch, M.: Myocardial infarct during the initial period. Circulatory arrest, Lille Med. **16**: 307-309, 1971.

Verska, J. J.: Potassium parenterally in treatment of ventricular arrhythmia, J.A.M.A. **219**:220, 1972.

Vic-Dupont, V.: Moral limits to resuscitation, Therapeutique **47**:501-503, 1971.

Vic-Dupont, V., et al.: Use of gentamicin in medical resuscitation, G. Ital. Chemioter. **16**:389-396, 1969.

Vidne, B., et al.: Venous pressure monitor, Surgery **67**:279-280, 1970.

Viel, B.: Coronary atherosclerosis in persons dying violently, Arch. Intern. Med. **122**:97-103, 1968.

Viglietto, A., et al.: Our experience with methicillin-ampicillin combination in resuscitation, Rass. Int. Clin. Ter. **51**:227-236, 1971.

Viljoen, J. F., et al.: Propanolol and cardiac surgery, J. Thorac. Cardiovasc. Surg. **64**:826-830, 1972.

Virtanen, K. S., and Halonen, P. I.: Total heart block as a complication of gout, Cardiology **54**: 359-363, 1969.

Vlahovitch, B., et al.: Les angiographies sous pression dans la mort du cerveau avec arrêt circulatoire encéphalique, Neurochirurgie **17**: 81-96, 1971.

Vogel, J., et al.: Direct current defibrillation during pregnancy, J.A.M.A. **193**:70, 1965.

Voight, G. C.: Death after intravenous diphenylhydantoin, Mod. Med. **37**:136, 1969.

Volkov, A. V.: Effect of glucocorticoids on outcome of resuscitation after prolonged periods of clinical death produced by rapid exsanguination. Fed. Proc. (Suppl.) **25**:496-498, 1966.

Vol'pert, E. I., et al.: Sudden death from ventricular fibrillation and resuscitation in myocardial infarct, Kardiologiia **7**:21-26, 1967.

Vol'pert, E. I., et al.: Outcomes of resuscitation in acute myocardial infarct, Kardiologiia **10**: 69-73, 1970.

Von Maur, K., et al.: Hypersensitive carotid sinus syncope treated by implantable demand cardiac pacemaker, Am. J. Cardiol. **29**:109-110, 1972.

Voss, D. M., and Magnin, G. E.: Demand pacing and carotid sinus syncope, Am. Heart J. **79**: 544-547, 1970.

Wade, O. L.: Movements of the thoracic cage and diaphragm in respiration, J. Physiol. **124**: 193-212, 1954.

Wagner, G. S., et al.: The use of drugs in achieving successful DC cardioversion, Progr. Cardiovasc. Dis. **11**:431-442, 1969.

Wakabayashi, A., et al.: Heparinless total left heart bypass with induced ventricular fibrillation, Am. J. Surg. **122**:243-248, 1971.

Wakabayashi, A., et al.: Pulsatile pressure-regulated coronary perfusion during ventricular fibrillation, Arch. Surg. **105**:36-42, 1972.

Wallace, A. G., et al.: Coronary care units, their goals, current experience and future, Cardiology **50**:337-351, 1967.

Wallace, H. W., et al.: The stubborn pacemaker catheter, Surgery **68**:914-915, 1970.

Walsa, R.: Resuscitation, cerebral death, and organ transplantation, Orv. Hetil. **111**:3003-3010, 1970.

Walter, C. W.: Safe electric environment, Bull. Am. Coll. Surg. **54**:177-190+, 1969.

Walter, P. F., et al.: Transient cardiac arrhythmia detection, Mod. Med. **38**:84, 1970.

Waltz, A. G.: Studies of the cerebral circulation: what have they taught us about stroke? Mayo Clin. Proc. **46**:268-273, 1971.

Wangensteen, S. L., et al.: The effect of external counterpressure on the intact circulation, Surg. Gynecol. Obstet. **127**:253-258, 1968.

Wangensteen, S. L., et al.: Detrimental effect of the G-suit in hemorrhagic shock, Ann. Surg. **170**:187-192, 1969.

Warbasse, J. R., et al.: Lactic dehydrogenase isoenzymes after electroshock treatment of cardiac arrhythmias, Am. J. Cardiol. **21**:496-503, 1968.

Ward, J. M., et al.: Effects of morphine on the peripheral vascular response to sympathetic stimulation, Am. J. Cardiol. **29**:659-666, 1972.

Warner, W. A., et al.: Ventricular fibrillation and catecholamine responses during profound hypothermia in dogs, Anesthesiology **33**:43-51, 1970.

Watkins, D. H.: Surgical management of pump failure of the heart, Surg. Gynecol. Obstet. **128**: 1304-1305, 1969.

Watson, C. C., et al.: Evaluation of pacing for heart block in myocardial infarction, Br. Heart J. **33**:120-124, 1971.

Wax, S. D., et al.: Evaluation of antifibrillatory agents and catecholamines by a physiologic method, Surg. Forum **19**:149-151, 1968.

Webb, W. R., and Howard, H. S.: Restoration of function of the refrigerated heart, Surg. Forum **8**:302-306, 1958.

Weber, A.: Calcium and the heartbeat, Heart Bull. **19**:31-33, 1970.

Wee, A. S.: Work after myocardial infarction, Singapore Med. J. **9**:178-181, 1968.

Wegrzyn, B., et al.: Emergency cardioversion, Kardiol. Pol. **12**:91-95, 1969.

Weighing plastic heart against clinical rules, Med. World News **10**:6-7, 1969.

Weil, M., et al.: Shock following acute myocardial infarction, Prog. Cardiovasc. Dis. **11**:1-17, 1968.

Weinberg, S. L.: Current status of instrumentation systems for the coronary care unit, Prog. Cardiovasc. Dis. **11**:18-28, 1968.

Weinstein, P.: The cardiovascular importance of the thrombosis of the central retinal vein, Acta Med. Acad. Sci. Hung. **26**:78-81, 1969.

Weirich, W. L., et al.: Control of complete heart block by the use of an artificial pacemaker and a myocardial electrode, Circ. Res. **6**:410-415, 1958.

Weiss, W. A.: Intravenous use of lidocaine for ventricular arrhythmias, Anesth. Analg. **39**:369-381, 1960.

Weisse, A. B., et al.: Relative effectiveness of three antiarrhythmic agents in the treatment of ventricular arrhythmias in experimental acute myocardial ischemia, Am. Heart J. **81**:503-510, 1971.

Weisz, G. M., et al.: Cause of death in fat embolism, Chest **59**:511-516, 1971.

Wells, P. H., et al.: Cardiac function after prolonged storage in an intermediate biologic host, J. Thorac. Cardiovasc. Surg. **62**:869-879, 1971.

Westin, B.: Infant resuscitation and prevention of

mental retardation, Am. J. Obstet. Gynecol. **110:** 1134-1138, 1971.

When is death? Citation **20:**76-77, 1969.

White, M., et al.: Multiple transmyocardial puncture revascularization in refractory ventricular fibrillation due to myocardial ischemia, Ann. Thorac. Surg. **6:**557-563, 1968.

White, R. J.: Effect of potassium supplements on the exchangable potassium in chronic heart disease, Br. Med. J. **3:**141-142, 1970.

White, R. J., et al.: Preservation of viability in the isolated monkey brain utilizing a mechanical extracorporeal circulation, Nature **202:**1082-1083, 1964.

White, R. J., et al.: Mechanical circulatory support of the failing brain, Trans. Am. Soc. Artif. Intern. Organs. **14:**349-351, 1968.

Whitlow, B.: Extreme measures to prolong life, J.A.M.A. **202:**226-227, 1967.

Wholey, M. H., et al.: A pulsatile intra-aortic balloon for ventricular assist: experimental arteriographic observations, Radiology **91:**493-496, 1968.

Why did the heart stop? Dis. Chest. **56:**370, 1969.

Wiener, L., and Dwyer, E. M., Jr.: Electrical induction of atrial fibrillation. An approach to intractable atrial tachycardia, Am. J. Cardiol. **21:**731-734, 1968.

Wiggers, C. J.: The physiological bases for cardiac resuscitation from ventricular fibrillation. Method for serial defibrillation. Am. Heart J. **20:** 413-422, 1940.

Wikland, B., et al.: Atrial fibrillation and flutter treated with synchronized DC shock. A study on immediate and long-term results, Acta Med. Scand. **182:**655-671, 1967.

Wilcken, D. E., et al.: Glucagon in resistant heart-failure and cardiogenic shock, J. Lancet **760:** 1315-1318, 1970.

Wild, J. B.: Emergency care of ventricular standstill, Nurs. Times **67:**734-735, 1971.

Wild, J. B., and Grover, J. D.: The fist as an external cardiac pacemaker, Lancet **2:**436-437, 1970.

Willanger, R., et al.: A neuropsychological study of cerebral anoxic sequelae of cardiac arrest, Acta Neurol. Scand. **46**(Suppl.)**:**103+, 1970.

Williams, C. D., et al.: Long-term management of cardiac pacemakers with a systemic approach to malfunction, Surgery **66:**644-654, 1969.

Williams, C. L., and Woods, L. P.: Experimental resection of myocardial infarction, Ann. Thorac. Surg. **10:**334-339, 1970.

Williams, E. R.: Cardiogenic syncope and epilepsy, Postgrad. Med. J. **43:**677-679, 1967.

Williams, R. B., Jr., et al.: Cardiac complications of tricyclic antidepressant therapy, Ann. Intern. Med. **74:**395-398, 1971.

Willis, H. P.: The nurse in the mobile ICU, Nurs. Times **64:**1617, 1968.

Willman, V. L., et al.: Neural responses following autotransplantation of the canine heart, Circulation **27:**713, 1963.

Wilson, H. E.: Cardiac resuscitation, Texas Med. **65:**67-71, 1969.

Wilson, R. F., et al.: Eight years of experience with massive blood transfusions, J. Trauma **11:** 275-285, 1971.

Wilson, R. F., et al.: Hemodynamic changes, treatment, and prognosis in clinical shock, Arch. Surg. **102:**21-24, 1971.

Windsor, H.: Cardiac arrest, Med. J. Aust. **2:** 1120, 1968.

Winkelvoss, E., et al.: Extrathoracic heart massage, Z. Aerztl. Fortbild. (Jena) **60:**889-900, 1966.

Winship, D. H., et al.: Ventricular aneurysms in old infarctions, Mod. Med. **37:**114-115, 1969.

Winsor, T.: Electrolyte abnormalities and the electrocardiogram, J.A.M.A. **203:**109, 1968.

Winter, P. M., et al.: Hyperbaric treatment of cerebral air embolism during cardiopulmonary bypass, J.A.M.A. **215:**1786-1788, 1971.

Winters, W. L., Jr., et al.: Diazepam. A useful hypnotic drug for direct-current cardioversion, J.A.M.A. **204:**926-928, 1968.

Witherspoon, C. D.: Resuscitative management of life-threatening emergencies, Pa. Med. **72:**49-52, 1969.

Witte, A. A.: A review of cardiac resuscitation in a general hospital, J. Am. Osteopath. Assoc. **70:** 123-130, 1970.

Wittenberg, S. M., et al.: Cardioversion and digitalis. IV. Effect of beta adrenergic blockade, Circulation **39:**29-37, 1969.

Wojtasik, W., et al.: Resuscitation in a case of ventricular flutter and fibrillation in a patient with WPW syndrome, Wiad. Lek. **22:**823-827, 1969.

Wolf, S.: The end of the rope: the role of the brain in cardiac death, Can. Med. Assoc. J. **97:** 1022-1025, 1967.

Wolf, S.: The turned-off heart, Med. Times **96:** 132-146, 1968.

Wolfe, W. G., et al.: A pathological study of unsuccessful cardiac resuscitation, Arch. Surg. **96:**123-126, 1968.

Wolff, G. A., et al.: A vulnerable period for ventricular tachycardia following myocardial infarction, Cardiovasc. Res. **2:**111-122, 1968.

Wolff, G. A., et al.: The navy's first coronary care unit: a review of 16 months' experience, Milit. Med. **134:**431-436, 1969.

Wolfson, B., et al.: Cardiac arrest following minor

surgery in unrecognized thyrotoxicosis: a case report, Anesth. Analg. (Cleve.) **47:**672-676, 1968.

Wolfson, S. K., Jr., et al.: The bioautofuel cell: A device for pacemaker power from direct energy conversion consuming autogenous fuel, Trans. Am. Soc. Artif. Intern. Organs **14:**198-203, 1968.

Wood, R. A.: Sinoatrial arrest: an interaction between phenytoin and lignocaine. Br. Med. J. **1:**645, 1971.

Woody, N. C., et al.: Direct digital intratracheal intubation for neonatal resuscitation, J. Pediatr. **73:**903-905, 1968.

Woolf, P. D.: Glucagon and the failing heart, Ann. Intern. Med. **73:**493-494, 1970.

Wright, B. D., et al.: Respiratory alkalosis, hypokalemia, and repeated ventricular fibrillation associated with mechanical ventilation, Anesth. Analg. (Cleve.) **48:**567-573, 1969.

Wukasch, D. C., et al.: The "stone heart" syndrome, Surgery **72:**1071-1080, 1972.

Wyant, G. W.: Malignant hyperpyrexia, Surgery **71:**473-474, 1971.

Yahr, W. Z., et al.: Cardiogenic shock: dynamics of coronary blood flow with intraaortic phase-shift balloon pumping, Surg. Forum **19:**142, 1968.

Yahr, W. Z. et al.: Intra-aortic phase-shift balloon-pumping in cardiogenic shock laboratory and clinical observations, Med. Ann. D.C. **38:**237-242 passim, 1969.

Yamada, E. Y., and Fukunaga, F. H.: Cardiopulmonary complications of external cardiac massage, Hawaii Med. J. **29:**114-117, 1969.

Yamaguchi, Y., et al.: Arterial-alveolar carbon dioxide gradient after cardiac resuscitation, Jap. J. Anesthesiol. **18:**14-22, 1969.

Yamamoto, K.: Experimental study of open heart surgery under circulatory arrest during profound hypothermia using extracorporeal circulation in dogs—the effect of circulatory arrest on myocardial metabolism, Acta Med. (Fukuoka) **38:**436-451, 1968.

Yamamoto, M., et al.: Evaluation of sudden heart arrest, Sanfujin Jissai **17:**405-410, 1968.

Yashon, D.: Clinical, chemical, and physiological indicators of cerebral non-viability in circulatory arrest, Trans. Am. Neurol. Assoc. **95:**31-35, 1970.

Yashon, D., et al.: Pressure and electrical correlates indicating cerebral viability during cardiac arrest and resuscitation, Trans. Am. Neurol. Assoc. **94:**350-353, 1969.

Yashon, D., et al.: Electrocortigraphic limits of cerebral viability during cardiac arrest and resuscitation, Am. J. Surg. **121:**728-731, 1971.

Yashon, D., et al.: Intracranial pressure during circulatory arrest, Brain Res. **31:**139-150, 1971.

Yasutomi, T.: Countermeasure for sudden cardiac arrest, Iryo **21:**1077-1086, 1967.

Yates, A. J.: Intra-arterial balloon tamponade, Surgery **6:**634-636, 1969.

Yatteau, R. F.: Radar-induced failure of a demand pacemaker, N. Engl. J. Med. **283:**1447-1448, 1970.

Yeboah, E. D., et al.: Acute renal failure and open heart surgery, Br. Med. J. **1:**415, 1972.

Ygge, J., et al.: Counterpulsation aids patient with myocardial infarct, Mod. Med. **37:**87, 1969.

Yigitbasi, O., et al.: Ventricular fibrillation: a delayed complication of direct current shock. Cardiology **51:**307-309, 1967.

Yokoyama, M., et al.: Transient hypopotassemia and ECG changes following hemodilution perfusion, Arch. Surg. **104:**640-643, 1972.

Youmans, C. R., Jr., et al.: Cardiac pacemaker no contraindication to ECT, Mod. Med. **38:**120, 1970.

Youmans, J. R., et al.: Efficacy of carbon dioxide in the treatment of cerebral ischemia, Surg. Forum **19:**425-426, 1968.

Yu, P. M.: Prehospital care of acute myocardial infarction, Circulation **45:**189-204, 1972.

Yusa, T., et al.: General anesthesia for a patient with past history of paroxysmal ventricular fibrillation, Jap. J. Anesthesiol. **20:**669-675, 1971.

Zacouto, F., and Amsellem, A. I.: On the development of assisted circulation, Biol. Med. (Paris) **60:**14-34, 1971.

Zapanta, E., and Pitts, F. W.: Cardiac arrest after medication through central-venous catheter, J. Neurosurg. **31:**695-697, 1969.

Zeichen, R., et al.: Hypokalemic heart arrest in primary aldosteronism (Conn's syndrome), Munch. Med. Wochenschr. **110:**700-702, 1968.

Zierott, G.: Resuscitation of the blood circulation, Ther. Ggw. **110:**1118-1130, 1971.

Zimmerman, T. S., et al.: Pulmonary embolism and unexpected death in supposedly normal persons, N. Engl. J. Med. **283:**1504-1505, 1970.

Zinn, M. B.: Management of cardiac arrhythmias in acute myocardial infarction, Texas Med. **65:**58-62, 1969.

Ziolkowski, J., et al.: Sudden cardiac arrest treated successfully with prolonged massage, Wiad. Lek. **20:**1715-1717, 1967.

Zipes, D. P.: Treatment of arrhythmias in myocardial infarction, Arch. Intern. Med. **124:**101-109, 1969.

Zoll, P. M.: Resuscitation of the heart in ventricular standstill by external electric stimulation, N. Engl. J. Med. **247:**768-771, 1952.

Zoll, P. M.: Rational use of drugs for cardiac arrest and after cardiac resuscitation, Am. J. Cardiol. **27:**645-649, 1971.

Zoll, P. M., et al.: Treatment of Stokes-Adams disease by external electric stimulation of the heart, Circulation 9:482-493, 1954.

Zoll, P. M., et al.: Treatment of unexpected cardiac arrest by external electric stimulation of the heart, N. Engl. J. Med. **254:**541-546, 1956.

Zoll, P. M., et al.: Long-term electric stimulation of the heart for Stokes-Adams disease, Ann. Surg. **154:**330-346, 1961.

Zoll, P. M., et al.: Ventricular fibrillation—a risk of fixed-rate pacemakers? Circulation **41**(**Suppl. 3**): 209, 1970.

Zuckermann, C.: Cardiac arrest and resuscitation, Clin. Lab. (Zaragoza) **76:**321-332, 1963.

Zuckerman, W., et al.: Clinical application of demand pacing, Ann. N. Y. Acad. Sci. **167:**1055-1059, 1969.

Zumino, A. Z. P., et al.: Effect of ischemia and low-sodium medium on atrioventricular conduction, Am. J. Physiol. **218:**1489-1494, 1970.

Zywicka-Twarowska, I., et al.: Effects of reanimation of the severely asphyxiated newborn infants: its evaluation and development. In: Proceedings of the symposium on intrauterine dangers to fetus, Prague, 1966, Excerpta Medica, pp. 505-509.

INDEX

A

A-B-C's of basic life support, 634, 877
A.C.D. solution (sodium citrate, citric acid, and dextrose), 769
Acetylcholine, 61, 358, 503
  as cardioplegic agent, 769, 778
  cholinesterase, 201-202, 206, 209
  mechanism of action, 61
  relationship to sodium with potassium, 205
  stone heart and, 401
  vagal stimulation and, 205
  ventricular fibrillation and, 490
Acidosis
  base-buffer solution, 206
  cardiogenic shock and, 406
  and catecholamines, 404, 406, 496
  and conductivity, 40
  drowning and, 378
  effect on heart, 40
  fibrillatory threshold, 783
  hemorrhage, 10
  metabolic, 10-11, 23-24, 206, 226, 283, 357, 383, 463, 677, 703
    during hypothermia, 779
    and ultrastructural damage, 703
  pharmacology of, 493-497
  and potassium levels, 197
  and pressor amines, 477
  respiratory, 49, 170
    hypercapnia, 270
    prevention of, 40-41, 206
  sodium bicarbonate and, 23, 383, 461-462, 495-496, 896; see also Sodium bicarbonate
  THAM, 206, 213, 496-497, 509
  ventricular fibrillation and, 205, 206, 346
Aconitine, 214
Adams-Stokes disease, 357, 414, 499, 716
  diagnosis, 126
  effect of atropine in prevention, 44
  ephedrine and, 505
  isoproterenol and, 485
  obstructive jaundice and, 144-147
  postural hypotension and, 299
  progressive external ophthalmoplegia, 51
  recurrent defibrillation and, 357, 361
  tumor, 222

Adams-Stokes disease—cont'd
  vagal stimulation, 147
  vagotomy and, 147
  ventricular fibrillation and, 249, 289
Adenochrome, 769
Adenosine triphosphate, 30, 65, 190, 192, 217, 247, 690, 712, 865
Adrenalin; see Epinephrine
Adrenergic mechanisms in production of ventricular fibrillation, 212
Aerobic glycolysis, 12, 687, 705
Agonal state, 7, 8-9
Air embolism; see Embolism
Airway; see also Artificial respiration
  Don Michael, 645-648, 890
Alkalosis
  fibrillatory threshold, 346
  metabolic, 11, 23
Allopurinal, 712
Alternating current, defibrillation by, 337, 338-340
AMBU bag, 263, 526, 614, 659, 729, 889
Ambulance resuscitation, 611-622, 641, 869
  airway patency, 270-272, 614
  arrhythmias during, 611, 616
  attendants, training of, 616
  emergency communication, 567, 617, 621, 624
  equipment, 903
  mobile intensive care unit, 76, 601-610, 618
  mobile life support unit, 904
  myocardial infarction management and, 611
  National Highway Traffic Safety Administration recommendations, 613-614
  prognosis, 835
  suction equipment, 612, 613-614
  supportive equipment, 903
  training of emergency medical technicians, 615-616
  by two people, 641
  vehicle types, 612-613, 618-621
  ventricular defibrillation and, 374, 611, 624
American Heart Association, Standards for CPR and ECC, 867-909
  recommendations of, 868, 906-907
American Red Cross, 616
Amicar, 461
ε-Aminocaproic acid (Amicar) for excessive fibrinolysis, 461

974